This book is dedicated to Ellen Levine Ebert, Sophie Ross Loosen, Alison Nurcombe, and Hannah Leckman.

Contents

Authors

Richard Balon, MD
Professor of Psychiatry and Behavioral Neurosciences
Associate Director of Residency Training
Department of Psychiatry and Behavioral
    Neurosciences
Wayne State University School of Medicine
Detroit, Michigan
Internet: rbalon@wayne.edu
Sexual Dysfunction and Paraphilias

William Bernet, MD
Professor of Psychiatry
Director, Vanderbilt Forensic Services
Vanderbilt University School of Medicine
Nashville, Tennessee
Internet: william.bernet@vanderbilt.edu
Child Maltreatment, Gender Identity Disorder, and
    Forensic Psychiatry

Wade Berrettini, MD, PhD
Karl E. Rickels Professor of Psychiatry
Director, Center for Neurobiology and Behavior
Department of Psychiatry
University of Pennsylvania School of Medicine
Philadelphia, Pennsylvania
Internet: wadeb@mail.med.upenn.edu
Psychiatric Genetics

Dan G. Blazer, MD, MPH, PhD
J. P. Gibbons Professor of Psychiatry and Behavioral
    Sciences
Vice Chairman for Education and Academic Affairs
Department of Psychiatry and Behavioral Sciences
Duke University School of Medicine
Duke University Medical Center
Durham, North Carolina
Internet: blaze001@mc.duke.edu
Psychiatric Epidemiology

Michael H. Bloch, MD
Albert J. Solnit Child and Adult Integrated
    Training Program
Child Study Center
Yale University School of Medicine
New Haven, Connecticut
Internet:michael.bloch@yale.edu
Tourette Disorder and Obsessive–Compulsive Disorder
    in Children and Adolescents

William V. Bobo, MD
Assistant Professor in Clinical Psychiatry
Department of Psychiatry
Vanderbilt University School of Medicine
Nashville, Tennessee
Internet: william.v.bobo@Vanderbilt.Edu
Schizophrenia

David A. Brent, MD
Endowed Chair in Suicide Studies and Professor of
    Psychiatry, Pediatrics, and Epidemiology
University of Pittsburgh School of Medicine
Department of Psychiatry
Western Psychiatric Institute and Clinic
Pittsburgh, Pennsylvania
Internet: BrentDA@upmc.edu
Depressive Disorders in Children and Adolescents and
    Pediatric Bipolar Disorder

Catherine Chiles, MD
Associate Clinical Professor of Psychiatry
Department of Psychiatry
Yale University School of Medicine
New Haven, Connecticut
Internet: catherine.chiles@yale.edu
Consultation–Liaison Psychiatry

Camellia P. Clark, MD
Assistant Adjunct Professor of Psychiatry
Department of Psychiatry
University of California, San Diego School of
    Medicine
San Diego, California
Internet: cclark@vapop.ucsd.edu
Sleep Disorders

Kenneth A. Dodge, PhD
William McDougall Professor of Public Policy and
    Professor of Psychology and Neuroscience
Director, Center for Child and Family Policy
Duke University
Durham, North Carolina
Internet: dodge@duke.edu
Developmental Psychology

Michael H. Ebert, MD
Associate Dean for Veterans Affairs and
    Professor of Psychiatry
Yale University School of Medicine
Chief of Staff, VA Connecticut Healthcare System
West Haven, Connecticut
Internet: Michael.Ebert@va.gov
The Psychiatric Interview and Eating Disorders

S. Hossein Fatemi, MD, PhD
Professor of Psychiatry, Pharmacology, and
    Neuroscience
Department of Psychiatry
University of Minnesota Medical School
Minneapolis, Minnesota
Internet: fatem002@umn.edu
Schizophrenia

Charles V. Ford, MD
Professor of Psychiatry
Department of Psychiatry and Behavioral
    Neurobiology
University of Alabama School of Medicine at
    Birmingham
Birmingham, Alabama
Internet:cford@uabmc.edu
*Somatoform Disorders and Factitious Disorders and
    Malingering*

Sandra L. Friedman, MD, MPH
Director, Neurodevelopmental Disabilities,
    Children's Hospital Boston/Harvard
Assistant Professor of Pediatrics
Harvard Medical School
Boston, Massachusetts
Internet: Sandra.friedman@childrens.harvard.edu
Intellectual Disability

J. Christian Gillin, MD (posthumous)
Formerly Professor of Psychiatry, University of
    California, San Diego, School of Medicine
Director, Mental Health Clinical Research Center,
    VA San Diego Healthcare System
San Diego, California
Internet: fgillin@ucsd.edu
Sleep Disorders

Harry E. Gwirtsman, MD
Associate Professor of Psychiatry
Department of Psychiatry
Vanderbilt University School of Medicine
VA Medical Center, Psychiatry Service
Nashville, Tennessee
Internet: harry.gwirtsman@vanderbilt.edu
Eating Disorders

Stephan Heckers, MD
James G. Blakemore, Professor of Psychiatry and
    Professor of Radiology
Chair, Department of Psychiatry
Vanderbilt University School of Medicine
Vanderbilt Psychiatric Hospital
Nashville, Tennessee
Internet: stephan.heckers@vanderbilt.edu
Schizophrenia

William A. Hewlett, PhD, MD
Associate Professor of Psychiatry and Pharmacology
Director of the Obsessive Compulsive Disorder
    (OCD)/Tourette Syndrome Program
Department of Psychiatry
Vanderbilt University School of Medicine
Psychiatric Hospital at Vanderbilt
Nashville, Tennessee
Internet: william.a.hewlett@vanderbilt.edu
Obsessive–Compulsive Disorder

Steven D. Hollon, PhD
Professor of Psychology (Arts and Sciences)
Professor of Psychology and Human Development
Associate Professor of Psychiatry
Vanderbilt University
Nashville, Tennessee
Internet: steven.d.hollon@vanderbilt.edu
Behavioral and Cognitive-Behavioral Interventions

David S. Janowsky, MD
Professor of Psychiatry
Department of Psychiatry
University of North Carolina at Chapel Hill School
    of Medicine
Chapel Hill, North Carolina
Internet: david_janowsky@med.unc.edu
Personality Disorders

Douglas Christian Johnson, PhD
Associate Research Scientist
Yale University School of Medicine and the National
    Center for PTSD Clinical Neurosciences Division
West Haven, Connecticut
Assistant Professor, Department of Psychiatry
University of California-San Diego and San Diego
    VA Healthcare System
San Diego, California
Internet: douglas.johnson@yale.edu
Posttraumatic Stress Disorder and Acute Stress Disorder

Yifrah Kaminer, MD, MBA
Professor of Psychiatry
Co-Director of Research
Division of Child and Adolescent Psychiatry
Department of Psychiatry & Alcohol Research
    Center
University of Connecticut School of Medicine
University of Connecticut Health Center
Farmington, Connecticut
Internet: Kaminer@psychiatry.uchc.edu
Substance-Related Disorders in Adolescents

Robert A. King, MD
Professor of Child Psychiatry
Yale University School of Medicine
Medical Director
Tourette's/OCD/Anxiety Disorder Clinics
Yale Child Study Center
New Haven, Connecticut
Internet: robert.king@yale.edu
Suicidal Behavior in Children and Adolescents

Howard S. Kirshner, MD
Professor, Vice-Chair of Neurology
Vanderbilt University Medical Center
A-0118 Medical Center North
Nashville, Tennessee
Internet: Howard.Kirshner@vanderbilt.edu
Delirium, Dementia, and Amnestic Syndromes

John H. Krystal, MD
Robert L. McNeil Jr., Professor of Psychiatry and
    Clinical Pharmacology
Deputy Chair for Research
Department of Psychiatry
Yale University School of Medicine
Connecticut Mental Health Center
New Haven, Connecticut
Internet: john.krystal@yale.edu
Posttraumatic Stress Disorder and Acute Stress Disorder

Joseph A. Kwentus, MD
Clinical Professor, Department of Psychiatry and
    Human Behavior
University of Mississippi School of Medicine
Jackson, Mississippi
Internet: jkwentus@precise-research.com
Delirium, Dementia, and Amnestic Syndromes

James F. Leckman, MD
Neison Harris Professor of Child Psychiatry,
    Pediatrics, and Psychology
Director of Research
Yale Child Study Center
Yale University School of Medicine
New Haven, Connecticut
Internet: james.leckman@yale.edu
*Tourette Disorder and Obsessive–Compulsive Disorder
    in Children and Adolescents*

Elizabeth L. Leonard, PhD
Lecturer in Psychiatry
Beth Israel Deaconess Medical Center
Harvard Medical School
Boston, Massachusetts
Internet: Elizabeth_leonard@hms.harvard.edu
Intellectual Disability

James W. Lomax, MD
Professor and Associate Chair
Director of Educational Programs
Karl Menninger Chair of Psychiatric Education
Menninger Department of Psychiatry and
    Behavioral Sciences
Houston, Texas
Internet: jlomax@bcm.tmc.edu
Psychodynamic and Social Interventions

Peter T. Loosen, MD, PhD
Professor Emeritus of Psychiatry
Department of Psychiatry
Vanderbilt University School of Medicine
Nashville, Tennesssee
Internet: ploosen@gmail.com
Mood Disorders

Peter R. Martin, MD
Professor of Psychiatry and Pharmacology
Director of the Division of Addiction Medicine,
Addiction Psychiatry Training Program, and
    Vanderbilt Addiction Center
Department of Psychiatry
Vanderbilt University School of Medicine
Vanderbilt Psychiatric Hospital
Nashville, Tennesseee
Internet: peter.martin@vanderbilt.edu
Substance-Related Disorders

Brett McDermott, MD
Associate Professor of Child and Adolescent
    Psychiatry
Director, Mater Child and Youth Mental Health
    Service
Department of Psychiatry
The University of Queensland
Mater Health Campus
South Brisbane, Queensland, Australia
Internet: Brett.McDermott@mater.org.au
*Posttraumatic Stress Disorder in Children and
    Adolescents following a Single-Event Trauma*

—

Herbert V. Meltzer, MD
Bixler/May/Johnson, Professor of Psychiatry and
    Professor of Pharmacology
Director of the Psychosis Program
Department of Psychiatry
Vanderbilt University School of Medicine
Psychiatric Hospital at Vanderbilt
Nashville, Tennessee
Internet: herbert.meltzer@vanderbilt.edu
Schizophrenia

James E. Mitchell, MD
Christoferson Professor and Chair
Department of Clinical Neuroscience
University of North Dakota School of Medicine and
    Health Sciences
President and Scientific Director, Neuropsychiatric
    Research Institute
Fargo, North Dakota
Internet: Mitchell@medicine.nodak.edu
Eating Disorders

Polly Moore, PhD, RPsgT
Director of Sleep Research
California Clinical Trials
San Diego, California
Internet: polly.moore@cctrials.com
Sleep Disorders

James L. Nash, MD
Associate Professor of Psychiatry Emeritus
Department of Psychiatry
Vanderbilt University School of Medicine
Nashville, Tennessee
Internet: james.nash@vanderbilt.edu
Psychodynamic and Social Interventions

Barry Nurcombe, MD
Professor of Child and Adolescent Psychiatry
Departments of Paediatric Medicine and Psychiatry
    and Neuroscience
University of Western Australia, Perth, Western
    Australia
Professor Emeritus of Psychiatry
The University of Queensland, Herston,
    Queensland, Australia, and Vanderbilt
University School of Medicine
Nashville, Tennessee
Internet: bnurcombe@uq.edu.au
*Clinical Decision-Making in Psychiatry, The
    Psychiatric Interview, Diagnostic Encounter for
    Children and Adolescents, Diagnostic Evaluation for
    Children and Adolescents, Diagnostic Formulation,
    Treatment Planning, and Modes of Treatment in
    Children and Adolescents, Preventive Psychiatry,
    Dissociative Disorders, Motor Skills Disorder and
    Communication Disorders, Oppositional Defiant
    Disorder and Conduct Disorder, Anxiety Disorders
    in Children and Adolescents, Developmental
    Disorders of Attachment, Feeding, Elimination, and
    Sleeping, and Psychological Reactions to Acute and
    Chronic Systemic Illness in Pediatric Patients*

John I. Nurnberger Jr., MD, PhD
Joyce and Iver Small Professor of Psychiatry
Professor of Medical and Molecular Genetics and
    Medical Neuroscience
Director, Institute of Psychiatric Research
Indiana University School of Medicine
Indianapolis, Indiana
Internet: jnurnber@iupui.edu
Psychiatric Genetics

Lisa Pan, MD
Research Fellow, Department of Psychiatry
University of Pittsburgh School of Medicine
Pittsburgh, Pennsylvania
Internet: thomasla@upmc.edu
Depressive Disorders in Children and Adolescents

Raymond J. Pan, MD
Research Fellow, Department of Psychiatry
University of Pittsburgh School of Medicine
Pittsburgh, Pennsylvania
Internet: panrjmd@gmail.com
Pediatric Bipolar Disorder

Howard B. Roback, PhD
Professor of Psychiatry and Psychology
Department of Psychiatry
Vanderbilt University School of Medicine
Nashville, Tennessee
Internet: howard.roback@vanderbilt.edu
Psychological and Neuropsychological Assessment

Robert M. Rohrbaugh, MD
Associate Professor and Director of Medical Studies
Department of Psychiatry
Yale University School of Medicine
Associate Chief and Director of Education and
    Training
Psychiatry Services VA Connecticut Healthcare
    System
VA Hospital
West Haven, Connecticut
Internet:robert.rohrbaugh@va.gov
Emergency Psychiatry

Lucy Salomon, MD
Consultant in Psychiatry
Nantucket Cottage Hospital
Nantucket, Massachusetts
Internet: slmnlucy@nantucket.net
Adjustment Disorders

Ronald M. Salomon, MD
Associate Professor of Psychiatry
Department of Psychiatry
Vanderbilt University School of Medicine
Nashville, Tennessee
Internet: ron.salomon@vanderbilt.edu
Adjustment Disorders

R. Taylor Segraves, MD, PhD
Professor of Psychiatry, Case Western Reserve
    University School of Medicine
Chair, Department of Psychiatry
MetroHealth Medical Center, Cleveland
MetroHealth Medical Center
Cleveland, Ohio
Internet: rsegraves@metrohealth.org
Sexual Dysfunction and Paraphilias

Michael J. Sernyak, MD
Professor of Psychiatry, Department of Psychiatry
Yale University School of Medicine
Chief of Psychiatry Service and Mental Health
    Service Line Manager
VA Connecticut Healthcare System
West Haven, Connecticut
Internet: michael.sernyak@va.gov
Emergency Psychiatry

Richard C. Shelton, MD
James G. Blakemore, Research Professor of
    Psychiatry and Professor of Pharmacology
Vice Chair for Research
Department of Psychiatry
Vanderbilt University School of Medicine
Nashville, Tennessee
Internet: richard.shelton@vanderbilt.edu
*Psychopharmacologic Interventions, Other Psychotic
    Disorders, Mood Disorders, and Anxiety Disorders*

Deborah R. Simkin, MD
Adjunct Associate Professor and Residency Director
Department of Psychiatry
University of South Alabama College of Medicine
Mobile, Alabama
Clinical Assistant Professor
Florida State Medical School
Destin, Florida
Internet: Deb62288@aol.com
Substance-Related Disorders in Adolescents

Steven M. Southwick, MD
Professor of Psychiatry
Department of Psychiatry
Yale University School of Medicine
VA Connecticut Health Care System
West Haven, Connecticut
Internet: steven.southwick@va.gov
Posttraumatic Stress Disorder and Acute Stress Disorder

Thomas J. Spencer, MD
Associate Director, Clinical and Research Program in
    Pediatric Psychopharmacology
Massachusetts General Hospital
Associate Professor of Psychiatry
Harvard University Medical School
Boston, Massachusetts
Internet: spencer@helix.mgh.harvard.edu
Attention Deficit Hyperactivity Disorder

Ludwik S. Szymanski, MD
Director Emeritus of Psychiatry
Institute for Community Inclusion
Children's Hospital, Boston
Associate Professor of Psychiatry
Harvard Medical School
Boston, Massachusetts
Internet: ludwik.szymanski@childrens.harvard.edu
Intellectual Disability

John W. Thompson Jr., MD
Vice-Chair, Professor, and Chief, Section of Adult
    Psychiatry
Director, Division of Forensic Neuropsychiatry
Department of Psychiatry and Neurology
Tulane University School of Medicine
New Orleans, Louisiana
Internet: jthomps3@tulane.edu
Impulse-Control Disorders

Travis Thompson, PhD
Professor of Pediatrics, Autism Program
University of Minnesota Medical School
Minneapolis, Minnesota
Internet: tithompson@comcast.net
Behavioral and Cognitive-Behavioral Interventions

Michael G Tramontana, PhD
Associate Professor of Psychiatry and Neurology
Department of Psychiatry
Vanderbilt University School of Medicine
Psychiatric Hospital at Vanderbilt
Nashville, Tennessee
Internet: michael.tramontana@vanderbilt.edu
*Diagnostic Evaluation for Children and Adolescents,
    Learning Disorders, and Motor Skills Disorder and
    Communication Disorders*

Fred R. Volkmar, MD
Director, Child Study Center
Chief, Child Psychiatry, Children's Hospital at Yale
Irwing B. Harris Professor of Child Psychiatry,
    Pediatrics and Psychology
Yale University School of Medicine
New Haven, Connecticut
Internet: fred.volkmar@yale.edu
Autism and the Pervasive Developmental Disorders

James S. Walker, PhD
Assistant Professor of Psychiatry, Neurology,
    and Psychology
Department of Psychiatry
Vanderbilt University School of Medicine
Nashville, Tennessee
Internet: James.S.Walker@Vanderbilt.edu
Psychological and Neuropsychological Assessment

Larry W. Welch, EdD
Consulting Psychologist
Social Security Administration
Medical Unit of Disability Determination Services
    of Tennessee
Kingston Springs, Tennessee
Internet: Larry.W.Welch@ssa.gov
Psychological and Neuropsychological Assessment

Daniel K. Winstead, MD
Robert G. Heath Professor and Chair, Department
    of Psychiatry and Neurology
Tulane University School of Medicine
New Orleans, Louisiana
Internet: winstead@tulane.edu
Impulse-Control Disorders

Thomas N. Wise, MD
Professor of Psychiatry and Behavioral Sciences
Johns Hopkins University School of Medicine
Chair, Department of Psychiatry
Behavioral Health Services
Inova Health System
Falls Church, Virginia
Internet: thomas.wise@inova.org
Consultation–Liaison Psychiatry

Preface

Current Diagnosis & Treatment: Psychiatry, Second Edition, reflects the current dynamic state of psychiatric knowledge. New discoveries from the basic biomedical and psychological sciences are having a major impact on psychiatric practice today. The task is to translate these new discoveries into a form useful to clinicians. This text is intended to be practical, succinct, and useful for all health care professionals who encounter and provide care for individuals with psychiatric symptoms and behavioral disturbance.

The field of psychiatry has undergone a gradual change in the last several decades. It has moved from a body of medical and psychological knowledge that was theory-bound, to an empirical approach that is more flexible with regard to reasoning about etiology. This change came about as it became apparent that developments in neurobiology, genetics, and cognitive and developmental psychology would make unanticipated inroads into our understanding of the etiology and pathogenesis of psychiatric syndromes. Furthermore, a more flexible philosophy evolved regarding the description and definition of psychiatric syndromes. Some syndromes have indistinct boundaries and shade into each other. In addition, the idea of discovering a single underlying biochemical characteristic of a psychiatric syndrome, which would in turn clarify the diagnostic description and predict treatment, was recognized as being hopelessly simplistic. Moreover, through the complexity of behavioral genetics, we now understand that those genotypes which are becoming highly significant in understanding psychopathology and developmental psychology may lead to unexpected phenotypes which do not fit our current conception of the psychiatric syndromes.

Section I of *Current Diagnosis & Treatment: Psychiatry, Second Edition*, identifies some of the major tributaries of scientific knowledge that inform the current theory and practice of psychiatry and also presents techniques for the evaluation of psychiatric patients. Section II presents the diagnosis, phenomenology, and psychopathology of the major adult psychiatric syndromes and their evidence-based treatments. Section III presents the same material for the major syndromes seen in child and adolescent psychiatry. Section IV presents specialized settings for diagnosis and treatment in psychiatry.

Current Diagnosis & Treatment: Psychiatry, Second Edition, is written from an empirical viewpoint, with recognition that the boundaries of psychopathological syndromes may change unexpectedly with the emergence of new knowledge. Eventually, the accumulation of new knowledge will sharpen our diagnostic techniques and improve the treatment of these illnesses that have such a high impact on normal development, health, and society.

Acknowledgments

We wish to thank Ellen Levine Ebert for her editorial assistance in the preparation of the text, Louise Bierig for her thoughtful developmental editing, and Anne Sydor for her leadership and advice throughout the process.

Michael H. Ebert, MD
Peter T. Loosen, MD, PhD
Barry Nurcombe, MD
James F. Leckman, MD
November 2007

SECTION I

Psychiatric Principles and Practice

Clinical Decision Making in Psychiatry

1

Barry Nurcombe, MD

■ THE PURPOSE OF CLINICAL REASONING

It is through clinical reasoning that clinicians collect, weigh, and combine the information required to reach diagnosis; decide which treatment is required; monitor treatment effectiveness; and change their plans if treatment does not work. The study of clinical reasoning, therefore, concerns the cognitive processes that underlie diagnosis and the planning and implementation of treatment.

Diagnosis has three purposes: to aid research, to summarize information, and to guide treatment. For clinicians, the chief purpose of diagnosis is to summarize information in such a way as to guide treatment. In one approach to diagnosis, the clinician matches a pattern of clinical phenomena elicited from the patient against the idealized patterns of disease entities and chooses the diagnosis that best fits. In another approach, the clinician attempts to understand the particular environmental, biological, psychological, and existential factors that have both led to the current problem and perpetuated it. The first approach, therefore, seeks commonality and lends itself to generic treatment planning. The second approach stresses uniqueness and the adaptation of treatment to the individual. In good clinical practice the two approaches are complementary.

■ CLINICAL REASONING & ACTUARIAL PREDICTION

Diagnosis and treatment are risky ventures, fraught with the possibility of error that can have serious consequences. How can error be minimized? On the one hand are the clinicians who, having elicited information that is generally both incomplete and inferential, diagnose patients and use subjective probabilities to predict outcome. On the other hand are the psychological actuaries who regard natural clinical reasoning as so flawed as to be virtually obsolete and who seek to replace it with reliable statistical formulas.

A considerable amount of research has been conducted into the fallacies and biases that can lead clinicians astray. For several reasons, such research has had little effect on clinical practice. Actuarial experiments sometimes seem artificial, or even rigged (against the clinician), and may be dismissed as irrelevant. Clinicians are prone to concede that others may make a particular mistake in reasoning but they themselves are unlikely to do so. Indeed, clinicians often have a degree of self-confidence that enables them to survive in an uncertain world, and they are not likely to accept their defects unless they see a practical remedy. Finally, clinicians may fear that, if tampered with, their mysterious diagnostic skills will evaporate and be replaced by computing machines.

Table 1–1. Common Errors in Clinical Reasoning

If a set of clinical findings (F) matches a textbook syndrome (D), clinicians are apt to diagnose it without sufficiently taking P(D) and P(F) into account.
Clinicians must often rely on their subjective estimations of P(D) and P(F). They tend to be overconfident concerning the accuracy of these estimations.
Clinicians may overestimate P(D) as a result of recent experience (e.g., reading a journal article). Thus, exotic disorders may be overdiagnosed.
Clinicians are conservative. Despite corrective feedback, they are slow to correct their subjective base-rates.
Clinicians are prone to rely too much on confirmatory data, whereas negative evidence is more powerful.
Early preference for a particular diagnostic hypothesis may be hard to dislodge and can deflect the subsequent collection or evaluation of evidence.

■ RESEARCH INTO CLINICAL REASONING

There are three types of research into clinical reasoning: clinical judgment, decision theory, and process tracing. **Clinical judgment research** attempts to identify the criteria used by clinicians in making decisions. **Decision theory** explores the flaws and biases that deflect accurate clinical judgment. **Process tracing** elucidates the progressive steps of naturalistic reasoning. The first two types are statistical and prescriptive, the third is normative.

CLINICAL JUDGMENT & DECISION THEORY

According to the "lens" model of clinical judgment, each patient exhibits a set of symptoms, signs, or criteria that the clinician weighs and combines to reach a decision (e.g., whether the patient is at risk for suicide or whether he or she should be hospitalized). Researchers attempt to "capture the policy" of the expert decision maker in order to construct mathematical models that replicate clinical judgment.

Given the fuzzy nature of clinical data, medical decisions have to be probabilistic. Accordingly, decision theorists base their research on Bayes' theorem. This theorem states that P(D/F) (the probability that a diagnosis is present given a clinical finding) is a function of P(F/D) (the probability that a finding will be associated with that diagnosis), P(D) (the probability of the diagnosis in that population), and P(F) (the probability of the finding in that population). Thus,

$$P(\text{D/F}) = \frac{P(\text{F/D}) \times P(\text{D})}{P(\text{F})}.$$

The intuitive clinician gauges P(F/D) from theoretical knowledge and experience. However, P(F/D) must be combined with the local base rates for both the disease and the finding—base rates that are often unknown or ignored by the clinician. Unfamiliarity with Bayes' theorem and other biases can introduce several errors into clinical reasoning (Table 1–1).

Decision theory has been applied most often to convergent problems, for example, whether or not to hospitalize a patient. The better choice should be the one that has the highest expected utility. **Expected utility** is the product of the probability of an outcome and its subjective utility (e.g., how highly the patient or physician values that outcome). Consider the following case:

A 14-year-old girl is evaluated in a pediatric hospital ward after she has taken an overdose of 50 acetaminophen tablets. She has made one previous suicide attempt. The recent suicide attempt occurred after she was rejected by a boyfriend. The patient is emotionally labile and clinically depressed. She is hostile to her mother and refuses to agree to a "no-suicide contract." The consequences of hospitalizing the patient versus not hospitalizing her but referring her for outpatient treatment can be represented in Figure 1–1. The clinician is expected to opt for the choice that leads to the greater expected utility.

However, clinical decisions are usually more complex than can be represented by a simple decision tree of the type shown in Figure 1–1. Multiple branching yes–no decision trees have been constructed to aid diagnostic decision making (see, e.g., Appendix A in *Diagnostic and Statistical Manual of Mental Disorders,* fourth edition [DSM-IV]) and to encode expert treatment decisions. Utility and probability are also important considerations when cost–benefit analyses are undertaken, for example, concerning the desirability of mass screening procedures.

Research has shown that clinicians do not always follow the expected utility model. For example, decision making may be biased by the readiness with which a particular outcome can be remembered, particularly if it has

Action	Outcome	Probability	Utility
Hospitalizing	Death	0	0
	No change or worse	.3	0
	Lost to treatment	.1	0
	Improved	.6	100
Not Hospitalizing	Death	.01	0
	No change or worse	.4	0
	Lost to treatment	.3	0
	Improved	.2	100

Expected utility of hospitalizing =
$(0 \times 0) + (.3 \times 0) + (.1 \times 0) + (.6 \times 100) = 60$

Expected utility of not hospitalizing =
$(.01 \times 0) + (.4 \times 0) + (.3 \times 0) + (.2 \times 100) = 20$

Figure 1–1. Expected utility estimation.

had an emotional impact on the clinician (e.g., a patient's recent suicide). Decision making is also affected by the way problems are presented. For example, a treatment that saves 800 lives out of 1000 may be preferred to one that sacrifices 200 out of 1000 (although the two situations are equivalent in risk). Furthermore, the probability of an outcome can sometimes affect the subjective estimation of its utility, whereas theoretically the two should be independent.

American Psychiatric Association: *Diagnostic and Statistical Manual of Mental Disorders,* 4th edn. Text Revised. American Psychiatric Association. 2000.

Schwartz S, Griffin T: *Medical Thinking.* Springer Verlag, 1986.

Weinstein MC et al.: *Clinical Decision Analysis.* WB Saunders, 1980.

PROCESS TRACING

Comparing experts with novices, researchers have traced the steps of naturalistic reasoning in areas such as chess, physics, mathematics, neurology, family practice, internal medicine, radiology, and psychiatry. A chess expert, for example, has built up from experience the memory of perhaps 50,000 chessboard patterns. Each pattern is

Table 1–2. Decision Pathway Toward Diagnosis

1. Communicate and elicit pertinent data.
2. Perceive salient cues.
3. Evaluate the significance of salient cues.
4. Make clinical inferences.
5. Assemble significant cues and clinical inferences as a clinical pattern.
6. On the basis of the pattern, generate an array of categorical and dynamic diagnostic hypotheses.
7. Design an inquiry plan and search for both disconfirmatory and confirmatory evidence.
8. On the basis of new evidence, progressively revise, rule out, or rule in the diagnostic hypotheses.
9. Reach a diagnostic conclusion.

associated with possible moves. Rapid pattern matching dynamically linked to good choice of next move explains the capacity of the chess expert to play and defeat many novices simultaneously. Thus, pattern recognition is linked to strategic option choice. The expertise of the diagnostician is similar: The recognition of an incomplete clinical pattern that matches, in part, the memory of a diagnostic syndrome is linked to tactical choices for eliciting, evaluating, and integrating further evidence to solve the diagnostic puzzle.

Clinical reasoning is a species of "bounded rationality" in which the clinician converts an open problem (i.e., a "problem space" with no clear endpoint) into a series of closed problems ("small worlds"), each with a hypothesized endpoint. In other words, the open problem is reframed as an array of closed problems that organize the search for evidence. The entire process depends on general cognitive ability and specific experience with the kind of problem space in question. Furthermore, diagnosis is not a static endpoint but rather a dynamic way station on the road to treatment. The decision pathway toward diagnosis is shown in Table 1–2 and is described in more detail in the sections that follow.

Eliciting & Perceiving Salient Cues

Even before the patient is seen, the clinician may have gathered cues, for example, from the referring agent. As the patient enters the office, before the interview begins, the clinician scans the patient's eyes, face, skin, clothes, gait, coordination, posture, and voice in order to perceive salient cues (e.g., "pale, elderly, frail, shabbily dressed, worried-looking woman using a walking stick, favoring her left leg"). The clinician must be alert to pertinent cues, distinguishing them from the immense amount of noise in the perceptual field. Initially, the net is cast widely so as to maximize the chance of correctly recognizing salient cues, perhaps at the expense of perceiving data

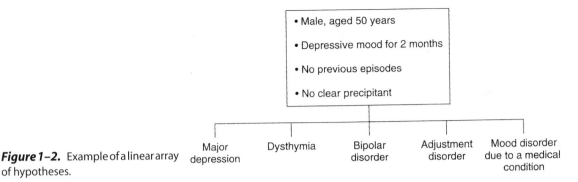

Figure 1–2. Example of a linear array of hypotheses.

that turn out to be irrelevant. As the diagnostic process proceeds, however, the gathering of evidence becomes more and more focused.

The patient sits down and the interview begins. The clinician's demeanor, receptiveness, and empathic communication encourage the patient to tell his or her story. More cues are elicited from the patient's spontaneous account of self.

Evaluating Cues & Making Inferences

Out of the enormous amount of noise, the experienced clinician knows what to look for. Freckles, for example, are less likely to be pertinent than are blue lips (although, in certain circumstances, freckles could be relevant). Blue lips, however, must be evaluated before they are regarded as significant (i.e., abnormal). Has the patient been eating berries, or is the blueness circulatory in origin? If the blueness is circulatory in origin, is it due to central or peripheral dysfunction?

If a patient says that people are talking about him or her, the clinician must decide whether this complaint is based on reality, whether it is an exaggeration of reality, or whether it is based on a false conviction (i.e., a delusion). The experienced clinician makes tentative inferences, at first, which he or she is prepared to revise if subsequent information does not bear them out.

Assembling Cues & Inferences as a Clinical Pattern

Soon after the clinical encounter has begun, the clinician begins to form cues and inferences into tentative patterns that form the gist of clinical reasoning; for example, (1) potentially lethal suicide attempt; (2) angry, depressed, disheveled adolescent girl lying in a hospital bed; (3) uncooperative and dismissive toward the examiner; (4) said to have made one previous suicide attempt (the time and lethality of which are uncertain at this point). The efficiency and accuracy of pattern discernment distinguishes the expert from the novice, as does the efficiency with which the expert matches clinical patterns, incom-

plete though they may be, against his or her memory of diagnostic syndromes.

Generating Categorical & Dynamic Hypotheses

The pattern prompts hypotheses, and hypotheses organize the subsequent clinical inquiry. The capacity of working memory limits the array of hypotheses to between four and six. The array of hypotheses may be linear or hierarchical (see Figures 1–2 and 1–3 for examples). Hypothetical reasoning prevents premature closure on one diagnosis and spares short-term memory by dividing the information derived from cues and inferences into strategic units, from each of which a systematic search for evidence can be planned. Hypotheses are open to revision in the light of new information derived from the inquiry process.

The diagnostic hypotheses generated are usually a mixture of categorical and dynamic types. **Categorical hypotheses** are expressed in terms of DSM-IV or a similar taxonomy. **Dynamic hypotheses** (e.g., "vulnerability to rejection related to abandonment by father") operate in parallel with categorical hypotheses and are not exclusive of them.

Designing an Inquiry Plan & Searching for Evidence

The inquiry process (i.e., history, mental status examination, physical examination, laboratory testing, special investigations, and information from collateral sources, past records, and consultations) has two aspects: **standard** and **discretionary**. Clinicians standardize their data collection (e.g., past medical history, mental status examination), casting the net widely to gather important cues and evidence in people from particular age, ethnic, or social groups. For example, questions about substance abuse, physical and sexual abuse, suicidal ideation, and antisocial behavior are virtually obligatory for adolescent patients. Similarly, certain urine and blood chemistry and hematologic tests may be part of a standard screen for

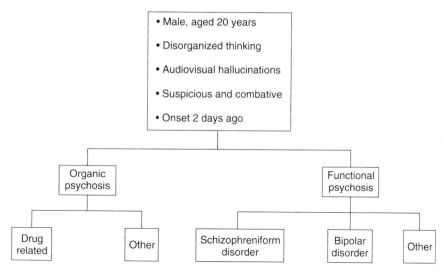

Figure 1–3. Example of a hierarchical hypothesis.

hospitalized patients. For the most part, however, the inquiry plan is discretionary. It is designed to elicit information relevant to the array of diagnostic hypotheses.

Revising, Deleting, or Accepting Hypotheses

Modifications of the standard history, mental status examination, and physical examination are determined by the diagnostic hypotheses. For example, if lead poisoning is hypothesized (e.g., as a cause of childhood hyperactivity), the clinician will inquire about the child's physical environment (e.g., exposure to old paint, batteries, or tetraethyl lead), examine the child's teeth and gums, and test the child's blood and urine. The inquiry plan yields data that complete the clinical pattern from which the preliminary hypotheses were derived and allows the clinician to disconfirm hypotheses or to refine them.

Reaching a Diagnostic Conclusion

When enough evidence has been gathered, the clinician weighs and summarizes the evidence supporting or refuting hypotheses that have not already been rejected. Sometimes, a single diagnosis is insufficient, and two or more diagnoses are required to account for a heterogeneous pattern of clinical features. Next, the clinician expands the diagnosis, combining dynamic and categorical diagnoses in a diagnostic formulation (see Chapter 36).

Cox K: Perceiving clinical evidence. *Med Educ* 2002;36:1189.

Dowe J, Elstein A: *Professional Judgment.* Cambridge University Press, 1988.

Elstein AS, Shulman LS, Sprafka SA: *Medical Problem Solving.* Harvard University Press, 1978.

Eva LW: What every teacher needs to know about clinical reasoning. *Med Educ* 2004;39:98.

Groves M, O'Rourke P, Alexander H: Clinical reasoning: The relative contribution of identification, interpretation, and hypothesis errors to misdiagnosis. *Med Teach* 2003;25:621.

Kushniruk AW, Patel VL, Marley AA: Small worlds and medical expertise. *Int J Med Inform* 1998;49:255.

■ THE STRATEGY OF CLINICAL REASONING

Diagnostic reasoning is a feed-forward, feedback hypothetico-deductive process involving cue recognition, clinical inference, hypothesis testing, inquiry planning, the search for evidence, the reaching of a diagnostic conclusion, and diagnostic formulation. In order to support the complexity of this process, the diagnostician must do several things (Table 1–3).

Nurcombe B, Gallagher RM: *The Clinical Process in Psychiatry.* Cambridge University Press, 1986.

■ FLAWS

Flexible and efficient though diagnostic reasoning may be, it is subject to a number of flaws (heuristic errors

Table 1–3. The Strategy of Diagnostic Reasoning

Tolerate uncertainty, avoid premature closure, and consider alternatives.

Separate cue from inference; be able to refer inferences to the salient cues from which they were derived.

Be aware of personal reactions to the patient.

Be alert for fresh evidence, particularly evidence that demands a revision or deletion of a hypothesis or diagnosis.

Value negative evidence above positive evidence.

Be prepared to commit to a diagnosis when enough evidence has been gathered.

Table 1–4. Potential Flaws in Diagnostic Reasoning

Only a limited number of hypotheses can be dealt with.

Subjective probabilities may be inaccurate (e.g., because of recent vivid experience).

Clinicians may lack a systematic inquiry plan.

Clinicians may fail to test all hypotheses in an impartial manner.

Clinicians may fail to refine or discard hypotheses in accordance with the evidence.

Clinicians may rely on a natural inclination to prefer confirmatory to disconfirmatory evidence.

Clinicians may be reluctant to commit to a diagnostic conclusion.

and biases) that are a consequence of the fact that the human computer has inherent capacity limitations and is vulnerable to interference by intrinsic and extrinsic factors.

The diagnostician's judgment can be clouded by fatigue or illness. Clinical judgment can also be biased when the clinician has an emotional reaction to the patient based, for example, on unresolved conflict from his or her own childhood experience (i.e., countertransference).

As mentioned earlier in this chapter, no more than four to six diagnostic hypotheses can be juggled at one time because the capacity of short-term memory is limited. This limitation is even more evident in the case of dynamic hypotheses, in which case the clinician will, unfortunately, often be satisfied with a single hypothesis, failing to consider alternatives.

The human computer is more impressed by information and hypotheses that appear early in the diagnostic encounter and is relatively less efficient at accounting for later data, especially if subsequent data run counter to first impressions. However, the expert clinician is able to adjust initial hypotheses in response to new information and to discard them when they no longer fit. Expert radiologists, for example, know where to look, what to see, and how to frame an anomalous pattern conceptually. They then engage in "top-down–bottom-up" recursive thinking, testing their initial flexible hypotheses against the details of the radiologic film and progressively adjusting or discarding their hypotheses in accordance with the evidence.

In the same way, the expert psychiatrist quickly discerns significant cues, makes tentative inferences, and assembles a dynamic pattern that allows efficient hypothesis generation. From these hypotheses, he or she begins recursive hypothesis testing, seeking both standard and discretionary data. Table 1–4 lists the chief potential flaws in this process.

CONCLUSION

Even after training, experience, and self-reflection, the clinician's reasoning is not perfectible. How can it be improved? No contemporary computer can match the skill of the expert clinician in recognizing and weighing cues and inferences, and assembling efficient patterns. However, computers excel at storing information, generating extensive arrays of hypotheses, calculating Bayesian probabilities, avoiding judgment biases, and ensuring that inquiry plans will be systematic. In the future, when base-rate probabilities are better understood, computers will become indispensable to accurate diagnosis and treatment planning. Self-report questionnaires, structured interviews, and search protocols could also enhance the reliability and comprehensiveness of data collection.

Although computers, questionnaires, standard interviews, and inquiry protocols can supplement the human computer, they cannot, as yet, replace it. Whether they will ever be able to do so is conjectural. Until then, they should be regarded as potential aids to the clinical decision maker, not rivals.

Psychiatric Epidemiology

Dan G. Blazer, MD, PhD

■ THE BIOPSYCHOSOCIAL MODEL & THE WEB OF CAUSATION

The late George Engel promulgated a theoretical model, based on general systems theory, of the etiology of mental disease that remains central to epidemiologic investigations into the twenty-first century. Research demonstrates that unitary explanations are not adequate to explain disease etiology or thus inform appropriate prevention and treatment strategies. Engel suggested an interrelatedness among biological, psychological, and social factors. Biological factors include hereditary, anatomic, and molecular factors and those factors related to gender, age, and ethnicity. Psychological factors include temperament, personality, motivation, emotion, attention, and cognition. According to Engel's theory, social factors included family, society, culture, and environment; other authors would include religious and spiritual as well as economic factors in this group. Engel also believed that the physician's contribution, through a psychosocial presence, to this "collaborative pathway to health" was often inseparable from that brought by the patient. From this perspective, psychiatric epidemiologists explore the frequency, distribution, outcome, and causation of psychiatric disorders. Identifying a case becomes the first task of the epidemiologist. An essential component of all these uses is the determination of valid **denominators** to compare the characteristics of populations with and without disease. For example, to determine the **prevalence** of a case (i.e., the frequency of the case in a given population at a given point in time) one must know the number of persons both with and without the disorder in the population. To determine the **incidence** of a case (the number of new cases that emerge in the population over a given interval (usually 1 year), one must know the number of people in the population at the beginning of an interval who do not experience the disorder. A list of key terms in epidemiology can be found in Table 2–1.

In recent years, psychiatric epidemiologists have recognized that cases often occur simultaneously in the same person (the cases are **comorbid**). Recent studies have emphasized not only the prevalence and incidence of individual cases but also comorbid cases.

Engel GL: The clinical application of the biopsychosocial model. *Am J Psychiatr* 1980;137:537–544.

Lilienfeld DE: Definitions of epidemiology. *Am J Epidemiol* 1978; 107:87.

CONCEPT OF THE "CASE"

The *Diagnostic and Statistical Manual of Mental Disorders,* fourth edition, Text Revised (DSM-IV-TR), and other psychiatric diagnostic systems disaggregate psychiatric disorders into discrete cases. For example, either an individual meets criteria for a diagnosis of major depressive disorder or he or she does not. To identify a case, one must have criteria for identifying cases, but these criteria may vary from one nomenclature to another. For example, the criteria for a case in DSM-IV-TR differ from those in DSM-III in some circumstances.

The use of the concept of a case in epidemiology makes it easier for practicing clinicians to interpret the types of studies performed by epidemiologists, although by arbitrarily assigning an individual to a category of either "case" or "noncase," one loses considerable data. Several early epidemiologic studies were cognizant of this dilemma and attempted to assign patients to groups based on how well they met the predetermined criteria for each group; these researchers recognized that the ability of clinicians to assign individuals as either cases or noncases was not perfect and was more applicable to a probability function than to a simple yes or no decision. Similarly, the use of symptom rating scales does not require that an individual be assigned to a case or noncase category but rather permits the assessment of depressive psychopathology as a continuum. (Examples of "case finding" in psychiatric epidemiology are provided below in the description of individual studies.)

American Psychiatric Association: *Diagnostic and Statistical Manual of Mental Disorders,* 4th edn. Text Revised. American Psychiatric Association, Washington DC 2000.

Table 2–1. Key Terms in Epidemiology

Prevalence: The frequency of a given disorder in a population at a particular point of time (i.e., it is the ratio of the number of cases of a disorder in the population divided by the number of persons in the population). Although community surveys take time to complete (usually 3 months to 1 year), it is assumed that the results of such studies estimate the frequency of a disorder within a population (usually given as a percentage) on a given day. In some cases, prevalence is measured not as the frequency on a given day but as the frequency of all cases of the disorder that are present during some interval of time, such as 1 month or 1 year.

Denominator: In the prevalence ratio, the denominator is the number of persons in the population. This number becomes important because the prevalence may vary depending on the population from which cases are selected. For example, the denominator may be all persons in a community, all females in a community, all persons attending a clinic, all persons 65 years of age or older attending a clinic, or all African Americans in the community. For each denominator, prevalence may vary.

Incidence: The likelihood, over a period of time (usually 1 year), that an individual who is free from a given disorder will develop it. For example, if 1000 persons are free of a disorder on January 1 and 100 develop the disorder during the next 12 months, then the incidence of that disorder is 10%. In most cases, incidence is much lower than prevalence, and, naturally, because incidence reflects a rate, the collection of data at two or more points in time is necessary to determine incidence.

Risk: The likelihood that an individual will experience a psychiatric disorder. In this sense, risk is basically a measure of incidence.

Risk factor: Any factor that may increase the likelihood that a person will develop a psychiatric disorder. For example, it is known that female gender, younger age, lower socioeconomic status, and being divorced are risk factors for developing major depression. A risk factor may not necessarily be causal.

Risk profile: The array of risk factors associated with a specific disorder.

Relative risk: The increased (or decreased) risk for developing a disorder among persons with a risk factor, compared to persons without a risk factor.

Comorbidity: The presence of at least two distinct disorders in the same individual, each with its own etiology, presentation, and course.

OTHER EPIDEMIOLOGIC CONCEPTS

To discern the relationship(s) between factors that contribute to the emergence of a case, epidemiologists explore what has been described as the **web of causation**. The concept of a web of causation is that specific relationships, such as the relationship between social stressors and a mental disorder, may be connected through a variety of intervening variables that interrelate in a way best illustrated by a web consisting of nodes (etiologic factors) and strings (interrelationships of these etiologic factors). For example, genetic factors may lead to endophenotypes (such as dysfunction of a neurotransmitter system), which lead to intermediate phenotypes (such as a depressed mood), which in turn are shaped by the social environment of the individual. Social factors, in turn, may alter genetic expression. Epidemiologic studies assist investigators in sorting out the different nodes and interactions within this web of causation.

According to Morris, epidemiology has several vital uses: (1) study of the historical health of communities and the estimation of morbidity for different disorders, (2) assessment of the efficiency of health programs and services, (3) determination of individuals **at risk** of acquiring a disease or disability in all their various presentations, (4) identification of syndromes as the unified collection of related signs and symptoms, and (5) assist-

ing in " . . . the search for the causes of health and disease." Proper epidemiologic studies can promote sound health policy, enable more rational health care planning, and facilitate cost-effective prevention and treatment.

MacMahon B, Pugh TF, Ipsen J: *Epidemiological Methods.* Little, Brown, 1960.

Morris JN: *Uses of Epidemiology.* Williams & Wilkins, 1964.

▮ HISTORICAL PERSPECTIVE

FIRST GENERATION STUDIES

The earliest formal psychiatric epidemiologic studies were undertaken during the first part of the twentieth century. They were generally of limited scale, relied on institutional records, and used small groups of informants for their data. These were "convenience" studies in which, instead of initiating the surveys themselves, epidemiologists assembled health data from those persons who had already received treatment for a medical problem or had committed suicide. Faris and Dunham's relatively large pre–World War II study examined the geographic distribution of patients with mental disorders in mental hospitals in the Chicago area. They found that manic–depressive illness was distributed equally throughout the geographic area, whereas schizophrenia clustered in the lower socioeconomic areas.

SECOND-GENERATION STUDIES: THE STIRLING COUNTY & MIDTOWN MANHATTAN STUDIES

In comparison to pre–World War II investigations, the studies that followed World War II took advantage of the considerable health information gathered on the military forces during the war. This was the beginning of the "community survey" era of epidemiology. Postwar studies—such as the Stirling County (Nova Scotia) Study, the Midtown Manhattan Study, and the Baltimore Study of mental illness in an urban population—were second-generation studies that attempted to determine the prevalence rates of mental illness in community residents with the help of nonpsychiatrist clinical interviewers. The postwar studies examined general health as well as psychiatric disorders and tended to gather and interpret rates of symptom presentation in groups rather than assess the presence of discrete cases. The gathering of often-isolated symptoms, or the finding of psychopathology or emotional illness by using the data collection system of the World War II era, was not helpful to health planners or policymakers.

Contributing to the ascension of psychiatric epidemiologic research during the early postwar period was the realization that the increase in mortality and morbidity associated with chronic disease (including that of mental disorders) was more important than was the mortality and morbidity associated with acute, generally infectious, disorders. Difficulty with case identification in the community continued to preclude the determination of prevalence rates for specific clinical disorders.

The initial paradigms for these newer studies were often quite different. The Stirling County Study attempted to determine rates for qualitatively different disorders as well as for overall impairment. The Midtown Manhattan Study assumed that mental disorders were on a continuum and—reflecting the thinking at that time (that mental illness differed in degree and not kind)—that all clinical manifestations of illness could be evaluated in terms of functional impairment. The overall prevalence of psychiatric impairment from both of these studies was approximately 20%. Leighton and colleagues demonstrated in Stirling County that the mental illness of the individual could be influenced, for benefit or detriment, by the attributes of the community, thus ushering in an emphasis, during the late 1950s and early 1960s, on social psychiatry.

THIRD-GENERATION STUDIES

Third-generation epidemiologic studies were based on more advanced epidemiologic and statistical techniques and on a move toward scientific or evidence-based medicine. These studies began with the important development of operational criteria for mental disorders (specifically DSM-III). Newer methodological techniques helped address the increasing need for more exact rates of specific disorders for specific persons in specific settings. Indeed, effective treatment has been shown to be related directly to accurate and thus specific assessment and diagnosis. Similarly, appropriate mental health policy planning for the unique health needs of persons with various psychiatric disorders depends greatly on an accurate and precise definition of boundaries between disorders. Further, research into the etiology and thus effective treatment and, it is hoped, eventual prevention of psychiatric disorders must derive from the specificity of operational criteria. Otherwise, the blurring that has occurred between symptom patterns can lead only to similar blurring in the assessment of treatment and prevention effectiveness.

The American Psychiatric Association's DSM-III was a clear departure from its predecessors in that the specificity and boundaries that demarcated a foundation of this evolving instrument led to specific case and noncase determinations. Many etiologic assumptions in DSM-II that were not demonstrated by empirical research were abandoned in DSM-III. Although interview instruments have been derived from each of these criteria sets, the Diagnostic Interview Schedule (DIS), associated with the development of DSM-III, was the first instrument designed for use by (trained) lay interviewers in community-based epidemiologic studies, a decision based on cost–benefit considerations. The DIS became the preferred instrument for use in most large epidemiologic studies during the 1980s, such as the epidemiologic catchment area (ECA) study (see next section).

THE NATIONAL INSTITUTE OF MENTAL HEALTH'S EPIDEMIOLOGIC CATCHMENT AREA STUDY

The National Institute of Mental Health's ECA study was the most comprehensive and sophisticated epidemiologic study accomplished in its time in the United States. When it was undertaken between 1980 and 1984, its purpose was to provide the best estimates, for the United States, of the prevalence of alcohol and drug abuse and other mental disorders, based on a formalized criteria set (DSM-III) rather than global impairment. Unlike previous studies, this investigation included not only data from institutional and community samples but also longitudinal data and information on disease severity. The

ECA investigators explored the specific demographic, biological, psychosocial, and environmental factors that might influence the presence and the severity of a mental disorder (i.e., the biopsychosocial model). The study not only allowed investigators to follow up on possible clinical change but also assessed the service utilization of both mental health and general health services. The ECA study has assisted greatly in the planning for future health care service needs including physical resources, financing, personnel, and educational requirements. The ECA study also confirmed the capability of DSM-III criteria to discriminate among mental disorders and generally helped sharpen the nosology of mental illness.

Although the methodology of the ECA study was a great improvement on previous work, the use of DSM-III as the basis for case identification tended to emphasize reliability rather than validity. DSM-III diagnostic criteria, in contrast to DSM-II criteria, were intended to enhance diagnostic reliability, which, although necessary, is insufficient to establish diagnostic validity. Further, because lay interviewers were employed in the ECA study, indepth, qualitative data could not be collected.

Compared to previous surveys, the ECA study found lower rates of virtually all disorders, except for phobic disorders (as can be seen in Table 2–2). Women exhibited higher rates of mental disorders than did men, although there were important differences in the rates for specific disorders. Men had higher rates of substance abuse and antisocial personality disorder, and women had significantly higher rates for anxiety-based, affective, and somatization disorders. Men and women exhibited similar rates for schizophrenia and manic episodes. The ECA study showed that individuals with comorbid conditions were more likely to receive treatment than were those with a single disorder; yet, less than one third of persons with mental illness, a substance abuse disorder, or both received any treatment. An important methodological finding was that, in comparison to international studies (after adjusting for differences in diagnostic categories and time frames), disease rates based on the DIS were found to be essentially compatible with previous epidemiologic studies based on the PSE.

THE NATIONAL COMORBIDITY STUDY AND ITS REPLICATE

The National Comorbidity Study (NCS) was the first attempt in the United States to estimate the prevalence of specific psychiatric disorders, with and without comorbid substance abuse, in a national population sample. The NCS was designed to further the findings of the ECA study, but in contrast to the ECA study (which was drawn from local and institutional groups), the NCS had a national focus. The NCS sought risk factors as well as

prevalence and incidence rates, in contrast to the ECA study, which focused only on the latter. Table 2–2 provides comparison data from the two studies. With its national focus, the NCS made possible regional comparisons, including rural and urban differences, and it was possible to establish, on a national basis, more precise investigations into unmet mental illness treatment needs. Furthermore, the NCS was referenced to the DSM-III-R rather than DSM-III and also contained some questions that would allow comparison to the future DSM-IV and the *International Classification of Diseases,* 10th edition (ICD-10). The NCS found a higher prevalence of mental disorders in the U.S. population, and this prevalence was aggregated in approximately one sixth of the population (i.e., in individuals who had three or more comorbid disorders).

In the NCS, risk profiles were constructed for depression alone and when found in association with other psychiatric disorders: 4.9% of persons studied were found to have current major depression (i.e., within the last 30 days) and 10.3% to have major depression within the past 12 months (see Table 2–2). The lifetime prevalence of depression was 17.1%. Risk factors for both current and lifetime depression were as follows: being female; having a lower level of education; and being separated, widowed, or divorced. The NCS investigators fielded a new survey between 2001 and 2003 (the NCS Replicate) and found even higher 1-year prevalence of specific psychiatric disorders: major depression (6.7), bipolar disorder I and II (2.6), dysthymic disorder (1.5), generalized anxiety disorder (3.1), panic disorder (2.7), obsessive compulsive disorder (1.0), alcohol abuse (3.1), alcohol dependence (1.3), posttraumatic stress disorder (3.5), and a diagnosis of any disorder (26.2). The rates for all time frames and the demographic distributions in the NCS and NCS-R were higher than those found in the ECA study. The fact that a different method of case identification was used probably explains most of the difference in prevalence between the NCS and the ECA study. The sample from the NCS was younger, and younger persons are known to have a higher prevalence of major depression. The NCS also suggested that although "pure" depression may have a strong biogenetic contribution, comorbid depression may be more environmentally determined. Furthermore, as in the ECA study and other international investigations, more recent birth cohorts were found to be at increased risk for major depression.

Many explanations have been offered for the striking finding of high estimates of childhood depression and the unexpectedly low estimates of depression in the elderly: methodological limitations including the bias found in diagnostic instruments for the assessment of psychopathology in both children and the elderly, differential morbidity, faulty sampling, response-biased

Table 2–2. Comparison Data from the NCS and ECA Study[1]

Disorder	Prevalence Rates (12 months)	
	NCS (12 months)	ECA Study
Any disorder	27.7	20
Substance abuse disorders	16.1	N/A
Alcohol abuse and dependence	10.7 dependence only	6.8
Drug abuse and dependence	3.8 dependence only	2.41
Schizophrenia/schizophreniform disorders	0.5 (0.1)	1.0
Affective (mood) disorders	8.5	5.1
Manic episode	1.4	
Major depressive episode	7.7	2.7
Dysthymia	2.1	2.3
Anxiety disorders	11.8	N/A
Social Phobia	6.4	6.2
Panic	1.3	0.9
Obsessive-compulsive disorder	N/A	1.65
Antisocial personality disorder (life time)	4.8	1.2
Cognitive impairment	N/A	1.3

[1]ECA study data are from Robins LN, Regier DA (eds). *Psychiatric Disorder in America.* New York, The Free Press. NCS data are from Kessler RC, McGonagle KA, Zhao S, et al: Lifetime and 12-month prevalence of DSM-III psychiatric disorders in the United States. Results from the National Comorbidity Survey. *Arch Gen Psychiatry* 51: 8–19, 1994.
N/A, not available.

memory, institutionalization, and selective migration. Some or all of these explanations may play a role.

Continued investigation of the NCS data, building on the findings of the Medical Outcome study (which showed that depressive symptoms themselves were a significant risk factor for other diseases found that major and minor depression were not distinct entities but were actually on a continuum. Further, and also using the NCS data, the lifetime prevalence of major and minor depression associated with seasonal affective disorder (SAD) was found to be much lower (1%) than that found in previous studies. This was probably because the instrument used more accurately reflected DSM-III-R criteria for SAD. Another study, using the NCS data, found a significant lifetime association between panic disorder and depression in patients who first present with panic disorder and a less powerful but statistically valid association for those who first present with depression. An investigation from Germany, using the revised version of the Composite International Diagnosis Interview on a community sample of adolescents and young adults, found that agoraphobia and panic disorder had "marked differences in symptomatology, course, and associated impairments" and were not necessarily linked, a finding at odds with some earlier studies. If confirmed, this study, which used a more sophisticated epidemiologic design than was available in much earlier studies, will demonstrate a more precise separation between several disorders previously considered to be closely related. This finding may lead to a more definitive basis for both prevention and treatment strategies.

More narrowly focused epidemiologic studies have contributed to increased understanding of psychiatric disorders associated with social conditions. Through a population survey, Breslau and colleagues demonstrated that posttraumatic stress disorder occurred in 9.2% of the population following exposure to trauma. Not only was this prevalence lower than that reported previously, but the most common trauma experienced was the unexpected death of a loved one, not the usually reported combat, rape, or other serious physical assault. Bassuk and colleagues investigated the prevalence of mental illness and substance abuse disorders among homeless and low-income housed mothers, compared to the prevalence of these disorders among all women in the NCS, and found the prevalence of trauma-related disorders among poor women to be significantly higher than that found among women in the general population.

American Psychiatric Association: *Diagnostic and Statistical Manual of Mental Disorders,* 3rd edn. American Psychiatric Association, 1980.

Bassuk EL et al.: Prevalence of mental health and substance use disorders among homeless and low-income housed mothers. *Am J Psychiatry* 1998;155:1561.

Blazer DG, Kessler RC, Swartz M: Epidemiology of recurrent major and minor depression with a seasonal pattern. The National Comorbidity Survey. *Br J Psychiatry* 1998;172:164.

Breslau N et al.: Trauma and post traumatic stress disorder in the community: The 1996 Detroit Area Survey of Trauma. *Arch Gen Psychiatry* 1998;55:626.

Faris R, Dunham H: *Mental Disorders in Urban Areas.* Chicago: University of Chicago Press, 1939.

Kessler RC et al.: Lifetime and 12-month prevalence of DSM-III-R psychiatric disorders in the United States. Results from the National Comorbidity Study. *Arch Gen Psychiatry* 1994;51:8.

Kessler RC et al.: Prevalence, correlates, and course of minor depression and major depression in the National Comorbidity Survey. *J Affect Disord* 1997;45:19.

Kessler RC et al.: Prevalence, severity, and comorbidity of 12-month DSM-IV disorders in the National Comorbidity Survey replication. *Arch Gen Psychiatry* 2005;62:617.

Kessler RC et al: Lifetime panic-depression comorbidity in the National Comorbidity Survey. *Arch Gen Psychiatry* 1998;55:801.

Leighton DC et al.: *The Character of Danger: Psychiatric Symptoms in Selected Communities.* Basic Books, 1963.

Pasamanick B et al.: A survey of mental disease in an urban population. *Am J Public Health* 1956;47:923.

Robins L, Regier D: *Psychiatric Disorders in America: The Epidemiologic Catchment Area Study.* New York: The Free Press, 1991.

Robins L, Helzer J, Croughan J: Diagnostic Interview Schedule: Its history, characteristics and validity. *Arch Gen Psychiatry,* 1981;38:381–389.

Strole L, Fisher AK: *Mental Health in the Metropolis: The Midtown Manhattan Study.* McGraw-Hill, 1982.

Wittchen HU, Reed V, Kessler RC: The relationship of agoraphobia and panic in a community sample of adolescents and young adults. *Arch Gen Psychiatry* 1998;55:1017.

RURAL–URBAN DIFFERENCES & THE SOCIAL DRIFT HYPOTHESIS

Another important finding of most epidemiologic studies is that the prevalence of some mental disorders, particularly schizophrenia, has been found to be higher in urban and industrialized areas than in rural areas. A number of explanations for this finding have been suggested: social migration (the downward drift of persons and families experiencing schizophrenia to lower socioeconomic levels), inbreeding among the mentally ill, and the greater availability in urban areas of services for the chronically mentally ill. These differences may also reflect the comparative integration and stability of rural areas. Leighton and colleagues, in their study of rural Nova Scotia, found that depression (and other psychiatric disorders) were more common for all ages in "disintegrated" communities. Given the recent emphasis on the genetic basis of many psychiatric disorders, more research must be done on the degree of possible inheritance of these disorders in populations, and on the social drift hypothesis, before firm conclusions can be reached.

Leighton AH: *My Name is Legion.* New York: Basic Books, 1959.

MENTAL DISORDER, PHYSICAL HEALTH, & SOCIAL FUNCTIONING

A survey of the point prevalence of schizophrenia within three regions of Scotland was undertaken in 1996, replicating a similar survey conducted in 1981. In comparison to the 1981 study, the patients studied in 1996 had both more positive and negative symptoms and more nonschizophrenic symptoms. Some of the symptoms encountered involved physical health.

An increasing number of epidemiologic studies have demonstrated that depression is a serious illness in its own right and that depressive disorder, and depressive symptoms without a formal depressive disorder being present, can have a serious impact on the general physical health of an individual. The Medical Outcome study looked carefully at this association by evaluating processes and outcomes of care for patients with the chronic conditions of hypertension, diabetes, coronary heart disease, and depression. Patients with either a current depressive disorder or depressive symptoms in the absence of a disorder tended to have worse physical health, poorer social role functioning, worse perceived current health, and (perceived) greater bodily pain than did patients without a chronic depressive condition. Further, the poor functioning associated with depression or depressive symptoms was equal or worse than that associated with eight major medical conditions, and the effects of depressive symptoms and chronic medical conditions were addictive. For example, the combination of advanced coronary artery disease and depressive symptoms was associated with roughly twice the reduction in social functioning than was found with either condition alone. These authors and subsequent studies concluded that it was important to correctly assess and treat depression in all health care settings in order to improve overall patient outcome, reduce patient and family suffering, and reduce societal costs. The Medical Outcome study was one of the first to directly compare the social and occupational costs of physical and psychiatric disorders, emphasizing that psychiatric disorders are a major public health concern. More recent research has extended these findings.

Spitzer and colleagues found that depression, anxiety, somatoform disorders, and eating disorders were associated with considerable impairment in health-related quality of life scales. As in the Medical Outcome study, impairment was found in patients with subclinical symptoms and in those with clinically diagnosable disorders. Mental disorders appeared to contribute to overall impairment to a greater degree than did medical conditions.

From 1982 to 1996, the comorbidity of physical and psychiatric disorders was studied in an unselected 1966 northern Finland birth cohort. In comparison to individuals without a psychiatric diagnosis, psychiatric patients were found to have been hospitalized more frequently for injuries, poisonings, or indefinite symptoms. Men were more commonly hospitalized with a variety of gastrointestinal and circulatory disturbances; women with a comorbid psychiatric disorder were more commonly hospitalized with respiratory disorders, vertebral column disorders, gynecologic disorders, or induced abortions. Epilepsy, nervous and sensory organ disorders in general, and inflammatory disorders of the bowels were more common in patients with schizophrenia as compared to those without the disease. The National Treatment Outcome Research Study, the first large-scale prospective, multisite treatment outcome study of drug users in the United Kingdom, found an extensive range of psychological and physical health problems among this population. Studies looking at the comorbid features of physical and psychological health have consistently demonstrated a high correlation, and these findings have given leaders in the health, social service, and criminal justice systems impetus to plan integrated approaches to this vulnerable, and at least dually afflicted, population.

Gossop M et al.: Substance use, health, and social problems of service users at 54 drug treatment agencies. Intake data from the National Treatment Outcome Research Study. *Br J Psychiatry* 1998;173:166.

Kelly C et al.: Nithsdale Schizophrenia Surveys. 17. Fifteen year review. *Br J Psychiatry* 1998;172:513.

Makikyro T et al.: Comorbidity of hospital-treated psychiatric and physical disorders with special reference to schizophrenia: A 28 year follow-up of the 1966 Northern Finland General Population. *Public Health* 1998;112(4):221–228.

Spitzer RL, Kroen Ke K, Lirzan M, et al.: Health related quality of life in primary care patients with mental disorders, *J Am Med Assoc* 1995;274: 1511–1517.

Wells KB et al.: The functioning and well-being of depressed patients. *J Am Med Assoc* 1989;262:914.

CONCLUSION: EPIDEMIOLOGY, ETIOLOGY, & PUBLIC HEALTH

Epidemiology places psychiatric disorders in a broad context, which is not always apparent with individual patients. This comprehensiveness is the basis of the biopsychosocial model. Three kinds of factors may be operative: those that promote vulnerability (or indeed resilience), those that "release" symptoms at a particular time, and those that determine how long a particular disorder will last. Koopman (1996) adds that there is now a shift to studying complex systems that create patterns of disease. Such studies are conducted by the comprehensive monitoring of individuals as individuals and when they interact with others and their environment.

Research by Kendler and colleagues (1993), investigating the risk factors for depression among twins, is among the first of an increasing number of epidemiologic studies based on an integrated biopsychosocial approach. Henderson (1996) extends this approach along the causal continuum in a slightly different way, noting that "the concept of populations having different frequency distributions of morbidity, not just different prevalence rates for clinical cases, carries with it the implication that some factor or factors are pushing up the over-all distribution in some groups, but not in others." He suggests that there may be some instrumental "force" in the environment that promotes disease. According to Susser and Susser (1996), epidemiology historically offered the paradigm of the "black box," in which exposure was related directly to outcome, without much interest (and thus investigation) into contributing factors or pathogenesis. Moving toward a more fundamental, comprehensive, and integrative goal, these authors would suggest the alternative paradigm of "ecoepidemiology" or the study of "causal pathways at the societal level and with pathogenesis and causality at the molecular level." Among the lessons that may be drawn then are (1) that intervention by those in health policy and practice must involve a population-based strategy rather than a singular focus on afflicted or vulnerable individuals, (2) that the web of causation is multidimensional, and (3) that theory and practice are interdependent.

Korkeila and colleagues (1998) investigated factors predicting readmission to a psychiatric hospital during the early 1990s in Finland. Frequently admitted patients were found to be an identifiable group with three defining characteristics: previous admissions, long length of stays, and a diagnosis of psychosis or personality disorder. This study was particularly important because it reconfirmed earlier work that showed that, in this era of an emphasis on community care, there may be a small group of patients who, with the current treatment strategies available, may always need frequent or longer hospital treatment.

Public health prevention and treatment strategies drawn from any research must be carefully and critically constructed. This will not be easy. Intervention with individuals and even populations of individuals may be both more difficult and less effective when the real ". . . target is a social entity with its own laws and dynamics." To begin to address these issues of profound complexity and increasing topical relevance, many authors have strongly supported the reintegration of population-driven epidemiology into public health. Adding support and some urgency to this drive has been the advent of managed care, which has created information needs that only more

sophisticated epidemiologic investigations can address. Questions on specific treatments for specific patient populations in specific settings; the effectiveness of various forms of health care, including management and finance strategies; and the relentless quest for ways to improve quality while simultaneously attending to related costs will all require methodologically sound investigations.

Henderson AS: The present state of psychiatric epidemiology. *Aust N Z J Psychiatry* 1996;30:9.

Kendler KS et al.: The prediction of major depression in women: Towards an integrated etiologic model. *Am J Psychiatry* 1993;150:1139.

Koopman J: Comment: Emerging objectives and methods in epidemiology. *Am J Public Health* 1996;86:630.

Korkeila JA et al.: Frequently hospitalized psychiatric patients: A study of predictive factors. *Soc Psychiatry Psychiatr Epidemiol* 1998;33:528.

Susser M, Susser F: Choosing a future for epidemiology. I. Eras and paradigms. *Am J Public Health* 1996;86:668.

Psychiatric Genetics

John I. Nurnberger, Jr., M.D., Ph.D., & Wade Berrettini, M.D., Ph.D

■ METHODS IN PSYCHIATRIC GENETICS

A scientific revolution has occurred in the field of genetics with the advent of molecular biological techniques. Using these techniques, genes influencing risk for many neuropsychiatric diseases have been identified: initially Mendelian single gene conditions such as Huntington disease were resolved; in the last few years complex genetic conditions such as alcohol dependence have yielded specific genes. Some of this work has been facilitated by the study of endophenotypes or biologic vulnerability markers.

CLINICAL EPIDEMIOLOGY: TWIN, FAMILY, AND ADOPTION STUDIES

Three types of population genetic studies—twin, family, and adoption studies—are conducted to ascertain whether a particular human phenomenon is substantially genetically influenced.

Twin studies are based on the fact that monozygotic (MZ) or identical twins represent a natural experiment in which two individuals have exactly the same DNA sequence for each of their genes. This is in contrast to dizygotic (DZ) or fraternal twins who share 50% of their DNA sequences and are no more genetically similar than any pair of siblings. A phenomenon that is influenced by genetic factors should be more "concordant" (similar) in MZ twins compared to DZ twins.

Family studies can answer three critical questions concerning the inheritance of a disorder:

Are relatives of an affected subject at **increased risk** for the disorder compared to relatives of control subjects?

What other disorders may share a common genetic vulnerability with the phenomenon in question?

Can a specific mode of inheritance be discerned?

A family study typically begins with a **proband** or initially ascertained patient, whose relatives are then studied.

Nurnberger Jr JI, Wiegand R, Bucholz K, et al.: A family study of alcohol dependence: Coaggregation of multiple disorders in relatives of alcohol-dependent probands. *Arch Gen Psychiatry* 2004;61:1246–1256.

Adoption studies: In adoption studies the risk for the disorder may be evaluated in four groups of relatives: the adoptive and biological relatives of affected adoptees and the adoptive and biological relatives of control adoptees. If the disorder is heritable, one should find an increased risk among the biological relatives of affected subjects, compared to the other three groups of relatives. One can also compare risk for illness in adopted-away children of ill parents versus adopted-away children of well parents.

Segregation analysis may be used to determine whether the pattern of illness in families is consistent with a specific mode of transmission. This is most useful for conditions in which a single gene accounts for a substantial portion of the variance. Most major psychiatric disorders do not appear to fall in this category.

Some of the complexities of major psychiatric disorders are as follows:

Variable penetrance (some individuals with a genetic predisposition will not manifest the disease)

Phenocopies (individuals without a genetic predisposition who manifest the symptoms of the disease)

Genetic heterogeneity (more than one type of genetic cause can produce the same syndrome)

The diagnostic boundaries of a syndrome may be uncertain.

Pleiotropy (one gene may be expressed in different ways in different persons).

Linkage Analysis

At any genetic locus, each individual carries two copies (**alleles**) of the DNA sequence that defines that locus. One of these alleles is inherited from the mother and the other from the father. These alleles will be transmitted with equal probability (i.e., 1/2), one of the two alleles to each offspring. If two genetic loci are "close" to each other on a chromosome, their alleles tend to be inherited together (not independently) and they are known as "linked" loci. During meiosis, crossing over (also known as **recombination**) can occur between homologous chromosomes, thus accounting for the observation that alleles at linked loci are not **always** inherited together.

The rate at which crossing over occurs between two linked loci is directly proportional to the distance on the chromosome between them. In fact, the genetic distance between two linked loci is defined in terms of the percentage of recombination between the two loci (this value is known as **theta**). Loci that are "far" apart on a chromosome will have a 1/2 chance of being inherited together and they are not linked. Thus, the maximum value for theta is 0.5, while the minimum value is 0. Linkage analysis is a method for estimating theta for two or more loci.

The probability that two loci are linked is the probability that theta <0.5. The probability that the two loci are not linked is the probability that theta = 0.5. Thus, a LOD (logarithm of the odds ratio) score is defined as

LOD score

$$= \log_{10} \left[\frac{\text{probability that a family has theta} < 0.5}{\text{probability that a family has theta} = 0.5} \right].$$

Although it is possible to perform such calculations by hand (see Ott, 1985), LOD scores are usually calculated using computer programs, such as GENEHUNTER or Merlin. Since a LOD score is a log value, scores from different families can be summed. For complex conditions, collections of affected sib pairs may be studied rather than large families. A LOD score of 1.0 indicates that linkage is 10 times more likely than nonlinkage. For simple genetic conditions, a LOD score of three or greater is evidence for linkage, while a score of −2 or less is sufficient to exclude linkage for the sample studied. For disorders with more complex forms of inheritance (including most psychiatric disorders), a higher positive LOD score is required (3.6 for definite linkage and 2.2 for suggestive linkage).

Lander E, Kruglyak L: Genetic dissection of complex traits: Guidelines for interpreting and reporting linkage results. *Nat Genet* 1995;11(3):241–247.

McQueen MB, Devlin B, Faraone SV, et al.: Combined analysis from eleven studies of bipolar disorder provides strong evidence of susceptibility loci on chromosomes 6q and 8q. *Am J Hum Genet* 2005;77:582–595.

Association Studies

In association studies one compares allele frequencies for a given locus in two populations, one of which is composed of unrelated individuals who have a disease, while the "control" population is usually composed of ethni-cally similar unrelated persons who do not have the disease. If a particular allele commonly predisposes individuals to the disease in question, then that allele should occur more frequently in the disease population, compared to the control population.

There are potential pitfalls to the case-control association approach. The locus chosen for study must predispose to illness. Thus, loci chosen for association studies are often known as candidate genes. If the locus does not predispose to illness, then the results of an association study should be negative. However, false positive results can occur if the two populations are not carefully matched for ethnic background. One alternative control group is the parents of affected individuals (the alleles *not* transmitted to the affected child compose the "control group"—this is known as the Transmission Disequilibrium Test or TDT).

Schulze TG, McMahon FJ: Genetic association mapping at the crossroads: Which test and why? Overview and practical guidelines. *Am J Med Genet* 2002;114(1):1–11.

High-Risk Studies

Biochemical studies of individuals with psychiatric diseases are always confounded by the issue of disease effects: are biochemical differences between affected individuals and controls related to the cause of the disorder, or are they related to the effects of the disorder (or its treatment)? When investigating possible biochemical differences for a genetic disease, this difficult issue can be addressed by studying a group of individuals (usually adolescents or young adults) who are at high risk to develop the disorder under study (usually because they have parents and/or other relatives with the disorder). The high-risk group may then be followed over time to assess whether the biochemical abnormalities observed are truly predictive of the disease.

Schuckit MA, Smith TL, Chacko Y: Evaluation of a depression-related model of alcohol problems in 430 probands from the San Diego prospective study. *Drug Alcohol Depend* 2006;82(3):194–203.

MOLECULAR GENETIC METHODS

Simple sequence repeat (SSR) markers, also known as **microsatellites** represent a group of polymorphisms based upon a variable number of a repeated sequence. However, in the case of SSR markers, the repeated sequence consists of 2–5 nucleotides. The repeated sequence is often—$(CA)_n$—,—$(AG)_n$—, or—$(AAAT)_n$—, although other SSR sequences have been described. The region containing the SSR is amplified by using a thermostable DNA polymerase in a **polymerase chain reaction (PCR)**. Microsatellites are commonly used to test linkage.

A different class of DNA markers, **single nucleotide polymorphisms (SNPs)**, are usually used to detect association. An SNP is variation at one base in a DNA sequence (e.g., compare GATACA with GATGCA, in which the fourth nucleotide can be either "A" or "G"). It is estimated that there are ~3 million common SNPs in the human genome, evenly distributed across the 3 billion bases of the human genome.

SNP detection is now highly automated, permitting the determination of more than one million SNP genotypes on each DNA sample, via DNA "chips" (microscope slide shaped devices) to which are attached up to one million oligonucleotides (short fragments of DNA sequence ~20–30 bases in length). These oligonucleotides each permit the determination of the presence of an allele at a single SNP. This advance now permits **genome-wide association** studies for complex disorders, in which the frequency of alleles at each of the one million SNPs are compared in large groups of cases and controls.

Wellcome Trust Case Control Consortium: Genome-wide association study of 14,000 cases of seven common diseases and 3,000 shared controls. *Nature* 2007;447:661–678.

AFFECTIVE DISORDERS

1. Genetic Epidemiologic Studies

A. FAMILY STUDIES

Family studies in affective disorder have continually demonstrated an aggregation of illness in relatives (Table 3–1). In a study at NIMH, 25% of the relatives of bipolar (BP) probands were found to have bipolar or unipolar (UP) illness, compared to 20% of relatives of UP probands and 7% of relatives of controls. In the same study, 40% of the relatives of schizoaffective probands demonstrated affective illness at some point in their lives. These data demonstrate increased risk in relatives of patients. They also show that the various forms of affective illness appear to be related in a hierarchical way: relatives of schizoaffective probands may have schizoaffective illness themselves, but are more likely to have BP or UP illness. Relatives of BP probands have either BP or (more likely) UP illness.

Age of onset may be useful in dividing affective illness into more genetically homogeneous subgroups. Early-onset probands have an increased morbid risk of illness in relatives in some data sets. Other **subphenotypes**, such as cycling frequency and comorbid anxiety disorders or substance use disorders, have also been studied.

A birth cohort effect was observed in several family studies, with an: an increasing incidence of affective illness among persons born more recently. The cohort effect was observed among relatives at risk to a greater degree than in the general population. The reasons for this increase in incidence are not yet clear.

B. TWIN STUDIES

Twin studies show consistent evidence for heritability. On the average, MZ twin pairs show concordance 65% of the time and DZ twin pairs 14% of the time.

C. ADOPTION STUDIES

Several adoption studies have been performed in the area of affective illness. The results have been generally consistent with genetic hypotheses.

2. The Affective Spectrum

Following are the types of affective disorders and other disorders that are genetically related:

BPI—Classic "manic–depressive illness" with severe mania, generally including episodes of major depression as well.

BPII—This disorder is genetically related to BPI and UP. There is some evidence in recent family studies for an excess of BPII illness in relatives of BPII probands. It has been demonstrated that BPII tends to be a stable lifetime diagnosis, that is, patients do not frequently convert to BPI.

Table 3–1. Steps Involved in the Detection of Polymorphisms

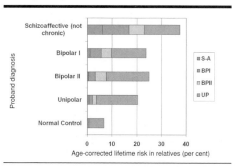

Table 3–2. Concordance Rates for Affective Illness in Monozygotic and Dizygotic Twins[*,†]

	Monozygotic Twins		Dizygotic Twins	
Reference	**Concordant Pairs/ Total Pairs**	**Concordance (%)**	**Concordant Pairs/ Total Pairs**	**Concordance (%)**
Luxenberger (1930)	3/4	75.0	0/13	0.0
Rosanoff et al. (1935)	16/23	69.6	11/67	16.4
Slater (1953)	4/7	57.1	4/17	23.5
Kallman (1954)	25/27	92.6	13/55	23.6
Harvald and Hauge (1965)	10/15	66.7	2/40	5.0
Allen et al. (1974)	5/15	33.3	0/34	0.0
Bertelsen (1979)	32/55	58.3	9/52	17.3
Totals	95/146	65.0	39/278	14.0

[*]Data not corrected for age. Diagnoses include both bipolar and unipolar illness.
[†]Full references are found in Nurnberger et al., 1994.

Rapid cycling—Rapid-cycling BP illness has been the subject of great theoretical and clinical interest. A link with thyroid pathology has been proposed. Rapid-cycling appears to arise from factors which are separable from the genetic vulnerability to BP illness and which do not lead to aggregation within families. However "rapid switching" of mood, which is related, appears to be familial.

UP mania—This entity includes BPI patients with no history of major depression. This group is not distinguishable from other BPI patients on the basis of family pattern of illness.

Cyclothymia—This condition of repetitive high and low mood swings, generally not requiring clinical attention, is probably genetically related to BP disorder.

Schizoaffective disorder—A group of patients with intermittent psychosis during euthymia have an increase in affective illness and schizophrenia in relatives. This group may have the highest genetic load (total risk for affective or schizophrenic illness in relatives) of any diagnostic category. They may carry genes related to both BP illness and schizophrenia. Patients with chronic psychosis and superimposed episodes of mood disorder confer risk for both chronic psychosis and mood disorder to relatives but have less overall genetic load.

Schizophrenia—An overlap in linkage areas and vulnerability genes has been identified in recent years; some of this overlap may relate to genes involved in glutamate neurotransmission.

Eating disorders—Family studies of anorexia and bulimia have generally found excess affective illness in relatives. Relatives of anorexics may have similar risk for affective disorders to that of relatives of BP probands.

Attention-deficit disorder—Children with this disorder appear to have increased depression in their relatives. The opposite has not been demonstrated (BP/UP probands have not been reported to have increased risk of attention deficit disorder in their offspring).

Alcohol dependence—There may be overlapping vulnerability traits. Alcoholism appears to be comorbid with UP and BP disorders (each appears to confer an increased risk for the other within individuals). There is some evidence that alcoholism with affective disorder may itself aggregate within families.

3. Linkage Studies

Linkage has been demonstrated on 4p, 6q, 8q, 13q, 18p, 18q, and 22q. Other areas are "close" to significant (e.g., 12q, 21q, and Xq).

4. Endophenotypes

A number of endophenotypic markers have been suggested, including:

REM sleep induction by cholinergic drugs,
white matter hyperintensities on MRI,
amygdala activation on fMRI,
hippocampal size,
response to tryptophan depletion, and
response to sleep deprivation.

5. Gene expression studies

Studies have begun on genome-wide gene expression in animal models of affective disorder, in brain samples from autopsy studies of patients with mood disorders, and in peripheral tissues such as blood. These studies should be helpful in identifying candidate genes for mood disorders.

6. High-Risk Studies

More offspring of patients than controls have a diagnosed Axis I disorder. Offspring of BP parents may be more prone to respond to dysphoric feeling states with "disinhibitory" behavior.

7. Association/Candidate Gene Studies

Numerous candidate gene studies are now in the literature for BP illness. A few genes have emerged with replicated findings, or positive meta-analyses from multiple studies. We will feature these here.

G72—This gene is one of the two implicated together in association studies on chromosome 13q. The gene G30 is a DNA sequence that is reverse-transcribed within G72. The association was first identified by Hattori et al. (2003) after work by Chumakov and colleagues in schizophrenia. It has been replicated by three other independent groups. The most recent work shows association not only with BP illness, but also with a subset of subjects who have schizophrenia with clear mood episodes. The function of G72 (also sometimes referred to as DAOA) may be to, oxidize serine, a potent activator of glutamate transmission via a modulatory site on the NMDA (n-methyl-d-aspartate) receptor. Inadequate DAOA function might be hypothesized to lead to problems in modulating the glutamate signal in areas of the brain such as the prefrontal cortex. Evidence from animal studies suggests that glutamate antagonists have antidepressant effects, and that depression is associated with inadequate modulation of glutamate neurotransmission. However a recent study suggests that the major role of G72 may be in maintaining neuronal structure.

Brain-derived neurotrophic factor (BDNF)—This gene is a candidate based both on position (11p14, near reported linkage peaks in several family series) and function (as a neuronal growth factor, it is implicated in several recent theories of depression and BP mood disorder). BDNF has shown significant association with BP illness in three independent reports in family-based data, but not in several case-control series. Two reports have suggested association in child/adolescent-onset BP disorder, and two additional series show association in rapid-cycling BP patients. Several studies have shown that an-

tidepressant administration is associated with increased central BDNF levels in experimental animals, and administration of BDNF itself has been associated with antidepressant-like activity. Depression has been postulated to be associated with decreased neurogenesis in the hippocampus, which is dependent on neurotrophic factors, including BDNF. Mood stabilizing medications used in BP illness are thought to have neuroprotective effects.

Disrupted in schizophrenia 1 (DISC1)—This gene on chromosome 1q was identified in a Scottish family with a genetic translocation and with multiple cases of psychiatric disorders, primarily schizophrenia. However DISC1 variants were associated with mood disorders in family members as well. Later studies in an independent series of BP patients in Scotland were positive for association as well. A study in Wales of schizoaffective patients showed a linkage peak in the same chromosomal location. This gene is expressed in multiple brain regions, including the hippocampus, where it is differentially expressed in neurons. It is associated with microtubules; in mice, disruption of DISC1 leads to abnormal neuronal migration in the developing cerebral cortex. DISC1 appears to interact with phosphodiesterase 4B, which may play a role in mood regulation.

5HTT, MAOA, COMT—These three genes have been shown in meta-analyses to be associated with BP disorder, even though no strong effects have been shown in any one study. The effect size for each appears to be in the range of 10–20% increase in risk. Each of these genes is associated with other behavioral phenotypes, and each has been reported to interact with environment to increase the risk of specific disorders (major depression, antisocial personality disorder, and schizophrenia respectively). Recent data in BP illness are more positive for 5HTT than for MAOA or COMT.

P2RX7 (aka P2X7, P2X7R)—This gene on 12q24 was identified in a French–Canadian case-control series following linkage studies using large pedigrees from the same population. It is a calcium-stimulated ATPase. The data are suggestive, but await replication in an independent study.

GRK3—This is the only candidate identified using animal model studies (a mouse model employing methamphetamine). The original gene expression studies were followed up by association studies in several samples as well as expression studies in human lymphoblasts. This gene participates in the down-regulation of G-protein coupled receptors.

8. Empirical Data for Genetic Counseling

Molecular genetic studies hold great promise in the future for families with affective disorder, particularly BP disorder. However genetic counseling currently is based on empirical risk figures.

The lifetime risk for severe (incapacitating) affective disorder is about 7%. Risk is increased to about 20% in first-degree relatives of UP patients, and 25% in first-degree relatives of BP. It appears to be 40% in relatives of schizoaffective patients. The risk to offspring of two affectively ill parents is in excess of 50%. Overall risk figures appear to be rising in recent years, but more so in relatives of patients than in the general population (keeping at about a 3:1 ratio). Average age of onset is about 20 for BP disorder and 25 for UP.

Craddock N, Forty L: Genetics of affective (mood) disorders. *Eur J Hum Genet* 2006;14(6):660–668.

Holmans P, Weissman MM, Zubenko GS, et al.: Genetics of recurrent early-onset major depression (GenRED): Final genome scan report. *Am J Psychiatry* 2007;164(2):248–258.

Schulze TG, Hedeker D, Zandi P, et al.: What is familial about familial BP disorder? Resemblance among relatives across a broad spectrum of phenotypic characteristics. *Arch Gen Psychiatry*. 2006;63(12):1368–1376.

ALCOHOLISM
1. Epidemiologic Genetic Studies

A. Twin Studies

Twin studies tend to show heritability of drinking behavior and heritability of alcoholism. A Finnish twin study included interview data on 902 male twins between 28 and 37 years of age. Heritability was 0.39 (i.e., about 39% of the variance between members of a twin pair is due to genetic factors) for frequency of drinking and 0.36 for amount consumed per session. A second Finnish study involved several thousand pairs of twins in the state twin registry. Overall heritability for total alcohol consumption was 0.37 in males and 0.25 in females. A study in which 572 twin families from the Institute of Psychiatry register were examined found that additive genetic factors accounted for 37% of the variance in alcohol consumption among drinkers, when pedigree data are considered together with twin data and the effect of shared environment on twin concordance is accounted for. The critical data from these three large twin studies are strikingly similar, at least in males.

Twin studies of alcoholism itself have generally shown heritability. Kaij studied registration of twin subjects at the Swedish County Temperance Boards. Such registration implies that a complaint was made about a person's behavior while drinking, either by the police or a third party. This would not generally include alcoholics who are socially isolated, though they might be significantly impaired. The registration information was followed up with personal interviews of probands and cotwins. In a total of 205 twin pairs, proband-

wise concordance was 54.2% in MZ's and 31.5% in DZ's (*p* <.01). Concordance rates in MZ's increased with the severity of the disturbance. A reanalysis of these data shows heritability to vary from 0.42 to 0.98, the more serious forms of alcoholism being more heritable.

Kendler conducted a population-based study of female twin pairs from the Virginia twin registry. Personal interviews were completed on 1033 of 1176 pairs. MZ concordance varied from 26% to 47% (depending on whether a narrow or broad definition of alcoholism was used) while DZ concordance ranged from 12% to 32%. The calculated heritability was 50–61%. This suggests a substantial genetic influence for alcoholism in women.

B. Adoption Studies

Goodwin compared 55 adopted-away male children of an alcoholic parent with 78 adoptees without an alcoholic parent. The groups were matched by age, sex, and time of adoption. The principal finding was that 18% of the proband group were alcoholic compared with 5% of the controls (*p* <0.02). This study also compared adopted-away sons of alcoholics with sons of alcoholics raised by the alcoholic parent. There was no difference.

Bohman used state registers in Stockholm to study 2324 adoptees born in that city between 1930 and 1949. Male adoptees whose fathers abused alcohol (excluding those who were also sociopathic) were more likely to be alcoholic themselves (39.4% vs. 13.6%, p <0.01) compared with adoptees without an alcoholic (or sociopathic) father. Cloninger, Bohman, and Sigvardsson postulated a familial distinction of alcoholics: a milieu-limited (type I) and a male-limited (type II) group. Type I alcoholics usually have onset after age 25, manifest problems with loss of control, and have a great deal of guilt and fear about alcohol use. Type II alcoholics have onset before age 25, are unable to abstain from alcohol, and have fights and arrests when drinking, but less frequently show loss of control and guilt and fear about alcohol use. Cloninger reanalyzed the Stockholm Adoption data using these specified categories. He showed that type I alcoholics were significantly greater in prevalence only among those adoptees with both genetic and environmental risk factors (i.e., alcoholism in both biologic and adoptive parents). Type I was the most common type of alcoholism; however, it was present in 4.3% of controls with no risk factors. Type II alcoholism was present in only 1.9% of the controls but in 16.9–17.9% of adoptees with genetic risk factors. The presence or absence of environmental risk factors (alcoholism in adoptive parents) did not appear to make a difference.

Bohman extended this finding to women adoptees, identifying as particularly important the incidence of alcoholism in the biologic mothers of these adoptees.

C. FAMILY STUDIES

There is a concentration of alcoholics in the families of alcoholic probands. Cotton (summarizing 39 studies on families of 6251 alcoholics and 4083 nonalcoholics) reports an overall prevalence of 27.0% alcoholism in fathers of alcoholics and of 4.9% in mothers; 30.8% of alcoholics had at least one alcoholic parent. The same preponderance of alcoholism was not seen in the parents of comparison groups of patients with other psychiatric disorders. The studies of nonpsychiatric controls reviewed in the same study show alcoholism rates of 5.2% in fathers and 1.2% in mothers. A recent report from the Collaborative Study of the Genetics of Alcoholism (COGA) shows significant coaggregation of drug dependence, mood disorders, and anxiety disorders as well as alcohol dependence in the relatives of persons with alcohol dependence.

2. Disorders Genetically Related to Alcoholism

Winokur reported an increased prevalence of depression in the female relatives of alcoholics, roughly comparable to the increased prevalence of alcoholism in male relatives. Some forms of illness may result from shared vulnerability factors. Recent studies suggest that comorbid disorders (including alcoholism and affective illness) themselves run in families.

Bohman and Cloninger observed that adopted-away daughters of type II (male-limited) alcoholics manifest no increase in alcoholism but do show an increase in somatization disorder.

It is not possible to conclude at this time that a single genetic predisposing factor is manifest as either alcoholism or sociopathy (antisocial personality disorder). However, some sociopathic alcoholics may transmit both alcoholism and sociopathy as part of the same syndrome.

Earls reported an increase in the *Diagnostic and Statistical Manual of Mental Disorders,* third edition (DSM-III) behavior disorder in general (attention deficit disorder with hyperactivity, oppositional disorder, and conduct disorder) in the offspring of alcoholic parents. The risk is greater for offspring of two alcoholic parents than for those of one alcoholic parent.

3. Linkage Studies

Several linkage studies have been completed in sizeable populations. Genes predisposing to alcohol dependence appear to be located on chromosomes 1, 2, 4, 7, and 16.

4. Association Studies

GABRA2—Variants in GABRA2 on chromosome 4p have been shown by Edenberg and colleagues in COGA to be associated with the power of **beta** oscillations in the EEG (which are inversely related to inhibitory neuronal activity in the cortex) and to alcohol dependence. This association has now been replicated by four other groups. GABRA2 appears to be particularly strongly related to problems with impulse control; the risk allele is also seen in adolescents with conduct disorder and in alcohol dependent persons who are drug dependent. Other GABA receptor genes such as GABRG3 may also be associated with alcohol dependence.

ADH4—ADH (alcohol dehydrogenase) is the major metabolic enzyme for alcohol, catalyzing its breakdown into acetaldehyde, which is then further metabolized by aldehyde dehydrogenase (ALDH). Both ADH and ALDH have variants associated with the "flushing" reaction to alcohol (a feeling of warmth accompanied by reddening of the skin and sometimes nausea and tachycardia). These variants are most common in East Asian populations. They tend to protect against the development of alcohol dependence. In recent studies, single nucleotide polymorphisms in some of the ADH enzymes (genes for several isoenzymes of ADH are located on chromosome 4q) have been associated with alcohol dependence in Caucasian populations and in Native Americans. The strongest finding is in ADH4, which appears to be associated with the early onset of regular drinking.

CHRM2—The M2 muscarinic receptor gene on chromosome 7q was associated with alcohol dependence and major depression in the COGA study, an association that has been replicated. The association with depression recalls the cholinergic-adrenergic balance hypothesis of Janowsky and colleagues from the 1970s (in which a relative increase in central cholinergic activity is associated with depression and a relative increase in central adrenergic activity with mania).

hTAS2R16—This gene, located under the same linkage peak on 7q as CHRM2, codes for a bitter taste receptor. Variants are associated with alcohol dependence, which is consistent with studies showing that relative sensitivity to sweet taste is related to alcohol acceptance in rodent models. The risk gene variant is much more common in African Americans than in European Americans.

DRD2—Originally reported about a decade ago, the literature on DRD2 is still controversial. A meta-analysis of 21 studies shows an increased risk of alcoholism of 50–100% for persons carrying the A1 allele. However, recent work has questioned whether this polymorphism may actually be reflecting variation in a gene next to DRD2.

5. Etiologic Marker Studies

Major areas of concentration in the search for a potential biologic trait marker of alcoholism include the following: (1) enzymes of alcohol metabolism and other enzymes;

(2) EEG and evoked potentials before and after alcohol; (3) psychologic/psychophysiologic differences; and (4) behavioral and neuroendocrine responses to alcohol.

Alcohol is metabolized primarily in the liver by alcohol dehydrogenase (ADH) and aldehyde dehydrogenase (ALDH). Four isozymes of ALDH are known. Three are found in the cytoplasm and one (ALDH2) in the mitochondria. It is the latter that is probably responsible for most acetaldehyde metabolism in vivo. The ALDH2 enzyme is lacking in about 50% of Japanese and apparently in other Oriental groups as well. Such people are subject to the "flushing" reaction from alcohol (similar to a disulfiram reaction). Alcohol elimination is not different in such subjects; however, the alcoholism rate is significantly diminished.

A poorly synchronized resting EEG (lower alpha) has been thought to be related to a predisposition for alcoholism. Change in alpha rhythm following alcohol is more concordant in MZ than DZ twins (as are multiple other EEG parameters). Change in alpha rhythm following alcohol was also found to differentiate young adult subjects at high risk for alcoholism from controls.

Measurements of event-related potentials have shown smaller P300 waves following visual stimuli in 7–13-year-old sons of alcoholics compared to controls. The EEG/ERP area remains one of the more promising in the field of pathophysiologic markers for alcoholism. Schuckit has studied behavioral and neuroendocrine responses to alcohol infusion in a series of high-risk populations. Offspring of alcoholics displayed less subjective intoxication, than controls. A follow-up shows that decreased subjective intoxication is correlated with later development of alcoholism in sons of alcoholics.

Summary

There appear to be hereditary factors operative in normal drinking behavior and in vulnerability to alcohol abuse. The "flushing" reaction to acetaldehyde is one of the clearest instances of a pharmacogenetic variant that influences human behavior, though even here the interaction between genotype and environment in different ethnic groups may result in very different outcomes. Alcoholism clearly runs in families. It is more often manifest in men than in women. The familial preponderance is primarily genetic and the differentiation by gender is primarily the result of sociocultural factors. There may be two distinct types of alcoholism with different patterns of inheritance, type I (or milieu-limited) and type II (or male-limited). Type II alcoholism is more severe and more likely to be strongly influenced by major gene effects. Genetic markers for the vulnerability to alcoholism have yet to be verified. Of most interest are studies suggesting EEG/ERP differences in those at risk, the studies showing decreased responsiveness to alcohol in those at risk, and the neurochemical investigation of appropriate animal models of alcoholism. The recent single gene findings for GABRA2, ADH4, and CHRM2 have provided a stimulus for additional studies of the presumed functional consequences of these genetic variants in alcohol dependent subjects.

Dick DM, Jones K, Saccone N, et al.: Endophenotypes successfully lead to gene identification: Results from the collaborative study on the genetics of alcoholism. *Behav Genet* 2006;36(1):112–26.

Nurnberger JI, Jr., Bierut LJ: Seeking the connections: Alcoholism and our genes. *Scientific Am* 2007;296(4):46–53.

ALZHEIMER DISEASE

Genetic etiologies are clear for some forms of Alzheimer disease. The specific genes that influence vulnerability have been identified (Table 3–3). Epidemiologic studies, however, do not show high heritability of the disorder. This is partially attributable to multiple etiologic, environmental as well as genetic factors. It is also related to the variable age of onset of the condition. Early-onset cases are more likely to be hereditary, and may be determined by single genes. Later-onset cases are more likely to be multifactorial. Important genetic factors in late-onset cases may be obscured by the fact that mortality from other causes decreases familial aggregation.

TWIN STUDIES

A total of 81 twin pairs, where at least one member is affected with Alzheimer disease (AD), have been reported in the literature. The MZ concordance rate

Table 3–3. Genes Implicated in Alzheimer Disease

Chromosomal Location	Clinical Correlate	Frequency	Gene Name	Reference
21q	Early onset	Rare	APP	Goate et al., 1991
1	Early onset	Rare	Presenilin II	Levy-Lahad et al., 1995.
19	Late onset	Common	ApoE	Strittmatter et al., 1993
14	Early onset	Rare	Presenilin I	Schellenberg et al., 1992

(approximately 45%) is not different from the DZ concordance rate (approximately 35%) in these studies.

FAMILY STUDIES

Most of the relatives of later-onset AD probands will have died of other causes before passing the age of risk. However, the risk to siblings of probands (with an affected parent) whose age of onset was less than 70 years is close to 50%. The morbid risk may be 40% for first-degree relatives at age 90. Heun reported a 30% incidence of dementia in first-degree relatives of Alzheimer's probands compared to 22% in controls.

A subset of early-onset AD cases is highly familial. At least some AD cases (primarily those with later onset) are sporadic.

LINKAGE AND ASSOCIATION STUDIES

In 1987, St. George-Hyslop et al. reported linkage of familial AD to RFLP markers on chromosome 21. The peak LOD score (4.25) suggested a causative gene near these markers. Subsequently, certain isolated, rare AD families have been found to have a point mutation in the gene for amyloid precursor protein. These studies suggest that abnormalities in this gene (which produces a proteinaceous material found to accumulate in the extracellular space in brains of persons with AD) can cause the disease by itself. Another cause of early-onset familial Alzheimer's is a gene on chromosome 14. Additional families are linked to a gene on chromosome 1. The genes on chromosome 1 and 14 code for proteins named presenilins and appear to be highly homologous.

Many late-onset families show linkage to a region of chromosome 19 coding for lipoprotein E (usually abbreviated as ApoE), which is also implicated in cardiovascular illness. One copy of the E4 allele will increase risk fourfold compared to that with E2. Two copies of E4 increase risk by a factor of eight. It is not clear at this time whether E4 is a risk factor for all ethnic groups and families or just in selected populations. The molecular mechanisms for the Alzheimer's vulnerability genes are now the subject of intense investigation. There is reason to suspect that they all affect the accumulation of amyloid.

Grupe A, Abraham R, Li Y, et al.: Evidence for novel susceptibility genes for late-onset Alzheimer's disease from a genome-wide association study of putative functional variants. *Hum Mol Genet* 2007;16(8):865–873.

Murrell JR, Price B, Lane KA, et al.: Association of apolipoprotein E genotype and Alzheimer disease in African Americans. *Arch Neurol* 2006;63(3):431–434.

ANTISOCIAL PERSONALITY DISORDER

EPIDEMIOLOGIC STUDIES: TWIN STUDIES

In a Danish twin study, 32.6% (28/86 pairs) of MZ twins were concordant for criminal behavior, compared to 13.8% (21/152 pairs) of DZ twins ($p < 0.001$). In a Norwegian twin study, Dalgard and Kringlen found a higher MZ concordance (25.8%) for crime compared to DZ concordance (14.8%), but this failed to reach statistical significance ($p = 0.11$).

Schulsinger and Crowe conducted adoption studies of antisocial personality disorder (AP). In these early studies, there was a consistent observation that the adopted-away offspring of AP biologic parents had a higher risk for antisocial behavior than did control adoptees. For example, 6/46 adoptees of female felons met criteria for AP compared to 0/46 control adoptees. In this study, outcome was unrelated to the length of time the adoptees remained with their biologic mothers. In Schulsinger's study of 57 adoptee AP and 57 control probands, AP was found among 3.9% (12/305) of biological relatives of AP adoptees, compared to 1.4% (4/285) of biological relatives of control adoptees, a highly significant difference. If only the fathers were considered, 9.3% of probands' biological fathers (5/54) received a diagnosis of AP compared to 1.8% of the biological fathers of control adoptees. In a larger study, using adoption and criminal registries, Mednick reported that when neither the biologic nor adoptive parents had been convicted, adoptees had a conviction rate of 13.5%. If only the adoptive parents were convicted, the adoptee conviction rate rose to only 14.7%. If only the biologic parents were convicted, the adoptee conviction rate was 20%. When both sets of parents had been convicted, the conviction rate for adoptees was 24.5%. The risk for conviction in a male adoptee increased as a function of the number of convictions in the biological and adoptive parents.

These findings were confirmed in a later study of criminality in a cohort of adoptees from Stockholm. Both genetic and "postnatal" influences were detectable in the risk for AP. When postnatal factors predisposed to criminality, 6.7% of male adoptees were criminal compared to 2.9% of male adoptees with nonpredisposing postnatal and genetic backgrounds. When the genetic background, but not the postnatal environment, was predisposing, 12.1% of male adoptees were criminal compared to 2.9% of control male adoptees. When both genetic and postnatal backgrounds were judged to predispose to criminal behavior, 40.0% of male adoptees were criminal. These results are consistent with the additive effects of genes and postnatal influences. The environmental influences implicated were multiple foster homes (for men) and extensive institutional care (for women).

EPIDEMIOLOGIC STUDIES: FAMILY STUDIES

Of 223 male criminals, 80% were found to have a diagnosis of AP in a study by Guze. Sixteen percent of interviewed male first-degree relatives also had this diagnosis, while only 2% of female relatives had AP, compared to 3% and 1% in the relatives of controls. Increased rates of alcoholism and drug abuse were also found among the first-degree relatives of these criminals.

A family study of 66 female felons and 228 of their first-degree relatives revealed increased rates for AP (18%), alcoholism (29%), drug abuse (3%), and hysteria (31%), all the hysteria occurring in the female relatives. Predictably, male relatives had a threefold increase in AP (31%) compared to the female relatives (11%). The increased risk for AP among first-degree relatives of female felons (31%) compared to the risk for relatives of male felons (16%) may be related to a greater genetic and social predisposition in the families of the female felons.

CYTOGENETIC STUDIES

Several reports have suggested that the prevalence of XYY males in prisons and penal/mental institutions is higher than the prevalence in the general population. The XYY karyotype is associated with slightly lower than normal intelligence, tall stature, and cystic acne. This karyotype is found in approximately 1/1000 of male newborns. Hook found XYY in 1/53 of 3813 males in 20 penal/mental institutions. Witkin surveyed all tall Danish men from a birth cohort, finding 12/4139 (0.29%) who had the XYY anomaly. Five of these 12 XYY men had a criminal record, primarily petty criminality. Witkin suggests that lower than average intelligence may account for the excess of criminal activity among XYY males. This karyotype does not seem to be associated with a predisposition to impulsive violence, as once thought.

Biological Markers

Nielsen identified a variant of the tryptophan hydroxylase gene (which codes for the synthetic enzyme for serotonin) associated with low 5-hydroxyindoleacetic acid (5-HIAA) in cerebrospinal fluid and suicide attempts in violent criminal offenders. Goldman replicated this finding. This deserves follow-up using family-based association methods, though it is now clear that brain serotonin is almost exclusively produced by another metabolic enzyme (TPH2). Low 5-HIAA has been associated with impulsivity and violence in experimental colonies of rhesus monkeys. A Dutch family was reported with lowered monoamine oxidase A activity caused by a point mutation on the eighth exon of the MAOA gene. Males with this mutation (both MAO genes are on the X chromosome) show impulsive aggression, arson, attempted rape, and exhibitionism. It is likely that other familial monoamine defects will be found to be associated with aggressive behavior.

Brunner HG, Nelen M, Breakefield XO, et al.: Abnormal behavior associated with a point mutation in the structural gene for monoamine oxidase A. *Science* 1993;262(5133):578–580.

Higley JD, Linnoila M: Low central nervous system serotonergic activity is trait like and correlates with impulsive behavior. A nonhuman primate model investigating genetic and environmental influences on neurotransmission. *Ann N Y Acad Sci* 1997;836:39–56.

Lappalainen J, Long JC, Eggert M, et al.: Linkage of antisocial alcoholism to the serotonin 5-HT1B receptor gene in 2 populations. *Arch Gen Psychiatry* 1998;55(11):989–994.

ANXIETY DISORDERS

The increased familial risk for anxiety disorders has been known for over 100 years. Family studies of panic disorder using modern criteria are often complicated by comorbidity with social phobic disorder and generalized anxiety disorder. One family study of pure panic disorder probands found a significantly higher risk of panic episodes among first-degree relatives compared to relatives of controls. There was a fivefold increase in risk for any anxiety disorder. Similarly, an increased (11.6%) risk for agoraphobia has been reported for the relatives of agoraphobic probands, compared to 1.9% for relatives of panic probands and 1.5% for control probands. A study of simple phobia found an increased risk (31%) for simple phobia among relatives of probands with that diagnosis (but no other anxiety disorder) compared to relatives of well probands (11%). A family history study of social phobia demonstrated that relatives of phobic probands are at increased risk for this disorder (6.6%) compared to relatives of panic disorder probands (0.4%) or relatives of controls (2.2%).

A separate genetic transmission for generalized anxiety disorder has not been established. In a family study, Noyes found that relatives of probands had a greater risk than relatives of controls, but this risk is not greater than the risk for relatives of panic disorder probands. Conversely, a separate study reported similar risks for generalized anxiety among relatives of panic disorder probands and relatives of probands with generalized anxiety. Thus, while there is some evidence for familial transmission of generalized anxiety, the transmission may not be specific. In summary, family studies provide evidence that some anxiety disorders are transmitted separately. This is best established for panic disorder and least so for generalized anxiety.

TWIN STUDIES

In a Norwegian sample, the concordance of all anxiety disorders for MZ twins (34.4%) was significantly greater than that for DZ twins (17.0%).

Hamilton and colleagues reported a syndrome linked to chromosome 13q; the complex phenotype included anxiety disorders and urinary tract dysfunction.

Crowe RR, Goedken R, Samuelson S, et al.: Genomewide survey of panic disorder. *Am J Med Genet* 2001;105(1):105–109.

Hamilton SP, Fyer AJ, Durner M, et al. Further genetic evidence for a panic disorder syndrome mapping to chromosome 13q. *Proc Nat Acad Sci USA.* 2003;100(5):2550–2555.

ATTENTION DEFICIT DISORDER

Early family studies of attention-deficit disorder noted alcoholism and sociopathy in male relatives and hysteria in female relatives. This same constellation was not manifest in the adoptive parents of adopted ADD children.

Family studies suggest that antisocial personality aggregates in the relatives of ADD children, specifically when the children have conduct or oppositional disorder. Biederman and colleagues found rates of affective illness increased in relatives of their group. ADD itself was also increased in relatives. ADD and antisocial behavior tended to occur together.

Deutsch et al. have reported on the association of minor physical anomalies with ADD. The relationship is consistent, with a genetic latent trait model (an underlying autosomal dominant gene producing either ADD, physical anomalies, or both). Mutations in the gene for the thyroid hormone receptor have been found in one group of subjects with ADD. More recent studies in large cohorts have reported association with several dopamine-related genes, including the dopamine transporter and DRD4.

Asherson P, Brookes K, Franke B, et al.: Confirmation that a specific haplotype of the dopamine transporter gene is associated with combined-type ADHD. *Am J Psychiatry* 2007;164(4):674–677.

Khan SA, Faraone SV: The genetics of ADHD: A literature review of 2005. *Curr Psychiatry Rep* 2006;8(5):393–397.

Todd RD, Huang H, Smalley SL, et al.: Collaborative analysis of DRD4 and DAT genotypes in population-defined ADHD subtypes. *J Child Psychol Psychiatry* 2005;46(10):1067–1073.

AUTISM (PERVASIVE DEVELOPMENTAL DISORDER)

The pooled frequency of autism in sibs is about 3%, which is 50–100 times the population rate. Folstein and Rutter reported an MZ concordance of 36% and a DZ concordance of 0%. When the phenotype was expanded to include language and cognitive abnormalities, concordance rates were 82% and 10%. This sample of twins, though carefully selected, was small, but the essential conclusions regarding heritability have been confirmed in later studies.

A segregation analysis in a series of multiplex families was consistent with autosomal recessive inheritance. However, the excess of affected males in the sample suggested sex-specific modifying factors.

What is striking about the genetics of autism is its association with multiple single-gene disorders. The most clearly documented of these disorders is the fragile X syndrome. Perhaps 8% of autistic subjects have the cytogenetic fragile X; 16% of fragile X males are autistic. There are also probable associations between autism and tuberous sclerosis, neurofibromatosis, and phenylketonuria. A variety of other reports of chromosomal anomalies and single-gene associations with the autistic syndrome have been reported.

A number of genome-wide genetic surveys of the autistic phenotype have been reported. All these studies have examined affected pairs of siblings where both twins have a narrowly defined phenotype of autism or where one sib has the narrowly defined autistic phenotype and the other has a defined pervasive developmental disorder. A consistent finding is seen on the long arm of chromosome 7 from 7q22-qter. Folstein reported that the linkage on 7q was specific to families in which the proband had a specific language disorder (usually reading difficulty along with later-onset autism). It is notable that the linked region includes the gene recently dubbed "speech 1" also known as FOXP2 and known to be a transcription factor), which was recently found to be associated with specific language disorder.

A significant site has been found on chromosome 2q32. Other statistically suggestive regions found to date are on chromosomes 5q14, 13q21, and 16p13.3, and near the centromere of chromosome 19.

An autistic phenotype found in individuals with the chromosomal duplications of Prader-Willi/Angelman syndrome on 15q11-q13 has focused considerable research in this region of the genome. Interest has concentrated on the GABRB3 receptor gene in 15q12. GABRB3 shows peak expression both temporally and spatially during pre- and early postnatal murine brain development.

Due to the finding of hyperserotonemia in a proportion of autistic children, it has been suggested that the serotonergic system may play an important role in the etiology of the disease. There are conflicting results regarding the genetic involvement of the serotonin transporter.

Recent data suggests involvement of several of the neuroligin and neurexin proteins (involved in synaptic structure) in genetic predisposition to autism. As more single gene findings emerge, the genetic structure of autism appears quite complex, with cytogenetic abnormalities, common gene variants and rare variants all represented.

Autism Genome Project Consortium: Mapping autism risk loci using genetic linkage and chromosomal rearrangements. *Nat Genet* 2007;39(3):319–328.

Sebat J, Lakshmi B, Malhotra D, et al.: Strong association of de novo copy number mutations with autism. *Science* 2007; 316(5823):445–449.

DRUG DEPENDENCE

GENETIC EPIDEMIOLOGY: ADOPTION STUDIES

In an adoption study of drug abuse, 443 adoptees from Iowa were studied; half were selected for psychopathology in biologic parents and the other half matched for age and sex. Parents were not directly examined but information from adoption records was available. Forty adoptees manifested drug abuse of one kind or another. Antisocial behavior in a biologic relative predicted drug abuse in the adoptee. Alcohol problems also predicted drug abuse in the absence of antisocial behavior. The environmental factors implicated included divorce and significant psychiatric pathology in the adoptive parents.

In an adoption study of smoking behavior, using a large Swedish cohort, the authors observed that adoptees' status (e.g., current or heavy smoker) is associated with their siblings' smoking status. Surprisingly, adoptees' smoking status was not predicted by their biologic or adoptive parents smoking status.

GENETIC EPIDEMIOLOGY: TWIN AND FAMILY STUDIES

A study of the Vietnam Era Twin Registry revealed evidence for a common genetic factor operating across pharmacologic classes. These authors also found evidence for class-specific genetic factors, especially in opioid dependence, similar to results of a family study. Abuse and dependence for six different classes of drugs was assessed in an adult male twin cohort of Virginia residents (~1200 twin pairs). The authors report the detection of a common genetic influence for use and abuse/dependence, across the pharmacologic classes of drugs of abuse, as well as pharmacologic class-specific genetic factors predisposing to use. A single common environmental factor predisposed to illicit use. These results confirm their earlier study of female–female twin pairs. Since these were two population-based twin studies, there were few opioid dependent cases and few cocaine dependence cases, a cautionary note. The relatively clear conclusion from these twin, family, and adoption studies is that there are general genetic factors increasing risk for addiction to multiple drugs of abuse, and there are pharmacologic-class specific genetic factors that appear to increase risk predominantly for addiction to a single pharmacologic class of drugs (e.g., opioids).

LINKAGE STUDIES

Two linkage studies of opiate dependence have been published, both of which implicate areas on chromosome 17q.

Multiple linkage studies of nicotine dependence have been published in the last 5 years. While many loci have been nominated, most LOD scores have been below genome-wide significance, and confirmation has been less frequent than hoped. There are several promis-

ing findings, however. Saccone combined two linkage scans of Australian and Finnish smokers to report a LOD score > 5 (genome-wide significant p value = 0.006) at ~25 cM on chromosome 22.

ASSOCIATION STUDIES

Recent genome-wide association studies by Bierut of ~1100 nicotine dependent probands and ~900 controls identify the alpha 5 nicotinic cholinergic receptor cluster (including the alpha 5, alpha 3 and beta 4 receptor subunit genes) as associated with nicotine dependence. These results implicate biologically plausible candidate genes. One implicated SNP is a mis-sense variation in the alpha 5 subunit gene. Multiple other candidate genes are expected to emerge from more intensive analysis of these data.

Association studies of candidate genes for nicotine, stimulant (including cocaine), or opioid dependence have nominated literally dozens of alleles as risk factors. Most will eventually prove to be false positives, but, since odds ratios may be less than 1.5 for true positives, large-scale studies in multiple ethnic populations are needed.

Bierut LJ, Madden PA, Breslau N, et al.: Novel genes identified in a high-density genome wide association study for nicotine dependence. *Hum Mol Genet* 2007;16:24–35.

Gelernter J, Panhuysen C, Wilcox M, et al.: Genome-wide linkage analysis of heroin dependence in Han Chinese: Results from wave one of a multi-stage study. *Am J Med Genet B Neuropsychiatr Genet* 2006;141(6):648–652.

Saccone SF, Pergadia ML, Loukola A, et al.: Genetic Linkage to Chromosome 22q12 for a Heavy-Smoking Quantitative Trait in Two Independent Samples. *AJHG* 2007;80:856–864.

EATING DISORDERS

A. FAMILY STUDIES

Controlled family studies have been conducted over the past two decades. These studies suggest that there is considerable familial aggregation. Table 3–4 summarizes the results from these studies. It is difficult to estimate precisely the risk to first-degree relatives because the control samples are not sufficiently large to detect more than one to two affected relatives of controls. However, the overall pattern suggests substantial risk, almost certainly greater than 10 and perhaps much larger. There are increased rates of AN among first-degree relatives of DN probands, and increased rates of BN among first-degree relatives of AN probands. This clustering of eating disorders in families of AN and BN individuals provides strong support for familial transmission of both disorders.

B. TWIN STUDIES

There have been a number of twin studies of AN. However, many of the studies were small and often had methodological weaknesses. If one examines the twin

Table 3–4. Family Studies of Anorexia Nervosa

Study	Risk for AN Among First-Degree Relatives of	
	AN Probands	**Control Women**
(Gershon, 1983)	2.0% ($N = 99$ relatives)	0% ($N = 265$ relatives)
(Logue et al., 1989)	1.3% ($N = 153$ relatives)	0% ($N = 103$ relatives)
(Strober et al., 1990)	4.1% ($N = 387$ relatives)	0% ($N = 703$ relatives)
(Herpertz-Dahlmann, 1988)	4.3% ($N = 69$ relatives)	0% ($N = 69$ relatives)
(Lilenfeld et al., 1998)	1.1% ($N = 93$ relatives)	0% ($N = 190$ relatives)
(Strober et al., 2001)	3.4% ($N = 290$ relatives)	0.3% ($N = 318$ relatives)
Mean	3.1% (34/1091 relatives)	0.06% (1/1648 relatives)

studies with the largest number of subjects and most appropriate methodology, mean concordance rates are 64% for MZ twins and 14% for DZ twins. Differences between these rates suggest a modest additive heritability with a large influence of nonadditive genetic and/or shared environmental factors. More recent studies have used structural models to estimate the fraction of risk attributable to additive genetic factors. The estimates of heritability range from 0.48 to 0.76. These studies are summarized in Table 3–5.

One of the first twin studies of eating disorders described pairwise concordance of 56% in MZ and 5% in DZ pairs (71% and 10% with probandwise figures). Family history assessment (including additional informant data from parents) showed that 4.9% of the female first-degree relatives and 1.16% of the female second-degree relatives had had anorexia at some point in their lives, a risk considerably higher than the reported population prevalence. The MZ cotwins were much more similar in "body dissatisfaction," "drive to thinness," weight loss, length of amenorrhea, and minimum body mass index. Estimates indicate that roughly 58–76% of the variance in the liability to AN, and 54–83% of the variance in the liability to BN, can be accounted for by ge-

netic factors. Although the confidence intervals on these estimates are wide, consistent findings across studies support moderate heritability of these traits. For both AN and BN, the remaining variance in liability appears to be due to unique environmental factors (i.e., factors that are unique to siblings in the same family) rather than shared or common environmental factors (i.e., factors that are shared by siblings in the same family).

Eating disorder symptoms themselves also appear to be moderately heritable. Twin studies of binge eating, self-induced vomiting, and dietary restraint suggest that these behaviors are roughly 46–72% heritable. Likewise, pathological attitudes such as body dissatisfaction, eating and weight concerns, and weight preoccupation show heritabilities of roughly 32–72%. Taken together, findings suggest a significant genetic component to AN and BN as well as the attitudes and behaviors that contribute to, and correlate with, clinical eating pathology.

C. MOLECULAR STUDIES

The first AN linkage scan was based on ~200 multiplex kindreds and revealed a locus on 1p (NPL score = 3.5 at D1S3721, 72.6cM; Grice et al., 2002). Additional genotyping in the region resulted in an increased NPL score of

Table 3–5. Genetic and Environmental Variance in Anorexia Nervosa, as Estimated from Twin Studies

Study	Country	Additive Genetic	Family Environment	Residual
Wade et al., 2000	USA	.58 (.33–.84)	0	.42 (.16–.68)
Klump et al., 2001	USA	.76 (.35–.95)	0	.24 (.05–.65)
Koortegaard et al., 2001	Denmark	.48 (.28–.65)	0	.52
Bulik et al., 2006	Sweden	.56 (0–.87)	.05 (0–.64)	.38 (.13–.84)

95% CI in parentheses.

3.91 at 72.0 cM. Analysis of diagnostic phenotypes, using obsession scale scores and drive for thinness scores as covariates, revealed additional linkage peaks. SNP genotyping at several candidate genes (HTR1D, HCRTR1 and OPRD1) revealed limited evidence for association with the HTR1D and OPRD1 genes (Bergen et al., 2003). These observations were confirmed in an independent population of AN individuals (Brown et al., 2007).

The first BN linkage scan was based on ~300 multiplex families and yielded a genome-wide significant LOD score of 2.92 on chromosome 10p. When analysis was restricted to those ~133 multiplex kindreds characterized by self-induced vomiting, the LOD score increase on 10p to 3.39. A promising candidate gene within the 10p linkage peak is glutamic acid decarboxylase (GAD2), a gene implicated in obesity.

Many family-based and case-control association studies of monoamine-related, obesity-related, and neurotrophin-related genes have been published in the past 10 years. These have been small, underpowered, and limited in the numbers of genes (and variants within genes) tested. More recently larger samples sizes have been employed in candidate gene studies, using collaborative, multisite approaches. For example, it was reported that the Met allele of a mis-sense variation in the BDNF gene was associated with AN in Spanish patients. Subsequently, this was confirmed (Ribases et al., 2005) in European collaborative samples totaling greater than 1500 patients.

Bergen AW, van den Bree MBM, Yeager M, et al.: Candidate genes for anorexia nervosa in the 1p34–36 linkage region: Both serotonin 1D and delta opioid receptors display significant association to anorexia nervosa. *Mol Psychiatry* 2003;8:397–406.

Brown KM, Bujac SR, Mann ET, et al.: Further Evidence of Association of OPRD1 & HTR1D Polymorphisms with Susceptibility to Anorexia Nervosa. *Biol Psychiatry* 2007;61:367–373.

Grice DE, Halmi KA, Fichter MM, et al.: Evidence for a susceptibility gene for anorexia nervosa on chromosome 1. *Am J Hum Genet* 2002;70(3):787–792.

Ribases M, Gratacos M, Fernandez-Aranda F et al.: Association of BDNF with restricting anorexia and minimum body mass index: A family-based association study of eight European populations. *Eur J Hum Genet* 2005;13:428–434.

MENTAL RETARDATION
1. Epidemiologic Studies

Twin studies (performed 40–60 years ago) show an MZ concordance of 100% ($N = 83$) and a DZ concordance of 55% ($N = 10$). These would undoubtedly be performed today with separation according to specific causal factors. Adoption studies have not been performed.

Recurrence risk for siblings of a retarded child has been estimated to range from 9.5% to 23% depending on severity of the disorder and the mother's reproductive history. For mothers who have already had more than one retarded child, the risk is 25–50% for sibs.

2. Specific Etiologic Causes

Many medical syndromes are manifest as mental retardation, such as specific errors of metabolism and chromosomal anomalies. Polani estimated that of the 4% of human conceptions that are chromosomally abnormal, 85–90% are selectively eliminated as spontaneous abortions. Of live births, 6% may have a genetic or developmental abnormality of some type; 0.5% survive with chromosomal abnormality; 4% with another developmental anomaly; and 1.5% with a single gene disorder. Among single gene causes of mental retardation, Koranyi listed five dominant diseases (tuberous sclerosis, neurofibromatosis, Sturge–Weber disease, von Hippel-Lindow, and craniosynostosis), and four recessive diseases (Hurler–Hunter disease, galactosemia, G-6 phosphodehydrogenase deficiency and familial hypoglycemia), as well as three recessive aminoaciduria and three lipid-related disorders. Many more are listed in McKusick's compendium *Mendelian Inheritance in Man*.

Down syndrome accounts for MR in 1.5 persons per 1000 and is the most common single cause of the condition. The prevalence of Down's varies greatly and is primarily determined by maternal age. Familial microcephaly is present in about 1/40,000 births but may account for a significant proportion of MR because of its effects in heterozygotes (see below). Fragile X syndrome accounts for about 0.5/1000, and other X chromosome syndromes for another 1/1000. All metabolic causes together are responsible for 1/1000 and chromosomal abnormalities for 3/1000.

A. DOWN SYNDROME

This condition, well studied, is accounted for by a triplication of genetic material on chromosome 21. The area is being localized more and more precisely using molecular techniques combined with cytogenetics. It is probable that sections of 21q22.2 and 21q22.3 are involved, though 21q21 may also be implicated. The areas involved include genes for amyloid and superoxide dismutase. The ETS-2 proto oncogene is near this area as well, and its presence may be related to the well described increased incidence of leukemia in persons with Down syndrome and their relatives. Human 21q21–22.3 is homologous to portions of mouse chromosome 16. A mouse model of Down has been described based on a laboratory-generated reciprocal translocation involving this area.

The reasons for triplication or nondisjunction in Down's are not entirely clear. The likely etiologic factors are environmental rather than genetic. Vulnerability for the condition does not seem to be inherited. A small proportion of Down's patients have a translocation rather than a triplication.

As noted above, the clearest correlate is maternal age. Yet it has been known for some years that the origin of the nondisjunction might be paternal as well as maternal. Serum markers contribute to prenatal determination (decreased alpha-fetoprotein and estriol and increased human chorionic gonadotropin), and aid in the selection of women for referral to amniocentesis.

It has been reported that a familial association exists between Alzheimer's and Down's, but this is unlikely to be generally true. Recent studies suggest that triplication of a critical region on chromosome 21 is not likely to be the sole cause of clinical variation in Down syndrome, and that other genomic areas are probably important as well.

B. Fragile X Syndrome

Fragile X syndrome is named after a cytogenetic observation; cultured cells from some patients show chromosomal breakage under appropriate conditions. There are actually multiple "fragile sites" on human chromosomes. The fragile X (breakage at Xq27.3) is merely the best known. The syndrome itself was originally described by Martin and Bell who described a large pedigree with mental retardation segregating in an x-linked recessive pattern.

Fragile X is the most common form of X-linked MR and is, in general, the most common heritable form of MR (Down's being genetic but not inherited). It is estimated that 1/850 persons carry the defect. Of those, 4 out of 5 males will express the clinical phenotype as compared with 1 out of 3 females (some homozygotes are nonpenetrant and some heterozygotes are penetrant). Genetic tests are now available to determine carrier status in nonpenetrant individuals. The precise genetic error in the Xq27.3 region is now known to be a triplet repeat of variable length. Increased numbers of repeats (associated with greater severity of illness) occur as the gene is passed to succeeding generations. When the number of repeats exceeds a threshold, clinical manifestations are seen.

Most female Fragile X heterozygotes do not have MR. However schizotypal features are seen in about one third of a sample of carriers, and there is an association with affective disorders as well. Some subjects with fragile X develop an autistic syndrome.

Raymond FL, Tarpey P: The genetics of mental retardation. *Hum Mole Genet* 2006;15(2):R110–116.

Sutherland GR, Baker E: The clinical significance of fragile sites on human chromosomes. *Clin Genet* 2000;58(3):157–161.

OBSESSIVE–COMPULSIVE DISORDER
1. Epidemiologic Research
Twin Studies

There are no large twin studies of OCD. Rasmussen and Tsuang reviewed reported series and noted that 32 of 51 (63%) MZ pairs were concordant. Lenane studied 145 first-degree relatives of 46 children with OCD. Of the 90 parents personally evaluated, 15 (17%) received a diagnosis of OCD, compared to 1.5% of the parents of 34 conduct-disordered children who served as a control group. The 17% prevalence rate is significantly higher than the population prevalence rate of about 2%. Fathers were three times as likely as mothers to receive a diagnosis of OCD. Of the 56 siblings personally evaluated, three (5%) met criteria for OCD. When age-correction was applied, the rate rose to 35%. This figure should be viewed with caution because of the magnitude of the age correction for siblings. It should be noted that all probands had severe childhood-onset OCD, and were referred to the authors for treatment. It is possible that childhood-onset OCD represents a more severe form of the OCD spectrum. Nevertheless, this carefully conducted family study reveals an increased risk of OCD among the first-degree relatives of OCD probands.

When OCD occurs in the familial context of Tourette syndrome, it may be part of the spectrum of Tourette syndrome. However, most OCD occurs in individuals who have no first-degree relatives affected by Tourette's. Occasionally, an individual destined to develop Tourette's will present with symptoms of OCD, and the motor tics appear subsequently. These patients are often diagnosed as having OCD until motor tics develop.

OCD appears to be familial and single gene identification studies are proceeding. Several avenues of research suggest a serotonergic abnormality for OCD patients. Recent data from Goldman shows a rare mutation in the serotonin transporter associated with obsessive–compulsive disorder in a single pedigree. An association was also recently reported with oligodendrocyte lineage transcription factor 2 (OLIG2).

Chacon P, Rosario-Campos MC, Pauls DL, et al.: Obsessive-compulsive symptoms in sibling pairs concordant for obsessive-compulsive disorder. *Am J Med Genet B Neuropsychiatr Genet* 2007;144(4):551–555.

Samuels J, Shugart YY, Grados MA, et al.: Significant linkage to compulsive hoarding on chromosome 14 in families with obsessive-compulsive disorder: Results from the OCD Collaborative Genetics Study. *Am J Psychiatry* 2007;164(3):493–499.

Stewart SE, Platko J, Fagerness J, et al.: A genetic family-based association study of OLIG2 in obsessive-compulsive disorder. *Arch Gen Psychiatry* 2007;64(2):209–214.

SCHIZOPHRENIA

A. TWIN STUDIES

MZ twin concordance is greater than DZ twin concordance in each study of schizophrenia, consistent with genetic hypotheses. Second, the heritability of broadly defined schizophrenia is greater than the heritability of strictly defined schizophrenia. This is consistent with a spectrum concept: some individuals with the genetic loading for schizophrenia manifest a different condition. Third, the amount of discordance is considerable; even in MZ twins using a broad definition of illness the discordance is 51%.

A series of nine MZ twins with schizophrenia who were raised apart from infancy was described. Three were completely concordant and three were partially so.

Twin study paradigm to generate data regarding environmental effects in schizophrenia—Examining age of onset in the Maudsley Hospital twin series, it was found that there was a high incidence of illness in the second of a pair of twins within 2 years of onset in the first twin. Further categorizing the group on the basis of whether the twins lived together or apart, he found the 2-year incidence to be primarily in those living together. That is, twins living together are concordant in age of onset, while twins living apart do not. This intriguing finding suggests an environmental factor.

B. FAMILY STUDIES

Pooled European family study data show an age-corrected morbid risk of 5.6% in parents, 10.1% in siblings, and 12.8% in children. The lower rate in parents is thought to be related to a relative decrease in fertility among schizophrenic patients. The general population figure concerning risk for schizophrenia is about 1%; thus, all classes of first-degree relatives of schizophrenic patients have a clear increase in prevalence. The risk for offspring of two schizophrenic parents is difficult to estimate because of the small number of cases. It is probably between 35% and 45% (in pooled data it is 46.3%). Among second-degree relatives (uncles, aunts, nephews, nieces, grandchildren), half-siblings, and cousins, the risk is 2–4%.

Thus, close relatives of schizophrenic patients have about a five- to tenfold excess risk for the illness. The risk diminishes in more distant relatives. A further group of first-degree relatives appear to develop "schizophrenic spectrum" disorders (see below). Nevertheless, the majority of close relatives of schizophrenics are psychiatrically normal.

There is no strong evidence for genetic determination of the conventional subtypes of schizophrenia (hebephrenic, catatonic, and paranoid forms). Though there is significant concordance in MZ twins for subtype, this does not hold true in family studies.

The question of the distinctness of schizophrenia and affective disorders is not settled. In a large family study using lifetime diagnoses and separately examining relatives of probands with schizophrenia, chronic schizoaffective disorder, acute schizoaffective disorder, BP affective disorder, UP affective disorder, and controls, it was concluded that there was evidence for overlap in genetic liability. Specifically, an increase in UP disorder was seen in all groups of relatives of patients. Relatives of schizoaffective probands (both chronic and acute) showed both an excess of affective disorders and an excess of chronic psychoses. However, BP probands did not show an excess of schizophrenic relatives, and schizophrenic probands showed no excess of BP relatives. The most parsimonious explanation of these data is that there is a "middle" group of disorders (schizoaffective) that is genetically related to both schizophrenia and affective illness, and that it may not be possible to separate the groups on clinical criteria.

With regard to mode of transmission, the available data have been analyzed extensively. The results have generally been interpreted as favoring a multifactorial rather than a single-locus model.

C. ADOPTION STUDIES

The adoption study methodology was first applied to schizophrenia ~40 years ago. It was reported that there is an excess of schizophrenia in the adopted-way offspring of schizophrenic women compared to control adoptees. A series of large, systematic studies were carried out by Kety and Rosenthal, who analyzed adoption and psychiatric hospitalization registries in Denmark. In the later studies, subjects were directly interviewed. In all studies, adoptees were separated from their biologic parents at an early age and adopted by non relatives. It was found that there were more schizophrenia and schizophrenia spectrum disorders in the biologic relatives of schizophrenic adoptees than in the biologic relatives of psychiatrically normal adoptees. The prevalence of psychiatric illnesses in the adoptive relatives of the two groups was comparable but small.

The frequency of schizophrenia spectrum disorders is higher in adopted-away offspring of schizophrenic parents than in the adopted-way offspring of normal parents. All of these studies have been criticized on the grounds of selection bias and the validity of diagnosis, and comparisons. However, further independent analysis of the data has confirmed the results: that is, biologic relatives of schizophrenics who have not shared the same environment have a significantly higher prevalence of schizophrenia and schizophrenic spectrum disorders than do biologic relatives of comparable control groups.

D. SPECTRUM STUDIES

Thirty percent of first-degree relatives of schizophrenic patients have associated disorders. The particular DSM-III-R diagnostic categories that seem to be implicated are paranoid personality and schizotypal personality. Schizotypal personality disorder is most likely part of the schizophrenia spectrum, with suggestive evidence for paranoid and schizoid as well. A separate entity characterized by paranoid delusions only (simple delusional disorder) may also exist, for which the inheritance is independent of that for schizophrenia and affective disorder.

E. MOLECULAR STUDIES

Multiple linkage scans of the schizophrenic genome have been conducted, using DSM-III-R, DSM-IV, IDC and/or RDC criteria. These linkage scans have been the subject of meta-analyses in which available data have been combined using different methods. Results are only partially convergent. Genomic regions implicated in the meta-analyses include 1q, 5q, 6p, 6q, 8p, 13q, 15q and 22q. Several of these regions will be discussed below with a focus on those that contain highly promising candidate genes.

On chromosome 6p, there is evidence that alleles of the dysbindin (DTNBP1) gene are associated with schizophrenia, although there are some negative reports (for review see Ross et al., 2006). Multiple haplotypes have been associated with schizophrenia in these reports. There is evidence that dysbindin levels are reduced in postmortem schizophrenia brains. An SNP in the 3'UTR of the dysbindin gene may mediate the reduced expression of dysbindin. At least one dysbindin risk haplotype may be associated with decreased cognitive ability. There may be some overlap between psychotic BP disorder and schizophrenia in terms of dysbindin risk alleles.

An 8p candidate gene, neuregulin 1 (NRG1), is associated with schizophrenia (Steffansson et al., 2002). While there is substantial evidence for the role of NRG1 in the genetics of schizophrenia, other investigators (some employing multiplex samples with positive linkage signals in the region) have not confirmed the association of NRG1 with schizophrenia. Others have found evidence for an association of NRG1 alleles with psychotic BP disorder, suggesting a genetic overlap between this entity and schizophrenia.

Alleles at G72 and G30, two novel genes on 13q32 are associated with schizophrenia in multiple populations (for review see Li and He, 2007). G72 and G30 overlap and orient in opposite directions on 13q32. G72 is a primate-specific gene possibly expressed in the caudate and amygdala; (however, some researchers have not been able to detect mRNA in postmortem human brain). Using yeast two-hybrid analysis, evidence for physical interaction was found for G72 and D-amino-acid oxidase (DAO). DAO oxidizes D-serine, a glutamate receptor modulator. Coincubation of G72 and DAO in vitro revealed a functional interaction, G72 enhancing the activity of DAO. As a result, G72 has been named D-amino-acid oxidase activator (DAOA). Associations between DAOA and schizophrenia have been reported in samples from China, Germany, Ashkenazi Jews, South Africa, and the United States. Childhood-onset schizophrenia has been associated with DAOA in a small sample. Various risk alleles and haplotypes have been reported in schizophrenia.

Curiously, independent datasets suggest that the G72 locus contributes to the risk for BP disorder. No clear functional variation has been established.

Several other candidate genes have been implicated repeatedly in the etiology of schizophrenia, including RGS4, COMT, and DISC1, for which a translocation (with a breakpoint at the DISC1 gene) segregates with multiple behavioral disorders in a Scottish family (for review see Mackie et al., 2007).

Endophenotypes in Schizophrenia

The concept of endophenotypes in psychiatric disorders has been developed over the last several decades. The term defines an illness-related characteristic, observable through biochemical testing or microscopic examination. A valid endophenotype should be more closely related to more pathophysiologic genes for the nosologic category, compared to the entire symptom syndrome in a nosologic category.

The utility of endophenotypes in psychiatric research is now more appreciated, because we have a more accurate understanding of the genetic complexity of operationally defined disorders in the current psychiatric nosology. Endophenotypes should create more homogeneous subtypes, which may cut across the current nosologic boundaries. In that case, more rapid advances can be made in understanding these disorders at the molecular level.

CRITERIA FOR AN ENDOPHENOTYPE

Criteria for an endophenotype have been derived.

It must be associated with illness in the general population;

It should be stable and state-independent. In other words, it must be observable despite the fact that the patient is in partial or complete remission;

It should be heritable;

It should segregate with illness within families.

Among kindreds in which the proband has the endophenotype, it should be observable at a higher rate among unaffected family members compared to the general population.

There are many reports of attentional deficit measures in schizophrenia. An endophenotype that has been studied extensively in schizophrenia is "working memory." This term can be defined as the "holding of information in consciousness, in preparation for complex processing." Working memory can be assessed through multiple different mental tasks, such as N back, Wisconsin Card Sort, and reverse digit span. Deficits in working memory have been described as an endophenotype for schizophrenia. The fraction of individuals with schizophrenia who are designated as having abnormal working memory varies with the tests employed, the sample, and the definition of abnormal (e.g., 1.5 or 2 standard deviation units below the mean for controls). If consideration is given only to studies of large numbers of cases and controls, most reports find 25–50% of persons with schizophrenia as falling in the variably defined "deficit range" for working memory.

Several lines of evidence suggest that working memory deficits are in part heritable. Twin studies of subjects unaffected and discordant for schizophrenia who are MZ and DZ twin pairs indicate that genetic influences in schizophrenia-related working memory deficits are prominent. Multiple studies suggest that a small fraction of the variance in working memory scores is explained by a functional mis-sense SNP (Val/Met) in the COMT gene.

Compared to controls, working memory deficits are more common among the unaffected relatives (compared to controls) of schizophrenic individuals who have deficits themselves. The effect size for this observation is relatively small; substantial sample numbers are required to have adequate power. If only those studies which examined at a minimum more than 50 relatives and 50 controls are considered, the preponderance of data suggests that unaffected relatives of schizophrenic individuals have some of the neuropsychological deficits seen in affected persons. However, there is a negative publication bias, and a great variety of neuropsychological measures have been used (Wisconsin Card Sort, digit span, trail making, tests of verbal and spatial fluency, etc.). The effect size is not large, as evidenced by the fact that many smaller studies have found no significant difference between the relatives of schizophrenic individuals and controls.

The preponderance of data suggests that neuropsychological/cognitive deficits in schizophrenia are present more often among affected persons, compared to controls. There are data to indicate that the measures are heritable. Finally, most larger studies find that the nonpsychotic relatives of schizophrenic individuals score comparably poorly on neuropsychological tests. The different measures of neurocognitive functioning may be valid endophenotypes for schizophrenia.

A promising endophenotype for schizophrenia is an abnormality of the P50 auditory evoked potential. The P50 wave is a positive deflection on by scalp electrodes occurring 50 milliseconds after an auditory stimulus, typically a single click. When two such clicks are presented, (the second, 200 milliseconds or more after the first), the amplitude of the P50 wave after the second click is normally reduced, in comparison to the amplitude of the wave after the first click (see figure below). This phenomenon is considered by some to be an electrophysiologic signature of sensory gating. In some subjects with schizophrenia, the amplitude of the P50 wave for the second click is similar to the amplitude after the first click, as shown below. This has been interpreted as a defect in sensory gating. (Figure 3–1)

The P50 abnormality is found more often among individuals with schizophrenia, compared to controls, although this has not been universally confirmed. The abnormality is also found more frequently among the relatives of persons with schizophrenia, compared to controls. Based on twin studies, it is partially heritable. Heritability is also implied by reports that DNA sequence polymorphisms in and near the alpha 7 nicotinic receptor subunit gene on chromosome 15 explain some of the variance in the P50 abnormality. The chromosome 15 location is a confirmed linkage region for schizophrenia, lending interest to this line of investigation.

While there is ample evidence that the P50 is under partial genetic control, there is substantial evidence that P50 parameters are influenced by environmental forces. Nicotine can "normalize" an abnormal P50 test. This finding becomes more intriguing when it is recalled that about 80% of individuals with schizophrenia are daily smokers. Furthermore, atypical antipsychotic medications can "normalize" abnormal P50 testing. These results indicate a critical point when endophenotypes are considered: environmental influences must be considered, not only as sources of variance (e.g., experimental error, circadian variation, influence of personal habits such as nicotine and caffeine intake), but also as clues to the pathways from gene variants to endophenotypes, or from endophenotypes to key symptom clusters.

In summary, genetic studies of schizophrenia have identified numerous promising candidate genes through linkage and association approaches. These include DAOA, NRG1, dysbindin, DISC1, RGS4, COMT and others. Research has revealed several promising endophenotypes, particularly auditory evoked potential abnormalities and neurocognitive deficit.

Li D, He L: G72/G30 genes and schizophrenia: A systematic meta-analysis of association studies. *Genetics* 2007;175(2):917–922.

Mackie S, Millar JK, Porteous DJ: Role of DISC1 in neural development and schizophrenia. *Current Opin Neurobiol* 2007;17:95–102.

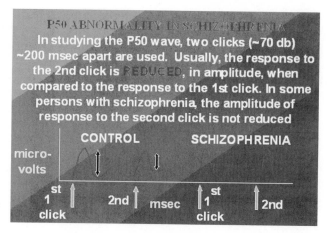

Figure 3–1. "Sensory Gating" Abnormality in Schizophrenia

Ross CA, Margolis RL, Reading SA, Pletnikov M, Coyle JT: Neurobiology of schizophrenia. *Neuron* 2006;52:139–153.

Stefansson H, Sigurdsson E, Steinthorsdottir V, et al. Neuregulin 1 and susceptibility to schizophrenia. *Am J Hum Genet* 2002;71:877–892.

SOMATIZATION DISORDER

In a family history study, Coryell evaluated first-degree relatives of 49 probands with Briquet syndrome. First-degree relatives of non-Briquet syndrome hysteria and affective disorder probands formed the control groups. The risk for a complicated medical history was 8.0% in the first-degree relatives of Briquet syndrome probands compared to control values of 2.3% and 2.5% respectively.

In a family study of Briquet syndrome, Guze and colleagues reported a significantly increased risk for Briquet syndrome among the first-degree female relatives of Briquet syndrome probands (7/105), compared to female relatives of control probands (13/532). Additionally, they reported an increased risk for antisocial personality among the male (18/96) and female (9/105) relatives of the Briquet syndrome probands, compared to the risk for male (44/420) and female (14/532) relatives of controls.

Torgersen studied 14 MZ twin pairs and 21 DZ twin pairs in which one member had a somatoform disorder (somatization disorder, conversion disorder, psychogenic pain disorder or hypochondriasis). 29% of MZ twin pairs were concordant for somatoform disorder compared to 10% of DZ twin pairs. This difference was not significant.

ADOPTION STUDIES

In an analysis of a large Swedish adoption cohort, Sigvardsson identified a set of discriminant function variables that distinguished female adoptees with repeated brief somatic complaints and psychiatric disability ("somatizers") from other female adoptees. In a subsequent analysis, Bohman divided somatizers into two groups, "high-frequency somatizers" (those who have high prevalence of psychiatric, abdominal, or back complaints) and "diversiform somatizers" (those who have a lower frequency of complaints, but multiple, highly variable symptoms). Thirty percent of the high-frequency somatizers had histories of alcohol abuse and/or criminality (based upon the national registries for these behaviors). Their male biological relatives were at increased risk for violent criminal behavior and alcohol abuse. For both types of somatizers, a cross-fostering analysis provided evidence for both congenital and postnatal influences on the development of somatoform disorder. These studies suggest a familial connection between some types of somatoform disorder, alcoholism, and criminality. Torgersen makes the appropriate point that not much research has been carried out in this area in recent years the reason for this is not clear.

Guze SB. Genetics of Briquet syndrome and somatization disorder. A review of family, adoption, and twin studies. *Ann Clin Psychiatry* 1993;5(4):225–230.

Torgersen S. Genetics and somatoform disorders. *Tidsskr Nor Laegeforen* 2002;122(14):1385–1388.

TOURETTE SYNDROME

Epidemiologic Research

A. TWIN STUDIES

Price studied 43 pairs, 30 MZ and 13 DZ same-sex pairs. MZ twin concordance was 77% for any tics, compared to 23% for DZ twins. For Tourette disorder proper, the MZ concordance rate was 53%, compared to the DZ rate of 8%. These are all significant differences.

Table 3–6. Family Study Data for Genetic Counseling*

Family History*	Unselected General Population Risk	Increased Risk for Offspring
Unipolar disorder (UP)	6%	2-fold (16%) for UP 4-fold (4%) for BP
Bipolar disorder (BP)	1%	9-fold (9%) for BP 2-fold (16%) for UP
Schizophrenia (SZ)	1%	10-fold (10%) for SZ 2-fold (15%) for UP
Alcoholism	5% males, 1% females	5-fold (27% for males, 5% for females)
Panic disorder	0.5%	12-fold (6%)
Tourette's syndrome	0.25%	100-fold (25%)
Alzheimer's disease	3%	5-fold (15%) at age 75
Attention-deficit/hyperactivity disorder	3%	5-fold (15%)
Anorexia nervosa	0.5%	10-fold (5%)

*These data assume that only one parent is affected.

Pauls studied 338 biological relatives of 38 Tourette disorder probands, 21 adoptive relatives and 22 relatives of normal controls. Among the biological relatives, 8.3% had Tourette disorder, while 16.3% had chronic tics and 9.5% had OCD. These risks are all significantly greater than the risks for the 43 relatives of controls.

Segregation analyses have fit both single locus models and polygenic models to the familial pattern of this disorder.

B. Linkage Studies

A collaborative effort to use systematic genomic screening to find genes causing Tourette's has been underway for several years. Recent results implicate chromosome 2p. Rare mutations in the dendritic growth protein SLITRK1 (chromosome 13q) have been associated with this condition.

GENETIC COUNSELING

Empirical data for genetic counseling is summarized in Table 3–6. These data assume that the other parent is unaffected. The percentages in parentheses after the family history provide the unselected general population risk. For example, the general population lifetime risk for UP illness (defined narrowly) is 8%. If a subject has a parent with UP depression, the lifetime risk is double that of the general population (16%). Such individuals are also at fourfold increased risk for BP illness.

Some illnesses have narrow age-at-onset distributions in the general population. For example, first episodes of BP illness almost always occur before age 60. Fully 50% of BP individuals have their initial episode (depressive or manic) prior to age 20. This should be considered in a general way when assessing risk. For example, an unaffected 40-year-old son of a parent with BP illness has already passed through most of the age at risk, and thus, his risk is substantially less than 9%. An estimate of 2% would be more accurate in this case.

It is anticipated that genotypic methods will be adapted for use in genetic counseling in the coming years. Such methods are not yet widely applicable aside from use in certain unusual families with single gene conditions. Most experts feel that genotypic screening for persons with multifactorial disorders would still be premature; however some products are already on the market, and it seems likely that the predictive power of such methods will approach clinical utility within the next decade.

Nurnberger JIJr, Bierut LJ. Seeking the connections: Alcoholism and our genes. *Scientific Am* 2007;296(4):46–53.

Tsuang D, Faraone SV, Tsuang MT. Psychiatric genetic counseling. In: Floyd EB, David JK (eds). *Psychopharmacology: The Fourth Generation of Progress.* New York: Raven Press, 1995. Available at http://www.acnp.org/g4/GN401000181[no page range]

The Psychiatric Interview[1]

Barry Nurcombe, MD, & Michael H. Ebert, MD

4

Human behavior is complex. When it becomes dysfunctional because of environmental stress or brain disease it can mystify the inexperienced clinician. This is especially true of neurobehavioral disorders, which involve neuropsychiatric changes in cognition and emotion that overlap the boundary of psychiatry and neurology. The clinician must appreciate and assess the signs and symptoms of neurobehavioral disorder with the same discernment as in physical syndromes such as myocardial infarction or infectious disease.

This chapter describes the psychiatric history and mental status examination (MSE), in the conduct of an effective psychiatric interview. The steps of the interview process are described along with the techniques the clinician must master in order to elicit information relevant to a diagnostic formulation in an orderly, reliable, and comprehensive manner. The components of the psychiatric history and the MSE are described in accordance with the stages of the interview during which they would usually be obtained.

What can be achieved at the initial psychiatric interview? The outcome depends on the situation in which it is conducted and what the physician and the patient are seeking. For example, a brisk, focused interview in an emergency room contrasts with the more extensive survey appropriate to an outpatient clinic. Both types of interview differ from what is possible at the bedside of a patient who is severely ill in a medical or surgical ward. Despite these observations, fundamental issues can be addressed to varying degree in any clinical situation, as illustrated in Table 4–1. We return to these issues in our discussion of the elements of the psychiatric history.

THE STAGES OF THE PSYCHIATRIC INTERVIEW

Inception

If the interviewer works in a clinic, at the opening of the psychiatric interview he or she goes to the waiting room,

introduces himself or herself to the patient, accompanies the patient to the interview room, and shows him or her to a seat. After taking identifying data from the patient, the interviewer can tell the patient what he or she already knows. This approach avoids unnecessary mysteries and clears the way for action. Consider the following example:

> Psychiatrist: Your parents came to see me yesterday. They told me they're worried because your schoolwork has fallen off, although you've always been a good student; you've dropped most of your friends; and you seem to have become depressed. Last week they found one of your assignments in which you spoke about suicide. They think you may need help for an emotional problem.
>
> Patient (a 16-year-old boy): So?
>
> Psychiatrist: So they asked you to see a psychiatrist. I get the impression you're not too happy about that.
>
> Patient: No.
>
> Psychiatrist: Maybe we can start by you telling me how you feel about it.

Interviews are not always conducted in an office; they may be transacted beside a patient's bed, or between pieces of equipment in the examination room of an emergency clinic, or even while driving a car. Wherever they occur they include a pattern to the beginning, a certain formality. The interviewer introduces himself or herself, says why he or she is there, and invites the patient to respond by telling his or her story. If the patient does not want to do so, the interviewer helps the patient to explain why.

Reconnaissance

The interviewer helps the patient tell his or her story as spontaneously as possible. He or she listens and does not interrupt any more than is necessary to keep the story flowing. The interviewer does not rush the reconnaissance nor try to direct it prematurely. If all the interviewer does is ask direct questions, all he or she will get is answers. Open-ended probes should be used as much as possible. The more leading the probe, the less valid

---

[1] Some of this material also appears in Nurcombe B, Gallagher RM: *The Clinical Process in Psychiatry: Diagnosis and Management Planning.* Cambridge University Press, 1986. Reprinted with the permission of Cambridge University Press.

Table 4–1. Issues to be Addressed in the Psychiatric Interview

Chronology of events and development of symptoms; subjective concerns of the patient; and concerns of patient's family, friends, neighbors, or employers
Insight, judgment, and motivation for treatment
Precipitation of illness and relevant stressors
Predisposition and family history of psychiatric illness
Presentation
Previous psychiatric illness and behavioral problems
Previous psychiatric treatment and/or mental health intervention

the response, unless the issue in question is a simple, unequivocal one. The facilitating techniques we describe later in this chapter are particularly appropriate for the reconnaissance stage.

Detailed Inquiry

After the patient has finished his or her story, the interviewer seeks further information about the present illness, past illness, medical history, early environment, education, and other relevant matters from the psychiatric history. A full detailed inquiry will take several interviews, but a scanning of the features most important for a provisional diagnosis can be accomplished within an hour.

Table 4–2 lists the content of the psychiatric history. The order suggested in the table should not be followed blindly. The interviewer should be prepared to deal with topics in whatever sequence is natural. In accordance with the case, some areas will be emphasized and others pursued in less detail.

Detailed inquiry involves questioning, but the questions are kept as open ended as possible at the outset,

Table 4–2. Content of the Psychiatric History

Identifying data
Presenting problem
History of present illness
History of past psychiatric illnesses
Medical history
History of drug or alcohol intake or of antisocial behavior
Early development and childhood environment
Educational history
Vocational history
Family history
Sexual history
Marital history
Characteristic coping mechanisms, values, ideals, aspirations

moving from general to specific as more detail is required. Compare the following questions:

- How are things in your marriage?
- How are things between you and your wife?
- How do you and your wife get on?
- Is your marriage a happy one?
- Do you love your wife?

This approach is similar to the way a surgeon approaches a guarded section of a painful abdomen: from the outside in. Direct questions provoke circumscribed responses and are most appropriate to issues of fact (e.g., What year were you married?).

Some issues are left to a later time after a therapeutic alliance has developed. Unless the patient presents his or her sexual life as a problem at the outset, an exploration of this area is usually postponed.

Transitions

The interviewer never moves abruptly from one topic to another. Change should be signaled. For example, the psychiatrist could say, "Okay. I'd like to go on from there to something else. Could you tell me about the jobs you've had? What did you do after you left school?"

Standard Versus Discretionary Inquiry

Part of the detailed inquiry is standardized, including questions obligatory for patients of a given age, in a specific clinical situation, or as part of a minimum database. The components of a standard inquiry should be defined for each clinical setting. The rest of the detailed inquiry is largely discretionary and involves the eliciting of evidence supporting or refuting the diagnostic hypotheses generated after reconnaissance.

ELEMENTS OF THE PSYCHIATRIC HISTORY

We now discuss the components of the psychiatric history, which are shown in Table 4–1. Each issue addressed in Table 4–1 must be addressed and the information related to one of the categories shown in Table 4–2.

The Present Illness

An accurate psychiatric history is the guide to diagnosis, intervention, and treatment. To this end, it is useful to define the present episode with its precipitants and then determine whether the present episode constitutes a discrete psychiatric illness or an episode in a chronic psychiatric illness that can be documented chronologically.

Some patients present a variety of subjective concerns. Others have a more focused complaint and can identify particular issues as problematic. Whatever the problem(s) for which the patient or his or her associates seek help, the clinician attempts to delineate them; to understand how the patient experiences them; and to ascertain their duration, onset, development, and persistence.

Precipitation of Illness & Relevant Stressors

If the problems had an onset, the interviewer attempts to determine whether the patient experienced physical or psychosocial stress at that time. The mere coincidence of stress and onset does not substantiate a causal association; indeed, causation remains speculative in some cases. Causation is supported, however, if the patient previously had a breakdown when exposed to a similar stress or if the patient's account of the stress indicates its personal significance.

Some stressors have universal impact. Others are highly idiosyncratic, and painstaking work may be required before they can be unraveled in psychotherapy. In some cases it is an open question whether an event was a true precipitant, or secondary to a disorder in its early stages, or mere coincidence.

Previous Psychiatric Illness & Behavioral Problems

The interviewer considers the following questions in evaluating the patient for previous psychiatric illness and behavioral problems: Has the patient had any problems of a similar nature in the past? What precipitated them, if anything? Has the patient had any other emotional disorders or physical symptoms related to tension? Has the patient had, or does he or she have, physical or neurologic disease that could contribute to the present problem? Does the patient have, or has he or she had, personal habits (e.g., substance abuse) that could cause, precipitate, or complicate the present problem?

Previous Psychiatric Treatment & Mental Health Intervention

The interviewer should be aware of any therapeutic interventions prior to the current evaluation, including formal psychiatric treatment (or treatment by another mental health professional), emergency evaluations, hospitalizations, or mental health treatment rendered by a primary care physician. The clinician who carried out the treatment and the treating facility should be identified, as should the approximate date(s) and duration of treatment. The patient's response to each pharmacologic agent and associated side effects should be documented. The type, duration, and results of psychotherapy should be identified. The interviewer will usually verify and amplify this information by requesting records from previous treating professionals and facilities, with appropriate written consent from the patient.

Predisposition & Potentials

The interviewer considers the following questions in evaluating the patient for predisposition to and family history of psychiatric illness: What kind of person was the patient before he or she became ill? What biopsychosocial strengths and weaknesses predisposed the patient to breakdown? These questions require a comprehensive evaluation, and it is unrealistic to expect all of this information to be elaborated in a single interview. However, important pieces of the jigsaw puzzle are usually available, if the interviewer keeps his or her eyes and ears open. The interviewer can seek information about the following additional questions: What personal and environmental strengths, resources, and liabilities are apparent at the present time? What has the patient got going for him or her now? What holds the patient back? What hurdles does he or she face? An inventory is required of the patient's physical, intellectual, emotional, and social assets and deficiencies. This inventory is crucial to the design of an individualized plan of management.

Presentation

The interviewer considers the following questions in evaluating the patient's current presentation for treatment: Why does the patient seek help now? Is the patient being seen at the onset of a disorder or later, either when a relatively defined pattern of symptoms has developed or after the patient has recovered partially but remains troubled by residual difficulties? Did the patient come of his or her own accord, or was he or she persuaded to do so? Did others bring in the patient for treatment? Why?

Insight, Judgment, & Motivation for Treatment

The interviewer considers the following questions in evaluating the patient's insight, judgment, and motivation for treatment: Does the patient think he or she is unwell? Does the patient think he or she has been referred inappropriately? The patient may be correct. If the patient recognizes his or her own disturbance, does he or she have any idea of its nature or cause? How realistic are these notions?

What kind of help does the patient seek, if any? Is this in line with what is advisable, appropriate, or feasible? Is the patient troubled by doubts concerning his or her problem and the kind of treatment he or she will receive? Fears of craziness or of exotic psychiatric treatments are likely to be inflamed by deep-seated anxieties about helplessness and victimization. These fears are often aggravated by images derived from family or cultural values, including those depicted in the media. It is better that such concerns be expressed as soon as possible and corrected when they are the result of misinformation.

Family History

The family history is an important component of the initial interview. It helps to understand the patient's family structure and the family influences that were brought to bear on the patient's growth and development. It documents the patient's genetic predisposition to psychiatric illness. This initial inquiry is the beginning of a genogram that can be developed in more detail in subsequent interviews. The initial interview should identify each family member for one or two generations and also identify individuals with psychiatric illness for at least two generations. This line of questioning is subtle because of social stigma and the natural reluctance of individuals to disclose family problems. It is desirable to inquire about the presence of psychiatric illness in several ways. The interviewer may begin with an open-ended question such as inquiring whether any family member has had emotional or behavioral problems. Follow-up questions can include whether any family member has been treated by a behavioral health provider and whether anyone in the family has been hospitalized for psychiatric illness.

Social History

The social history should be elicited in the first diagnostic interview, even if time does not permit a full exposition of this subject. This part of the initial interview informs the examiner of the social, cultural, and family structural influences that contribute to the patient's personality, values, and social integration. Open-ended questions that invite the patient to describe the structure and membership of the nuclear and extended family is a good start. Often the description will be colored by feelings and attitudes toward each person that can be explored in depth in a subsequent interview. Marriages, children, divorces, major illnesses, and deaths within the immediate family should be documented as part of the social history. This part of the interview can be interwoven with the family history of illness, particularly psychiatric illness. The social history is often ignored in initial psychiatric interviews, but the absence of this information limits the diagnostic formulation.

Educational and Occupational History

The initial diagnostic interview should include a brief educational and occupational history. During this part of the interview, the diagnostician is forming a time line to register major events in the patient's life and evaluating

developmental milestones. The educational history helps to give a developmental history extending through the second decade of life, as well as an indirect indication of intellectual capacity and social adjustment. Interruptions in education are often a sign of emerging psychopathology or a discrete behavioral setback or crisis. The occupational history is valuable life history information, but can also indicate periods in a person's life when an acute psychiatric illness occurred or when the gradual development of psychopathology altered a person's life, including his ability to work. Choices of educational and occupational paths may provide a window into understanding a patient's personality, motivation, identification with people who are important to the patient, and family values and influences.

A military history is important when it is relevant to the patient's life. Major psychiatric illnesses often present for the first time under the stress of military service when the individual is in his late teens and early twenties. Military health care provides substantial documentation of symptoms in an acute psychiatric illness, diagnosis, and response to treatment. If an individual has a medical discharge from the military, the documentation of the illness is very useful data for diagnostic impression, treatment response, and prognosis.

Legal History

A legal history is relevant in an initial psychiatric interview if the interviewer infers that it may be important for the diagnostic impression. To omit this inquiry because it is a difficult subject is an error if it turns out that the diagnostic formulation hinges on this aspect of the history. The content of this history can include lawsuits, divorce and custody disputes, bankruptcy, arrests, convictions, and imprisonment.

Forming Hypotheses

Throughout the initial interview, the diagnostician is working to form hypotheses about the etiology of the current problem under evaluation. This involves an acquired skill set that involves memory, a questioning technique that draws the patient out in a nonintimidating manner, a capacity to convey empathy, and an ability to make each part of the interview productive in terms of information gathering, while also building an alliance with the patient. It is reasonable to take occasional notes, but it is a poor technique to look at a written document constantly instead of the patient. Likewise, it is poor technique to follow a rigid interview outline and not follow leads that the patient offers when they occur. It is precisely this mixture of structure and completeness in acquiring clinical data, combined with spontaneity in following psychodynamic leads and continually forming hypotheses about the patient's defining life events and diagnosis, that constitutes a skill acquired gradually by the experienced clinician.

MSE: CONTENT, PURPOSE, & FORMAT

The MSE is a set of systematic observations and assessments undertaken by a diagnostician during the clinical interview. Properly conducted, the MSE provides a detailed and systematic description of the patient at that time, information essential to the consolidation of those patterns of clues and inferences that are required for the generation of diagnostic hypotheses. The MSE, guided by the hypothetico-deductive approach to diagnosis, is an essential part of the subsequent inquiry plan. In this section we offer a comprehensive description of the components of the MSE. In regard to a particular patient—and in accordance with the clinical context, background information, and psychiatric history—the interviewer will apply the MSE tactically, pursuing brief, comprehensive, or discretionary lines of inquiry, as warranted.

The Need for Standardization

Because the MSE, like the psychiatric history, should involve routine and discretionary lines of inquiry according to the context of assessment and the diagnostic hypotheses being entertained, it should not be standardized as a whole. Instead the separate observations and assessments that compose the MSE should be standardized. The techniques of eliciting data should be formalized, the phenomena in question clearly defined, and the weight to be placed on each phenomenon clarified.

Reliability

The **reliability** of a test refers to the likelihood (usually expressed as a correlation) that similar results will be obtained on retesting (**test–retest reliability**) or that similar results will be obtained by different observers (**interrater reliability**). Test–retest reliability applies to relatively stable characteristics such as the use of language; it is not to be expected in characteristics (e.g., mood) that are potentially changeable and often linked to a current situation.

When psychiatrists test for the patient's abstracting ability, for example, by asking the patient to explain proverbs in his or her own words, how certain can the psychiatrist be that the clinical test is a true measure of the ability in question? In other words, what is the **validity** of the test? Over the years, a set of informal mental state assessments has accumulated but in some instances their validity is questionable. When we describe any clinical test in this chapter, we will consider its validity along with the mental faculties required for adequate performance on the test.

Types of MSEs

A. BRIEF SCREENING MSE

When a patient has been referred to an ambulatory clinic for a situational or personality problem, and none of the indications for a comprehensive screening examination pertain (see next section), a brief, informal screen is sufficient. The brief screening MSE is completed during the inception, reconnaissance, and detailed inquiry stages of the psychiatric interview. In particular, the interviewer notes the patient's general appearance, motor behavior, quality of speech, relationship to the interviewer, and mood. From the patient's demeanor, conversation, and history, the interviewer makes inferences about consciousness, orientation, attention, grasp, memory, fund of information, general intellectual level, language competence, and thought process. Abnormal thought content is not investigated unless clinical clues indicate the need for such discretionary inquiry (e.g., into hallucinations, obsessions, depersonalization). Physiologic functions (e.g., sleep, appetite, libido, menstrual cycle, energy level) and insight should always be assessed.

B. COMPREHENSIVE SCREENING MSE

The interviewer should be alerted to the need for a comprehensive screening MSE whenever there is a reasonable possibility that the patient has psychosis or primary or secondary brain dysfunction. Table 4–3 summarizes the settings and clues that mandate a comprehensive MSE. If the clinician has any doubts, the comprehensive screen should be completed.

Components of the MSE

Table 4–4 summarizes the areas to be covered in the MSE. The following sections describe these areas in more detail:

A. APPEARANCE & BEHAVIOR

From the moment the interviewer first greets the patient, he or she will be aware of the patient's appearance. The interviewer should try to describe it in detail before drawing inferences from it. What is the patient's physique and habitus? Is there evidence of weight loss or gain? Does the patient have any conspicuous marks or disfigurement? The interviewer should describe the patient's face and hair. Does the patient look ill? What is the expression of the eyes and mouth? Does the patient appear to be in touch with the surroundings? Is the patient clean and neat, or does he or she exhibit deficiencies in personal hygiene revealed by poor grooming of the skin, hair, or nails? How is the patient dressed? Is the patient's clothing neat? Is it appropriate or peculiar? After the interviewer describes these characteristics, he or she determines whether an inference may be made about

Table 4–3. Indications for a Comprehensive Screening Mental Status Examination

The patient is seen in a hospital emergency room or crisis clinic; is being managed on a nonpsychiatric ward and has been referred for consultation; or is being admitted to a psychiatric unit.

The patient is older than 40 years.

The patient has a history of psychiatric disorder, substance abuse, organic brain disorder, or physical disorder that could affect brain function.

The patient's personal habits, memory, concentration, or grasp have deteriorated recently.

The patient or other informant presents clinical clues that suggest current mood disorder, psychosis, or organic brain dysfunction (e.g., persistent or intermittent depression, withdrawal, elation, overactivity, bizarre ideation, hallucinations, delusions, ideas of influence and reference, headaches, loss of memory and grasp, disorientation, disordered language, headaches, seizures, motor weakness, tremor, or sensory loss).

Physical examination indicates or suggests brain dysfunction.

In forensic referrals, when mental competence or legal insanity are in question.

the kind of "statement" the patient is attempting to make with his or her attire.

The interviewer notes general overactivity or underactivity, abnormalities of posture, gross incoordination, or impairment of large muscle function. What is the patient's gait like and how does he or she sit? The interviewer notes any abnormalities of finer movement and posture, such as tremor, tics, or fidgeting.

Stereotypies are organized, repetitive movements or speech or perseverative postures. They are usually associated with schizophrenia, particularly the catatonic type. A striking variant of postural stereotypy is **waxy flexibility,** in which the patient will remain indefinitely in a position into which the interviewer places him or her (e.g., standing on one leg). Other disorders of movement associated with catatonia include a stiff expressionless face; facial grimacing or contortions; stiff, awkward, or stilted body movement; and unusual mannerisms of expressive movement or speech. The latter should not be confused with the gracelessness of someone who is socially anxious. The interviewer also notes whether the patient exhibits any rituals such as a need to touch objects repetitively, as in obsessive–compulsive disorder, or any habits such as nail biting, thumb sucking, lip licking, yawning, or scratching.

Table 4–4. Sections of the Mental Status Examination

A. Appearance and behavior
B. Relationship to the interviewer
C. Affect and mood
D. Cognition and memory
E. Language
F. Disorders of thought
G. Physiologic function
H. Insight and judgment

The interviewer attends to the accent, pitch, tone, and tempo of the patient's speech, paying particular attention to unusually high or low pitch and abnormal tone, as in the high-pitched "squawking" monotone sometimes encountered in children with early infantile autism.

In mutism, which may occur in advanced brain disorder, severe melancholia, catatonia, or conversion disorder or in the elective mutism of negativistic children, the patient is unable or unwilling to utter anything. In conversion disorder, mutism is less common than is aphonia, in which the patient is able to speak only in a hoarse whisper.

B. Relationship to the Interviewer

The interviewer should infer the quality of the patient's relationship by how he or she behaves and by what he or she says. The relationship may be constant, it may vary with the topic being discussed, or it may be influenced by other factors. These factors may remain obscure if they are unexpressed (e.g., when the patient is privately amused by an auditory hallucination). The interviewer should note whether this is the case.

Affective states are difficult to assess, aside from noting whether they are inconstant or are apparently influenced by obscure factors. The interviewer draws on a number of behavioral clues to assess the quality of the patient's relationship and mood. As a rule, the more inferential the judgment, the more unreliable the conclusion. Interviewers may differ in their inferences concerning a patient's affect, especially when it is unstable, ambiguous, complex, or shielded by interpersonal caution.

The interviewer's behavior will inevitably affect the ebb and flow of the patient's feelings. The patient may be responding appropriately to the interviewer's friendly approach (or rudeness, for that matter). He or she will also be responding to highly idiosyncratic internal predispositions. For example, a patient may harbor mingled anxiety and deference for somebody he or she perceives as a threatening authority figure who must be placated.

Given the fallibility of inference, the interviewer is well advised to stick closely to observations and be able to cite them. This skill requires training. The beginner may be overly impressed by brilliant intuitive leaps; the expert heeds intuition but realizes how unreliable it is. The beginner grasps for, and holds firmly to, an inference, sometimes in spite of contrary evidence. The expert makes the inference, cites the clues on which it is based, can offer alternative explanations, and discards the inference for a better one if contrary evidence emerges.

The quality of the patient's eye contact is of great importance in gauging affective states. Negativistic patients, especially those with catatonia, may avert their gaze from the interviewer. Children with early infantile autism characteristically demonstrate eccentricities of eye contact, for example, staring "through" the interviewer or averting their gaze from him or her. A delirious patient whose sensorium is impaired may stare into space, as may a melancholic or schizophrenic patient whose thoughts are dominated by gloomy ruminations or delusional preoccupations. Intermittent staring is a feature of different forms of epilepsy. The interviewer notes whether the patient's attention can be captured, albeit briefly. If not, the interviewer should suspect an organic brain disorder.

Some patients stare at the interviewer intently. He or she should distinguish the wide eyes of awe or fear from the narrowed slits of hypervigilant suspiciousness. Other patients make hesitant eye contact, particularly when they are embarrassed about what they are saying. Not all patients with shifty gaze are liars, and some prevaricators have learned to deliver their lines without batting an eyelash.

The impact of the eyes on interpersonal relations cannot be overestimated. The configuration of supraorbital, circumorbital, and facial musculature; eyelids; palpebral fissure; gaze; depth of ocular focus; pupil size; and conjunctival moisture combine to produce a range of social signals of great significance for interpersonal dominance, competition, attraction, hostility or avoidance, the initiation and punctuation of conversation, and the feedback a person requires to know how the other person has responded to what one has said.

Eyes and face are combined with body posture and movement in a gestalt. The face provides the clues to remoteness, bewilderment, and perplexity, whereas the whole body is involved in tenseness (e.g., clenched fists, sweaty palms, stiff back, leaning forward), restlessness, preoccupation, boredom, and sadness.

The patient may be uncommunicative or, in the extreme, quite mute. In contrast, he or she may be friendly and communicative, even loquacious or garrulous. Patients convey antagonism by hectoring; by being uncooperative, impertinent, or condescending; or even by making direct threats, criticizing, or verbally abusing the interviewer. In contrast, by tone of conversation and demeanor, the patient can convey respect, deference, anxiety to please, or ingratiation. The interviewer notes and describes the following attitudes in the patient: shyness, fear, suspiciousness, cautiousness, assertiveness, indifference, passivity, clowning, interest in the interviewer, clinging, coyness, seductiveness, or invasiveness.

C. AFFECT & MOOD

Affect refers to a feeling or emotion, experienced typically in response to an external event or a thought. The patient's relationship to the interviewer is a particular manifestation of affect. Affects are usually associated with feelings about the self or about others who are of personal significance to the individual. Less often, an affect is experienced alone, as though adrift from its reference point. Affect is the conscious component of a monitoring system that signals whether the individual is on track toward a personal goal; whether he or she is obstructed, frustrated, or prevented from achieving the goal; or whether he or she has already attained it. Compare, for example, the anticipatory pleasure at preparing to meet someone beloved; the anxiety and fear at seeing the beloved with a serious rival; the rage and despair of loss; and the exaltation of reunion. Similar, though more complex, affects may attend mountain climbing, solving mathematical puzzles, or giving birth. Whatever the goal, its remoteness, proximity, loss, repudiation, attainment, or inaccessibility are all accompanied by self-monitoring affect.

In contrast to an affect, which may be momentary, **mood** refers to an inner state that persists for some time, with a disposition to exhibit a particular emotion or affect. For example, a mood of depression may not prevent an individual from deriving momentary diversion from a joke; however, the expression of gloom, sadness, or desolation returns and prevails. Affects and mood are inferred from the patient's demeanor and spontaneous conversation. A general query such as "How are you feeling, now?" or "How have your spirits been?" can be helpful. The interviewer should try to avoid leading questions such as "Do you feel depressed?"

Demeanor and affect usually coincide, but sometimes they do not. For example, a stiff smile can mask anxiety or depression. If the interviewer suspects this to be the case, he or she can offer an indicating or clarifying interpretation to help the patient recover suppressed emotion, such as "I notice that even though you speak of sad things, you are smiling" or "It's hard to smile when you feel bad inside."

The interviewer describes in the mental status report the general qualities of the patient's emotional expression. Particular morbid affects or moods are noted. For example, is the patient **affectively flat,** that is, emotionally dull, monotonous, and lacking in resonance? This presentation is characteristic of chronic schizophrenia and dementia. Is the patient **emotionally constricted,** with a narrow range of affect, as in obsessional or schizoid personality? Does the patient exhibit **inappropriate or incongruous affect,** in that it is not in keeping with the topic of conversation?

Does the patient show evidence of **lability,** suddenly changing from neutral to excited or from one emotional pole to the other? Lability is often associated with emotional intemperateness, an abrupt unreflective expression of heightened emotion (e.g., excited anticipation, affection, irritation).

The interviewer notes the presence of **histrionic affect,** the blatant but rather shallow expression of emotion often observed in those who exaggerate their feelings in order to avoid being ignored and who need to capture, or who fear to lose, the center of the interpersonal stage. Histrionic affect is often encountered in people with histrionic, narcissistic, or borderline personality disorder.

Morbid euphoria, a sense of well-being expressed in inexorable good spirits, is encountered in hypomania or mania and less commonly in schizophrenia and organic brain disorder. Frontal lobe dysfunction, characteristic of neurosyphilis, disseminated sclerosis and after traumatic brain injury, may be associated with fatuous joking and lack of foresight. Silliness is sometimes encountered in histrionic or immature people overwhelmed by the enormity of a difficult situation. Morbid silliness is also characteristic of some disorganized schizophrenic patients.

As it becomes exaggerated, euphoria merges into elation and excitement; although the manic patient commonly also exhibits irritation if obstructed or thwarted. An extreme and transcendent exaltation of mood may be observed in the ecstatic states rarely associated with acute schizophreniform or schizophrenic disorders and epilepsy.

Apathy, a pervasive lack of interest and drive (also known as **anergia**), may be observed in patients with preschizophrenic, schizophrenic, depressive, and organic brain disorders. The apathetic patient has little or no enthusiasm for work, social interaction, or recreation. Anergia is usually associated with a decrease in sexual activity. **Anhedonia,** a subjective sense that nothing is pleasurable, is commonly associated with anergia and is observed in preschizophrenic, schizophrenic, and melancholic patients. **Excessive fatigue,** which may be manifest as hypersomnia, is associated with many disorders such as organic brain disorder, schizophrenia, anxiety disorders, depressive disorders, and somatization disorder.

When applied to an affect or mood, **depression** refers to a pervasive sense of sadness. Depression is often related to a life event involving loss, rejection, defeat, or disappointment. It may be associated with tearfulness and anger about the event. In severe depression or melancholia, the patient feels emotionally deadened or empty, the world stale and unprofitable, and the future hopeless. The patient is preoccupied with dark forebodings and may be agitated by persistent self-recrimination about past misdeeds. Diminished concentration and a slowing of thinking and movement characteristically accompany depressed affect and gloomy ruminations. In some patients agitated depression is associated with psychomotor restlessness. Severe depression has important somatic features, including characteristic posture and facies, headache, irritability, precordial heaviness, gastrointestinal slowing, anorexia, weight loss, loss of sexual interest, and insomnia. Depression typically has a diurnal variation: Dysphoria, hopelessness, and agitation are worse in the morning, and the patient brightens up by evening.

The interviewer will readily recognize **open anger** and **irritability.** These feelings may be quite understandable in the context of the patient's circumstances. Morbid anger, however, is defined by its pervasiveness, frequency, disproportionate quality, impulsiveness, and uncontrollability. Morbid anger is associated with organic brain disorder, usually in the form of catastrophic reactions to frustration, especially when the patient can no longer complete a familiar or easy task. Abnormal anger is also associated with some forms of epilepsy; personality disorders of the aggressive, antisocial, borderline, or paranoid type; attention-deficit and disruptive behavior disorders of childhood; drunkenness; paranoid disorders; hypomania or mania; and intermittent or isolated explosive disorders.

Controlled hostility may be expressed as sullenness, uncooperativeness, superiority, or mockery. It can be helpful to invite the patient to express anger or resentment directly and to define its origin. This is particularly the case with adolescents. When working with adolescents, the interviewer might consider saying, "Whenever I ask you a question, you close up. Something about being here is making you pretty uptight. Can you tell me what it is?"

Anxiety and **fear** refer to the subjective apprehension of impending danger, together with widespread manifestations of autonomic discharge (e.g., dilated pupils; cold, sweaty palms; tachycardia; tachypnea; nausea; bowel hurry; urinary urgency). Fear has an object: the need to defend oneself against uncertain odds (e.g., a charging bull, a near accident in an automobile). Anxiety is associated with the threat to an essential value, for example, being attached to someone beloved, not being a coward, being successful, or being highly regarded. Direct action (i.e., fight or flight) can eliminate fear, whereas the adaptive solution to anxiety is likely to require planning and persistence. Anxiety and fear are biologically advantageous because they signal the need for constructive responses.

In morbid anxiety, affect is cast adrift from its moorings, either to float free or fasten on a substitute, phobic object or situation (e.g., heights, a particular animal, elevators, enclosed spaces, being fat). Morbid anxiety appears disproportionate or eccentric and is recognized as pathologic by the patient and others. Many of the disorders of thought content (described later in this chapter) can be regarded as unconsciously determined, pathologic mechanisms that detach anxiety from its object or block and divert it at its origin.

D. Cognition & Memory

Table 4–5 lists the cognitive functions that can be assessed in an MSE. We describe them in more detail in the following sections:

1. Level of consciousness & awareness—The psychiatrist may be asked to consult on a comatose or stuporous patient, if a nonorganic cause is hypothesized. **Coma** is a state of nonawareness from which the patient cannot be aroused. Diminished awareness is called semicoma or **stupor,** in which case the subject is temporarily rousable (e.g., by pain or noise) but reverts to stupor when the stimulus ceases. In stupor, eye movements become purposeful when the painful stimulus is applied, and wincing or pupillary constriction may occur, but the patient remains akinetic and mute. Stupor and coma occur in primary neuronal dysfunction (e.g., Alzheimer disease), secondary neuronal dysfunction (e.g., metabolic encephalopathy), supratentorial lesions (e.g., infarction, hemorrhage, tumor), subtentorial lesions (e.g., infarction, hemorrhage, tumor, abscess), and psychiatric disorder (e.g., dissociative disorder, depression, and catatonia).

Psychogenic coma is suggested by normal vital and neurologic signs, resistance to opening the eyes, normal pupillary reactions, and staring (rather than wandering) eyes. Swallowing, corneal, and gag reflexes are usually intact, and electroencephalography and oculovestibular reflexes are normal. Intravenous barbiturate may increase verbalization in psychogenic stupor. It depresses awareness further in organic conditions.

Torpor denotes a lowering of consciousness short of stupor. Awareness is narrowed and restricted, and apathy, perseveration, and psychomotor retardation are observed, but the more dramatic phenomena of delirium (i.e., illusions, hallucinations, and agitation) are lacking. Torpor is associated with severe infection and multiinfarct dementia.

In **twilight or dreamy states,** restricted awareness is manifested as disorientation for time and place, with reduced attention and impaired short-term memory. In addition, the patient may have the sense of being in a dream.

Delirium is a common condition in medical and surgical wards. It is caused by a diffuse cerebral dysfunction of acute or subacute onset and fluctuant or reversible course. After prodromal restlessness and insomnia, delirium typically presents with obtundation, emotional lability, and visual illusions. The clinical features tend to worsen at night ("sundowning"), with insomnia, agitation, hallucinations, and delusions. So-called quiet deliria are common, with little more to note than clouding of consciousness, mild disorientation for time and place, and reduced concentration. Restlessness, tremor, asterixis (irregular, asymmetrical jerking of the extremities), myoclonus, and disturbance of autonomic function are also common. Patients vary in their psychological reactions to delirium: depressive, paranoid, schizophreniform, anxious, and somatoform responses may be encountered. Delirious patients may be fearfully or combatively hypervigilant, or torpid and apathetic.

Visual illusions, which are characteristic of delirium, involve the patient misinterpreting moving shadows, curtains, and surrounding bedroom furniture. Physical sensations may also be misperceived. For example, the patient may mistake abdominal pain for the knives of malefactors and tinnitus for radio waves. If poorly systemized delusional beliefs arise, the patient may act on them, seeking escape or defense. Visual hallucinations are more common than auditory hallucinations in delirium. Visual hallucinations are sometimes playful (e.g., animals romping), sometimes personal (e.g., the face of a dead relative), or sometimes horrible or threatening (e.g., dismembered bodies, accidents). They are most evident at night and can be provoked when the eyes are closed, especially when the orbits are pressed. Affect is usually labile in delirium, but persistent blunting, anxiety, suspiciousness, hostility, depression, or euphoria may be encountered and is usually congruent with the prevailing illusions or hallucinations.

Delirious patients may exhibit wandering attention and concentration; their thinking may become disconnected or incoherent and their memory impaired. These patients sometimes confabulate, linking memories out of correct sequence. Subtle restriction of consciousness often occurs during acute anxiety and results in vagueness or amnesia for traumatic experiences. Rarely, the amnesia is accentuated. The patient may wander off in a daze, turning up in an emergency room unaware of his

---

Table 4–5. Cognitive Functions

Level of consciousness and awareness
Orientation, attention, and concentration
Memory
Information
Comprehension
Conceptualization and abstraction

Table 4–6. Clinical Tests of Orientation

Time
Hour
Day
Date
Month
Year
Place
Building
City
State
Person
Name
Address and telephone number
Age
Occupation
Marital status

Table 4–7. Clinical Tests of Attention and Concentration

Subtract sevens or threes, serially, from 100.
Reverse the days of the week or months of the year.
Spell simple words backwards (e.g., *world*).
Repeat digits (two, three, four, or more) forward and
    backward.
Perform mental arithmetic (Number of nickels in $1.35?
    Interest on $200 at 4% for 18 months?).

or her name or address. This is known as **dissociative fugue state** and should be differentiated from epilepsy or postictal conditions.

2. Orientation, attention, & concentration—Disorders of orientation are most often involved when the sensorium is clouded, as in torpor, obtundation, dreamy states, delirium, or fugue. Orientation is usually lost in the following order: time, place, and person. Disorientation for time and place usually indicates organic brain disorder. Disorientation for personal identity is rare and is associated with psychogenic or postictal fugue states, other dissociative disorders, and agnosia (loss of the ability to recognize sensory inputs). The interviewer assesses the patient's orientation by asking him or her for the information listed in Table 4–6. The reliability of the clinical assessment of orientation is high, but its predictive validity is uncertain.

Attention is involved when a patient is alerted by a significant stimulus and sustains interest in it. Concentration refers to the capacity to maintain mental effort despite distraction. An inattentive patient ignores the interviewer's questions, for example, or soon loses interest in them. The distractible patient is diverted from mental work by incidental sights, sounds, and ideas.

Table 4–7 describes simple clinical tests for attention and concentration. These tests have high reliability but little validity. Primarily they test the ability to concentrate. A patient's ability to answer arithmetic questions requires not only concentration but also intelligence and education. Errors are common and are related to psychiatric disturbance, socioeconomic status, intelligence, and the patient's ability to cope with an interview situation. The procedure helps to identify organic brain disorder but has little diagnostic specificity.

3. Memory—Memory has several stages. Information must first be registered and comprehended. It is then held in short-term storage. If the material is to be retained beyond immediate recall, a more durable memory trace is formed. Memory traces in long-term storage will decay, consolidate, or become simplified and schematized, partly as a result of subsequent experience. Long-term memories are retrieved or recalled from storage by tagging a pattern of sensory phenomena and matching it with long-term memory schemata.

In clinical practice, abnormal memory is manifest as **amnesia** (memory loss) or **dysmnesia** (distortion of memory). Psychogenic amnesia occurs in several forms. During and after severe anxiety, memory is likely to be defective. Some people have the ability to repress unwelcome anxiety-laden ideas; their memory is thereby rendered patchy or selective. In dissociative disorders, such as psychogenic amnesia and fugue, the patient usually loses memory for a circumscribed period of time during which profoundly disturbing events took place. Less commonly the amnesia is generalized (i.e., total) or subsequent (i.e., amnesia for everything after a particular time).

In addition to displaying generalized amnesia, patients in a psychogenic fugue state may travel a distance from home and assume a new identity. Often it is unclear in such cases whether unwitting self-deception or conscious imposture are involved.

Organic amnesia occurs in acute, subacute, and chronic forms. After acute head trauma, **retrograde amnesia** (loss of memory of past events) is likely to occur as a result of a disruption of short-term memory. The extent of **anterograde amnesia** (inability to form new memories) after head trauma is an index of the severity of brain injury. Amnesia also occurs in association with alcoholism (i.e., blackouts) and after acute intoxication, delirium, or epileptic seizures.

Subacute amnesia (the amnestic syndrome) occurs in Wernicke encephalopathy, a disease caused by thiamine deficiency and encountered most commonly after alcohol abuse. Wernicke encephalopathy is characterized by conjugate gaze ophthalmoplegia, nystagmus, ataxia, and delirium. After the delirium clears, most patients experience a residual Korsakoff syndrome with disorganized

Table 4–8. Clinical Tests of Memory

Testing immediate recall

Repeat digits forward and backward. (Present digits at 1-second intervals. The average adult performance is up to six forward and four backward.)

Repeat three unrelated words (e.g., *apple, table, grass*) immediately.

Repeat three three-part words (e.g., 33 *Park Avenue, brown mahogany table, 12 red roses*).

Testing recent memory

Repeat the three one-part phrases after 1, 3, and 5 minutes.

Repeat the three three-part phrases after 1, 3, and 5 minutes.

Recall events in the recent past (e.g., a chronological account of the present illness, the last meal, an account of how the patient got to the office, the names of the physicians and nurses who are caring for the patient in the hospital).

Repeat this sentence: *One thing a country must have to become rich and great is a large, secure supply of wood.*

Recount the following story with as many details as possible:

William Stern/a 63-year-old/state representative/ from Walton County,/ Utah,/ was planning his reelection campaign/ when he began experiencing chest pain./ He entered Logan Memorial Hospital/ for 3 days of medical tests./A harmless virus was diagnosed/ and he, his wife,/ Sandra,/ and their two sons,/ Rick and Tommy,/ hit the campaign trail again. (The average patient should be able to reproduce 8 of the 15 separate ideas in this paragraph. Less adequate performance suggests defective recall of information that requires hierarchical analysis, short-term memory storage, and sequential recall.)

Testing remote memory

Recall parents' names, date and place of birth, graduation dates, age and year of marriage, and occupational history.

---

memory in an otherwise clear sensorium. Patients with Korsakoff syndrome have difficulty recalling events from before the onset of the encephalopathy. They also experience severe impairment of the ability to lay down new memories after the encephalopathy. The retrograde amnesia affects the patient's ability to remember the precise order in which events occurred. The anterograde amnesia, however, tends to be even more marked; the most severely affected patients, for example, are unable to store new information. As a consequence, these patients are often disoriented for place and time and may confabulate to fill the memory gaps. Thus, the characteristic pattern of Korsakoff syndrome is of amnesia, disorientation, confabulation, a facile lack of concern, and a tendency to get stuck in the one groove of thought (**perseveration**). Chronic amnesia, as in dementing illnesses, extends back for years. Recent memory is lost before remote memory.

Disorders of recognition include déjà vu, déjà vécu, and psychotic misidentification. **Déjà vu** and **déjà vécu** are common and normal, particularly in adolescents. They involve the sudden uncanny feeling that one has experienced the present situation, or heard precisely the same current conversation, on a previous occasion. These phenomena are associated with anxiety and less commonly with temporal lobe epilepsy. **Psychotic misidentification** may occur in schizophrenia. These patients describe familiar people as strangers or claim to recognize people they never met. Patients with Capgras syndrome regard familiar individuals (such as family members) as doubles or impersonators of themselves.

Disorders of recall include retrospective falsification and confabulation. All people indulge at times in **retro-**spective falsification, embellishing the past to present a more appealing, tragic, or amusing impression. Histrionic people sometimes invent such an extensive and impressive past that they are drawn into imposture. Depressive individuals find sin, failure, and occasion for self-recrimination in their unexceptional lives. After recovery from psychosis, patients often repress their memories of illness and retain only bland or vague reminiscences of the acute disorder. It is inadvisable to ask them to recall their experiences in detail.

A **confabulation** is a false memory that the patient believes is true. Confabulations may be quite detailed, but they are often inconsistent and fanciful. Confabulations commonly fill memory gaps, especially in the amnestic syndrome. Some schizophrenic patients confabulate, spinning complicated fantasies about telekinesis, extrasensory perception, nuclear radiation, and the like. It is difficult to draw the line between confabulation and deception in the hysterical impostor or the dramatic abnormal illness behavior of the patient with Munchausen syndrome.

Table 4–8 lists the clinical tests for immediate, recent, and remote memory. These tests have good test–retest and interrater reliability. Their validity is affected by intelligence and age and by emotional states such as depression and to a lesser extent anxiety. The most useful tests for detecting organic lesions appear to be orientation, delayed recall, sentence repetition, and general information.

4. Information—The patient's fund of general knowledge depends on education and current interest in

Table 4–9. Clinical Test of Information

Name the last four presidents, starting with the current president.
Name the mayor, state governor, and state senators.
Name four large United States cities.
Discuss four important current events.
For what are these people famous: George Washington, Christopher Columbus, William Shakespeare, Albert Einstein?

Table 4–10. Clinical Tests of Conceptualization and Abstraction

1. How are the following pairs similar or alike?
   a child and a dwarf
   a tree and a bush
   a river and a canal
   a dishwasher and a stove
2. How are the following pairs different?
   a lie and a mistake
   idleness and laziness
   poverty and misery
   character and reputation
3. What is the meaning of the following proverbs? (Ask the patient if he or she has heard them before.)
   "A rolling stone gathers no moss."
   "People who live in glass houses should not throw stones."
   "Strike while the iron is hot."

contemporary affairs. Table 4–9 provides a clinical test of information. Organicity is suggested if the patient makes 12 or more mistakes ($\varepsilon = 60\%$) on this test. If administration is standardized, reliability is high. The test is quite useful as an estimate of organicity, although it does not assess a unitary cognitive function.

5. Comprehension—A patient's comprehension is evaluated by his or her grasp of the importance of the immediate situation. For example, does the patient know why he or she is where he or she is? Does the patient appreciate that he or she is ill or in need of treatment? Does the patient understand the purpose of the examination?

There are no tests for comprehension. It is evaluated as the interview proceeds. Although comprehension is often disturbed in delirium and dementia, for example, there is no evidence that this disturbance contributes anything to the diagnosis of organicity beyond what is provided by other tests of the sensorium (i.e., orientation, concentration, memory).

6. Conceptualization & abstraction—Simple levels of conceptualization are assessed by testing the patient's capacity to discern the similarities and differences between sets of individual words. The patient's capacity to abstract is tested by asking the patient to discern the meaning of well-known metaphorical statements (Table 4–10). The tests listed in Table 4–10 have poor reliability and validity. They are affected by intelligence, educational level, culture, and age and have little discriminating power. The tests do not effectively detect organicity. Research has shown that clinicians using these tests could not distinguish between manic patients, schizophrenic patients, and creative writers. They are of most use when they tap unmistakable formal psychotic thought disorder. Consider the following examples:

A young man with disorganized and accelerated thinking responds thus to the proverb "People in glass houses should not throw stones": "Oh yeah. My California uncle passed the shotgun out the windows and started firing!"

To the proverb "A rolling stone gathers no moss," he answers, "Put a few pebbles in your mouth when you're hiking. You'll go a few more miles."

Another young patient, who has the delusion that he is Christ, responds to the glass houses proverb as follows: "Those who know that it has been seen what they have done—and believe me it has all been seen—let him who is without sin cast the first stone. Okay? That's what I believe it means."

The same patient responds to the rolling stone proverb in this way: "If you can continue to move and always move and always follow yourself and no one else, you'll never have the evil one within yourself."

Unfortunately the sample of thinking provoked by these tests is usually so small, and its pathology so equivocal, that these tests are of dubious virtue.

E. LANGUAGE

Language is a system of communication that is also used as a tool of thought. Language facilitates thinking by the way semantics hierarchically organizes ideas and concepts and by the way in which syntax indicates the relationship between those ideas and concepts.

Language competence is assessed from the patient's speech during the psychiatric interview. Any history of spoken or written language difficulty, or any observation of clumsy articulation, disordered rhythm, and difficulty in the understanding or choice of words, should be noted and investigated further. **Language comprehension** is tested by asking the patient to point to single objects, and then to point to a number of objects in a particular sequence. The interviewer may also ask the patient to perform a series of actions in an arbitrary sequence (e.g., "Touch your nose with your right index finger, then point that finger at me, then put it behind your back."). **Language expression** is evaluated by asking the patient to repeat words, phrases, and sentences and to name correctly a number of objects. Expression and comprehension are evaluated by asking the patient to read a passage aloud and to answer questions about it. Asking the patient to take dictation tests graphic language. Any errors and slowness in performance should be noted. The following sections describe some common disorders of language.

1. Aphasia—Aphasia is a dysfunction in the patient's ability to express himself or herself. The three most common forms of aphasia are all manifest as difficulty in repeating words or phrases. In **Broca aphasia,** comprehension is relatively intact but expression dysfluent, sparse, telegraphic, and full of circumlocution. In **Wernicke aphasia,** comprehension is affected. Expression, though fluent, rambles, lacks meaning, and is full of errors to which the patient seems oblivious. In **conduction aphasia,** comprehension is intact, expression is fluent but full of errors and pauses, and repetition is difficult; however, reading is relatively intact.

2. Muteness—Muteness is seldom found in neurologic disease, except in the acute phase, in seizure disorder, or in advanced cerebral degeneration. The aphasic patient is never mute. Muteness is much more commonly a sign of melancholia, stupor, catatonia, somatoform disorder, dissociation or negativism in children (i.e., elective mutism).

3. Schizophrenic language—The psychiatrist's main diagnostic problem is to differentiate schizophrenic language from the "jargon" of Wernicke aphasia. Schizophrenic patients tend to be heedlessly bizarre in thought content; aphasic patients are more aware of their errors and are more likely to use substitutions to overcome their language defects. The confused speech of schizophrenic patients is known as **word salad.** It may be so chaotic as to be barely comprehensible.

4. Paralogia—Paralogia, or talking past the point, occurs when the patient gives answers that are erroneous but reveal knowledge of what should be the correct answer. For example, the interviewer may ask, "How many legs has a cow?" and the patient responds, "Five." Talking past the point occurs in Ganser syndrome (also called the syndrome of approximate answers). It is most likely to be observed in individuals who regard hospitalization for insanity as preferable to incarceration for crime.

5. Neologisms—Neologisms are new words coined by the patient. They are often condensations of ideas that attempt to capture the ineffable. Neologisms are most common in schizophrenia; they must be distinguished from aphasic paraphasia, and circumlocution, to which the patient resorts in order to overcome expressive difficulty. Sometimes a neologism reveals that the patient has been "derailed" by the sound or sense of an associated word or idea. At other times, neologisms are a response to hallucinations or a defense (in a private code) against

the intrusion by the interviewer upon the patient's privacy.

F. Disorders of Thought

Pathology of thought may be found in the process, in the form, or in the content of thinking. The process and form of thinking may be disordered in terms of tempo, fluency (including continuity and control), logical organization, and intent. Normal thinking is characterized by reasonable but not excessive speed, and a smooth and continuous flow from one idea to the next. Normal thinking has clear goal-direction, organization, and consensual logic in the links between, and the sequence of, its constituent ideas.

In psychological illness, particularly the turmoil associated with psychoses such as schizophrenia and mania, any or all of the above characteristics may be disorganized. Pathologic thinking can be sluggish, headlong, disconnected, meandering or halting, and prone to lose its track, wander off at tangents, or follow an illogical line.

Abnormal thinking can be experienced by the thinker as invasive, inserted, or controlled by alien forces (**thought insertion**). It can also be sensed as leaking, stolen, lost, or broadcast from the mind into the outside world (**thought withdrawal** or **broadcasting**). Finally, the psychotic thinker, oblivious to or unconcerned about the need to make sense, may lose contact with the audience or use language defensively as a mocking camouflage.

1. Abnormalities of thought process & form

i. Tempo— Thinking is accelerated in **flight of ideas,** which may reach such a pitch that goal direction is lost and the connection between ideas is governed not by sense but by sound or idiosyncratic verbal or conceptual associations. Alliteration, assonance, rhyme (**clang associations**), and punning may determine the torrent of ideas that is distracted readily by internal or environmental stimuli. Flight of ideas is usually associated with **pressured speech** and may be experienced by the patient as racing thoughts. Flight of ideas is characteristic of mania, but it may occur also in excited schizophrenic patients, especially those in acute catatonia. In hypomania the flight of ideas is less marked, the tempo being accelerated but the associations less disorganized.

The tempo of thinking may be slowed in **retardation of thought,** especially in major depression. The patient often complains of fuzziness, woolliness, and poor concentration. Response time to questions is increased. There are long silences during which the patient may lose the thread of the conversation. In the extreme, retardation of thought becomes mutism or even stupor.

ii. Fluency— In **circumstantiality,** although the goal direction of thinking is retained, associations meander into fruitless, overly detailed, or barely relevant byways. The listener may feel impelled to hurry the speaker along. Circumstantiality is said to be characteristic of some epileptic patients whose peculiar combination of pedantry, perseveration, religiosity, and cliché lend their thinking a so-called "viscous" quality.

Perseveration refers to a tendency to persist with a point or theme, even after it has been dealt with exhaustively or the listener has tried to change the subject. It is also observed, for example, when a child fixedly repeats one aspect of a drawing, leaving multiple lines or dwelling on the shading in an exaggerated manner.

iii. Continuity— In **thought blocking,** the patient's speech is interrupted abruptly by silences that last less than a second or much longer, even a minute or more. During the pause the patient's eyes often flicker, particularly if he or she is listening to an auditory hallucination. Sometimes the patient becomes mentally blank. Blocking is often precipitated by questions or ideas that have personal significance, particularly if their import is threatening. Blocking is an uncommon but striking sign. It tends to be identified far too often, the observer mistaking the retarded thinking of a depressed or preoccupied patient for the abrupt roadblock of the true phenomenon. It is almost pathognomonic of schizophrenia but must be differentiated from the absences of petit mal epilepsy, the hesitation caused by anxiety, and the peculiar mental fixity associated with amphetamine intoxication.

During the period of blocking, intermediate associations may be lost, and the patient recommence on an apparently different track **(tangential thinking).** This can give rise to a phenomenon known as the **knight's move in thought:** The listener can sometimes intuit how the patient got from A to E and realizes that the unspoken intermediate associations (B, C, and D) were quite indirect. On other occasions, the patient's thinking appears subject to **derailing** (jumping the track to proceed on a different subject), particularly when a sore point has been touched on. Patients are often aware of disturbances in the continuity of their thinking and will describe how their thoughts become paralyzed, interrupted, or jumbled.

iv. Control— Akin to the subjective phenomena described in the previous section is the patient's sense that speed, direction, form, or content of thought are out of control. Complaints such as "confused," "racing thoughts," "unable to concentrate," "scatterbrained," "jumbled," and "going crazy" often reflect the subjective perception of pathologically accelerated, dysfluent, or discontinuous thinking.

Sometimes schizophrenic patients report that their thinking is controlled by external forces or people, for example, by means of radio waves or other transmissions. Thinking may be perceived as directed by the external agency, or particular thoughts experienced as having been implanted by it. This is known as **thought insertion** or **thought alienation.**

In **thought deprivation** or **thought broadcasting,** the patient senses that ideas are leaking out of the mind, being stolen by others, or being broadcast via radio or television. The perception that the television picks up and repeats one's thoughts may provoke a grandiose or persecutory delusional misinterpretation.

v. Logical organization— Psychotic thinking may reflect a deterioration in the capacity to think formally or logically. Commonly, the schizophrenic patient uses a private logic, with overpersonalized concrete symbols. Within this logical framework, conceptual boundaries are blurred, and the thinking patterns are metaphorical and idiosyncratic, almost as if they emerged directly from a dream-state. Thus, to the observer, when such thoughts are expressed, they appear on the surface to be diffuse, bizarre, and lacking in clarity. However, it is possible to interpret their meaning in the context of the patient's personal situation, and the issues that he or she is struggling with.

vi. Intent of communication— The conventional purpose of discourse is to communicate, but the clinician may be misled by the intentions of a schizophrenic patient. The schizophrenic patient may attempt to remain private or to deride the clinician, subtly, by conversing in an obscure, remote, supercilious, attacking, mocking, or farcical manner.

2. Abnormalities of thought content—Several disorders are virtually defined by the presence of abnormalities of thought content. In many instances the patient will complain of these phenomena (e.g., a phobia of heights); in other cases the patient appears to have accepted an eccentric idea (e.g., the delusion of being a reincarnation of Christ) and to be acting accordingly. Abnormal thought may be divided into the following categories: abnormal perceptions, abnormal convictions, abnormal preoccupations and impulses, and abnormalities in the sense of self.

i. Abnormal perceptions— Perception is physical sensation given meaning, the integration of sensory stimuli to form an image or impression, in a manner or configuration influenced by past experience. Perception may be increased or decreased in intensity. **Heightened perception** occurs in delirium, mania, after hallucinogens, and in the rare ecstatic states that occur as part of acute schizophrenia or "transported" hysterical trances. **Dulled perception** occurs in depression and organic delirium.

In **derealization,** the external world seems different, changed, vague, unreal, or distant. This symptom is common during adolescence, in association with **depersonalization,** the sense that one is distanced from the environment or a spectator of one's own actions. It is also associated with anxiety or dissociative disorders, depression, schizophrenia, organic brain disorder, and after hallucinogen use. In **synesthesia,** the subject perceives color in response to music, for example. It is a common psychedelic experience.

Time may be experienced as accelerated under the influence of hallucinogens, in mania, or during an epileptic aura. Time may seem slowed or stopped in depression or epilepsy. In some conditions, time seems to lack continuity and the subject feels uninvolved in the temporal stream. This is particularly likely to be encountered in depersonalization, amnestic syndromes, depression, schizophrenia, or toxic-confusional states.

An **illusion** is sensory stimulation given a false interpretation, that is, a false perception. Illusions are most likely to occur when the mind is under the sway of an emotionally determined ideational "set" (e.g., vigilance for an intruder), when sensory clarity is reduced (e.g., at night), or when both sets of circumstances are operating (as when a frightened elderly patient has both eyes bandaged following ophthalmic surgery). Illusions are common in delirium and may be visual (e.g., fluttering curtains seen as intruders), auditory (e.g., a slamming door interpreted as the report of a pistol), tactile (e.g., skin sensations thought to be caused by vermin), gustatory (e.g., poison detected in the taste of food), kinesthetic (e.g., flying), or visceral (e.g., abdominal pain thought to be caused by ground glass). Illusions may also occur in hysteria, depression, and schizophrenia, particularly when perception is subordinated to a delusional idea (e.g., of guilt or persecution) or an emotion of great force (e.g., abandonment or erotic yearning).

A **hallucination** is a false perception that occurs in the waking state in the absence of a sensory stimulus. It is not merely a sensory distortion or misinterpretation, and it carries a subjective sense of conviction. A true hallucination appears to the subject to be substantial and to occur in external objective space. In contrast, a normal mental image is insubstantial and experienced within internal subjective space. Deafness, tinnitus, or blindness, usually in association with dementia or delirium, may determine the modality of hallucinations.

Sensory deprivation experiments have produced visual and auditory hallucinosis in many subjects. Hallucinosis and delirium following cataract operation probably acts by the same mechanism, especially in association with dementia. Diencephalic and cortical disease may be associated with hallucinations (usually visual). Tumors of the olfactory or basal temporal regions may cause olfactory hallucinosis, for example, as an aura. Hallucinations, especially visual in modality (though sometimes vestibular and kinesthetic), are common in the delirium caused by toxins (e.g., drugs, hallucinogens, alcohol, toxins), fever, cerebro-vascular disease, and central degenerative disorders. Hallucinations may also be a prominent feature of the uncommon schizophrenia-like psychosis

associated with epilepsy. Aside from these medical circumstances, hallucinations are common and normal, especially in some people, when falling asleep (hypnagogic) or waking (hypnopompic). Severe sleep deprivation can cause hypnagogic hallucinosis.

Hallucinations can be auditory, visual, olfactory or gustatory, tactile, or somatic. In form, they may be amorphous, elementary, or complex. They may be experienced as emanating from inner or outer space and, if from outside, from near or far. Hallucinations may be unsystematized, appearing to have no link to life circumstances, or systematized and part of a causally interconnected delusional world.

Auditory hallucinations may be inchoate (e.g., humming, rushing water, inaudible murmurs), fragmentary (e.g., words or phrases such as "fag," "get him," or "beastly") or complex. Typically the schizophrenic patient locates complex hallucinations in inner or outer space, as a voice or voices speaking to or about him or her. The voice may be soothing, mocking, disparaging, or noncommittal. Sometimes the voice echoes the patient's thoughts or comments neutrally on his or her actions. Sometimes the voice orders the patient to perform actions, or puts thoughts into his or her head, a perception verging on thought insertion. The voice may be perceived as coming from the radio or television, from outside the window, or even from a distant place. In alcoholic hallucinosis, typically, a conspiracy of threatening whisperers plan to injure the patient, provoking the patient to self defense or flight.

Visual hallucinations vary from elemental flashes of light or color, as in disorders of the visual pathways and cortex, to well-formed scenes of people, animals, insects, and things. In delirium, insects or other small objects may be seen moving on the bed or in the surroundings. Lilliputian hallucinations, of little people on the bed, for example, occur in delirium and other organic brain syndromes. Complex audiovisual hallucinations may occur in temporal lobe epilepsy. In general, visual hallucinosis suggests acute brain disorder rather than functional psychosis and tends to occur in a setting of confusion or obtundation. Sometimes, however, a schizophrenic patient will report visual hallucinations (e.g., trips in flying saucers) aligned with his or her prevailing delusions. The visual hallucinations of hysteria or dissociative disorder have a pseudo-hallucinatory (i.e., "unreal", "as though") quality and sometimes represent the intrusive memory of a traumatic event, as when a war veteran reexperiences a battle incident.

Olfactory and gustatory hallucinations (e.g., burning rubber, steak and onions) may occur in epilepsy. Schizophrenic patients may perceive gas being pumped into their bedrooms by persecutors or may think they taste poisonous substances in their food. Melancholic patients may be conscious of the stench of corruption rising from their unworthy bodies or may complain of the changed, metallic, tasteless quality of their meals.

Tactile hallucinations are characteristic of cocaine and amphetamine intoxication, the patient being distracted by the sensation of insects crawling on the skin. Schizophrenic patients may detect the effect on the skin of radioactivity beamed at them from a hostile source.

Somatic hallucinations occur in schizophrenia, whereby genital, visceral, intracerebral, or kinesthetic sensations are often referred to the influence of persecutors or machines. The melancholic patient may have the sense of having no stomach, with food dropping from the throat into a void.

In schizophrenia, or under the influence of hallucinogens, the patient may have the uncanny sense that somebody, a presence, is behind him or her. This can occur in states of extreme fear, but it may become a central feature of schizophrenia, in the guise of the Doppelgänger or Horla, a hallucinatory double of the self who always lurks just behind the periphery of vision.

ii. Abnormal convictions— A **delusion** is a false belief not susceptible to argument and inconsistent with the subject's sociocultural background. Bordering on delusion is the **overvalued idea,** a notion eccentric rather than false but likely to become a governing force in the patient's life.

It is not always easy to draw the line between an eccentric individual, somebody who holds unfamiliar views that are nevertheless consistent with a different sociocultural system, and a deluded person. Indeed, some people drift across the misty boundaries between these categories. An active delusion, however, is rigid, unshakable, and self-evident. It dominates the subject's life, subordinating all other matters. It is private, idiosyncratic, egocentered, and inconsistent with the common experience of people from the same background. A delusion, therefore, isolates the subject from others and alienates them from him or her.

Severe sensory deprivation, or exhaustion and physical privation, may lead to delusional misinterpretation, often associated with wish-fulfilling hallucinations. A delusion can act as a transcendental escape from an existential wasteland. This is the ground from which cosmic, messianic, and redemptive delusions grow.

As for the content of delusions, the commonest are of persecution, jealousy, love, grandeur, disease, poverty, and guilt. **Delusions of persecution** are most frequently encountered in schizophreniform disorders or schizophrenia, paranoid disorders, organic mental disorder (especially alcoholic hallucinosis, amphetamine delirium or delusional disorder, other hallucinogenic syndromes, epilepsy, and all forms of delirium) and, less commonly, in melancholia or during transitory psychotic breaks in the life-course of patients with borderline personality. The patient may perceive others as talking conspiratorially about him or her (delusions of reference) or spying on him or her. External agencies (e.g., communists, FBI, freemasons) are regarded as acting in concert and disconcerting the subject with radiation, poisonous gases, radio and television, intruders, assassins, and so on. The patient often alludes to the use of tape recorders, cameras, and other surveillance paraphernalia. Delusions of poisoning, particularly by the spouse, are sometimes encountered.

Delusions of jealousy occur in the same syndromes as delusions of persecution but are especially likely in association with alcoholism in men. In that case, delusions of marital infidelity (possibly related to alcohol-related sexual impotence) are characteristic, the patient closely scrutinizing his partner and her belongings for evidence of adultery.

Delusions of grandeur occur in mania, schizophrenia, paranoid disorders, and organic delusional syndromes (e.g., neurosyphilis). In mania and organic grandiosity, the patient's megalomania (e.g., of being God, the governor, the Virgin Mary, Napoleon) are in line with his or her general high spirits. In schizophrenia and paranoid disorders, an inflated sense of importance may be reinforced by auditory hallucinations and the grandiosity of a delusional explanation for ideas of persecution: Why else would important agencies (e.g., the FBI, the Vatican, the PLO) be persecuting the patient?

Erotic delusions (erotomania) are more common in female schizophrenic or paranoid patients. A lonely person develops a crush on another, often a celebrity or prominent citizen. Fantasies evolve into delusions, and the subject bombards the other person with telephone calls and messages. The failure of the loved one to reciprocate is put down to conspiratorial forces that stand in the way of destiny. In schizophrenia, the patient may receive erotic hallucinations from the beloved.

Somatic delusions, usually of disease or ill health, occur in many psychiatric disorders. Schizophrenic patients may have bizarre complaints, possibly in an attempt to explain somatic hallucinatory experiences, for example, of blood running backward in the head, of radiation being trained on the genitals by an outside agency, or of objects placed inside the body by malevolent forces. In melancholia, the patient may have delusions of being dead (no blood in the body), of the internal organs rotting away, or of the brain being destroyed by syphilis, in retribution for an unpardonable sin. The boundary between hypochondriasis, disease phobia, and disease conviction on the one hand and somatic delusions on the other may be difficult to define.

Melancholic patients are prone to **delusions of poverty** and **delusions of nihilism.** The future is hopeless, the present desolate, the patient destitute and abandoned to a bleak fate. Depressive patients may also complain of inordinate guilt, the most extreme punishments being meted out to them for unremarkable, ancient transgressions.

iii. Abnormal preoccupations & impulses— A **phobia** is a morbid and irrationally exaggerated dread that focuses on a particular object, situation, or act (see Chapter 19). Phobias differ from generalized anxiety in their focused quality, although a diffuse anxiety state sometimes precedes a phobic disorder. The patient is aware of the exaggerated, irrational nature of a phobia and regards it as symptomatic. The patient often tries to avoid the phobic situation or is compelled to perform actions (such as hand washing) in order to eradicate the object of the fear, or atone for tabooed action.

An **obsession** is a persistent idea, desire, image, phrase, or fragment of music that cuts into the stream of conscious thinking. The patient recognizes the alien nature of the obsession and attempts to resist it, without success. The obsession often presses the subject to perform compulsive acts, to relieve anxiety. The key characteristics of obsessions are their persistent, irresistible, imperative nature; their ego-alien quality; and their repetitiousness. Obsessional symptoms have been reported after encephalitis. They occur in the premonitory phase of schizophrenia or as part of a major depression (e.g., the patient may experience persistent ruminations that old tax returns were in error and that ruin will result). Obsessive–compulsive symptoms are most characteristic of the anxiety disorder that bears the same name (see Chapter 21).

Impulsions differ from compulsions in that the former are less likely to be resisted, and they are episodic rather than repetitious, although the distinction may be blurred at times. Impulsions tend to occur in externalizing personalities, whereas compulsions are more typical of inhibited, constricted people. Impulsions cause difficulty for others and may lead to legal entanglements. Impulsive acts often spring from an emotional setting of anger, anxiety, frustration, rejection, sadness, or humiliation, particularly when the subject is disinhibited by alcohol. Common impulsions include violent assault, fast driving, excessive drinking or eating, gambling, sexual assault, sexual exhibitionism, shoplifting, stealing, and fire-setting. Sudden, episodic, if not explosive, onset is the hallmark of these phenomena. The subject does not or cannot exercise inhibition or self-control. Desire short circuits thought, leading to action without reflection.

iv. Abnormalities of the sense of self— The normal person has a sense of selfhood composed of the following elements: a sense of existing and being involved in one's own body and activity; a sense of personal continuity in time between past, present, and future; a sense of personal integrity; and a sense of distinction between self and outside world. In psychiatric disorders, any or several of these phenomena may be disturbed. For example, the individual may feel uninvolved in his or her own body or actions, like a spectator looking at another person (as in depersonalization); the individual's sense of temporal continuity may be dislocated, with the past and future seeming remote and the present but a series of disconnected scenes; the individual's ego may feel as though it is falling apart, shedding, fragmented, or split in two; or the difference between the self and other persons or objects may have become blurred.

The sense of depersonalization, often associated with derealization, occurs in adolescence, epilepsy, dissociative disorders, schizophrenia, and depression. Adolescents in severe emotional turmoil sometimes develop a sense of discontinuity, disintegration, and dedifferentiation. These symptoms are very common after ingestion of hallucinogens (and may be reexperienced as flashbacks) and in reactive psychosis, schizophreniform disorder, or schizophrenic disorders.

G. PHYSIOLOGIC FUNCTION

Sleep disturbances are often encountered in psychiatric practice. Sleep deprivation may precipitate or accentuate psychiatric disorder. Sleep disturbance may be a prodrome, a symptom, or a sequel of psychiatric disorder. Many psychopharmacologic agents also affect sleep. See Chapter 27 for more on sleep disorders.

Appetite may be increased in depression (especially dysthymic personality) and after psychotropic drug medication. Eating binges (not necessarily determined by increased appetite) may occur in bulimia nervosa as a condition separate from, in alternation with, or following, anorexia nervosa (see Chapter 26).

Anorexia and weight loss can occur in almost any stress condition but are particularly likely in major depression, paranoid schizophrenia, somatoform disorders, alcoholism or drug addiction, and, of course, anorexia nervosa. A comprehensive physical screening investigation is always required when anorexia and weight loss are present.

Sexual desire may be increased in mania, in some forms of acute schizophrenia, and in narcissistic or borderline personality under stress. Sexual behavior may be disinhibited after alcohol or drug ingestion, in delirium, or in organic dementia. Sexual desire is decreased by any debilitating disorder, by anxiety, worry, tiredness, age, poor nutrition, and lack of affection for the partner. It is usually reduced by depression, schizophrenia, alcoholism, substance abuse, and by neuroleptic, antihypertensive, and antidepressant medication.

Absent, irregular, infrequent, and scanty menstrual periods may occur in psychiatric disorder, particularly in depression, anorexia nervosa, anxiety disorders, schizophrenia, and substance abuse. Any condition that reduces total body fat to below 14%, in the female, produces anovulation and amenorrhea. Dysmenorrhea, dyspareunia, vaginismus, and other pelvic complaints are common in somatoform disorders, and in abnormal illness behavior generally, but a discretionary physical screen is required before a stress-related condition is diagnosed. See Chapter 25 for a more complete discussion of sexual dysfunctions.

Any or all body systems may be accelerated in the hyperdynamic states of anxiety, delirium, mania, and catatonic excitement or slowed in the general hypomotility of depression, organic dementia, and hypothyroidism. The patient's level of energy, or fatigue, may also be affected by disorders with accelerated or sluggish mental processes. Anergia, weakness, or obscure bodily discomfort are encountered frequently in somatoform disorders.

H. INSIGHT & JUDGMENT

1. Insight—The patient's attitude or insight into the illness has several aspects. For example, does the patient recognize that he or she has a problem? Does he or she identify the problem as personal and psychological in nature? Does he or she understand the nature and cause of the illness? Does he or she want help and, if so, what kind of help?

The hypomanic patient has no problem. He or she feels very well (e.g., high-spirited, amusing, energetic, expansive, and optimistic). The manic or schizophrenic patient may view the problem as external (i.e., other people or agencies are stupidly obstructive or malevolent). Many patients with externalizing personality disorders (e.g., borderline, antisocial, narcissistic) blame others for their predicament.

Sophisticated patients, particularly those who have undergone previous treatment, may have considerable knowledge of the formal diagnosis and the theoretical or actual causes of their disorder. Indeed, sometimes this causes problems in treatment: Other mental health professionals who develop psychiatric illness are notoriously difficult to manage for this reason.

The patient may be aware of having a problem but want no help, or he or she may want help of a particular sort or from a particular kind of clinician. Whenever this is reasonable and feasible, it should be arranged. The patient's desires should be respected as much as possible in the negotiation phase of the clinical process.

2. Judgment—The interviewer can ask the patient one of the following questions to test judgment: What would you do if you found a stamped, addressed envelope in the street? Why are there laws? Why should promises be kept? Good judgment requires intact orientation, concentration, and memory. There is no evidence that a finding of poor judgment adds anything to diagnosis beyond that provided by the detection of deficits in the lower-order functions, such as accomplishing household chores, maintaining personal hygiene, or selecting appropriate attire.

Termination

A psychiatric interview may last 15 minutes or go on for much longer. The usual time is about 50 minutes: Long enough for a rapid survey but not so long as to exhaust the patient. The interviewer can signal the approach of the conclusion by saying, for example, "Our time is almost finished, and there are a few things we need to discuss."

A concluding summary of the material points of the interview can be very helpful. It allows the patient to correct or modify misinterpretations and leads naturally into the interviewer's plan for what happens next—another interview, for example, or special investigations.

PRACTICAL MATTERS

Facilitating the Interview

If an interview is to achieve its purpose (i.e., to gather information), the interviewer must develop an atmosphere favoring the expression of ideas, feelings, and attitudes. The patient must develop a sense of trust and confidence in the interviewer, in order to be as spontaneous as possible. He or she will thereby see the interview as encouraging participation and collaboration toward a therapeutic end, through free expression and self-exploration.

What can the interviewer do to promote trust, spontaneity, and free expression? The interviewer must accept the patient, without moral judgment. If he or she cannot do so, it is better to be honest about it and refer the patient to another physician. Anybody can help somebody, but nobody can help everybody. If a patient angers, repels, or frightens the interviewer, and the feeling persists, the interviewer should seek help from a colleague.

The interview is facilitated if the interviewer understands the patient and conveys this understanding by facial expression, intonation, and well-timed reflections of the content and emotion behind the patient's story. The deepest affective understanding is empathy, that is, **feeling with**, or sharing the feelings of, the patient. It contrasts with sympathy, which is a **feeling for** the patient.

The open-ended style of questioning described earlier in this chapter as being most appropriate to reconnaissance and detailed inquiry helps to convey the spirit of collaboration, free expression, and self-exploration. An atmosphere of trust is fostered if the interviewer is relaxed and receptive, not preoccupied, rushed, abrupt, or irritable. Interviewers will likely adapt to their own purposes the techniques of others that have impressed them.

Interview Setting

A skilled interviewer can be effective walking along a corridor, playing catch, or sitting by the side of a bed. Nevertheless, offices are preferable to closets, and chairs are an improvement over packing boxes. If the interviewer has the opportunity, he or she should arrange the interview room to take advantage of its size, proportions, furnishings, and design.

The fundamental principles are simple. The room should be large enough to fit the patient, a desk, chairs, and other equipment, without crowding the interviewer. It is desirable, though not always possible, to have enough room and seating to accommodate the patient and four others, particularly if the interviewer plans to see families as well as individuals. The arrangement of the desk and chairs should allow entry and egress, but the interviewer should not sit between the patient and the door. He or she should try not to interview people from across a desk. Harsh lighting should be avoided. The patient should not be blinded by glare shining directly from a window or a lamp. The chairs should be comfortable, and the interviewer should not tower over the patient. The interviewer should not leave the patient stranded in the middle of the room; people feel less exposed with something solid behind them. The interviewer should not sit too close (i.e., knee to knee) or too far away. He or she should be near enough to make arm contact by leaning forward.

Interview Techniques

The interviewer should encourage free expression during the reconnaissance and detailed inquiry stages of the psychiatric interview. He or she does so by the setting provided, the atmosphere created, and the interview techniques used. The interviewer should be at ease with these techniques, and they should be used naturally, without flamboyance or stiltedness. If a particular technique does not suit the interviewer, he or she should not use it; an alternative should be found that conveys the same spirit and has a similar purpose.

The following are examples of useful techniques: Attentive listening, subtle vocal and nonvocal encouragement, support and reassurance, the reflection of feeling, gentle indication, and judicious paraphrasing.

Having invited the patient to tell his or her story, the interviewer waits and listens. He or she does not stare but meets the patient's gaze from time to time to indicate he or she is following. The interviewer's intent but relaxed posture indicates involvement. If the interviewer takes notes, they are brief and unobtrusive.

While the flow of associations proceeds, the interviewer need do little but maintain relaxed concentration, signaled by posture, eye contact, and subtle nonvocal or vocal encouragement. A nod or an "uh-huh" or "mm-mm" at strategic points may be all that is needed. Sometimes, when the flow seems to waver or slow, it is very effective to pick up and repeat a significant phrase or the last word the patient has said. But the interviewer should

not be mechanical and should not do something unless it feels natural.

The interviewer needs to be alert to the patient's reactions, particularly to changes in voice intonation and speech tempo, tensing of facial muscles, alterations of skin color, and moistening of conjunctivae, which herald a flush of anxiety or anger or a sudden feeling of sadness.

How does the interviewer handle silences? If the patient is thinking fruitfully, all the interviewer need do is wait. Similarly, if the patient has broken down in tears, it may be better to wait calmly until the patient can continue. If the silence occurs when the patient has lost track of or has confused feelings about the topic, the interviewer can facilitate associations with a subtle oral reflection, picking up a key word, phrase, or idea from the recent conversation and repeating it gently, sometimes with a questioning intonation. Oral reflection is also useful to help circumstantial patients get back on track.

The reflection of feeling is a variant of the technique of oral reflection. The interviewer picks up and echoes feelings explicit or implicit in what has been said but that have been expressed incompletely up to that point.

Transference & Countertransference

Transference refers to the unreasonable displacement of attitudes and feelings that originated in childhood to people in the here and now. This phenomenon is particularly likely to affect the doctor–patient relationship when patients are made vulnerable by fear, anxiety, guilt, despair, or hope.

Note the term "unreasonable" in the definition. The patient who is upset by overt rudeness is not displaying transference. However, if the patient is angered because the interviewer has a mustache or wears pearls, it is apparent that something is being added to an objectively neutral situation.

The patient may unconsciously regard the physician as a parent or a sibling, casting him or her in a caring or antagonistic role. Some examples of the commonest roles are of nurturing mother, demanding mother, protective father, punitive father, and rivalrous sibling. Sometimes older patients will relate to the physician as though they themselves were parents, reversing the roles.

How can the interviewer recognize transference? When the patient is exceptionally deferential, hanging onto the interviewer's opinions, singing his or her praises to others, or is easily slighted by a brief or delayed appointment, the interviewer may suspect a positive transference. When the patient is unexpectedly hostile, suspicious, or competitive, and there is no reasonable explanation for such antagonism, a negative transference is likely.

It is not difficult to imagine how a positive transference can become eroticized, the patient falling in love with an idealized parental figure. Most of these infatuations are transitory, like the crushes of adolescence. If the interviewer recognizes them and responds in a professional manner, they will go no further. Occasionally, however, unscheduled visits, notes, telephone calls, unasked for gifts or seductive dress indicate that the matter is more serious. The interviewer may need to consult a psychiatric colleague to decide how to proceed. The interviewer should not respond impulsively, out of fear or affront, lest a vulnerable patient be hurt.

Transference has its counterpart in a physician's **countertransference,** which occurs when a physician irrationally transfers to a patient his or her attitudes and feelings derived from childhood experiences. Psychiatric interviewers must be alert for countertransference. They should suspect it whenever they have powerful feelings of affection, protectiveness, fear, frustration, irritation, hatred, or erotic excitement toward a patient; when they very much look forward to the next appointment; or when they cannot tolerate a particular patient. If the interviewer recognizes these feelings, they will be much less likely to respond impulsively with rejection, flight, or self-indulgence. Once again, the interviewer should seek the help of a colleague or group of colleagues if he or she is unsure how to proceed in the patient's best interests.

There is no need to be embarrassed by transference or countertransference. Experienced clinicians know that these emotional displacements are ubiquitous and inescapable. They are most likely to be problematic when the interviewer is overworked, preoccupied, or rendered emotionally vulnerable by the vicissitudes of his or her personal life. The interviewer must look after himself or herself physically and emotionally and should do the best he or she can to have a fulfilling life outside of medicine itself.

STRUCTURED INTERVIEWS AND RATING SCALES

There is a role for standardized rating scales and structured interviews in developing a psychiatric history and evaluating changes in psychopathology while a patient is under treatment. However, these instruments are rarely appropriate to substitute for a traditional psychiatric interview in clinical practice. Screening questionnaires are used in primary care practice or in identifying psychopathology in large populations. Examples are depressive screening instruments in primary care and posttraumatic stress disorder screening instruments in military populations.

Diagnostic rating scales are used to identify specific psychiatric disorders in epidemiological studies and large scale clinical trials. Specific training is required to administer these scales to obtain appropriate validity and reliability. The Present State Examination was developed to standardize psychiatric diagnosis in international epidemiological studies, such as those conducted by the World Health Organization. The Composite International Diagnostic Interview was developed by the World Health Organization using items from the Present State Examination. The Diagnostic Interview Schedule is an epidemiological instrument designed to be used by nonclinicians in large scale epidemiological studies to develop diagnoses found in DSM-IV, Research Diagnostic Criteria, and Feighner criteria. The Schedule for Affective Disorders and Schizophrenia was developed by Endicott and Spitzer to differentiate between affective disorders and schizophrenia in a standardized manner for clinical research. The Structured Clinical Interview for Axis I DSM-IV Disorders was developed to arrive at Axis I diagnoses according to DSM-IV. It is widely used in clinical trials and epidemiological studies.

Symptom-based scales are designed to measure change in a particular symptom or a syndrome-based group of symptoms, rather than establish a diagnosis in the framework of a particular diagnostic system. These scales can be useful in clinical practice to document, objectively and quantitatively, the change in response to a therapeutic intervention or simply change over time. They can be self-rating scales completed by the patient or rater-administered scales completed by the clinician. Obviously, the disadvantage of self-rated scales is the reliability of the measurement.

The Brief Psychiatric Rating Scale measures major psychotic and nonpsychotic symptoms in patients with a major psychiatric disorder. It is a widely used rater-administered scale for evaluating baseline psychopathology and treatment response, particularly in inpatient populations. The Hamilton Rating Scale for Depression is one of the most widely used rater-administered scales for assessing symptoms of depression and measuring their change over time. It is frequently used in clinical trials. The Beck Depression Inventory and the Zung Depression Scale are both self-rating scales that are frequently used to evaluate severity of depression in patients engaged in treatment. The Zung scale is also used as a screening instrument for depression. The Hamilton Rating Scale for Anxiety is a frequently used rater-administered scale for evaluating the severity of anxiety symptoms. There are a variety of symptom-based scales designed to be used in child psychiatric disorders, substance-abuse disorders, and geriatric psychiatric syndromes. The reader is directed to the bibliography for further details in these areas.

CONCLUSION

The purpose of the psychiatric interview is to obtain information from the patient about the presenting problem and its precipitation and about previous disorders, predisposition, biopsychosocial strengths and limitations, reason for the current presentation, insight, and desire for help. The psychiatric history covers topics that range from identifying data to coping mechanisms. The four stages of the interview—inception, reconnaissance, detailed inquiry, and termination—are adapted to different topics.

In the inception stage, the interviewer makes introductions, gets the patient or family seated, takes identifying information, and summarizes what he knows. The quality of the interview is enhanced if the interviewer creates an atmosphere of trust, spontaneity, and expressiveness by his or her acceptance, empathic understanding, open-ended style, and natural manner. The decor, lighting, furnishings, and arrangement of the room can also promote (or subvert) the desired atmosphere.

During the reconnaissance stage, the interviewer helps the patient describe the presenting problem and its precipitation and development.

During the detailed inquiry, routine and discretionary, the interviewer explores past illness; early development and environment; later educational, occupational, social, and marital history; interests, values, and aspirations; habitual coping style; family history; and mental status.

During the interview, the clinician fosters free expression and association by being attentive and by using certain techniques such as vocal and nonvocal encouragement, support and reassurance, reflection of ideas or feelings, indication of inconsistencies, and paraphrasing.

The clinician will seldom, if ever, need to turn over every stone and pebble in this chapter. What is required is a set of criteria to decide whether comprehensive or brief discretionary screening MSE is indicated.

At termination, the interviewer summarizes the interview and negotiates with the patient over what the next step should be.

Carlat DJ: *The Psychiatric Interview.* Philadelphia: Lippincott Williams & Wilkins, 1999.

Colby KM: *A Primer for Psychotherapists.* New York: Ronald Press, 1951.

Guze BH, Love MJ: Medical assessment and laboratory testing in psychiatry. In: Sadock BJ, Sadock VA (eds). *Comprehensive Textbook of Psychiatry,* 8th edn. Philadelphia: Lippincott Williams & Wilkins, 2005, pp. 916–928.

Maj M, Gaebel W, López-Ibor JJ, Sartorius N: *Psychiatric Diagnosis and Classification.* New York: Wiley, 2002.

Othmer E, Othmer SC, Othmer JP: Psychiatric interview, history and mental status examination. In: Sadock BJ, Sadock VA (eds). *Comprehensive Textbook of Psychiatry,* 8th edn. Philadelphia: Lippincott Williams & Wilkins, 2005, pp. 794–826.

Sadock BJ: Signs and symptoms in psychiatry. In: Sadock BJ, Sadock VA (eds). *Comprehensive Textbook of Psychiatry,* 8th edn. Philadelphia: Lippincott Williams & Wilkins, 2005, pp. 847–859.

Sajatovic M, Ramirez LF: *Rating Scales in Mental Health.* Hudoon OH: Lexi-Comp Inc., 2001.

Scheiber SC: The psychiatric interview, psychiatric history, and mental status examination. In: Hales RA, Yudofsky SC, Talbott JA (eds). *The American Psychiatric Press Textbook of Psychiatry,* 2nd edn. Washington DC: American Psychiatric Press, 1994, pp. 187–220.

Diagnostic Encounter for Children and Adolescents

5

Barry Nurcombe, MD

I. INTERVIEWING PARENTS

INITIAL CONTACT

Children are usually referred to psychiatrists by their parents or caregivers. Parents should be made aware that a collaborative approach to diagnosis and treatment is essential and that their children older than 3 years of age should be prepared for the diagnostic encounter. The initial contact is usually made over the telephone by the parent or referring agent. The importance of the impression made at that first contact cannot be underestimated. The initial intake staff member gathers identifying information and a brief history of the presenting complaint. Emergency situations must be dealt with at once and urgent situations within 24 hours. Table 5–1 lists situations, roughly in the order of frequency, that require immediate evaluation.

SEQUENCE OF INTERVIEWS

If the initial interview is prompted by a crisis, or if the family has come a long distance, the clinician should see the whole family together. Even if there is no crisis, some clinicians still favor interviewing the whole family first whereas others prefer interviewing the parents first, before interviewing the child or adolescent at a separate later interview. Even if the parents are separated or divorced, it is preferable to interview both parents, unless the tension between them would be unmanageable. Other clinicians prefer to interview an adolescent first, before interviewing the parents. In any case, the clinician should try to avoid having the child wait anxiously in the waiting room while lengthy parent interviews are conducted. At some point, the parents will need to be interviewed to obtain a detailed history (see "Interviewing Parents" section) and

the family interviewed together to throw light on family dynamics (see "Interviewing Families" section).

INTAKE QUESTIONNAIRES & CHECKLISTS

Important data can be collected even before the first interview. For example, the parent can complete a Child Behavior Checklist and a developmental history form. Teacher versions of the Child Behavior Checklist can also be obtained if the child's behavior in school is an important issue. Previous mental health evaluations, psychological reports, medical records, and school records are also available in some cases. Thus, the clinician can focus during the parent interview on the developmental issues and symptom patterns that emerge from the preliminary data.

PURPOSE OF THE PARENT INTERVIEW

The initial parent interview serves several purposes. Most important, it helps the clinician form an alliance with the parents, and it helps the parents prepare the child for the next interview. The clinician can use the parent interview to obtain a formal history of the child's presenting problem, medical history, early development, school progress, and peer relations as well as information on the child's recreational activities and interests, home and family environment, and family history. The clinician can also gather from this interview information about parent–child relations and communication, the parents' child-rearing techniques and methods of discipline used, and the family's values and aspirations. The clinician can gather information on the parents' current marital relationship and its development and can ascertain how the parents understand the child's problem and the kind of help they are seeking.

Table 5–1. Situations Requiring Immediate Evaluation

Suicidality
Homicidal impulses
Dangerous assaultiveness
Dangerous risk-taking (e.g., running away from home)
Drug or alcohol intoxication
Psychotic thought disorder (e.g., hallucinations, delusions)
Impending parental breakdown related to the child's disruptive behavior
Recent trauma (e.g., as a result of rape or civilian catastrophe)
Recent loss with abnormal grief reaction
Acute school refusal
Suspension or expulsion from school
Police involvement
Physical deterioration in a patient known to have an eating disorder

---

SEQUENCE OF THE PARENT INTERVIEW

The parent interview proceeds through four key stages: (1) inception, (2) reconnaissance, (3) detailed inquiry, and (4) termination.

Inception

The interviewer begins by greeting the parents in the waiting room and ushering them into the office, indicating where they should sit. The interviewer then tells the parents what he or she already knows and invites them to tell their story.

Reconnaissance

The interviewer should let the parents proceed at their own pace without interruption other than to facilitate the flow of associations or clarify issues. As the story unfolds, the interaction between them is observed. Do they support each other? Does one parent do most of the talking? Do they interrupt or contradict each other? Which issues evoke the most emotion from them? Do they express warmth, humor, coolness, detachment, remoteness, tension, irritation, or hostility? If one parent becomes upset, how does the other respond?

Detailed Inquiry

After the parents have finished their story, the areas listed in the next several sections are explored. These areas should be surveyed in a standard diagnostic inquiry, and particular areas should be explored in depth according to

the diagnostic hypotheses triggered by the clinical pattern that is emerging.

A. THE PROBLEM

When did the problem first appear? Did its onset coincide with a physical or psychosocial stressor? How has the problem evolved? Is the problem persistent or intermittent? If intermittent, do exacerbations coincide with vicissitudes in physical health or the environment (e.g., family, school, peer relations)? What have the parents done about it? Are there any other problems in the child's behavior at home, at school, with siblings, or with peers?

B. REFERRAL

Who referred the parents? Why do they come now? How do they feel about it? Have they sought help before? If so, from whom, and how effective was the help? What kind of help do they expect now?

C. MEDICAL HISTORY

Has the child had any significant physical illness, physical disability, surgery, accidents, or hospitalizations? If so, at what age, what was the duration, and did any adverse psychological reactions occur? Has the child sustained any head injuries or had seizures, syncope, headaches, eye symptoms, abdominal or limb pains, nausea or vomiting, or prolonged or frequent absences from school? Has the child had previous psychological disturbances? If so, what were the cause, treatment, and outcome? Is the child currently taking any medication? Does he or she have significant allergies?

D. DEVELOPMENTAL HISTORY

1. Pregnancy—What were the circumstances surrounding conception of the child (e.g., motivation, acceptance, convenience, emotional turmoil, reaction of in-laws)? What was the nature of the marital relationship during pregnancy? Did the parents have a sex preference? How was the mother's physical and emotional health during pregnancy? Did she have toxemia, eclampsia, kidney disorder, hypertension, or febrile illness? Were any X-rays taken during pregnancy? Did she take prescribed or over-the-counter medications, tobacco, alcohol, or illicit drugs during pregnancy, and if so, how much and how often? Did she experience excessive nausea, vomiting, or vaginal bleeding during pregnancy? How was she prepared for labor?

2. Delivery—Did the mother have a normal confinement? Was the child born at term? How long did labor last? What was the nature of the delivery? Did any complications occur? How soon did the mother see the infant after delivery? What were the mother's initial thoughts on seeing the infant?

3. Neonatal status—What was the infant's birth weight, maturity, and physical condition? Was the infant in intensive care? If so, for how long? What was the method of feeding? How well did the infant gain weight as a neonate? Did the infant have problems with asphyxia, cyanosis, jaundice, convulsions, vomiting, rigidity, or respiratory disorder?

4. Feeding—Was the child breastfed? If so, for how long? Was formula used? When were solids introduced? How well did the child gain weight? Did the child have problems with vomiting, diarrhea, constipation, colic, food allergies, or eczema? Did later conflicts over eating occur (e.g., refusal to eat, bulimia, hoarding)? What are the child's current eating habits?

5. Motor development—At what age (in months) did the child first hold his or her head erect, sit alone, stand, and walk alone? How is the child's coordination (gross and fine)? Is the child right- or left-handed? Does the child have repetitive movements or mannerisms?

6. Speech development—When did the child first use single words, two- and three-word phrases, and sentences? Did the child have trouble with faulty articulation or stammering? How mature is the child's current language, vocabulary, and syntax? Is the child able to carry a conversation?

7. Sphincter control—When did the child first learn to control his or her bladder and bowels? What method of training was used? How did the child respond to training (e.g., with resistance or acceptance)? Did the child regress during training? Has the child had problems with enuresis or encopresis?

8. Sleep—Has the child had sleep problems in the past? What are the child's current sleep habits (e.g., is the child a deep sleeper, restless, or insomniac)? Does the child have fears of the dark or of being alone? Does the child sleepwalk, rock head or body, have nightmares or night terrors, or resist going to bed?

9. Sexual development—Did the child display early sexual curiosity or sex play? Has the child received sex education? Has the child begun to menstruate, or have nocturnal emissions? Does the child masturbate? What is the child's gender-role identification? Is he or she interested in the opposite sex? Has the child experienced any sexual trauma?

E. Educational Progress

1. Academics & activities—What schools has the child attended? What grade is the child in now? Who are the child's teachers? How is the child's current academic performance? Does the child have any learning problems or any need for special education or tutoring? Does the child participate in school sports and activities?

2. Behavior—How are the child's relationships with peers and teachers? How does the child respond to school

rules? What is the child's capacity to concentrate? Does the child have problems with truancy, fear of going to school, or school refusal? Has the child bullied others or been the victim of bullying? What is the child's attitude toward homework? Does the child exhibit any antisocial behavior at school? Does the child have any history of drug or alcohol use or abuse?

3. Ambitions & involvement—What are the child's ambitions? Is the child involved in social and recreational activities?

F. Home Environment

1. Physical arrangement—Where is the home located? What is the neighborhood like? What are the neighbors like? How is the home laid out? What are the sleeping arrangements? Does the home have inside and outside spaces for play? Are the parents satisfied with the domestic arrangements?

2. Schedule—What is the child's typical weekday and weekend schedule, from rising to retiring?

G. Parent–Child Relationships

1. Child's behavior—How was the child's early temperament (i.e., easy or difficult)? Has this changed with age? What is the child's general mood? What is the child's capacity for affection, tolerance for frustration, and proneness to tantrums? Is the child aggressive, resentful, fearful, or timid; depressed; sociable; and accepting of limits, rules, and discipline? How does the child respond to punishment (i.e., by being stubborn or compliant)?

2. Parenting methods—What methods do the parents use to set limits and discipline the child? Are these methods applied with consistency? How much time does the family spend together (i.e., father–child, mother–child, entire family)?

3. Attitudes & conflicts—What are the child's attitudes toward each parent (e.g., closeness, mutual understanding)? Do conflicts about dependence and independence exist between the child and parents?

H. Social Relationships

1. Siblings & peers—How are the child's relationships with siblings and peers? Does the child tend to be a leader, a follower, or a protector? Is the child overly dependent?

2. Games—Is the child able to win or lose at games? What are the child's favorite games?

3. Social behavior—Does the child exhibit any antisocial behavior? How are the child's relationships with authority figures?

I. FAMILY BACKGROUND

1. Parents—What is each parent's age, occupation, and physical and mental health? What is each parent's drug and alcohol intake? What are the age, health, and occupations of both sets of grandparents? What are each parent's family, educational, and occupational backgrounds? Pay particular attention to the emotional climate of each parent's family of origin, the relationship between the parents and their parents, the parents' schooling, and their occupational histories. What is the family history of psychiatric disorders, mental retardation, learning problems, substance abuse, antisocial behavior, or physical illness?

2. Marital history—Were the parents married previously? How did they meet, and what was their courtship like? Were they both accepted by their respective in-laws? What were the early years of marriage like (e.g., sexual adjustment, division of labor, management of money, method of settling interparental disputes)? Is there a history of competition, unfulfilled needs, hostility, abuse, or separations? How effective is each parent's parenting ability? What is their capacity for affection? What is their motivation for childcare and childrearing?

3. Siblings—How old is each of the child's siblings? What is the current health of each sibling? How does each sibling do in school or in his or her occupation? What is each sibling's overall personality? How does each sibling relate to the child?

4. Family values—What is the family's ethnic or sociocultural background? Is there a relative emphasis on conformity or independence, authority or freedom, warmth or coolness, control or expression? What are the family's religious, moral and esthetic values? Does the family put an emphasis on education, piety, money, success, prestige, or gender differentiation?

5. Family & community—How involved is the family in school activities, religious organizations, cultural bodies, and civic affairs?

Termination

At the end of the parent interview (usually one or two 2-hour interviews), the information gathered is summarized. The parents should be invited to add anything they think is important and to correct any misinformation. The interviewer should then tell them when he or she wants to see the child and the family again.

Lewis M, King RA: Psychiatric assessment of infants, children and adolescents. In: Lewis M (ed). *Child and Adolescent Psychiatry.* Philadelphia: Lippincott Williams & Wilkins, 2002, pp. 525–543.

Nurcombe B: The diagnostic encounter in child psychiatry: Data gathering. In: Nurcombe B, Gallagher RM (ed). *The Clinical Process in Psychiatry.* New York: Cambridge University Press, 1986, pp. 460–506.

Simmons JE: *Psychiatric Examination of Children,* 2nd edn. Philadelphia: Lea & Febiger, 1974.

II. EVALUATING INFANTS

PURPOSE OF THE INFANT EVALUATION

The psychiatric evaluation of infants and their parents is designed to yield information concerning the following: the nature and development of the problem perceived by the parents; the child's developmental history; the parent's history (e.g., early relationships, prior experience with children, knowledge of child development, marital relationship, and medical and psychiatric history); parent–child interaction; infant development and attachment; and the parents' perception of the infant.

Information on these matters is gathered by interviewing the parent, observing the infant, observing the interaction between parent and infant, and if necessary, conducting standardized assessments.

INTERVIEWING THE INFANT'S PARENTS

Infants and their parents are usually referred by a pediatrician because of disturbances in regulation (e.g., insomnia, excessive crying, feeding problems, head banging), social disturbances (e.g., interactional apathy or negativism, traumatic separation, excessive separation anxiety), psychophysiologic disturbances (e.g., failure to thrive, vomiting), or developmental delay.

It is debatable whether, at the first interview, the parents should be interviewed alone or together with the infant. The infant's presence is likely to generate historical information from the parents that might otherwise be missed. However, a number of interviews will be required, observation of parent–child interactions will always be necessary, and the aim of the interview will not be achieved unless a working alliance is formed.

The interview begins with introductory questions about family structure and dates of birth and quickly proceeds to a history of the problem. The following questions could be asked: When did the problem begin? How has it evolved? What is the problem now? What have the parents done about it? How do they account for it? Why do they come for help now? What do they want from the clinician?

Next, the clinician elicits the infant's developmental history, including the circumstances surrounding, and the reaction of both parents to, conception, pregnancy, delivery, and early infant care. The child's medical history will also be gathered.

As the alliance deepens, the clinician elicits information about the parents' relationships with their own parents and siblings, their prior experience of childcare, their knowledge of child development, their preconceptions about being a parent, and their expectations about the baby (and whether these expectations have been borne out). The history and current status of the marital relationship will also be explored. If other individuals provide a significant amount of the infant's care, they should also be interviewed.

The clinician seeks to identify critical dynamic sequences of behavioral interaction (e.g., the mother becomes anxious, disorganized, and angry if the baby refuses to eat), looking for connections between present emotional interactions and past significant relationships and events.

◼ OBSERVING THE PARENT–INFANT INTERACTION

During the interview, parents should be encouraged to attend to the infant's needs, for example, consoling, changing, or feeding the infant, if necessary. Parents will also be asked to play with the child. Parent–child dyads can then be observed with regard to the quality of attachment, the vigilance of the parents concerning the infant's safety, the parents' attunement to and effectiveness in responding to the infant's need states, the quality of parent–child play, parental teaching ability, parental control, the affective tone of the interaction, and infant temperament. The clinician should remember that he or she is observing only brief samples of dyadic behavior. By seeking a working alliance and putting the parents at ease, the clinician can try to ensure that the samples of behavior observed are representative.

The next several sections describe specific observations about the parent–child interaction that the clinician can make during the infant evaluation.

1. Attachment—How close is each dyad? Are they, for example, detached or clinging, or able to separate sufficiently to allow the infant to explore? Does the infant seek body or eye contact with the parent? Does contact with the parent reassure the child, or is the infant inconsolable? Does the infant explore the surroundings recklessly, confidently, cautiously, or not at all? Does the infant get pleasure from the exploration? How does he or she respond to separation? How does the parent feel about it?

2. Protection—Is the parent vigilant, overprotective, or careless in regard to the infant's reckless, cautious, or confident exploration? Or does the parent strike a good balance, given the infant's apparent temperament? How does the parent feel about the infant's exploration?

3. Regulation of Need States—Is the parent attuned to the infant's needs concerning hunger, discomfort, pain, or stimulation? Does the parent know when to stimulate the infant, when to back off, and when and how to console the infant? Does the parent make effective use of eye contact, soothing voice, smiling, facial movement, wrapping, touching, holding, rocking, nursing, and dorsal patting or rubbing in stimulating or consoling the infant? How does the infant respond to the parent's ministrations?

4. Play—Do parent and infant play together in a manner appropriate to the infant's developmental level? Do parent and infant enjoy the playful interaction?

5. Teaching—If the infant is old enough, ask the parent to teach him or her to stack blocks or solve a puzzle. Does the parent make effective use of modeling and language? Does the infant imitate the parent? Does the parent allow the infant sufficient opportunity for trial and error to solve a problem independently?

6. Control—Does each parent maintain calm, confident control of the infant, or is the parent helpless, passive, inconsistent, disorganized, explosive, punitive, or overly controlling? How effectively does the parent communicate in words? How does the infant respond? In response to the parent's attempts to control his or her behavior, is the infant heedless, provocative, negativistic, passive, disorganized, or biddable?

7. Emotion—What is the affective tone of the interaction? Is the infant generally happy, angry, sad, neutral, affectively "empty," or unresponsive? What is each parent's emotional state? Are the members of the dyads attuned to each other? If the infant becomes upset, is he or she able to regain equanimity in a reasonable time?

8. Temperament—Temperament refers to relatively enduring characteristics of the infant's behavioral response to the internal and external environments. Despite limitations in the duration and representativeness of the behavioral sample elicited, the clinician may be able to make observations concerning the infant's activity level, tendency to approach or withdraw from people, adaptability to new situations, affective intensity, mood, persistence with tasks or play, sensory threshold, and distractibility.

■ STANDARDIZED TESTING

Through standardized testing, the clinician can explore hypotheses generated from the history and observation of parent–infant interaction. Tests are available, for example, with regard to infant psychomotor development, parent–infant interaction, infant attachment, quality of the home environment, infant temperament, and the parent's working model of the infant. Although some of these tests are best regarded as research instruments, several may have clinical utility. Furthermore, parents can be involved in the data-gathering process of many of these tests, with potentially great educational benefit.

A. DEVELOPMENTAL LEVEL

Tests of infant development have only modest predictive validity with regard to tested intelligence in later childhood. There is increasing evidence that intellectual development is characterized by individual differences and discontinuity rather than a smooth progression. Early infant development tests must be applied too soon to tap those elements of intelligence (e.g., language-based cognitive skills) that are highly responsive to the home environment. Nevertheless, if the infant tests very low in some or all developmental domains, the clinician should be concerned.

1. Brazelton Neonatal Behavioral Assessment Scale—The Brazelton Neonatal Behavioral Assessment Scale (NBAS) was designed for use with the full-term neonate, but it has also been modified to apply to high-risk infants. The NBAS is usually administered 3 and 9 days after birth. It surveys reflexes and behavioral responses in such a way as to yield a profile of social interactiveness, state control, motoric behavior, and physiologic response to stress. It has modest predictive power with regard to later developmental measures.

2. Bayley Scales of Infant Development (2–30 months)—The Bayley Scales assess development in three domains: mental (perception, memory, problem solving, communication), psychomotor (gross and fine motor), and behavior (the affective responses of the infant). This test uses a structured play approach.

3. Infant Muller Scales of Early Learning (0–38 months)—The Infant Muller Scales of Early Learning assess gross motor development, visual reception, visual

expression, language reception, and language expression. The scales are useful in following the progress of children who are thought to have specific areas of developmental delay.

4. Other instruments—The Transdisciplinary Play-Based Assessment and the Connecticut Infant–Toddler Developmental Assessment Program involve the parents with the clinical team in the collection of data on different domains of development.

B. PARENT–CHILD INTERACTION

The Greenspan–Lieberman Observation System for Assessment of Caregiver Interaction During Semistructured Play and the Parent–Child Early Relationship Assessment rate interactive behavior from videotaped samples of free or semistructured play. Parental detachment, emotional negativity, lack of vocal contact, lack of visual contact, and inconsistency, for example, can be detected, along with infant detachment, negative affect, inattention, and defects in motor and communication skills.

C. INFANT ATTACHMENT

The best-known measure of infant attachment is the Strange Situation (12–24 months). In this technique, the infant–parent dyad is exposed to a series of brief episodes involving gradually increasing stress, as the parent stays with the child, leaves, returns, and leaves; a stranger joins the child; and the parent finally returns. The child's behavior during the two reunion episodes is classified as secure, insecure–avoidant, insecure–resistant, or disorganized. Disorganized behavior is particularly likely to be associated with serious environmental pathology and poor outcome.

D. HOME ENVIRONMENT

The Home Observation for Measurement of the Environment (two versions: 0–3 years, 3–6 years) assesses the quality of intellectual stimulation in the home by rating the parent's involvement with and responsiveness to the child, the organization of the home environment, and the provision of a variety of play materials.

E. INFANT TEMPERAMENT

The Revised Infant Temperament Questionnaire asks the parent to rate the infant in nine domains of temperament and allows the infant to be categorized as easy, slow to warm up, difficult, intermediate low, or intermediate high. This instrument is a measure of parental perception of the infant and is influenced by the parent's personality.

F. THE PARENT'S WORKING MODEL OF THE CHILD

The Working Model of the Child Interview is a research instrument with potential clinical applicability. It is a structured interview that explores topics such as the child's development, the parent's perception of the child's

Table 5–2. The NCCIP Classification of Infant Disorders

Disorder of social development and communication
   Autism
   Atypical pervasive developmental disorder
Psychic trauma disorder
   Acute, single event
   Chronic, repeated
Regulatory disorder
   Hypersensitivity type
   Under-reactive type
   Active-aggressive type
   Mixed type
   Regulatory-based sleep disorder
   Regulatory-based eating disorder
Disorders of affect
   Anxiety disorder
   Mood disorder
      Prolonged bereavement
      Depression
      Labile mood disorder
      Mixed disorder of emotional expressiveness
      Deprivation syndrome
Adjustment reaction disorders

personality and behavior, and the parent–child relationship. The parent's responses are rated on a number of scales (e.g., coherence, richness, flexibility, intensity), and the parental model of the child is classified as balanced, disengaged, or distorted.

DIAGNOSTIC FORMULATION & TREATMENT PLANNING

The diagnostic hypotheses generated during the parent interview are tested and refined during the observation of parent–infant interaction, and when required, through the use of standardized tests. If no pediatric examination has been completed, or if specialized pediatric consultation is required, this will be requested. The current problem is classified, for example, according to the NCCIP scheme (Table 5–2). Next a diagnostic formulation is completed and a treatment plan designed (see Chapter 36), and the diagnosis and plan are discussed with the parents as the clinician seeks to consolidate the working alliance preparatory to the treatment phase.

Clark R, Paulsen A, Conlin S: Assessment of developmental status and parent–infant relationships. In: Zeanah CH (ed). *Handbook of Infant Mental Health.* New York: Guilford Press, 1993, pp. 191–209.

Gillam WS, Mayes LC: Clinical assessment of infants and toddlers. In: Lewis M (ed). *Child and Adolescent Psychiatry.* Philadelphia: Lippincott Williams & Wilkins, 2002, pp. 507–524.

Hirshberg LM: Clinical interviews with infants and their families. In: Zeanah CH (ed). *Handbook of Infant Mental Health.* New York: Guilford Press, 1993, pp. 173–190.

Lamb ME et al.: Infancy. In: Lewis M (ed): *Child and Adolescent Psychiatry.* Philadelphia: Williams & Wilkins, 1996, pp. 241–270.

National Center for Clinical Infant Programs: *Diagnostic Classification of Mental Health and Developmental Disorders.* Washington DC: Zero to Three. NCCIP, 1994.

III. INTERVIEWING CHILDREN

PURPOSE OF THE CHILD INTERVIEW

Depending on the child and the clinical circumstances, an interview with a child of 4–11 years of age has a number of purposes. The interview can help the clinician ascertain how the child feels about being interviewed and what the child believes to be the purpose of the interview. It can also help to correct misapprehension and orient the child to the interview. The interview can be used to determine whether the child recognizes that a problem exists and, if so, what accounts for it. In terms of aiding the diagnosis, the interview can be used to complete a mental status examination; to explore the child's self-concept and perceptions of the key figures in his or her world (e.g., family, friends, authorities); to assess the child's intellectual, language, emotional, social, and moral development; and to gauge the effectiveness of the child's coping mechanisms. Finally, the interview can be used to establish a working alliance and to assess the child's capacity to benefit from treatment.

FACTORS AFFECTING THE CHILD INTERVIEW

Although the primary purpose of the interview is diagnostic, it is artificial to separate diagnosis from treatment. Adverse impressions formed early can impede or obstruct therapy; in contrast, if an alliance is formed early, the child will be more willing to return for treatment.

The type of interview that evolves depends on the child's developmental level, personality, and expectations; the environment in which the interview takes place; the interviewer's personality and interactive style; and the goals of the interview. For example, a preschool child is likely to express ideas and feelings through actions rather than words. In contrast, a mature 11-year-old child may be able to converse throughout the interview. Most children mix play with conversation. The clinician must, therefore, combine observation, play, and conversation in different degrees with children of different maturity levels.

The well-adjusted child is likely to be reticent about sharing very personal matters with a stranger, unless he or she accepts the need to do so. The psychologically disturbed child may be even more inhibited; initially, such children may express fantasies, secrets, or private fears indirectly. In contrast, some disorganized, emotionally needy younger children have such poor defenses that they release a torrent of psychopathologic material before they have established a trusting relationship with the examiner.

The child's expectation of the interview greatly influences its course. Children seldom come to a psychiatrist of their own accord, and the individuals who bring them may not have prepared them well. Children may enter the interview hostile, fearful, bewildered, apathetic, or even eager for help. Younger children commonly fear bodily invasion (e.g., injections) or are concerned that the physician will expose secret inferiorities or shameful memories. Some children are afraid that they will be induced to talk about matters so frightening that they have never talked about them before. Adolescents universally have a fear of being rendered helpless. Children with a history of antisocial behavior may expect a tricky cross-examination. Children with learning problems may be afraid of being exposed as dunces. The experienced interviewer can often anticipate these fears and deal with them early in the interview.

Office Environment

Although an experienced clinician can be surprisingly effective in unpromising surroundings, adequate space and equipment are helpful. Some clinicians have access to separate playrooms with extensive equipment and fittings, but many arrange their own offices to interview children.

An ideal room will be large enough to have a carpeted section for seated interviewing, a section with linoleum-tiled floor suitable for play, and a small table and chairs. Play equipment should be stored in a lockable cupboard that has additional space for materials associated with particular patients who are in therapy. Otherwise, the equipment is communal. An inquisitive child can be told that the play material belongs to the office and may not be taken away.

With regard to play equipment, it is preferable to err on the side of frugality. Clinicians should remember that equipment is a means to the development of a relationship and the expression of thoughts and feelings. The less clutter, the more the child must draw from inside. A list of basic equipment would include the following: easel, newsprint paper and felt pens, blocks, assorted toy wild and domestic animals, matchbox cars, dolls (representing parents, brother, sister, baby, grandparents, together with nurse and doctor), one or two stuffed animals, a rubber ball, a pack of playing cards, and a set of checkers. Clinicians can add to this list other items (e.g., puppets, toy pistols, board games, dolls' house furniture, plastic construction models), guided by their interest and what seems to work best for them. Clinicians should avoid games that preclude fantasy, such as chess or Scrabble. Finger paints, poster colors, and Play-Doh are suitable only for fully equipped playrooms, but clinicians may wish to keep a soccer ball, a football, and a baseball and gloves for outdoor play.

Clinicians should not be anchored to the office. An occasional visit to a soda fountain, outdoor construction site, nursery, or gymnasium can be very useful, especially with highly active youngsters who find a restricted office environment tedious.

Style of the Interview

The goals of the interview shape its style. Sometimes it is essential to obtain from the child a detailed account of a past event, especially in medicolegal situations. Such situations are much less common than those in which clinicians can allow the interview to evolve as the interaction dictates.

Two polar interviewing styles are exemplified by the relatively **unstructured approach** and the highly **structured interview.** Structured interviewing may be valuable for research purposes, but it is not recommended for regular clinical interviewing.

A **semistructured interview** involves the application of a flexibly and sensitively applied systematic approach. The interview should be organized in accordance with a hypothetico-deductive strategy, but it should not compromise a positive relationship for the sake of extracting information. In most cases, two or three 1-hour interviews are required in order to gather enough information to reach a reliable diagnosis.

Clinicians who wish to work with children should enjoy being with children. They should be sufficiently in touch with the past to be able to recapture and empathize with the sadness, anger, frustration, bewilderment, and enthusiasms of childhood. Clinicians should be warm, accepting, and supportive but neither overly identified with the child nor intolerant of children's natural messiness. Some interviewers are active, engaging, and direct. Some are very quiet, saying no more than is necessary to keep the child's conversation flowing. Some use humor to relax the anxious child. All should be unhurried, with no axe to grind; children are very perceptive of intolerance or irritation cloaked by a falsely bright exterior. The best interviewer is a kind of catalyst—able to attend when the child is freely associating or playing, able to interpolate a comment or question to restart a stalled interview, able to get down on the floor and play with the child when it is appropriate to do so, but capable of setting reasonable limits. Skillful clinicians inject only as much of themselves into the situation as necessary to allay the child's anxiety and promote his or her self-expression.

Clinicians should reflect on their personal responses to each patient. When these responses are dominant, inexorable, and overly generalized, they disrupt the empathic acceptance required for effective interviewing. They can vary from intellectualization and boredom when confronted by an inarticulate child, to the need to rescue a troubled child from what are perceived as villainous parents. The rescuer is likely to set up an unproductive tug-of-war with parents. Others are prone to reductionistic thinking, avoiding close contact with the child and withdrawing into their particular theoretical preference (e.g., neurobiology, systems theory, psychoanalytic theory, cognitive–behavioral theory).

■ CONDUCTING THE CHILD INTERVIEW

Guidelines

The interviewer should not wear a white coat; it signals needles to some children. Clothing should enable the interviewer to sit on the floor if needed. The interviewer should not whisper to the parents about the child in the child's presence. He or she should speak openly, or leave comments to a later time.

The interviewer should try to avoid taking notes during the interview. A few key phrases may be jotted down to provide reminders of the sequence of events. The interviewer then may dictate his or her memory of the interview as soon as it is finished.

Special Considerations

The cardinal aim of the first interview is to help the child relax with the interviewer and to lay the foundation of trust. Nothing should be allowed to compromise this aim, because without trust little can be achieved. If trust does develop, the interviewer will be able to clarify the purpose of the interview, ascertain whether the child perceives problems in his or her life, evaluate the child's affect and capacity to relate to the interviewer, and catch a glimpse of his or her family life. Further specific features of the child's history and mental status can often wait for a second or third interview, unless the child is especially cooperative at the initial interview, or unless the matter is urgent.

The mere expression of feeling without reflection or understanding is not helpful. The child who breaks things or attacks the interviewer is likely to be terrified or overcome with remorse. In any case, he or she will be reluctant to return. The following rule may bear repeating to the child: "You may say or do what you want, except you must stay with me for the whole time, and I will not allow you to break things or hurt yourself or other people." This precaution needs to be stated only if the child seems likely to infringe on the implicit rule.

At the start of the interview, the interviewer should go into the waiting room and greet the parents and child. He or she should sit beside the child and offer an introduction. The interviewer should tell the child that together they will talk, draw, and play for about an hour and then should invite the child into the interview room. If the child is resistant, the interviewer should wait briefly to see if the parents can reassure the child. If this does not work, the parents may be asked to bring the child into the room, indicating that they will be leaving when the child is comfortable. Usually, the parents can leave after a short time, at a signal from the interviewer. If not, it is seldom necessary for the parents to be present for more than one or two interviews.

For the younger child, the interviewer will have set out suitable play materials in the interview room. The child of 9 or 10 years of age can be ushered to an appropriate chair. The interviewer can begin by asking older children why their parents asked them to come and how they feel about it. If the child cannot say, the interviewer should tell the child what he or she already knows and ask for the child's personal reaction to this information. If the child is younger, he or she may be invited to use the play equipment. The interviewer should not push the child. The play theme should emerge on its own. The interviewer may then gently test the child to see whether he or she is prepared to talk.

Questions to Ask

If the child is comfortable conversing with the interviewer, the topics listed in Table 5–3 can be touched on. These topics flow in a natural sequence from neutral to personal. The first seven topics, though informative, are essentially ice-breakers. The last four topics require reflection and are likely to be more difficult for the child.

Table 5–3. Issues Covered During the Child Interview

Content Category	Issues Covered
Attendance	Reason for and feelings about attendance.
School	School, class, teacher. Best and least liked teachers. Reasons? Best and least liked subjects. Reasons? School grades and homework. Liking for other school activities. Reasons? Changes of school? Reasons?
Neighborhood	Neighborhood, social groups, clubs.
Recreation	Hobbies, talents. Best liked activity. Reasons? Sports.
Social relationships	Best friend. Reason best friend is liked? Enemies. Reasons enemies are disliked? Experiences of persecution or scapegoating.
Leadership/ambitions	Opportunities and aspirations for leadership. Ambition with regard to occupation, marriage, and family.
Illness	Recent illnesses, experiences of hospitalization.
Domestic arrangements	House: layout, yard space, bedroom. Chores. Parents, siblings, pets. Family activities most enjoyed. Relationship between parents, alliances within the family, and conflicts within the family.
Fantasy	Dreams, good and bad. Three wishes. What would the child do with $1,000,000? Mutual story-telling. Drawings: of the family doing something together, of a person, of "something nice" and "something nasty."
Symptoms	Fears, anxiety, obsessions, compulsions, dissociative phenomena, depression, depersonalization. If indicated, hallucinations, ideas of reference, delusions, concerns about death, suicidal ideation, difficulty controlling anger, and antisocial behavior.
Insight	Understanding of the reason for attendance. Understanding of the nature of the problem. Desire for help.

However, the list should not be followed rigidly; rather, the topics can be explored in a discretionary manner. One child may be disposed to give a detailed account of peer and family relations, another will provide little on anything beyond neutral topics, and a third will prefer to play with toys and to converse intermittently about them.

Children are relatively more concrete than adolescents. They have difficulty understanding abstractions, taking an objective view of themselves or others, and accurately timing past events. Questions should not be framed in a leading or suggestive manner (a caution that applies particularly in medico-legal situations). Children are confused by complex or compound questions: One idea to one question is best. The interviewer should avoid asking children "Why?" because it puts them on the defensive. Consider the following example:

Patient: The other kids pick on me.
Clinician: Why?
Patient: I don't know. They're mean.

The clinician might have asked the following questions: What do they say? What do they do? How do you feel about it? What do you do about it? When a child uses an unusual word or phrase, particularly if it has an "adult" quality, do not assume it has the same meaning for the child that it has for you. Inquire further.

The interviewer should avoid trying to ferret out the truth from a child who has been involved in antisocial behavior. Instead he or she should try to get in touch with the child's feelings about the situation and what led up to it. It can sometimes be useful to gently point out discrepancies or inconsistencies to an older child who is apparently fabricating a story.

When the interviewer introduces matters that have an anxiety-laden connotation, especially if they seem to imply that the child is "weird" or unique, it can be helpful to associate the issue with the difficulties of other children in similar circumstances. These are known as **buffer comments.** Consider the following example:

Clinician: I see a lot of kids here who have problems after their parents get divorced. Some of them can't help blaming somebody. I wonder if you ever felt like that.

Ending the Interview

At the end of the interview, the clinician should recapitulate with the child what they have both learned about the child's reasons for being seen and how he or she feels about it. If another interview is planned, the interviewer should indicate when it will be. Children should not be asked if they would like to return for another visit. The child may be taken back to the parents in the waiting room. Whispered hallway consultations with the parents should be avoided. If urgent consultation with the parents is needed at that time, the interviewer should conduct the discussion briefly in the interview room, preferably with the child present.

INTERPRETING CHILDHOOD FANTASY

The interpretation of childhood play and fantasy is a specialized skill requiring theoretical knowledge and supervised practical experience. It is important to know the normative fantasies of children of different ages. For example, 4-year-old children often have fantasy themes concerning omnipotence, loss of approval, bodily injury, and curiosity about body differences and functions. By 5–6 years of age, children have an emerging capacity for guilt following transgressions. The polarities of love and hate, kindness and cruelty, death and rebirth are of-

ten expressed in fantasy. By 7–8 years of age, children have a fear of injury, particularly in competitive interaction with peers. There are emerging fears of inferiority in comparative strength, speed, beauty, or intelligence, and a concern with rules and conformity. Gender-role differences are also important. By 9–10 years of age, children have a capacity for guilt and internal conflict, but morality tends to be black and white. Children may be normally preoccupied with the themes of television shows and cartoons, particularly those themes having to do with heroic invulnerability, pursuit and rescue, transgression and punishment. Gender-role differences become more imperative as adolescence approaches.

The clinician should not be surprised if an 8-year-old child prefers to draw with paper and pencil than with poster colors or finger paints. No particular importance should be attached to the observation that a 4-year old enjoys constructing towers and knocking them over or that a 6-year old recounts episodes of "Spiderman." The trick is to recognize deviations from, distortions of, or immaturity in, the normative phase-related themes discussed in this section. Children struggling to cope with unresolved inner conflicts concerning self-control, dependence and independence, activity and passivity, recklessness and injury, male and female, transgression and punishment, invulnerability and helplessness, and dominance and submission are likely to express these themes in play over and over again. It is the idiosyncratic details; the repetitiousness; and the distorted, deviant, or grossly immature theme that should alert the interviewer to fantasy material of diagnostic importance.

Lewis M, King RA: Psychiatric assessment of infants, children, and adolescents. In: Lewis M (ed). *Child and Adolescent Psychiatry: A Comprehensive Textbook.* Philadelphia: Lippincott Williams & Wilkins, 2002, pp. 525–543.

Simmons JE: *Psychiatric Examination of Children,* 3rd edn. Philadelphia: Lea & Febiger, 1981.

IV. INTERVIEWING ADOLESCENTS

PURPOSE OF THE ADOLESCENT INTERVIEW

The initial psychiatric interview of an adolescent has three general purposes: (1) establishing the possible diagnoses, (2) providing therapeutic intervention, and (3) creating a foundation for psychiatric treatment. The first purpose is to establish the possible diagnoses. The interview of the adolescent is only one part—perhaps the most important part—of the full diagnostic process, which also includes interviewing the parents and may include psychological testing, laboratory tests, a physical examination, and the gathering of information from outside sources.

The second purpose for the initial interview is to provide some form of therapeutic intervention. After a single conversation this intervention is not likely to constitute a cure but may simply be a sense of relief for the adolescent to get something off his or her chest. The youngster may leave the appointment with a sense of satisfaction that somebody is making an effort to listen to his or her grievances or with a sense of hope that there will be a way to solve a particular problem over a period of time.

The third purpose of the initial interview is to create a foundation for a continuing course of psychiatric treatment. It is the time to start negotiating the alliance between the therapist and the adolescent. That is, the interviewer communicates that he or she will try to understand the youngster's point of view, even if he or she does not agree with it. The interviewer will promote the interests of the patient in both the short term (e.g., resolving an immediate impasse or conflict) and the long term (e.g., defining and encouraging goals and aspirations). At the same time the interviewer will help the adolescent acknowledge and accept his or her responsibilities to family and community.

■ FACTORS AFFECTING THE ADOLESCENT INTERVIEW

Although the diagnostic process can be both productive and enjoyable, it is frequently a difficult experience for both the interviewer and the interviewee. A physician who feels perfectly comfortable and competent in dealing with an adult patient may become frustrated and tongue-tied when he or she tries to develop a conversation with a 14-year-old adolescent. It is almost always possible to establish rapport and collect information from adolescents, despite the tension and suspicion that may be sensed by both parties.

The physical setting of the interview is important. The office does not need to be fancy, but it should be comfortable and pleasant, relatively soundproof, and located far enough from the waiting room to create a sense of privacy.

Style of the Interview

The general manner in talking with adolescents should be relaxed and informal. It is good to have a sense of humor. Stuffiness creates distance; arrogance invites sarcasm; authoritarianism invites defiance. Being informal and friendly does not mean that the interviewer should become chummy and ingratiating. Teenagers want some degree of social distance between themselves and adults.

Should the interviewer initially meet with the parents, with the teenager, or with the entire family together? It depends on the presenting problem and the circumstances of the interview, but the most common format is for the interviewer to go to the waiting room, introduce himself or herself to both the patient and the parents, ask the patient to come with him or her to the office, and indicate that he or she will meet with the parents in a little while. The purpose, of course, is to communicate to the teenager that this meeting is for the teenager. It is helpful to know the parents' primary concerns ahead of time, which can be learned at the time the appointment is set up or perhaps through an intake questionnaire.

Some adolescents are cooperative, talkative, and quite aware of the purpose of the meeting. In that case, the patient may be perfectly willing to launch into a discussion of the reason for the evaluation. Other youngsters are embarrassed, guilty, or defensive. In that case, it is usually preferable initially to avoid the topics that are most difficult and to spend some time talking about subjects that are important but not as threatening. This part of the interview is an opportunity to take an interest in the patient's general life experience, not just in the immediate problem area. By the end of the meeting, the interviewer should know about the teenager's assets and successes as well as his or her problems.

Asking direct questions may not be the best way to elicit information. Teenagers become defensive almost automatically when they hear questions like "Where did you go?" and "Why did you do it?" Instead of asking, "Why did you steal that car?" the interviewer might say, "Tell me what you were thinking about when you were driving the car."

The interviewer may wish to propose other forms of communication, in addition to the usual dialogue. It might be helpful to ask the youngster to draw a picture of what happened or what he or she observed. The teenager may be able to communicate through dolls or puppets. Young adolescents may be more comfortable with play materials that are typically used with younger children. However, the interviewer should be careful not to insult a more mature teenager by suggesting that he or she use the dolls that are in the office.

Interviews Are Like Poetry

The communications of teenagers and all patients can be considered on several levels. The **content** refers to the actual meaning of the words involved. For example, a youngster may relate a significant fact, that he is failing the ninth grade for the second time. The **form** of the communication refers to the manner in which the statement is made. The statement may be anything from quite coherent to very illogical, simple or convoluted, accompanied or not by inappropriate affect. For example, the boy who was failing the ninth grade repeatedly may announce it with undue bravado, rather than with the contrition one would expect. The **meaning** of the statement may go beyond the conscious, literal words of the content. For example, the meaning of failing the ninth grade twice may be a terrible feeling of pessimism and hopelessness. Finally, communication may be considered from the point of view of **transference.** That is, the youngster may assume that the interviewer will berate him for failure in the same way that his parents did.

Countertransference

The interviewer should examine his or her own feelings toward the patient and the patient's family. These feelings, called **countertransference,** can promote or impede the progress of the evaluation. For instance, the clinician investigating a case of alleged child abuse may be horrified at the youngster's suffering and outraged at the father who allegedly caused it. The interviewer's outrage may interfere with his or her objectivity.

Barker P: *Clinical Interviews with Children and Adolescents.* New York: WW Norton & Company, 1990.

Bernet W: Humor in evaluating and treating children and adolescents. *J Psychother Pract Res* 1993;2:307.

Katz P: Establishing the therapeutic alliance. *Adolesc Psychiatry* 1998; 23:89.

Meeks J, Bernet W: *The Fragile Alliance.* Melbourne FL: Krieger Publishing, 1990.

■ CONDUCTING THE ADOLESCENT INTERVIEW

It is advisable for the interviewer to develop and follow a fairly consistent format in interviewing adolescents. Such a format helps the interviewer remember to touch on a number of important areas in addition to the topic that is of most immediate interest. The interviewer should follow a regular format but be flexible and ready to improvise. As the interviewer moves from one topic to the next, he or she should use transitions and keep the youngster informed about why a particular subject is being discussed. For example, the interviewer could say, "Now I want to ask you some questions about your family, so that I know who everybody is."

Starting the Interview

One way to start the interview is to ask the youngster whose idea it was to come for the appointment. That may lead to a discussion of the chief complaint and the present illness.

If the patient is defensive, the interviewer can invite the patient to tell about school, which is usually a nonthreatening subject. The patient can describe his or her schedule, comment on specific subjects studied, and talk about what he or she thinks is the best part and the worst part of school. A discussion of the patient's ideas about what he or she will be doing after high school graduation gives an indication of the patient's level of optimism and his or her ability to engage in long-range planning.

Collecting Information

The interviewer might ask whether other children in the patient's school get in trouble and what happens to them, which is an opportunity for the youngster to talk about the various bad things that a child might do without necessarily attributing any of it to himself or herself. The discussion of other children in school leads naturally to the topic of peer relationships. Most teenagers can relate what they enjoy doing with friends and also what they may like to do by themselves.

Talking about enjoyable activities gives the adolescent an opportunity to tell about special interests, abilities, hobbies, music, and television. The interviewer can ask about the television shows that the youngster enjoys and ask whether he or she can relate what happened during specific episodes. Not only does this test the patient's memory and ability to organize a narrative, but the youngster may project his or her own issues and concerns onto favorite television shows.

Another useful topic is the youngster's version of his or her health history, because he or she may have interesting and unusual notions about illnesses and operations he or she has had. The health history leads to other areas, such as substance abuse. The interviewer should ask specifically about use of tobacco, alcohol, marijuana, cocaine, hallucinogens, and inhalants. The health history also leads to a discussion of sexual activities and related issues, such as sexually transmitted diseases.

It is always important for the youngster to tell about his or her family: the names of family members, their ages, what kind of work they do, whether they have had serious illness or problems. It might be useful to ask what the parents do when the youngster has been particularly good or particularly bad. The interviewer could ask if the parents are unusually strict, which leads to questions about emotional abuse and physical abuse.

Incorporating the Mental Status Examination

One way to blend the history and the mental status examination is to take an **inventory of affects.** The interviewer may ask the patient to tell about a time when he or she was particularly happy, a time he or she was worried, a time he or she was frustrated, and so on. The interviewer may ask about a time that something funny or silly happened or ask the patient to relate a favorite joke.

If the patient has been depressed, the examiner should ask about suicidal thoughts and behaviors, which are not unusual among adolescents (see Chapter 39). Sometimes it is preferable to be indirect, using questions such as, "Have you ever known anybody who was suicidal?" "Did your friend ever do anything to actually hurt himself?" or "Did anything like that ever happen to you?" Teenagers should be encouraged to tell a parent or other adult if they have persistent or serious suicidal thoughts. If suicidality is a serious concern, this would be a good time to tell the youngster about both confidentiality and the exceptions to confidentiality. Most youngsters find it reassuring (rather than threatening) to learn that the new doctor will keep them safe by discussing dangerous or risky impulses with their parents.

Depending on the differential diagnoses that the interviewer is considering, it may be appropriate to ask the patient about psychotic processes such as delusions, hallucinations, thought insertion and removal, and ideas of reference. Because many adolescents like to demonstrate what they know about psychological phenomena, it is possible to ask a series of questions such as, "Do you know what a hallucination is?" "Can you give me an example of a hallucination?" "Have you ever known anybody who hallucinated?" and "Does that ever happen to you?"

Getting to the Point of the Interview

The interview should not end without addressing the issue or the behavior that led to the referral in the first place. Almost always, that topic will come up at some point during the interview—at the outset of the interview; during the discussion of the patient's school activities, friends, medical history, and family; or through questions related to mental status. Occasionally the patient is so defensive, embarrassed, or simply lacking in insight that he or she seems to avoid the basic reason for the evaluation. Perhaps the parents have brought the youngster because of their concerns about inappropriate sexual behaviors, bizarre obsessive preoccupations, or persistent antisocial conduct. In such cases, the patient may be strongly motivated to keep the interviewer busy discussing other topics. If the youngster seems to be avoiding the subject, the in-

terviewer can bring it up by saying, for example, "Your mom told me on the phone that you have been taking three or four showers every day. Can you tell me about that?" The interviewer can explain that he or she needs to hear the whole story, including the adolescent's side of the story, in order to be of help.

Ending the Interview

After collecting this information, the clinician may want to summarize his or her understanding of the most significant topics. This summary communicates to the patient that the interviewer has tried to understand the situation from the patient's point of view and also allows the patient to make additions or corrections.

It is good to end the initial interview on a positive note. For example, the interviewer can comment positively on the youngster's plans for the future, make specific suggestions regarding the patient's presenting problems, or simply say that the interviewer has enjoyed the meeting.

The end of the initial interview is also an appropriate time to touch on the subject of confidentiality. Because the interviewer is about to meet with the patient's parents, he or she might say, "We have talked about a lot of things today. Is there anything you said that I should not discuss with your folks?" This is a concrete way of communicating that the material discussed in therapy is generally confidential. The patient's answer may tell a lot about his or her relationship with the parents, and it also protects the therapist from making some blunder with the parents early in the relationship with the family. The interviewer can add that he or she would need to tell the parents if the patient appeared to be at risk for self-harm or for harming another person.

American Academy of Child and Adolescent Psychiatry: Practice parameters for the psychiatric assessment of children and adolescents. *J Am Acad Child Adolesc Psychiatry* 1997;36:4S.

Kalogerakis MG: Emergency evaluation of adolescents. *Hosp Community Psychiatry* 1992;43:617.

■ STRUCTURED DIAGNOSTIC PROCEDURES

Clinical information regarding adolescents may also be collected through structured interviews and standardized inventories. These tools are commonly used in clinical research and epidemiologic studies, but they may be useful in clinical practice in some circumstances. These structured procedures are not required for a satisfactory diagnostic interview of an adolescent but may increase the sensitivity of the evaluation in some cases. See Chapter 35 for more information on structured interviews. Another instrument is the Child Behavior Checklist, a questionnaire regarding symptoms and behaviors that may be completed independently by the father, mother, and adolescent. The responses are compared to normative data, and the patient is scored along internalizing and externalizing symptom clusters.

Weist MD, Baker-Sinclair ME: Use of structured assessment tools in clinical practice. *Adolesc Psychiatry* 1997;21:235.

V. INTERVIEWING FAMILIES

IMPORTANCE OF THE FAMILY INTERVIEW

The family (considered in its broadest sense to include the combined nuclear and extended family system) is the developmental matrix for every child's behavior: normal and symptomatic. This universal principle is the basis of family interviewing. The family interview provides a rapid and efficient method of diagnosis and treatment in child and adolescent psychiatry.

Family diagnosis is concerned with the prevailing condition of the family. Family assessment is the process of gathering information about that condition. Although the clinician endeavors to understand each individual, family interviewing concerns the patterns of interaction of those individuals.

The symptomatic behavior of the child or adolescent may not be the source of the family's problems, but rather its result. In children and adolescents, symptoms are shaped by the family matrix in which they start and are perpetuated. Symptoms in young people develop as their hereditary endowment is shaped by their experiences in the family environment. Pathologic behavior can be interpreted as a strategy for survival in a maladaptive family system.

These concepts are embodied in family systemic thinking in four ways: (1) symptoms reflect family relationship disturbances and not simply deviant behavior; (2) if the patient is approached as the exclusive repository of pathology, much diagnostic and therapeutic leverage is lost; (3) functional psychopathology can be fully understood only in context of the family; and (4) if the dysfunctional family matrix can be changed, the child's or adolescent's symptoms may change.

There is much debate in the field of family therapy concerning the classification of family psychopathology. A discussion of the various approaches is beyond the scope of this chapter.

PURPOSE OF THE FAMILY INTERVIEW

The family interview can provide important interactional data complementing individual interviews and contributing to diagnosis and treatment planning. The goals of the family interview are as follows: to gather a comprehensive history of the present illness, to observe and assess pathogenic family interactions, to determine whether the child's disturbed behavior stems from pathologic family interactions, to formulate a family diagnosis and design a treatment plan, to promote the family's understanding and motivation for treatment, and to negotiate a therapeutic alliance concerning the diagnosis and treatment plan.

CONTENT OF THE FAMILY INTERVIEW

Table 5–4 lists the topics commonly covered in a family interview. Steirlin et al. consider it desirable that all members of the family be present at the family interview. Clinicians may find this unfamiliar, but it is surprisingly easy to accomplish. Frequently a sibling will provide the key to a therapeutic dilemma, saving hours of diagnostic time. Table 5–5 lists the aspects of family interaction that can be observed in a family interview.

The parents and the clinician often have a justifiable concern that children should not be unnecessarily burdened with the problems of marital discord; however, such problems are already part of the children's experience. Siblings are part of the family and are consciously or unconsciously aware of their parents' or siblings' difficulties. Because the family's problems are never discussed in a way that leads to resolution and reconciliation, they tend to encourage unhealthy fantasy or promote feelings of insecurity. The first interview with the whole family may offer a chance for relief. At last, long-concealed doubts, anger, and differences can be aired, and children's fears that they are the cause of their parents' difficulties allayed.

Children can offer valuable help to the clinician in his or her efforts to establish contact with the family. Younger

Table 5–4. Issues Covered During the Family Interview

Content Category	Issues Covered
Explicit information	What are the chief complaints of the family and the patient? ("Patient" denotes the identified patient; however, the symptomatic child often turns out to be quite adaptable and is the symptom bearer for an even more disturbed family system.) How do family members understand the present problem? How does the patient see it? Have organic factors been considered (hereafter, it will be assumed that these have been ruled out)? Why does the family come in at this time? What is the background of the problem? How has the family attempted to solve this problem in the past? What are the family's expectations of the interview? What are their motivations and resistances?
Background information	Perinatal and childhood development Current medical problems and medications Past medical and psychiatric illnesses and hospitalizations Family medical and psychiatric history Family demographics Family's employment, educational, housing, and financial status Legal problems of family and patient, past and present
The patient's relationships	With peers (Is the patient gregarious? Popular? Friendly? A loner? Combative?) With teachers and school personnel (Is the patient an academic success or failure? Compliant? Oppositional?) With siblings (Is the patient cooperative? Antagonistic?) With parents and extended family (Are family relationships close? Harmonious? Frictional? Distant? Hostile?) Are supportive aunts, uncles, or grandparents available?
Family's relationships	With the community, such as church and school (Is the family connected? Participative? Isolated? Aloof?) With extended family (Is the family cordial? Warm? Welcoming? Distant? Cold? Rejecting?) With friendship networks (Is the family rewarding? Congenial? Conflictual? Isolated?)

children, especially, are relatively untouched by convention and social inhibitions and can become the therapist's ally. While fearful and guilt-laden parents may find it hard to be open about their differences, small children are often quick to come to the central problem. Take, for example, a family with two boys, aged 5 and 7 years. The older child has various physical symptoms and is physically immature and severely hyperkinetic. The parents complain vigorously about their son, but when questioned about what makes the symptoms better or worse, their answers are vague. Further, they appear guarded about their relationship and the family's emotional climate. Tactful questioning is to no avail. As the parents attempt to sustain a bland facade, the younger child suddenly says, "But you're always fighting!" Thereafter, it develops that the patient's symptoms are worst in the evenings and over the weekends when the parents are together and quarreling. In this family, marital conflict was the heart of the problem. In subsequent therapeutic sessions, if the conflict can be dealt with constructively, the parents will communicate better and the child's hyperactivity is likely to improve.

It is appropriate to honor legitimate wishes for privacy. For example, when parents want to discuss sexual problems, the children may be asked to wait in a playroom.

■ CONDUCTING THE FAMILY INTERVIEW

Haley has proposed four stages for the initial interview: (1) introduction, (2) problem identification, (3) family interaction, and (4) conclusion.

Table 5–5. Aspects of Family Interaction Observed in the Family Interview

Aspects of Family Interaction	Questions to Consider
Overall family communication	Are family members harmonious? Cooperative? Irritable? Immature?
Parental interaction	Are the parents close? Encouraging independence? Responsible? Congenial? Remote? Unstable? Frictional?
Parent-child interaction	Are the parents appreciative? Accepting? Supportive? Respectful of privacy? Critical? Neglectful? Discouraging independence? Intrusive? Do exclusive alliances exist (e.g., overly close mother and overly dependent child, excluding father)?
Sibling interaction	Interviews that include the patient's siblings can provide crucial data. Is the patient treated as the perfect child? Is the patient being scapegoated (i.e., blamed for the family's problems)? Do the siblings accept the blaming or try to defend the patient?
Extended family interaction	Does the patient have a supportive aunt, uncle, or grandparent who resists the pathogenic atmosphere of the nuclear family? Is the mother so attached to her own mother that she is more like a child herself? Is the father's anger toward a family member taken out on one of the children?

Introduction

In the introduction, the clinician greets the family members, learns their names, and sets them at ease. The clinician gives recognition and status to every family member through direct interaction with each of them. He or she explains the rationale for involving all members of the family, for example, by saying, "The more members of the family I see, the more they can help me to help Billy. Besides, I can get much more information more quickly." The clinician acknowledges family members' apprehensions and provides support. He or she avoids guilt-inducing statements by reframing the problem, for example: "Society is sometimes critical of these problems, but I can see you've done the best you could in the face of many difficulties." Finally, he or she observes the patterns of power and affiliation as they are revealed, for example, where family members sit and who speaks out.

Problem Identification

In the problem identification stage, the clinician elicits a statement of the problem from each member of the family. Labels attached to people are transformed into relationship questions (e.g., the statement "She's spoiled" elicits from the clinician, "I see, who spoils her the most?"). Statements that are too long or too short are controlled (e.g., with responses such as "Excuse me. I need to interrupt you Mary, so I can hear what Tom has to say" or "I'm surprised Mr. Smith. You must have noticed more than that."). At the end of this stage, the clinician elicits from a family member a summary of the problem (e.g., "Mr. Smith would you summarize the problem as we've been discussing it?").

Family Interaction

In the family interaction stage, the clinician has two members talk with each other about the problem (e.g., "Talk directly to your wife about this, instead of telling me."). The discussion may be interrupted to bring other family members into the conversation (e.g., "They seem to be stuck. Why don't you help them out?"). The seating arrangement may be changed in order to alter interactive patterns (e.g., "Mom, I'd like you to sit by Dad and give Billy a bit more space on the sofa."). The interviewer may reframe the family views of reality, for example, by emphasizing a family member's good intentions or recasting symptoms as having a positive function in the family (e.g., "What do you think might happen if they didn't have you to worry about?").

CONCLUSION

In the conclusion, the clinician provides a summary in such a way as to engender hope (e.g., "Most families have some periods of difficulty with their teenagers, and they get past them."). The clinician provides encouragement so as to increase motivation for treatment. Humor may be useful. The clinician invites questions to increase understanding, outlines a treatment plan, and arranges further sessions with key family members, as necessary.

■ A CASE STUDY

The identified patient, Billy, has been referred because of school refusal in second grade. He is 6 years old and is accompanied by his parents and two older siblings.

Billy's symptoms, which began shortly after his father lost a middle management job as a result of corporate downsizing, have worsened over an 8-month period, despite efforts to help him by family and school. After Billy's father lost his job, the parents began to quarrel. Billy is most likely to refuse to go to school when parental friction is greatest.

Early in the history-taking part of the interview, the parents begin to argue about the facts. Billy leaves his chair, huddles under his mother's arm, starts to suck his thumb, and distracts the parents. The father then turns his anger on Billy, yelling, "Stop bothering your mother and get back to your chair!" Billy looks stunned and starts to cry. At this point, the mother, pampering Billy, angrily criticizes the father for being too harsh. The father, wounded, withdraws into sullen silence, drawing the two older children into the confusion. Billy's older brother supports the father. His sister supports her mother. The parents are heartened by their children's support and relax. Billy goes back to his chair. Calm is restored. The interview resumes, but the same pattern recurs three more times in the course of the interview.

Family Assessment

Family assessment elucidates the family's relationship patterns. Billy's family responds to distress with a blindly repetitive pattern. The pattern fails to relieve the distress. Assessment leads to treatments aimed at pathogenic interaction patterns, in order to change the problematic behavior.

1. Explicit information—The family's complaint is Billy's school refusal, which is seen as Billy's problem. Because Billy's symptoms clearly began at a time of family stress (i.e., father's job loss), an organic cause is unlikely. The family comes in now because Billy's symptoms have become worse. Their goal is to relieve Billy's symptoms.

2. Background information—A history of unremarkable childhood development is obtained. Billy had the usual childhood diseases without hospitalizations. There are no current medical problems. The family medical and psychiatric history is unremarkable.

3. Family demographics—This is an educated, middle-class family. Its finances are threatened because of the father's unemployed status. There are no legal problems.

4. Patient's relationships—The patient's relationships with peers and teachers are limited by his school refusal. He is immaturely attached to his mother, distant from his father, and detached from his siblings.

5. Observational data—The emotional climate in this family is conflictual and immature. The parental interactions are hostile and childlike, with incessant squabbling. The mother's interactions with the patient are smothering and infantilizing, excluding the father. The father displaces his anger at his wife onto Billy. Billy responds to his parents' quarreling with intrusive, protective, self-defeating behavior, showing little evidence of comfortable distance or a respect for family privacy. The older siblings take sides in ways that split the family and encourage the parents to abdicate their responsibilities as parents. The oldest son's alliance with his father sets him against his mother. The daughter's alliance with her mother sets her against her father. At the first sign of friction between his parents, Billy steps in and distracts them but remains "caught in the middle" throughout the interview. Repeatedly, and at considerable cost to himself, he absorbs the painful, angry tension between his parents, each time restoring the family to a temporary balance.

Family Diagnosis

Although Billy is the youngest, he is the pivotal family member. He has been given the power to regulate the expression of his parents' unresolved conflicts. Parental conflicts are detoured through him, overwhelming him and leaving him little emotional energy to cope with school. Although the parents behave in stereotyped, immature ways, the children can be seen as taking care of them. Their caretaking puts them in parental roles toward their parents, reversing the normal generational hierarchy. Rather than settling differences in healthy ways, Billy's parents rely on their children for support and protection. Rewarded by his parents for soaking up their pain, Billy is predisposed to future self-defeating behavior. Moreover, his normal maturation is blocked. As things stand, should he extricate himself from his key peacekeeping position, his parents would suffer. Billy's school refusal is greatest when the parental friction is greatest. He unwittingly stays home to protect his parents from hurting each other.

As the identified patient, Billy plays a vital role in his family. His symptoms stabilize the transactions between his parents. By focusing on his problems, his parents avoid their own. While the other family members are stuck in unchanging roles, Billy maintains a delicate balance between going to school and staying home to protect his parents from themselves. In this way, he signals not only his own distress but the family's as well and is instrumental in getting help for the whole system.

Family Treatment

Family treatment often seeks to restructure pathogenic family relationships, thus eliminating the need for the identified patient's role. In this case, Billy's parents lack relationship skills and cannot cope with the family crisis. After establishing rapport and trust, the clinician could refer the family to family therapy. The goal of family therapy would be to help the parents resolve their marital issues with a more appropriate caretaker (i.e., the therapist). The children could then be excused from the treatment and from their dysfunctional supportive roles. As Billy's parents stop drawing him into their conflicts, his school refusal would probably abate within a few weeks, without further medical intervention.

Beavers WR, Hampson RB: *Successful Families: Assessment and Intervention.* New York: WW Norton & Company, 1990.

Glick ID, Clarkin JF, Kessler DR: *Marital and Family Therapy,* 3rd edn. New York: Grune & Stratton, 1987.

Gurman AS, Kniskern DP: *Handbook of Family Therapy.* Vol 2. Levittown PA: Brunner/Mazel, 1991.

Josephson AM: Family therapy. In: Lewis M (ed). *Child and Adolescent Psychiatry: A Comprehensive Textbook.* Philadelphia: Lippincott Williams & Wilkins, 2002, pp. 1036–1054.

Kerr M, Bowen M: *Family Evaluation.* New York: Norton, 1988.

Psychological and Neuropsychological Assessment

James S. Walker, PhD, Howard B. Roback, PhD, & Larry Welch, EdD

■ PSYCHOLOGICAL EVALUATION IN THE PSYCHIATRIC CONTEXT

Psychological evaluation in the psychiatric context generally refers to measurements from psychological testing (in addition to the utilization of information from the history and traditional mental status examination), made for the purpose of helping delineate and clarify a patient's psychopathology. Psychological testing is frequently requested to address specific clinical issues such as the patient's need for hospitalization, personality factors complicating Axis I symptoms, the possible presence of malingering, identification of major therapeutic issues, the patient's potential for suicide, his or her primary defense mechanisms and coping style, and the most appropriate discharge options. The child psychiatrist may need to rule out neurodevelopmental disorders such as mental retardation with cognitive testing. Questions a psychiatrist may ask in a neuropsychological referral are typically related to the role of possible central nervous system dysfunction in a patient's pathology and its impact on daily functioning. For example, does a patient have dementia or pseudodementia, is a patient's behavioral or emotional dyscontrol the result of personality factors or impaired central nervous system mechanisms that modulate such reactions, and what is the extent of organic damage and associated cognitive impairment? In addition to clarifying the diagnosis and assisting in treatment planning, psychological testing can play an important role in outcome assessment by helping to document the effectiveness of the treatment provided to a given patient.

The psychiatrist's ability to call upon and utilize psychological consultation on complex clinical cases in the course of practice leads to many diagnostic advantages over relying upon interview and observations alone, particularly in today's health care environment that emphasizes documentation. Further, having an understanding of a patient's personality structure, amenability to treatment, and verbal skills, for example, are extremely useful

in deciding whether psychosocial treatments or pharmacological treatment alone would be the preferred treatment modality. The demonstration of treatment effectiveness by measurably positive changes on symptom report scales is important documentation for insurance companies, managed care corporations, and patient consumers. The measurement of a patient's tendency to deliberately exaggerate or to experience somatoform symptoms is often critical in the medicolegal context. Similarly, the measurement of cognitive skills and deficits adds a dimension to the psychiatrist's understanding of the patient's abilities, whether it be the identification of precocity in a preschooler or dementia in an aged professional who is reluctant to retire despite complaints from clients and business partners.

MEASUREMENT CONCERNS

The selection of tests to address given referral questions is determined according to whether they satisfactorily meet key psychometric standards. Psychological tests are typically norm-referenced, that is, the score of an individual patient is compared to the average of the standardization sample, the group of persons to whom the test was initially administered, and who were carefully chosen as being representative of the population of interest (e.g., patients with a diagnosis of bipolar I disorder). The test procedures themselves are also standardized. While informal bedside testing can be adapted to one's personal style and has the flexibility of incorporating items specific to the referral questions, standardized testing implies uniformity of test administration, scoring, and interpretation.

Standardization contributes to the test's reliability, that is, it must be internally consistent and produce the same or similar results if given to the same individual at different times. For example, if a medical school applicant scores in the 98th percentile on the Medical College Admissions test (MCAT) on Saturday and in the 60th percentile on Monday using the same test version or an equivalent form, the measure is said to be unreliable because little confidence can be put in either score. The useful psychological test must ultimately also have validity, the most important criterion for a test: the degree to which the test actually measures what it claims to be measuring. The validity of a test can be assessed in a number of different ways. It can be measured against an external, well-accepted criterion (criterion validity). For example, with regard to its criterion validity, does the MCAT score actually predict medical student performance as measured by relevant external criteria, such as grades, faculty evaluations, and successful completion of training? Does a test for obsessive–compulsive disorder (OCD) correctly identify most patients who have been diagnosed as meeting OCD criteria by multiple raters? Criterion validity is assessed by calculating the test's sensitivity (its ability to correctly classify a patient as having the condition of interest), and its specificity (its success in correctly classifying patients without the condition). Another type of validity, content validity, involves a systematic analysis of the individual items comprising the test in order to determine how well the items sample the behavior domain under study. For example, a measure of depression should consist of items that sample all major aspects (e.g., cognitive, physiologic, and behavioral) of the construct with respect to their relative importance. A test must also have ecological validity, the degree to which the test genuinely reflects cogent, real-world realities and behavior. For example, an elderly patient may perform very poorly on a test of mental arithmetic skills, but the score may bear little relationship to her ability to balance a checkbook if she can compensate for her concentration problems by using the aid of pencil and paper. The utility of a test is another key characteristic, referring to its unique usefulness in answering the relevant referral questions and contributing to the desired outcome. The tests described in this chapter are among those that have withstood scrutiny over time and demonstrated their utility in psychiatric practice.

■ PERSONALITY AND BEHAVIORAL ASSESSMENT

Interest in personality assessment predates the scientific advances in psychological testing. Throughout the ages, people have evaluated their own conduct and the actions of others for the purpose of understanding and predicting behavior. Scientific personality testing has its origins in the study of individual differences through psychological measurement.

Contemporary personality and behavior measures are typically described as being either objective or projective in type. The use of the term "objective" implies that responses are objectively scored and interpreted according to normative data. Examples of the former include comprehensive objective personality tests, behavioral rating scales, and actuarial assessment techniques. We have selected examples of these types of objective personality and behavioral instruments for discussion, as they are the ones the psychiatrist is most likely to encounter in clinical practice. That is, when referring patients for personality testing, there will be a greater likelihood that many of the following will be administered and discussed in the psychologist's report. There will also be a parallel discussion of projective tests.

COMPREHENSIVE OBJECTIVE PERSONALITY TESTS

Comprehensive personality tests are structured paper-and-pencil self-report instruments whose items are answered in a standard format (e.g., true–false). Usually the patient is the respondent, though some tests utilize the input of significant others. They are scored in a quantitative manner, and resulting numerical scores are subjected to statistical analyses. Typically, a profile is generated that contrasts the patient's scores with those of the normative sample. Normative data are provided in the test manual, as are reliability and validity information.

Minnesota Multiphasic Personality Inventory-2

The Minnesota Multiphasic Personality Inventory-2 (MMPI-2) is the most frequently used personality inventory in clinical practice. In the 1930s, psychiatrists and psychologists had to rely almost exclusively on interview procedures to assist them in making clinical decisions. Starke Hathaway and Charley McKinley, a psychologist–psychiatrist collaborative team at the University of Minnesota, published the original MMPI in 1943. It was developed entirely from an empirical perspective, with response items chosen solely on the basis of their ability to distinguish among cohorts of psychiatric patients with given disorders. This 566-item true-false test was designed to yield 10 clinical subscales: Hypochondriasis, Depression, Hysteria, Psychopathic Deviate, Masculinity–Femininity, Paranoia, Psychasthenia, Schizophrenia, Hypomania, and Social Introversion. For ease of communication, each scale was given an associated number. For example, Hypochondriasis = 1, Depression = 2, and so forth. Psychologists typically refer to these numbers when discussing an MMPI profile among themselves, as many scale names are clinically outdated (e.g., Psychasthenia). In addition, there are multiple validity scales available which measure the respondent's test-taking attitude (e.g., defensiveness, exaggeration of symptoms). Sets of items selected for inclusion in the test's final version differentiated a specific clinical sample (e.g., depressed patients on the Depression subscale) from the normal subjects who comprised the standardization group.

The MMPI was revised in 1989 as the MMPI-2, which consists of 567 self-descriptive statements. In the revision, several original items were reworded or deleted, and statements focusing on suicide, substance abuse, and related matters were added. The revised version also includes a standardization sample that is more representative of the U.S. population (based on census data). In 2003, an extensive project was completed that restructured the clinical scales of the MMPI-2 and anchored them in an empirically derived factor structure. Another extensive revision of the MMPI-2 is reportedly soon to be published, reducing its length and revising the primary clinical scales. These changes guarantee that the MMPI-

2 and its successors will continue to play an important role in the assessment of psychopathology, though its evolution as an instrument raises many questions about validity and utility that will need to be addressed by careful research.

Interpretation of the MMPI-2 is based primarily on a profile analysis consisting of two or three highest scale elevations. Scales with T scores of 65 or above are considered clinically significant. Abnormally low scores are interpretable. Numerous books are available to help the clinician interpret specific code types. The basic profile form of a hand-scored MMPI-2 is shown in Figure 6–1. The patient's profile suggests a depressive disorder with possible cognitive changes or even psychotic involvement (elevated Depression and Schizophrenia scales) in an individual who is overly dependent, self-centered, and naïve

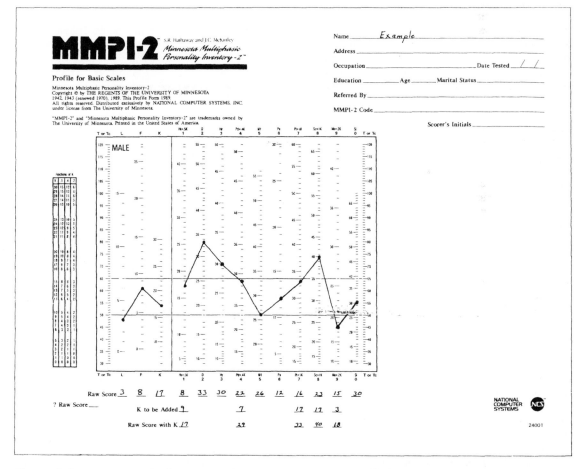

Figure 6–1. Minnesota Multiphasic Personality Inventory-2 (MMPI-2) Profile for Basic Scales. (Copyright © 1989 the Regents of the University of Minnesota. All rights reserved. "MMPI-2" and "Minnesota Multiphasic Personality Inventory-2" are trademarks owned by the University of Minnesota. Reproduced by permission of University of Minnesota Press.)

about their own feelings and motivations (elevated Hysteria scale).

Personality Assessment Inventory

The Personality Assessment Inventory (PAI) was constructed in 1991 by Leslie Morey, then a professor of psychology at Vanderbilt University, with the goal of closely corresponding to contemporary psychiatric concepts and diagnostic nomenclature, such as found in the *Diagnostic and Statistical Manual of Mental Disorders* (DSM). The test consists of 344 items answered on a four-point Likert-type format: totally false, slightly true, mainly true, and very true. In addition to the 11 clinical scales (diagnosis), there are 5 treatment consideration scales (prognosis), 2 interpersonal scales (social support), and 4 validity scales. The clinical scales are Somatic Complaints, Anxiety, Anxiety-Related Disorders, Depression, Mania, Paranoia, Schizophrenia, Borderline Features, Antisocial Features, Alcohol Features, and Drug Features. An important feature of the PAI scales is that they are further divided into subscales that reflect specific components or subtypes of a given disorder. For example, a patient's specific manifestation of anxiety may be as excessive worry and concern (i.e., cognitive) rather than trembling hands (e.g., physiologic). The treatment scales (Suicidal Ideation, Treatment Rejection, Nonsupport, Stress, Aggression) also provide the clinician with pertinent information for treatment planning, an especially useful feature of this test.

Applications and Limitations of Comprehensive Personality Tests

The MMPI-2 and PAI are two important objective personality inventories for diagnostic classification and treatment planning. The empirically developed MMPI-2 is used primarily for spotlighting acute psychiatric (Axis I) issues and for identifying patients' psychopathological patterns that may not be explicitly apparent to either the patient or the clinician. The PAI is a more "face-valid" test; that is, the scales correspond, often very explicitly, with current psychiatric (DSM) conceptions of Axis I disorders and Axis II personality disorder criteria. Though designed to be an improved MMPI-2, most clinicians who have used both have found each to contribute uniquely useful information to the assessment process, as reflected by the immense popularity of both instruments.

There are several advantages to using comprehensive personality measures. They are relatively simple to administer. The arduous task of data entry, scoring, and calculating scales may be accomplished by computer. Test manuals provide standardization and psychometric information (e.g., validity and reliability data) for the user, as well as guidance in clinical interpretation. Comprehensive personality instruments also have limitations. They are primarily behavioral in content and may provide inadequate information about the respondent's underlying motives or psychodynamics. For example, two patients may produce identical profiles indicating that they feel depressed and anxious. In one case the symptoms may be the result of acute situational stress (e.g., financial reversals), whereas in the other case, the symptoms may be long-standing and connected to historical issues, such as unresolved childhood trauma. Further, the prescribed objective response method (e.g., true-false or four-point scale) prevents patients from elaborating or qualifying their responses.

Butcher JN, Dahlstrom WG, Graham JR, Tellegen A, Kaemmer B: *MMPI-2 (Minnesota Multiphasic Personality Inventory-2: Manual for Administration and Scoring, Revised Edition.* Minneapolis, MN: University of Minnesota Press, 1989.

Morey LC: *An Interpretive Guide to the Personality Assessment Inventory (PAI).* Odessa, FL: Psychological Assessment Resources, 1996.

Tellegen A, Ben-Porath S, McNulty JL, Arbisi PA, Graham JR, Kaemmer B: *The MMPI-2 Restructured Clinical (RC) Scales.* Minneapolis, MN: University of Minnesota, 2003.

BEHAVIOR RATING SCALES

Behavioral rating scales are objective scales that may be self-administered or, especially when used with children or severely impaired individuals, rely on the reports of knowledgeable informants. These scales usually focus upon a single disease construct (e.g., depressive symptoms, obsessive–compulsive symptoms, PTSD symptoms) or upon a set of specific behaviors of interest in a given population, such as ratings of childhood behavioral problems. The scale's scores are then typically compared to normative data in the form of averages or cutoff points identified by research as optimal in predicting a given criterion. Behavior rating scales tend to be more focused on a given set of behaviors or symptoms, or are developed on a given subpopulation (e.g., children, PTSD victims) than comprehensive personality tests. As such, they may be more limited in scope, but may assist the clinician in specifically elucidating a patient's clinical presentation in a more complete fashion.

The chapters in this volume on child assessment reference some of the most widely used comprehensive child behavior rating scales (e.g., Child Behavior Checklist). Adaptive behavior rating scales for children and adults, such as the Vineland Adaptive Behavior Scale, provide standardized procedures for assessing functional abilities, key to the assessment of mental retardation, and other developmental disorders. These tests, and ones like them, are in reality collections of multiple behavior rating scales that are conormed on a single population and designed to tap several domains of behavior.

Beck Depression Inventory

One of the most widely used rating scales is the Beck Depression Inventory, now in its second version. Though often used to aid in diagnosing depression, its major utility is in measuring the severity of self-reported depressive symptoms, and in describing the particular manifestation of depression in a given patient. It contains self-rating items of all the DSM criteria of depression, as well as other changes commonly experienced in depressive patients. A simple glance at the rating form yields a wealth of information, such as the overall severity of the symptoms, and whether the patient's symptoms are more physiological, cognitive, or mood-oriented in nature.

Applications and Limitations of Behavior Rating Scales

Many advantages of behavioral rating scales have already been mentioned. They represent powerful tools in assessing the severity of psychiatric disorders and in illuminating the nature and characteristics of many behavioral syndromes. The sheer wealth of scales is almost bewildering: for nearly any given disorder, the clinician or researcher will have an array of well-researched instruments from which to choose. Their utility is in great demand whenever objective, repeatable, quantifiable data are required to assess patients' progress in treatment, the efficacy of new research treatments, or the measurement of quality outcomes.

Their very specificity unfortunately contributes to some of their disadvantages. By focusing only on a given syndrome or symptom cluster, the use of a targeted rating scale may serve to mask initial diagnostic errors because symptoms from other syndromes may not be assessed. Perhaps their greatest weaknesses are apparent in the forensic assessment context. In most cases, the scales are so transparent ("face-valid") that it is easily apparent to the respondent exactly what disorder or set of behaviors is being assessed by the scale. Few of the measures have acceptable validity indexes to identify the impact of potentially defensive responding or malingering. Even unintentional false reporting, such as by a frustrated parent who is at wit's end over a child's disruptive behavior, or a parent who is determined to cast their child's conduct problems in an acceptable light by over-endorsing depressive symptoms, can muddy the conclusions. In sum, the utility of these scales is quite limited in the forensic realm, and are best used in the context of a comprehensive, multimodal assessment.

Beck AT, Steer RA, Brown GK: *BDI-II Manual.* San Antonio, TX: Psychological Corporation: 1996.

Bellack AS, Hersen M: *Behavioral Assessment: A Practical Handbook,* 4th edn. Upper Saddle River, NJ: Allyn & Bacon, 1998.

ACTUARIAL ASSESSMENT TECHNIQUES

Actuarial measures are assessment methods based purely on given patient characteristics, demographic information, and historical data that are mathematically combined to make probabilistic classifications of patients (e.g., risk of violence or likelihood of responding favorably to a given type of treatment). However, for many clinicians, the thought of basing treatment or placement decisions on actuarial descriptors or cut scores may seem foreign, if not repellent. Yet there are psychiatric evaluation contexts that sometimes require the input of such techniques. For example, the psychiatrist who assesses a patient's suicide risk by asking about history of prior attempts, current plans, intentions, means, age, level of stress, and religiosity is in fact using an informal analogue of an actuarial process to make a critical determination. Attempts to more rigorously codify systems for assessing suicidal risk have met with some success (e.g., Suicide Potential Scale).

Actuarial techniques are most often appropriate in clinical situations in which a decision must be made in one direction or the other, regardless of the quality of the data, because of the gravity of the potential outcomes. In addition to suicide risk, the most common situations requiring an estimate of risk usually revolve around violent behavior. Multiple actuarial rating systems have been researched and developed in this area, including aids to the evaluator involved in assessing risk of sexual reoffending (e.g., STATIC-99), risk of suicide (e.g., Suicide Potential Scale), and risk of violent reoffending in individuals with a known history of violence (e.g., Violence Risk Assessment Guide, or VRAG).

Violence Risk Assessment Guide

The latter technique, the VRAG, is the product of an extensive research program on violent offenders in a maximum-security institution in Ontario. The VRAG represents a typical actuarial procedure. The patient is rated on several static dimensions, such as the nature of their offense, the presence of a psychotic disorder, age, presence of childhood conduct disorder, and several other variables. The patient is also subjected to an interview with the Hare Psychopathy Checklist, a semistructured interview technique designed to identify the degree of a patient's psychopathy, or tendency to demonstrate personality characteristics shown to be related to serious acts of violence (see Table 6–1).

The patient's overall score is then compared to a sample of offenders with a known recidivism rate, and a probability value of future reoffending is assigned. While marked by a large error rate, this method is considerably superior to nonquantitative clinical judgments of violence risk made by psychologists and psychiatrists. This

Table 6–1. Hare's Characteristics of Psychopathy

Superficial	Glib, slick, and smooth in social interactions.
Grandiose	Possessing an inflated sense of importance and self-assuredness
Lack of remorse	Unconcerned about others' distress, disdainful of victim's feelings
Lack of empathy	Unable to place oneself in the inner world of another person, callous
Pathological conniving	Deceitful, shrewd, cunning, manipulative
Impulsive	Acts without considering consequences, reckless, displays anger with little provocation
Sensation seeking	Pathological need for excitement and a sense of risk
Lack of responsibility	Parasitic lifestyle, promiscuous sexual behavior, failure to meet obligations
Lack of goals	Aimless lifestyle, no sense of purpose
Juvenile delinquency	Pattern of rights violations beginning in childhood or adolescence
Adult sociopathy	A diverse pattern of adult antisocial behaviors, career criminality

and similar methods are now commonly used in forensic consultation, and have been accepted for use by the courts in multiple court decisions.

Applications and Limitations of Actuarial Methods

The advantages to the psychiatrist in utilizing these actuarial methods, when available, are considerable. In addition to providing a check on personal biases and minimizing the inherent inaccuracy of general impressions based on a global impression of the patient, professional risk issues are minimized. By definition, these techniques represent the standards generally accepted by the mental health community, and thus would presumably serve as a powerful protective measure in the unhappy event of liability litigation following a patient committing a violent act. Disadvantages include the fact that the error rates of these methods, though superior to clinical judgment, remain very high. Presumably, many more predictive factors or combinations thereof need to be identified in order to reduce the error rate. Such methods also do not usually take into account dynamic factors such as availability of treatment, compliance with treatment, intrapersonal changes due to the consequences of past acts of violence, or the impact of supervision and scrutiny, to name a few. Consequently, actuarial analysis is best employed as an adjunct to, not a replacement for, comprehensive psychological or psychiatric assessment.

Cull JG, Gill WS: *Suicide Probability Scale Manual.* Los Angeles, CA: Western Psychological Services, 1991.

Hanson RK, Thornton D: *The Static-99: Improving Actuarial Risk Assessments for Sex Offenders.* User Report 99–02. Ottawa: Department of the Solicitor General of Canada (www.sgc.gc.ca).

Hare RD: *The Hare Psychopathy Checklist-Revised.* Toronto, ON: Multi-Health Systems, 1991.

Quinsey VL, Harris GT, Rice ME, Cormier CA: *Violent Offenders: Appraising and Managing Risk.* Washington, DC: APA Books, 1998.

PROJECTIVE PERSONALITY TESTS

As opposed to objective personality testing, in projective personality testing, the individual is provided unstructured test stimuli (e.g., inkblots, incomplete sentences, pictures of human figures) and required to give meaning to them. The theoretical assumption is that the patient's responses reflect primarily a "projection" of the individual's inner needs, motivations, defenses, and drives. That is, tests are intended to elicit a projection of unconscious material from the subject's inner life. In theory, the manner in which the patient organizes and perceives the ambiguous test stimuli reveals something about his or her distinctive personality. There are objective scoring systems for some projective tests, such as the Exner Comprehensive Scoring System, one of the most sophisticated and widely used for the Rorschach. However, some clinicians prefer to make psychodynamic interpretations from the thematic content of the patient's Rorschach responses, arguing that they are achieving a much richer understanding of the patient than that provided through more sterile numerical analysis of the person. Proponents of objective personality inventories often criticize their counterparts who favor projective testing for not meeting higher standards of validity, reliability, and standardization. Many clinicians, however, utilize a test battery of both objective and projective tests when performing a psychological workup on a patient. Such a strategy will likely result in a more comprehensive evaluation of a

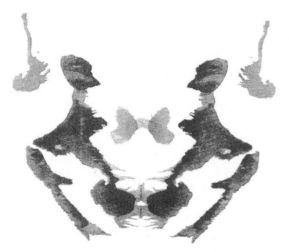

Figure 6–2. Rorschach Test Plate 1, by Rorschach H. (Copyright © 1921, 1948, 1994 by Verlag Hans Huber AG, Bern, Switzerland. Reproduced by permission.)

patient and provide more confidence in replicated findings from different types of test stimuli. Three of the projective tests that have stood the proverbial "test of time" are the Rorschach Inkblot Test, the Thematic Apperception test (TAT), and the Sentence Completion test (SCT).

Rorschach Inkblot Test

The Rorschach Inkblot Test was the creative effort of a Swiss psychiatrist, Hermann Rorschach, who first published the test in 1921. Out of several hundred inkblot configurations, he selected 10 cards because of the variety of responses they elicited. Five of the bilaterally symmetrical inkblots are achromatic, two have additional spots of red, and three combine several colors (Figure 6–2).

During the test administration, the examiner asks the patient what each card looks like (i.e., "What might this be?"). The examiner then records the patient's responses verbatim, the time it takes to generate responses, and any nonverbal reactions. After the responses are compiled, the examiner asks the patient to go through the cards again. This is referred to as the inquiry phase. In the latter phase, the examiner is attempting to identify the factors influencing the response—what parts of the blot are used and what features made the blot look a certain way (e.g., color, movement, texture, shading, and form). All of these factors are interpretable. For example, perception of movement (e.g., the percept of a bird in flight) is considered to relate to the richness of an individual's fantasy life. The form determinant (e.g., how closely the response corresponds with the selected area of the inkblot) is believed to indicate an individual's reasoning

powers and reality testing. Persons with good psychological functioning tend to have refined and differentiated perceptions, whereas the perceptions of psychologically impaired persons generally fit poorly with the form of the blot associated with their response. Color responses are believed to reflect the emotional life of the respondent. For example, pure color responses (i.e., the blot color itself stimulates the respondent's associative process) are considered to reflect an individual with poorly integrated emotional reactions. Location choice (e.g., the area of the blot where the respondent associates his or her response) is also considered to reflect something about one's personality. For example, an emphasis on very small details is considered to reflect an individual who has a very critical attitude or is overly concerned with trivialities.

Responses are analyzed in terms of the number that fall into various categories (e.g., movement, form, location), the normative frequency of these categories for different clinical groups, and the relationships among determinants (i.e., ratios such as percentage of conventional form). Psychodynamically oriented examiners also interpret the content of responses in terms of symbolic meaning (e.g., perception of an island may reflect a sense of isolation). When interpreted within the respondent's specific experiences, the latter analyses are believed to reveal a great deal about an individual's unique personality style.

A number of Rorschach scoring and interpreting systems have been developed since its inception. Irving Weiner and John Exner have attempted to put contemporary Rorschach assessment on a psychometrically sound basis. For instance, the Exner Comprehensive Scoring System emphasizes structural rather than thematic content of responses. This complex scoring system involves categorizing responses in an objective manner by converting them into ratios, percentages, and other indices. Interpretations are primarily data based rather than theoretically based. The Exner system has been well received by the current generation of Rorschach testers whose graduate training has emphasized the importance of psychometric standards in assessment.

Thematic Apperception Test

The TAT was developed in 1943 by Harvard psychologist Henry Murray. The test consists of 29 pictures and one blank card. The cards have recognizable human figures (Figure 6–3), and the patient is asked to generate a story of what is happening in the scene. The subject is asked to tell what led up to the situation, what the people are thinking and feeling, and how the situation will end. There is significant variability in the scoring of TAT responses. Some examiners prefer a more intuitive approach to understanding the psychodynamic implications of a story; others favor a more complex scoring

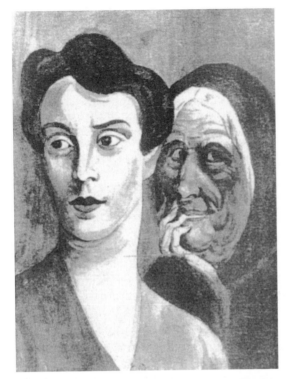

Figure 6–3. Card 12F from the Thematic Apperception Test. (Reprinted by permission of the publishers from Henry A Murray, Thematic Apperception Test, Plate 12F, Cambridge, Mass.: Harvard University Press, Copyright © 1943 by the President and Fellows of Harvard College, © 1971 by Henry A Murray.)

system (e.g., Murray's drive system analysis). In the former case, the psychologist attempts to identify significant emotions and attitudes projected onto the cards. Each card is intended to elicit information about a specific type of relationship (e.g., child–mother, child–father) or an important psychological area (e.g., sexuality). Themes that recur with unusual frequency are judged to reflect prominent psychological needs. As on the Rorschach, the examiner records the verbatim responses of the examinee for later analysis. Because of their real-life content, TAT stimuli are less ambiguous than are Rorschach cards.

Sentence Completion Tests

Like the Rorschach and the TAT, SCTs are used frequently in personality assessment. They generally consist of a number of incomplete sentences (e.g., I feel guilty when . . . .) that are completed by the patient. They are intended to provide information about the respondent's interpersonal attitudes and relationships, personality style,

and other issues that are important to the examiner. The referral questions will help determine which one of several different published SCT versions is used in a given case. Many psychologists would agree that the SCT is more likely a semiprojective test because the items are more transparent than are the Rorschach inkblots and the TAT cards. As psychologists who have reviewed these instruments have pointed out, incomplete sentences are among the least researched of projective methods. They appear to persist because, like a slot machine, there is an intermittent payoff in their usage. It may be that some patients are more comfortable communicating information to the clinician in a written form than they are in the face-to-face conversational context.

Application of Projective Personality Tests

Psychodynamically oriented psychologists use the Rorschach as part of a test battery for evaluating clinical issues such as the degree of a patient's cognitive–perceptual pathology. For example, to evaluate whether a patient has a low-grade thought disorder, the psychologist may examine the Rorschach protocol in terms of idiosyncratic responses with a distorted form level. Further, persons with a thought disorder often emit three types of pathologic responses: (1) confabulated whole responses (using a single detail as a basis for an entire response, for example, "This looks like a whisker, so the rest of the card is a cat's face."); (2) fabulized combinations (making one incongruous concept out of two percepts in close physical proximity, for example, "This looks like a bridge and this looks like legs, so this area is a bridge with legs."); and (3) contaminated responses (seeing two different things at the same blot area and then fusing them together, for example, "This is a dog. It's a bug. No, it's a dog-bug."). In these responses, the patient is demonstrating inadequate conceptual boundaries, as well as confusion in thought, perception, and reasoning. The Rorschach is also useful for generating hypotheses about the individual's personality style; however, psychologists often look for collateral support for their inferences about personality style in the patient's objective personality data, interview statements, and case history. The TAT and the SCT are used primarily to generate hypotheses about an individual's family and social relationships, areas of conflict, and related Axis II issues.

Advantages and Limitations of Projective Personality Tests

Some controversy surrounds the use of projective personality tests. Many clinicians find the instruments described here as highly useful for diagnostic purposes and for evaluating personality functioning. However, results of studies examining the psychometric properties of these tests at best have yielded equivocal results, perhaps with the exception of elements of the Exner Comprehensive Scoring System for the Rorschach Inkblot Test. Nonetheless, a sizable number of clinicians continue to argue that projective personality tests should not be subject to standard psychometric evaluation and that such attempts are damaging to the potential richness of these methods for understanding an individual's distinctive personality. It is highly unlikely that these differences will be resolved anytime soon.

Exner JE: *The Rorschach, Basic Foundations and Principles of Interpretation,* 4th edn. New York: John Wiley & Sons, 2002.

CLINICAL DECISION MAKING IN PERSONALITY ASSESSMENT

Following the gathering of test data, the psychologist analyzes the materials for purposes of clinical decision making and prediction, and endeavors to address the specific referral questions. If testing included both objective and projective measures, then the examiner performs two functions—one being that of the psychometrist or actuary who minimizes subjective interpretation, and the other that of the clinician who relies heavily on clinical interpretation and behavioral observations. The objective of such a dual role is to use separate data points as a means of cross-validating the ultimate conclusions. For example, if a patient scores several standard deviations above the mean on the MMPI Schizophrenia scale, the clinician anticipates bizarre responses (e.g., contaminated responses) on the Rorschach, and would expect behavioral observations to support the presence of disordered thought and behavior. If these assumptions are correct, then there is increasing support for the presence of a psychotic adjustment. If not, then an alternative explanation is sought.

After analyzing the data, the psychologist communicates the findings, resulting clinical impressions, and any treatment recommendations to the referring psychiatrist in the form of a psychological test report. The report is crafted to communicate a meaningful picture of the patient in a format most useful for the referring physician. For example, a psychodynamically oriented psychiatrist generally prefers a report that helps him or her better understand the patient from that perspective. A psychiatrist whose practice is primarily medication focused may prefer a report that focuses on specific symptoms, suggested by objective testing, that the psychiatrist can address pharmacologically. The psychiatrist may also ask that a patient be retested after treatment to assess quantitatively the effectiveness of his or her intervention. With the psychiatrist's approval, the psychologist will review test findings with the patient. However, psychotherapy-oriented psychiatrists often prefer to have their patients discover insights for themselves, rather than from reading the psychological report.

An example of a psychological test report follows. A pretest interview was conducted with the patient, as with all testing cases. The goals of the interview are to establish rapport, gain clinically useful information, and address any concerns that the patient may have about the evaluation.

Psychological Test Report

The patient is the 19-year-old son of a hard-driving and successful attorney living in a medium-sized southeastern city. The patient's father was very concerned about his son's suspension from an Ivy League college for academic reasons. According to the father, the patient appeared depressed, withdrawn, and somewhat uncommunicative since his return home. He sought only minimal contact with long-time friends attending a local college. The patient's inability to hold down a job as a salesman in a small store owned by a family friend was embarrassing to the patient's parents. His father consulted with a physician friend who recommended that the patient be referred to a psychiatrist for a formal evaluation. The psychiatrist requested a testing consult from a clinical psychologist.

Tests Administered—MMPI, Wechsler Adult Intelligence Scale-Revised (WAIS-R), PAI, TAT, Suicide Probability Scale (SPS), SCT, Rorschach Inkblot Test

Background—The patient, a 19-year-old single male, was referred by his psychiatrist for psychological evaluation. The focus of this assessment was to explore whether the patient's recent emotional, academic, occupational, and social dysfunction are related to individual or family dynamic issues or are a manifestation of some other more malignant underlying pathology.

Interview—The patient reported that he was suspended by his university for academic failure after one semester but hoped to reenroll this coming fall. He noted that, despite experiencing no academic difficulties in high school, "a lot of stuff happened at [college]." He specified that motivational difficulties (inability to get out of bed) and increasing alcohol abuse contributed to his academic troubles. He denied the use of other illicit substances. He added that he initially was comfortable with the move away from home and family to a new city and college dorm life. However, he then became progressively more isolated, socially disconnected, and lonely. The patient claimed, "Even in a room full of people I would feel left out." He further qualified that such a situation did not always distress him, as he sometimes preferred to remain aloof, withdrawn, and to "wallow in my misery." He claimed that his pattern of isolation was long-standing, but not as frequent or severe as it became in college. He admitted to periods of depressed mood of varying severity, during which his preference for isolation was enhanced. The patient endorsed passive thoughts of suicide in the past but denied urges to act on impulses for self-harm or elaboration of a plan to do so.

The patient revealed a number of idiosyncrasies centering around social interaction. For example, he admitted to often pretending that one of his friends or acquaintances is riding in the car with him, or sitting in his bedroom with him, and he will rehearse how he would act if the person were really present. He acknowledged that such fantasy is much less threatening than social reality, as it "gives me an idea of what I'd be like in front of others and helps me boost my self-image."

He mentioned that his deflated self-image and low self-esteem have troubled him throughout his life. He claimed that he continually worries "if I'm good enough" and that he will "mess up." The patient stated that his parents, especially his father, often reacted to his mistakes with "a lot of yelling and shouting, and making me feel guilty." He described his relationship with his parents and only sister to be much like his social experiences, characterized by a lack of connectedness and belongingness. In reference to his father, the patient said, "I have no real connection, I guess; I don't identify with him and don't even really talk to him." However, the patient added that his father had "smoothed out" after having a heart attack a few years earlier, resulting in him being more talkative than volatile. Still, the patient denied the growth of a close emotional bond with his father.

The patient was employed by a local sporting goods store after being dismissed from college, but he was fired because of "disagreements with the boss." He stated that he is not presently in a romantic relationship but has been in the past. Interestingly, he described past sexual experiences as "emotionally confusing," adding, "I want more than just a squeeze toy, I want someone I can talk to."

Test Findings

Intelligence—The patient achieved an estimated Full Scale intelligence quotient (IQ) score of 105 on selected subtests of the WAIS-R, which places him in the average range of intellectual functioning. His Verbal scale IQ score of 107 and Performance scale IQ score of 102 are also within the average range. Although the patient's Verbal–Performance IQ score discrepancy (5 points) is not diagnostically significant, his inter- and intratest scatter suggests the likelihood of a disruption in cognitive functioning. This is further indicated by the pattern of WAIS-R subtests on which he performs best (Vocabulary, Information) and worst (Comprehension, Similarities, and Digit Symbol). Based on these findings, one would anticipate that academically he performed best on

courses depending on long-term memory (e.g., history) and poorest on those requiring complex abstraction and new learning. His social judgment is also likely poor. Finally, it appears that his cognitive inconsistency has resulted in lower-than-expected IQ scores.

Personality—On objective testing (MMPI, PAI), the patient's profiles consistently suggest someone emphasizing his problems, perhaps making a "plea for help" in the midst of intense psychological turmoil. His MMPI profile is invalid because of excessive endorsement of pathologic items. That is, he overstated his symptoms to an unusual degree. His PAI profile is remarkable for symptoms of depression, anxiety, and assent to disturbed thought processes. Individuals with similar profiles often experience feelings of hopelessness, worthlessness, and personal failure. Their affective distress is often accompanied by a backdrop characterized by social isolation and detachment. They typically have few interpersonal relationships that could be described as deep, close, and supportive. These individuals experience great ambivalence between urges to fulfill unmet needs for affiliation and belongingness and the threatening anxiety they feel related to intimate involvement.

The patient's scores on both the SPS and PAI Suicidal Ideation Scale indicate that he is experiencing intense and recurrent thoughts related to suicide. He should be considered at serious risk for self-harm.

Projective test results also suggest that the patient is experiencing substantial psychological turmoil at this time. Numerous responses on the Rorschach reflect inner disharmony, intense anger, and a possibly burgeoning paranoid cognitive process. A review of his Rorschach protocol reveals descriptors such as "frightening" and "menacing" to card 3 (see Figure 6–2) and "mad," "angry," "being attacked," "decaying," and "about to collapse" to other cards. These projections lead to speculation that the patient is externalizing the emotions and sense of deterioration that he is experiencing internally. The lack of human content perceived on the Rorschach suggests that the patient has likely established a wall between himself and others and is experiencing significant social isolation.

The patient's TAT scenarios provide rich themes of disruptive relations with each parent figure. The patient described a card depicting a father–son interaction as "two ships passing in the night as the father has no awareness or insight into the son's emotional needs." To the family card, he referred to the figures as immersed in their own activities while the son is left to feel "lonely, depressed, and unneeded." He responded to the mother–son card with a scenario in which the child is confused as to what he needs to do to gain his parents' approval or positive attention. Of concern, the patient responded with an upbeat theme of contentment to a TAT card that often generates depressive and sometimes suicidal scenarios.

On the SCT, the patient also provided prominent themes of detachment from parental figures, loneliness, rumination, and social isolation. Most alarming is "Sometimes . . . I think about my own funeral." After the four SCT stems "I am," the patient responds: "lost," "worried," "alone," and "exhausted."

Clinical Impressions—Although the patient denied suicidal ideation or impulses on interview, test results (SPS, PAI, TAT, SCT) consistently suggest that he may be experiencing severe and recurrent thoughts related to self-harm at this time. Close monitoring of the patient in this regard is indicated, with consideration of future hospitalization if warranted. His tendency for isolation and excessive rumination, his apparent perplexity and apprehension about his own functioning, his lack of perceived support, and his age all combine to make him a worrisome patient.

The patient's overall personality test data (including Rorschach perceptions of "decay" and things "collapsing") likely reflect on the patient's own subjective experience of decline. The patient appears preoccupied with his symptoms and failures to the extent that he has lost all interest in others. So apprehensive is this morbid self-concern that the patient appears to be exhibiting profound passivity and social lethargy and, for all practical purposes, appears to be approaching virtual immobility. The patient reported spending much of his day in his room, withdrawn from peer or substantial familial interaction. We would also anticipate that he is moving in the direction of the bottom of the mood cycle with recurring self-annihilative thought content.

On the SPS he responded that he feels he cannot be happy no matter where he is and that the world is not worth continuing to live in. His morbidly depressed feeling tone may reflect grieving over loss of functioning or a component of a possible schizoaffective disorder. We suspect that the patient was able to function academically in a highly structured high school environment but was also perceived as "odd" by teachers and peers. However, the transition to a less-structured college situation may have highlighted how poor his adjustment actually was. Further complicating the situation are his family dynamics, which leave him feeling even further disconnected and unsupported. A major concern in this case is that the patient may be developing a chronic pattern of apathy, dysfunction, severe social disruption, and peculiarity. That is, an evolving schizophrenic or schizoaffective disorder cannot be ruled out.

In addition to pharmacologic management of his cognitive and affective disturbances, some important practical issues will need to be addressed. The patient reported that he anticipates returning to college in the fall. It is difficult at this point to envision that being anything other than another failure experience. He will likely have significant difficulty in attention, persistent concentration, and processing of complex intellectual tasks. If his condition is stabilized by medication, a less severe transition might be considered. For instance, living at home and taking a significantly reduced college course load at a less academically stressful local institution might be worth a try. However, even that might prove a stretch.

An alternative would be referral to a vocational rehabilitation service that could evaluate and direct the patient to an appropriate training or work situation that would be low pressure and highly structured. The patient would likely confront serious difficulties if he tried on his own to enter a competitive work environment. However, with his family background, if he chose the latter option, a job such as a clerk in a hospital medical records' division might be a consideration. Perhaps this option would be more attractive to him and his high-achieving family than would blue-collar work. Further, it would entail relatively limited public contact.

■ TRADITIONAL COGNITIVE TESTING

Traditionally, psychologists have been relied upon to measure cognitive constructs such as intelligence, academic skills, and language abilities. The development of intellectual assessment methods in the early part of the twentieth century, with the subsequent development of standardized assessment methods for a whole range of cognitive functions, added immeasurably to clinical psychiatry's and psychology's understanding of mental retardation and other neurodevelopmental disorders.

Intellectual and academic skills testing is most often sought during childhood development, though at times intellectual functions are also examined in adults. Some common referral questions include:

1. Is this child mentally retarded?
2. Does the patient meet the criteria for an academic skills disorder?
3. Is this child's learning problems due to overall cognitive deficiency, or to attentional and behavioral problems?
4. Is the patient likely to succeed in college?
5. What is the patient's preferred learning style?
6. Does this person have the capacity to parent a child without assistance?

A wide range of psychological tests exists to examine intelligence, academic skills, and other cognitive abilities. The most widely used intellectual tests are the Wechsler series of comprehensive intelligence tests. The Wechsler tests, produced by Harcourt Assessments, are available in different versions for testing throughout the lifespan: preschool (Wechsler Preschool and Primary Scale of Intelligence, 3 years to 7 years 3 months), childhood (Wechsler Intelligence Scale for Children-IV, ages 6 (through 16), and adulthood (Wechsler Adult Intelligence Scale-III, ages 16 through 84). This test in its various forms also often serves as a major portion of most neuropsychological assessments (see below). Another popular comprehensive intelligence test with a venerable history is the Stanford Binet series of intelligence tests, now in its fifth version.

These and other intelligence tests generally provide a composite standard score, known as the intelligence quotient (IQ) that represents the patient's overall performance on the test as compared to others of the same age group. IQ scores are typically expressed as a standard score in which 100 is the mean, with a standard deviation of 15. Thus, a Wechsler Full-Scale IQ score of 115 would correspond to a percentile of 84. A Wechsler Full-Scale IQ of 70 (2nd percentile) represents the traditional margin between individuals considered to be mentally retarded and those not so classified. Of course, scores between one and two standard deviations below the mean reflect a degree of subaverage function, and scores in this range raise the possibility of the DSM classification of "Borderline Intellectual Function."

In addition to a composite score, intelligence tests yield component summary scores reflecting specific areas of function, such as verbal abilities. In the case of the WISC-IV, for example, the Verbal Factor score is a summation of the patient's scores on the subtests tapping general knowledge and verbal expression (Information, Similarities, and Comprehension). Other summary scores, depending on the test used and the theory of its author, include "Performance IQ," or visual-perceptual-motor skills, processing speed, memory, quantitative skills, and sequential versus simultaneous processing.

The Wechsler tests each contain similar subtests that make up the overall tests. It is of course not legally permissible or wise to publish exact intelligence test items. Figure 6–4 provides a set of sample items that are very similar to items found on the Wechsler series of tests, and should convey to the reader a sense of the tasks offered to the patient. General fund of knowledge is assessed on the Information subtest, whereas expressive word knowledge is tapped by the Vocabulary subtest. The Arithmetic subtest measures the patient's ability to compute numerical problems mentally. Digit Span assesses the patient's ability to complete number repetitions forward and backward, thus tapping simple auditory focusing. The pa-

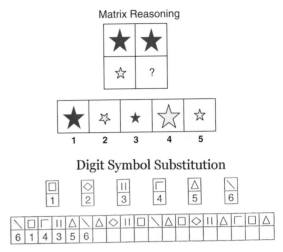

Figure 6–4. Simulated items similar to those in the *Wechsler Intelligence Scales for Adults and Children.* (Copyright © 2005 by Harcourt Assessment, Inc. Reproduced with permission. All rights reserved.)

tient's social judgment and reasoning are evaluated on the Comprehension subtest, on which interpretation of proverbs is also required. On the Similarities subtest, the patient is asked to explain how opposite or unrelated objects (e.g., an orange and a peach) are alike in some obvious or abstract way (e.g., both fruits). The Picture Completion subtest is a visual analysis task in which the patient indicates the essential missing parts of pictures (e.g., a handle on a car door). The Picture Arrangement subtest requires the patient to create a logical sequence for cartoon-like cards that tell a story. On the Block Design subtest, a nonverbal test of abstraction, the patient must use colored blocks to replicate in three dimensions a two-dimensional construction shown on a card. The Object Assembly subtest requires the patient to place jigsaw puzzle pieces together to form familiar objects. The Digit Symbol subtest requires the patient to match numbers to symbols, measuring speed of visual processing. Other subtests found on the WAIS-III include Matrix Reasoning (an untimed test of visual analysis and nonverbal reasoning), Letter–Number Sequencing (a test of working memory and mental control), and Symbol Search (a test involving visual scanning speed and accuracy).

Examination of a patient's performance on summary scores, as well as on individual subtests, can yield a wealth of data about cognitive strengths and weaknesses, learning style, and areas of clinical deficit. For example, a relatively low score on verbally mediated tasks may raise the likelihood of a verbal academic skills disorder, a paucity of educational or cultural learning experiences, or even an aphasic syndrome.

EXHIBIT D

Sample – Paraphrased Wechsler-like Questions

Information

1. How many wings does a bird have?
2. How many nickels make a dime?
3. What is steam made of?
4. Who wrote "Tom Sawyer"?
5. What is pepper?

Comprehension

1. What should you do if you see someone forget his book when he leaves a restaurant?
2. What is the advantage of keeping money in a bank?
3. Why is copper often used in electrical wires?

Arithmetic

1. Sam had three pieces of candy and Joe gave him four more. How many pieces of candy did Sam have altogether?
2. Three women divided eighteen golf balls equally among themselves. How many golf balls did each person receive?
3. If two buttons cost $0.15, what will be the cost of a dozen buttons?

Similarities

1. In what way are a lion and a tiger alike?
2. In what way are a saw and a hammer alike?
3. In what way are an hour and a week alike?
4. In what way are a circle and a triangle alike?

Vocabulary

This test consists simply of asking, "What is a _____?" or "What does _____ mean?" The words cover a wide range of difficulty.

Figure 6–4. *(Continued)*

Academic skills disorders are defined by DSM as a learning impairment that is associated with significantly worse performance on an academic skill than would be expected based on a patient's intelligence. Thus, psychological testing is a necessity for the accurate assessment of such cases. For example, the expected reading level of a young man with an average IQ of 105 would likewise be 105. If his reading score departed significantly from this figure, such as falling in the 70's, the possibility of a reading skills disorder should be entertained. Child psychologists have at their disposal an array of academic skills tests, usually termed "achievement tests," to assess such academic skills as reading, writing, spelling, and mathematical skills. Many of these tests are very sophisticated and comprehensive, allowing for precise diagnosis not only of the overarching academic skills disorder, but also its particular expression in a given child or adult. For example, it is often possible not only to diagnose a reading disorder, but also to determine whether the reading problem is primarily due to failure to identify the word or to comprehend and retain the words' contents.

Sattler JM: *Assessment of Children: Cognitive Applications,* 4th edn. San Diego: Jerome M Sattler, 2001.

■ NEUROPSYCHOLOGICAL ASSESSMENT

Neuropsychological assessment refers to the application of standardized measurement techniques to determine the relationship between brain impairment and its cognitive and behavioral concomitants. Interest in cases that focus on the interface between psychiatry and neurology provided the impetus for the modern clinical development of neuropsychology as an important subspecialty within clinical psychology. The clinical neuropsychologist is typically a clinical psychologist who is also trained in the neurosciences and clinical neurology. The application of standardized cognitive measurement techniques to brain-behavior relationships has proved a useful and often determinative source of information in individuals with neurodevelopmental disorders and acquired brain dysfunction. The American Academy of Neurology (1996) has produced official guidelines affirming the value of neuropsychological assessment in the practice of neurology.

Neuropsychological assessment in the psychiatric setting is often indicated when questions about cognition or brain-behavior relationships are raised during the course of the psychiatric evaluation that are not explicable by history, mental status observations, radiological techniques, or laboratory techniques alone. The neuropsychologist is typically called upon when a complex set of symptoms and behaviors dictates indepth measurement and observation of an individual's neurocognitive function and/or neurobehavioral characteristics.

Once used primarily to help identify focal brain lesions, the role of neuropsychology in diagnosis has diminished somewhat with the advent of advanced neuroradiological techniques. However, neuroimaging may provide equivocal results in many instances of diffusely based disorders (e.g., hypoxic–anoxic dementia, neurotoxic exposure, early dementia). Magnetic resonance imaging (MRI) techniques may detect gross structural damage but not changes at the molecular or cellular level. Under such circumstances, neuropsychological testing may provide a more sensitive measure of brain function. For example, neuropsychological testing is useful in distinguishing between early dementia and those symptoms of depression that mimic cognitive impairment. Because these conditions may be present simultaneously, sorting out the relative contribution of each can help indicate appropriate treatment. Depressed elderly patients perform differently on neuropsychological tests than do patients with irreversible cognitive deficits, although the deficits may be indistinguishable on mental status examination. Indepth neuropsychological testing can lead to a better perspective of the patient's effort and level of energy, frequency of giving up on more difficult items, attempts to minimize deficiencies, and patterns of strengths and weaknesses.

Psychiatrists and psychologists are often called upon to estimate whether a brain-injured individual has returned to a prior level of function, such as when confronted with the question of whether the patient can return to work. This is also an issue of great interest in many medicolegal situations, such as the estimation of compensable impairment in workers' compensation injuries, or damage liability in personal injury cases. For example, after receiving a left frontal contusion, a law student may expect to encounter difficulty in classes that tap verbal reasoning, whereas a skilled machinist might be just as debilitated from a comparable right-hemisphere lesion. Examination of these referrals often hinges upon comparison of current test results with premorbid abilities. Premorbid function can be assessed informally by taking a careful history including prior educational achievement, occupations, daily activities, hobbies, and personal achievements. Both actuarial and assessment techniques also exist that allow for estimation of prior function. Prior intelligence can be predicted within a degree of error by mathematical regression techniques, utilizing demographic information such as educational level, occupational history, age, and region of the country. Reading ability is highly resistant to most acquired cognitive disorders, with the exception of course of alexia. Thus, reading skill is a good marker of prior function. Other cognitive skills that can be assessed with the neuropsychological evaluation tend to remain constant, even with significant cortical insults. The most powerful techniques are those which mathematically combine both psychometric data with demographic estimation techniques (e.g., Wechsler Test of Adult Reading, Oklahoma Premorbid Intelligence Assessment).

Referral for assessment of patients in the acute recovery process from stroke or traumatic brain injury can assist with treatment planning regardless of whether diagnosis is an issue. However, within the first few days or weeks of recovery from acute compromise in ability, as occurs with head injury or stroke, a comprehensive evaluation may not be appropriate for two reasons. First, data may not be reliable because of disruption of attentional mechanisms and, therefore, may not reflect the patient's true capacities at the time of testing. Second, until the patient has stabilized and begun to reach a plateau of recovery, limited predictive value can be gathered from testing. For example, the prognostic value of testing a patient at 3 weeks after cessation of drinking will more accurately predict long-term recovery than will similar testing done at 3 days. In degenerative illnesses (e.g., dementia), repeated longitudinal evaluations are essential for accurate diagnosis and tracking of symptom progression. Differential diagnosis is sometimes not possible without follow-up testing, in which case the first evaluation serves as a baseline.

In variable or ongoing illness, such as multiple sclerosis or epilepsy, timing is also essential in that the referring psychiatrist must have an idea of whether a recent exacerbation has occurred. Also, fatigue, anxiety, and performance inconsistencies due to recent seizures, motivational problems, and lack of tolerance in brain-compromised patients must be considered in the referral process. These issues are critical because results will have varying prognostic value depending on the point at which the patient is evaluated.

Another important set of referral questions addresses the patient's level of residual functional capacity after recovery. Normal resumption of activities of daily living, socialization, and performance in work-like settings may not be possible depending on age, course of illness, severity of injury, and the presence of concomitant psychiatric illness. These are functional questions that may be best answered by a combination of assessment techniques, including administering formalized tests (see next section), observing the patient in demanding environments, interviewing the family, and taking a complete history of illness.

American Academy of Neurology: Assessment: neuropsychological testing of adults: Considerations for neurologists. *Neurology,* 47, 592–599, 1996.

Heilman KM, Valenstein E (eds): *Clinical Neuropsychology,* 4th edn. New York: Oxford University Press, 2003.

NEUROPSYCHOLOGICAL ASSESSMENT INSTRUMENTS

The most recent version of a popular handbook for neuropsychologists reviews more than 160 tests that have found their way into common use among neuropsychologists (Strauss et al., 2006), and these are only a small subset of the tests available commercially or in the research literature. Instead of attempting to present specific tests

to the reader, categories and representative examples of neuropsychological tests will be described here, in order to convey a sense of the range and utility of neuropsychological testing.

Intelligence Tests in Neuropsychological Assessment

As noted above, a comprehensive intelligence test, usually the Wechsler test appropriate to the age of the patient, often serves as the backbone of most neuropsychological evaluations. Comprehensive intelligence tests have the advantage of carefully developed norms and the fact that they tap many key neurocognitive abilities (e.g., verbal expression, processing speed, visual analytic skills). Due to the development of the standardization samples on these tests, it is also possible to account for the expected effects of such variables as educational level and ethnicity, if desired. A disadvantage is the fact that comprehensive IQ scores and summary index scores tend to be resistant to changes caused by neurocognitive disorders. Partially, this is due to the fact that neurocognitive disorders rarely cause generalized dysfunction except in more severe cases. Also, intelligence tests are not weighted heavily with executive function and memory tests, the tests shown to be most sensitive to cortical dysfunction. Indeed, it is not unusual for an early- to mid-stage Alzheimer's patient to be relatively debilitated due to memory loss, but score near normal limits on most sections of the WAIS, or for a Pick's Disease patient to exhibit grossly inappropriate behavior but have an average or better IQ.

Folstein Mini-Mental State Examination

The Folstein Mini-Mental State Examination (MMSE) is a universally recognized neuropsychological test that is widely used by psychiatrists, psychologists, neurologists, and geriatric practitioners. This test taps several cognitive functions including orientation, word memory, naming, verbal comprehension, writing, and drawing. Benefits of the MMSE are the instant recognizability of the test and the fact that so many clinicians across differing disciplines can readily interpret its scores. Unfortunately, it is short on items tapping executive function, and its memory section, as generally administered, is crude. The MMSE is often supplanted with tests that have additional memory and executive items to allow for greater sensitivity to senile dementia and a broader range of assessed functions (e.g., Modified MMSE; Dementia Rating scale).

Halstead-Reitan Neuropsychological Test Battery

The Halstead-Reitan Neuropsychological Test Battery (HRNTB) contains many of the most commonly used neuropsychological tests. It originated from the work of Ward Halstead, who in 1947 at the University of Chicago, published his observations of several hundred case studies of patients who had frontal lobe damage. By using 10 scores, Halstead blindly distinguished patients with confirmed brain lesions from control subjects. Ralph Reitan, a student of Halstead's, modified the battery in 1955 to identify lateralizing features of patient performances such as motor deficits expected in subtle stroke, the effect of temporal lobe epilepsy on memory, and the loss of abstraction ability associated with frontal damage. Reitan also modified the original battery to include tests that would accurately measure aphasia and variations of normal aging. The battery often had limited utility other than in merely determining the presence of organicity before other techniques (e.g., neuroimaging) were available to do so. From continued use of the battery over the decades, three of the original ten scores were dropped because of questionable validity.

Currently, the Halstead Impairment Index is the most widely accepted global measure of brain dysfunction in neuropsychology. Most normal subjects are able to pass 60–100% of the tests included in the Index. Patients who have moderate impairments may be within the normal range on only 30–60% of the tests, and those with severe dysfunction on less than 30%. The Index includes seven scores within the following five subtests:

1. Category Test—The Category Test is an abstract reasoning task consisting of 180 items. The patient is required to use mental flexibility and problem solving to form concepts, utilizing feedback from the examiner about the accuracy of their attempts.

2. Tactual Performance Test—The Tactual Performance Test is a test requiring the integration of multiple cognitive skills: spatial skills, spatial memory, dexterity, processing speed, and planning ability. The patient is blindfolded and placed before a board with cutouts into which blocks can be inserted. The patient is then asked to place the blocks in the cutouts, first using the dominant hand, then the nondominant hand, then both. Then the patient is asked to draw a representation of the board from memory. Since more than 40% of the brain's processing power is devoted to visual processing, removal of vision presumably cripples the efficiency with which the patient can approach the task. For the brain-injured patient, excessive time is often required to complete this task. The lateralized nature of the test allows for some comparison of relative hemispheric efficiency.

3. Finger Tapping Test—Finger tapping is a test of fine motor speed. Five consecutive 10-second trials are obtained with the dominant and nondominant index fingers, and then compared to norms. Injury to either region of motor cortex, as well as injuries affecting overall cortical efficiency, can result in degraded scores on this task.

4. Rhythm Test—The Rhythm test originated from the Seashore Measures of Musical Talent test, in which the patient is asked to differentiate between 30 pairs of rhythmic patterns. These pairs are presented in rapid succession on a tape recorder, and the patient must distinguish whether they are the same or different.

5. Speech Sounds Perception Test—The Speech Sounds Perception Test involves 60 spoken nonsense words that are administered by audiotape. The patient is required to underline the corresponding printed response on an answer sheet, measuring verbal discrimination and sustained attention.

General Neuropsychological Deficit Scale

In addition to the seven scores provided by five Index subtests, other subtests from the HRNTB are used to represent patients' performances on the General Neuropsychological Deficit scale (GNDS). Subtests used to contribute to this scale, in addition to those in the Index, include the Lateral Dominance examination, Grip Strength, the Sensory–Perceptual examination, Tactile Form Recognition, the Trail-Making Test Parts A and B, and the Aphasia Screening test. The GNDS, much like the Impairment Index, provides a global impairment rating but takes into account 42 variables, thus increasing reliability. Clinical judgment also allows the clinician to take into account variables in the interpretation of data related to level and pattern of performance, pathognomonic signs and laterality."

Heaton RK, Miller SW, Taylor MJ, Grant I: *Revised Comprehensive Norms for an Expanded Halstead-Reitan Battery: Demographically Adjusted Neuropsychological Norms for African American and Caucasian Adults.* Odessa, FL: Psychological Assessment Resources, Inc. 2004.

Reitan R, Wolfson D: *The Halstead-Reitan Neuropsychological Test Battery: Theory and Clinical Application.* Tucson, AZ: Neuropsychology Press, 1993.

Strauss E, Sherman EMS, Spreen O: *A Compendium of Neuropsychological Tests: Administration, Norms, and Commentary, 3rd edn.* New York: Oxford University Press, 2006.

FUNCTIONS MEASURED IN NEUROPSYCHOLOGICAL ASSESSMENTS

Sensorimotor Functions

Many neuropsychologists administer a partial neurological examination as part of their overall assessment. Depending on the referral questions, the sensorimotor assessment may include informal testing of olfactory function, visual fields, auditory perception, stereognosis (tactile appreciation of objects), and cerebellar function (e.g., heel-to-shin testing, alternating hand movements). As mentioned above, standardized testing of strength, motor speed (hand and foot tapping), and fine motor control are generally a component of the examination.

Attention and Concentration

After assuring an adequate level of consciousness, assessment of attention provides fundamental information as to whether evaluation of other cognitive domains, such as intelligence, memory, or language, will be valid. Further, because the ability to focus and maintain attention is highly sensitive to many acute and ongoing conditions (e.g., alcohol withdrawal, intoxication, delirium), a stable, chronic process may be affected less than will a recent or changing one. At the most basic level, this domain measures the patient's ability to attend to incoming information without being distracted. Examples of simple attentional tasks include digit repetition or visual tapping span, requiring forward or backward sequencing of auditory or visual stimuli.

Sustained attention, known as vigilance or continuous performance, is another type of attention. Attention Deficit Hyperactivity Disorder (ADHD) is a disruptive behavior disorder in which individuals have a great deal of difficulty avoiding distractions and maintaining appropriate, goal-directed behavior. A newer area of cognitive assessment that shows great promise for practitioners who work with ADHD children and adults is continuous performance testing for sustained attention (e.g., Conners Continuous Performance Test, Test of Variables of Attention). Continuous performance tests are most often computer-administered, and generally exist in either visual or auditory formats. In the visual modality, the child (or adult) is asked to sit before a computer screen and to respond to one type of stimulus, while suppressing responses to another. The tests go on for several minutes, and the boring nature of the task tends to elicit omissions and variable response times from individuals with attentional deficits. While only limited success has been achieved with these tests as diagnostic instruments for ADHD, they are quite successful in measuring the effectiveness of psychostimulant medication on individuals known to have ADHD. As such, an assessment using these tests can allow the psychiatrist to avoid the use of costly and potentially risky psychostimulant medications among patients who are unresponsive to its effects. These tests are also widely used by neuropsychologists to assess the attentional abilities of brain-injured patients.

Figure 6–5 represents the attempt of a right parietal stroke patient to complete a sustained visual attention task, the Mesulam Visual Cancellation Task, revealing neglect in the left visual field. This patient resumed driving after her stroke, but she likely contributed to an accident when she pulled into traffic and was struck by a car she did not see on the left side. Similar lateralized inattention may occur in other modalities (e.g., tactile) when patients have focal lesions.

Learning and Memory

Compromise of memory is the most common patient complaint and referral question for neuropsychological testing. Milder memory problems, or problems with visual memory may not be readily apparent on screening tasks such as the MMSE. Because memory is not a static or unitary process, careful assessment can help to characterize variations in performance, which can have diagnostic value. Patients who have anterograde amnesia, or faulty learning of new material or events after the onset of their disorder, have more difficulty consolidating their learning experiences into longer storage. Retrograde amnesia, or the inability to retrieve remote memories, is less prominent in organic memory loss, especially if the onset is sudden, as in head injury. However, certain chronic conditions and disease processes, such as Korsakoff's syndrome and Alzheimer's disease, may produce a more dense retrograde amnesia. Memory is often evaluated in the mental status examination by assessing orientation, current events, and recall of words or objects. Although screening is sometimes adequate to determine the presence of a gross dementia, full neuropsychological evaluation can detect whether the difficulty is with encoding, storage, or retrieval mechanisms, and whether the impairment is associated more with one modality than another (e.g., verbal or visual).

The most widely used global memory test is the Wechsler Memory Scale (WMS), now undergoing its most recent revision, which will result in the WMS-IV. These tests yield memory quotients similar to IQ scores (expected mean is 100; standard deviation is 15). It provides for evaluation of immediate memory, delayed memory, and working memory skills, in both visual and verbal modalities.

Language

Testing for aphasia is a necessary part of diagnosis and treatment planning in some developmental and learning disabilities, progressive disorders (e.g., dementia, tumor), or recovery from an acute injury such as stroke or head injury. Impairment of language on a gross level is often more noticeable because of the frequent need for clear communication. However, subtle language deficits can go undetected in informal conversation and occasionally in more formal assessment. At the very least, language screening should include tasks to measure quality of spontaneous speech, naming, comprehension, repetition,

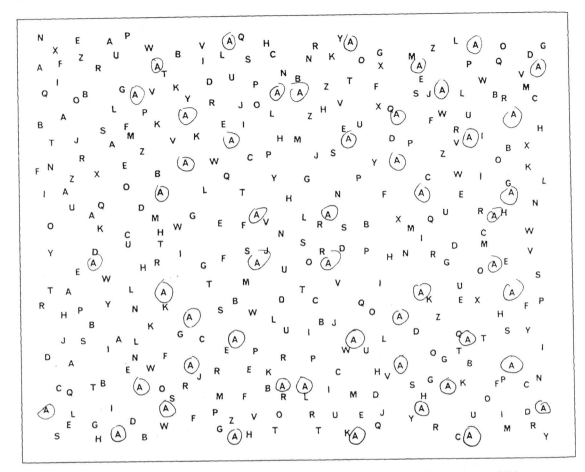

Figure 6–5. The Visual Cancellation Task from Mesulam (1986) showing neglect of target letters (A's) on extreme left. (Reproduced by permission of FA Davis Co.)

reading, writing, calculation, and left–right orientation. Naming, the most sensitive element of most underlying language disturbances, is often measured through confrontational naming tasks such as the Boston Naming Test, a 60-item test of picture identification. Well-studied aphasia screening batteries include the Boston Diagnostic Aphasia examination and the Western Aphasia Battery. If the neuropsychological assessment confirms the presence of aphasia, a speech language pathology evaluation may be required to plan detailed treatment.

Executive Functions

Executive functions refer to cognition and personality skills that are integrative in nature, allowing the person to attend to salient stimuli while disregarding others, maintain situational awareness, plan, reason hypothetically, solve problems, self-monitor demands and emotional

reactions; in short, executive function is composed of all metacognitive and emotional processes that serve to help the person adapt to the environment or reach an overarching goal. Though many of these functions are partly if not primarily subserved by the frontal lobes, their complex nature generally requires the entire brain working in concert for maximal success, thus the descriptive term "integrative functions" is also often used. Neuropsychological functioning under the rubric of executive tasks includes abstraction, problem solving, set generation and sequencing, ability to maintain or terminate behaviors, and ability to plan and organize. These functions are mediated by the frontal lobes. Personality characteristics having to do with judgment, social appropriateness, inhibition versus impulsivity, and motivation are also at least partially related to frontal activity. The most famous example of an organically driven personality change is that of Phineas Gage, a railroad worker in the 1880s, who sustained a traumatic injury to the frontal lobes when a tamping iron was blown through his head. This formerly docile, responsible worker became irascible, foul-mouthed, and disinhibited. As his reckless and menacing behavior continued, his coworkers described him as "no longer Gage."

Specific tasks that are frequently used to study the integrity of the frontal systems include the Wisconsin Card Sorting Test. This procedure provides an index of how well the examinee can formulate hypotheses and solve problems. Cards are matched by principles that are not stated directly, and the patient must shift cognitive sets as the rules for sorting change without forewarning. Other good measures of executive functioning include Controlled Oral Word Fluency, which requires verbal set generation (e.g., words beginning with certain letters), the Category test (concept formation), and the Trail-Making Test (measuring visual shifting and sequencing).

Visuospatial Functioning

Visuospatial functioning measures both the patient's ability to function within his or her environment with regard to recognition of objects and his or her construction and perception of spatial relations. Such abilities are important in daily activities that require the patient to recognize faces and remember geographic location and spatial orientation and in procedural learning tasks such as driving a car. Because patients with progressive neurologic disorders such as Alzheimer's disease or right hemisphere strokes are particularly susceptible to deficits in this area, careful testing will be able to determine whether the patient is likely to encounter problems in getting lost or living independently. Figure copying, clock drawing, visual organization of parts to whole, facial recognition, and map orientation are samples of tasks used to assess this domain.

Mesulam M: *Principles of Behavioral Neurology.* Philadelphia, PA: FA Davis Co, 1986.

Tranel D: Neuropsychological assessment. *Psychiatr Clin N Am* 1992; 15:283.

CLINICAL DECISION MAKING IN NEUROPSYCHOLOGICAL ASSESSMENT

Before the psychiatrist or neurologist can be assured of the diagnosis of dementia or other acquired cognitive disorders, most often a host of alternative diagnoses must be ruled out. For depression, delirium caused by physical illness or medication effects, a recent but recovering brain insult (e.g., closed head injury), recent seizures, and malingering are only a few possible explanations for apparently impaired function or transiently deficient test scores. In cases of documented brain compromise

from treatable conditions, the psychiatrist may wish to begin appropriate therapy (e.g., treatment of depression in pseudodementia). If cognitive recovery is less than expected, follow-up neuropsychological examination or referral for further neurodiagnostic procedures may be warranted.

In some cases, neuropsychological evaluation may provide the only means for detecting alteration or recovery in brain function in more subtle disorders. Additionally, an estimate of the patient's capacity to return to normal work and social activities will be addressed most effectively in an open dialogue with the referring psychiatrist. The following case example illustrates the need for such close communication.

Neuropsychological Evaluation Report

A 23-year-old single female was seen in psychotherapy for depression, which was thought to be a reaction secondary to an unwanted pregnancy. Although distinct neurovegetative signs were absent, the patient's family noticed that she was socially withdrawn and had lost interest in usual activities. She had difficulty initiating behavior and spent most of her day appearing "bored," according to her concerned family. She spent most of her time sitting motionless in front of the television. Although she did not exhibit improvement from psychotherapy, sessions were continued. The patient's development of severe headaches was thought to be related to depression. When she developed a slight right facial droop, language abnormalities, and a right hemiparesis, she was referred for organic workup, including neuropsychological testing. Examination revealed an expressive aphasia, slowness in initiating activity, poor planning ability, decreased judgment, and a marked visual neglect on the right visual field. This finding coincided with her clock drawing (Figure 6–6A), which showed obvious right-sided neglect due to the frontal mass shown on MRI (Figure 6–6B). On surgical removal, the mass was found to be a rare meningioma.

ASSESSMENT OF MALINGERING

The possible presence of faked or exaggerated symptoms for personal gain is a vital threat to the validity of any examination, mental or medical. Numerous studies have shown that malingering is common among psychiatric and neurological patients who are referred for psychological or neuropsychological evaluation and also engaged in litigation, workers' compensation actions, or disability insurance findings. Most studies suggest a 30–50%

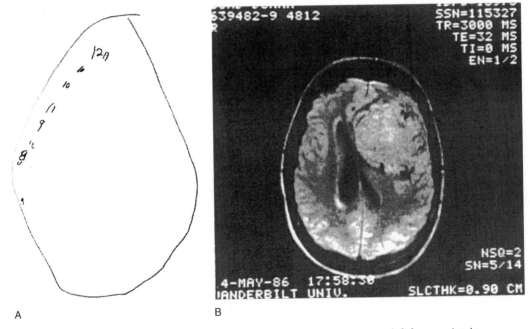

Figure 6–6. (A) Clock drawing showing neglect of right side. (B) MRI showing left front parietal tumor.

proportion of malingering patients among such referrals. Even young children have been shown in research studies to be able to successfully mislead skilled clinicians. The prospect that one out of every two or three medicolegal patients is feigning or exaggerating is a sobering one, and one whose implications are arresting for the average clinician who prefers to take care of patients rather than systematically investigate the validity of the patient's complaints. The situation is seen to be even more complex when one considers that in the course of everyday practice, the potential agenda of some patients may not be apparent for weeks until a letter arrives from an insurer or the local disability determination office.

Patients often malinger physical disorders, pain, psychosis, posttraumatic stress disorder, severe depression, panic disorder, seizures, and memory deficits, to name a few feigned presentations. Disorders that are episodically manifested, such as panic attacks or seizures, represent a unique challenge to the clinician because of the relative lack of power of the mental status examination. In our experience, memory deficits are often feigned, presumably because it seems to many patients that loss of memory would be easy to both describe and feign on examination, though these expectations are in fact inaccurate.

The most powerful tool the clinician has in identifying malingered disorders is thorough knowledge of, and experience with, the disorder in question. It is a challenge for most patients to learn what symptoms to report to feign a given disorder, and an even greater challenge to

convincingly produce facsimiles of symptoms upon mental status examination. For this reason, referrals to rule out malingering should preferably be sent to clinicians who are very experienced with the disorder in question. The patient suspected of feigning schizophrenia should be referred to a specialist in psychotic disorders, and the apparently head-injured patient to a clinician with extensive experience with patients who have experienced mild, moderate, and severe head injuries.

Another powerful tool to detect malingering is psychological assessment. Many standardized psychological assessment techniques are now available for assessing many malingered disorders. Referral to a psychologist, or neuropsychologist in the case of suspected malingered dementia, presents several advantages to the psychiatrist or neurologist. The quantitative nature of the results yields an ability to report more precisely and convincingly the impression of malingering. It is much better, in our experience, to be able to report that "Test X indicated a 95% probability of malingering," than to have to base such a grave determination on clinical observations and judgment alone. Deferring the question to a referral source allows the clinician to maintain some professional distance from the situation, perhaps allowing a therapeutic relationship with the patient to be maintained, even if the conclusion is adverse. And finally, malingering tests are much more successful at detecting exaggeration or malingering when the patient is very clever, has been coached, or is claiming subtle deficits or symptoms.

VERBAL SUBTEST

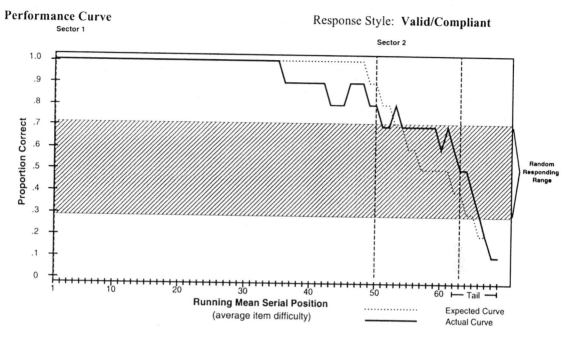

NONVERBAL SUBTEST

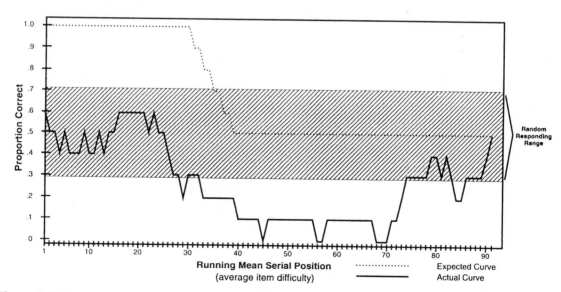

Figure 6–7. Test profiles from the Validity Indicator Profile, showing both effortful and invalid performances. (Copyright © 1997, 2003 by NCS Pearson, Inc. VIP Performance Curve reproduced by permission of the copyright holder.)

DETECTION OF MALINGERED PSYCHIATRIC SYMPTOMS

The MMPI-2 and the PAI, discussed previously, both contain scales designed to detect the exaggerating or the overly defensive patient. Much more research has been done with the MMPI-2 in this area, making it the better choice if only one test can be administered. Scales have been developed for the MMPI-2 to assess wholesale endorsement of unusual symptoms (F scale, F [B] scale); endorsement of unusual symptoms rarely endorsed even by an inpatient psychiatric population (F [p] scale), and to identify patients who are feigning physical debility (Fake Bad scale), just to name a few. The MMPI-2 also has a scale that identifies persons who are presenting themselves as unusually virtuous (Lie scale), and several scales of defensiveness, or tendency to deny negative or unhealthy characteristics.

Another test used to identify individuals feigning psychiatric problems is a structured interview technique, the Structured Interview of Reported Symptoms (SIRS). Developed by Rogers (1991), the SIRS provides for systematic assessment of common patterns of responses and behaviors in malingering patients, such as assent to absurd symptoms, improbable combinations of symptoms, and differences between item endorsement and observable behaviors. The SIRS was designed to minimize false positives, that is, to avoid identifying individuals as malingering who are not feigning mental illness. As such, it fails to identify a proportion of malingerers, but is very successful in given forensic populations where patients often grossly overendorse symptoms while faking psychosis or other debilitating syndromes.

DETECTION OF MALINGERED COGNITIVE DEFICITS

Many patients present with malingered memory or reasoning deficits. Intellectual, neuropsychological, and other cognitive tests can be easily compromised by poor effort, and often such lack of effort is intentional. Without formal testing for malingering, low test scores or apparent dementia on mental status examination may inaccurately result in classifications of patients as demented or mentally retarded. Even children have been shown to be able to successfully feign cognitive deficits.

Cognitive malingering tests utilize several different strategies to detect feigned cognitive problems, and fortunately knowledge of these strategies does not always subvert the tests, even in clever and well-informed patients. One set of tests utilizes floor effect tests, that is, tests that appear to be difficult but in fact are nearly always successfully performed even by individuals with moderate cognitive impairment. The malingering patient often scores well below the expected level as compared to genuinely impaired patients, thus allowing a probabilistic determination of malingering to be made.

Forced choice tests are another strategy, often combined with the strategy above. These tests utilize the fact that forcing the patient to guess between two dichotomous responses, one correct and the other incorrect, results in a known expected value if the patient has no ability in that area at all: 50%. If a patient scores significantly worse than he or she would by flipping a coin, then strong evidence of malingering is produced. In that circumstance, the only credible explanation is that the patient must have known the right answer, since the wrong one was so often chosen. When failed, these tests provide the strongest evidence of malingering. The technique is also adaptable to a wide variety of possibly malingered conditions, e.g., blindness, tactual imperception, deafness. Unfortunately, very few malingers fail forced choice tests, presumably recognizing that a higher level of performance would be the norm even for a severely impaired individual.

An example of a widely used test that combines both forced-choice and floor effect features is the Test of Memory Malingering (TOMM). This test is composed of fifty pictures, which are shown to the patient in repeated trials. The patient is tested by being given a dichotomous choice between each correct picture and a foil. The patient's score yields a classification of likelihood of malingering. If the patient scores below chance levels, a precise probability rating can be assigned demonstrating the certainty level of malingering beyond any reasonable question.

Other cognitive malingering tests utilize known principles of learning or test taking to identify unusual patterns of test performance. For example, even individuals with severe memory impairment tend to respond with significantly more correct answers when they are given recognition choices. Another principle is that, on average, the patient should score better on easier items than on more difficult ones, and that once a patient's level of ability has been exceeded, further answers should have no greater accuracy than chance. The Validity Indicator Profile is a successful test utilizing this principle. Figure 6–7 shows two VIP profiles in which the patients' accuracy of responses is charted. The first profile represents an honest, effortful profile on the verbal portion of the VIP. The patient successfully gets most of the easier items correct, then a point is reached at which mistakes are made. Eventually the patient is able to perform no better than chance. On the Nonverbal subtest, however, the patient is malingering. The patient fails many items, even though the profile shows that he can pass more difficult items successfully. These results are consistent with a patient feigning reasoning problems, but presenting with intact language function, a common combination among sophisticated malingerers feigning disability.

Frederick RI: *Validity Indicator Profile Test Manual.* Minneapolis National Computer Systems, 1997.

Rogers R: *Clinical Assessment of Malingering and Deception, 2nd edn.* New York: Guilford Press, 1997.

Tombaugh TN: *Test of Memory Malingering.* North Tonawanda, NY: Multi-Health Systems, 1996.

CONCLUSION

This chapter has attempted to provide the reader with an introduction to psychological evaluation techniques that are relevant to psychiatry. Psychological testing often provides clinicians with greater diagnostic confidence than interview data alone. It is uniquely useful for comprehensively describing personality styles, diagnosing syndromes dependent upon psychometric data (e.g., mental retardation, academic skills disorders), comprehensively describing a patient's neurocognitive functions, and identifying malingering patients.

Psychological testing referrals from medical specialties other than psychiatry are becoming much more commonplace. Internists and orthopedists typically refer for psychological testing patients with pain complaints for which no organic basis can be detected, or for which the complaints are far in excess of what one would anticipate from physical findings. Transplant surgeons want information about an individual's cognitive ability to follow a complex medical regimen and how personality factors may affect treatment compliance. Neurologists and neurosurgeons utilize neuropsychological evaluation in differentiating the relative contributions of neurologic and psychological factors in a patient's behavioral symptoms. Contemporary personality and neuropsychological techniques are linked closely to advances in statistical methodology. The increasing partnership between quantitative psychology and psychological assessment holds promise for improving our understanding and measurement of complex human behavior.

Diagnostic Evaluation for Children and Adolescents

Barry Nurcombe, MD, Michael Tramontana, PhD

7

Based on the diagnostic hypotheses (generated, tested, and refined during history taking), the mental status examination, and the observation of family interaction, the inquiry plan proceeds to physical examination and, if required, to laboratory testing, special investigations, consultations, and psychological testing.

Figure 7–1 summarizes the flow of clinical reasoning from history taking, mental status examination, the generation of diagnostic hypotheses, through physical examination and special investigations, the refinement of the clinical pattern, secondary diagnostic hypotheses, psychological testing, and the diagnostic conclusion, to the diagnostic formulation and treatment plan.

■ I. CHILD MENTAL STATUS EXAMINATION

■ PURPOSE OF THE CHILD MENTAL STATUS EXAMINATION

The child mental status examination is a set of systematic observations and assessments that provide a detailed description of the child's behavior during the diagnostic interview. Combined with the history and physical assessment, the mental status examination yields evidence that helps the clinician to refine, delete, or accept the diagnostic hypotheses generated during the diagnostic encounter (see Chapter 34), and to decide whether special investigations are needed in order to test particular diagnostic hypotheses. Thus, the mental status examination is an integral part of the inquiry plan. In accordance with the diagnostic hypotheses and the inquiry plan, the mental status examination may be brief or comprehensive, but it always incorporates both standard and discretionary probes.

The mental status examination of the adolescent is similar to that of the adult (see Chapter 4). However, the examination of children is sufficiently different to warrant separate discussion. Many of the observations required to complete the mental status examination are made in the course of the semistructured interview with the child (see Chapter 5). Other observations, such as the clinical tests that screen cognitive functions, are part of a standardized set of questions.

■ AREAS ADDRESSED BY THE MENTAL STATUS EXAMINATION

Table 7–1 lists the areas covered by the mental status examination. For the most part, the first five areas are noted as the interview proceeds, whereas the last five require special questions.

Appearance

Note the following: height, weight, nutritional status; precocious or delayed physical maturation or secondary sexual characteristics; abnormalities of the skin, head, facies, neck, or general physique; personal hygiene and grooming; and style and appropriateness of dress.

Motor Behavior

Observe the following: general level of physical activity (e.g., hyperkinesis, hypokinesis, bradykinesis), in comparison with others of the same age; abnormalities of gait, balance, posture, tone, power, and fine and gross motor coordination; abnormal movements (e.g., tremor, twitching, shivering, tics, fidgeting, choreiform movements, athetoid movements, motor overflow); mannerisms, rituals, echopraxia, or stereotyped movements; motor impersistence; or pronounced startle response.

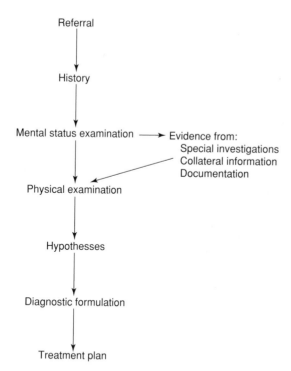

Referral

↓

History

↓

Mental status examination → Evidence from:
Special investigations
Collateral information
Documentation

↓

Physical examination

↓

Hypotheses

↓

Diagnostic formulation

↓

Treatment plan

Figure 7–1. The process of clinical reasoning.

Voice, Speech, & Language

Listen for the following: accent; abnormality in pitch, tone, volume, phonation, or prosody (e.g., squawking, shouting, whispering, monotony, hoarseness, scanning, high-pitched voice); abnormality in the amount of speech (e.g., mute, impoverished, voluble, loquacious) or its tempo (e.g., slowed, accelerated); abnormal rhythm (e.g., stuttering); abnormal articulation (e.g., dyslalia); unusual or inappropriate use of words (e.g., idioglossia, profanity); echolalia; abnormal syntax; and impairment in expressive or receptive language (e.g., difficulty finding words).

Table 7–1. Areas Covered by the Mental Status Examination

Appearance
Motor behavior
Voice, speech, and language
Interaction with the examiner
Mood and affect
Cognitive functions
Thought processes
Thought content
Fantasy
Insight

Interaction with the Examiner

Note the patient's eye contact (e.g., eyes averted, unfocussed, staring). Is the child friendly and cooperative, or resistant, oppositional, shy, or withdrawn? Is he or she assertive, aggressive, impudent, sarcastic, cynical, fearful, clinging, inhibited, indifferent, clowning, invasive, coy, or seductive? Is the child a reliable informant?

Mood & Affect

In demeanor and conversation, does the patient show evidence of a persistent abnormality of mood or of poor emotional regulation? For example, is there evidence of anxiety, tension, rage, depression, elevation of mood, silliness, apathy, or anhedonia? Is the child emotionally labile, or conversely, does he or she exhibit a restricted range of affect? Which topics evoke the most intense emotion?

Cognitive Functions

Cognitive screening tests do not replace formal psychological testing. They serve as rapid clinical screens to determine whether formal testing is required. The following areas should be tested: attention, orientation, memory (immediate, recent, remote), judgment, abstraction, and intelligence (see Panels I–VI). Do not proceed with the tests described in the accompanying panels unless the patient has demonstrated a basic familiarity with numbers, letters, and words (see Table 7–2).

Thought Processes

Is there evidence of abnormal tempo, with flight of ideas or acceleration, slowing, or poverty of thought processes? Does the stream of thought lack clear goal direction, with vagueness, incoherence, circumstantiality, tangential thinking, derailment, or clang associations? Is the normal continuity of associations disrupted by perseveration, circumlocution, circumstantiality, distractibility, or blocking? Is there evidence of impairment in logical or metaphorical thinking, for example, in a blurring of conceptual boundaries or abnormally concrete thinking?

Table 7–2. Prescreening Questions for Cognitive Testing

Area	Ask Patient To
Numbers	Count from 1 to 20
Letters	Recite the alphabet
Words	Point to his or her nose, mouth, chin, neck, and knees

I. ASSESSMENT OF ATTENTION

Clinician: "Listen carefully. I'm going to say some numbers, but sometimes I'll say a letter instead.
Say Yes! each time you hear me say a letter instead of a number."
Recite the following at the rate of one item per second:

1 2 3 D 9 8 A 4 E Z 6 1 5 9 T 3 B 8 2 Q 7 3 2 J L 4 8 2 C

Evaluation:
Record number of errors of omission: _____
Record number of errors of commission: _____
Total: _____

Clinician: "Listen again. This time I'm going to say some letters, but sometimes I'll say a number instead. Say Yes!
each time you hear me say a number instead of a letter."
Recite the following at the rate of one item per second:

B K L 4 O(oh) 6 P M 9 C N F O(oh) P 6 S 1(one) E G 3 J H U 0(zero) 9 6 W T 5

Evaluation:
Record number of errors of omission: _____
Record number of errors of commission: _____
Total: _____

Serial sevens. *Clinician:* "Can you subtract 7 from 100? What is 100 minus 7?" *If correct, say:* "Good. I want you
to count backwards, taking 7 from 100, then 7 from 93, as far back as you can." *(Record response)*

Correct answer: 93, 86, 79, 72, 65, 58, 51, 44, 37, 30, 23, 16, 9, 2

Evaluation:
Record time (seconds) taken to reach final number: _____
Record number of errors: _____

If the subject cannot subtract 7 from 100, try serial threes.

Serial threes. *Clinician:* "Can you subtract 3 from 20? What is 20 minus 3?" *If correct, say:* "Good. I want you to
count backwards, taking 3 from 20, then 3 from 17, as far back as you can."
(Record response).

Correct answer: 17, 14, 11, 8, 5, 2

Evaluation:
Record time (seconds) taken to reach final number: _____
Record number of errors: _____

II. ASSESSMENT OF ORIENTATION

Ask the patient the following questions:

Time:

"What is the day of the week?"
"What is the date?"
"What season is it?"
"What time is it?"
"How long have we been talking here?"

Place:

"What is this place?"
"What kind of place is this?"
"How did you get here?"
"How far is this place from your home?"

Person:

"Tell me your name."
"What school do you go to?"
"What grade are you in at school?"
"Who am I?"
"What is my job?"
"Why have you come to see me?"

Evaluation:

Record number of accurate responses: —————

III. ASSESSMENT OF MEMORY

Recent Memory

Clinician: "Now I will give you three things to remember, and in a few minutes I will ask you to recall what they are. John Smith, 500 Kings Highway, Green." *After five minutes, say:* "Please repeat those three things."

Evaluation (choose one):

Accurate
Needs prompting
Cannot repeat any
Refused

Clinician: "Now keep those things in your mind until I ask you for them again."

Immediate Memory

Clinician: "I want you to listen carefully and repeat these numbers after me." *Speak at the rate of one number per second. Continue upward until the patient fails. Record the last accurate repetition.*

8
4 3
3 9 6
4 2 1 9
8 5 1 9 2
9 3 5 2 8 6
7 5 8 3 9 2 4

Evaluation (record number):

Unable
Refused

(continued)

III. ASSESSMENT OF MEMORY (*continued*)

Clinician: "Now please repeat these numbers backward." *Continue upward until the patient fails. Record the last accurate repetition.*

> 3
> 9 1
> 4 7 3
> 5 8 2 9

Evaluation (record number):

> Unable
> Refused

Clinician: "Now, what were those three things I asked you to remember?"

Correct answer: John Smith, 500 Kings Highway, Green

Evaluation (choose one):

> Refused
> None correct
> Parts of A *or* B correct, only
> Parts of both A *and* B correct
> C correct, only
> Two fully correct, only
> Two out of three correct
> Three correct

Remote Memory

Clinician:

> "What is your address?"
> "What is your telephone number?"
> "Where were you born?"
> "What is the date of your birthday?"
> "What is your mother's name?"
> "Where was she born?"
> "What is the date of your mother's birthday?"
> "What is your father's name?"
> "Where was he born?"
> "What is the date of your father's birthday?"

Evaluation:

> Record number of accurate responses: ————

IV. ASSESSMENT OF JUDGMENT

Clinician: "Suppose the teacher had her back to the class and someone else flicked a rubber band at you. What would you do?"

Wait for spontaneous answer and record it.

If no answer is given, offer the following prompts:
> "Ignore it?"
> "Raise your hand to tell the teacher?"
> "Go after the one that threw it?"

Clinician: "Suppose you were out walking and you saw smoke pouring out of the roof of a house on your street. What would you do?"

Wait for spontaneous answer and record it.

IV. ASSESSMENT OF JUDGMENT (*continued*)

If no answer is given, offer the following prompts:
> "Arouse someone in the house and tell them?"
> "Ring a fire alarm?"
> "Run home and tell your mother?"
> "Ignore it?"

Clinician: "Imagine you were walking home from school and a girl in front of you dropped her purse without knowing it. What would you do?"

Wait for spontaneous answer and record it.
If no answer is given, offer the following prompts:
> "Tell her or give it back?"
> "Ignore it?"
> "Look inside?"
> "Keep it?"

V. ASSESSMENT OF ABSTRACTION

Clinician: "Tell me how these two things are alike:"

> wood and coal
> apple and peach
> ship and automobile
> iron and silver
> baseball and orange
> airplane and kite
> ocean and river
> penny and quarter

Clinician: "Do you know what a proverb is?" *(If not, discontinue.)* "Good. Tell me, in your own words, what these proverbs mean."

> A stitch in time saves nine.
> People in glass houses should not throw stones.
> A rolling stone gathers no moss.

Clinician: "Tell me the meaning of the following words:" *Read out loud, ceasing after five consecutive items are incorrect:*

orange	roar	scorch
envelope	muzzle	brunette
straw	haste	peculiarity
puddle	lecture	priceless
tap	mars	regard
gown	skill	disproportionate
eyelash	juggler	shrewd
		tolerate

(continued)

V. ASSESSMENT OF ABSTRACTION (*continued*)

Evaluation:

Number Correct	Vocabulary Age
5	6 years
6	6 years 8 months
7	7 years 4 months
8	8 years
9	8 years 8 months
10	9 years 4 months
11	10 years
12	10 years 8 months
13	11 years 4 months
14	12 years
15	13 years 3 months
16	14 years
17	14 years 3 months
18	14 years 6 months
19	14 years 9 months
20	Average adult

VI. DRAWING ABILITY

Clinician: *Use a No. 2 pencil with eraser on 8 × 11 blank paper. Instruct the patient as follows:* "On this piece of paper, I would like you to draw a whole person. It can be any kind of person, just make sure it's a whole person and not a stick figure or a cartoon figure." *For a young child who does not understand "person":* "You may draw a man or woman, a boy or girl." (*There is no time limit.*)

Evaluation: One point (3 months) is given for each item. Multiply the total number of correct items by 3. This is the patient's "drawing age" in months. Quote drawing age in years and months. Calculate the patient's "drawing quotient" as follows:

(Drawing age/Chronological age) × 100

Each feature present:

Head	Ear	Shoulders	Leg
Eye	Hair	Arm	Foot
Nose	Neck	Hand	Heel
Mouth	Trunk	Finger	Clothing

Details:

Pupil	Nostrils	Hands distinct from arms
Eyebrow	Two-dimensional nose	Arm joints
Eyelash	Hair more than on crown	Leg joints

Correct number of features:

Two eyes	Ten toes
Two ears	Two articles of clothing
Two hands	Four articles of clothing
Ten fingers	Costume complete

(continued)

VI. DRAWING ABILITY (*continued*)

Relatively correct location:
    Symmetrical features
    Ears in correct position
    Neck continuous with head
    Arms from shoulders

    Legs attached to trunk
    Opposition of thumb
    joints shown

Proportional size:
    Head more than circle
    Eye longer than high
    Body longer than head

    Fingers longer than wide
    Arms in proportion
    Legs in proportion

In profile:
    Eyes glance to front
    Forehead shown
    Chin projection shown
    Profile
    Correct profile

Thought Content

From the history given by the parents, the intake questionnaires and checklists, and free discussion with the child, the clinician will have generated hypotheses that can be tested by direct probes concerning clinical phenomenology. The following symptoms may not be routinely checked unless there are good hypothetico-deductive reasons for doing so: anxiety, separation anxiety, school refusal, panic attacks, phobias, obsessions, compulsions, impulsions, delusions, hallucinations, ideas of reference, ideas of influence, thought alienation, thought-broadcasting, depersonalization, déjà vu, derealization, suicidal ideation, impulses to injure the self or others, preoccupation with somatic functioning, somatic symptoms, stealing, fire setting, truancy, and fighting. In contrast, suicidal ideation, self-injury, assaultive impulses, substance abuse, physical or sexual abuse, risk taking, and antisocial behavior must always be inquired about when diagnostic evaluations are undertaken with adolescents.

Fantasy

The child's fantasy is elicited through play, drawing, and storytelling. By his or her unobtrusive interest, the clinician can facilitate the child's fantasy and encourage the child to express it. Table 7–3 lists a variety of techniques that can be used to elicit fantasy.

Insight

Is the child aware that he or she has a problem? If so, how is the problem conceptualized? Does the child want help for the problem?

■ STRUCTURED INTERVIEWING

Semistructured playroom interviews with children 7–12 years of age have been found to have a test–retest reliability of 0.84 and an interrater reliability of 0.74, with regard to the detection of abnormality. However, interviewers who are unaware of the parents' perception of the child's problems tend to underestimate abnormality in comparison with parent reports of child behavior.

In order to compensate for the potential unreliability of unstructured or semistructured interviewing, a number of structured interviews have been introduced. As a rule, these interviews are too cumbersome for everyday clinical work; however, they are widely used to standardize subject selection in research studies. Arguably, semistructured and structured interviewing complement each other: The semistructured interview yields information mainly about the child's perception of self and environment, whereas the structured interview focuses on symptomatology. When reliable diagnostic categorization is the overriding consideration, structured interviews such as those described in this section are clearly preferable. It should be remembered, however, that with children younger than 10–12 years of age, the reliability of direct questions concerning symptomatology is affected by the fact that children are limited in their capacity to be objective about themselves. Furthermore, emotionally disturbed preadolescents tire if exposed to long, tedious interviews and may become careless in their answers. Table 7–4 provides more detailed information on these instruments.

Table 7–3. Techniques to Elicit Fantasy

After the child has drawn a person, ask him or her the following types of questions:

Is that person a man or a woman, a boy or a girl?
How old is he/she?
What is he/she doing in that picture?
What is he/she thinking about?
How does he/she feel about it?
What makes him/her happy?
What makes him/her sad?
What makes him/her mad?
What makes him/her scared?
What does he/she need most?
What's the best/worst thing about him/her?
Tell me about his/her family?
What will he/she do next?

Use the Kinetic Family Drawing test:

a. Ask the child to draw his or her family doing something together.
b. Note who the child puts in the family; the proximity of the figures; the coherence of or separations between group members; the relative importance and power of the family members; and their apparent emotions, attachments, rivalries, and so on.
c. Ask the child to explain the drawing, saying what the family members are doing, thinking, and feeling, and what the outcome will be. Base your questions, in part, on discretionary probes derived from the dynamic hypotheses you have generated.

Ask the child to draw "something nice" and "something nasty." Consider using the following questions as icebreakers:

What would you do if you had a million dollars?
If you had three wishes, what would they be?
If you were wrecked on a desert island, who (and what) would you like to have with you?
Ask the child to tell you about (good/bad) dreams he or she has had recently.
Ask the child for the earliest thing he or she can remember, and for his or her earliest memory about his or her family.

A. DIAGNOSTIC INTERVIEW FOR CHILDREN AND ADOLESCENTS (DICA)

DICA is a semistructured interview that uses a modular technique, organized by diagnostic syndrome. Parent, child, and adolescent versions are available. Clinical judgment is required at several decision points; otherwise, lay interviewers can administer DICA. A computerized version is available for recording and scoring results. DICA has reasonable validity comparing pediatric and psychiatric referrals (especially in academic and relationship problems).

B. DIAGNOSTIC INTERVIEW SCHEDULE FOR CHILDREN (DISC)

DISC is a highly structured interview that is organized by topic, in a manner close to a natural free-flowing interview. It is mainly epidemiologic in purpose. Parent and child versions are available, and clinical judgment is not required. DISC has reasonable validity comparing pediatric and psychiatric referrals. Diagnoses are generated by computer algorithm.

C. SCHEDULE FOR AFFECTIVE DISORDERS AND SCHIZOPHRENIA FOR SCHOOL-AGE CHILDREN (K-SADS)

K-SADS is a semistructured instrument that has been used extensively in child psychiatry research. Parent, child, and epidemiologic versions are available. Clinical judgment is required. The same clinician interviews the parent and the child and attempts to resolve discrepancies in their reports. This interview was originally developed to identify children with affective disorder. It now emphasizes affective, anxiety, and schizophrenic disorders. It is scored manually, and diagnosis is reached from summary ratings. Pilot validity data come from follow-up, treatment change, and biological correlate studies.

D. CHILD ASSESSMENT SCHEDULE (CAS)

CAS is a semistructured interview that has been used with both children and adolescents. Parent and child versions are available. Interviewer training is required. Interview items are grouped by topic (e.g., school, peers, family), not syndrome. CAS does not cover posttraumatic stress

Table 7–4. Structured Interviews in Child and Adolescent Psychiatry

Instrument	Target Age (years)	Time Needed (minutes)	Reliability
Diagnostic Interview for Children & Adolescents (DICA)	6–17	60–90	Interrater and test–retest reliabilities are acceptable Parent–child agreement: 0–0.87 on specific items (k = 0.76–1.00 for anxiety and conduct disorders)
Diagnostic Interview Schedule for Children (DISC)	9–17	60–90	Interrater reliability: 0.94–1 for symptoms Test-retest reliability for parents: .9 (symptoms), 0.76 (syndromes); for children aged 14–18: 0.8 (symptoms), 0.36 (syndromes) Parent–child agreement: 0.27 (greatest for disruptive symptoms, less for depression or anxiety)
Schedule for Affective Disorders and Schizophrenia for School-Age Children (K-SADS)	6–18	180	Interrater reliability: .65-.96 (syndromes) Test-retest reliability: variable, 0.09–0.89 (symptoms), 0.24–0.7 (syndromes) Parent-child agreement: 0.08–1.00 (symptoms)
Child Assessment Schedule (CAS)	7–17	45–75	Interrater reliability: 0.73 (for content, less for diagnosis); higher for hyperactivity and aggression (0.8), less for anxiety (0.6)
Interview Schedule for Children (ISC)	8–17	90–120	Interrater reliability: 0.64–1.0 Parent–child agreement: 0.2–0.95 (symptoms), 0.32–0.86 (syndromes), lowest for subjective symptoms
Child & Adolescent Psychiatric Assessment (CAPA)	8–18	90–120	Not available

disorder, dissociative disorder, or adolescent schizophrenia. Its pilot validity was estimated by comparing inpatients, outpatients, and normal subjects.

E. INTERVIEW SCHEDULE FOR CHILDREN (ISC)

ISC was designed originally for a longitudinal study of depressed children and may be most useful for the diagnosis of depression. Parent and child versions are available. ISC requires clinical skill, judgment, and training.

F. CHILD AND ADOLESCENT PSYCHIATRIC ASSESSMENT (CAPA)

CAPA is intended for use in both clinical and epidemiologic settings. Parent and child versions are available. It starts with an unstructured discussion and proceeds to a systematic inquiry into a broad range of symptoms for which an extensive glossary is available. It contains psychosocial and family functioning sections. Lay or clinician interviewers can administer it, and it is scored by computer algorithm.

Angold A, Costello AJ: Structured interviewing. In: Lewis M (ed). *Child and Adolescent Psychiatry: A Comprehensive Textbook.* Philadelphia: Lippincott Williams & Wilkins, 2002, pp. 544–554.

Lewis M, King RA: Psychiatric assessment of infants, children, and adolescents. In: Lewis M (ed). *Child and Adolescent Psychiatry: A Comprehensive Textbook,* 3rd edn. Philadelphia: Lippincott Williams & Wilkins, 2002, pp. 525–543.

Simmons JE: *Psychiatric Examination of Children,* 3rd edn. Philadelphia: Lea & Febiger, 1981.

■ II. PHYSICAL EXAMINATION, LABORATORY TESTING, & SPECIAL INVESTIGATIONS

■ PHYSICAL EXAMINATION

Usually, a physical examination has already been completed by the child's pediatrician. If not, the clinician

Table 7–5. Physical Examination Items Deserving Special Attention

Growth parameters: height, weight, and head circumference plotted on standard curves
Minor physical anomalies (associated with developmental problems such as hyperactivity):
Abnormally small or large head
"Electric" hair (fine, dry hair standing upright from the scalp)
Epicanthic folds (skin folds in the upper internal eyelid)
Hypertelorism (eyes deep-set and widely separated)
Low-set, malformed, asymmetrical ears with adherent earlobes
High palate
Furrowed tongue
In-curved little finger
Long third toe
Syndactyly
Gap between first and second toes
Other head, face, or body dysplasias that might indicate a congenital disorder (e.g., signs of fetal alcohol syndrome)

should refer the family to the primary physician. In some circumstances, however, it is important that the child psychiatrist complete the physical examination. Table 7–5 lists those aspects of the physical examination to which the clinician should pay particular attention.

Table 7–6 lists symptoms that could be referable to the central nervous system and indicate the need for a neurologic examination. The psychiatrist can perform a brief, routine neurologic screen during the interview by observing the child's speech, gait, posture, balance, gross and fine motor tone, power and coordination, facial symmetry, and ocular movements and by checking for tics,

Table 7–6. Symptoms that Indicate the Need for Neurologic Examination

Headache
Visual impairment
Deafness
Tinnitus
Poor balance
Episodic disruption of consciousness
Memory defects
Intermittent confusion
Anesthesia
Paresthesia
Motor weakness
Impaired coordination
Abnormal movements
Recent loss of sphincter control

Table 7–7. Extension of the Neurologic Examination

Domain	Functions or Abnormalities
Cranial nerves	Movement of eyes, face, and tongue Pupillary reflexes Visual fields Hearing
Motor power and tone	Shoulder Elbow Wrist Hand Knee Ankle
Reflexes	Biceps Triceps Supinator Patellar Ankle Plantar
Fundi	Papilledema Anterio-venous abnormalities Abnormal pigmentation

Note: Leave the examination of the reflexes and fundi to the end.

tremor, clonus, or choreiform movements of the fingers and hands. Table 7–7 lists extensions to the routine screen that can be implemented by baring the child's feet and forearms.

Some child psychiatrists avoid physical examination. The clinician may worry that an upsetting physical examination will impede a positive relationship or tilt the spontaneous development of the child's transference. There may be some point to these considerations, but the potential benefits of a nonintrusive physical examination outweigh its disadvantages.

Soft or nonfocal signs are phenomena thought to have no clear locus or origin, to be developmentally normal up to a certain age, and to reflect uneven neurologic maturation in older children. Table 7–8 lists commonly identified neurologic soft signs. Can these signs be consensually identified and elicited in a standard manner? Do they have significant test–retest and interrater reliability? Do they occur frequently enough in an at-risk population to make them worth eliciting? Are they singly or in clusters associated with disorders such as learning disability, attention-deficit/hyperactivity disorder, or schizophrenia? Do they predict which hyperkinetic children will respond to stimulant medication? For none of these questions is there a clear answer.

Table 7–8. Neurologic Soft Signs

Choreiform or athetoid movements, especially of the out-stretched fingers and hands

Dysdiadochokinesia (difficulty performing rapid alternating movements)

Dysgraphesthesia (difficulty interpreting a figure traced on the palm of the hand)

General clumsiness

Synkinesis (the tendency for other parts of the body to move in unison when one part is moving)

Pincus JH: Neurological meaning of soft signs. Pages 573–581 in Lewis M (ed). *Child and Adolescent Psychiatry: A Comprehensive Textbook,* 3rd edn. Philadelphia: Lippincott Williams & Wilkins, 2002, pp. 573–581.

■ SPECIAL INVESTIGATIONS

The routine use of special investigations for all referred adolescents is not justified. Before ordering a consultation, test, or special investigation, the clinician should consider whether it is a screen inquiry that has a reasonable chance of yielding important information in the clinical population in question (e.g., routine drug or pregnancy testing for hospitalized adolescents) or, in the case of a discretionary probe, whether the particular inquiry could conceivably rule out (or help to rule in) a diagnostic hypothesis. Table 7–9 lists the types of consultations and special investigations often used in child and adolescent psychiatry.

Table 7–9. Common Consultations and Special Investigations

Consultations
Pediatric consultation
Neurologic consultation
Other specialist consultations (e.g., speech pathology)

Special investigations
Laboratory testing (e.g., blood, urinalysis, electrolytes, liver function, thyroid function, urine drug screening, and genetic screening)
Acoustic and ophthalmologic examination
Electroencephalography
Neuroimaging
Psychological testing

■ CLINICAL SITUATIONS LIKELY TO REQUIRE SPECIAL INVESTIGATIONS

The clinician must rule out physical disease by the judicious ordering of specific consultations, tests, or investigations in suspicious clinical situations. Table 7–10 lists the clinical situations in which organic causes must be ruled out.

Acute or Subacute Disintegration of Behavior and Development

After a period of normal or relatively normal development, the child may fail to make developmental progress and lose recently acquired skills such as sphincter control, coordination, dexterity, attention and concentration, memory, language, capacity for problem solving, school performance, emotional control, and social competence. In some cases, the child may demonstrate abnormal motor patterns, hallucinations, delusions, and disorganization of thinking. Table 7–11 lists organic causes that must be excluded.

Acute Psychotic Episode

The child or adolescent may become mentally disorganized, socially inappropriate, affectively incongruent, or emotionally labile and report audiovisual hallucinations, illusions, ideas of reference, and delusions of persecution or grandeur. Sometimes the patient becomes mute, immobile, posturing, apparently self-absorbed, assuming odd postures of the arms, head, and trunk. The following disorders must be excluded: substance-induced psychotic disorder (using urine and blood toxicology) and psychotic disorder due to general medical condition (which requires pediatric consultation and tests specific to hypothesized medical conditions such as hyperthyroidism, hypersteroidism, neurologic disorder).

Anorexia or Weight Loss

The child or adolescent may lose weight markedly as a result of voluntary restriction of food intake. The following conditions should be ruled out: chronic systemic infection (especially tuberculosis); systemic malignancy (especially pancreatic, mediastinal, retroperitoneal, pulmonary, lymphatic, or leukemic malignancy); hypothalamic or pituitary tumor (using skull X-rays, computed tomography [CT] scan, tomogram of sella turcica, or magnetic resonance imaging [MRI]); diabetes mellitus

Table 7–10. Clinical Situations Likely to Require Special Investigation

---

Acute or subacute disintegration of development and behavior, with loss of previously attained developmental milestones, deterioration in school performance, and the emergence of erratic aggressive behavior, clinging dependency, or confusion

Acute psychotic episode

Anorexia or weight loss

Attention-deficit, hyperactivity, and impulsivity, especially if of recent or sudden origin

Delay in speech and language development, loss of previously acquired speech and language, or the recent emergence of deviant speech or language

Depression, especially if associated with slowed thinking, deterioration of concentration, vagueness, and fatigue

Episodic or progressive lapses or deterioration of awareness with dreaminess; obtundation; defect in the sensorium; and perhaps, subjective depersonalization, derealization, and hallucinosis

Episodic violence out of proportion to the apparent precipitant, often with memory gaps or amnesia for the episode

General or specific learning problems (e.g., in reading, writing, or calculation)

Localized or generalized abnormal movements that may be associated with vocal abnormalities

Pervasive developmental impairment (especially if associated with an uneven profile of abilities)

Sleep disturbance or excessive drowsiness

Somatoform symptoms of recent onset that mimic a physical disorder but are not consistent with the typical pattern of physical disorder

---

(using urinalysis and glucose tolerance testing); hyperthyroidism (using thyroid function tests); and drug addiction (using toxicology screens).

Headache

The chief causes of headache in childhood are migraine and tension headaches. Migraine is episodic and can be associated with vertigo, unexplained vomiting and abdominal pain, and, rarely, with hemiplegia, temporary episodic impairment of receptive or expressive language, and confusion. Tension headaches are commonly of daily occurrence and difficult to localize. Headaches due to raised intracranial pressure tend to be worse upon wakening or to wake the child, and to be associated with vomiting, papilledema, cranial nerve dysfunction, sluggish papillary reflexes, and visual impairment. Seizure related headache can be ictal or postictal. Specialist consultation is required if the clinician suspects an organic cause of headache.

Attention-Deficit, Hyperactivity, and Impulsivity

Before or after starting school, the child may demonstrate poor concentration, distractibility, and a tendency to impulsiveness, with or without hyperactivity and learning problems. Table 7–12 lists organic causes that must be excluded.

Delay in Speech and Language Development

The child may manifest a relative delay in comprehending speech or in expressing and correctly enunciating words, phrases, and sentences. Table 7–13 lists organic causes that must be excluded.

Depression

The child or adolescent may become underactive or overactive; insomniac or hypersomniac; impaired in thought tempo, concentration, and energy; readily provoked to tantrum or weeping; socially withdrawn; or preoccupied with thoughts of low self-esteem, guilt, and loss. The differential diagnosis includes virtually any physical disorder that could sap energy, impair thinking, and disrupt the capacity to cope.

The following general systemic diseases should be excluded: malignancy, chronic infectious disease, viral infection (e.g., influenza, infectious hepatitis, infectious mononucleosis), hypothyroidism, hypoadrenalism, chronic anemia, and subnutrition (e.g., anorexia nervosa). Chronic intoxication with anticonvulsants or sedatives must be excluded (using urine drug screens and blood levels), as must degenerative central nervous disease (using central nervous system examination, specific tests for the systemic diseases being excluded, CT scan, or MRI).

It is often difficult to determine to what degree a child's depression is part of a pathophysiologic process or to what degree it represents a secondary psychological reaction to loss of function, hospitalization, restriction of freedom, lack of stimulation, or loneliness.

Episodic or Progressive Lapses or Deterioration of Awareness

The patient, usually an adolescent, may experience recurrent episodes during which he or she has a sense of being

Table 7–11. Excluding Organic Causes of Disintegration of Behavior and Development

Possible Organic Cause	Special Investigations
General systemic disease	
Thyroid disorder	Thyroid function tests
Adrenal insufficiency	Adrenal function tests
Porphyria	Examination for urinary porphyrins
Disseminated lupus erythematosus (LE)	Examination for LE cells
Wilson's disease	Serum ceruloplasmin
Toxic factors	
Delirium due to systemic infection, electrolyte abnormality, or physiologic toxins	Electroencephalography; specific biochemical, bacteriologic, or virologic tests
Drugs (e.g., intoxication with sympathomimetic drugs, anticholinergic drugs, hallucinogens, or anticonvulsants; withdrawal from sedatives)	Urine drug screen, blood toxicology
Central nervous system disease	
Seizure disorder	Electroencephalography with nasopharyngeal electrodes, telemetry
Space-occupying lesion	Skull X-ray, CT scan, MRI
Herpes encephalitis	Electroencephalography, examination of cerebrospinal fluid, immunologic testing
Metabolic or subacute viral encephalitis	Electroencephalography, examination of cerebrospinal fluid, immunologic testing
Degenerative diseases	Urine amino acids, electroencephalography, MRI, biopsy
Demyelinating disease	MRI
Leukemic infiltration of central nervous system	Examination of blood and cerebrospinal fluid

Table 7–12. Excluding Organic Causes of Attention-Deficit, Hyperactivity, and Impulsivity

Possible Organic Cause	Special Investigations
Hyperthyroidism	Thyroid function tests (if there is other evidence of hyperdynamic cardiovascular function and sympathetic overactivity)
Plumbism	Urine lead levels, examination of blood for stippled cells, X-rays of long bones
Seizure disorder	Electroencephalography with nasopharyngeal leads
Sleep apnea	Otorhinolaryngologic examination, sleep electroencephalography and observation
Sydenham's chorea	Blood antistreptolysin-O antibody titer

Table 7–13. Excluding Organic Causes of Speech and Language Development Delay

Possible Organic Cause	Special Investigations
Deafness	Acoustic testing
Palatal abnormality	Physical examination
Cerebral palsy	Neurologic examination
Mental retardation	Physical examination, psychological testing
Seizure disorder	Electroencephalography
Aphasia	Consult with speech pathology, neuropsychological testing
Developmental articulatory dyspraxia	Consult with speech pathology and pediatric neurology
Pervasive developmental disorder	See Table 35-11

abruptly altered, different, or unreal and of observing the self as a spectator. The adolescent may perceive that the world is unreal and different or that conversations and scenes have been experienced previously in precisely the same manner. The following organic causes must be excluded: seizure disorder (using electroencephalography), cardiac arrhythmia (using electrocardiology), narcolepsy (using electroencephalography), migraine, and hallucinogenic drug use (using urine drug screen).

Episodic Violence

The child or adolescent may periodically lose control, assault others, or destroy property. Violent behavior may be unheralded but it usually arises from an emotional context of tension with or without alcohol or drug intake and is disproportionate to the apparent provocation. The individual may or may not have a conduct disorder. The following disorders must be excluded: temporal lobe seizures (using electroencephalography with nasopharyngeal leads), herpes encephalitis (using electroencephalography, immunologic study, and examina-

tion of cerebrospinal fluid for viral culture and immunology), drug effects (e.g., alcohol, phencyclidine, hallucinogens, amphetamine) (using urine drug screen), and idiosyncratic reaction to alcohol (using patient's history).

General or Specific Learning Problems

The child or adolescent may manifest a general or specific difficulty in learning, particularly in reading, writing, written expression, calculation, or spatial skills. Table 7–14 lists organic causes that must be excluded.

Localized or Generalized Abnormal Movements

The child or adolescent may manifest repetitive movements that may or may not be partly or wholly under control. The following disorders must be excluded: attention-deficit/hyperactivity disorder, tic disorder, Sydenham's chorea (using antistreptolysin-O titer), Huntington disease, Wilson disease, paroxysmal choreoathetosis, dystonia musculorum deformans,

Table 7–14. Excluding Organic Causes of Learning Problems

Possible Organic Cause	Special Investigations
Visual defect	Test visual acuity and visual fields; ophthalmoscopy
Deafness	Acoustic testing
Cerebral palsy	Neurologic examination
Mental retardation	Physical examination, psychological testing
Seizure disorder	Electroencephalography
Dementia due to intracranial space—occupying lesion or cerebral degeneration	Neurologic examination: skull x-rays, CT scan, MRI
Inability to pay attention in class because of debilitating illness, fatigue, hunger, pain, or drug use	None

Table 7–15. Excluding Organic Causes of Pervasive Developmental Impairment

Possible Organic Cause	Special Investigations
Hearing impairment	Acoustic testing
Aphasia	Speech pathology consultation, language testing
Seizure disorder	Electroencephalography
Chromosomal anomaly	Chromosome analysis (especially if the child looks dysplastic)
Metabolic disorder	Tests for amino acids in the urine (especially phenylketonuria)
Intracranial lesion	Skull X-ray, CT scan, MRI (only if an intracranial space-occupying lesion or demyelinating disease is suspected)
Herpes encephalitis	Virologic studies of the cerebrospinal fluid, immunologic testing (if there has been an acute or subacute regression), electroencephalography

cerebellar tumor or degeneration, and drug effects (e.g., caffeinism, extrapyramidal side effects of neuroleptic medication).

Pervasive Developmental Impairment

During infancy or afterward, the child may manifest a severe arrest or retardation of language, intellect, and social development. Additional features may include unexplained episodes of panic or rage, marked resistance to environmental change, hyperactivity, repetitive motor phenomena, and deviant speech and language. The onset may be in early infancy (before 30 months) or afterward (up to about 7 years). Sometimes the child regresses from a state of relatively normal development to a state of developmental impairment. More often, the child's abnormal development becomes evident gradually. Several organic causes must be excluded (Table 7–15).

Sleep Disturbance or Excessive Drowsiness

The child may present with hypersomnia, insomnia, nightmares, night terrors, restless sleep, or sleepwalking. Table 7–16 lists organic causes that must be excluded.

Somatoform Symptoms

The child or adolescent may develop a set of symptoms that mimic physical disorder. Common conversion symptoms are loss of consciousness, loss of phonation, motor impairment, abnormal movements, seizures, special sensory defect, anesthesia, pain, loss of balance, bizarre gait, or gastrointestinal complaints such as vomiting and abdominal pain. Conversion disorder can mimic many physical conditions. The inquiry plan should both exclude the hypothetical physical disorder and establish positive criteria for conversion (i.e., emotional trauma coinciding with onset; pattern of symptoms representing the patient's naive idea of pathology; contact with a

Table 7–16. Excluding Organic Causes of Sleep Disturbance or Excessive Drowsiness

Possible Organic Cause	Special Investigations
Seizure disorder	Electroencephalography (including polysomnography)
Delirium (e.g., in acute febrile illness or toxic states)	Electroencephalography
Narcolepsy	Electroencephalography
Intoxication with or withdrawal from sedative, opiate, anticonvulsant, neuroleptic, or antidepressant drugs	Urinary drug screen
Hypoglycemia	Blood sugar (e.g., insulinoma)
Sleep apnea	Polysomnography, otorhinolaryngologic examination
Any debilitating disease, especially disease associated with chronic hypoxia (e.g., congenital heart disease, pulmonary insufficiency, anemia)	None

Table 7–17. Excluding Disorders Likely to be Mistaken for Conversion Disorder

Possible Organic Cause	Special Investigations
General systemic disease	
Disseminated lupus erythematosus (LE)	Examination for LE cells
Hypocalcemia	Blood calcium
Hypoglycemia	Blood sugar (e.g., insulinoma)
Porphyria	Urinary porphyrins
Central nervous system disease	
Multiple sclerosis	Neurologic examination, MRI
Movement disorders (chorea, dystonia musculorum deformans, Tourette's syndrome, Wilson's disease)	None
Spinal cord tumor	Neurologic examination, radiography, MRI
Intracranial space–occupying lesion (especially in brain stem, cerebellum, frontal lobe, or parietotemporal cortex)	Neurologic examination, skull radiography, CT scan, MRI
Seizure disorder	Electroencephalography
Migraine	None
Dystonic reactions produced by neuroleptic drugs	None

model for the disease; pattern of symptoms fulfilling a communicative purpose; secondary gain for the patient in the form of nurturance, security, or avoidance of difficulty; and a pattern of symptoms and signs inconsistent with physical disease). Table 7–17 lists the physical disorders especially likely to be mistaken for a conversion disorder.

Gillberg C: Part III: Assessment. In: Gillberg C (ed). *Clinical Child Neuropsychiatry.* New York: Cambridge University Press, 1995, pp. 295–322.

Neeper R, Huntzinger R, Gascon GG: Examination I: Special techniques for the infant and young child. In: Coffey CE, Brumback RA (eds). *Textbook of Pediatric Neuropathology.* Washington, DC: American Psychiatric Press, 1998, pp. 153–170.

III. PERSONALITY EVALUATION

PURPOSE OF THE PERSONALITY EVALUATION

Questions that come to the attention of clinicians often relate to differential diagnosis (i.e., whether a patient is more appropriately assigned one *Diagnostic and Statistical Manual of Mental Disorders,* fourth edition [DSM-IV] diagnosis as opposed to another). However, even in this age of managed care and associated limitations on testing, psychologists are still occasionally asked to perform evaluations that characterize the patient beyond this reductionistic level and that describe the patient's resources and liabilities, underlying conflicts, stress tolerance, and so on. Indeed, many psychologists take the position that in order to effectively assign a specific diagnostic label it is frequently necessary to understand the functioning of the whole person.

TYPES OF PERSONALITY EVALUATIONS

Personality evaluation can be divided into three main areas. These include behavior rating scales used to assess a patient's overt behavior and, by extension, psychological functioning; projective tests ordinarily used to describe a patient's underlying concerns, issues, perceptions of other people, and self-attributions (the "content" of the mind, if you will); and structural tests used to characterize the patient's psychological structure, including coping resources, typical defensive tactics, capacity for intimacy, and reasoning capacity (the "form" of the mind). A fourth

Table 7–18. Types of Personality Evaluation

Evaluation Type	Function	Examples
Behavior rating scales	Describe an individual's functioning in everyday life	Achenbach's Child Behavior Check List
Projective tests	Characterize an individual's underlying concerns	Incomplete Sentences Test Thematic Apperception Test
Structural tests	Depict a person's personality	Rorschach Inkblot Test Minnesota Multiphasic Psychiatric Inventory-A (MMPI-A) Millon Adolescent Personality Inventory
Specific diagnosis scales	Assess an individual's functioning with respect to a specific diagnosis	Children's Depression Inventory Revised Child Manifest Anxiety Scale

group of scales is used to assess the patient's functioning with respect to a specific diagnosis, such as depression. Table 7–18 summarizes these scales.

Behavior Rating Scales

Behavior rating scales are used both by psychologists and by clinicians, including child psychiatrists. They describe a patient's functioning in everyday life, as a step toward understanding the patient. Perhaps the most well-known of such scales is Achenbach's Child Behavior Checklist. This scale requires a parent to respond to questions related to the child's social functioning and behavioral problems. On the basis of these responses, the child is rated on a number of symptom groupings, or factors, that can be divided into two categories: those that reflect internalizing psychopathology (e.g., sadness, withdrawal, anxiety) and those that reflect externalizing psychopathology (e.g., temper outbursts, demandingness, stubbornness). Such rating scales, although perhaps limited in the amount of information obtained from the respondent, are useful in that they provide psychologists with data derived from a careful observer, namely, the parent.

Projective Tests

Projective measures assume that a subject projects unconscious issues, themes, and expectancies onto an ambiguous external stimulus, thereby providing the diagnostician with meaningful clinical data. Traditionally, such techniques have been organized on the basis of their assumed depth of exploration. For example, the Incomplete Sentences Test, which requires a patient to complete sentence stems such as "I like" or "My mother," is assumed to gather information of which the patient is reasonably conscious or aware. Alternatively, the Thematic Apperception Test may evoke material that is deeper and less obvious in meaning to the patient. However, the latter task is hampered by the fact that such information is generally quite symbolic in nature and hence

is open to misinterpretation on the part of the examiner. Moreover, data derived from projective testing often has limited connection to the specific question being posed by the referral source, which often relates to distinguishing between competing diagnostic possibilities or characterizing a patient's psychological assets and liabilities.

The reader may note that in discussing projective measures, we have yet to describe the Rorschach Inkblot Test. During the past 15 years or so, there has been much discussion of the nature of the Rorschach task. Various authors have noted that, in fact, there are two essential Rorschach functions. First, the Rorschach may serve as a projective measure, evoking material that leads us to define a person's idiosyncratic or specific concerns, fears, conflicts, or interests. For example, an abused teenage girl may provide the response "two men killing a little girl," emphasizing the degree to which this particular person fears or anticipates that aggressive males may victimize her.

Second, various authors have said that the real strength of the Rorschach task lies not in its projective function but in its use as a means of evoking behavior that can illuminate the patient's personality structure. For example, regardless of the particular content of a given protocol, one might assess the degree to which the outlines of a patient's perceptions match the outlines of the test stimuli, based on a consensus of others. Weakness in this regard may be interpreted as an impairment in perceptual accuracy or reality interpretation. Likewise, responses may be assessed with respect to unrealistic reasoning (e.g., "looks like a bat because it's green"). In general, most contemporary research and clinical work on the Rorschach relates to this use as a perceptual–cognitive task, as opposed to a stimulus to fantasy.

Structural Tests

The Rorschach may be viewed as a structural task in the above-described manner. That is, information provided on this measure can be used to paint a picture of an individual quite apart from his or her worries, concerns, or problematic issues. In addition to the Rorschach, the Minnesota Multiphasic Personality Inventory-Adolescent (MMPI-A) is frequently administered to young patients. A revision of the MMPI-2 for adolescents, this scale involves the original set of basic scales, which assess functioning along dimensions such as depression, hypochondriasis, rebelliousness, and social introversion. The test is published with information permitting scoring on various subscales that compose the basic scales. Finally, content scales are provided that are, for the most part, rationally derived groupings of items relating to matters such as obsessiveness, family problems, and school problems. MMPI-A administration and interpretation proceeds much like the relevant scale for adults. The patient is asked to complete almost 500 questions, and responses are then interpreted based on patterns of scale elevations.

The MMPI-A cannot be administered to children under the age of 13 years. Instead, an MMPI-like technique, the Personality Inventory for Children, may be administered. This test requires a knowledgeable adult, preferably the primary caregiver, to characterize the child by answering over 400 questions. The responses can be scored to provide information in areas such as depression, somatic problems, delinquency, withdrawal, and so on. Both the MMPI-A and the Personality Inventory for Children contain validity scales to evaluate the respondent's response set (i.e., attempts to provide an unrealistically positive or negative impression).

The Millon Clinical Multiaxial Inventory was originally published as an alternative to the MMPI, which was considered to be weak in several areas. For example, the MMPI has been considered excessively Axis I oriented, neglecting factors such as personality styles and disorders that may lay the groundwork for the development of Axis I features, such as affective disorders, anxiety disorders, and so on. Millon's tests also offer a different definition of scale elevations. Millon has made the point that in view of the differing base rates for different forms of psychopathology, the traditional mode of interpreting personality scales is insufficient. The Millon Adolescent Clinical Inventory provides more of a focus on Axis II disorders.

Specific Diagnostic Scales

In this era of managed care, an emphasis has been placed on the definition of very specific questions for the psychologist to address. Thus, scales assessing specific clinical entities are becoming used much more frequently than before. Traditional measures (e.g., the Beck Depression Inventory) are often used. So too are versions adapted for younger patients such as the Children's Depression Inventory. The Revised Child Manifest Anxiety Scale is also used frequently.

Archer RP: *MMPI-A: Assessing Adolescent Psychopathology.* Mahwah NJ: Lawrence Erlbaum Associates, 1992.

Exner JE: *The Rorschach: A Comprehensive System.* New York: John Wiley & Sons, 1993.

Millon T: *Toward a New Personology.* New York: John Wiley & Sons, 1990.

Developmental Psychology

8

Kenneth A. Dodge, PhD

■ DEVELOPMENTAL CONCEPTS

The concept of development is the backbone of modern behavioral science. Psychiatric practitioners and behavioral scientists are concerned primarily with change, its origins, and its control. **Developmental psychology** is the scientific study of the structure, function, and processes of systematic growth and change across the life span. Systems of classification of behavior (including psychiatric nosology) take into account not only contemporaneous features and formal similarities among current symptoms and syndromes but also past qualities, immediate consequences, long-term outcome and likelihood of change (naturally or through treatment).

Whereas developmental psychology is concerned with species-typical patterns of systematic change (and central tendencies of the species), the discipline of **developmental psychopathology** is concerned with individual differences and contributes greatly to the understanding of childhood disorders.

The organizing framework of developmental psychopathology is a movement toward understanding the predictors, causes, processes, courses, sequelae, and environmental symbiosis of psychiatric illnesses in order to discover effective treatment and prevention. This movement is guided by in a developmental framework that integrates knowledge from multiple disciplines (e.g., psychobiology, neuroscience, cognitive psychology, social psychology) and levels of analysis (e.g., neuronal synapse, psychophysiologic response, mental representation, motor behavior, personality pattern). The relationship between developmental psychology and developmental psychopathology is reciprocal: The study of normal development gives context to the analysis of aberrations, and the study of psychopathology informs our understanding of normative development.

A developmental orientation forces a scholar to ask questions that move beyond the prevalence and incidence of disorders. Table 8–1 lists some of these questions.

THE ORTHOGENETIC PRINCIPLE

The **orthogenetic principle** proposes that development moves from undifferentiated and diffuse toward greater complexity, achieved through both differentiation and consolidation within and across subsystems. The newborn infant is relatively undifferentiated in response patterns, but through development achieves greater differentiation (and less stereotypy) of functioning. Each period of development is characterized by adaptational challenges resulting from environmental demands (e.g., a mother who has become unwilling to breast-feed) and from emerging internal influences across subsystems (e.g., growing recognition of the self as able to exert control). The challenges are best conceptualized not as mere threats to homeostasis; rather, change and the demand for adaptation define the human species, and challenges push the individual toward development. The inherent adaptational response of the species is toward mastery of new demands. The mastery motive is as yet unexplained by science, although it is characteristic of the human species (see "Adaptation and Competence" section later in this chapter).

Thus, development is characterized by periods of disruption in the homeostasis of the organism brought on by new challenges, followed by adaptation and consolidation until the next challenge is presented. The adaptive child uses both internal and external resources to meet a challenge. **Successful adaptation** is defined as the optimal organization of behavioral and biological systems within the context of current challenges. Adaptation requires the assimilation of past organizational structures to current demands as well as the generation of new structures equipped to meet the demands.

Piaget described two types of change: **assimilation,** which involves incorporation of the challenge into existing organizational structures (e.g., an infant might treat all adults as the same kind of stimulus); and **accommodation,** which involves reorganization of the organism's structures to meet the demands of the environment (e.g., a developing infant learns to discriminate among adults and to respond differently to different adults) (see

Table 8–1. Questions Related to a Developmental Orientation

How and why do some at-risk individuals become psychologically ill, whereas others do not?
How do the capacities and limitations of the human species at various life stages predispose individuals to disorder? (For example, why are females at relatively high risk for depression during adolescence?)
How do genes and the environment interact to produce psychopathology?
How are various disorders related developmentally? (For example, how does oppositional defiant disorder lead to conduct disorder, which leads to antisocial personality disorder?)
Where are the natural boundaries between normal and abnormal?
Are there critical periods, and if so, why? (For example, why is a high lead level in the blood more detrimental early in life?)
What does the concept of multifactorial causation imply for the likely success of intervention?

"Organismic Theory" section later in this chapter). Accommodation is more complex than assimilation, but successful adaptation requires a balance of both.

Maladaptation, or incompetence in responding to challenge, is characterized by the inadequate resolution of developmental challenges (as in the psychoanalytic concept of fixation). Maladaptation may be evidenced by developmental delays or lags, such as the continuing temper tantrums of an emotionally dysregulated child beyond the period when such behavior is normative. At any phase, the organism will manifest some form of regulation and functioning, even if it is not advantageous for future development. Thus, the child's tantrums might serve to regulate both a complex external environment of marital turmoil and an internal environment of stress. However, suboptimal regulation will prevent or hamper the individual from coping with the next developmental challenge.

Sometimes, apparently effective responses to a particular challenge lead to maladaptation at a more general level. Consider a toddler who responds to the withdrawal of a mother's undivided attention by ignoring her. Although this pattern of response may mean calmer evenings temporarily, the toddler will be ill equipped to respond to other challenges later in development. Consistent social withdrawal may cause the child to fail to acquire skills of assertion; however, continued ignoring of the mother may lead to a phenotypically distinct response in the future (e.g., depression in adolescence). Thus, the orthogenetic principle calls to mind the functioning of the' entire organism (not merely distinct and unrelated subsystems) and the readiness of that organism to respond to future challenges.

Lerner, RM (ed): Theoretical models of human development. In: *Handbook of Child Psychology,* Vol 1. New York: Wiley, 2006.

MAJOR PRINCIPLES OF ONTOGENY & PHYLOGENY

Cairns and Cairns outlined seven principles that characterize the human organism in interaction with the environment over time: conservation, coherence, bidirectionality, reciprocal influence, novelty, within-individual variation, and dynamic systems. The first principle is that of **conservation,** or connectivity in functioning across time. Even with all the pressure to change, social and cognitive organization tends to be continuous and conservative. The constraints on the organism and the multiple determinants of behavior lead to gradual transition rather than abrupt mutation. Observers can recognize the continuity in persons across even long periods of time; that is, we know that a person remains the same "person." For Piaget, who began his career by writing scientific papers on the evolution of mollusks, this within-person continuity principle is consistent with his view that species-wide evolution is gradual. Piaget believed that development within individuals reflects development of the species (i.e., ontogeny recapitulates phylogeny).

The second principle is **coherence**. Individuals function as holistic and integrated units, in spite of the multiple systems that contribute to any set of behaviors. One cannot divorce one system from another because the two systems function as a whole that is greater than its component parts. This fact is another conservative force, because an adverse effect on one part of a system tends to be offset by compensatory responses from other parts of the system. This phenomenon applies to all human biological systems and can be applied to psychological functioning.

The third principle is a corollary of the second: Influence between the organism and the environment is **bidirectional**. The person is an active agent in continuous interaction with others. Reciprocal influences are not identical; rather, at each stage of development, the person organizes the outer world through a mental representational system that mediates all experience with the world. Nevertheless, reciprocity and synchrony constrain the person, and the relative weight of these constraints varies at different points in development. At one extreme, it is possible to speak of symbiosis and total dependency of the infant on the mother; at the other extreme, behavior geneticists refer to genetic effects on environmental variables (such as the proposition that genes produce behavior that leads to the reactions that one receives from others in social exchanges).

Another corollary of the second principle is the principle of **reciprocal influence** between subsystems within the individual. Behavioral, cognitive, emotional, neurochemical, hormonal, and morphologic factors affect each other reciprocally. Mental events have biological implications and vice versa. Among the most exciting research directions in developmental psychopathology has been afforded by the technology of functions magnetic resonance imaging (fMRI), which enables the understanding of how environmental stimuli and behavioral displays are mediated through brain activity.

The fifth principle of ontogeny is that **novelty** arises in development. Change is not haphazard. The forces of reciprocal interaction within the individual and the environment lead not only to quantitative changes in the individual but also to the emergence of qualitatively distinct forms, such as locomotion, language, and thought. These changes represent growth rather than random events, in that previous forms typically remain and are supplemented by novel forms.

The sixth principle of phylogeny is that of **within-individual variation** in developmental rates across subsystems. Change within a subsystem occurs nonlinearly, as in language development or even physical growth. Some of this nonlinearity can be explained by species-wide phenomena, such as puberty, but much of it varies across individuals. In addition, rates of change vary within an individual across subsystems. Consider two young children, identical in age. Child A may learn to crawl before child B, but child B might catch up and learn to walk before child A. Likewise, child B might utter a recognizable word before child A, but child A might be talking in sentences before child B. This unevenness within and across individuals characterizes development and makes predictions probabilistic rather than certain. Some of the variation is attributable to environmental factors that have enduring personal effects (such as the lasting effects on cognitive achievement of early entry into formal schooling) or biological factors that have enduring psychological effects (such as the effect of early puberty on social outcomes), whereas other factors may have only temporary effect (such as efforts to accelerate locomotion onset) or no effect at all.

Finally, according to the seventh principle, development is extremely sensitive to unique configurations of influence, such as in **dynamic systems.** Growth and change cannot be reduced to a quantitative cumulation of biological and environmental units. Also, development is not simply hierarchical, with gradual building of functions on previous ones. Rather, development often follows a sequence of organization, disorganization, and then reorganization in a different (possibly more advanced) form. In physical sciences, this principle is called **catastrophe theory**, reflecting the hypothesis that during the disorganization, events are literally random. But re-organization occurs eventually, in lawful and predictable ways.

Dynamic systems theory incorporates several postulates about growth and change. First, change occurs nonlinearly. Second, minor quantitative changes can lead to dramatic qualitative changes in state. Consider how flow of water from a spigot changes from a succession of droplets to a stream or how water itself turns to ice. These major qualitative shifts occur in a regulated way with only minor qualitative changes in a parameter. Third, microlevel events that occur repeatedly often precipitate macrolevel changes in an organism's state.

Granic and Patterson (2006) have described how dynamic systems theory contributes to our understanding of the development of serious conduct disorder. Early difficult temperament and minor conduct problems sometimes shift dramatically to serious violence and antisocial personality disorder through a series of subtle changes in the microlevel characteristics of a parent–child relationship. Coercive exchanges, positive reinforcement, and capitulation by one party at a microlevel can lead a child to emerge from the interaction with macrolevel changes in the propensity for antisocial behavior in other relationships.

Cairns RB, Cairns BD: *Lifelines and Risks: Pathways of Youth in Our Time.* New York: Cambridge University Press, 1994.

Granic I, Patterson GR: Toward a comprehensive model of antisocial development: A dynamic systems approach. *Psychol Rev* 2006;113(1):101.

AGE NORMS

A simple but powerful developmental concept that has affected psychiatric nosology is that of **age norms**. Rather than evaluating a set of behaviors or symptoms according to a theoretical, absolute, or population-wide distribution, diagnosticians increasingly use age norms to evaluate psychiatric problems. Consider the evaluation of temper tantrums. In a 2-year-old child, tantrums are normative, whereas in an adult, angry outbursts could indicate an intermittent explosive disorder or antisocial personality. More subtle examples affect the diagnosis of many disorders in the *Diagnostic and Statistical Manual of Mental Disorders,* fourth edition (DSM-IV), such as attention-deficit/hyperactivity disorder, mental retardation, and conduct disorder. With regard to major depressive episodes and dysthymic disorder, age-norming has resulted in consideration of different symptoms at different ages in order to diagnose the same disorder (e.g., irritability and somatization are common in prepubescent depression, whereas delusions are more common in adulthood). DSM-IV explicitly requires consideration of age, gender, and culture features in all disorders, suggesting the importance of evaluating symptoms within the context of their expression.

The importance of age-norming suggests the need for empirical studies of symptoms in large epidemiologic samples and the linking of research on normative development to psychopathology. In this way, developmental psychopathology is similar to psychiatric epidemiology (see Chapter 5). Despite the increased emphasis on age-norming, ambiguity pervades current practice. DSM-IV defines disorders in terms of symptoms that are quantified as "often," "recurrent," and "persistent" without operational definition. Some clinicians intuitively contextualize their use of the term "often" relative to a child's agemates (so that "often displays temper tantrums" might mean hourly for a 2-year-old child and weekly for a teenager), whereas other clinicians do not (so that "often" has the same literal meaning across all ages). The "specific meaning of these terms is not clear in the context of some DSM-IV disorders. Complete age-norming might imply the removal of all age differences in prevalence rates (reducing disorder merely to the statistical extremes of a distribution at an age level), whereas complete neglect of age norms implies that at certain ages a disorder is ubiquitous. To resolve these problems, developmental researchers need to learn which patterns of symptoms ought to be examined epidemiologically, and psychopathologists need to compare their observations to empirical norms.

American Psychiatric Association: *Diagnostic and Statistical Manual of Mental Disorders,* 4th edn. Washington DC: American Psychiatric Association, 1994.

DEVELOPMENTAL TRAJECTORIES

Diagnosticians must consider not only the age-normed profile of symptoms but also the developmental trajectories of those symptoms (both age-normed and individual). For example, consider three 10-year-old children who exhibit aggressive behavior. As depicted in Figure 8–1, child A has displayed a relatively high rate of aggression historically, but the trajectory is downward. Child B has displayed a constant rate of aggressive displays, and child C's aggressive displays have accelerated geometrically. Which child has a problematic profile? The diagnostician will undoubtedly want to consider not only current symptom counts (in relation to age norms) but also the developmental trajectory of these counts (and the age norm for the trajectory). Child C might be most problematic because of the age trend, unless this trend were also age normative (e.g., some increase in delinquent behavior in adolescence is certainly normative). In contrast, child B's constant pattern might be problematic if the age-normed trend were a declining slope.

Some DSM-IV disorders explicitly take into account the trajectory of an individual's symptoms. For example, Rett's disorder, childhood disintegrative disorder, and

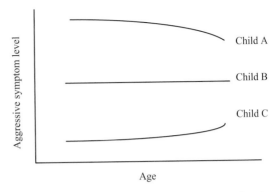

Figure 8–1. Three hypothetical developmental trajectories for aggressive behavior.

dementia of the Alzheimer's type involve deviant trajectories. The diagnosis of other disorders may require trajectory information that is not yet available. This information must be based on longitudinal study of individuals and not cross-sectional data, because only longitudinal inquiry allows for the charting of growth curves within individuals over time. Population means at various ages indicate little about within-individual changes. Population-wide symptom counts might grow systematically across age even when individual trajectories are highly variable.

Recent advances in quantitative methodology have enabled researchers to identify trajectories of development that mark different risk. Growth curve analyses are being used to identify predictors of trajectories so that dimensions can forecast future change in behavior based on normative profiles.

Costello EJ: Developments in child psychiatric epidemiology. *J Am Acad Child Adolesc Psychiatry* 1989;28:836.

Nagin DS: Analyzing developmental trajectories: A semi-parametric, group-based approach. *Psychol Methods* 1999;4:139.

THE BOUNDARY BETWEEN NORMAL & ABNORMAL

One of the tenets of developmental psychology is that a knowledge of normal development informs psychopathology partly because the boundaries between normal and abnormal are sometimes vague, diffuse, or continuous. Many disorders (e.g., conduct disorder, dysthymic disorder) are defined on the basis of cutoffs in dimensional criteria rather than on qualitative distinctions that are more easily recognizable. Criteria such as "low energy" and "low self-esteem" (for dysthymic disorder) and "marked or persistent fear" (for social phobia) are matters of degree. One of the central questions is where to locate the boundary between normal and abnormal when the criteria of psychopathology are dimensional.

In some cases, the boundary is arbitrary. In other cases the "true" boundary might be identified on the basis of three considerations: (1) a noncontinuous pattern of the distribution of scores, (2) a qualitatively distinct change in functioning that accompanies a quantitative difference in a score, or (3) unique etiology at the extreme of a distribution.

The first consideration is whether the population of scores is distributed normally with a single mode or bimodally with an unusually large number of cases at one extreme. A large number of cases at one extreme would suggest that a second causal agent is operating, beyond whatever agent caused the normal distribution. A second causal agent might suggest a deviant (i.e., psychopathologic) process. Consider the relation between the intelligence quotient (IQ) score (a continuous measure) and mental retardation. The distribution of IQ scores in the U.S. population is not normal. Far more cases of IQs below 70 occur than would be expected by a normal distribution. Thus, the distinction between normal and abnormal IQ scores is not merely one of degree.

The second consideration is whether qualitative differences in functioning occur with quantitative shifts in a criterion. For example, if a decrement of 10 IQ points from 75 to 65 makes it significantly more difficult for a child to function in a classroom than a decrement from 100 to 90, then a case can be made for locating the cutoff point near an IQ of 70.

The third consideration is the possible distinct etiology of scores at an extreme end of the distribution. A single set of causes will ordinarily lead to a normal distribution of scores. A disproportionate number of scores at an extreme often suggests a separate etiology for those scores. In the case of IQ scores, one set of forces (e.g., genes, socialization) leads to a normal distribution, whereas a second set of forces (e.g., Down syndrome, anoxia, lead toxicity) leads to a large number of cases at the low extreme.

Cicchetti D, Toth SL: Developmental psychopathology and preventive intervention. In: Renninger KA, Sigel IE (Vol eds). *Handbook of Child Psychology* 2006, p. 497; New York.

MULTIPLE PATHWAYS

A vexing problem highlighted by research in developmental psychology is that some disorders involve multiple etiologic pathways. The principles of equifinality and multifinality, derived from general systems theory, hold for many disorders. **Equifinality** is the concept that the same phenomenon may result from several different pathogens. For example, infantile autism results from congenital rubella, inherited metabolic disorder, or other factors. **Multifinality** is the concept that one etiologic factor can lead to any of several psychopathologic outcomes, depending on the person and context. Early physical abuse might lead to conduct disorder or to dysthymic disorder, depending on the person's predilections and the environmental supports for various symptoms; poverty predisposes one toward conduct disorder but also substance abuse disorder.

The diversity in processes and outcomes for disorders makes the systematic study of a single disorder difficult. Unless scholars consider multiple disorders and multiple factors simultaneously, they cannot be sure whether an apparent etiologic factor is specific to that disorder. Inquiry into one disorder benefits from a conceptualization within a larger body of development of normal adjustment versus problem outcomes. The broad coverage of developmental psychology provides the grounding for inquiry into various disorders.

Rutter M: Psychosocial resilience and protective mechanisms. In: Rolf J, Masten AS, Cicchetti D, Nüchterlein K, Weintraub S (eds). *Risk and Protective Factors in the Development of Psychopathology.* New York: Cambridge University Press, 1990.

BIOSOCIAL INTERACTIONS

The discovery of biosocial interactions in psychiatric disorders has been labeled one of the most important discoveries on all of science in the past decade. Not only are multiple distinct factors implicated in the genesis of a disorder, the profile of factors often conspires to lead to psychopathologic outcomes. Empirically, this profile is the statistical interaction between factors (in contrast with the main effects of factors). Thus, a causal factor might operate only when it occurs in concert with another factor. For example, the experience of parental rejection early in life is a contributing factor in the development of conduct disorder but only among that subgroup of children who also display a biologically based problem such as health difficulties at the time of birth. Likewise, health problems at birth do not inevitably lead to conduct disorder; the interaction of a biologically based predisposition with a psychosocial stressor is often required for a psychopathologic outcome.

Caspi et al. (2002) hypothesized that risk for conduct disorder grows out of the early experience of physical maltreatment, but only among a subpopulation characterized by polymorphism in the gene encoding the neurotransmitter-metabolizing enzyme monoamine oxidase A (MAOA). They found that physically maltreated children with a genotype conferring high levels of MAOA expression were less likely to develop antisocial problems than children without this genotype. These findings help us understand why not all victims of maltreatment grow up to victimize others, and they also indicate that environmental experiences may be necessary to potentiate the action of a genotype.

The same group of researchers has discovered a biosocial interaction in the development of depressive disorder. Life stressors precipitate the onset of depressive episodes, but only among a subpopulation characterized by a functional polymorphism in the promoter region of the serotonin transporter (5-HT T) gene. Individuals with one or two copies of the short allele of the 5-HT T promoter polymorphism exhibit more depressive symptoms, diagnosable depression, and suicidality in response to stressful life events than individuals homozygous for the long allele. The importance of biosocial interactions suggests the importance of examining multiple diverse factors simultaneously, both in empirical research and clinical practice.

Caspi A, McClay J, Moffitt TE, et al.: Role of genotype in the cycle of violence in maltreated children. *Science* 2002;297:851.

Caspi A, Sugden K, Moffitt TE, et al.: Influence of life stress on depression: Moderation by a polymorphism in the 5-HTT gene. *Science* 2003;301:386.

CRITICAL PERIODS & TRANSITION POINTS

A **critical period** is a point in the life span at which an individual is acutely sensitive to the effects of an external stimulus, including a pathogen. Freud argued that the first 3 years of life represent a critical period for the development of psychopathology, through concepts such as regression, fixation, and irreversibility. The concept of critical stages gained credence with studies of social behavior in animals by the ethologist Lorenz and the zoologist Scott. This concept is part of several central theories of social development, such as Bowlby's attachment theory (discussed later in this chapter). The rapid development of the nervous system in the first several years, coupled with relatively less neural plasticity in subsequent years, renders this period critical. The effects of exposure to lead and alcohol, for example, are far more dramatic when the exposure occurs in utero or in early life.

A variation of the concept of a critical period is the hypothesis of gradually decreasing plasticity in functioning across the life span. As neural pathways become canalized, mental representations become more automatic and habits form. However, the notion of the primacy of early childhood has been thrown into question by empirical data that indicate greater malleability in functioning than was previously thought. Rutter, for example, suggests that a positive relationship with a parental figure is crucial to the prevention of conduct disorder and that this relationship can develop or occur at any point up to adolescence, not just during the first year of life.

Some developmental psychologists have argued for other critical periods in life, such as puberty and giving birth as critical periods for the development of major depressive disorder in women, although this assertion has been contested. Critical periods might be defined not only by biological events but also by psychosocial transitions. Developmental psychologists have increasingly recognized the crucial role of major life transitions in altering developmental course, accelerating or decelerating psychopathologic development, and representing high-risk periods for psychopathology. These **transition points** include but are not limited to entry to formal schooling, puberty and the transition to junior high school, high school graduation and entry into the world of employment, marriage, birth of children, and death of loved ones (particularly parents or spouse). These transitions have been associated with elevated risk for some forms of psychopathology. One task of developmental psychologists is to discover which life transitions are most crucial and how these transitions alter the course of development of some but not other forms of psychopathology.

Kandel ER, Hawkins RD: Neuronal plasticity and learning. In: Broadwell RD (Vol ed). *Decade of the Brain. Vol 1: Neuroscience, Memory, and Language.* Washington DC: Library of Congress, 1995.

IMPORTANCE OF CONTEXT

One of the most important contributions of developmental psychology has been the discovery that patterns of behavior, and of process–behavior linkage, vary across contexts. In the context of U.S. society, a child who is teased by peers might find support for retaliating aggressively, whereas the same teasing experience in Japanese society might cause shame, embarrassment, and withdrawal. Thus, reactive aggressive behavior might be stigmatized as psychopathology in one culture but not another. Context shapes single behaviors and may also shape patterns of psychopathology.

Context also provides the frame or ground through which individual behaviors are given meaning. For example, a child interprets a parent's discipline in relation to norms that are observed culture-wide. In cultures that endorse the use of corporal punishment as appropriate, a child who is punished in this manner (at mild, nonabusive levels) is not at particularly high risk for anxiety problems or conduct problems. However, in cultures that do not endorse this type of parenting, a child who is corporally punished is likely to interpret it as a signal that the parent rejects the child as aberrant or is an aberrant parent, and either interpretation is likely to lead to anxiety and conduct problems.

Context can be defined at many levels, from discrete situational features to broad cultural features and from internal states such as mood to external factors such as geography or time of day. Bronfenbrenner's continuum of environmental contexts forms the basis of his ecological theory (discussed later in this chapter).

Bronfenbrenner U: *The Ecology of Human Development: Experiments by Nature and Design.* Cambridge, MA: Harvard University Press, 1979.

Dodge KA, Coie JD, Lynam D: Aggression and antisocial behavior in youth. In: Damon W (Series ed), Eisenberg N (Vol ed), *Handbook of Child Psychology, Vol. 3. Social, Emotional, and Personality Development,* 6th edn. New York: Wiley, 2006, pp. 719–788.

Lansford JE, Chang L, Dodge KA, et al.: Physical discipline and children's adjustment: Cultural normativeness as a moderator. *Child Dev* 2005;76(6):1234–1246.

ADAPTATION & COMPETENCE

Research in developmental psychology has sometimes enabled sharper distinctions between normal and abnormal (such as when a genetic marker of a disorder is identified), but more often it has articulated the continuity between normal and abnormal. Research has suggested that disorders might be defined less by noncontextualized behavioral criteria (e.g., a score on an IQ test) and more by an assessment of the individual's level of adaptation and functioning. This concept has been embraced by the term **competence,** or adaptive functioning, which is the level of performance by an individual in meeting the demands of his or her environment to the degree that would be expected given the environment and the individual's age, background, and biological potentials.

Empirical research has shown that measures of childhood social competence are important predictors of adolescent psychiatric disorders, including conduct disorder and mood disorders. Impaired social competence is a premorbid marker for the onset of schizophrenia and is a predictor of relapse.

The concurrent importance of adaptive functioning is so obvious that this concept has become part of the diagnostic criteria for some disorders. For example, a diagnosis of mental retardation requires impairment in adaptive functioning above and beyond the score on an IQ test. A diagnosis of generalized anxiety disorder requires impairment in social functioning in addition to the absolute pattern of anxiety. A diagnosis of obsessive–compulsive disorder requires marked personal distress or significant impairment in functioning. Some broad definitions of mental disorder are based on a general assessment of an impairment in adaptive functioning due to cognitive or emotional disturbance.

Kazdin AE: *Conduct Disorders in Childhood and Adolescence.* Thousand Oaks, CA: Sage, 1995.

Kupersmidt JB, Dodge KA (eds): *Children's Peer Relations: From Development to Intervention.* Washington, DC: American Psychological Association, 2004.

RISK FACTORS & VULNERABILITY

Epidemiologic and developmental researchers have introduced the notion of **risk factors** to identify variables known to predict later disorder (see Chapter 5). A risk factor is defined by its probabilistic relation to an outcome variable, without implying determinism, early onset of disorder, or inevitability of outcome. Risk factors are either markers of some other causal process or causal factors themselves. One goal of developmental research is to determine the causal status of risk markers. As noted earlier in this chapter, social competence, or level of adaptive functioning, is a broad risk factor for many disorders, but empirical research must determine whether this factor merely indicates risk that is caused by some other factor (e.g., genes) or constitutes a contributing factor in itself.

Risk factors often accumulate in enhancing the likelihood of eventual disorder. For example, the probability of conduct disorder is enhanced by low socioeconomic status, harsh parenting, parental criminality, marital conflict, family size, and academic failure. The number of factors present seems to be a stronger predictor of later disorder than is the presence of any single factor, suggesting that causal processes are heterogeneous and that risk factors cumulatively increase vulnerability to a causal process.

The concept of **vulnerability** has been applied to individuals who are characterized by a risk factor. Many empirical studies of the development of disorder use samples that are defined by a risk factor (such as offspring of alcoholics and first-time juvenile offenders); however, it is not clear that the causal and developmental factors are similar in disordered individuals who come from high-risk and low-risk populations.

Biederman J, Milberger S, Faraone SV, et al.: Family-environment risk factors for attention-deficit hyperactivity disorder. *Arch Gen Psychiatry* 1995;52: 464.

Cicchetti D, Cohen DJ (eds): *Developmental Psychopathology,* Vols. 1–3. New York: Wiley, 2006.

MEDIATORS & PROCESS

Developmental psychologists study the causal process through which disorder develops. The identification of a risk factor does not necessarily imply a causal process for these reasons: (1) a risk factor might be a proxy for a causal factor and empirically related to a disorder only because of its correlation with this causal factor (the so-called third-variable problem), (2) a risk factor might

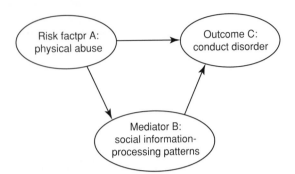

Figure 8–2. Mediation of the effect of physical abuse on the development of conduct disorder.

occur as an outcome of a process that is related to a disorder rather than as the antecedent of the disorder, or (3) a risk factor might play a causal role in a more complex, multivariate process. Indeed, individuals who are predisposed to a disorder often select environments that are congruent with the disorder. The environment might appear to "cause" the disorder but instead merely be a marker of risk. Therefore, developmental psychologists often attempt to understand the process through which risk factors are related to eventual disorder. The factors that are identified as intervening variables in this process are called **mediators,** or variables that account for (or partially account for) the statistical relation between a risk factor and a disorder.

Four empirical steps are required to demonstrate at least partial mediation (Figure 8–2). First, risk factor A must be empirically related to outcome C (i.e., there must be a phenomenon to be mediated, called the **total effect**). Second, A must be related to mediator B. Third, B must be related to C. Finally, in a stepwise regression or structural equation model analysis, when B has been added to the prediction of C, the resulting relation between A and C (called the **direct effect)** must be reduced significantly from the original bivariate relation. The difference between the total effect and the direct effect is called the **indirect effect**, that is, the magnitude of the mediation of the effect of A on C by B.

An example (depicted in Figure 8–2) is the biased pattern of social information-processing that often results from an early history of physical abuse. Early abuse (A) is a known risk factor for the development of conduct disorder (C) (i.e., it is statistically correlated with later conduct disorder, but many abused children do not develop this disorder nor do all persons who have conduct disorder show a history of abuse). Early abuse is also correlated with the development of a social information-processing pattern (B) of hypervigilance to threatening cues, perceiving the social world as a hostile and threatening place, and poor social problem-solving

skills. These mental factors (B) are associated statistically with later conduct disorder (C) and account for about half of the effect of early abuse (A) on later conduct disorder (C).

Baron RM, Kenny DA: The moderator-mediator variable distinction in social psychological research: Conceptual, strategic, and statistical considerations. *J Pers Soc Psychol* 1986;51:1173.

Dodge KA, Pettit GS: A biopsychosocial model of the development of chronic conduct problems in adolescence. *Dev Psychol* 2003;39(2):349.

MODERATORS & PROTECTIVE FACTORS

Rutter found that the effect of a risk factor on a disorder can vary across contexts, populations, or circumstances. That is, the magnitude of an effect might be reduced (or enhanced) under different conditions. For example, the effect of early harsh discipline on the development of conduct disorder is reduced under circumstances of a warm parent–child relationship. This phenomenon is called a **moderator effect** and is defined by a significant interaction effect between a risk factor and a moderating factor in the prediction of a disorder.

Moderator variables have also been called **protective**, or **buffering**, factors. A protective factor protects, or buffers, the individual from the pathogenic effects of a risk factor. Intelligence and a positive relationship with a caring adult have been the most commonly studied protective factors for a variety of disorders. One remaining question is whether protective factors operate more strongly in high-risk than in low-risk groups; that is, if a variable buffers both low-risk and high-risk groups from risk, it is not clear whether that variable would be defined as a protective factor (or simply another predictor variable).

Rutter M, Sroufe LA: Developmental psychopathology: Concepts and challenges. *Dev Psychopathol* 2000;12:265–296.

INTERVENTION & PREVENTION AS EXPERIMENTS

There is a reciprocal relation between the scientific study of behavior in developmental psychology and the application of scientific principles to psychiatry. Concepts from developmental psychology have been applied in psychiatric practice, but psychiatric intervention can also be viewed as a field experiment to test hypotheses about behavioral development. Systematic intervention and prevention can be viewed as experiments to test basic principles. In fact, given the complexity of human behavioral development and the ethical restraints against known iatrogenic manipulations, clinical practice may be the most powerful scientific tool available to test hypotheses from

Table 8–2. General Developmental Theories

Theory	Key Concepts	Criticisms
Temperament theory	Traits, genetic origins of behavior	Imprecise measurement, static view of human beings
Organismic theory	Stages of development, transformational role	Empirical refutation
Attachment theory	Patterns of relationships, working models	Too much emphasis on destiny from infancy
Social learning theory	Observational learning, imitation, reinforcement	Exclusive emphasis on environmental influences and cognitive mediation
Attribution theory	Mental heuristics, causal influences	Lack of emphasis on development, too narrow
Social information-processing theory	Mental processes during social interaction	Nonbiological
Ecological theory	Levels of systems	Vague and not falsifiable

developmental psychology. Thus, the relation between these disciplines is reciprocal, and communication between the disciplines must be preserved.

Cicchetti D, Toth SL: Developmental psychopathology and preventive intervention. In: Renninger KA, Sigel IE, (Vol eds). *Handbook of Child Psychology*, 2006, p. 497, New York: Wiley.

GENERAL DEVELOPMENTAL THEORIES

Seven major theories of development are listed in Table 8–2, along with key concepts and criticisms of each theory. These theories, along with their applications, are described in detail in the sections that follow.

TEMPERAMENT THEORY

Since the "human bile" theories of ancient Greeks, scholars have speculated that persons are born into the world with varying predispositions to behave in particular ways, called **traits**. Trait theorists have postulated a variety of dispositional tendencies, from Eysenck's neuroticism and extraversion to the "Big Five" traits of agreeableness, openness, extraversion, neuroticism, and conscientiousness. In developmental inquiry, temperament theory has received the greatest attention. It has been hypothesized that infants are born with biologically based temperaments that vary on a continuum from difficult to easy. This trait is evidenced in ease of early care, including feeding, soothing, and cuddling. As children grow older, these differences are evidenced in ease of manageability (e.g., the temper tantrums of 18-month-old children and the behavior difficulties of the preschool period). The trait of difficultness has been hypothesized as a risk factor for conduct disorder. Empirical studies have found significant but modest support for this hypothesis. Prospective studies indicate that infants characterized as difficult are

indeed at risk for conduct problems in the early school years, but the relation is somewhat weaker (although still present) for predictions from infancy to adolescence.

A different temperament theory, proposed by Kagan, has focused on the continuum of biological inhibition as the marker variable. Some infants regularly withdraw from novel social stimuli (**inhibited pattern**) whereas others seek out social stimulation (**uninhibited pattern**). Optimal levels of inhibition may fall between these extremes. Highly inhibited infants exhibit separation anxiety from parents and are likely to grow into shy, fearful, and withdrawn children. They are thought to be at risk for panic disorder in adulthood. Inhibited individuals demonstrate an increase in heart rate and stabilization of heart rate variability in response to a stress challenge. Individuals vary systematically in the degree to which the hypothalamus, pituitary gland, and adrenal gland (called the HPA axis) respond with glucocorticoid secretion during stress. Inhibited children have a lower threshold of sympathetic nervous system response and display a greater rise and stabilization of heart rate than uninhibited children exhibit. This pattern acts as a traitlike temperamental characteristic throughout life that may be associated with symptoms of anxiety.

Another postulate of temperament theories is that temperament elicits environmental treatment that perpetuates behavior consistent with that temperament. For example, it is hypothesized that "difficult" children elicit harsh discipline, which exacerbates difficult behavior, whereas inhibited children seek secure environments that pose minimal challenge and risk. Plomin has shown through twin and adoption studies that environmental experiences have a heritable component; that is, inherited genes lead either to behavior patterns that elicit environmental reactions or to behaviors that seek particular environments, a phenomenon known as niche-picking.

Applications of the Theory

Most temperament theorists recognize the importance of both inherited and environmental sources of development, so this theory has spawned empirical research directed toward understanding how these forces interact. It may be that infants with a particular temperament will develop more favorably under certain environmental conditions than others, and the task of inquiry is to identify optimal temperament-environment matches. Researchers are examining whether temperamentally difficult (or highly inhibited) infants develop more favorably under conditions of environmental restraint and structure or flexibility and freedom.

Another application has been to encourage research on the process through which genetic effects may operate on human development, thus informing the age-old debate between the influence of nature and nurture on human behavior (see Chapter 6).

Criticisms of the Theory

One problem with research on temperament theory has been the reliance on parents for assessments of temperament. Parents may be biased or inaccurate, or they may lack a broad base of knowledge of other infants. A parent's perceptions about his or her child may be legitimate factors in the child's development, but these perceptions confound information about the child's actual behavior with the parent's construal of the behavior. Direct observational measures of behavior have been developed to assess temperament, as have measures of biological functions, including heart rate reactivity, cortisol secretions, and skin conductivity. These measures also show some stability across time and some predictive power, but the number of studies is small and the statistical effects weak.

Another problem is the difficulty of distinguishing genetic–biological features from reactions to environmental treatment. A 6-month-old infant brings both a genetic heritage and a history of environmental experiences to current interactions. Even biological measures (e.g., resting heart rate, cortisol levels) have a partial basis in past social exchanges, so that the task of sorting genetic from environmental sources in biobehavioral measures is difficult.

Rothbart MK, Bates JE: Temperament. In: Eisenberg N (ed). *Handbook of Child Psychology*, Vol. 3. New York: Wiley, 2006, p. 99.

ORGANISMIC THEORY

No one has had more influence in developmental psychology than Piaget. The coherence of behavior across diverse domains and the tendency for changes in abilities to occur simultaneously across domains form the basis of the organismic theory of Piaget and others such as Gesell, Werner, and Baldwin. This theory attempts to describe general features of human cognition and the systematic changes in thought across development. The organizing principle in organismic theory is **structure**, which is a closed system of transformational rules that govern thought at a particular point in development. Consider the 5-year-old girl who observes one row of nine beads placed near each other and a second row of six beads stretched across a greater distance than the first row. Even though the girl has counted the beads in each row and knows that nine is greater than six, in response to the question, "Which row has more beads?" she will answer, "The row with six beads." Moreover, the girl will see no contradiction in her answer. According to Piaget, this nonobvious phenomenon occurs because the girl's structural transformation law is to consider the whole of a stimulus, not each part separately. The child's rule structure is closed; that is, it is internally consistent and not easily altered by external contradictions.

Piaget hypothesized that infants are born with a general wiring for a crude set of transformational rules common to all sensorimotor coordination. These rules are part of the evolutionary inheritance of the human organism. Development occurs over a 12- to 15-year period in nonlinear chunks, called **stages**. Within each stage, functioning is internally consistent and stable (called an **equilibrium**). Change from one stage to the next occurs as a result of interaction between the child and the realities of the environment. When contradictory realities accumulate sufficiently, change occurs rapidly and globally. As discussed earlier in this chapter, processes of change involve assimilation and accommodation. Assimilation is the act of interpreting environmental experiences in terms that are consistent with existing rule structure (a form of generalization), whereas accommodation is the act of altering rule structures to account for environmental experience (a form of exception noting). Children engage in both assimilation and accommodation in order to maintain coherence (and the perception of consistency), until their overgeneralizations and exceptions become so contradictory that they must create higher-level, more flexible, novel structures that account for the contradictions of earlier stages. When a novel structure (i.e., a new set of rules) is achieved, **equilibration** consolidates the rules until contradictions accumulate to set the scene for the next stage change. Piaget's four broad stages of cognitive development are (1) the sensorimotor period, (2) the preoperational stage, (3) the concrete-operational stage, and (4) the period of formal operations.

Applications of the Theory

Many of Piaget's concepts continue to have heuristic value even today and to provide hypotheses relevant to psychopathology. The notions of egocentrism, the invariant sequences of skill acquisition, and increasing differentiation (i.e., development rather than mere change) provide hypotheses regarding the behavior of children who have conduct problems and of adolescents who are lagging developmentally. Furthermore, Piaget's discoveries of the limits of young children's abilities have inspired cognitive educational strategies.

Criticisms of the Theory

Even though Piaget's influence has been tremendous, crucial features of organismic theory have been refuted. Children have repeatedly been shown to be more competent than Piaget suggested they could be at a particular age. Piaget's proposed cross-domain universality in type of thought has been shown to be false, suggesting to some scholars that the stage concept is faulty. It has been replaced by concepts of learning strategies, information-processing patterns, and the parsing of multiple components in complex task completion.

Piaget J: Piaget's theory. In: Kesson W (ed). *Handbook of Child Psychology. Vol 1: History, Theory, and Methods,* 4th edn. New York: John Wiley & Sons, 1983.

ATTACHMENT THEORY

Bowlby generated a theory of attachment that has had enormous influence in contemporary developmental psychology. According to Bowlby, infants are born with innate tendencies to seek direct contact with an adult (usually the mother). In contrast to Freud's perspective that early attachment-seeking is a function of a desire for the mother's breast (and food), Bowlby argued that attachment seeking is directed toward social contact with the mother (the desire for a love relationship) and driven by fear of unknown others. By about 6–8 months of age, separation from the mother arouses distress, analogous to free-floating anxiety. The distress of a short-term separation is replaced quickly by the warmth of the reunion with the mother, but longer separations (such as those occur in hospitalization or abandonment) can induce clinging, suspicion, and anxiety upon reunion. Similar effects are seen in older children until individuation occurs, at which point the child is cognitively able to hold a mental representation of the mother while she is gone, enabling the child to explore novelty.

Bowlby hypothesized that individual differences exist in patterns of parent-infant relationship quality and that the infant acquires a mental representation (or working model) of this relationship that is stored in memory and carried forward to act as a guiding filter for all future relationships. This working model of relationships generalizes to other contexts and allows future interactions

Table 8–3. Attachment Types and Associated Working Models and Outcomes

Attachment Type	Working Model	Outcome
A: Avoidant	Fearful	Risk
B: Secure	Exploration with confidence	Healthy
C: Ambivalent	Panicky distress and anger	Risk
D: Disorganized	Great distress	Risk

to conform to the working model, thereby reinforcing the initial representation of how relationships operate. Thus, the quality of the initial parent-infant relationship has primary and enduring effects on later adjustment, relationships, and parenting.

Individual differences in attachment patterns have been assessed through a laboratory procedure called the Strange Situation, devised by Ainsworth. The parent and 12-month-old child are brought to an unfamiliar room containing toys, after which a stranger enters. The parent then leaves the room for a short period, followed by a reunion. The child's behavior, especially toward the parent upon reunion, is indicative of the quality of the overall parent-child attachment. Attachment classifications are summarized in Table 8–3.

About two thirds of children fit the "secure" response pattern (type B), in which they demonstrate distress when the parent leaves and enthusiasm (or confident pleasure) upon her return. An "avoidant" response pattern (type A) involves little distress and little relief or pleasure upon reunion with the parent. A "resistant or ambivalent" response pattern (type C) involves panicky distress upon the parent's departure and emotional ambivalence upon reunion (perhaps running toward the parent to be picked up but then immediately, angrily struggling to get down). Recently, scholars have identified a fourth class of response, "disorganized" (type D, empirically linked to early physical or sexual maltreatment), in which the child's behavior involves great distress and little systematic exploration or seeking of adults.

Applications of the Theory

Follow-up studies have shown that these patterns of attachment are somewhat stable over time (although not strongly correlated across relationships with different adults) and predictive of behavioral adjustment in middle childhood. Infants of types A, C, and D are all at risk for later maladjustment, although more specific patterns of outcome for each type have not been detected reliably. Developmental scholars have created methods for assessing relationship quality and working models at older ages and have related these assessments to current behavioral functioning.

Criticisms of the Theory

Critics of attachment theory suggest that the initial relationship does not determine destiny as strongly as Bowlby argued, and that long-term predictive power is due partly to consistency in the environment that led to the child's initial response pattern. Attachment theory has been used to condemn the practice of early out-of-home daycare (because it interferes with the development of a secure attachment with the mother), even though most studies find little long-term effect of such care after other confounding factors (e.g., economics, family stability, stress, later caregiving) are controlled. More broadly, the reversibility of the effects of early social deprivation and trauma remain controversial. The current general conclusion is that even though early experiences shape later experiences through the filter of mental representations, the plasticity of the human organism is greater than previously hypothesized, but only up to a point.

Ainsworth MDS et al: *Patterns of Attachment.* Hillsdale, NJ: Lawrence Erlbaum Assoc, 1978.
Bowlby J: *Attachment and Loss. Vol 3: Loss, Sadness, and Depression.* New York: Basic Books, 1980.

SOCIAL LEARNING THEORY

Bandura's social learning theory, though acknowledging the constraints of biological origins and the role of neural mediating mechanisms, emphasizes the role of the individual's experience of the environment in development. Other learning theories are based on the organism's direct performance of behaviors, whereas social learning theory posits that most learning occurs vicariously by observing and imitating models. For survival and growth, humans are designed to acquire patterns of behavior through **observational learning**. Social behavior in particular is a function of one's social learning history, instigation mechanisms, and maintaining mechanisms.

Four processes govern social learning: (1) attention, which regulates exploration and perception; (2) memory, through which observed events are symbolically stored to guide future behavior; (3) motor production, through which novel behaviors are formed from the integration of constituent acts with observed actions; and (4) incentives and motivation, which regulate the performance of learned responses. Development involves biological maturation in these processes as well as the increasingly complex storage of contingencies and response repertoires in memory.

Instigation mechanisms include both biological and cognitive motivators. Internal aversive stimulation might activate behavior through its painful effect (on hunger, sex, or aggression). Cognitively based motivators are based on the organism's capacity to represent mentally future material, sensory, and social consequences. Mentally represented consequences provide the motivation for action.

Maintaining mechanisms include external reinforcement (e.g., tangible rewards, social and status rewards, reduction of aversive treatment), punishment, vicarious reinforcement by observation, and self-regulatory mechanisms (e.g., self-observation, self-judgment through attribution and valuation, self-applied consequences). Development in social learning theory is decidedly not stage-like and has few constraints. For example, Bandura argued that even relatively sophisticated moral thought and action are possible in young children, given relevant models and experiences.

Applications of the Theory

Social learning theory has been applied most effectively to aggressive behavior, where it has provided powerful explanations for the effects of coercive parenting, violent media presentations, and rejecting peer interactions on the development of chronic aggressive behavior. Furthermore, it provides the basis for most current behavior-modification interventions in clinical practice.

Criticisms of the Theory

Critics dispute the primacy of cognitive mediation in understanding learning effects and the relative emphasis on environment over genetic and biological influences.

Bandura A: *Social Foundations of Thought and Action: A Social Cognitive Theory.* Englewood Cliffs, NJ: Prentice-Hall, 1986.

ATTRIBUTION THEORY

The emphasis on cognition in social learning theory is largely consequence oriented (i.e., based on individuals' cognitions about the likely outcomes of their behavior). Attribution theory is more concerned with how people understand the causes of behavior. Its origins are in the naïve or common-sense psychology of Heider, who suggested that an individual's beliefs about events play a more important role in behavior than does the objective truth of events. For social interactions, an individual's beliefs about the causes of another person's behavior are more crucial than are the true causes. For example, in deciding whether to retaliate aggressively against a peer following a provocation (such as being bumped from behind), a person often uses an attribution about the peer's intention. If the peer had acted accidentally then no retaliation occurs, but if the peer had acted maliciously then retaliation may be likely. The perceiver's task in social exchanges is to decide which effects of an observed action are intentional (reflecting dispositions) and which are situational.

When judging whether another person's behavior (such as aggression) should be attributed to a dispositional rather than a situational cause, perceivers use mental heuristics, such as correspondent inference and covariation. Perceivers examine whether the person's actions are normative or unique (if unique, they may indicate a dispositional rather than situational cause). They examine the other person's behavioral consistency over time and distinctiveness across situations (if the behavior is consistent, it more likely reflects a disposition). Finally, they examine whether the action has personal hedonic relevance to the perceiver (if the action is relevant to the perceiver, perceivers tend to attribute dispositional causes).

These principles predict the kinds of causal attributions that people make about the events around them, the circumstances under which people will make errors in inference, and people's behavioral responses to events. Extensions of attribution theory have addressed differences in the causal attributions made by people about themselves versus others (actor–observer effects), the kinds of explanations that people give for their own behavior and outcomes (internal versus external attributions), and the circumstances under which people spontaneously make attributions.

Applications of the Theory

Attribution theory has been applied to problems in several domains of psychiatry and health. Studies have shown that attributions predict behavioral responses to critical events such as interpersonal losses and failure. People who attribute their failure to a lack of ability on their part are likely to give up and to continue to fail, whereas people who attribute their failure to a lack of effort are likely to intensify future efforts to succeed. People who regularly attribute their failures to global, stable, and internal causes (i.e., they blame themselves) are at risk for a mood disorder and somatization disorder. People who attribute their own negative outcomes to the fault of others are likely to direct aggression toward the perceived cause of the outcome (and to develop a conduct disorder). Interventions have been developed to help people redirect attributions more accurately or more adaptively, most notably in cognitive therapies for depression.

Criticisms of the Theory

Until recently, the problem of development was relatively ignored in attribution theory. Studies only recently have begun to address topics such as the age at which attributions come to be made spontaneously, the relevance of

spontaneous attribution tendencies for age differences in depression, and the experiential origins of chronic attributional tendencies.

Dodge KA. Translational science in action: Hostile attributional style and the development of aggressive behavior problems. *Dev Psychopathol* 2006;18:791.

SOCIAL INFORMATION-PROCESSING THEORY

The comprehensive extension of social learning theory and attribution theory is to consider all of the mental processes that people use in relating to the social world. Simon's work in cognitive science forms the basis for social information-processing theory. This theory recognizes that people come to social situations with a set of biologically determined capabilities and a database of past experiences (Figure 8–3).

They receive as input a set of social cues (such as a push in the back by a peer or a failing grade in a school subject). The person's behavioral response to the cues occurs as a function of a sequence of mental processes, beginning with encoding of cues through sensation and perception. The vastness of available cues requires selective attention to cues (such as attention to peers' laughter versus one's own physical pain). Selective encoding is partially predictive of ultimate behavior. The storage of cues in memory is not veridical with objective experience. The mental representation and interpretation of the cues (possibly involving attributions about cause) is the next step of processing. A person's interpretation of a stimulus is predictive of that person's behavioral response (e.g., a hostile attribution made about another's ambiguously provocative push in the back will predict a retaliatory aggressive response). Once the stimulus cues are represented, the person accesses one or more possible behavioral responses from memory. Rules of association in memory, as well as the person's response repertoire, guide this retrieval. For example, one person might follow the rule "when intentionally provoked, fight back"; whereas another person might follow the rule "when provoked, run away." Accessing a response is not the same as responding behaviorally, however, as in the case of a withheld impulse. The next step of processing is response evaluation and decision making, wherein the person (not necessarily consciously) evaluates the interpersonal, intrapersonal, instrumental, and moral consequences of accessed behavioral responses and decides on an optimal response. Clearly, evaluations that a behavior is relatively likely to lead to positive consequences are predictive of that behavioral tendency. The final step of processing involves the transformation of a mental decision into motor and verbal behavior.

Social information-processing theory posits that people engage in these mental processes over and over in real

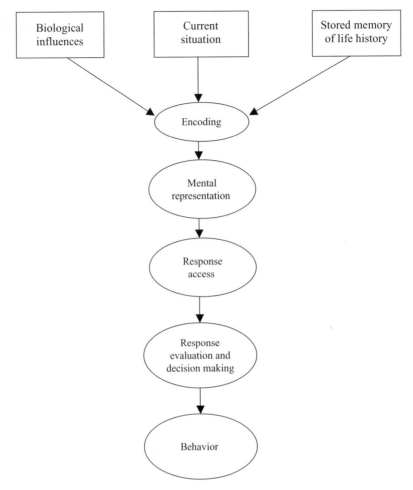

Figure 8–3. Social information-processing theory.

time during social interactions and that within particular types of situations, individuals develop characteristic patterns of processing cues at each step in the model. These patterns form the basis of psychopathologic tendencies. For example, in response to provocations, one person might regularly selectively attend to certain kinds of cues (such as threats), attribute hostile intentions to others, access aggressive responses, evaluate aggressing as favorable, and enact aggression skillfully. This person is highly likely to develop conduct disorder. Likewise, in response to academic failure, another person might selectively attend to his or her own contributing mistakes, attribute the outcome to personal failure, access self-destructive responses, evaluate all other responses as leading to further failure, and enact self-destructive responses effortlessly.

This person is likely to develop dysthymic disorder or major depressive disorder.

Applications of the Theory

Social information-processing theory has been used successfully to predict the development of conduct problems in children and depressive symptoms in adolescents. Not all individuals with conduct problems display the same deviant processing patterns at all steps of the model; however, most people with conduct problems display at least one type of processing problem. Some children with conduct problems show hostile attributional tendencies, whereas others evaluate the likely outcomes of aggressing as positive. These processing differences accurately predict subtypes of conduct problems: Children with hostile attributional tendencies display problems of reactive anger control, whereas children who make positive evaluations of the outcome of aggressing display instrumental aggression and bullying.

The development of processing styles has shed light on the development of psychopathology. For example, children with early histories of physical abuse are likely to become hypervigilant to hostile cues and to display hostile attributional tendencies. These tendencies predict later aggressive-behavior problems and account for the empirical link between early physical abuse and the development of aggressive-behavior problems.

Social information-processing theory has the potential to distinguish among types of psychopathology. In one investigation, groups of children with depressive, aggressive, comorbid, or no symptoms were found to display unique profiles of processing patterns. The aggressive group tended to attribute hostile intentions to others, to access aggressive responses, and to evaluate the outcomes of aggressing as favorable. The depressive group, in contrast, tended to attribute hostile intentions to others as well, but they also attributed the cause of others' hostile intentions to self-blame, and they accessed self-destructive responses and evaluated aggressive responses negatively.

Social information-processing theory has suggested interventions designed to help people construe situations differently and to act on the social world more effectively. For example, one intervention has been directed toward helping aggressive adolescents attribute interpersonal provocations in a less personalized and hostile way. This intervention has been successful in reducing the rate of aggressive behavior in these adolescents, relative to untreated control subjects.

Criticisms of the Theory

By focusing on in situ mental actions, processing theory relatively neglects enduring structural components of personality that are emphasized in psycho-analytic and Piagetian theories. Another criticism is that social information-processing theory locates the sources of deviant behavior in the individual, in contrast to the broader social ecology.

Dodge KA, Coie JD, Lynam D: Aggression and antisocial behavior in youth: In: Eisenberg N (Vol ed). *Handbook of Child Psychology: Vol. 3. Social, Emotional, and Personality Development.* New York: Wiley, 2006, p. 719.

ECOLOGICAL THEORY

Ecological theory evolved from the recognition that even though the environment has a major effect on develop-

ment, many models of development have limited generalizability across contexts. Consider, for example, classic studies by Tulkin and his colleagues on the effect of mother–infant interaction patterns on the infant's development of language and mental abilities. This effect is stronger among socioeconomic middle-class families than among lower-class families. Likewise, Scarr has found that the magnitude of genetic influences on intellectual development varies according to the cultural group being studied. Greater genetic effects are observed in middle-class white groups than in lower-class African American groups. Among lower-class families, different influences on development are operating. Findings such as these led ecological theorists such as Lewin, Bronfenbrenner, and Barker to conclude that models of development are bounded by the context in which they are framed.

Ecological theory suggests that process models of development have no universality; rather, they must be framed within the limits of a cultural and historical context. This theory must be distinguished from the radical postmodernist perspective that scientific principles have no objective basis. Ecological theorists conceptualize the environment systematically and attempt to understand how it affects development.

Bronfenbrenner has articulated an ecological model that includes developmental influences at the individual (person), person-by-environment (process), and context levels. He categorizes contextual settings into three types: microsystems, mesosystems, and exosterns. As discussed earlier in this chapter, the most proximal type is the microsystem, which includes the immediate physical and social environment. Examples of microsystems are homes, schools, playgrounds, and work places. Each microsystem has a structure and a set of rules and norms for behavior that are fairly consistent across time. Developmental scientists study processes within each of these settings, and ecologists warn them not to overgeneralize process phenomena from one microsystem to another.

The next type is the mesosystem, which is defined as a combination of microsystems that leads to a new level of developmental influence. For example, in understanding the effects of parental versus peer influences on adolescent development, one must consider not only each of the family and peer microsystems but also the effect of the combined mesosystem, that is, the effect of the conflict between the family's values and the peer group's values on the child's development.

The final type is the exosystem, a combination of multiple mesosystems. Research on the effects of maternal employment on child development has been enhanced by an understanding of this exosystem. That is, in order to understand how maternal employment affects a child's social development, one must understand not only the family and work context but also the cultural and historical contexts of women's employment.

Applications of the Theory

Ecological theory has led clinicians to question the generalizability of their practices across cultural, gender, and ethnic groups. Group-specific interventions are being developed. Ecological theory has also led to policy changes in the funding of research at the federal level, in that large research studies are now required to address questions of generalizability across groups. Finally, ecological theorists have pressed clinicians to consider the possibility that interventions at a broader level might exert a powerful effect at the microsystem level.

Criticisms of the Theory

Ecological theory is not a theory in the formal sense. Rather, it is a structured framework for identifying influences at numerous levels. Thus, it is not falsifiable. Its value is in alerting clinicians to factors that otherwise might be neglected.

Bronfenbrenner U, Morris PA: The bioecological model of human development: In: Lerner, RM (Vol ed), *Handbook of Child Psychology, Vol. 1: Theoretical Models of Human Development.* New York: Wiley; 2006, p. 793.

SYNTHESIS: DIATHESIS–STRESS MODELS & OTHER INTERACTIONIST THEORIES

It has been increasingly recognized that interactionist models of development apply to most forms of psychopathology. These models focus on the confluence of forces that must coalesce in order for a disorder to develop. The most basic of these models is the diathesis–stress model. A **diathesis** is a dispositional characteristic that predisposes an individual to a disorder. The disposition may be biological (as in a genetic predisposition for schizophrenia), environmental (as in poverty), or cognitive (as in low IQ). A disorder is probabilistically related to the presence of a diathesis, but the process of development of psychopathology requires that the individual with the diathesis also be exposed to a stressor, which, again, might be biological or environmental. Only those individuals with both diathesis and stressor are likely to develop the disorder.

Consider the diathesis–stress model of major depressive disorder. According to this model, individuals who display the cognitive diathesis of self-blame for failure are. at risk for the development of depression, but only if they subsequently experience a stressor that is linked to

the diathesis (such as failure). Statistically, this model hypothesizes an interaction effect, and it has been supported for a variety of problems, from depression to physical illness.

Theorists have noted that individual and environmental factors interact not only in static models such as the case of major depressive disorder but also over time in transactional models. These models articulate the reciprocal influences between person and environment and the unfolding of disorder across experience. Finally, theorists have come to recognize that the unfolding occurs in nonlinear, nonuniform ways that lead to qualitative changes in the individual, as in dynamic systems (see "Major Principles of Ontogeny and Phylogeny" earlier in this chapter). Dynamic systems models are borrowed from phenomena in physics to describe the development of novel behavior in infancy (such as the onset of locomotion and language) and have the potential to be applied to the development of novel deviant behavior in psychopathology.

Magnussen D, Stattin H: The person in context: A holistic-interactionist approach: In: RM Lerner (ed). *Handbook of Child Psychology, Vol. 1: Theoretical Models of Human Development.* New York: Wiley; 2006, p. 400.

LIFE-COURSE PROSPECTIVE INQUIRY

One of the most powerful methods in developmental clinical research is that of life-course prospective inquiry, closely linked to developmental epidemiology. By identifying an important sample (either a high-risk sample or a representative sample) and then following that sample with repeated assessments across time using hypothesis-driven measures, researchers have been able to identify risk factors in the development of a disorder, moderators of that risk, and mediating processes in the etiology of the disorder. Two such longitudinal studies are described in this section as examples of ongoing research in this field.

THE DEVELOPMENT OF DEPRESSION PROJECT

The Development of Depression Project has tested the diathesis–stress model of the development of major depressive disorder in adolescents. According to Garber, some children develop cognitive styles for attributing their failures and losses to internal, global, and stable characteristics of themselves, and they begin to have negative automatic thoughts in response to life events. Later, when confronted with failures and losses, these children are at elevated risk for developing major depressive disorder. It is the interaction of the cognitive diathesis and the life stressor, not either factor in isolation that leads to depression. In order to rule out competing hypotheses that cognitive styles or problem life events result from, rather than lead to, depression, a research design is needed that follows children across time.

The research strategy in this study was to identify a sample of children prior to adolescence; to assess cognitive diatheses, life events, family processes, and psychopathology in this sample at that time; and then to follow the children with repeated assessments throughout adolescence in order to determine which ones develop depression following common stressors of adolescent life.

At the first wave of assessment in sixth grade, 188 children and their parents were assessed for psychopathology, life events stressors, family processes, and most pertinent, the cognitive diathesis for depression. Analyses of the initial wave revealed that children of depressive parents demonstrated more subthreshold symptoms of depression and more negative attributional styles than did the children of nondepressed parents. Even though these findings are consistent with the hypothesized model, the critical test would come over time if initial depressive symptom levels could be controlled statistically to see whether attributional styles and life stressors interact to predict onset of depressive disorder. Annual follow-ups through young adulthood indicate that among those children who displayed at least some depressive symptoms, controlling for initial depressive symptom levels, the interaction of early cognitive diathesis and subsequent stressful life events significantly predicted later depressive symptom levels as determined by psychiatric interviews. That is, only those children with a combination of initial negative automatic thoughts and subsequent stressful life events showed elevated depressive symptoms later; all other groups showed lower levels of symptoms. This is a moderator effect: The cognitive diathesis moderates (or alters) the effect of stressful life events on depressive symptoms.

This prospective study has provided empirical support for a model in which early family interactions involving psychological control and lack of acceptance lead a child to develop cognitive styles of negative self-worth, negative automatic thoughts, and negative attributions for failure. Later, in adolescence, those children who show the unique combination of experiencing stressful life events and having negative automatic thoughts about those events are most likely to develop depression. This model integrates biological (genetic risk), family process, cognitive, and ecological (stressful life events) factors in the onset and course of depression. It also suggests three points for intervention with children who are at risk for depression. First, early family interactions involving acceptance and control might be targeted through parent training. Second, the child's cognitive styles might be addressed in brief preventive cognitive therapy. Third, the child's ecology might be modified by altering the child's exposure to stressful life events (or at least the child's experience of inevitable stressful events).

The findings of this seminal study have been used as the empirical basis for innovative intervention programs to prevent depressive disorder in early adolescents. Prevention scientists, including Gregory Clarke, Martin Seligman, Timothy Strauman, and Judy Garber, have developed individual- and group-based multisession programs designed to help adolescents alter their cognitive responses to failure, loss, and other stressors. Evaluation of these programs through randomized trials has revealed proximal success in altering targeted cognitive styles and distal success in preventing depressive symptoms in response to future stressors.

Hilsman R, Garber J: A test of the cognitive diathesis–stress model in children: Academic stressors, attributional style, perceived competence and control. *J Pers Soc Psychol* 1995;69: 370.

Horowitz JL, Garber J: The prevention of depressive symptoms in children and adolescents: A meta-analytic review. *J Consult Clin Psychol* 2006;74:421.

THE CHILD DEVELOPMENT PROJECT

The Child Development Project was initiated to understand the role of family experiences and patterns of social information processing in the development and growth of aggressive conduct problems and conduct disorder. The design is a developmental epidemiologic one: 585 preschool children at three geographic sites were selected randomly at kindergarten matriculation to participate in a 20-year longitudinal study. The hypotheses guiding the study were, based on the social learning theory in developmental psychology and the social information-processing theory in cognitive science, namely, that early family experiences of physical abuse and harsh discipline would predict later serious conduct problems; and that this relation would be mediated by the child's intervening development of problematic patterns of processing social information.

In-home family interviews and direct observations of family interactions provided information about the child's experience of physical abuse and harsh discipline in the first 5 years of life. About 12% of this random sample was identified as having experienced physical abuse at some time in their lives, a high rate that is consistent with national surveys of community samples. At subsequent annual assessments, video-guided interviews with each child provided measures of the child's patterns of social information processing. Finally, teacher ratings, peer nominations, direct observations, and school records provided evidence of externalizing conduct problems. The study followed this sample from preschool into high school.

Analyses indicated that the physically abused group of children had a fourfold increase in risk for clinically significant externalizing problems by middle school. This risk could not be statistically accounted for by confounding factors, such as socioeconomic status, child temperament, or exposure to other violent models. Thus, it seems that the experience of harsh parenting, especially if extreme, is partially responsible for conduct problems in some children.

Consistent with the original hypotheses, the physically abused children were also at risk for problems with social information processing. Specifically, physically abused children were relatively likely to become hypervigilant to hostile cues, to develop hostile attributional biases, to access aggressive responses to social problems, and to believe that aggressive behaviors lead to desired outcomes. Also consistent with hypotheses, children who demonstrated these processing patterns were likely to develop clinically significant externalizing problems in middle school and high school. Finally, the mediation hypothesis was supported, in that the child's social information-processing patterns accounted for about half of the statistical relation between early physical abuse and later conduct problems.

Lansford JE, Dodge KA, Pettit GS, Bates JE, Crozier J, Kaplow J: A 12-year prospective study of the long-term effects of early child physical maltreatment on psychological, behavioral, and academic problems in adolescence. *Arch Pediatr Adolesc Med* 2002;156:824–830.

CONCLUSION

Developmental psychology plays an important role in psychiatric science and practice. Concepts such as the orthogenetic principle, ontogeny, phylogeny, age-norming, and developmental trajectories can help the practicing psychiatrist to place a patient's current symptoms into developmental and ecological context. Common patterns in the development of psychopathology (e.g., biosocial interactions, multiple pathway models, mediational models, and bidirectional effects) enrich the psychiatrist's understanding of the etiology of psychiatric disorders.

Even though major developmental theories (e.g., temperament, attachment, social learning) have historical significance, most contemporary thinking is not directed at contrasting these theories at a macrolevel. Rather, it is understood that psychiatric phenomena usually involve complex interactions of factors at multiple levels. Current research is aimed at understanding how variables implicated by various theories interact to produce psychiatric disorder, rather than proving one general theory to be more meritorious than another.

The relation between developmental psychology and psychiatry is reciprocal. That is, knowledge gained from developmental theory and empirical findings has been useful to psychiatrists in both scientific understanding and practice, and the findings and concerns of psychiatrists have modified developmental theory and guided developmental empirical inquiry. These disciplines have been fused even more tightly in the emerging discipline of developmental psychopathology, which seeks to understand the etiology, process, and life-course of psychiatric phenomena.

Psychopharmacologic Interventions　9

Richard C. Shelton, MD

Most psychiatric disorders remain without well-established biological substrates; however, standardized diagnostic nosology has gained acceptance, primarily in the form of the *Diagnostic and Statistical Manual of Mental Disorders,* fourth edition (DSM-IV). As with other areas of medicine, there is no substitute for a careful diagnostic evaluation using externally validated diagnostic criteria. Whenever possible, the diagnostic evaluation should draw on a comprehensive database that includes family members, previous or concurrent providers, and other sources of information, and the evaluation should focus more on longitudinal data than just acute presentation.

■ PHARMACOKINETICS & PHARMACODYNAMICS

An understanding of the basic pharmacokinetics and pharmacodynamics of psychotropic drugs is required for their safe and effective utilization. With the exception of lithium (which is an element), most psychotropic drugs are lipophilic polycyclic amines. These drugs interact with neurotransmitter-binding sites, which confer their psychotropic effects. For example, most antidepressants act by allosteric binding to catecholamine- or indolamine-uptake binding sites (or with the monoaminergic catalytic enzyme monoamine oxidase), which enhances the synaptic availability of monoamines such as norepinephrine and serotonin. These effects can produce direct antidepressant actions but also may produce side effects such as nausea or nervousness. These drugs also interact with muscarinic cholinergic-binding sites, producing significant side effects such as dry mouth, blurred vision, and constipation, and with histamine-binding sites, producing drowsiness and weight gain. The relative profile of receptor binding affinities will allow the clinician to predict both the beneficial effects and side effects of specific drugs.

Most psychotropic drugs are fairly rapidly and completely absorbed from oral and intramuscular sites and, because of their relatively high lipid solubility, readily cross the blood–brain barrier. Intramuscular administration yields rapid absorption and distribution and bypasses first-pass hepatic metabolism. Therefore, plasma levels are achieved much more rapidly. Intramuscular delivery of antipsychotic drugs (e.g., haloperidol, olanzapine, ziprasidone) or antianxiety agents (e.g., lorazepam) are reserved primarily for the acute management of agitated and psychotic patients. An exception to this is the use of haloperidol or fluphenazine decanoate; both drugs are provided in oil suspension for long-term treatment of psychotic conditions. They require injection every 2–4 weeks and are given to patients who have problems with treatment compliance.

Most psychotropic drugs have high levels of protein (e.g., α_1 glycoproteins) binding. Notable exceptions include lithium and venlafaxine. Therefore, drug interactions could occur at the level of protein binding, in which case these drugs will displace (and be displaced by) other drugs with significant binding. This can result in unexpected toxicities; therefore, clinicians should take a careful drug history whenever they plan to prescribe a new drug to a patient.

With the exception of lithium, all psychotropic drugs are metabolized, at least in part, via cytochrome enzymes. After one or more metabolic steps, water-soluble products (e.g., glucuronides) are formed and eliminated via the kidney. Certain psychopharmacologic agents may induce or inhibit metabolism by cytochrome P-450 (CYP) enzymes. For example, car bamazepine can induce CYP 3A4, 2B1, and 2B2 enzymes, whereas certain serotonin selective reuptake inhibitor (SSRI) antidepressants may inhibit metabolism via CYP 2D6. These metabolic interactions must be considered when drugs are coadministered.

Most psychotropic drugs produce widely varying plasma levels, and monitoring may be helpful. However, plasma-level ranges are established only with certain tricyclic antidepressants (e.g., imipramine, desipramine, nortriptyline), with antipsychotics such as haloperidol and clozapine, and with lithium. Because of the narrow therapeutic index, plasma-level monitoring of lithium is part of accepted practice. With other drugs, where there are no established plasma level-response relationships, plasma-level monitoring can be used to check compliance or when severe side effects suggest abnormally increased levels. In addition, plasma levels may clarify a situation in which one drug may be increasing or decreasing the level of another. For example, an SSRI such as paroxetine may elevate plasma levels of other drugs that are metabolized by CYP 2D6 (e.g., haloperidol). Unexpected side effects could occur that would be clarified by a plasma-level measurement.

Nemeroff CB, DeVane CL, Pollock BG: Newer antidepressants and the cytochrome P450 system. *Am J Psychiatry* 1996;153:311.

Preskorn SH: Clinically relevant pharmacology of selective serotonin reuptake inhibitors: An overview with emphasis on pharmacokinetics and effects on oxidative drug metabolism. *Clin Pharmacokinet* 1997;32(Suppl 1):1.

Preskorn SH, Dorey RC, Jerkovich GS: Therapeutic drug monitoring of tricyclic antidepressants. *Clin Chem* 1988;34:822.

PHARMACOKINETICS IN SPECIAL POPULATIONS

Pharmacokinetics can differ by population. For example, children have a higher relative percentage of hepatic mass and a greater-than-expected elimination of drugs by first-pass metabolism. The elderly often have relatively reduced hepatic clearance and protein binding, which increases the relative plasma levels of most psychotropic drugs. Dosage adjustments must be made for differences in kinetics, and these adjustments should be based on research data, when available.

Pregnancy poses its own set of problems. Exposure of women of reproductive potential to psychotropic drugs raises the possibility of birth defects or spontaneous abortion should pregnancy occur. All women of reproductive potential should be counseled about pregnancy and drug exposure (i.e., to avoid pregnancy or to inform the physician before becoming pregnant). Lithium, anticonvulsant mood-stabilizing agents (e.g., carbamazepine or divalproex), and benzodiazepines have been associated with increased rates of specific birth defects and, generally, should be avoided, especially in the first trimester. The effects of antidepressants and antipsychotics are less clear, except for the case of paroxetine. Drugs should be withdrawn if possible; however, drug withdrawal is sometimes impossible. A risk–benefit analysis should be undertaken in which the potential risks of drug exposure are weighed against the hazards of no-drug therapy. Because the first trimester is the most important period of organogenesis, efforts should be made to avoid drug exposure during this period. Another consideration is that drugs may be withdrawn prior to delivery and reinstated afterward. This will help prevent untoward reactions such as excessive sedation, withdrawal, or discontinuation reactions in the newborn.

Nursing mothers generally can take psychotropics. Most drugs are excreted into breast milk, but the levels tend to be very low. The absolute short-term and long-term risks are unknown. An appropriate risk–benefit discussion should be undertaken with the patient.

Altshuler LL, Cohen L, Szuba MP, Burt VK, Gitlin M, Mintz J: Pharmacologic management of psychiatric illness during pregnancy: Dilemmas and guidelines. *Am J Psychiatry* 1996;153:592.

Ambrosini PJ: Pharmacotherapy in child and adolescent major depressive disorder. In: Meltzer HY (ed). *Psychopharmacology: The Third Generation of Progress.* Raven Press, New York: 1987, pp. 1247–1254.

Catterson ML, Preskorn SH, Martin RL: Pharmacodynamic and pharmacokinetic considerations in geriatric psychopharmacology. *Psychiatr Clin North Am* 1997;20:205.

Simeon JG: Pediatric psychopharmacology. *Can J Psychiatry* 1989;34: 122.

Stowe ZN, Owens MJ, Landry JC, Kilts CD, Ely T, Llewellyn A, Nemeroff CB: Sertraline and desmethylsertraline in human breast milk and nursing infants. *Am J Psychiatry* 1997;154:1255.

Vitiello B: Treatment algorithms in child psychopharmacology research. *J Child Adolesc Psychopharmacol* 1997;7:3.

PRINCIPLES OF PSYCHOPHARMACOLOGIC MANAGEMENT

Clinical practice involves establishing and maintaining an effective working relationship with a patient—the therapeutic alliance. This process requires the therapist and the patient to establish mutually acceptable goals and to agree on a plan to achieve these objectives. This is especially important in psychiatry because the beneficial effect of a drug may be delayed and because some patients may not have insight into their problem. The challenge of psychopharmacologic management is to maintain an effective working relationship with patients in the face of such obstacles.

The effective pharmacotherapist will maintain a broad biopsychosocial view of the patient's problem and will plan accordingly. Medications will help to address identified symptoms, but patients exhibit a wide array of problems, including psychosocial stressors (e.g., family and work issues) and more purely psychological factors that put the patient at risk for further problems. Pharmacotherapy, therefore, shares significant elements with psychotherapy. The pharmacotherapist must establish rapport and a working relationship with the patient, based on the expertise of the therapist and on mutual trust. The patient will depend on the therapist's ability to perform a risk–benefit analysis and to provide an adequate rationale for all elements of treatment. A therapeutic trial of medication may then be undertaken; however, this process of education and negotiation with the patient is an ongoing part of treatment.

Analyzing Risks & Benefits

The risk–benefit analysis considers many factors. The most basic of these factors is the presence of any medical or psychiatric contraindications to the use of a particular drug, including the potential for drug interactions. For example, although bupropion is an effective antidepressant, it generally is not given to patients who have a history of seizure disorder or a current psychotic condition because the drug has the potential to aggravate these problems. However, bupropion may be an especially good choice for patients who have erectile dysfunction. Alternatively, the pharmacotherapist may determine that medications are not required at all, preferring a course of individual or family therapy. The risk–benefit analysis involves the process of maximizing the potential benefit while minimizing the possible harm of pharmacotherapy.

Managing Nonresponse

Lack of complete response to a given treatment is common. The management of nonresponse should begin before treatment is initiated. The clinician should inform the patient of the possibility of nonresponse and the steps that might be taken in such a circumstance. Patients must be warned of the possible delay in response and of the importance of continuing compliance in face of incomplete improvement. If the response to treatment is inadequate, the clinician should review the treatment plan with the patient and explain to him or her the rationale for each next step. This review should always include the instillation of realistic hope. Suicidal potential must be evaluated as well.

Managing Side Effects

The review, documentation, and management of side effects is an important part of pharmacologic treatment. The clinician should warn patients of the possibility of side effects and should review with them those that are common. A general rule of thumb is that any side effect that occurs in 5% or more of patients in clinical trials should be discussed. However, the clinician should address any serious adverse experience, even those that might be rare, and should warn the patient that other unusual effects may occur. For example, although hypothyroidism is an uncommon outcome of lithium treatment, patients should be warned of this possibility. The clinician should review and document side effects with each patient and undertake a plan to manage unaccept-

able effects. Most side effects will improve with time, but noncompliance may be the price of ongoing serious problems. Each patient has his or her own tolerance for side effects, and the patient's tolerance must be considered. For example, sexual side effects of drugs may be completely unimportant for some patients (especially those with no current sexual partner) but critical for others. Further, sexual side effects may be unimportant in one phase of treatment and monumental in others (e.g., when a new relationship is established).

Laboratory evaluations may be required to determine if certain serious reactions have occurred (e.g., hepatotoxicity or nephrotoxicity). Certain drugs require regular plasma-level monitoring to provide the patient with a margin of safety. Biweekly white blood counts are an absolute requirement for clozapine therapy, and annual or biannual thyroid-stimulating hormone and creatinine tests may be performed for patients on lithium. Proper medication management requires regularly scheduled laboratory evaluations for many patients.

Addressing Concurrent Alcohol or Drug Use

Another safety issue is the concurrent use of alcohol or drugs of abuse. The clinician must take a careful drug and alcohol history; however, ongoing evaluation of the patient's drug and alcohol use also is required. In most cases, very modest alcohol use is allowed while a patient is taking psychotropic drugs; however, patients must be warned of potential drug interactions with alcohol with a potentiation of the sedative effects of both the prescribed medication and the alcohol. Alcohol should not be used concomitantly with sedative–hypnotic agents such as benzodiazepines.

Evaluating Response

The clinician should target specific symptoms as indicators of response to treatment. In the case of psychosis, the presence and severity of hallucinations, delusions, or agitation can be effective indicators of early response; however, a more comprehensive view of the patient's condition is required for longer-term management. This involves an ongoing evaluation of a variety of symptomatic domains, including cognitive and mood symptoms and social impairments. As a result, symptoms such as occupational impairment may be important indicators of the effectiveness of pharmacotherapy. Whatever the condition, the goal of pharmacotherapy is to minimize or eliminate symptoms and to return the patient to his or her maximal level of functioning. To this end, the clinician should review and document in each patient the change in a broad range of symptoms.

CONCLUSION

Psychopharmacotherapy ultimately represents a human endeavor in which the challenge to the clinician is the competent synthesis of the scientific basis of pharmacology with the psychosocial skills of the psychiatrist. The most successful pharmacotherapists have a thorough knowledge about the nature of psychiatric disorders, the mechanisms of drug action, and the applications of drug therapies, but they also have remarkable interpersonal skills in the management of patients. This integrative skill set in many ways defines competent contemporary psychiatry.

Marder SR: Facilitating compliance with antipsychotic medication. *J Clin Psychiatry* 1998;59(Suppl 3):21.

Behavioral and Cognitive–Behavioral Interventions

Travis Thompson, PhD, & Steven D. Hollon, PhD

◼ ROOTS OF BEHAVIORAL & COGNITIVE–BEHAVIORAL INTERVENTIONS

Although their roots can be found at the beginning of the twentieth century, modern behavioral and cognitive–behavioral therapies arose during the 1950s and early 1960s when the scientific study of behavior emerged as a subject with validity in its own right. Disordered behavior was no longer taken to be purely a symptom or indicator of something else going on in the mind. Of inherent concern was its relation to past and current environmental events thought to be causally related to that behavior. Methods developed in animal laboratories began to be tested—in laboratory, institutional, clinical, and school settings—with people who had chronic mental illness or intellectual disabilities and with pre-delinquent adolescents. Improvements in patient behavior and functioning were often striking. These changes took place against a backdrop of growing dissatisfaction with the prevailing notion that psychopathology typically arose from unobservable psychic causes that were assessed and treated using techniques that seemed to be based more on art than science. In addition, an accumulating literature of outcome studies revealed that much of the psychotherapy as it had been practiced until the early 1960s engendered very modest and largely unpredictable results. Thus, contemporary behavior therapies emerged from three distinct psychological traditions: classical or Pavlovian conditioning, instrumental or operant conditioning, and cognitive–behavioral and rational–emotive therapies.

CLASSICAL CONDITIONING

The first major perspective within learning theory approaches is typically referred to as **classical conditioning.** This perspective dates to the first decade of the twentieth

century and is largely attributed to the Russian neurophysiologist Ivan Pavlov. Pavlov was interested in studying the structure of the nervous system, in particular, simple reflex arcs between external events (**stimuli**) and an organism's behavior (**response**). He chose to study salivation in dogs in response to food and developed an apparatus that held the dogs suspended in a harness while a small amount of meat powder was deposited on their tongues. He would vary the amount and timing of the delivery of the meat powder and recorded the subsequent variation in the nature and amount of salivation.

What happened next confounded his simple neurologic experiments but opened the way to revolutionary new insights regarding how organisms learn to adapt their behaviors in response to novel environments. Pavlov found that, after a few trials, his dogs began to salivate when strapped into the harness, well in advance of any exposure to the meat powder on a particular trial. Naïve dogs placed in the harness for the first time did not salivate; experienced dogs that had been through the procedure earlier began to salivate well in advance of the delivery of the food. In effect, the dog's response came to precede the food stimulus, something that could not be explained in terms of a simple reflex arc.

Pavlov's genius lay in recognizing the importance of this observation. He shifted his attention from the study of simple reflex arcs to those conditions necessary to support changes in behavior as a consequence of prior experience, that is, **learning.** He sounded a bell to signal the start of a trial that was followed by the delivery of meat powder and found that he could reliably train the dogs to salivate to the sound of a bell and not to respond to other aspects of the experimental situation. In effect, he introduced a particularly salient stimulus that carried all the predictive information contained in the situation (ringing the bell predicted subsequent delivery of meat powder, whereas nothing happened until the bell was sounded); and the dogs came to salivate reliably only after the bell was rung. Once the bell was established as a particularly informative stimulus, he could occasionally omit the meat powder on subsequent trials, and the dogs continued to salivate to the sound of the bell.

This simple paradigm contained the key elements of classical conditioning. The meat powder represented what Pavlov came to call the **unconditioned stimulus.** All dogs with intact nervous systems salivate in response to meat powder being deposited on their tongues, whether they have any experience with that stimulus or not. Salivation represented the **unconditioned response.** The bell (or earlier, the entire experimental apparatus) represented the **conditioned stimulus.** Dogs do not naturally salivate to the sound of a bell, but they come to do so if it is paired with the meat powder (the unconditioned stimulus). Salivation to the bell alone represented the **conditioned response,** a learned response to an originally neutral stimulus that is not found universally among all members of the species.

Early Demonstrations in Humans

J. B. Watson, one of the leading figures in American psychology, recognized the potential relevance of classical conditioning as an explanation for the development of symptoms of psychopathology. Watson and a graduate student conducted a demonstration of how the principles of classical conditioning explicated by Pavlov could be extended to humans. In this study, Watson first showed that a 3-year-old boy called Little Albert had no particular aversion to a small white laboratory rat: He would reach for it and try to pet it, as young children are inclined to do. Watson and his assistant then placed a large gong out of sight behind Little Albert and sounded it loudly every time they brought the rat into the room. Although Little Albert had shown no initial aversion to the rat, he showed a typical startle response to the sounding of the gong (again, as most young children would). Before long, he became upset and burst into tears at the sight of the rat alone and would try to withdraw whenever it was brought into the room.

According to Watson, this study demonstrated that phobic reactions could be acquired purely on the basis of traumatic conditioning. Although Little Albert had previously been intrigued by the presence of the rat and showed no evidence of any fear in its presence, pairing of the rat (the conditioned stimulus) with the loud, unpredictable noise produced by the gong (the unconditioned stimulus) led him to become anxious and upset in the rat's presence (the conditioned response), just as he had naturally become upset by the sound of the gong (unconditioned response). He had not only acquired a fear response to the rat but also tried to escape from it or avoid exposure to it. According to Watson, Little Albert had acquired the two hallmarks of a phobia (unreasonable fear, and escape or avoidance behaviors) purely as a consequence of simple classical conditioning.

The next major study in the sequence was conducted by Mary Cover Jones in 1924. She reasoned that, if classical conditioning could produce a phobic reaction in an otherwise healthy child, the same laws of learning could be used to eliminate that reaction. She trained a young child to have a conditioned fear response to a small animal (a rabbit) and then proceeded to feed the child in the presence of the rabbit. She found that pairing of the conditioned stimulus (the rabbit) with a second, unconditioned stimulus (food)—which produced a different unconditioned response (contentment) that was incompatible with the first (anxiety)—came to override the original learning. The child began to relax in the presence of the rabbit and no longer showed the fear response that he had acquired earlier. Thus, Jones argued, she was able to provide relief via **counterconditioning**.

Despite these early demonstrations, it was several decades before behavioral principles were applied systematically to the treatment of psychiatric disorders. This delay resulted partly from the sense that these procedures were just too simplistic to be of practical use in the treatment of complex human problems. Required were methods based on these learning principles that could be adapted to deal with more complex problems of living. Andrew Salter provided the first such method. In a text that was ahead of its time, Salter described a series of procedures based on principles of conditioning that were suitable for addressing emotional and behavioral problems in human patients. Although that text attracted little attention when it was published in 1949, it described (in vestigial form) many of the strategies and procedures that would later be used in the clinical practice of behavior therapy.

Applications to Clinical Treatment

Joseph Wolpe provided the first coherent set of clinical procedures, based on principles of classical conditioning that had a major impact on the field. Wolpe had studied experimental neuroses in cats. In the course of his studies, which involved shocking animals when they tried to feed and observing the results of the conflict this produced, Wolpe replicated the essential features of Jones's earlier attempt to reduce a learned fear via the process of counterconditioning. He soon extended his work to people with phobic disorders and was able to reduce his patients' distress by pairing the object of their fear with an activity that reliably produced an incompatible response. Like Salter, he experimented with the induction of anger and sexual arousal before finally settling on a set of isometric exercises developed to help reduce stress in patients with heart conditions. This procedure, called **progressive relaxation,** consists of having patients alternately tense and relax different muscle groups in a systematic fashion and can lead to a state of profound relaxation. The isometric exercises could be paired with the presumably conditioned stimulus (whatever the patient feared) in order to have the new conditioned response (relaxation) override the existing arousal and distress that patients experienced in the presence of the phobic stimulus.

Wolpe called his approach **systematic desensitization.** In progressive relaxation training a hierarchy is developed that represents successive degrees of exposure to the feared object or stimulus. For example, a patient with fear of flying might be asked to visualize a variety of scenes that induce differing amounts of anxiety. Simply watching someone else board an airplane might induce only a minimal amount of anxiety, whereas boarding a plane oneself and flying through a thunderstorm would be expected to elicit more anxiety. Wolpe worked with the patient to develop a hierarchy of such imagined experiences and grade them on a scale from 0 to 100 in terms of how much distress they produced. He would then expose the patient to these stimuli (typically in imagination). He proceeded on to the next item in the hierarchy only when the client could tolerate a particular image without experiencing distress. If the patient started to become upset while visualizing an image, Wolpe would instruct the patient to stop the image and reinitiate the relaxation exercises until the feelings of arousal had passed. In this fashion, he systematically worked the patient through the hierarchy of representations of the feared object, proceeding as rapidly as the patient could without experiencing distress until the stimulus no longer elicited any anxiety.

Hundreds of studies have suggested that systematic desensitization (or its variants) is effective in the treatment of phobia and related anxiety-based disorders. Systematic desensitization has been applied widely to a host of problems and represents a safe and effective way of reducing anxious arousal in both adults and children. Major variations include substituting meditation or biofeedback for progressive relaxation as a means of producing the relaxation response (some people do not respond well to muscular isometrics) or arranging experiences in a graduated fashion. The basic approach appears to be robust to these minor modifications and is one of the few examples of a treatment intervention that is truly more effective than other interventions.

Extinction & Exposure Therapy

Despite its evident clinical utility, systematic desensitization is based on a misperception of the laws of classical conditioning. Classical conditioning is essentially ephemeral. Organisms stop responding to the conditioned stimulus when it is no longer paired with the unconditioned stimulus. Pavlov's dogs may have learned to salivate to the ringing of the bell, but if Pavlov kept ringing the bell after it was no longer paired with the meat powder, the dogs soon stopped salivating to its ring. This is referred to as the process of **extinction,** in which conditioned stimuli lose their capacity to elicit a response when they are presented too many times in the absence of the unconditioned stimulus.

This basic feature was considered so troublesome by early behaviorally oriented psychopathologists that they felt compelled to explain how such an ephemeral process could account for a long-lasting disorder such as a phobia (most phobias do not remit spontaneously over time). O. Hobart Mowrer solved the riddle when he postulated that phobic reactions essentially involve two learning processes: classical conditioning, to instill the anxiety response to a previously neutral stimulus; and operant conditioning, to reinforce the voluntary escape or avoidance behaviors that remove the patient from the presence of the conditioned stimulus before the anxious arousal can be extinguished. In essence, people who acquire a phobic reaction to a basically benign stimulus do not extinguish (as the laws of classical conditioning predict they should), because they do not stay in the situation long enough for classical extinction to take place.

This conclusion led some behavior theorists to suggest that although systematic desensitization was undoubtedly effective, it was unnecessarily complex and time consuming. The essential mechanism of change, they suggested, was extinction, not counterconditioning, and the only procedure needed was to expose the patient repeatedly to the feared object or situation. Of course, the therapist would also have to do something to prevent the patient from running away or otherwise terminating contact with the feared situation. Thus, according to exposure theorists, it was not necessary to ensure that patients experienced no fear in the presence of the phobic stimulus (as Wolpe claimed). Rather, all that was required was to get them into the situation and to prevent them from leaving until the anxiety had diminished on its own.

Several decades of controlled research have suggested that the extinction theorists were correct and that exposure (plus response prevention) is at least as effective as systematic desensitization and is more rapid in its effects. That does not necessarily mean that it is more useful than systematic desensitization in practice; many patients find exposure therapy very distressing and prefer the gentler alternative provided by systematic desensitization. Although exposure typically works more rapidly than does systematic desensitization (and both work more rapidly than do nonbehavioral alternatives), it often takes as long to persuade a patient to try exposure techniques as it does to complete a full course of systematic desensitization. Nonetheless, it is now clear that exposure (with response prevention) is a sufficient condition for symptomatic change and that Wolpe was in error when he suggested that allowing a patient to experience anxiety in the presence of the phobic situation delayed the process of change. Although patients who already have acquired a conditioned fear response will undoubtedly experience distress when exposed to the object of their fears, the fact that they become anxious during the course of that exposure neither facilitates nor retards the extinction process. (This is why most behavior therapists no longer use the term "flooding" to refer to exposure therapy; although it may be descriptive of the level of anxiety induced, it is misleading in that it seems to imply that the induction of anxiety is itself curative in some way.)

Exposure plus response prevention has a clear advantage over systematic desensitization (and virtually every other type of nonbehavioral intervention) in the treatment of more complex disorders related to anxiety. It appears to be particularly helpful in the treatment of obsessive–compulsive disorder (OCD) and severe agoraphobia. For example, treatment for a patient who has a fear of contamination and repetitive hand-washing rituals might involve having a therapy team spend a weekend locked in the patient's home, having the patient intentionally contaminate his or her hands and food with dirt (by shutting off the water to prevent hand washing). Similarly, a patient with severe agoraphobia would be encouraged to visit settings that he or she typically avoids (e.g., shopping malls or grocery stores) during the busiest times of the day and would be prevented (again by a therapy team or group) from leaving until his or her anxiety had subsided. Although systematic desensitization has had limited success with such severe disorders, the process of constructing and working through the literally dozens of hierarchies required typically makes the approach wildly impractical.

Summary

Strategies based on classical conditioning have been used in the treatment of depression, somatoform disorders, dissociative disorders, substance abuse, sexual difficulties, medical problems, and a variety of other disorders. In general, these approaches represent some of the most effective of the therapeutic interventions. As is the case with other types of behavioral strategies, they rest on a solid foundation of empirical work, much of it with nonhuman animals, and on the creative adaptation of those basic principles to human populations.

Kazdin AE, Weisz JR: *Evidence-Based Psychotherapies for Children and Adolescents.* New York: The Guilford Press, 2003.

Marks IM: *Fears, Phobias and Rituals.* Oxford, UK: Oxford University Press, 1987.

Rachman S, Hodgson RJ: *Obsession and Compulsions.* New York, NY: Prentice-Hall, 1980.

Wilson GT: Behavior therapy. In: Corsini RJ, Wedding D (eds). *Current Psychotherapies,* 5th edn. Itasca, IL: FE Peacock Publishing, 1995, pp. 197–228.

Wolpe J: *Psychotherapy by Reciprocal Inhibition.* Palo Alto, CA: Stanford University Press, 1958.

EMERGENCE OF INSTRUMENTAL & OPERANT LEARNING THEORY

As a graduate student at Columbia University, Edward Thorndike began a series of experiments that set a new course in the study of processes underlying behavior change and learning. He placed a cat in an enclosed chamber and attached a vertical pole in the center of the compartment to a rope that passed over several pulleys. When the cat bumped against the pole, the pole would tilt, causing the rope to open the door. The cat could then leave the compartment and drink milk from a nearby bowl outside the cage. At first, the cat seemed to move about unpredictably each time it was returned to the compartment. The time required for the cat to tilt the pole grew shorter on successive repetitions of the task, and the cat's method for opening the door on each trial became progressively similar to the method used on the preceding trial. The trial-by-trial record of time to escape from what Thorndike called his "puzzle box" was the first instrumental learning curve published in a scientific journal. Eventually, each cat quickly approached the pole—seemingly purposively—and tilted it to one side, opening the door. Thorndike described this as an **instrumental conditioning** process because the pole tilting was instrumental in releasing the cat from the chamber and permitting access to a reward. Thorndike's method differed from Pavlov's classical conditioning because no specific response was elicited by a conditioned stimulus. The form of each cat's behavior that tilted the pole was idiosyncratic and variable. There was nothing fixed about the behavior, as was typical of classically conditioned behavior. Thorndike's Law of Effect described the necessary and sufficient conditions for instrumental learning to occur.

Skinner & Operant Behavior

Whereas Thorndike studied the process of behavior change, three decades later, B. F. Skinner, a graduate student at Harvard University, was interested in discovering a method for identifying the functional components of sequences of behavior. Skinner was drawn to the writings of the physiologists Charles Sherrington and Ernst Magnus. Skinner was particularly taken with Sherrington's notion of the reflex arc. Skinner believed that psychologists had gotten seriously off on the wrong track by focusing on unobservable phenomenological events, which no amount of experimentation could verify, rather than following the example of physiology in studying observable events. Skinner wondered whether Thorndike's Law of Effect might explain how a single component could be isolated from the continuously free flowing activities of an organism, so that the component could be studied scientifically, much as Sherrington had done. Using a method very similar to Thorndike's, Skinner placed a rat in an enclosed chamber, and each time the rat depressed a telegraph key protruding through the wall of the chamber, a pellet of food dropped into a receptacle near the rat. The lever-pressing methods each rat used varied: most pressed with their paws, some pushed with their muzzles, and others held the telegraph key between their teeth and pulled down. All methods produced the same result—delivery of a pellet of food that the hungry rat seized and ate. Skinner said that the rat "operated" on its environment to produce reinforcing consequences, and the type of behavior was correspondingly called **operant behavior.**

In operant behavior, typically no stimulus was presented before an operant response that "caused" the behavior to occur (i.e., there was no conditioned stimulus). When Skinner analyzed the sequence of the rat's activities in an operant chamber, he found that after many repetitions when the rat approached the lever, depressed it, and heard the device click, which had been followed by food pellet presentation, the click sound produced by the lever press began to be rewarding without food pellet presentation. If a light were illuminated above the lever (indicating periods when food would be available), alternating with periods when the light was off (indicating lever presses would not produce food), soon the rat pressed nearly exclusively when the light was illuminated. The rat's behavior continued to be variable, changing from moment to moment even when the light was illuminated, unlike a classically conditioned reflex. Skinner called the food pellet a **reinforcer** and the light that signaled that operant responding would lead to reinforcer presentation, a **discriminative stimulus.** Skinner spelled out in surprisingly accurate detail laws of operant conditioning that have stood the test of time. Immediacy, magnitude, and intermittence of reinforcement affected the pattern of behavior maintained and also determined the persistence of behavior in the absence of reinforcement.

Skinner also observed that a stimulus repeatedly paired with food presentation (e.g., the "click" sound of the food pellet dispenser) came to serve as a reinforcer in its own right and would maintain considerable amounts of behavior over extended periods of time in the absence of primary reinforcement. Such previously neutral stimuli that took on reinforcing properties because of their pairing with primary reinforcers were called **conditioned reinforcers** or **secondary reinforcers**. Skinner recognized that, in most developed parts of the world, relatively limited aspects of human conduct seem to be directed toward seeking food or shelter. Instead, most human conduct seems to be governed by parent or teacher approval, threat of loss of affection, or symbols of recognition from employers or peers (e.g., paychecks, awards). Skinner reasoned that these reinforcers had developed their reinforcing properties (usually very early in an individual's life) from their repeated pairing with primary reinforcers. In short, they were powerful conditioned reinforcers. This observation led later educators, drug abuse counselors, psychologists, and psychiatrists working in applied settings to develop treatment methods based on conditioned reinforcers such as social approval or concrete objects paired with other reinforcers (e.g., check marks, stars, tokens, money).

Applications to Clinical Treatment

The practical utility of the operant apparatus and measurement approach was adopted quickly in experimental psychology, physiology, neurochemistry, pharmacology, and toxicology laboratories throughout the world. The methodology provided the springboard for the field of behavioral pharmacology, the study of subcortical self-stimulation, animal models of addictive behavior, and the study of psychophysics and complex human social behavior in enclosed experimental spaces. Skinner's pragmatic theory struck a popular chord with many young psychologists, special educators, and practitioners in training. In 1948, Sidney Bijou began an applied research program and experimental nursery school for children with intellectual disability at the Rainier School in Washington, applying operant principles. Bijou was joined by Donald Baer, a recent graduate of the University of Chicago, and they conducted seminal research on early child operant behavior. In 1953, Ogden Lindsley and Skinner began applying operant methods to study the behavior of patients with schizophrenia at Metropolitan State Hospital in Waltham, Massachusetts.

Several major events brought the emerging field of behavior modification to the attention of psychiatry. First, Teodoro Ayllon and Nathan Azrin were granted limited funds in 1961 for an experimental program to motivate and improve the functioning of a group of severely mentally ill, mostly schizophrenic, women who were institutionalized in Illinois. The program used a token reinforcement system originally developed by Roger Kelleher, who had studied the behavior of chimpanzees in laboratory settings. Tokens resembling poker chips were given to patients immediately after they completed agreed-upon therapeutic activities. Later the tokens could be exchanged for supplementary preferred activities or commodities. The changes in patient behavior were often dramatic and included markedly increased participation in therapeutic programs such as those aimed at employment, bathing, self-care, and related daily living skills.

Leonard Ullman headed a similar treatment unit in Palo Alto, California. Both programs operated on the principle that chronically mentally ill patients, primarily those with schizophrenia, had been largely unresponsive to conventional psychological therapeutic methods. Although older neuroleptic medications managed many of the florid symptoms of schizophrenia, they did little to increase the patients' general adjustment and often produced problematic side effects. These programs demonstrated that it was possible to use laboratory-based management methods to motivate patients with chronic schizophrenia, increasing their participation in hospital therapeutic programs and decreasing the amount of disturbed behavior. Although no one claimed these methods changed the underlying disorder, they were very effective tools for improving patient compliance and management.

A less frequently cited but still important study conducted during this era was Gordon Paul and coworkers' comparison of the effectiveness of a social learning theory approach to that of a more traditional milieu therapy approach to managing the behavior of patients with chronic mental illnesses in an institutional setting. It is the single best study of its kind, demonstrating persuasively the effectiveness of a behavior therapy strategy for activating socially resistant patients who have schizophrenia. It also carefully documented reductions in schizophrenic disorganization and cognitive distortion; improvements in normal speech and social interactions; reductions in social isolation; and greatly reduced aggressive, assaultive, and other intolerable behavior.

The second major event was the demonstration in 1963 by Ivar Lovaas, a clinical psychologist working at UCLA, that positive reinforcement methods could be used to teach children with autism a variety of skills. Until that time, there were no known effective treatments for autism. Lovaas worked with children who were mute and with echolalic children who had autism (labeled "schizophrenic children" at that time). These children were severely intellectually disabled, self-injurious, displayed severe tantrums, and were extremely noncompliant. Lovaas used a combination of hugs and praise, edible reinforcers, and highly controversial aversive stimulation techniques to reduce self-destructive behavior. In 1987, Lovaas published a report in which he used an intensive behavioral treatment regimen (40 h/wk of one-to-one contact), targeting language and social skills. He reported that 47% of the experimental group (9 of 19 children), functioned similar to typical peers after 2–3 years of treatment, compared with 2% of the control group. In 1993, he published a follow-up on those children at age 12 and found that of the nine children with best outcomes, eight continued to function in the normal range. Lovaas was the first researcher to document such marked improvement in such a large proportion of treated children with autism; however, other interventions using similar methods of behavior analysis appear to produce similar results.

The third major event that paved the way for modern behavior therapy methods was the work of Gerald Patterson and colleagues in developing a coercion model of the relationships between families and their children with conduct disorder. In the early and mid-1960s, Patterson began working with children of normal intelligence who displayed a wide array of predelinquent behavior. Some of the children displayed characteristics of attention-deficit/hyperactivity disorder, others seemed to have learning disabilities, and others were aggressive and noncompliant at home and school but exhibited no indications of other psychiatric or cognitive disability. On the basis of a series of laboratory and clinical studies, Patterson and his colleagues proposed that children who had conduct disorder and their families gradually learn a set of mutually coercive relationships based on interpersonal aversive stimulation and avoidance. On the basis of this model, he developed a behavioral treatment method drawing on basic operant methods (i.e., positive social and tangible reinforcement and loss of reinforcement resulting from behavior problems, both of which were based on unambiguous and consistent contingencies). He combined these techniques with what would later be called cognitive–behavior therapy methods (i.e., the use of verbal self-instruction to mediate behavior change).

Finally, in the late 1960s and early 1970s several large-scale programs were developed that applied operant behavioral principles in residential services for people with intellectual disability. These early institution-based programs paved the way for subsequent community-based service and treatment programs for people with intellectual disability, especially those with significant behavior problems.

Cooper JO, Heron TE, Heward WL: *Applied Behavior Analysis*, 2nd edn. New York: Prentice Hall, 2006.

Lord C, McGee J (eds): *Educating Children with Autism*. Washington DC: Commission on Behavioral and Social Sciences and Education of the National Academy of Sciences, 2001.

Patterson GR, Gullion ME: *Living with Children; New Methods for Parents and Teachers*. Champaigne, IL: Research Press, 1968.

Skinner BF: *Science and Human Behavior*. New York, NY: Macmillan, 1953.

COGNITIVE & COGNITIVE–BEHAVIORAL INTERVENTIONS

One of the major changes in behavioral approaches in the past several decades has been the emergence of the cognitive and cognitive–behavioral intervention. Based largely on social learning theory, these approaches posit that organisms are not just the passive recipients of stimuli that impinge on them but instead interpret and try to make sense out of their worlds. These approaches do not reject traditional classical and operant perspectives on learning; rather, they suggest that cognitive mediation plays a role in coloring the way those processes work in humans and other higher vertebrates.

Roots of Cognitive Therapy

The roots of cognitive therapy can be found in the early writings of the Stoic philosophers Epictetus and Marcus Aurelius, and in the later works by Benjamin Rush and Henry Maudsley, among others. It was Epictetus who, in the first century AD, wrote that "People are disturbed not by things, but the view which they take of them." Benjamin Rush, the father of American psychiatry, wrote in 1786 that by exercising the rational mind through practice, one gained control over otherwise unmanageable passions that he believed led to some forms of madness. A century later, Henry Maudsley reiterated the notion that it was the loss of power over the coordination of ideas and feelings that led to madness and that the wise development of control over thoughts and feelings could have a powerful effect. In modern times, Alfred Adler's approach to dynamic psychotherapy was cognitive in nature, stressing the role of perceptions of the self and the world in determining how people went about the process of pursuing their goals in life. George Kelly is often accorded a central role in laying out the basic tenets of the approach, and Albert Bandura's influential treatise on learning theory provided a theoretical basis for incorporating observational learning in the learning process.

Modern Approaches

Modern cognitive and cognitive–behavioral approaches to psychotherapy got their impetus from two converging lines of development. One branch was developed by theorists originally trained in dynamic psychotherapy. Theorists such as Albert Ellis, the founder of rational–emotive therapy, and Aaron Beck, the founder of cognitive therapy, began their careers adhering to dynamic principles in theory and therapy. They became disillusioned with that approach and came, over time, to focus on their patients' conscious beliefs. Both ascribe to an ABC model, which states that it is not just what happens to someone at point A (the antecedent events) that determines how the person feels and what he or she does at point C (the affective and behavioral consequences) but that it also matters how the person interprets those events at point B (the person's beliefs). For example, a man who loses a relationship and is convinced that he was left because he is unlovable is more likely to feel depressed and fail to pursue further relationships than one who considers his loss a consequence of bad luck or the product of mistakes that he will not repeat the next time around. Both theorists work with patients to actively examine their beliefs to be sure that they are not making situations worse than they necessarily are. Ellis typically adopts a more philosophical approach based on reason and persuasion, whereas Beck operates more like a scientist, treating his patients' beliefs as hypotheses that can be tested and en-couraging his patients to use their own behavior to test the accuracy of their beliefs.

The other major branch of cognitive–behaviorism involves theorists originally trained as behavior therapists who became increasingly interested in the role of thinking in the learning process. Bandura and Michael Mahoney represent two exemplars of this tradition, as do other theorists such as Donald Meichenbaum and G. Terence Wilson. These theorists tend to stay closer to the language and tenets of traditional behavior analysis and are somewhat less likely to talk about the role of meaning in their patients' responses to events. They are also as likely to focus on the absence of cognitive mediators (i.e., covert self-statements) as on the presence of distortions. For example, Meichenbaum developed an influential approach to treatment, called self-instructional training, in which patients with impulse-control problems are trained to modulate their own behavior via the process of verbal self-regulation.

These approaches focus on the role of information processing in determining subsequent affect and behavior. Beck, for example, has argued that distinctive errors in thinking can be found in each of the major types of psychopathology. For example, depression typically involves negative views of the self and the future; anxiety, an overdetermined sense of physical or psychological danger; eating disorders, an undue concern with shape and weight; and obsessions, an overbearing sense of responsibility for ensuring the safety of oneself and others. Efforts to produce change involve having the patient first monitor fluctuations in mood and relate those changes to the ongoing flow of automatic thoughts, subsequently using one's own behavior to test the accuracy of these beliefs. For example, a depressed patient who believes that he or she is incompetent will be asked to provide an example of something he or she should be able to do but cannot. The patient is then invited to list the steps that anyone else would have to do to carry out the task. The patient is then encouraged to carry out those steps just to determine whether he or she is as incompetent as he or she believes (typically, the patient is not).

Similarly, patients with panic disorder often misinterpret innocuous bodily sensations as signs of impending physical or psychological catastrophe, such as having a heart attack or "going crazy." The therapist provides a rationale that stresses the role of thinking in symptom formation and encourages the patient to test his or her belief in the imminence of the impending catastrophe by inducing a panic attack right in the office. As the patient experiences extreme states of arousal and panic with no subsequent consequences (i.e., neither dying nor "going crazy"), he or she comes to recognize that the initial arousal is not a harbinger of impending doom (as first believed), and the patient no longer begins to panic at the occurrence of arousal. In essence, like the behavioral approaches based on classical conditioning, modern cognitive and cognitive–behavioral interventions emphasize the curative process of exposing oneself to the things one most fears as a way of dealing with irrational or unrealistic concerns.

These approaches are well established in the treatment of unipolar depression, panic disorder, social phobia, generalized anxiety disorder, and bulimia. For these disorders, cognitive and cognitive–behavioral interventions appear to be at least as effective as other competing alternatives (including medications) and quite possibly more enduring. There are consistent indications that cognitive–behavioral therapy produces long-lasting change that reduces the likelihood that symptoms will return after treatment ends. The evidence is mixed with respect to substance abuse, marital distress, and childhood conduct disorder, although at least some indications are promising. Cognitive and cognitive–behavioral interventions are typically not thought to be particularly effective in patients who have formal thought disorder, although recent studies suggest that such interventions may reduce delusional thinking in psychotic patients who receive neuroleptic drugs.

Beck AT: *Cognitive Therapy and the Emotional Disorders.* Madison, CT: International Universities Press, 1976.

Ellis A: *Reason and Emotion in Psychotherapy.* New York: Lyle Stuart, 1962.

Hollon SD, Beck AT: Cognitive and cognitive behavioral therapies. In: Lambert MJ (ed). *Garfield and Bergin's Handbook of Psychotherapy and Behavior Change: An Empirical Analysis,* 5th edn. New York: Wiley & Sons, 2004, pp. 447–492.

Meichenbaum D: *Cognitive-Behavior Modification: An Integrative Approach.* New York: Plenum Publishing Corp, 1977.

O'Donohue WO, Fisher JE, Hayes SC: *Cognitive Behavior Therapy: Applying Empirically Supported Techniques in Your Practice.* New York: Hoboken, NJ: Wiley, 2003.

■ FUNDAMENTAL ASSUMPTIONS OF THERAPIES BASED ON LEARNING THEORY

Several basic assumptions are common to most learning-based interventions. Perhaps most fundamental is that the behavior of the individual who has been referred for psychiatric treatment is of concern in its own right. Behavior is not necessarily an indication of pathology at some other level of analysis (e.g., brain chemical or psychic). Pathologic behavior is often seen as the result of the demands of the environment in which the person is living, working, or going to school (or, in the case of the cognitive approaches, the person's perception of the environment). What appears to be pathologic may be a person's best adaptation to an impossible situation given the person's cognitive or personality limitations (e.g., living with alcoholic parents, residing in an abusive institutional or community residential setting, interacting with people who do not use the same communication system).

Although major mental illnesses have neurochemical substrates, much of the pathologic behavior observed by psychiatrists has been learned in much the same way that normal behavior is learned. Pathologic behavior generally follows the same scientific laws as normal behavior. Vulnerability to learning pathologic behavior is shaped by the biological substrate of inherited traits and neurochemical predispositions upon which the collective history of experiences is imposed. Individual differences in normal and pathologic behavior are attributable to dispositions created by variations in genetic makeup or differences in histories that predispose an individual to differences in motivation. Some people, by virtue of their genetic and associated neurochemical makeup, are prone to respond to mild, negative comments by other people as though such comments were aversive and to be avoided at all costs. Others, with different genetic makeup and correspondingly different neurochemical predisposition, may be largely impervious to similar negative reinforcers and cues. The former individuals are prone to develop avoidant behavior and extreme anxiety, whereas the latter individuals tend to be insensitive to aversive social situations.

In the early days of behavior modification and behavior therapy treatments, targets of treatment were often circumscribed responses (e.g., nail-biting, failing in school, encopresis). Since then, researchers have recognized that narrowly defined instances of pathologic behavior (i.e., presenting symptoms) are usually members of larger classes of problematic responses. The treatment task is not to treat the isolated behavior (e.g., arguing with parents or making self-deprecating remarks) but rather to identify the factors that determine the likelihood that any one of an entire class of responses may occur. Such factors could include, for example, the child having no legitimate mechanism for determining what is going on in his or her life, combined with parental submission to unpleasant, coercive responses. Failure to assess properly the full breadth of the members composing a functional response class could lead to symptom substitution. For example, the successful reduction of arguing by a defiant teenager by implementing a behavioral contract limited to arguing will, in most instances, lead to the emergence of other defiant behaviors (e.g., staying out beyond curfew, experimenting with alcohol). The task is to identify a broader class of problem behavior, develop hypotheses concerning the purposes served by that class of behavior, and then develop an intervention plan that makes the entire class of behavior ineffective and unnecessary.

Most of the causes of pathologic behavior are found in the relation between the individual, the environmental antecedents, and the consequences of his or her actions. An individual's history creates the context within which current environmental circumstances serve as either discriminative stimuli (e.g., a spouse coming home late from work) or conditioned negative reinforcers (e.g., threatened disapproval). An individual's history could also establish the motivational framework that governs most of the individual's actions. As a result, assessment usually requires obtaining information from the individual or other informants about events taking place in the individual's natural environment in order to obtain valid data concerning the circumstances surrounding the pathologic behavior. The meaning of an environmental cue or a putative motivating consequence is determined contextually. Whether a social stimulus is alarming, neutral, or positive will depend on the person's history and the circumstance in which the stimulus is being experienced. Similarly, a consequence can be positive, neutral, or negative depending on the individual's history and the circumstance in which the consequence is encountered. Thus, Thorndike's original Law of Effect has been contextualized. Whether this contextualization is conceptualized as residing in the cognitive domain or in the observable environment is a matter of some theoretical dispute, but the learning-based approaches emphasize idiosyncratic experience as the shaper of behavioral proclivities.

Bandura A: *Principles of Behavior Modification.* Austin, TX: Holt, Rinehart & Winston, 1969.

Craighead WE, Craighead LW, Ilardi SS: Behavior therapies in historical perspective. In: Bonger BM, Buetler LE (eds). *Comprehensive Textbook of Psychotherapy: Theory and Practice.* Oxford, UK: Oxford University Press, 1995.

Kazdin AE: *History of Behavior Modification: Experimental Foundations of Contemporary Research.* Baltimore, MD: University Park Press, 1978.

Krasner L: History of behavior modification. In: Bellack AS, Hersen M, Kazdin AE (eds): *International Handbook of Behavior Modification and Therapy,* 2nd edn. Springer Publishing Corp, 1990, pp. 3–25.

■ COMBINATIONS WITH MEDICATION

Many of the disorders treated with behavioral or cognitive–behavioral therapy can also be treated pharmacologically, although some cannot. In some disorders, a combination of drugs and behavioral (or cognitive–behavioral) therapy is more effective than either alone. For example, stimulant medication and cognitive behavior therapy produces greater behavioral improvements than either treatment alone among many children with ADHD. Combined treatment for depression retains the rapidity and robustness of the medication response and the enduring effects of cognitive or behavioral treatment. Despite the theoretically based concerns of advocates for each approach, one modality rarely interferes with the other, although such interference sometimes occurs. For many disorders, there simply are not adequate data to guide clinical practice; we often know that both modalities are effective in their own right but do not know whether their combination enhances treatment response.

Drugs and other somatic interventions appear to be essential to the treatment of the more severe disorders, particularly those that involve psychotic symptoms. Nonetheless, behavioral and cognitive–behavioral interventions can often play an important adjunctive role. Recent studies indicate that D-cycloserine administered during exposure therapy for phobias facilitates extinction of the exaggerated fear response to the phobic stimulus. Antipsychotic medications remain the most effective means of reducing the more florid symptoms of psychosis, and the newer, atypical antipsychotics show promise in relieving the negative symptoms of schizophrenia. Rehabilitation programs based on behavioral skills training appear to help redress impairments in psychosocial functioning in such patients and may allow the use of newer low-dose neuroleptic medications (see Chapter 16). Lithium and anticonvulsants provide the most effective means of treatment of the bipolar disorders, but cognitive–behavioral therapy can enhance compliance with drug therapy (see Chapter 18).

The relative importance of pharmacotherapy is less pronounced among even the more severe, nonpsychotic disorders and quite possibly is nonexistent among the less severe disorders. Cognitive therapy appears to be about as effective as pharmacotherapy for all but the most severe nonbipolar depressions and may be more enduring in its effect (see Chapter 18). Exposure-based therapies are quite helpful in reducing compulsive rituals in OCD (see Chapter 21) and behavioral avoidance in severe agoraphobia (see Chapter 19). Such therapies are often combined with medication to treat these disorders. Cognitive–behavioral therapy appears to be at least as effective and possibly longer-lasting than pharmacotherapy in the treatment of panic disorder and social phobia (see Chapter 19), and the same can be said with respect to the treatment of bulimia (see Chapter 26). Exposure-based treatment is clearly superior to pharmacotherapy (or any other form of psychotherapy) in the treatment of social phobia. There is little evidence that drugs are particularly helpful in the treatment of the personality disorders (see Chapter 30); however, a dialectic type behavior therapy appears to reduce the frequency of self-destructive behavior in patients with borderline personality disorder.

In general, the more severe the psychopathologic disorder, the greater the relative efficacy of pharmacotherapy and the more purely behavioral the psychosocial intervention should be. Medications are often useful to control disruptive symptoms, but behavioral interventions (especially operant ones) are uniquely suited to promoting new skills or restoring those that have been lost to illness or institutionalization. Behavioral interventions based on classical conditioning are particularly helpful in reducing undesirable states of arousal and affective distress; cognitive interventions reduce the likelihood of subsequent relapse by correcting the erroneous beliefs and attitudes that contribute to recurrence. These strategies rarely interfere with one another. It is often useful to combine them in practice to achieve multiple ends.

Klerman GL et al.: Medication and psychotherapy. In: Bergin AE, Garfield SL (eds). *Handbook of Psychotherapy and Behavior Change,* 4th edn. Hoboken, NJ: John Wiley & Sons, 1994, pp. 734–782.

Panksepp J: *Textbook of Biolocial Psychiatry.* New York: Wiley-Liss, 2003.

Reiff MI and Tippin S: *ADHD: A Complete and Authoritative Guide.* Elk Grove Village, IL: American Academy of Pediatrics, 2004.

■ COMBINED INTERVENTIONS IN DEVELOPMENTAL DISABILITIES

Behavioral interventions can be highly effective in improving the quality of life for people who have developmental disabilities and display serious behavior problems. Sometimes behavioral methods are insufficient by themselves. Psychopharmacologic treatments can control psychopathologic symptoms and behavior in some people with intellectual and related disabilities (e.g., attention deficit hyperactivity disorder, major depression, bipolar disorder, anxiety disorder, schizophrenia) in nondevelopmentally delayed individuals.

In elucidating how psychotropic drugs reduce problem behavior, it is helpful to examine the behavioral as well as the neurochemical mechanisms of drug action. Behavioral mechanisms refer to psychological or behavioral processes altered by a drug. Neurochemical mechanisms refer to the receptor-level events that are causally related to those changed behavioral processes. Some psychopathologic problems are associated so frequently with specific developmental disabilities that pharmacotherapy is among the first treatments to be explored. Anxiety disorder, especially OCD, is commonly associated with autism and Prader-Willi syndrome. Anxiety disorder manifests itself as ritualistic, repetitive stereotypic

motor responses (e.g., rocking or hand-flapping) and rigidly routinized activities (e.g., repeatedly lining up blocks, insisting that shoe laces be precisely the same length) that, if interrupted, provoke behavioral outbursts or tantrums. Selective serotonin reuptake inhibitors alleviate agitation, anxiety, and ritualistic behavior, such as skin-picking and self-injurious behavior. At times, aggression results from an anxiety disorder. For example, a patient with autism who has severe anxiety may strike out against others who are crowding too closely, in order to keep them at a distance. Fluvoxamine reduces anxiety and the need for increased social distance, thereby diminishing the need to strike out against others to keep them at a distance. Aggression, in this example, serves as a social avoidance response that fluvoxamine renders unnecessary. The behavioral mechanism of action is the reduction of anxiety and associated avoidance. The neurochemical mechanism is thought to be mediated by inhibition of serotonin reuptake with increased binding to the serotonin-2 receptors.

An individual with autism or intellectual disability who strikes his or her head in intermittent bouts throughout the day may do so because head blows cause the release of β-endorphin, which binds to the μ-opiate receptor, thereby reinforcing self-injury. In this way, a self-addictive, vicious cycle is established and maintained and through years of repetition becomes a firmly entrenched behavioral pattern. An opiate antagonist, such as naltrexone, blocks the reinforcing effects consequent to the binding of β-endorphin to the opiate receptor. Naltrexone reduces self-injurious behavior in approximately 40% of patients, primarily in those engaging in high-frequency, intense self-injury directed at the head and hands. Evidence indicates that elevated baseline levels of plasma β-endorphin after bouts of self-injury are predictive of a therapeutic response to naltrexone.

Repetitive self-injurious behavior, such as head banging and self-biting, can be treated effectively with complementary behavioral and pharmacologic strategies, as described in the following case example.

A 13-year-old boy with autism and severe intellectual disabilty and had no communication system at baseline. An observational functional assessment of the boy's self-injurious behavior in his natural environment (a special education classroom) indicated that approximately two thirds of this behavior was motivated by the desire to obtain attention or to escape from situations he did not like or found disturbing. Self-injury dropped 50% from baseline during the first naltrexone treatment phase. Next the patient was taught to use pictorial icons to make requests and indicate basic needs to others around him (Figure 10–1). His self-injury dropped subsequently by another 50% (i.e., a reduction of a total of 75% from

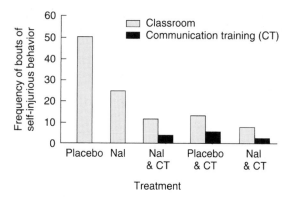

Figure 10–1. Efficacy of treatment for self-injurious behavior. Nal, naltrexone.

baseline) when communication treatment was initiated. On follow-up 1 year later, during which time naltrexone treatment had continued, the boy's self-injurious behavior had dropped to nearly zero. In this case, naltrexone blocked the neurochemical reinforcing consequences of self-injury, and communication training provided an appropriate behavioral alternative to indicate basic needs and wants. In short, combined treatment produced complementary, additive salutary effects.

Emerson E, Hatton C, Parmeter T, Thompson T (eds): *International Handbook of Applied Research in Intellectual Disabilities.* Chichester, UK: John Wiley & Sons Ltd., 2004.

Kelley ME, Fisher WW, Lomas JE, Roy Q, Sanders RQ: Some effects of stimulant medication on response allocation: A double-blind analysis. *J Appl Behav Anal* 2006;39:243–247.

Thompson T, Moore T, Symons F: Psychotherapeutic medications and positive behavior support. In: Odom S, Horner R, Snell M, Blacher J, (eds). *Handbook on Developmental Disabilities.* New York, NY: Guilford Press, 2007.

CONCLUSION

Modern behavioral and cognitive–behavioral interventions emphasize the role of learning and adaptation to the environment in shaping and maintaining normal life functions and in the emergence of maladaptive symptomatology. These interventions treat behavior as important in its own right and often seek to change instances of disordered behavior by the application of clearly articulated, basic principles of learning. There are three fundamental, interrelated perspectives: classical conditioning, which emphasizes the learning of associations between classes of stimuli; operant conditioning, which emphasizes the learning of relations between behaviors and their consequences; and the cognitive perspective, which emphasizes the role of idiosyncratic beliefs and misconceptions in coloring each of the two earlier perspectives. Learning-based approaches have sparked a major revolution in the treatment of psychiatric disorders. Each perspective can point to notable gains. Behavioral approaches can often be combined beneficially with medication and should be part of the armamentarium of any well-trained clinician.

Psychodynamic and Social Interventions

11

James L. Nash, MD, & James W. Lomax, MD

Many medical and perhaps most psychiatric conditions cannot be eradicated totally. The affected individual must often learn to manage a protracted or chronic condition. The scope of medical, surgical, and psychiatric intervention is therefore appropriately not limited to acute pathologic states in which a definitive therapy is applied and the person is restored to perfect function. Humans are subject to a multitude of adverse influences, both external and internal. Whether these adverse influences are from bad luck, bad genes, bad environment, or simply the effects of aging, suffering is inherent in the human condition, and the individual must learn to manage personal suffering. It is appropriate that physicians provide others with assistance in the management of suffering. Analogously, psychotherapy often is focused on modifying the patient's overall pattern of adaptation to life (personality). As Cloninger and others (1993) note, personality is best considered as an interactive combination of factors that are gene-based and relatively immutable with factors stemming from the nonshared environment. While the expressive psychotherapies may make some modifications in character as defined, there is very little that a psychological intervention can do to alter the gene-based expressions, which are conceptualized as "temperament" (novelty seeking, harm avoidance, reward dependence, and persistence). Thus, the psychotherapist must help the person accommodate to the more gene-based temperaments so that they are expressed in ways that create less havoc or irritation for the person's relational world.

Psychotherapeutic treatment is an important weapon in the armamentarium of the physician and a necessary component of the management strategy of many and diverse forms of human suffering. It is both common knowledge and the finding of considerable research that human suffering is eased by the ministrations of another caring human being. In psychotherapy, this easing of suffering is conceptualized to be a product of "the therapeutic relationship." For example, children learn to comfort themselves via the comforting presence of their mothers, participation in therapy groups may enhance the immune response of patients who have malignant melanoma, and

patients who have schizophrenia and who receive psychotherapy in addition to psychopharmacologic agents spend less time hospitalized.

Physicians need to learn the principles of psychotherapeutic management of human suffering in the interest of easing their patients' pain and transferring to them an improved ability to self-manage. It is not clear that a particular type of psychiatric disorder (e.g., depression) should necessarily be treated with a particular type of psychotherapy (e.g., interpersonal psychotherapy). Individual human suffering is so unique, and the life circumstances of any individual so varied, that psychotherapy must perforce be custom designed, at least in part. It is therefore more important to learn to conduct a coherent and useful psychotherapeutic experience for a patient than to learn one narrowly defined therapeutic style and expect all patients to fit its Procrustean bed.

This chapter is also concerned with another form of management: that of the physician's career and life. A real and multifaceted peril coexists with the many blessings and pleasures that derive from the privilege of knowing other humans so intimately and from the position of power and influence that physicians hold in their patients' lives. Physicians are subject not only to the same suffering that afflicts all people but also to the various forms of exquisite and potentially devastating suffering that can follow when mischief infects the physician–patient bond. In order for physicians to lead long, happy, productive professional lives, they must learn not only to manage their patients' care but also to manage their relationships with their patients. The term "secondary traumatic stress" refers to the therapist's suffering that specifically relates to patients with posttraumatic stress disorder. However, suffering is a part of good physicianship in treating a variety of other diagnostic categories as well. By the attentive acquisition of the principles of professional life management, physicians can largely avoid a chronic state of fear of their patients. Physicians' fear of patients derives from several related sources: (1) the patient will cross some boundary and render the physician uncertain how to behave. This leads the physician to an inability to be natural; (2) the patient will commit some act of aggression against the physician (sue him or her) because of some dissatisfaction; (3) empathic connection to any suffering patient is inherently a source of pain and sometimes almost diagnostic of certain types of psychopathology (the "praecox feeling" associated with treating individuals with schizophrenia.) Fear of patients is learned in residency training and must be unlearned in order for the physician to have a comfortable professional life. Fearful physicians cannot be creative, convey hope, or model joy in living. By doing three things the physician can come to enjoy life and the practice of the Art to which Hippocrates referred: (1) by understanding the nature of human vulnerability, both one's own and that of the patient; (2) by understanding the mechanisms whereby patients construct their experience of the physician and vice versa; and (3) by learning to apply the concepts of empathy, transference, and boundaries.

Cloninger CR, Surakic DM, Przyeck TR: A psychobiological model of temperament and character. *Arch Gen Psychiatry* 1993;50: 975–990.

Weingarten K: *Common Shock*. New York: Dutton Press, 2003, pp. 102–105.

DEFINITION OF PSYCHOTHERAPY

Psychotherapy can be defined in general terms as the use of verbal means to influence beneficially another person's mental and emotional state. Such a definition does not concern itself with training of the therapist and does not distinguish the activities of a well-intentioned friend from those of a paid professional. Psychotherapy will be understood here to refer to a process wherein an individual (the patient) participates in a structured encounter or series of encounters with another person who—by dint of training, licensure, certification, and ethical proscription— is qualified to influence the mental state of another in a way that decreases the suffering and/or increases the psychological, interpersonal, and behavioral options of the patient. There is no fundamental difference between the patient and the therapist other than the training of the therapist for the role. This point is made to emphasize that a psychotherapist is not superior to the patient, even though the therapist is the party responsible for the management of the therapeutic relationship. The patient may be inclined to think of the therapist as superior, but the therapist must avoid this prejudice. Nevertheless, the difference inherent in the training and preparation for the role is crucial.

QUALIFICATIONS OF A PSYCHOTHERAPIST

Personal Traits

Although training is the chief distinguishing feature of a psychotherapist, it alone cannot make a good psychotherapist out of every individual. The potential psychotherapist is an individual who is fascinated by the human condition and is not consciously exploitative, significantly emotionally handicapped, or impulsive. Intelligence is important, but more important are thoughtfulness and sensitivity. Some individuals may be said (semifacetiously) to be "too normal" to be psychotherapists. By this, it is meant that some energetic and optimistic people become quickly impatient with others' foibles. Other individuals have no diagnosable psychiatric conditions but do have strongly developed personality traits (pessimism, narcissism) or cognitive styles (suspicious, histrionic) that deter the patient. Some individuals represent a potential danger, both to themselves and to the patient, if allowed to assume the psychotherapist's role. This group includes the charismatic leader and (in contrast) the emotionally needy or love-starved individual. These individuals have powerful personal agendas that overshadow the patient's needs.

Training

Psychoanalytic institutes have, over decades, evolved a tripartite structure of training that can be criticized on various grounds but that is in principle fundamentally sound and provides a prototypical model. Ideally, a psychotherapist has first passed through some sort of screening to assess personal attributes as outlined in the preceding section. Other qualifications are generally specified (a particular terminal degree), but these requirements are usually in the interest of turf definition and are arbitrary. Having satisfied a training body that one is of reasonable character and is trainable, the student therapist then enters a course of theoretical study, supervised practice, and personal therapy experience. The length and content of such a training program varies considerably in practice. Some training programs emphasize theory; others emphasize the acquisition of specific skills and attitudes. The length of a training program (some months to many years) is a function of the ideals and scope of the learned method (a skill to be acquired or an identity to be forged). Mechanisms are in place to weed out candidates who do not pass muster and to graduate those who have achieved competence. Graduates are eligible to present their work to a national oversight organization that qualifies training programs, sets standards for the profession, admits new graduates into the profession, and requires its members to be accountable to its standards.

There are many such programs in the United States, although most are dedicated to teaching a specific psychotherapeutic discipline. Within these disciplines, the student is expected to master a particular body of theoretical knowledge. This knowledge, in conjunction with the student's personal therapy experience, is intended to provide a framework for understanding another's experience and for structuring therapeutic interventions while avoiding self-serving exploitation of the patient. In practice, a great deal of psychotherapy undoubtedly is practiced by individuals who have had less training than the ideal version outlined here. A typical psychiatric residency training program, for instance, does not require its graduates to have had a personal psychotherapy experience. Some therapists practice various forms of psychotherapy with little training and in an unregulated way.

Robertson MH: *Psychotherapy Education and Training: An Integrative Perspective.* Madison, Connecticut: International Universities Press 1995.

Rogers CR, Dymond R: *Psychotherapy and Personality Change.* Chicago: University of Chicago Press, 1954.

■ MAJOR FORMS OF PSYCHOTHERAPY

There may be hundreds of forms of psychotherapy; considerable overlap exists, however, among the legitimate forms because the general principles on which they are based are mostly agreed upon. The different forms of psychotherapy place special emphasis on one or another general principle. Whether a given therapy is significantly different from another, or more the brainchild of its originator, is often a matter of debate.

Four major forms of psychotherapy result from the different ways workers conceptualize the nature and development of psychic distress: dynamic, experiential–humanistic, cognitive–behavioral, and eclectic or integrated.

Dynamic Psychotherapies

The dynamic psychotherapies are based on the belief that much of human behavior, especially that which is troublesome to the individual, is motivated by psychological factors outside of the individual's awareness, including mental blind spots for both the therapist and the patient. One is compelled, therefore, to maintain self-defeating perspectives, and repeat ultimately unsuccessful and maladaptive behaviors, for unknown (unconscious) reasons. Defense mechanisms operate to stabilize the individual's emotional state, but the price paid for this stabilization may be high. The development of these problematic behaviors, personality traits, affect states, and other symptoms is generally understood to have occurred because of some unfortunate mix between the individual's inherent traits (intelligence, temperament) and the caregiving surround (developmental interferences) into which he or she has been thrust. In the dynamic therapies, improvement is measured by improved function in various realms of the person's life and by results from the new understandings gained in the context of a therapeutic relationship with the therapist. Traditionally, the dynamic therapies have been seen to exist along a somewhat artificial continuum with support at one end and insight at the other. Developments over the past 20 years have placed increased emphasis on the quality of the therapist–patient relationship as a central factor in a beneficial therapy experience.

Experiential–Humanistic Psychotherapies

The experiential–humanistic models of psychotherapy attempt to eliminate the objectivist perspectives seen as inherent in psychodynamic models and replace them with perspectivalist attitudes. That is, the individual's lived experience is viewed as the most, or only, important consideration. No attempt is made to decode the patient's distorted vision of the therapist in order to reconstruct an infantile experience, presumed to be repressed but inferred by the therapist based on knowledge of the universal phases of development. These therapy approaches take the patient's experience, including the patient's experience of the therapist, at face value. Psychopathology is viewed as resulting from the failure of caregivers to provide the empathic responsiveness necessary for the development of a self-structure that organizes experiences in the most adaptive way. The therapist will play a wider array of roles than in the more classically dynamic approaches, determined by the patient's needs and characteristics. Therapeutic effects derive from the formation of a personal narrative that, in the atmosphere of a new self-object experience (patient with therapist in a safe, gratifying, and development-enhancing relationship), allows for a reordering of the processing of personal experience.

Cognitive–Behavioral Psychotherapies

Cognitive–behavioral models of psychotherapy view psychopathology as the result of faulty thinking (cognitions) based on illogical beliefs. Various forms of mental illness (anxiety, inhibitions, depression) result from the powerful influence of these cognitions, for which there is understood to be little or no rational basis. Little time is spent attempting to explain the etiology of these beliefs, and the concept of a dynamic unconscious is seen as unnecessary. The patient's unsubstantiated beliefs ("others would be better off if I were dead") are challenged, with more adaptive beliefs implicitly or explicitly suggested and supported. The patient is thereby persuaded to discard irrational perspectives on the world ("no one will want you if you are not perfect") and replace them with more realistic, validated beliefs. Although other psychotherapies frequently include cognitive elements, the behavioral components of cognitive–behavioral therapy (flooding, blocking) involve action interventions that carry these methods into a clearly different realm (see Chapter 10).

Eclectic or Integrated Psychotherapies

In the practice of psychotherapy, most patients and clients receive a therapy that is an amalgam of the dynamic, experiential–humanistic, and cognitive–behavioral perspectives. This is not due to an inherent difficulty in staying within the confines of a particular method. It arises from the failure of each of the methods to account for the multifaceted presentation of human psychopathology. Unless he or she is immune to the possibility of reductionism, views therapy as a *tour de force*, or simply elects to ignore certain material, the therapist will recognize that each patient presents clinical material best handled by first one and then another perspective.

It would be ludicrous to attempt to paint a picture of a typical psychotherapy patient. The following case is presented to illustrate the typical complexity of the clinical picture that confronts the psychotherapist, and the usefulness of being familiar with a range of theoretical perspectives and techniques:

The patient was an early-middle-aged mother of two healthy children. She was an intelligent, sensitive, and kind woman who had been married for 15 years to a hard-working man who she felt did not understand her. Indeed, he was frustrated by her manifest pessimism, her guilt, and her inability to enjoy the many fruits of their hard work. She was chronically depressed, anxious, phobic, and compulsive. She was also hypochondriacal, sexually unresponsive, and indecisive. Her father died when she was 12 years old, a critical time in a girl's life. Her older brother had sexually abused her, and her sister had committed suicide. As the eldest girl in the family, she had been assigned domestic responsibilities inappropriate to her age following her father's death. The first-born brother's presence, however, stood between her and a sense of specialness. She grew up embittered and

thinking that she was not, and never would be, "good enough." Her sense of self was defined by her failures. Her successes were discounted as aberrations.

Although the patient might have benefited from pharmacotherapy, she said that she did not wish to take medication. She wanted a psychotherapy experience that would help her learn to enjoy her life more and unlock what she experienced as untapped potential. She feared that she might be contaminating her children's worldview, and she felt she was being unfair to her husband and restricting their life together. She saw her problem as chronic and severe and worried that she might one day follow her sister's suicidal path, an act that, for her family's sake, she desperately wanted to avoid.

In planning a psychotherapy for this patient, the therapist was struck by the myriad symptoms she exhibited, noting that all were in the "neurotic" sphere. She did not abuse substances and had no psychotic thought content. She seemed to experience both irrational thoughts and personal isolation. Her low self-esteem was related to chronic abusive experiences, and her guilty fears and inhibitions suggested unconscious themes of an oedipal nature. The pervasiveness of the patient's suffering and the history of her personal losses suggested that short-term work would not be effective and might even be damaging. A purely cognitive approach seemed inappropriate given the patient's overwhelming symptomatology: It would not address her many interpersonal needs. An open-ended and eclectic therapy seemed indicated.

Gabbard GO: *Psychodynamic Psychiatry in Clinical Practice,* 4th edn. Washington: American Psychiatric Publishing, Inc., 2005.

Gill MM: *Psychoanalysis in Transition: A Personal View.* New York: Analytic Press, 1994.

Stolorow RD, Atwood GE, Brandchaft B: *The Inter-Subjective Perspective.* Northvale, NJ: Jason Aronson, 1994.

■ EXPECTATIONS OF PSYCHOTHERAPY

Patients approach psychotherapy with a mixture of hopes and expectations, many of which are conscious and some of which are unconscious. Some of the patient's goals are reasonable and some are not. Patients do not intend to be unreasonable; their demands are a function of their neediness and their lack of information, including information about subjective experiences, which are vastly different from their own (cross cultural matches between patient and therapist). Therapists have knowledge, acquired through training and experience, of what is and is not attainable from psychotherapy. The therapist's ambitions and goals for the therapy may not, however, coincide with the patient's. More mature and experienced therapists become increasingly confident in the usefulness of a psychotherapy experience, while simultaneously becoming impressed with the unpredictable and nonspecific nature of the benefit. They understand the importance of allowing the patient to use therapy in a uniquely personal and creative way.

Therapists themselves are not immune to influences that induce them to place unreasonable expectations on therapy. These influences include pressures to move more quickly, more efficiently, and more definitively. The therapist may unwittingly accept the often somewhat seductive plea or demand to become a magician whose aims are accomplished by special power, not hard work. Some therapists feel apologetic for their limitations, ashamed of their imperfections, and guilty about their fees. These vulnerabilities, which signal a need for supervision or personal treatment, may combine with the patient's unreasonable demands to create an "unholy alliance" in which goals are implied but never stated, boundaries are fluid, and roles are not defined.

Patients and therapists should agree explicitly on the goals of the work they are performing mutually. If goals are not made explicit, they will likely become idiosyncratic and immeasurable as well as unreasonable and probably unattainable. Goals can be changed; indeed, it is good practice to compare notes from time to time, especially in a longer treatment, in order to assure that patient and therapist are still on the same track. In any event, one goal should always be to provide the patient with a positive, useful experience. The therapist may be the first significant other in the patient's life who has not wished to exploit the patient, or who has genuinely wished to hear and understand the patient. Such quite general influences may nevertheless be profoundly salutary. It is not necessary for "structural" change to be a goal of a therapy. Although some would distinguish between psychotherapy (change) and a supportive relationship (change not a requirement), setting any specific change as a goal runs the risk of dooming the treatment to failure and thus to its being seen as a negative event in the patient's life. Humans, most especially neurotic ones, are resistant to change. Neurosis is understood to describe the mind in conflict with itself over two opposing wishes—those that are reasonable and those that are unreasonable, or the wish to please versus the wish to oppose (Table 11–1) and suffering is experienced as the result of the conflict. Most humans will, regrettably, tend to continue to suffer rather than let go of one or the other wish. A positive experience with the therapist will likely have a continuing effect on the patient long after the treatment is ended, and changes will likely occur, albeit out of sight of the therapist.

Table 11–1. Patients in (or Entering) Psychotherapy

Reasonable wishes

To achieve more mature development (e.g., decrease emotional investment in parents and increase independence of function, decrease self-absorption and increase awareness of needs of others)

To restructure ways of organizing experience, including changing cognitive style and irrational beliefs

To decrease fear of one's own thoughts and feelings with less reliance on immature coping mechanisms

To increase communication skills in situations in which former limitations were the result of past untoward experiences leading to pathologic character structures

Unreasonable wishes

To become completely well-adjusted; mythically perfect; free of irrational, embarrassing, or shameful thoughts or feelings

To be changed without active effort

To have one's past erased, or be transformed in the present, for example, to become the therapist's child

■ THE PSYCHOTHERAPEUTIC PROCESS

PATIENT SELECTION & THERAPY PLANNING

What principles should guide the therapist in deciding whom and how to treat? Many individuals may be recognized as needing therapy, in the sense that their loved ones or personal acquaintances recognize them as suffering or causing others to suffer. Needing therapy in this sense is not the same as having the potential to use a psychotherapy experience. The process of assessing the likelihood that a prospective patient can benefit from psychotherapy of any type begins with the first encounter (often via the telephone) and should continue until therapist and patient are ready to close the evaluation phase and begin the treatment.

The first level of screening involves the question of need for hospitalization or the likelihood that hospitalization will be necessary in the near future. Although many of the principles discussed here are applicable to inpatients, psychotherapy other than crisis intervention therapy is not feasible in the face of active psychosis or immediate suicide threat. Similarly, a patient who is in the throes of active substance abuse or who is currently involved in a legal proceeding probably should be referred to a specialized help provider.

The telephone call may be used to screen out patients who might become involved in an encounter with a therapist that will be frustrating and essentially a waste of the patient's time and money. The patient should be asked how he or she came to call the particular therapist, in the interest of assessing what the patient likely knows about how the therapist works, and should be told what fees will be charged. The therapist should consider the following questions: Does there seem to be a beginning goodness-of-fit in that the referral makes sense? What is the nature of the complaint? Is the problem within the competence or interest range of the therapist? Does the prospective patient indicate a degree of reflectiveness, or is there excessive, needful demandingness or entitlement? Does the patient "hear" the therapist during the phone call? The patient should be informed that there will be a professional fee charged for the evaluation session. This serves as a useful screen for motivation and ensures that the therapist will be compensated for the time spent, even if the patient elects not to return. Obviously, this strategy applies only in a fee-for-service setting.

An initial phone call need not be lengthy, but it can be useful, and the patient should not be scheduled for a first visit unless the therapist feels a sense of enthusiasm about working with the patient. The patient may also have some questions for the therapist, which should neither threaten nor offend the therapist.

Occasionally, the patient will ask the therapist a question that will indicate that referral to a colleague, or simply a refusal, is the best strategy. Although some questions may need to be answered, others may seem so provocative or challenging that they alarm the therapist. It is better not to begin working with a patient in the first place than to have to refer the patient to another therapist after treatment has begun.

FIRST SESSION: EVALUATING THE PATIENT

The prospective patient is told that one session will be scheduled for an evaluation of the problem. At the end of that hour, the therapist and patient will compare notes and discuss options. Treatment has at this point not been offered and no such contract has been entered into. A first psychiatric session will generally be a mixture of medical interviewing, with a focus on the symptom picture and the patient's mental status, and open-ended interviewing, wherein the patient is given an opportunity not only to be heard but also to demonstrate ease with carrying the conversation. Given a reasonably cooperative patient, the first session should yield three things: (1) an Axis I diagnosis, if any; (2) a sense of goodness-of-fit between patient and therapist; and (3) an ever-growing sense in the therapist of "getting it," that is, of the patient's story beginning to make sense according to the therapist's understanding of the nature and development of psychopathology often conceptualized in reference to one or more clinical "models of the mind."

If the therapist is to plan a psychotherapy experience for the patient, an understanding of what is "wrong" with the patient must be developed. This extends beyond a clinical diagnosis and addresses the question of how psychotherapy will be designed to enable the patient to do a needed body of psychological work. The straightforward and succinct statement that forms in the therapist's mind is a basic version of the elaborate psychodynamic formulations from the heyday of psychoanalysis. It becomes the skeleton on which the flesh of the therapy will be hung. In the absence of the therapist's ability to explain to an observer (or to the patient) what he or she proposes to do and why or, better yet, what the therapist and patient will do together and why, it is likely that a kind of "chronic undifferentiated psychotherapy" will be undertaken. Such an enterprise will be unfocused. It may be pleasant, but it will lack thrust.

It bodes well for psychotherapy when the prospective patient engages the therapist in a personal way. Psychotherapeutic work in the realm of what has traditionally been referred to as the transference adds immediacy and zest to the treatment. Psychotherapy can be done without working with the patient's experience of the therapist, but such treatments are more sterile, intellectual, and distant. However, some patients cannot work effectively in this manner. Patients with narcissistic personality disorder, especially, need a considerable period of time before they feel comfortable revealing what to them represent humiliating notions about actually needing the therapist. The therapist cannot force transference into the foreground, but it can be a powerful tool when the patient will allow its use.

As the time allotted for the first evaluation session draws to a close, a number of complex and interlocking issues come to the forefront. If the evaluator is a psychiatrist, then four decisions must be made: (1) Is hospitalization indicated? If so, the whole psychotherapy matter will probably be tabled. The administrative details of getting the patient hospitalized become the focus of attention. (2) Is a different immediate intervention demanded by the patient's condition? If the therapist is required immediately to assume the role of active change agent (by prescribing psychotropic medication), certain other roles will be less easily established in the future. (3) How comfortable does the therapist feel about having "gotten it?" Generally, the patient will want to feel that the time has been well spent and that the therapist is forming a clear understanding of the patient's situation. The patient does not, however, want to experience the therapist as having decided too quickly about diagnosis and treatment. This will lead the patient to be suspicious of the therapist from the beginning. (4) Does the therapist feel that a therapeutic fit is likely to happen and is worth pursuing, or should this session be the last? Referral for whatever reason is best done at the time of the first visit.

A recommendation of no treatment should remain a possibility in the therapist's mind. If, however, the therapist is beginning to understand the patient and imagine a potential contract for a therapy, it is appropriate near the end of the first hour for the therapist to share with the patient reflections on the interview so far. This preliminary interpretive statement should be followed by the patient's invited response. Asking the patient if he or she has any preformed ideas about what the therapist might do to be helpful is often a useful strategy at this time. These exchanges will set the stage for an agreed-upon second evaluative session that explores areas that both parties feel are important but for which no time is left. In most cases the therapist can reassure the patient that things should be clear, both for therapist and patient, by the end of a second interview, and that a recommendation for treatment will be discussed at that time. The second interview should be scheduled sooner rather than later, preferably within less than 1 week. Patients who have made the decision to seek help generally have delayed for some time, but having begun the process, hope that it will move swiftly.

Gedo JE: A psychology of personal aims. In: *Beyond Interpretation.* New York: International Universities Press, 1979, pp. 1–25.

Dilts SL: *Models of the Mind: A Framework for Biopsychosocial Psychiatry.* Philadelphia: Brunner-Routledge, 2001.

SECOND SESSION: PROCESS & CONTRACT

A second evaluation hour is necessary for several reasons. The therapist may not be ready to present the patient with a therapy recommendation because the formulation is incomplete, or he or she may not want to rush the patient or may want to test the patient's reaction to the first session. Will the patient be able to share thoughts and reactions to the first hour? Will the patient feel better already, more hopeful of an improved future? Was there evidence of self-reflection that generated fresh associations?

The therapist may begin the second session with a statement that it will be useful to explore further a number of areas, but first, what were the patient's thoughts and reactions to the first hour? An important clue to the patient's psychological mindedness may be gleaned from an invitation by the therapist for the patient to say "where the session went" after the initial appointment had ended. Such early alliance building demonstrates that much of the responsibility for the treatment rests with the patient. The patient will often tell the therapist that he or she feels better or will report that new information has been recalled. An exploration of this material generally will enable the therapist to call attention to areas noted after the first session that need exploration, with the upcoming therapy recommendation clearly in mind. If left unexplored, these areas (substance abuse, legal trouble, and experience with other therapists) may erupt later as major obstacles.

The therapist is also considering further the nature of the problem and the type of treatment to be recommended. This will inevitably result in a compromise between what is ideal and what is feasible. The therapist needs to know the patient's capacity to fund therapy, ability to conform to the therapist's work schedule and office hours, and ways of handling separations. The therapist is also assessing how easily the patient talks, and about what. Patients who wish to discuss situational issues may need more time between sessions to allow events to occur. Patients who have strong reactions to the therapy encounters may have difficulty waiting for the next session. Patients who live some distance from the therapist's office, or who must exert considerable effort to get back and forth, will have trouble sustaining their initial enthusiasm. How much is the patient suffering? How motivated does the patient seem to be to initiate change? How stable and supportive is the patient's social support network? Does the patient have the ways and means to effect change? At least a rudimentary developmental history of the patient (if not taken in the first session) is often invaluable for the development of the therapeutic contract.

By the midway point of the second session, an experienced therapist will generally feel comfortable with an extraordinary amount of important information. A less experienced therapist may wish to obtain supervision at this point, but the seasoned therapist will have assessed and decided upon three key issues: (1) whether or not to prescribe medication; (2) whether tests (psychological, chemical, neuropsychological) are needed; and (3) what type of psychotherapy to recommend and at what frequency.

These issues are matters of the utmost importance to the patient's life and to other lives that psychotherapy will affect. The therapist is now poised to make recommendations that will have such an impact on the patient as to be remembered possibly for the rest of the patient's life. The patient may need help in sorting through the most salient implications. If third-party payment will be used, does the patient understand that confidentiality cannot be complete and that the future may bring difficult questions regarding history of treatment? Can the patient defer making significant life decisions that could negatively affect the course and outcome of psychotherapy? What are the dynamic forces at work between the patient and most significant other over the need for and possible result of therapy? The need for informed consent is great in the case of the potential psychotherapy patient, who may have little appreciation of what is about to be undertaken.

The therapist will then tell the patient precisely what is being recommended and why. Three areas must be covered: (1) the name of the psychotherapy, its rationale, its frequency, its anticipated length, and its cost; (2) the hoped-for outcome of the treatment, couched in terms that express optimism for realistic and attainable goals, and the likelihood of that outcome; and (3) alternative treatments, their anticipated length and costs, and their risks and likely outcome.

A schedule for visits will be negotiated, and a clear description will be provided of procedures regarding payment of the bill, appointment cancellation and lateness on the part of the patient or the therapist, and vacations. A standard written policy statement may be used. If third-party payment or certification procedures (health maintenance organizations [HMOs]) will be a part of the picture, these procedures, including the provision of a diagnosis, should be outlined clearly. The therapist should explain to the patient the diagnosis and should tell the patient what is expected of him or her during the treatment and what can be expected of the therapist. Some issues may be addressed only when they arise and become integrated into the context of the treatment. These issues include details such as telephone calls, chance meetings outside the office, and what names will be used.

By the end of the second session, the therapist and the patient may look forward with optimism and anticipation to the beginning of a psychotherapeutic endeavor between an informed patient and a therapist who knows where things are headed. The framework of treatment has been carefully built. Both parties know what to expect. Therapy is off to a good start.

BEGINNING OF PSYCHOTHERAPY

It can be said justifiably that therapy has been underway since its conception as a thought in the patient's mind, and certainly since the patient's first encounter with the therapist. Nevertheless, the therapist has made a point of separating evaluation from treatment, because of the wish not to enter into a formal medico-legal contractual responsibility for the patient's ongoing welfare (beyond handling any immediate needs the patient may have) until he or she is confident that the treatment is manageable. The treatment phase has now been launched, and the therapist becomes concerned with those phenomena that characterize the opening phase.

Whatever goals for the treatment enterprise the patient and therapist have agreed upon, the therapist knows that there is one overarching goal: to provide the patient with an experience that will enable some measure

of healing to occur. The therapist cannot will the patient into mental health, and the patient may find that personal resistances to change are too great to overcome. The therapist is confident, however, that careful attention to the application of considered strategies and tactics, informed by a detailed understanding of the nature of the patient's psychopathology against the background of his or her unique developmental experiences, and delivered with skill and sensitivity, will, over time, create a healthy atmosphere that the patient will use to the best possible advantage. To this end, the therapist considers the various or predominant role(s) to be played and the basic interventions to be undertaken. Staying in role, and consistently and effectively intervening over time, the therapist will have a corrective effect. The therapist must have the emotional well-being and personal attributes to make this possible.

Whatever the nature of the therapy, the opening phase is understood to involve two parts. First, the patient passes through the stages of engagement into the therapy process. The signs of the patient becoming "in therapy" will vary according to the structure of the particular therapy being used. In psychodynamic therapy, for instance, patients might be said to be "in therapy" when they begin to attach emotional importance to the therapist as a real person or to the nature of the intersubjective experience of patient and therapist. In therapy designed along more educational or supportive lines, the patient may report having been reflecting on the last session and provide additional thoughts about it. In some cases, the engagement will be revealed in a dream or in an unconscious but undeniable act of resistance.

After engagement has occurred, the second part of the opening phase plays out, with the unfolding and illumination before the eyes of the patient and the therapist of the nature of the problem. The way the problem is conceptualized is intensely personal. It is worked out between the patient and the therapist in language to which they will refer by mutual agreement. This language is a derivative of the blending of the therapist's methods of organizing the experience of the therapy with the patient's organization of the experience. The words used to describe the nature of the problem will reveal the predominant theoretical orientation of the therapist merging with the narrative that the patient is constructing. Once the problem has been defined in this mutual and cocreated manner, the opening phase is over.

MIDDLE PHASE OF PSYCHOTHERAPY

Before the middle phase of psychotherapy can begin, the alliance between patient and therapist must be established firmly and the core conflictual issue identified and agreed upon. The process of working through begins. The patient is confronted repeatedly with manifestations of problematic ways of organizing experiences and relating to others. In some therapies, this process occurs in the cauldron of the transference–countertransference. In other therapies in which the patient is unable to work with transference material, working through takes place once-removed, by examining relationships outside the therapy, both current and past. This confrontation has variable effects on the patient. There may be moments of new understanding and growth. There may be periods of flight away from the process via resistance maneuvers and regressive detours. The therapist's role is to "follow the red thread" of the patient's unconscious and automatic attitudes and behaviors and—through a mixture of empathic responsiveness, probing, clarifying, confronting, and interpreting—"hold the patient's nose to the grindstone" of the work of the treatment.

Many difficulties are encountered during the middle phase; some are inevitable and some are incidental to therapist error. All the desirable personal attributes and all the therapeutic competence that the therapist can muster will not ensure a smooth middle phase. Empathic failures by the therapist will lead to failures to intervene and to mismatches between patient need and therapist role selection. The therapist will lose sight of the patient's experience, and the patient's feelings will be hurt. A number of middle-phase problems are typical and are mentioned individually in the sections that follow.

A. ACTING OUT

The term "acting out" is used in different ways, but it is generally understood to refer to behavior that discharges the affects generated by the therapy process. A variety of behaviors are seen, involving both conscious and unconscious motivations. Individuals who are prone to impulsiveness or destructive behavior make relatively problematic psychotherapy subjects. The most flagrant behavior, such as substance abuse, suicide attempts, and middle-of-the-night phone calls, may be so difficult to manage as to make therapy impossible. If the therapist lacks the ability to bring administrative control to bear in order to preserve the treatment, he or she can be placed in the untenable position of being responsible for the patient's irresponsible acts.

Less dramatic forms of acting out must be recognized by the therapist, who should then confront the patient and bring the affects and associated thoughts into the therapy. The patient may quote the therapist to another person and arouse ire, especially if the other person is paying the bill. The patient may fail to pay the bill, miss sessions, cancel appointments, or be late; or the patient may make serious life decisions abruptly, especially regarding love relationships.

A single female mental health professional in her mid thirties sought treatment with a male therapist for recurrent major depression. She also described a disturbing behavioral propensity to make particularly poor choices for her romantic involvements. Her treatment involved pharmacotherapy for the depression and expressive psychodynamic psychotherapy. The latter was far more in-depth than her previous treatments, which were predominantly pharmacologically based. As the therapy unfolded, she began to recall experiences from her childhood, which involved sexually overstimulating "play" with a reclusive uncle who had been repeatedly entrusted with childcare and baby-sitting responsibilities. As this "play" was recognized as sexual exploitation, the patient increased the frequency of sessions in her therapy and became engaged in the therapy in a lively fashion. However, she soon found herself preoccupied with a female patient of hers who had characteristics of a borderline personality disorder. In a highly uncharacteristic manner, her preoccupation included urges to be involved in her patient's personal life in a way that would have clearly been both professionally damaging for the professional and disastrous for her patient.

The therapist suggested (interpreted) to his patient that she was displacing feelings of an erotic, loving transference relationship into the relationship with her female patient. This "displacement" was a compromise that transiently allowed her to feel less vulnerable, but also would result in the "punishment" she felt she deserved for her childhood sexual behavior with her uncle. Since their relationship was still rather early in its development, the therapist elected to communicate in a more direct and "educational" manner. The potential danger to his patient's professional well-being required greater and earlier activity than might be the case in a situation that did not involve such danger for the primary and secondary patients involved in this case.

Mutual analysis of these behaviors nearly always leads to an improved alliance and forward motion. Failure to confront the behavior retards or disrupts therapy.

The patient may demonstrate ego-syntonic acting out, in which he or she enacts unconscious themes through behavior that causes no harm. For example, the patient may come early for the appointment (the attendant hope being to see the therapist's other patients), or the patient may watch the clock so as not to overstay (the unconscious fear is of feeling dismissed). It is sometimes useful in therapy to look the gift horse in the mouth.

B. ACTING IN

Novice therapists are frequently troubled when patients do things in their presence that throw them off balance, disorient, or even frighten them. Many of these behaviors merely need to be experienced once in order to know how to handle them next time. Some behaviors may prompt the therapist to seek personal treatment.

A patient may put the therapist off balance by exhibiting overly familiar behavior. For example, a patient calls the therapist by her first name or asks to be called by his first name; a patient brings the therapist a small gift; or a patient asks personal questions about the therapist's life. The smooth management of these personal moments requires self-awareness, compassion, flexibility, and objectivity. It also requires factual knowledge of the nature of boundaries, boundary violations, and medical ethics, as well as theoretical knowledge of the nature of psychopathology and of the science of psychotherapy. Beginning therapists need regular forums in which they can process such events. Even very experienced therapists need access to consultation anytime they are inclined to engage in atypical therapeutic behavior or recognize that they are anticipating a "boundary crossing." In general, it is best to err on the side of awkward, stiff refusal than on the side of boundaryless permissiveness. One's technique will become smoother with time.

Some behaviors by the patient are more provocative and troublesome. For example, a patient asks for hugs or other personal contact or asks for a gift from the therapist; a patient wears revealing clothing or directly propositions the therapist; or a patient requests out-of-the-office contact. In such situations, the therapist should begin with gentle limit setting accompanied by sensible explanations. One does not say "I'd like to, but the ethics of my profession won't let me." One says, "Therapy is conducted through talk, not through action." (In psychoanalysis as opposed to psychotherapy, the therapist often will "interpret" the patient's behavior without any further elaboration, somewhat like a sports announcer's "calling the play by play." This use of words where there would more naturally be behavior is what led Freud to describe psychoanalysis as an endeavor for which there is "no model in other human relationships.") Occasionally a patient will persist, despite firm but gentle limit setting. The therapist then confronts the patient with his or her seeming inability to take no for an answer and invites an exploration.

A common behavior on the border between acting out and acting in involves encounters between the patient and the therapist's office personnel. The patient may pump the secretary for personal information about the therapist. The patient may attempt to befriend or even romance the office staff. These situations are easily dealt with when the staff is knowledgeable and well trained. Considerable trouble can result, however, when the office person has no understanding of the nature of a patient–therapist relationship or, even worse, harbors resentment toward the therapist–boss. Beginning therapists must take nothing for granted in the hiring and training of office personnel. Such individuals represent the therapist to the public, for better or for worse.

Gutheil TG, Gabbard GO: Misuses and misunderstandings of boundary theory in clinical and regulatory settings. *Am J Psychiatry* 1998;155(3):409–414.

C. STALEMATE

The term "stalemate" covers a variety of conditions, the essence of which is that the patient becomes dissatisfied with the therapy, makes no progress, and threatens to quit. This phenomenon has traditionally been seen from an objectivist perspective and understood as a manifestation of resistance (negative therapeutic reaction). More contemporary views of the therapy process interpret these states as commentaries on the nature of the relationship between the two parties. Active interpretation is usually required to restore the alliance and the therapy, and generally some degree of therapist self-disclosure involving the immediate interaction calls to the patient's attention the failure to get something from the therapist that the patient very much wants. It is not, of course, the gratification of these wishes that is the purpose of the therapy but rather their identification. Awareness and acknowledgment that the therapist plays an active role in the creation of the "analytic third" is necessary to uncover and illuminate these states of depletion in the patient. Using first person plural language ("We are having a problem.") when describing transferential problems and difficulties of the treatment is useful in communicating the therapist's awareness of his or her role in the creation of the therapeutic relationship.

D. THIRD-PARTY INTERFERENCES

Threatened spouses and parents are joined by third-party payers of all varieties in placing pressures on the very existence of psychotherapy. For example, an angry wife may request equal time to "set the record straight"; a jealous husband may knock on the door during a therapy hour; or an HMO may need more information before a claim for benefits can be processed. Sensitivity, flexibility, and strength are required of the therapist in order to protect the patient's confidentiality and preserve the life of the therapy.

E. OTHER NEGATIVE EFFECTS

Many complications are possible in psychotherapy. Constant pressure against the frame of a therapy is created by necessary restrictions. It is not easy to avoid boundary violations, but the task is made easier if the therapist has knowledge of behaviors that are considered to be boundary violations. Experience shows that it is folly to expect the patient to understand and control these matters. It is the therapist's responsibility.

The vulnerabilities of the psychotherapist are all too real, and patients can present many attractions to a therapist. The therapist is of course in danger of participating in boundary violations but is also vulnerable to painful affect states tied to the rigors and restrictions of the work. Commonly experienced signs of untoward therapist stress include excessive fatigue at the end of the day; depression, depletion, and having nothing left for life outside the office; inability to take time off ("dance of the hours"); or loss of objectivity and intemperate identification with the patient.

Rarely, the therapist will realize that a serious mistake has been made in the original conceptualization of the therapy and that the therapy should not be allowed to continue. It is better to interrupt treatment than to persist in the face of an untenable situation. The therapist may, for example, realize that the patient has been misdiagnosed and that significant antisocial elements are present. The patient may become engaged in behavior that runs counter to the contract or that the therapist finds intolerable (an HIV-positive patient who continues to expose unknowing partners). Consultation with a colleague may show the therapist the way out of the dilemma. If not, the only path may be to make alternative arrangements with careful consideration of the therapist's legal and ethical responsibilities.

In a gratifyingly high percentage of cases, when the patient–therapist fit has been a good one and the alliance has held together, the patient achieves most of the contracted-for goals. The patient is easier to be with, both for the therapist and significant others. The patient reports that life is better. Symptoms melt away, and characteristic ways of organizing experiences become less rigid and stereotyped. Relationships with other people improve. The patient begins to talk about life without the therapy, and the therapist begins to think that a successful ending for the therapy is in view. The middle phase is finished.

TERMINATION OF PSYCHOTHERAPY

The ending of a psychotherapy can occur under a variety of circumstances, some very satisfying for both parties, and some painful or traumatic, especially for the patient.

Termination by Mutual Agreement: Satisfied

In this situation, circumstances are optimal. The therapist and the patient are in agreement that the therapy should end because the work has gone well and the desired effect has occurred. If the therapy has been open ended, the classic phases of termination will be seen, colored by the patient's individual circumstances. The therapist will have begun to muse that termination has become a consideration, seeing that the patient is functioning well, both within and outside the therapy hour: There is no acting out, the original symptoms are no longer problematic, and the patient is being affirmed by the environment. When the patient raises the issue, it feels congruent to the therapist. It is discussed, and a mutually agreeable ending date is set. During the ensuing phase (brief or extended, according to agreement), a resurgence of symptomatology is typical, and the pain of loss of a relationship is experienced by both parties. The therapist knows the pain must be worked through by the patient and does not collude in any defensive maneuvers of the patient. The therapy ends on a bittersweet note, with recognition that good work was done and each party has devoted appreciated effort; but the work is over, and the patient is ready to move on. The therapeutic relationship is left intact. The therapist does not cross previously respected boundaries. The patient may well never return, but if the need arises, there would be no barriers.

Termination by Mutual Agreement: Elements of Dissatisfaction

More typical than the previously described ideal situation is one in which the patient and therapist agree to the ending of the therapy, but one or both feel a degree of dissatisfaction with what has been accomplished and would prefer to continue. The therapy may have been time limited from the beginning, either because the therapist conceptualized a time-limited treatment as optimal or because the patient had limited resources. Artificial limits may have been set by a managed care organization. Nevertheless, one or both parties may wish that either the therapeutic relationship or a new, personal relationship could continue when a useful change on the part of the patient seems highly unlikely. The patient and the therapist may agree that a hoped-for goal for the treatment will not be realized. These endings are painful to a degree, but they are not traumatic. The limitations of the experience are acknowledged, but there is a sharing in appreciation of the good work. The pain of separation is experienced, but there is no recrimination or bitterness.

Interruption of Psychotherapy: Disagreement

When one or both parties disagree with the ending of psychotherapy, the word "interruption" is a more descriptive designation than is "termination." The treatment is ending over the objections of one or both participants. For example, the patient announces the intention not to return, the patient is told that the therapist is leaving (relocating for a career move, rotating off residency service), or the financial support for the treatment is withdrawn unexpectedly. In these situations, psychological trauma will be experienced, generally more acutely by the patient, although losing a therapy case can be a staggering blow to a therapist's self-esteem. In any case, the nature of the felt trauma will be a function of the reason for the interruption and the psychological structure of the injured party.

When the patient leaves the therapist, it is important that the therapist remain in role. Although shocked, insulted, or frightened, the therapist must help the patient deal with the emotions surrounding the decision. Any impulse to counter with threats or dire predictions must be stifled, perhaps to be worked through in an ad hoc personal therapy encounter for the therapist. Because of the chronic nature of psychopathology, there is a good chance that the patient who interrupts therapy will seek therapy elsewhere, sooner or later. Therapists should always endeavor to make any encounter with a patient as therapeutic as possible.

When the therapist leaves the patient, the scene is ripe for damage to be inflicted on the patient, although the degree of damage can be controlled by sensitive and thoughtful management of the situation. To do so, the therapist must transcend the narcissistic investment in the reason for the interruption. The excitement one is feeling over an upcoming relocation or graduation or new baby will not be shared by the patient, informed or otherwise. The patient will feel variously bereft, abandoned, devalued, jealous, envious, or a plethora of other feelings determined by circumstances and character structure. The patient must be allowed to explore these states and express the attached affects. The therapist must remain in role, acknowledging nondefensively as many of the facts as is consistent with his or her established way of working. The patient's pain is not underestimated, and the patient's individuality is respected within reason as a schedule for the interruption is worked out.

In announcing the interruption, the therapist has two decisions to make: (1) when to announce it and (2) whether transfer to another therapist is indicated. Patients need adequate time to process an interruption, but announcing the interruption too soon may cause the remaining time to be a "lame duck" period in which little is accomplished. Likewise, the patient may be soothed to know that therapy will continue, but the new therapist will immediately assume great importance in the patient's mind even if never met, and this will distract the patient from dealing with feelings about the interruption.

In some cases, it will be obvious that further treatment will be needed, and the therapist will offer help in locating a replacement therapist. In these cases, the therapist can leave the interruption announcement until relatively late in the sequence, perhaps with only several sessions remaining. Other patients may not need a replacement therapist. The patient may be near enough to a termination that the work can be truncated. The patient may feel that transfer to a new therapist is not worth the trouble involved. The patient may wish to find further therapy in the future but wants to take a break from the process after the interruption. The therapy will profit from avoiding a premature and unilateral decision to recommend continued treatment. Such a recommendation may be more defensive against the therapist's guilt over leaving than it is sensitive to the patient's individuality. In such situations, where there is a good chance that the patient's therapy experience will end with the interruption, the therapist must give the patient more time. The therapist must assess the patient's record of dealing with separations. Some patients may need 6 months or more, and various tapering schedules and other modifications of the usual ways of working may be useful. Therapist inflexibility is usually experienced as damaging.

The management of an interruption or a termination requires sensitivity and skill. Having had the experience of being in therapy oneself adds immeasurably to the therapist's ability to be sensitive to the importance one attains in the eyes of the patient.

Gutheil TG, Gabbard GO: The concept of boundaries in clinical practice: theoretical and risk-management dimensions. *Am J Psychiatry* 1993;150:188.

Ogden TH: *Subjects of Analysis.* Northvale, NJ: Jason Aronson, 1994.

Strupp H, Binder J: *Psychotherapy in a New Key: A Guide to Time-Limited Psychotherapy.* New York: Basic Books, 1984.

■ CONCURRENT TREATMENTS

Individual psychotherapy as the sole therapeutic agent is the best treatment for many of the patients who present themselves to mental health professionals. Individuals with common personality disorders such as narcissistic personality and borderline personality, and those troubled by what may be called disorders of the spirit, are frequently best managed in the containing acceptance of an individual therapy. Such patients may seek psychotherapy from psychologists, social workers, and pastoral counselors, reasoning not only that such professionals are uniquely qualified to help them but also that psychiatrists will be either too expensive or disinterested in their problems. Although this recent historical development is unfortunate for the field of psychiatry, it is hoped that the recognition that psychiatry is in danger of "losing its soul" will spur the field to reclaim its place in the psychotherapy tradition.

Many patients, especially those encountered by psychiatrists, need more than individual therapy to manage their conditions. Depression seems to have replaced narcissism as the illness of our time, and combined psychotherapy and pharmacotherapy for mood disorders has become commonplace. In addition, a new recognition of the important role of supportive psychotherapy in the care of the seriously mentally ill has led to more collaboration between psychiatrists and nonpsychiatrist psychotherapists. Debates about whether psychotherapy can withstand the resistances set in motion by combined use of medication, and about whether the therapist should have a psychopharmacologist handle the medication, have been replaced by concerns over the impact of contemporary agents (fluoxetine) on the core of personality structure. Amidst this sea of change, however, it is easy to trivialize truths about the patient–therapist relationship. Fortunately the concept of dynamic pharmacotherapy has provided a framework within which to consider the positive and negative effects of combining psychotherapy and medication.

It is now well established that problems with medication compliance in patients who have chronic illnesses such as bipolar disorder and schizophrenia are common and costly realities in psychopharmacology. The sensitive application of psychotherapy by the psychopharmacologist makes for more successful pharmacotherapy. In contrast, therapists may be concerned that their psychotherapeutic zeal could bias them against potentially helpful biologic agents. This may lead them paradoxically to recommend medication too quickly. In many clinical situations the determination of the need for a psychopharmacologic agent is far from clear-cut. In these situations many patients do not want to take medication; they want the physician's time, person, and perceptual, conceptual, and executive skills. Many patients do not like the way medication affects them and fear that the doctor will lose interest in talking to them. Psychotherapists, including psychiatrists, commonly see patients who have been dissatisfied with their experience with a physician who seemed too quick to prescribe medication in lieu of engaging them in even a brief psychotherapy. Psychiatric treatment is clearly more satisfying to all concerned when the physician has the time and the freedom to prepare a truly customized treatment plan.

CONCLUSION

In undertaking to learn the basic principles of psychotherapeutic management, contemporary beginning psychiatric residents and medical students considering psychiatry as a career are inclined to question whether the effort is worthwhile. The ideas and the history of the field intrigue them, but they are overwhelmed by what seems a mysterious skill set, vast in scope and only slowly acquired. They question whether they will be "allowed" (by managed care organizations) to perform psychotherapy. They question whether they or their patients will be able to afford to spend an hour (or any significant portion thereof) together. Trainees at this level may be reminded that psychiatry as practiced in the emergency room of a city hospital at 3:00 AM, although necessary, represents only a small portion of the influence they can bring to bear on the toll taken by mental illness in our time. Advanced psychiatric residents quickly rediscover the lost soul of psychiatry and clamor for seminars and supervision in psychotherapy. They have learned again what was almost forgotten, what was almost buried under the avalanche of medical school facts and early residency sleepless nights. They rediscover the central role of relatedness in the definition of emotional well-being, and they learn to appreciate the pernicious impact of its loss in the manifestations of emotional despair. The road to the recovery of human relatedness is through the process of relatedness, and many times this requires a therapist. The quality and meaning of human life, both the professional's and the patient's, derive from relatedness. No amount of bottom-line accounting or conceptual reductionism can alter that truth.

Nemiah JC: The idea of a psychiatric education. *J Psychiatr Educ* 1981;5(3):183–194.

Diagnostic Formulation, Treatment Planning, and Modes of Treatment in Children and Adolescents

12

Barry Nurcombe, MD

■ DIMENSIONS OF THE DIAGNOSTIC FORMULATION

The diagnostic formulation summarizes and integrates relevant issues from the biopsychosocial, developmental, and temporal axes. The **biopsychosocial axis** refers to multiple systems, from molecular to sociocultural, that interact constantly and are manifest in current objective behavior and subjective experience. The **developmental axis** is applied to different levels of the biopsychosocial axis in order to determine whether each level is developmentally normal, delayed, advanced, or deviant. The **temporal axis** refers to the ontogenesis of the individual from his or her origins to the present and beyond.

Biopsychosocial Axis

Current functioning is the expression of multiple biopsychosocial levels within the patient, as he or she interacts with the physical, family, sociocultural, occupational, and economic environment. In order to evaluate present functioning, the clinician examines the levels and systems described in Table 12–1.

Developmental Axis

Each level of the biopsychosocial axis can be assessed with regard to what would be expected for that age. Some of these assessments (e.g., height, weight, head circumference) are very accurate. For others (e.g., intelligence), although a number of assessment instruments are available, existing measures represent a composite of skills potentially affected by extraneous factors (e.g., social class, motivation). For still others (e.g., ego defenses, working models of attachment), measurement techniques are relatively crude and the norms subjective.

Nevertheless, during interviewing and mental status examination, the clinician will scan the levels shown in Table 12–2 for delay, precocity, or deviation from the normal and, when appropriate, order formal special investigations.

Temporal Axis

All individuals have come from somewhere, exist where they are now, and are headed somewhere. Using the temporal axis, the clinician explores the unfolding of a problem up to the present time and attempts to predict where the patient is headed. The mileposts in this evolution can be classified, somewhat arbitrarily, in the following sequence: (1) predisposition, (2) precipitation, (3) presentation, (4) pattern, (5) perpetuation, (6) potentials, and (7) prognosis.

1. Predisposition—What early biological or psychosocial factors have stunted or deflected normal development, or rendered the patient vulnerable to stress? Table 12–3 lists several examples.

Given the current state of knowledge, it is often difficult or impossible to reconstruct these factors and their effects on the growing organism, particularly with regard to inherited vulnerability or propensity (e.g., as hypothesized for depressive disorder). However, postnatal deprivation or trauma may be recorded, for example, in the patient's medical record.

2. Precipitation—A precipitant is a physical or psychosocial stressor that challenges the individual's coping capacity and causes him or her to exhibit the symptoms and signs of psychological maladjustment. Table 12–4 lists several examples. A temporal relationship exists between the precipitant and the onset of symptoms. Sometimes the precipitant (e.g., parental discord) later becomes a perpetuating factor. Sometimes the precipitant is a reminder of a previous traumatic experience. Sometimes the precipitant ceases, and the patient returns to normal coping. Sometimes the precipitant ceases, but maladaptive coping persists or even worsens. In that case, perpetuating factors must be operating (see below).

Table 12–1. The Biopsychosocial Axis

Level	Systems Assessed
Physical level	Peripheral organ systems Immune system Autonomic system Neuroendocrine system Sensorimotor system
Psychological level	Information-processing systems Communication systems Social competence Internal working models of the self and others Unconscious conflicts, ego defenses, and coping style Patterns of psychopathology
Social level	Physical environment Family system (nuclear and extended) Sociocultural systems (peers, adults, school)

Not all current patterns of psychopathology have precipitants. Some psychopathologies (e.g., early infantile autism) may have evolved continuously since infancy or early childhood. The clinician should look for a precipi-

Table 12–3. Predisposing Biological and Psychosocial Factors

Genetic vulnerability or propensity
Chromosomal abnormality
Intrauterine insult or deprivation
Perinatal physical insult
Postnatal malnutrition, exposure to toxins, or physical trauma
Physical illness
Neglect or maltreatment
Parental loss, separation, or divorce
Exposure to psychological trauma

tant when normal functioning is succeeded by the onset of psychopathology.

3. Presentation—The clinician should consider why the family is presenting at this time. Is it, for example, that the child's behavior worries them or disrupts family functioning? Has the family's capacity to tolerate the child's behavior deteriorated? If so, why?

4. Pattern—The current pattern represents the current biopsychosocial axis. The clinician should evaluate the patient's current physical, psychological, and social functioning. To the extent that abnormalities in physical functioning (e.g., somatoform symptoms), information processing (e.g., amnesia), communication (e.g., mutism), internal models (e.g., self- hatred), coping style (e.g.,

Table 12–2. The Developmental Axis

Level	Systems Assessed	Assessment Method
Physical level	Peripheral organ systems (e.g., height, weight, head circumference)	Growth charts
	Sensorimotor system	Developmental assessment, neuropsychological testing
Psychological level	Information processing	Intelligence testing, special testing for memory and other cognitive functions, educational attainment testing, neuropsychological testing
	Communication	Speech and language assessment, neuropsychological testing
	Social competence	Behavioral observation, psychological testing
	Internal working models	Interviewing, personality testing
	Conflicts, defenses, coping style	Interviewing, behavioral observation, personality testing
	Symptom patterns	Interviewing, checklists, structured interviews
Social level	Family system, peer relations, school functioning	Family interviews, observations, checklists

Table 12–4. Examples of Precipitating Factors

Physical
- Physical illness
- Surgery
- Accidental injury

Psychosocial
- Civilian catastrophe
- War
- Parental conflict, separation, or divorce
- Loss of a loved one
- Rejection
- Academic stress
- Hospitalization

compulsive risk-taking), and social competence (e.g., social withdrawal) can be defined as psychopathologic phenomena, the clinician will assemble configurations of symptoms and signs that form categorical syndromes (e.g., residual posttraumatic stress disorder, dysthymia) and dynamic patterns (e.g., traumatophilia, introversion of aggression, unresolved conflict following trauma).

The clinician also evaluates the family, and the social, school, cultural, and economic environment in which the family lives. Table 12–5 lists the issues to consider in evaluating the quality of family interactions. The clinician also assesses the **acuity** of the problem pattern (i.e., its imminent danger to the patient and others), its **severity** (i.e., the levels of biopsychosocial functioning affected and the degree to which they are affected), and its **chronicity**.

5. Perpetuation—If the precipitating stress (e.g., parental conflict) does not dissipate, the child's maladaptation is likely to continue. If the stress is removed, the child is likely to spring back to normality. If not, the clinician must ask why not. The reason could be either within or outside the child.

Internal perpetuating factors can be biological or psychological. For example, overwhelming psychic trauma can trigger a train of unreversed biochemical derangements, involving catecholamines, corticosteroids, and endogenous opiates, that cause the numbing and hyperarousal associated with the traumatic state. Unresolved psychic trauma can also produce a personality that seeks compulsively to reenter traumatic situations, thus reexposing the self to victimization and further trauma.

External perpetuating factors include the reinforcement of child psychopathology that occurs in dysfunctional family systems, for example, the protective parent who shields a delinquent child from punishment, or the anxious, enmeshed parent who unwittingly reinforces a child's separation anxiety and school refusal.

6. Potentials—In addition to addressing psychopathology and defects, the clinician should consider the child's physical, psychological, and social strengths. A child with a learning problem may be talented at sports, or be physically attractive, or have a talented, supportive family. In treatment planning, the clinician must consider how strengths can be harnessed in order to circumvent or compensate for defects or problems.

7. Prognosis—The clinician should predict what is likely to happen with or without treatment, remembering that it is impossible to anticipate all the unfortunate and fortuitous happenstance that can block, divert, or facilitate a particular life trajectory.

■ THE DIAGNOSTIC FORMULATION: AN EXAMPLE

The clinician should summarize the diagnostic formulation in a succinct manner. Consider the following example:

> Susan is a 14-year-old adolescent who has a 2-month history of the following symptoms, which

Table 12–5. Factors Involved in the Quality of Family Interactions

The quality of communication about important matters between family members. Do they express their messages clearly and do they listen to and hear each other?

The capacity of family members to share positive and negative emotions. Are they able to praise and encourage each other? Can they express love? If they are angry with one another, can they say so without losing control?

The sensitivity of family members to each other's feelings. Are they aware when other family members are sad, upset, hurt, enthusiastic, or happy, and do they respond accordingly?

The capacity of the family to set rules and control behavior. Are they clear about rules and consistent in their following up of whether the rules are followed? If children must be disciplined, are penalties appropriate and timely?

The appropriateness and flexibility of family roles. Is it clear who does what in the family? If one family member is absent or indisposed, can other family members fill in?

The capacity of the family to solve problems and cope with crises. When the family is confronted with a problem, can family members work together to solve it?

were precipitated by her observation of a house fire in which the 4-year-old brother she was baby-sitting perished: traumatic nightmares, intrusive memories, frequent reminders, emotional numbing, avoidance of situations that remind her of the event, startle responses, irritability, depressive mood, social withdrawal, guilt, and suicidal ideation. She has acute posttraumatic stress disorder with complicated bereavement and secondary depression precipitated by psychic trauma.

Susan's physical health is good and her sensorimotor functioning intact. She is of low average intelligence and approximately 2 years retarded in reading, language, and mathematical attainment. She has very low self-esteem, views herself as the family drudge, and is resentful of her alcoholic father's domination of her mother and her siblings. She has a close relationship with a married sister.

Susan's symptoms are reinforced by her mother's bereavement and the family's emotional insensitivity and poor communication. This is a large family, in which Susan has played the role of parentified child, supporting the mother and taking responsibility for much of the housekeeping and child care. Susan was predisposed to develop a depressive trauma reaction by her long-standing (but suppressed) resentment at being the family drudge and at being the frequent target of her father's emotional abuse.

Susan has the following strengths and potentials: She has supportive friends; her older married sister is very helpful; and she enjoys child care.

Without treatment, the current posttraumatic stress disorder is likely to continue. There is a risk of suicide.

GOAL-DIRECTED TREATMENT PLANNING

The purpose of treatment can range from short-term crisis management to long-term rehabilitation, remediation, or reconstruction. For that reason, the goals of treatment will vary according to the level of care the patient is receiving. The following levels of care are provided in child and adolescent mental health services: very brief hospitalization, brief hospitalization, brief partial hospitalization, extended day programs, residential treatment, intensive outpatient care, and outpatient care (see Chap-

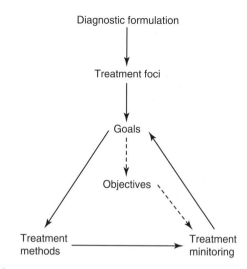

Figure 12–1. Goal-directed treatment planning.

ter 16). Very brief hospitalization (1–14 days) is suited to crisis alleviation and the reduction of acuity. Brief hospitalization (2–4 weeks) aims at stabilization, as do brief partial hospitalization programs. Residential treatment programs, extended partial hospitalization programs, and outpatient treatment have more ambitious goals related to remediation, reconstruction, or rehabilitation.

COMPONENTS OF GOAL-DIRECTED TREATMENT PLANNING

The essence of goal-directed planning is the extraction of treatment foci from the diagnostic formulation and the expression of the foci as goals and objectives, with predictions of the time required for goal attainment. On the basis of the goals, treatment methods can be selected. On the basis of the objectives, goal attainment (i.e., treatment effectiveness) can be monitored until the goal is attained and treatment terminated (see Figure 12–1).

Foci

Those problems, defects, and strengths that can be addressed, given the resources and time available, should be extracted from the diagnostic formulation. The clinician should not merely list behaviors in an unintegrated "laundry list." Pivotal foci, those internal or external factors that activate, reinforce, or perpetuate psychopathology, are especially important. For example, mother–child enmeshment may be the key to a problem of separation anxiety. A behavioral program for separation anxiety applied in the school setting will fail unless the clinician addresses the mother's involvement in her child's fear of leaving home.

Table 12–6. Categorization of Treatment Goals

Category	Example
Behavioral	Reduce the frequency and intensity of aggressive outbursts.
Educational	Remediate reading deficit.
Familial	Enhance quality of communication and emotional sensitivity between father and patient.
Medical	Stabilize diabetes mellitus.
Physical	Increase weight.
Psychological	Alleviate unresolved conflict concerning past physical abuse.
Social	Reduce the intensity and frequency of provocative behavior toward authority figures.

Goals

Goals indicate what the clinician or clinical team aims to achieve, at the given level of care, on the patient's behalf (Table 12–6). A goal is a focus preceded by a verb. The focus "depressive mood," for example, becomes "Alleviate depressive mood" when rewritten as a goal. As described in the introduction to this section, goals are categorized according to whether they promote crisis alleviation, stabilization, reconstruction, remediation, rehabilitation, or compensation. Crisis alleviation, stabilization, reconstruction, and remediation foci are preceded by verbs such as "alleviate," "ameliorate," "remediate," "eliminate," "reduce the intensity of," "reduce the frequency of," "stabilize," or "counteract." Rehabilitation and compensation goals are preceded, for example, by "enhance," "augment," "facilitate," or "increase the intensity/frequency of." Behavioral goals are best suited to crisis alleviation and stabilization settings (e.g., inpatient hospitalization).

Objectives

Goals assert what the clinician aims to do. Objectives indicate what the patient will (be able to) do, say, or exhibit at the end of that stage of treatment. Objectives should always be stated in behavioral terms. Goals and objectives may be intermediate (e.g., at the point of discharge from hospital) or terminal (e.g., at the end of outpatient treatment). Goals and objectives may be ambitious (e.g., "Resolve internal conflict regarding punitive father figure" or "The patient will be able to cooperate appropriately with his superior at work in the performance of his assigned tasks") or advisedly limited (e.g., "Gain weight. At the end of hospitalization, the patient will weigh 79 pounds").

Whereas goals take the long, abstract view, objectives indicate when enough is enough, making the clinician or team accountable, and alerting them when treatment is not progressing as well as anticipated.

Target Date

For each set of goals and objectives, a time is predicted. For example, the goal "Alleviate depressive mood and suicidal ideation" may have the objective "The patient will express no suicidal ideation spontaneously or during mental status examination for a period of 1 week." The clinician may predict that such a stabilization objective will be attained, for example, in 3 weeks.

Therapy

For each goal, the clinician selects a therapy or set of therapies, according to the following criteria: greatest empirical support, resource availability (i.e., clinical resources, time, finances), least risk, greatest economy (i.e., time, expense), and appropriateness to family values and interaction style.

The modes of therapy are discussed in the next section of this chapter. Do not confuse the term "objective" with a therapeutic strategy or tactic. An objective is the behaviorally stated endpoint of a phase of treatment. Treatment strategies or tactics (e.g., "Encourage father to attend patient's baseball games") represent the means of getting to the endpoint, that is, the adaptation of a particular intervention to the needs of the patient and family.

Treatment Monitoring

Objectives are the key to monitoring both the patient's progress and the treatment plan's effectiveness. Progress can be assessed by periodic milieu observations, mental status examinations, measurement of vital signs or other physical parameters, laboratory testing, standard questionnaires, rating scales, or psychological testing. To the extent that an objective can be measured, the measure should be stated (e.g., "The patient's score will drop to below 12 on the Conners Parent–Teacher Questionnaire"). Not all objectives can be measured numerically, and for some, subjective, qualitative monitoring is required. The clinician should not fall into the trap of deleting objectives that cannot be measured objectively. Some pivotal goals and objectives, particularly those related to psychodynamic or family systems issues, require qualitative monitoring; and ingenious assessments of dynamic issues can sometimes be planned. For example, the goal "Resolve conflict about past sexual abuse" could be monitored, for a particular patient, in terms of the frequency, duration, and acuity of dissociative episodes.

Revision

If progress stalls, the patient deteriorates, or unforeseen complications arise, the clinician or team will be alerted by the treatment monitors. Then a decision must be made. Continue? Change the goals? Modify the objectives? Reconsider the therapy? Periodic treatment monitoring (e.g., monthly for outpatient treatment, daily for inpatient or partial hospitalization) keeps the clinician or team accountable and prevents therapeutic drift.

Termination

When the objectives are reached, the patient is ready either to move on to the next phase or level of treatment or to terminate the treatment.

DISADVANTAGES & ADVANTAGES OF GOAL-DIRECTED TREATMENT PLANNING

Goal-directed treatment planning must be learned. It does not build on the naturalistic process of treatment planning (which usually starts from treatments rather than goals). It requires the clinician to be explicit about matters that are customarily avoided or blurred (e.g., target dates). Imposed on uncomprehending or resistant clinicians, goal-directed treatment plans are typically relegated to the status of irrelevant paperwork or to a mindless printout from a computerized treatment planning menu.

Goal direction has numerous advantages, however. It provides a common intellectual scaffolding with which a clinical team can plan. It serves notice to clinicians to monitor progress and review their plans if they are ineffective. It provides a useful basis for negotiating with families, obtaining truly informed consent, and facilitating or consolidating the treatment alliance. Finally, it is a potentially useful tool for utilization review and outcome research.

Nurcombe B: Goal-directed treatment planning and the principles of brief hospitalization. *J Am Acad Child Adolesc Psychiatry* 1989;27:26.

Nurcombe B, Gallagher RM: *The Clinical Process in Psychiatry.* Cambridge University Press, 1986.

■ TYPES OF TREATMENT

A sophisticated, multifaceted, individually designed management plan requires a comprehensive biopsychosocial, temporal, and developmental diagnostic formulation. The diagnostic formulation should be shared with the patient and parents at a special interview, and the parents' and patient's collaboration sought in following the goal-directed treatment plan.

In almost every case, a combination of techniques will be used in child and adolescent psychiatry because the biopsychosocial needs of patients demand a multifaceted treatment plan. For example, an adolescent hospitalized for anorexia nervosa is likely to require a combination of the following forms of therapy: (1) pediatric treatment to correct subnutrition and fluid and electrolyte imbalance, follow nutritional progress, and treat medical complications; (2) behavior modification to counteract voluntary restriction of food intake; (3) nutritional education; (4) individual expressive psychotherapy to provide insight and promote conflict resolution; and (5) family therapy to help the family undo the parent–child enmeshment and hidden interparental conflict that are commonly associated with this disorder.

There are three broad modes of treatment in child and adolescent psychiatry: **physical, psychological**, and **social**. Within each mode there are modalities (e.g., medication); within each modality there are techniques or classes (e.g., tricyclic antidepressant medication); and within each technique there are specific subtechniques, therapies, or agents (e.g., imipramine). Research into the treatment of child and adolescent psychiatric disorders has far to go. Even though few if any specific treatments have been established, evidence is gathering that some empirical treatments (e.g., clomipramine in obsessive–compulsive disorder) work better than placebo. Until more evidence is at hand, many of the indications for treatment described in the sections that follow are based on clinical experience rather than controlled experimentation. This chapter introduces readers to the broad range of modalities available. Subsequent chapters relate the details of treatment for particular conditions.

PHYSICAL TREATMENT

Electroconvulsive treatment is not used in child and adolescent psychiatry except perhaps in rare cases of adolescent catatonic schizophrenia unresponsive to antipsychotic medication. The only physical treatment of significance is psychopharmacology.

A. GENERAL PRINCIPLES OF PSYCHOPHARMACOLOGY

1 Before commencing pharmacotherapy, the clinician should obtain from the patient a full psychiatric and medical history, a medication history, and a history of allergic reactions; ascertain what other drugs the patient is currently taking; and ask whether the patient is using illicit drugs.

2 Psychopharmacologic treatment should always be part of a broader treatment plan derived from a diagnostic formulation.

3 Parents and child should be involved in the treatment plan; informed consent for pharmacologic treatment must be obtained; and parents and child should be educated about the nature, side effects, risks, and benefits of the medication proposed (and of the alternative treatments, if any).

4 Psychopharmacologic treatment targets symptoms, not disorders.

5 The clinician should ask the parents and child about misconceptions they may have of drug treatment in general or the particular pharmaceutical agent prescribed. For example, parents may be unnecessarily afraid that drug treatment will lead to addiction, whereas children may feel inferior if they must take drugs at school.

6 The clinician should seek a working alliance with responsible, informed parents and an educated patient.

7 When necessary, after getting permission, the clinician should form a working alliance with the school.

8 A medical examination, appropriate special investigations, and laboratory tests (including pregnancy testing in female patients) are required in order to rule out contraindicated conditions.

9 The clinician should quantify the targeted baseline symptom(s) and monitor progress with appropriate checklists or rating scales.

10 The clinician should select an appropriate drug according to the following criteria: least known risk and best evidence of efficacy. If possible, the clinician should follow FDA guidelines, but if not, he or she should make a rational choice based on available scientific evidence. If the choice is nonstandard, the clinician must document a risk–benefit analysis and ask for a consultation from a colleague.

11 It is advisable to start with a low dosage and increase it gradually until the symptoms remit, no further improvement accrues, the upper recommended dosage is reached, or complications occur.

Treatment should be continued at the lowest effective dosage.

12 The clinician should monitor side effects regularly.

13 Side effects (e.g., the sedative effect of antidepressant medication) can sometimes be used to treat other symptoms (e.g., insomnia).

14 The clinician should monitor serum levels if he or she is unsure whether the patient is receiving an adequate dose, or if there is a possibility that a toxic level of drug has been reached.

15 The clinician should prescribe medication for as short a period as possible. When medication is an adjunctive part of treatment, for example, it may be possible to discontinue it when psychosocial therapies are in place. "Drug holidays" are sometimes appropriate (e.g., when the child is out of school).

16 Polypharmacy should be avoided. The clinician should use drug combinations only after single appropriate drugs have been given an adequate trial and found ineffective.

17 When withdrawing medication, the clinician should usually taper the dosage, unless it is known that abrupt cessation is not dangerous.

B. CLASSES OF PSYCHOPHARMACOLOGIC AGENTS

The following classes of medication are used in child and adolescent psychiatry: psychostimulants, adrenergic agents, antidepressants, antipsychotics, mood regulators, anxiolytics, anticonvulsants, and miscellaneous agents.

Psychostimulants

The best-known psychostimulants are methylphenidate, dextroamphetamine sulfate, and adderall. They are the drugs of choice for treating attention-deficit/hyperactivity disorder and narcolepsy in childhood and adolescence, and possibly in preschool children. Magnesium Pemoline has fallen out of favor because it is potentially hepatotoxic. Atomoxetine, a presynaptic inhibitor of the noradrenaline transporter enzyme, has the advantages of requiring only once-per-day dosage. Slow-release forms of methylphenidate and dextroamphetamine are also available. Psychostimulants should be used with caution if the patient or family members have a history of substance abuse or antisocial behavior; if the patient has tic disorder, psychosis, liver impairment, growth failure, or a cardiac abnormality; or if the patient is pregnant. They should be used with caution if the patient is taking monoamine oxidase inhibitor (MAOI) medication. Common side effects are insomnia, irritability, anorexia, nausea, abdominal pain, and increased hyperactivity. Less common side effects are depression, social withdrawal, psychosis, tics, growth retardation, and hepatitis (pemoline). Psychostimulants should be monitored carefully if used in combination with anticoagulants, anticonvulsants, guanethidine, phenylbutazone, heterocyclic antidepressants (e.g., imipramine), sympathomimetics, or MAOIs. Patients taking psychostimulants should be monitored for involuntary movements, heart rate, and growth rate.

Adrenergic Agents

The most commonly prescribed adrenergic agents are clonidine and guanfacine. Both are often used in combination with methylphenidate in treating attention-deficit/hyperactivity disorder. Clonidine targets impulsivity and hyperactivity and has also been used in treating Tourette syndrome, opioid withdrawal, nicotine withdrawal, anxiety disorder, agitation, bipolar disorder, and posttraumatic stress disorder. Guanfacine targets inattention, impulsivity, and hyperactivity in attention-deficit/hyperactivity disorder. Clonidine should be used with caution if depression, a cardiovascular or renal disorder, or diabetes mellitus is present. Its main side effects are sedation, hypotension, headache, dizziness, gastrointestinal symptoms, and depression. Guanfacine, though less sedating, has similar side effects. Both drugs have a potential for augmenting the sedating effects of other central nervous system (CNS) depressants and for a hypertensive rebound after abrupt discontinuation.

Antidepressants

The antidepressants most often used in child and adolescent psychopharmacology are tricyclic antidepressants (TCAs) and selective serotonin reuptake inhibitors (SSRIs).

1. Tricyclic antidepressants—The most commonly prescribed TCAs are imipramine, amitriptyline, desipramine, nortriptyline, and clomipramine. These drugs are used to treat enuresis, attention-deficit/hyperactivity disorder, separation anxiety disorder, and posttraumatic stress disorder. Though formerly widely used in the treatment of depression in children and adolescents, empirical evidence for their effectiveness is lacking. Furthermore, TCAs have been possibly involved in several cardiotoxic deaths. Clomipramine is the drug of choice in treating obsessive–compulsive disorder and has also been used to treat trichotillomania. The TCAs are contraindicated if the patient is pregnant, has had a hypersensitivity reaction, or is taking an MAOI. They should be used with caution if the patient has schizophrenia or an epileptic, cardiac, or thyroid disorder. Side effects include increased pulse rate, cardiac conduction slowing, arrhythmia, and heart block; anticholinergic symptoms; anxiety, psychosis, mania, and confusion; seizures; insomnia; tics, tremor, and incoordination; skin rash; and photosensitivity. Sudden death has been associated with high dosages

of imipramine and desipramine, possibly because of cardiac conduction abnormalities. A baseline electrocardiogram (ECG) is indicated, and ECG monitoring is required at intervals as the dosage is increased. A complete blood count, differential diagnosis, pregnancy testing, and substance abuse history should be obtained, because when TCAs are taken along with marijuana and nicotine, their cardiac side effects may be aggravated. Plasma levels should be drawn 1 week after the last dosage increase. TCAs must be tapered when being discontinued.

2. Selective serotonin reuptake inhibitors—The members of the SSRI class currently most often prescribed in the United States are fluoxetine, sertraline, paroxetine, citalopram, and fluvoxamine. SSRIs are used for the treatment of depression, attention-deficit/hyperactivity disorder, obsessive–compulsive disorder, trichotillomania, anxiety disorder, eating disorder, posttraumatic stress disorder, drug craving, and self-injurious behavior. They are contraindicated if the patient has been taking MAOI drugs within the past 5 weeks, or if the patient is pregnant or has liver disease. There is heated debate about whether SSRIs can precipitate suicidal behavior in children and adolescents. This debate is, as yet, unresolved. Common side effects of SSRIs include gastrointestinal symptoms, nervousness, restlessness, insomnia, intensified dreaming, dry mouth, and sexual dysfunction. Less common side effects are excitability, mania, rash, hair loss, and seizures. The SSRIs interact with MAOIs, TCAs, lithium, and tryptophan and should not be prescribed with benzodiazepines or buspirone. Before administering an SSRI, the clinician should record the patient's vital signs, height, weight, and liver function, and test for pregnancy. Patients should be monitored at each visit for the emergence of mania and excitation, and every 3 months for height and weight. A medication trial of 6–8 weeks is required. SSRIs may be discontinued without tapering.

3. Other agents—Trazodone is a second- or third-line antidepressant with sedative side-effects. The indications for trazodone use in children and adolescents have not been established; but it has been used to treat depression associated with marked insomnia. Bupropion is a second- or third-line drug for treatment of major depressive disorder and possibly attention-deficit/hyperactivity disorder. Indications have not been established for children and adolescents. Nefazodone is seldom used because of the risk of central serotonin syndrome and hepatotoxicity. The best-known members of the monoamine oxidase inhibitor class are tranylcypromine, phenelzine, isocarboxazid, and moclobemide. Because of their potentially dangerous interaction with dietary tyramine and with a variety of other drugs, MAOIs are not recommended for treatment of disorders in children and adolescents. MAOIs are described in more detail in Chapter 9.

Antipsychotics

The most commonly prescribed antipsychotics were the phenothiazines, thioxanthenes, diphenyl-butylpiperidines, butyrophenones, dibenzoxazepines, and indolic compounds. However, atypical antipsychotic drugs (e.g., risperidone, olanzapine, quetiapine, ziprasidone, aripiprazole) have largely replaced them, except in the treatment of acute psychotic disturbance. Antipsychotics are indicated for the treatment of schizophrenia, delirium, and Tourette syndrome. They have also been used to alleviate self-injury and aggressiveness in pervasive developmental disorder and for nonspecific agitation. They are contraindicated if the patient has a history of hypersensitivity, agranulocytosis, or neuroleptic malignant syndrome. They should be used with caution in pregnant patients, in patients who are comatose, and in patients who are also taking CNS depressants. Clozapine is seldom used today because of the risk of blood dyscrasia, seizures, and hepatotoxicity. Antipsychotic agents are described in more detail in Chapter 9.

Mood Stabilizers

Lithium is indicated in the treatment of bipolar disorder in adolescents, and has been used in the treatment of bipolar disorder in children (to augment TCAs). It has also been used to treat bulimia and attention-deficit/hyperactivity disorder and to alleviate violent behavior. During adolescence, bipolar disorder can be difficult to distinguish from schizophrenia, schizoaffective disorder, and schizophreniform disorder. Adolescent patients who exhibit psychosis should be monitored carefully for mood disorder, and a trial of lithium should be considered. In adult psychotic patients, lithium potentiates neuroleptic medication and stabilizes mood. Lithium in combination with haloperidol alleviates explosive aggression in patients with conduct disorder. Lithium has been used to treat intractable attention-deficit/hyperactivity disorder, but its effectiveness is uncertain. Lithium may be useful, perhaps in combination with fluoxetine, in treating bulimia. Lithium is contraindicated if the patient has had a previous allergic reaction to the drug. It should be used with caution in pregnant patients and in patients who have severe dehydration; renal, cardiovascular, or thyroid disease; or diabetes mellitus. Lithium mobilizes calcium and may affect bone growth. Valproic acid appears to be as effective as lithium in juvenile mania. Lithium and valproic acid may be combined with antipsychotic medication (e.g., risperidone, quetiapine, or olanzapine) in the treatment of mania. Lithium and valproic acid are described in more detail in Chapter 9.

Anxiolytics

The anxiolytics formerly most commonly prescribed in child and adolescent psychiatry were benzodiazepines, antihistamines, and azapirones and propranolol. These drugs have been largely supplanted by the SSRIs.

Partly because of diagnostic confusion in the field of juvenile anxiety disorders and partly because of the paucity of controlled studies, knowledge concerning the indications for anxiolytics is patchy. SSRIs have been used to treat panic disorder, separation anxiety disorder, generalized anxiety disorder, posttraumatic stress disorder, obsessive–compulsive disorder, insomnia, sleepwalking, night terrors, and acute violent behavior. Anxiolytics are described in more detail in Chapter 9.

The high-potency anxiolytics alprazolam and clonazepam may be useful in treating panic disorder and agoraphobia. Lorazepam and oxazepam can be useful in the short-term treatment of agitation or acute violence. Buspirone causes less sedation and has less abuse potential than do benzodiazepines; it may be useful in treating generalized anxiety disorder and obsessive–compulsive disorder. Benzodiazepines should be used to treat insomnia only for relatively brief periods of time and only if the immediate benefits outweigh the risks of hangover and rebound insomnia.

Propranolol has been used with aggressive patients and in treating performance anxiety, generalized anxiety disorder, panic disorder, hyperventilation, posttraumatic stress disorder, withdrawal from alcohol, neuroleptic-induced akathisia, and lithium tremor.

Anticonvulsants

The anticonvulsants most often used in child and adolescent psychopharmacology are carbamazepine, valproic acid, and phenytoin. They have been used to treat alcohol withdrawal, trigeminal neuralgia, bipolar disorder, major depression, intermittent explosive disorder, attention-deficit/hyperactivity disorder, psychosis, enuresis, and night terrors. Carbamazepine and valproic acid may be used to supplement or replace lithium in treating refractory mania and as an adjunct to neuroleptic medication in the treatment of psychosis. Carbamazepine is a second-line drug in the treatment of depression. There is a need for controlled studies of the effectiveness of these three drugs in intermittent explosive disorder and conduct disorder. Carbamazepine is a drug of last resort in the treatment of attention-deficit/hyperactivity disorder. Anticonvulsant medication is contraindicated in patients with known hypersensitivity, bone marrow depression, liver disease, or renal disease; in pregnant patients; and in patients concurrently taking MAOIs. Anticonvulsants are described in more detail in Chapter 9.

Miscellaneous Agents

Opiate antagonists (e.g., naloxone, naltrexone) have been used to counteract self-injurious behavior in mentally retarded children and in children with early infantile autism. There are conflicting reports concerning the long-term benefit of naltrexone in these conditions. Triiodothyronine has been used to augment TCAs in treating adult major depression. There are no controlled studies of its use in juveniles. Despite initially promising data, the usefulness of fenfluramine in treating autistic disorder has not been confirmed.

Kutcher SP (ed): *Practical Child and Adolescent Psychopharmacology.* Cambridge, UK: Cambridge, 2002.

Pappadopulos EA, Guelzow ET, Wong C, Ortega M, Jensen PS: A review of the growing evidence base for pediatric psychopharmacology. *Child Adolesc Psychiatr Clin N Am* 2004;13:817–856.

Scahill L, Martin A: Pediatric psychopharmacology II. In: Lewis M (ed). *Child and Adolescent Psychiatry: A Comprehensive Textbook,* 3rd edn. Philadelphia: Lippincott, Williams & Wilkins, 2002, pp. 951–973.

PSYCHOLOGICAL TREATMENT

Psychological treatments include a variety of techniques that can be divided into four main groups: (1) individual psychotherapy, (2) behavior modification, (3) social and cognitive–behavioral therapy, and (4) remedial therapies and education.

A. INDIVIDUAL PSYCHOTHERAPY

The different forms of individual psychotherapy vary in accordance with four dimensions: (1) brief versus protracted; (2) supportive, directive, and reality-oriented versus expressive, exploratory, and oriented to unconscious material; (3) structured, interpretive versus unstructured, client-centered; and (4) play-oriented versus verbally oriented.

Supportive Psychotherapy

Supportive psychotherapy represents a loose collection of techniques without distinctive theoretical basis derived broadly from humanistic understanding and personal experience.

1. Aims—The aims of supportive psychotherapy are to (1) establish a close relationship; (2) define current problems; (3) consider and implement problem solutions; (4) avoid ego-alien, unconscious material; and (5) restore preexistent ego defenses.

2. Indications—Supportive psychotherapy is indicated for the treatment of adjustment disorders, temporary emotional crises due to situational stress, remitted psychotic disorders when the patient is in need of rehabilitative help, and substance use disorders.

3. Contraindications—Supportive psychotherapy should not be used to treat severe disorders that require more specific or more extensive therapy.

4. Dangers—Supportive psychotherapy is relatively safe except for the possibility of excessive dependency on the therapist. The development of an undesirably intense relationship with the therapist is a potential problem with any therapeutic technique, but it is more likely in intensive psychotherapy.

Client-Centered Therapy

Client-centered therapy is a form of play therapy or verbal psychotherapy in which the patient (client) is gently encouraged to explore personal feelings and attitudes. In client-centered therapy the therapist empathically reflects the feelings, explicit or implicit, in the patient's play and verbal or nonverbal communications. The pace of therapy is determined by the patient. Therapy is usually brief to intermediate in duration.

1. Aims—The aims of client-centered therapy are (1) to establish an empathic, accepting relationship and (2) to encourage self-exploration by judicious reflection of feeling.

2. Indications—Client-centered therapy is indicated for the treatment of adjustment reactions and mild anxiety disorders in children and adolescents. It is also useful for treating problems of adolescence that involve career choice, academic commitment, or mild identity confusion.

3. Contraindications—Client-centered therapy should not be used to treat severe disorders, especially psychosis or prepsychosis, conduct disorder, and borderline personality.

4. Dangers—Client-centered therapy could lead to excessive or unresolved dependence in some cases. Otherwise, it is relatively safe.

Exploratory Psychotherapy

Exploratory psychotherapy is a form of play therapy or verbal psychotherapy in which the patient's unconscious conflicts, usually in a specified area, are resolved by interpretations based on the patient's play or verbal and nonverbal behavior. It is usually extended in duration (6–12 months) and moderately intensive (1–2 times per week).

1. Aims—The aims of exploratory psychotherapy are (1) to establish a relationship, (2) recognize transference feelings, (3) help the patient to become aware of unconscious wishes and defenses by judicious interpretation, and (4) help the patient to terminate the relationship.

2. Indications—Exploratory psychotherapy is indicated for treatment of anxiety, somatoform, and dissociative disorders; personality disorders and interpersonal difficulties related to neurotic conflict; and trauma spectrum disorders.

3. Contraindications—Exploratory psychotherapy is contraindicated if the patient's ego strength is too fragile to cope with the emergence of traumatic material in the context of a close therapeutic relationship, or if the patient has a psychotic or prepsychotic disorder.

4. Dangers—Exploratory psychotherapy could provoke an intense transference reaction with severe emotional turmoil.

Interpersonal Psychotherapy

Interpersonal psychotherapy is a brief form of psychotherapy, which has been adapted for adolescents with major depression. Twelve weekly sessions are recommended, in accordance with a treatment manual. The interpersonal psychotherapist is an active, practical problem solver, focusing on the here-and-now. A variety of techniques are applied: psychoeducation, clarification, facilitating the expression of affect, communication analysis, problem solving, and decision analysis. Parents are involved in the initial and middle phases. Liaison with the school is encouraged.

1. Aims—In depression, the therapist aims first to provide education about the condition, then to relate depression to the interpersonal context. Problem areas are identified and a treatment contract set. In the middle stage of therapy, grief, role disputes and transitions, and interpersonal deficits are dealt with. The last four sessions focus on residual problems, reviewing progress, and relapse prevention.

2. Indications—Depressive disorders in adolescence.

3. Contraindications—As for exploratory psychotherapy.

4. Dangers—As for exploratory psychotherapy.

Child & Adolescent Psychoanalysis

Child and adolescent psychoanalysis is an extensive (e.g., 1–5 years) and intensive (e.g., 3–5 times per week) form of exploratory therapy in which a radical resolution of unconscious conflicts is sought through the exploration of a transference relationship between patient and analyst.

1. Aims—The aims of child and adolescent psychoanalysis are (1) to establish a relationship, (2) encourage spontaneous expression of thoughts and emotions (through play and conversation), (3) aid resolution of unconscious conflict by interpreting unconscious wishes and ego defenses, (4) support the patient in working through personal solutions to problems that have been rendered conscious in analysis, and (5) help the patient terminate the relationship.

2. Indications—Child and adolescent psychoanalysis is indicated for treatment of anxiety disorders, somatoform disorders, trauma spectrum disorders, and borderline personality disorder (if not severe).

3. Contraindications—Child and adolescent psychoanalysis should not be used to treat psychotic disorder, pervasive developmental disorder, conduct disorder, severe personality disorder, or other disorders in patients who cannot tolerate intimacy.

If psychoanalytic therapy is to succeed, the patient must have reasonable capacity to tolerate tension and intimacy, the ability to express emotions in words, the motivation to seek help, and considerable economic resources.

4. Dangers—The dangers of child and adolescent psychotherapy are similar to those associated with exploratory psychotherapy.

B. BEHAVIOR MODIFICATION

Behavior modification represents a group of loosely associated therapeutic techniques derived from the principles of learning.

1. Aims

i. Systematic desensitization—Exposing the patient to progressively more anxiety-provoking stimuli, while at the same time teaching him or her to relax, or pairing the phobic stimuli with a pleasant activity (such as eating), or associating the phobic stimuli with pleasant fantasy.

ii. Reinforcement of coping responses—Rewarding responses that counteract, or are incompatible with, the problem behavior.

iii. Exposure—Forced entry into the phobic situation and the prevention of avoidance.

iv. Shaping—Rewarding progressive approximations to desired responses, especially in habit training.

v. Token reinforcement—Poker chips, stars on a calendar, and the like can be exchanged at stipulated times for reward (e.g., money, privileges). The tokens are used for immediate reinforcement of desirable behavior.

vi. Aversion—Interrupting undesirable behavior (e.g., self-destructive head banging) by applying a noxious stimulus (e.g., an electric shock) whenever the undesirable behavior is expressed.

vii. Time-out—Deprivation of anticipated reinforcement (e.g., attention) by consistently isolating the child when the undesirable behavior (e.g., tantrums) is expressed.

viii. Massed practice—Multiple repetitions of an undesired behavior (e.g., a habit spasm) in order to weaken its association with an underlying emotional state (e.g., anxiety).

ix. Substitution—Replacing an undesirable behavior (e.g., smoking) with a neutral one (e.g., chewing).

2. Indications—Behavioral therapy is indicated for treatment of phobic disorders, eating disorders, oppositional defiant disorder, and preschool management problems (e.g., tantrums) as well as for habit training (e.g., functional enuresis or encopresis).

3. Contraindications—Behavioral therapy should not be used to treat psychosis or in situations in which the patient has transference fears of, or is resistant to, being controlled.

4. Dangers—Behavioral therapy could lead to deterioration or aggravation of the psychiatric condition (reported after implosion) or to the appearance of new undesirable behavior (e.g., if desensitization is too limited in scope).

C. Social & Cognitive–Behavioral Therapy

Social and cognitive–behavioral therapy is a group of techniques that focus on intermediate cognitive responses as the primary target for intervention, with the aim of changing behavior.

1. Aims

i. Participant modeling:—Combining the observation of a model that behaves in a desired way with the opportunity to practice the desirable behavior.

ii. Interpersonal problem-solving:—Teaching the patient to infer the causes and consequences of interpersonal events and actions, and to consider alternative solutions to interpersonal dilemmas.

iii. Cognitive–behavioral therapy:—Helping the patient to define and alter the self-defeating expectations and attitudes that underlie maladaptive behavior.

iv. Self-instruction training:—Teaching the patient to reflect upon a problem rather than act impulsively.

2. Indications—Social and cognitive–behavioral therapy is used to encourage behavior that will counteract a phobia, to overcome social impulsiveness or inhibition, to counteract the pessimism that predisposes an adolescent to depression, to replace motor impulsiveness with reflectiveness, or to counteract obsessive–compulsive behavior.

3. Contraindications—Social and cognitive–behavioral therapy should not be used to treat psychosis.

4. Dangers—Social and cognitive–behavioral therapy could lead to deterioration or aggravation of the psychiatric condition or to the appearance of new undesirable behavior if the therapy is too limited in scope.

D. Remedial Therapies & Education

Remedial therapies and education represent a large group of remedial or rehabilitative programs designed to help the child or adolescent overcome chronic physical, educational, or social handicap, or make the most of talents and potential strengths.

1. Aims—Remedial therapies and technologies have been developed for a variety of disabilities, including cerebral palsy, orthopedic handicap, blindness, deafness, aphasia, and learning disability.

These therapies may be provided in a separate institution (e.g., a school for the hearing impaired) or incorporated in a regular school program (i.e., in the case of mainstreaming). The contemporary trend is toward mainstreaming whenever possible.

2. Dangers—The child may be labeled and discriminated against in a separate (categorical) program, a disabled child's needs may overwhelm teacher and classmates in a mainstream program, or the child may not be accepted by unimpaired classmates.

SOCIAL TREATMENT

Group Therapy

In group therapy, groups of six to eight children or adolescents, with a group leader, meet at intervals between daily to once per week. Groups for preschool children emphasize social stimulation. Activity groups for latency-age children emphasize socialization. Groups for adolescents focus on mutual support and the sharing of common problems. Group therapy is often used as an adjunct to other forms of therapy (e.g., during hospitalization).

1. Aims—The aims of group therapy are (1) to provide social experience, (2) allow expression of feeling in an accepting environment, (3) foster awareness of common experience and allow the group to consider solutions to common problems, and (4) promote group cohesiveness (e.g., during hospitalization).

2. Indications—Group therapy is indicated during hospitalization of latency-age children or adolescents. It is useful for treating problems with social isolation and for helping adolescents who share the same problem (e.g., divorce, physical handicap, substance abuse).

3. Contraindications—Group therapy should not be used to treat disorders in patients who are disturbed by forced intimacy.

4. Dangers—Though it is not always possible, it is preferable for the group to be balanced, with a judicious combination of aggressive "instigators," compulsive "neutralizers," and dependent "followers." If there are too many aggressive children, the group will explode.

If there are too many neutralizers or followers, group process may stagnate.

Role Play

Role play is a subtechnique of group therapy, commonly used in hospital treatment, in which a recent social incident is reenacted. The role players usually are not the individuals who were involved in the incident, but those who were involved will help with the reenactment.

Role playing is used to help patients develop insight and consider common problems and alternative solutions. It can be used as a medium for cognitive–behavioral therapy.

Casework for Parents

Casework varies from intermittent contact with the patient's parents (in order to keep them informed about progress) to intensive therapy, for example, in regard to marital problems, child management, or health care.

1. Aims—Casework may be used to provide information, promote more consistent child management or health care, institute a behavior modification program at home, resolve marital problems, or prepare one or both parents for referral to another therapist.

2. Indications—Casework is indicated whenever the child is in intensive individual therapy, in order to keep parents aware and involved; and to facilitate behavior modification in the natural environment by enlisting the parents as agents of the therapeutic plan.

3. Contraindications—If parents are mutually antagonistic, they may need to be interviewed separately.

Conjoint Family Therapy

Conjoint family therapy is a form of group therapy in which the identified patient's whole family receives treatment. The family members meet with a family therapist (sometimes with male or female cotherapists) for intensive brief therapy (in order to facilitate crisis resolution) or for more extended periods of time (if radical changes in family interaction are proposed).

1. Aims—Conjoint family therapy is used to resolve family crises; to promote a common understanding of family problems; to consider alternative solutions to common problems, especially when the family has reached an impasse; to foster a common awareness of previously unexpressed family rules, roles, and expectations; and to alter long-standing maladaptive interaction patterns (e.g., coalitions, rifts, scapegoating, enmeshment, or skewing), promote clearer communication, and enhance the emotional sensitivity of family members.

2. Indications—Conjoint family therapy is indicated when the patient is recovering following hospitalization for severe mental illness and whenever the patient's problems are perpetuated by deleterious family interaction patterns.

3. Contraindications—Conjoint family therapy should be avoided or used with caution in the following situations: (1) when family members are excessively hostile or intrusive toward the patient; (2) when the parents are on the verge of separating; or (3) when the patient needs to become independent of the family system.

4. Dangers—Conjoint family therapy could result in the problem shifting to another family member, as the homeostasis of the family is changed when the designated patient improves. It could also accentuate a preexisting rift between the parents.

Psychiatric Hospitalization

Psychiatric hospitalization involves the placement of a severely disturbed child or adolescent in a psychiatric inpatient unit that has special programs and a therapeutic milieu designed for children or adolescents. The special program coordinates psychiatric, pediatric, psychological, nursing, educational, and occupational care and therapies. The placement may be brief (e.g., 1–2 weeks), intermediate (2–4 weeks), or extended (longer than 1 month) depending on the patient's needs.

1. Aims—Psychiatric hospitalization aims to separate a disturbed patient temporarily from the family; to stabilize suicidal, self-injurious, aggressive, or disorganized psychotic behavior; or to institute treatment programs that require complex coordination and intensive monitoring.

2. Indications—Psychiatric hospitalization is warranted when suicidal, aggressive, or disruptive behavior which is beyond the control of the family is caused by treatable mental illness (especially schizophreniform disorder, schizophrenia, posttraumatic stress disorder, eating disorder, and severe mood disorder). It may also be warranted when the child's severe emotional disorder is perpetuated by complex family interaction pathology or when comprehensive diagnostic evaluation of a complex case is needed, especially for cases that require the coordination of a number of specialties (e.g., an adolescent who has a chronic physical illness associated with a serious psychiatric disorder and family interaction problems).

Specific disorders warranting hospitalization include the following: depressed mood and suicidality secondary to emotional stress; severe anxiety, somatoform, and dissociative disorders; severe eating disorder; substance use disorder; organic mental disorder (e.g.,

Table 12–7. Safeguards Against the Dangers of Hospitalization

Clear but nonautocratic psychiatric leadership
Staff selected for defined but overlapping roles
Clarity of general aims and individual treatment goals
Good coordination of, and communication between, staff
A plan for postdischarge disposition
Family involvement in admission, diagnosis, management planning, and continuing treatment
An environment that, as far as possible, approximates that of the average child of that age (in schooling, social opportunity, and recreation) and that deemphasizes chronic invalidism
Partial hospitalization for less severely disturbed patients
Planned discharge to outpatient or partial hospital care as soon as possible
Good coordination between regional inpatient unit and community mental health agencies and clinicians

Table 12–8. Examples of Partial Hospitalization Programs

Pediatric hospital units for infants and children who have experienced physical neglect or abuse affecting physical health
Preschool daycare programs for children with special physical, educational, or psychological needs (e.g., culturally disadvantaged children or children with pervasive developmental disorders)
Residential units for children and adolescents with severe physical handicaps or disorders
Residential units for adolescents with substance dependence (usually emphasizing behavior control)
Residential units for adolescents with conduct disorder (usually emphasizing behavior control)
Residential units for the mentally retarded
Boarding schools for adolescents with learning and emotional problems

substance-induced delirium or hallucinosis); and pervasive developmental disorder (for diagnosis, behavioral analysis, and management planning in aggressive or self-injurious patients).

3. Contraindications—Psychiatric hospitalization should not be used to treat conduct disorder of the undersocialized, aggressive type without treatable comorbid psychiatric disorder or in some cases of personality disorder (especially of borderline type) in which there is a danger of reinforcing a patient's chronic sick role. Furthermore, it is contraindicated if hospitalization could cause alienation between the patient and his or her family.

4. Dangers—Psychiatric hospitalization may accentuate dependency and inadvertently train the child or adolescent to be a "patient." It may lead to scapegoating and permanent extrusion by an alienated family. Also, excessive pressure on inexperienced inpatient unit staff could lead to communication breakdown and deleterious effects on all patients. These dangers can be averted if the safeguards listed in Table 12–7 are implemented.

Specialized Partial Hospitalization or Residential Units

Residential programs are based usually on an educational or behavioral (rather than a medical) model, with programs designed for children or adolescents who have special problems. Partial hospitalization programs are based on a psychiatric inpatient model, except that the patient

returns home each night. In all cases, the child's or adolescent's problems are more severe or complex than can be dealt with in conventional outpatient treatment. Examples are given in Table 12–8.

Other Placements Away From Home
Other placements may involve temporary or permanent placement of a child or adolescent in a foster or group home. Options include (1) foster placement as a temporary expedient, while the parents and child are in treatment, preparatory to the return of the child; (2) permanent foster placement, with or without view to adoption, after disintegration of the home of origin or when the parents are unable to provide adequate care; (3) group home placement for children and adolescents who are emotionally too overreactive to cope with the emotional vicissitudes of foster home placement; and (4) community group homes designed to promote independent-living skills for mentally retarded adolescents or adolescents with pervasive developmental disorders.

Josephson AM (ed): Current perspectives on family therapy. *Child Adolesc Psychiatr Clin N Am* 2001;10:395–662.

Leventhal BL, Zimmerman DP (eds): Residential treatment. *Child Adolesc Psychiatr Clin N Am* 2004;13:237–440.

Lewis M: Treatment. Section 7. In: Lewis M (ed). *Child and Adolescent Psychiatry: A Comprehensive Textbook,* 2nd edn. Philadelphia Williams & Wilkins, 1996, pp. 765–934.

Remschmidt H (ed): *Psychotherapy with Children and Adolescents.* Cambridge, UK: Cambridge, 2001.

Weisz JR, Hawley KM, Doss AJ. Empirically tested psychotherapies for youth internalizing and externalizing disorders. *Child Adolesc Psychiatr Clin N Am* 2004;13:729–815.

Preventive Psychiatry

Barry Nurcombe, MD

13

THE PREVALENCE OF PSYCHIATRIC DISORDER IN CHILDREN AND ADOLESCENTS

In a survey of 52 studies, Roberts et al. (1998) found that the average prevalence of psychiatric disorder in children and adolescents was 15.8%, with a range of 11–22%.

Sawyer et al. (2000) surveyed a representative sample of 4500 Australian school children aged 4–17 years, using the Child Behavior Checklist (CBCL) (Achenbach, 1991), the Diagnostic Interview Schedule for Children (DISC-IV) (Shaffer et al., 2000), and the Child Health Questionnaire (CHQ) (Landgraf, et al., 1996). Adolescents aged 13–17 years also completed the Centre for Epidemiologic Studies Depression Scale (CES-D) (Radloff, 1977) and the Youth Risk Behavior System Questionnaire (YRBS) (Berener et al., 1995). Sawyer et al. found that 14.7% of children and 13.1% of adolescents were in the clinical range. Children and adolescents with mental health problems had a poorer quality of life, lower self-esteem, and worse school performance than those who did not have, and were a greater burden to their families. Adolescents with mental health problems reported high rates of suicidal behavior, smoking, drinking, and drug use. Few psychiatrically disturbed children were receiving any professional treatment, and those who did receive help usually obtained it from general practitioners, school counselors, or pediatricians. Very few had attended a specialized mental health service or clinician.

These sobering statistics indicate that, even if primary diagnostic and therapeutic services were effective, and even if the links between primary and specialized professional services were efficient, there are far too many seriously disturbed families for existing facilities to serve. Furthermore, there is little empirical support for different kinds of mental health treatment outside of laboratory studies (Weisz et al., 1995), and the dropout rate from community services is alarmingly high. For these reasons, the idea of prevention has been promoted. Prevention aims to avert or divert unfavorable developmental trajectories in such a way as to reduce the incidence or severity of psychopathology and promote mental health.

RISK FACTORS AND RESILIENCE

The **risk factors** known to be associated with later psychiatric disorders vary from **biological** (e.g., genetic or chromosomal abnormality; exposure to intrauterine toxins such as alcohol or nicotine; premature birth; exposure to toxins such as lead during early development; and chronic physical disability such as epilepsy or brain injury) and **temperamental** (e.g., behavioral inhibition or difficult temperament) to **familial** (e.g., parental depression, alcoholism and antisocial personality; disorganized infant–parent attachment; coercive child rearing; single-parent or blended families; marital discord and domestic violence; physical abuse, sexual abuse and neglect), **socioeconomic** (e.g., poverty; membership of a disadvantaged minority group) and **catastrophic** (e.g., civilian disaster or war).

Protective factors counterbalance risk. It is known, for example, that an easy, likeable temperament, above-average intelligence, good support from at least one parent, a cohesive family environment, and social capital in the form of good schools, adequate community resources for sport and skill-building, and good employment prospects protect otherwise vulnerable individuals from psychiatric disorders. Protective factors act by moderating the effect of risk factors or by promoting alternative, compensatory processes that enhance personal effectiveness and self-esteem.

Hypothetically, prevention might work by eliminating risk factors (e.g., the cessation of smoking or drinking during pregnancy), or decreasing their impact (e.g., reducing the incidence of premature birth by providing good antenatal care and nutrition for socially disadvantaged women) or by enhancing protective factors (e.g., providing good schools and social opportunities).

In reality, most outcomes have multiple determinants. Psychopathology following child sexual abuse, for example, is associated with three groups of **moderating factors**: antecedent factors such as the quality of child attachment prior to the abuse; the nature of the abuse experience—repeated, coercive, intrafamilial, genital penetration being the most adverse; and the quality of parental support after the child discloses the abuse. Moderating factors operate through **mediating factors,** for example: whether the child has sustained posttraumatic stress disorder; the child's attitude to self and others; and the child's coping methods (denial, dissociation, distraction, escape, and repetition–compulsion being the most pathogenic).

Preventive intervention that aims to reduce the incidence of psychopathology after child sexual abuse might therefore focus on improving the quality of family support to the child, treating parental psychopathology, counteracting the child's adverse attitudes to herself and others, helping the child to assimilate and cognitively reconstruct memories of abuse, treating posttraumatic stress disorder, and promoting healthy self-assertiveness and self-protection. Prevention which aims to stop sexual abuse from occurring in the first place relies upon promoting community awareness, teaching children to avoid or report perpetrators, and treating as soon as possible sexually abused boys, a proportion of whom will otherwise grow up themselves to be sexual perpetrators as adults.

Repucci et al. (1999) have reviewed the debate between those who advocate mental health promotion and competence building as the cornerstone of prevention and those who reject competence building and sociopolitical change in favor of reducing the risk of developing a DSM-IV-TR disorder. In other words, universal approaches to prevention are pitted against programs that target at-risk individuals or groups for intervention. This debate has not been resolved.

THE GOALS AND TYPES OF PREVENTION

Prevention refers to intervention that aims to eliminate, or reduce the incidence of, or ameliorate the severity of, general or specified psychopathology in the population as a whole or in particular groups that are at risk of developing psychiatric disorder or impairment.

Preventive intervention can be classified according to when in the course of the development of a psychiatric disorder the intervention is applied (Caplan, 1964). **Primary prevention** refers to intervention in normal populations to avert future mental ill health (e.g., school-based alcohol and drug education). **Secondary prevention** focuses on special at-risk groups in order to stave off the development of psychopathology (e.g., the treatment of sexually abused children). The term **tertiary prevention**

(the early treatment of patients with established psychiatric disorders) has fallen into disuse.

An alternative classification system has been proposed by the Institute of Medicine (Mrazek & Haggerty, 1994). **Universal prevention** is offered to the entire population of a particular area (e.g., good antenatal care). **Targeted prevention** is offered to particular groups. **Targeted indicated prevention** is directed at groups who are identified as being at risk by virtue of biological markers or symptom patterns (e.g., children with epilepsy, or highly aggressive preschool children). **Targeted selective prevention** is aimed at children who are at increased risk by virtue of their membership of a vulnerable subgroup (e.g., the children of highly stressed, economically disadvantaged, single mothers), or because they are experiencing or about to experience a life transition or stressful event (e.g., change of schools or divorce).

Prevention can also be classified in accordance with the **level** and **timing** of intervention. The level of intervention refers to whether the intervention is delivered to the individual, the family, the peer group, the school, the workplace, or the community as a whole. Timing refers to the developmental period when the intervention occurs: antenatal, infancy, preschool, middle childhood, adolescence, or adult.

Take, for example, the following program. Olds et al. (1986) successfully reduced the incidence of child maltreatment by delivering a nurse-home-visiting program to mothers who were at risk of abusing their children by virtue of adolescent pregnancy, poverty, and single parenthood. The program began antenatally and continued until the child was 2 years old. This was a primary, targeted, selective prevention of family-level type, delivered in the antenatal/infancy period.

DEVELOPMENTAL DISCONTINUITY, DIVERGENT DEVELOPMENT, AND EQUIFINALITY

Discontinuity refers to breaks or changes in development, which lead to a different outcome. For example, a number of studies have shown that a proportion of children who have been seriously sexually abused have no discernible psychopathology at the time of ascertainment. However, Gomez-Schwarz et al. (1990) found that, when assessed 18 months later, many previously asymptomatic children had serious psychopathology.

Divergent development refers to the way that a single stressor can lead to a variety of later outcomes (e.g., child sexual abuse is linked to disturbed self-concept, chronic emotional distress, self-harm, substance abuse, dissociative disorder, somatoform disorder, sexual problems, and revictimization or sexual perpetration in adulthood).

Equifinality or convergent development refers to the way that a variety of risk factors affecting the child at different periods of development can lead to the same outcome. For example, antisocial behavior in male adolescents is predicted by genetic background, disorganized attachment, coercive child rearing, aggressive behavior in early childhood, impaired verbal intelligence, learning problems, gravitation toward delinquent companions in late childhood, and early initiation into alcohol and drug use. Some of these risk factors may be causative whereas others represent points on the longitudinal development toward an undesirable end point.

It is important to determine whether a risk factor is **causal** (e.g., genetic factors in attention-deficit/hyperactivity disorder) or a **noncausal correlate** (e.g., abnormal saccadic eye movements in schizophrenia). Prevention should be aimed at those causal factors that are accessible for intervention. Furthermore, a single risk factor can play different parts in the causation of psychiatric disorder. Family dysfunction, for example, can precede and foreshadow sexual abuse, increase the likelihood that it will occur, be precipitated by the disclosure of abuse, and aggravate its effect (Spaccarelli, 1994).

The possibility of adverse and favorable **reciprocal interactions** should be considered. For example, premature children raised by disadvantaged parents are more likely to develop depressed intelligence and learning problems than are those raised in families that provide good social and language stimulation to the child during infancy and the preschool period. Preventive intervention might, for example, intervene to generate progressively more and more favorable interactions between premature child and mother.

■ EMPIRICALLY BASED PROGRAMS FOR THE PREVENTION OF CONDUCT DISORDER

To exemplify the reasoning behind prevention programs, the problem of conduct disorder and antisocial behavior will be discussed.

Conduct disorder is associated with four kinds of behavior: aggressiveness (intimidation, use of a weapon, cruelty, fire-setting, coercive sexual behavior); deceitfulness (lying, stealing); rule violation (refusal to follow the rules at home or school, running away from home, truancy, vandalism); and impulsiveness (explosive anger, thoughtless destructiveness). Early-onset conduct disorder is more common in boys and has a worse prognosis than the adolescent-onset variety. Conduct disorder is often preceded by oppositional-defiant disorder and, in 25% of cases, evolves into adult antisocial personality disorder, which is likely to be associated with serious criminal behavior. Since the prevalence of conduct disorder is high (about 5.5% in both sexes; 8.1% in boys; 2.8% in girls), any reduction in the number of those with the disorder would be likely to result in huge savings for the community by virtue of increased personal productivity, less crime, and sparing of the police, criminal justice, and correctional systems.

The following risk factors have been identified: genetic factors (e.g., the inheritance of callous, remorseless personality traits); disorganized parenting; parental depression, personality disorder, antisocial behavior, and substance abuse; disrupted attachment experiences; poor language stimulation and impaired verbal intelligence; child maltreatment; failed fostering; academic failure; school dropout; gravitation toward antisocial peers; and early introduction to alcohol and substance abuse. The influence of criminogenic environment is probably through the stress experienced by vulnerable parents in such circumstances and the malign influence of antisocial peers. These risk factors interact in a transactional, developmental cascade.

Hypothetically, intervention could begin in the antenatal period with the identification of vulnerable parents and the provision of supportive intervention; in the preschool era with the identification and treatment of depressed or disorganized parents with oppositional children and the provision of language enrichment education; and in primary school with identification of those at risk of dropping out of school, the availability of remedial education, and the promotion of therapeutic intervention for children with disruptive behavior. It is apparent that intervention has much less chance of success if the adolescent has dropped out of school and begun to associate preferentially with antisocial peers.

Infancy

The University of Rochester Nurse Visitation Program (Olds et al., 1986) compared the effect of four programs for antenatal women in a random controlled assignment design: level 1, information and support; level 2, free transport to antenatal and well-baby clinics; level 3, nurse home visiting; and level 4, nurse home visiting continuing regularly for 2 years. Adolescent antisocial behavior was averted, particularly in the level 4 program. For example, level 4 versus level 1 groups had 50% fewer arrests, 30% fewer convictions, and 10% fewer juvenile supervision orders. In earlier years, in level 4 families there were less child abuse, neglect, substance abuse, and parental crime, and fewer pregnancies.

The Pre-School Period

The High Scope Perry Preschool Project (Weikart & Schweinhart, 1992) targeted 3 to 4-year-old children with low intellectual performance from low-income families. The intervention involved language stimulation education and home visiting to promote parental involvement. At ages 19 and 24, the intervention group compared to controls had fewer school dropouts, less chronic offending, and fewer property and violent offences.

Middle Childhood

The "Fast Track" program (Conduct Problems Prevention Research Group, 1999) was a multicomponent, multisite intervention delivered to Grade 1 high-risk children, involving universal and selective programs. High risk was identified as aggression, poor problem solving, and parental problems. All children in a selected class experienced the PATHS program, to promote emotional understanding, problem solving, and emotional control. High-risk families received parent group, child social skills, and remedial teaching programs over 3 years. Modest results were found in intervention groups compared to controls in regard to "caseness."

Adolescence

Functional Family Therapy (Barton & Alexander, 1981), Multisystemic Therapy (Henggeler et al., 1998), and Treatment Foster Care (Chamberlain & Reid, 1994) are the only programs that have proven effective with conduct disordered adolescents. It is apparent that the longer the intervention is delayed, the more difficult (and expensive) it is to effect change.

■ THE CHARACTERISTICS OF SUCCESSFUL PREVENTIVE INTERVENTION PROGRAMS

Nation et al. (2003) reviewed prevention programs across four areas: substance abuse, risky sexual behavior, school failure, and delinquency and violence. The nine qualities that characterized programs that were effective, were as follows:

Comprehensiveness—Successful programs employ combinations of interventions to increase awareness and promote skills, and are directed at individual, family and school-system levels. Risk factors are addressed and protective factors enhanced or promoted.

Variation in teaching methods—Most effective programs emphasize skill building through interactive instruction and practical experience.

Adequate dosage—Good interventions last long enough and are sufficiently intense to have an effect: the greater the needs of the participants, the longer the duration of the program and the more intensive it must be. Booster programs are provided to enhance skills learned or to introduce new, developmentally appropriate skills.

Theoretical model—Effective interventions are grounded in explicit theoretical models of the interaction between risk and protective factors, and how these factors might be eliminated, ameliorated, or enhanced.

The promotion of positive relationships—Parent–child, child–teacher and peer relationships are addressed, and positive adult models (e.g., mentors) provided.

Appropriate timing—Effective interventions are delivered before the participants have developed the targeted problem to a full extent, thus giving the intervention the opportunity to alter pathogenic developmental trajectories. Furthermore, the intervention is developmentally appropriate; in other words, it is tailored to the cognitive and social development of the participants.

Sociocultural relevance—Intervention programs that reflect local community norms, cultural beliefs and practices increase the receptiveness of participants and families. Successful programs take into account the individual needs of participants. One-size-fits-all programs work best for those who least need them and may be actually harmful for those most in need of intervention.

Outcome evaluation—Effectiveness is based on evaluation, not anecdote or fashion. Good programs incorporate continuous quality improvement through the feedback of outcome data.

Staff training and support—Effective programs pay close attention to the selection, training, supervision and continuing support of staff. The opinions of staff should be sought concerning the implementation and evaluation of the program. High staff turnover, conflict, and demoralization sabotage effective intervention. Supervision and the provision of treatment manuals counteract the tendency of some staff to drift off the treatment model. In other words, an attempt is made to ensure that the program is delivered with fidelity.

THE NEED FOR RESEARCH

Excellent reviews of the effectiveness of preventive intervention have been provided by Durlak and Wells (1997), Carr (2002), and Reppucci et al. (1999).

In many prevention studies, the follow-up period has been too brief to assess the long-term impact of the intervention. Few researchers have attempted to replicate findings or to examine the validity of their programs in other populations or settings. More information is needed concerning the effect of the quality of implementation, particularly treatment fidelity, on outcome, and whether matching the program to the individual, developmental, and sociocultural characteristics of participants enhances effectiveness, and which of the components of the program are effective and essential.

In the future, programs will be based on explicit theoretical models derived from empirical research into how risk and protective factors interact in causal chains to produce undesirable outcomes. Intervention programs should have clear goals and objectives, operationalized intervention methods, treatment manuals to assure standardization, and multimodal outcome evaluation. Future studies should determine which participants benefit from the program, which do not benefit, and which are made worse.

PLANNING AN EFFECTIVE PROGRAM

The first requirement is to choose a problem which is serious and prevalent in the particular community. Are the community receptive to the idea of prevention or, if not, could prevailing attitudes be changed? The researcher should consider whether his or her interest in the problem and current position allow sufficient motivation, authority and time to get the job done.

The choice of a planning team is essential. Best of all are people who are known to have the skills (e.g., in particular intervention techniques, program design, or statistical analysis) required to form a balanced design team. Mavericks and egocentrists should be avoided; a high degree of collaboration is required.

Next, what is known about the risk and protective factors associated with the problem? Have any theoretical models been proposed? If so, which one best encompasses the interactive chain of factors that produces the undesirable outcome? If none of the available models is

adequate, an original model must be hypothesized as the basis for the design of the intervention.

The timing and level of the intervention must be chosen. Generally speaking, the earlier an adverse developmental trajectory can be diverted, the better. In general, targeted interventions are more effective than universal interventions. Universal interventions often fail to reach those most in need, and expend their energy on those who do not need them. However, effective universal educational programs can create a social environment favorable for targeted intervention. The program could be directed toward the individual, the family, or a social system such as a classroom, school, or workplace. Generally, multiple levels are preferable. Parent education and involvement are likely to enhance the effect of a child-directed program. If particular individuals should be targeted, what screening instruments are required?

The program should be suitable for the sociocultural or ethnic group for which it has been designed. Others who have implemented programs for the particular group should be consulted. A cultural consultant may be asked to join the team, and other team members and clinician implementers should be recruited, if possible, from the ethnic group involved.

How many subjects are required, and what is the power of the design to find a clinically significant effect? What evaluation instruments will be used, and for how long will results be followed up? What statistical techniques will be required to analyze the results? If possible, a statistical consultant should be a member of the research team.

What resources are needed in terms of staff, equipment, travel, etc.? What support will be needed from senior administrators (e.g., politicians, government department heads), local administrators (e.g., employers, school principals), and local staff (e.g., teachers, physicians, hospital staff) to recruit subjects and pursue the program? How will the program be advertised to those who need to know, for example, the parents of children to whom a program is to be offered? As many allies as possible should be attracted. Journalists can be very helpful. The preventive researcher should never refuse an opportunity to speak about the program on radio, television, or in the press. A program website can be designed to publicize the program and disseminate information (e.g., through progressive bulletins) about the problem it addresses.

The costs of the project should be carefully estimated and funding sought. The program will usually need to be piloted, if possible, to eliminate mistakes and to refine the intervention. If possible, clinician implementers should be recruited from existing staff. Thus, it will be a community-based rather than a laboratory study, and the results will have more ecological validity. If support is sought from a research-funding agency, the design of the program should include a well-chosen control group, random assignment if feasible, comprehensive outcome measures, a power analysis, and pilot data.

If subjects are to be recruited from schools or health agencies, for example, top-level and local authority and support will be needed. However, referral sources often forget about intervention projects, particularly if their staff changes. They will need to be reminded through regular visits, written information, and scientific presentations.

All long-term projects are affected by attrition due to change of residence, parental or child resistance to the program, or premature self-termination. If possible, it is desirable to include self-terminators in the outcome evaluation.

At the outset, as the project proceeds, and when it has been evaluated, information should be disseminated about the problem in general, the nature of the project, and the results of the intervention. The target audiences are the politicians and administrators from whom authority and funding has been obtained, the local managers from whom collaboration is sought, referral sources, and the general public.

COST-EFFECTIVENESS AND COST–BENEFIT ANALYSES

The aim of prevention is to intervene early in order to avert later more serious problems. School dropout, adolescent pregnancy, juvenile delinquency, drug abuse, suicide in adolescence or young adulthood, and posttraumatic adjustment problems, for example, are serious social problems. Not only do they limit personal productivity, but they can also become arduous (if not impossible) to reverse or control. Antisocial behavior, for example, requires expensive (and largely ineffective) control and management by the police, probation, and correctional systems. It is reasonable, therefore, to ask whether the cost of prevention (and its likelihood of success) is less than the cost of the undesirable outcome. Durlak (1997) points out that there is no standard procedure for cost analysis: No agreement about what is a cost, or what is a benefit, or how to compare them. Furthermore, costs vary with the setting of implementation.

Yates (1998) has described the mathematical principles of **cost-effectiveness analysis** (CEA) and **cost–benefit analysis** (CBA). CEA compares costs to outcomes as they are measured in human services and social science assessments. CBA compares costs to program outcomes that are measured in the same units as costs (e.g., dollars). **Cost-offsets** are funds that other agencies or individuals will not have to spend because of what an in-

tervention will accomplish. For example, for each child diverted from antisocial behavior as an adult, there are cost-offsets for the police, and correctional and health systems. **Benefits** are the resources generated by the program (e.g., the income earned by individuals who might otherwise have been incarcerated).

The CEA and CBA compare costs and outcomes separately, or combine them in the form of a single index such as a ratio. Ratios of benefits divided by costs are easy to present and comprehend. If benefits exceed costs, a program is potentially supportable. Lipsey (1984) surveyed delinquency prevention programs and found benefit–cost ratios varying from 0.17 to 8.79. Many analyses, however, fail to include personal benefits accruing from successful intervention such as improved quality of life. It is difficult to attach a dollar value to such an outcome. The Quality of Life Index (Miller and Galbraith, 1995) was designed to do so.

In CEA a detailed list is provided of all costs and benefits, some expressed in monetary terms (e.g., wages), and others in descriptive form (e.g., the hours required to complete an intervention program, or greater vocational attainment). External benefits (e.g., reduction of insurance premiums, or fewer motor vehicle accidents) should also be considered.

Durlak (1997) points out a danger: Politicians and administrators may be so concerned by the cost of an intervention that they ask for it to be curtailed in intensity, duration, or quality. It is often a mistake to do so. It could be argued that token or emasculated programs do little good and can ultimately do harm if it is found that time and money has been ineffectually expended.

THE ETHICS OF INTERVENTION

It is important not to claim more benefit from a proposed prevention program than it can deliver. Unfulfilled promises lead to the disillusionment of referring agents, clinicians, funding agencies, and the public. Programs that have no empirical basis (e.g., those that rely upon education alone) should not be supported. Researchers and administrators have the responsibility to ensure that the scarce amount of money available for prevention (said to be no more than 3% of the United States health budget) is well spent.

THE FUTURE

To date, no preventive programs have tackled the major DSM-IV categories of schizophrenia, bipolar disorder, manic depressive disorder, or obsessive–compulsive disorder. The prevention of these conditions will require greater knowledge of their genetics and the gene–environment interactions that predict them. Most preventive programs today target risky behavior (e.g., smoking, drinking, drug use, unprotected sexual activity, school dropout, suicidal behavior), parenting problems (e.g., coercive parenting, parents at risk of physically abusing their children, maternal depression), problems associated with chronic physical illnesses (e.g., asthma and diabetes), the prevention of cognitive delay in premature infants or socially disadvantaged preschool children, and the prevention of psychopathology following psychological trauma.

Recent meta-analyses or reviews of the literature (e.g., Durlak and Wells, 1997; Reppucci, Woolard and Fried, 1999; Carr, 2002) make it clear that a number of primary and secondary prevention programs are both clinically effective and cost-effective. The programs that work have definable characteristics (e.g., an empirically based theoretical model; clear goals and objectives; standardized interventions; good staff training, supervision and support; outcome measurement). Universal programs are often of insufficient intensity and duration to reach those most in need.

In the future, the emphasis will pass to targeted programs that operate on multiple levels (child, family, school, workplace, and community), with sensitivity to the sociocultural group or groups involved. Funding bodies will increasingly demand that proposed prevention programs be empirically based, and that operating programs be accountable for their results.

The dissemination and adoption of effective research programs is a serious problem. Rotheram-Borus and Duan (2003) advise that private enterprise models of marketing and dissemination be adopted by prevention experts, and that experts collaborate with marketing organizations in disseminating their programs. Dissemination requires programs to be presented in such a way as to be acceptable to clinicians, the public, politicians, administrators, and funding bodies.

Achenbach TM: *Manual for the Child Behaviour Checklist/4–18 and 1991 Profile*. Burlington, VT: University of Vermont, 1991.

Barton C, Alexander JF: Functional family therapy. In: Gurman AS, Kniskern DP (eds). *Handbook of Family Therapy*, New York: Brunner Mazel, 1981, pp. 403–443.

Bor W: Prevention and treatment of childhood and adolescent aggression and antisocial behaviour: A selective review. *Aust N Z J Psychiatry* 2004;38:373–380.

Brener ND, Collins JL, Kann L, Warren CW, Williams BI: Reliability of the Youth Risk Behaviour Survey Questionnaire. *Am J Epidemiol* 1995;141:575–580.

Caplan G: *Principles of Preventive Psychiatry*. New York: Basic Books, 1964.

Carr A: *Prevention: What Works with Children and Adolescents?* Hove, UK: Brunner-Routledge, 2002.

Chamberlain P, Reid JB: Differences in risk factors and adjustment for male and female delinquents in treatment foster care. *J Child Fam Stud* 1994;3:23–39.

Conduct Problems Prevention Research Group: Initial impact of the fast track prevention trial for conduct problems: I. The high-risk sample. *J Consult Clin Psychol* 1999;67:631–657.

Durlak JA, Wells AM: Primary prevention mental health programs for children and adolescents: A meta-analytic review. *Am J Community Psychology* 1997;25:115–143.

Durlak JA: *Successful Prevention Programs for Children and Adolescents*. New York: Plenum, 1997.

Gomez-Schwartz B, Horowitz JM, Cardarelli AP, Souzier M: The aftermath of child sexual abuse: 18 months later. In Gomez-Schwartz B, Horowitz JM, Cardarelli, AP (eds). *Child Sexual Abuse, The Initial Effects*. Newbury Park, CA: Sage, 1990.

Henggeler SW, Schoenwald SK, Borduin CM, et al.: *Multisystemic Treatment of Antisocial Behavior in Children and Adolescents*. New York: Guilford, 1998.

Landgraf JM, Koetz L, Ware JE: *The CHQ User's Manual*, 1st edn. Boston, MA: The Health Institute, New England Medical Center, 1996.

Lipsey MW: Is delinquency prevention a cost-effective strategy? A California perspective. *J Res Crime Delinquency* 1984;21:279–302.

Miller TR, Galbraith M: Injury prevention counselling by pediatricians: A benefit-cost comparison. *Pediatrics* 1995;96:1–4.

Mrazek PJ, Haggerty RJ: Reducing the risk for mental disorder: Frontiers for preventive intervention research. Washington, DC: National Academy Press, 1994.

Nation M, Crusto C, Wandersman A, et al.: What works in prevention: Principles of effective prevention programs. *Am Psychol* 2003;58:449–456.

Nurcombe B, Bickman L, de Andrade A, et al.: Attrition from a community-based treatment program for sexually abused children and adolescents. *J Am Acad Child Adolesc Psychiatry* (submitted for publication).

Olds DL, Henderson CR, Chamberlin R, Tatelbaum R: Preventing child abuse and neglect: A randomised trial of nurse-home visitation. *Paediatrics* 1986;78:65–78.

Reppucci MD, Woolard JL, Fried CS: Social, community and preventive interventions. *Annu Rev Psychol* 1999;38:58–58.

Roberts RE, Attkisson CC, Rosenblatt A: Prevalence of psychopathology among children and adolescents. *Am J Psychiatry* 1998;155:715–725.

Rotheram-Borus MJ, Duan N: Next generation of preventive interventions. *J Am Acad Child Adolesc Psychiatry* 2003;42:518–526.

Sawyer MG, Kosky RJ, Graetz BW, Arney F, Zubruik SR, Baghurst P: The national survey of mental health and wellbeing: The child and adolescent component. *Aust N Z J Psychiatry* 2000;34:214–220.

Shaffer D, Fisher P, Lucas C, Dulcan MK, Schwab-stone M: NIMH Diagnostic interview schedule for children, version IV (NIMH DISC-IV): Description, differences from previous versions, and reliability of some common diagnoses. *J Am Acad Child Adolesc Psychiatry* 2000;39:28–38.

Sinclair MF, Christenson SL, Evelo DL, Hurley CM: Dropout prevention for youth with disabilities: Efficacy of a sustained school engagement procedure. *Except Child* 1998;65:7–22.

Spaccarelli S: Stress, appraisal, and coping in child sexual abuse: A theoretical and empirical review. *Psychol Bull* 1994;116:340–362.

Weikart DP, Schweinhart LJ: High/Scope Preschool Program outcomes. In: McCord J, Tremblay RE (eds). *Preventing Antisocial Behavior: Interventions from Birth through Adolescence.* New York: Guilford, 1992, pp. 67–68.

Weisz JR, Weiss B, Ham SS, et al.: Effects of psycotherapy with children and adolescents revisited: A meta-analysis of treatment outcome studies, *Psychol Bull,* 1995;117:450–468.

Yates BT: Formative evaluation of costs, cost-effectiveness and cost benefit: Cost procedure, process, outcome analysis. In: Bickman L, Rog D (eds). *Handbook of Applied Social Research Methods.* Thousand Oaks, CA: Sage 1998, pp. 285–314.

SECTION II

Psychiatric Disorders in Adults

<table>
<tr><td>

Delirium, Dementia, and Amnestic Syndromes

</td><td>

14

</td></tr>
</table>

Joseph A. Kwentus, MD, & Howard S. Kirshner, MD

INTRODUCTION

In everyday practice, psychiatrists serve as members of medical teams in providing treatment to patients who have delirium, dementia, or other cognitive disorders. Psychiatrists often see these patients in hospitals, nursing homes, and other institutional settings. A psychiatrist usually acts as a consultant to a primary care physician or to a hospital service. Psychiatrists help primary care physicians understand the degree to which medical illness contributes to psychiatric symptoms or confusion. Proper treatment of the medical problem may lead to substantial improvement in psychiatric or neurobehavioral symptoms. Psychotropic medication may be helpful in the management of the patient's illness. Psychiatrists must consider medical diagnoses, treatments, drug interactions, and side effects when they prescribe psychotropics as part of their role on the medical team.

Patients who have cognitive disorders are often unable to give a reliable history, and the history obtained from third parties usually does not totally reveal the diagnosis. The psychiatrist must rely heavily on data obtained from the physical examination and from laboratory tests, electroencephalogram (EEG) findings, and brain imaging. The medical model provides the most appropriate understanding of patient care in cases of delirium and dementia because the medical model stresses a biological etiology for the patient's symptoms. This approach helps the physician establish crucial links between the patient's medical pathology and the neurobehavioral or psychiatric

symptoms. Once links have been established, the psychiatrist can recommend drug therapy and psychotherapy integrated in a comprehensive medical treatment plan.

Patients with delirium and the behavioral complications of dementia often require complicated therapeutic regimens. In some older patients, treatment is not well tolerated and may produce cognitive changes. This is particularly true when patients are receiving treatment for medical disorders. The clinician should understand the behavioral side effects of medical therapies. Removing drugs that produce confusion can help reestablish cognitive function.

Psychiatrists may attempt to treat agitation or hallucinations by adding psychotropics, but these drugs may worsen the patient's condition. Psychiatrists must be prepared to analyze the possibility of multiple drug interactions before launching into psychopharmacotherapy.

Physicians who treat cognitive disorders need to cross the traditional boundaries between psychiatry and neurology. More often than not, older patients have multiple disorders. Delirium, dementia, and affective disorder often coexist. The psychiatrist should not only treat depression and other correctable disorders, but also determine the existence of dementia and establish a prognosis, in order to plan appropriate treatment.

The physician must educate the patient and the family about the nature of the specific illness and the rationale for treatment. Disease processes that cause cognitive deficits may be very complex. Families are often exceedingly anxious because they anticipate the need to accept change in a meaningful relationship. They demand answers. Serious social and financial hardships add to a sense of dread about the future. Most families benefit from a thorough explanation of the patient's condition. Ultimately, the physician must be prepared to explain the contribution made by the various disease processes. The physician must know how to deliver bad news so that family members can take proper steps to prepare for the future. In the process, families expect the physician to respect the dignity of the cognitively-impaired patient. Whenever possible, the psychiatrist must try to help the family salvage hope and meaning.

■ THE AGING BRAIN

Although organic mental disorders occur at any age, they are more common in older patients. As the number of elderly people increases, clinicians will more frequently encounter patients with these disorders. The diagnosis of cognitive disorders is more complex in older patients because physical problems interact with emotional and social factors. The psychiatrist must be familiar with the cognitive changes associated with normal aging before determining the impact of a neurological illness or a psychiatric disorder. Assessment of these patients requires meticulous attention to the mental status examination. If physicians are not thorough in the cognitive assessment of their geriatric patients, they may miss significant deficits, some of which may be treatable.

ANATOMY

Delirium, dementia, and memory disorders become more common with advancing age; as a person ages, the brain becomes more vulnerable to a variety of insults. Brain weight and volume attain their maximal values in teenage years, and the brain loses both weight and volume as it ages. Significant atrophy of the brain has begun by the time that most people reach their 60s. By the 10th decade, the ratio of the brain to the skull cavity has fallen from 93% to 80%. When cortical neurons decrease in number, the cortical ribbon thins. Large neurons decrease in number whereas the number of small neurons increases.

Normal aging and dementia affect specific areas of the brain, especially the association cortices of the frontal, temporal, and parietal lobes. The limbic system, the substantia nigra, the locus coeruleus, the hippocampus and the parahippocampal regions, and the deep frontal nuclei all exhibit a sizable loss of neurons. Despite the loss of neurons, the aged brain continues to undergo dynamic remodeling. In normal older people, dendrites in the hippocampal regions continue to show plasticity. When dendritic arborization fails, mental powers begin to decline.

The relationship between cognitive functions and the morphologic changes that occur as the brain ages is incompletely understood. The volume of the cerebral ventricles increases with age, but the range of ventricular size is greater in old age than in youth. Increases in the size of ventricles, sulci, and subarachnoid spaces are observed easily with modern imaging techniques.

On a microscopic level, lipofuscin granules collect in neurons of aging brains. Fibrous astrocytes increase in size and number. The hippocampus exhibits granulovacuolar changes. Senile plaques and neurofibrillary tangles may occur in the brains of normal older individuals. The number of plaques and tangles in normal brains is less than the number observed in the brains of patients with Alzheimer's disease (AD). The overlap between patients with seemingly normal cognition and those with mild AD, however, can be difficult to discriminate in an individual brain. Small infarcts and ischemic white matter lesions are observed in the brains of many normal older people, both at autopsy and in brain imaging studies.

PHYSIOLOGY & NEUROTRANSMITTERS

Aging brains have a diminished capacity to respond to metabolic stress. The brain's demand for glucose decreases. EEG activity slows. Blood flow declines, and oxygen use diminishes. Glucose metabolism is crucial because it contributes to the synthesis of the neurotransmitters acetylcholine, glutamate, aspartate, gamma amino butyric acid (GABA), and glycine. Effects of slight abnormalities in glucose metabolism are obvious even in the resting state. The senile brain shows impaired transmitter synthesis and reduced transmitter levels.

Acetylcholine has been studied because of its role in memory. Older people exhibit a decrease in the synthesizing enzyme for acetylcholine, choline acetyl transferase. Uptake of circulating choline into the brain decreases with age. Decreased levels of acetylcholine in the hippocampus may relate to age-related declines in short-term memory. In AD, damage to the ascending cholinergic system plays an important role in the loss of memory and in other cognitive deficits.

Decreased catecholamines are linked more closely to affective changes than to cognitive changes in older people. Noradrenergic cell bodies in the locus coeruleus appear to decline in number with aging, but concentrations of norepinephrine appear to remain normal in target areas. The synthetic enzyme tyrosine hydroxylase increases with aging, whereas the degradative enzyme monoamine oxidase increases. Research also suggests reduced serotonergic innervation in the aging neocortex.

Loss of dopaminergic innervation of the neostriatum is a prominent age-related change that corresponds with the loss of dopaminergic cell bodies from the substantia nigra. Age-related decreases in basal ganglia dopamine make older patients more sensitive to the side effects of neuroleptics. Dopaminergic innervation of the neocortex and the neostriatum are not affected.

Studies of the brains of older patients have revealed a decrease in norepinephrine, serotonin, acetylcholine, and dopamine receptors. A decrease in β-receptor density results in reduced cyclic adenosine monophosphate and decreased adaptability to the external environment.

In contrast, older patients exhibit an increase in benzodiazepine-GABA receptor inhibitory activity and an increased sensitivity to benzodiazepines.

The capacity of mitochondria declines with age. Mitochondrial oxidants may be the chief source of the mitochondrial lesions that accumulate with age. The brain becomes susceptible to injury by free radicals that damage mitochondrial DNA, proteases, and membranes. Free radicals are likely a major contributor to cellular and tissue aging.

COGNITIVE PERFORMANCE

Changes in cognitive performance related to aging vary greatly. Information processing, particularly verbal speed and working memory, show the most pronounced changes. The number of correct answers required for the same IQ score in a 70-year-old, as compared to a 25-year-old, is approximately 50%. On the other hand, some cognitive skills are resistant to aging. Vocabulary and ability to read quickly tend to remain preserved and can be used to estimate premorbid IQ in cognitively impaired senior citizens. Older people who possess highly developed cognitive abilities can mask memory defects for a time. This "cognitive reserve" is especially noted in topics related to the person's long-term reading. Even the Mini Mental State examination, a relatively crude test of cognitive function, shows major effects of education on performance. These resistant aspects of cognition are often referred to as "crystallized intelligence," as compared to the "fluid intelligence" of memory and attention that is less resistant to aging. These studies encourage all of us to stay mentally active, continue reading in our professional disciplines, as we age.

After age 70, brain functions and capabilities decline more rapidly. Cognitive decline related to aging produces impaired memory, diminished capacity for complex ideas, mental rigidity, cautious responses, and behav-

ioral slowing. Slowing of responses is the most consistent cognitive change. As a result, it takes longer to provide professional services to older people.

Physicians who spend sufficient time testing mental status in older individuals are more likely to obtain accurate results than physicians who rush through the examination. Given enough time, older people will complete the following tasks accurately: (1) random digits forward, (2) un-timed serial arithmetic problems, (3) simple vigilance tests, (4) basic orientation, and (5) immediate memory. Unfamiliar stimuli, complex tasks, and time demands cause difficulty for older people. When older patients are asked to reorganize material (e.g., repeating digits backward), they often become anxious. Immediate memory continues to be normal in most patients, but if the memory task calls for split attention or reorganization, older people will have a harder time. Whenever the items to be remembered exceed primary memory capability, seniors show a decrement in memory acquisition and retrieval. Seniors have more difficulty remembering names and objects when they are not in a familiar routine. They do poorly on memory tasks that involve speed, unfamiliar material, or free recall. Although older people have a hard time organizing information, their memory performance improves if they control the rate of presentation. Practice also improves performance. Cognition does not operate in isolation from personality or social relationships. Because learning and memories occur within a range of contexts, a more useful test is one that emphasizes real-life memory.

Seniors usually perceive themselves as less effective than when they were younger, a perception that affects performance. The memory complaints of older adults are often related to low self-confidence or other personality variables. As a result, when seniors experience an increase in self-esteem and motivation their objective performance also improves. Similarly, lack of confidence reduces cognitive expectations even further.

Bartus RT, et al.: The cholinergic hypothesis of geriatric memory dysfunction. *Science* 1982;217:408.

Budson AE, Price BH: Memory dysfunction. *N Engl J Med* 2005; 352:692–699.

Burke DM, McKay DG: Memory, language, and aging. *Phil Trans R Soc Lond B* 1997;352:1845–1856.

Cockburn J, Smith PT: The relative influence of intelligence and age on everyday memory. *J Geront* 1991;46:31–36.

Crum RM, Anthony JC, Bassett SS, Folstein MF: Population-based norms for the Mini-Mental State Examination by age and educational level. *JAMA* 1993;269:2386–2391.

Folstein MF, Folstein SE, McHugh PR: "Mini-Mental State": A practical method for grading the cognitive state of patients for the clinician. *J Psychiatr Res* 1975;12:189–198.

Hultsch DF, Dixon RA: Learning and memory in aging. In: Birren JE, Schaie KW (eds). *The Handbook of the Psychology of Aging*. San Diego: Academic Press, 1990, pp. 258–274.

Kirshner HS: Mild Cognitive Impairment: To Treat or Not to Treat. *Curr Neurol Neurosci Rep* 2005;5:455–457.

McCartney JR: Physician's assessment of cognitive capacity. Failure to meet the needs of the elderly. *Arch Intern Med* 1986;146:177.

Quinn J, Kaye J: The neurology of aging. *The Neurologist* 2001;7: 98–112.

Sacks O: A neurologist's perspective on the aging brain. *Arch Neurol* 1997;54:1211–1214.

Shimamura AP, Berry JM, Mangels JA, et al.: Memory and cognitive abilities in university professors. *Psychol Sci* 1995;6:387–394.

■ DELIRIUM

Delirium is one of the most dramatic presentations in psychiatry and neurology. Delirious patients become acutely agitated, disoriented, and unable to sustain attention, form memories, or reason. In the past, the term *delirium* was reserved for an agitated, hyperactive state, whereas *encephalopathy* applied to confusional states in which the level of consciousness was normal or depressed. Currently, no distinction is made between these two conditions. In fact, delirium is now synonymous with "acute brain syndrome," encephalopathy, acute confusional state, and toxic psychosis.

Delirium is an extremely common clinical problem in hospitalized patients. An estimated 30–50% of hospitalized elderly people become delirious, amounting to an overall incidence of about 10% of all hospitalizations. Delirium increases morbidity and mortality for any hospitalization, and the cost to society is enormous.

The definition of delirium from the DSM-IV follows, below. Delirium, like dementia, involves multiple cognitive functions, including attention, memory, reasoning, language, and executive function. In contrast to dementia, delirium typically develops relatively acutely and fluctuates more from hour to hour and day-to-day. Delirium involves alterations in level of consciousness, agitation and hypervigilance or drowsiness, disturbed perception (hallucinations, delusions), psychomotor abnormalities (restlessness, agitation), and autonomic nervous system hyperactivity (tachycardia, hypertension, fever, diaphoresis, tremor). All of these phenomena are less common in dementia.

 ESSENTIALS OF DIAGNOSIS

DSM-IV Diagnostic Criteria
Delirium Due to General Medical Condition

A. *Disturbance of consciousness (i.e., reduced clarity of awareness of the environment) with reduced ability to focus, sustain, or shift attention.*

B. *A change in cognition (such as memory deficit, disorientation, language disturbance) or the development of a perceptual disturbance that is not better accounted for by a preexisting, established, or evolving dementia.*

C. *The disturbance develops over a short period of time (usually hours to days) and tends to fluctuate during the course of the day.*

D. *There is evidence from the history, physical examination, or laboratory findings that the disturbance is caused by the direct physiological consequences of a general medical condition.*

Substance Intoxication Delirium
A–C. Same as above

D. *There is evidence from the history, physical examination, or laboratory findings of either (1) or (2):*

(1) *the symptoms of Criteria A and B developed during substance intoxication*

(2) *medication use is etiologically related to the disturbance*

Substance Withdrawal Delirium
A–C. Same as above

D. *There is evidence from the history, physical examination, or laboratory findings that the symptoms of Criteria A and B developed during, or shortly after, a withdrawal syndrome.*

(Reprinted with permission, from *Diagnostic and Statistical Manual of Mental Disorders*, 4th edn. Copyright 1994 American Psychiatric Association.)

General Considerations

A. EPIDEMIOLOGY

The prevalence of delirium in general hospital patients is 10–30%. Up to 50% of surgical patients become delirious in the postoperative period. Delirium accompanies the terminal stages of many illnesses. It occurs in 25–40% of patients who have cancer and in up to 85% of patients with advanced cancer. Close to 80% of terminal patients will become delirious before they die.

Distinguishing delirium from depression in this population is important because physicians can treat both conditions and improve quality of life for the terminally ill. Many patients today make living wills or assign loved ones a durable power of attorney for health care. By explaining the causes and treatment of delirium to family members, the physician empowers them to decide what is best for the patient.

Age is the most widely identified risk factor for delirium. Patients with dementia are at high risk for delirium. Forty-one percent of dementia patients have delirium on admission to the hospital. Twenty-five percent of patients who are admitted to the hospital with delirium will ultimately be diagnosed as having dementia. Other factors that predict delirium in hospitalized patients include: Prior brain disease, vision or hearing loss, presence of a fracture on admission, symptomatic infection, stress or major environmental change, neuroleptic, anticholinergic, sedative medications or substance use or withdrawal, sleep deprivation, and use of restraints, a bladder catheter, or any surgical procedure during the admission.

The incidence of delirium in nursing homes is also quite high. Because the onset of delirium is more insidious in seniors than in young people, there is an even higher probability that delirium will be overlooked in nursing homes. Illnesses such as unrecognized urinary tract infection may cause delirium. More serious, life-threatening illnesses can also present with delirium. Hospital staff must be trained to recognize delirium at an early stage so that they can identify and promptly treat the primary medical condition. Common causes of delirium in older people include hypoxia, hypoperfusion of the brain, hypoglycemia, hypertensive encephalopathy, intracranial hemorrhage, CNS infection, and toxic-confusional states. Even when delirium is recognized and treated promptly, it predicts future cognitive decline. Many elderly patients who have been delirious never fully recover.

B. Etiology

A variety of conditions lead to delirium. These conditions can be categorized into four major groups: (1) systemic disease secondarily affecting the brain, (2) primary intracranial disease, (3) exogenous toxic agents, and (4) withdrawal from substances of abuse. The *Diagnostic and Statistical Manual of Mental Disorders,* fourth edition (DSM-IV) classifies delirium according to the presumed etiology. If delirium is due to a systemic medical condition or to primary intracranial disease, then the medical cause is listed in the Axis I diagnosis. Substance-induced delirium and substance withdrawal delirium are classified separately. Substance-induced delirium includes delirium caused by toxins and by drugs of abuse. If the etiology is not found, the diagnosis is delirium not otherwise specified. In most clinical situations, delirium is caused by multiple factors.

1. Systemic disease—Delirium can be caused by any type of systemic disease. When a medical condition causes delirium, the primary disease has caused either failure in cerebral blood flow or failure in cerebral metabolism. Cardiac conditions cause delirium by decreasing cerebral perfusion. Patients who have experienced cardiac arrest, cardiogenic shock, severe hypertension, or congestive heart failure are at risk of delirium. Organ failure syndromes such as renal, hepatic, and respiratory insufficiency can all cause delirium. Endocrine and metabolic disturbances affect brain metabolism. Hyponatremia and hypoglycemia may be the most prevalent causes in this category. Hypothyroidism is a common endocrine factor.

Central nervous system (CNS) causes of delirium include vasculitis, stroke, and seizure. Paraneoplastic phenomena in the brain (e.g., limbic encephalitis) may cause altered mental status in cancer patients.

Nutritional status also contributes to delirium; the most notable examples are vitamin B_1 deficiency in alcoholic patients, vitamin B_{12} deficiency, and pellagra. Infections may affect the nervous system directly, as in meningitis and encephalitis, but more often they cause delirium indirectly through toxins. In elderly patients who have generalized sepsis or even local infections such as urinary tract infections, altered mental status may precede both fever and leukocytosis. Mental status change may be the only manifestation of infection. In at least half the cases, the cause of delirium is multi-factorial. Urinary tract infection, low serum albumin, elevated white blood cell count, and proteinuria are among the most significant risk factors. Other risk factors include hyponatremia, hypernatremia, severity of illness, dementia, fever, hypothermia, psychoactive drug use, and azotemia.

No matter what systemic illness causes delirium, the clinical consequences are stereotypical. The diverse insults that cause delirium appear to act via similar metabolic and cellular pathways. A cascade of pathology in central neurotransmitter systems destabilizes cerebral function. Factors include oxidative stress, reductions in dopamine, norepinephrine, and acetylcholine, changes in either direction in serotonin, depolarization of neurons, and effects of stress such as sympathetic discharges and activation of the hypothalamic–pituitary–adrenocortical system. Ultimately, dysfunctional second messenger systems may provide the cellular mechanism of metabolic delirium.

2. Primary intracranial disease—Delirium can be caused by lesions in a variety of brain regions. Vascular pathology is more likely to cause confusional states if lesions are present in the basal nuclei and thalamus. Bilateral lesions of the thalamus or caudate nuclei are especially associated with delirium. Delirium is also more likely to accompany strokes in patients with preexisting brain atrophy or seizures. In traumatic brain injury, deeper brain lesions are associated with longer periods of delirium. Frontal lobe syndromes can also mimic delirium.

3. Exogenous toxic agents—Delirium due to substances may occur as the result of substance abuse or as an undesirable effect of medical therapies. Patients with delirium may exhibit symptoms suggesting pathology in specific neurotransmitter systems. Delirium in substance abusers who overdose provides the best example of a neurotransmitter-specific delirium.

Stimulants act through dopamine and other catecholamine pathways. Stimulant overdoses can cause confusion, seizures, dyskinesia, and psychomotor agitation, however, the most common presentation is that of an agitated paranoid state. Patients with stimulant-induced delirium can be dangerous, to which the saying "speed kills" attests. People who abuse stimulants are involved in violent acts more often than are those who abuse other substances. The dopamine excess observed in stimulant-induced delirium may provide a model to understand delirium in other general medical conditions. The effectiveness of dopamine-blocking agents such as haloperidol in the treatment of delirium suggests that excess dopamine relative to acetylcholine may produce delirium in general medical conditions and in stimulant-induced delirium.

D-Lysergic acid diethylamide (LSD) causes a different form of delirium through its action on serotonin receptors. This hallucinogen causes intensification of perceptions, depersonalization, derealization, illusions, hallucinations, and incoordination. Patients with delirium due to medical conditions may also experience illusions and hallucinations. Serotonin systems also may be affected in these patients. Under certain circumstances patients who are taking selective serotonin reuptake inhibitor (SSRI) antidepressants, especially when combined with other serotonergic medications, develop the *serotonin syndrome*, of which delirium can be a prominent feature.

Disruption of pathways served by N-methyl-D-aspartate (NMDA), a subtype of glutamate receptor, induces patients who are intoxicated with phencyclidine to display yet another symptom complex. Phencyclidine overdose is well recognized because of its tendency to produce assaultive behavior, agitation, diminished responsiveness to pain, ataxia, dysarthria, altered body image, and nystagmus. The NMDA receptor is also involved in the biological effects of alcoholism, such as intoxication and delirium tremens. Ethanol-induced up-regulation of NMDA receptors may underlie withdrawal seizures. The NMDA receptor also mediates some of the more damaging effects of ischemia during a stroke. Stimulation of NMDA receptors can lead to permanent brain damage. For this reason, conditions that lead to NMDA stimulation should be treated promptly.

Activation of brain GABA receptors causes some manifestations of sedative or alcohol overdose. Sedative intoxication causes slurred speech, incoordination, unsteady gait, nystagmus, and impairment in attention or memory. Some manifestations of hepatic encephalopathy may be the result of excessive stimulation of GABA receptors. Delirium tremens occurs when insufficient stimulation of GABA receptors results from withdrawal from benzodiazepines or alcohol. Treatment with benzodiazepines improves delirium tremens.

Drugs that have anticholinergic properties are very likely to contribute to delirium. In hospitalized patients, symptoms of delirium occur when serum anticholinergic activity is elevated. Total serum anticholinergic activity also helps to predict which patients in intensive care units become confused. Symptoms of anticholinergic delirium include agitation, pupillary dilation, dry skin, urinary retention, and memory impairment.

Physicians must be cautious when prescribing psychoactive drugs to seniors. One of the most common causes of delirium is iatrogenic. Common agents such as digoxin may induce cognitive dysfunction in older people, even with therapeutic digoxin levels. In the intensive care unit, antiarrhythmic agents such as lidocaine or mexiletine may cause confusion. Among the narcotics, meperidine is particularly likely to cause confusion and hallucinations. Benzodiazepines, other narcotics, and antihistamines are also frequent contributors to delirium. In psychiatric patients, tricyclic antidepressants (TCAs) and low-potency neuroleptics are frequent contributors. Note that these drugs have anticholinergic properties, and agents such as benztropine or trihexyphenidyl, used to combat extrapyramidal effects are also anticholinergic. The list of other drugs that may induce confusion is extensive.

The misuse of psychoactive drugs causes as many as 20% of geropsychiatric admissions. The odds of an adverse cognitive response increase as the number of drugs rises. Adverse drug reactions are a source of excess morbidity in elderly patients. A high index of suspicion, drug-free trials, and careful monitoring of drug therapy reduce this problem. Occasionally, a specific antidote is available for a drug-induced delirium. Physostigmine may reverse anticholinergic delirium and is sometimes useful in treating TCA overdoses. Narcotic-induced delirium can be reversed with naloxone. Flumazenil is an imidazobenzodiazepine that antagonizes the effects of benzodiazepine agonists by competitive interaction at the cerebral receptor. Naloxone and flumazenil have short half-lives and may have to be readministered.

Boyer EW, Shannon W: The serotonin syndrome. *N Engl J Med* 2005;352:1112–1120.

Devinsky O, Bear D, Volpe BT: Confusional states following posterior cerebral artery infarction. *Arch Neurol* 1988;45:160–163.

Erkinjuntii T, et al.: Dementia among medical inpatients. *Arch Intern Med* 1986;146:1923.

Francis J, Martin D, Kapoor WN: A prospective study of delirium in hospitalized elderly. *J Am Med Assoc* 1990;263:1097.

Gibson GE, et al.: The cellular basis of delirium and its relevance to age-related disorders including Alzheimer's disease. *Int Psychogeriatr* 1991;3:373.

Gleckman R, Hibert D: Afebrile bacteremia. A phenomena in geriatric patients. *J Am Med Assoc* 1982;248:1478.

Inouye SK, Charpentier PA: Precipitating factors for delirium in hospitalized elderly persons. Predictive model and interrelationship with baseline vulnerability. *JAMA* 1996;275:852–857.

Inouye SK: Delirium in older persons. *New Engl J Med* 2006;354: 1157–1165.

Kirshner HS: Delirium and acute confusional states. In: Kirshner HS (ed). *Behavioral Neurology. Practical Science of Mind and Brain.* Boston, MA: Butterworth Heinemann, 2002, pp 307–324.

Kumral E, Ozturk O: Delusional state following acute stroke. *Neurology* 2004;62:110–113.

Lipowski AJ: Delirium (acute confusional states). *J Am Med Assoc* 1987;258:1789.

Mach JR, Jr., et al.: Serum anticholinergic activity in hospitalized older persons with delirium: A preliminary study [see comments]. *J Am Geriatr Soc* 1995;43:491.

Mesulam MM, et al.: Acute confusional states with right middle cerebral artery infarction. *J Neurol Neurosurg Psychiatry* 1976;39:84.

Packard RC. Delirium. *Neurologist* 2001;7:327–340.

Clinical Findings

A. BASIC EVALUATION

Although the evaluation of delirium entails the analysis of very straightforward data, physicians often miss the diagnosis. The physician must obtain a careful history, perform a relevant physical examination, conduct a mental status examination, and review the patient's medications and laboratory tests. Physicians who do not conduct a careful physical examination may overlook asterixis, tremors, psychomotor retardation, and other motor manifestations of delirium. An organized mental status examination is the cornerstone of the assessment. The clinician who makes assumptions about the patient's cognitive status will make mistakes. This is particularly true in patients who are apathetic. After the physician has assessed the patient's mental status, he or she should carefully review laboratory data and the patient's medications.

B. SIGNS AND SYMPTOMS

The essential feature of delirium is an alteration in attention associated with disturbed consciousness and cognition. One of the most disconcerting clinical characteristics of delirium is its fluctuating course. Symptoms are everchanging. The patient's mental status varies from time to time. Cognitive deficits appear suddenly and disappear just as quickly. Patients may be apathetic at one moment, yet a short time later they may be restless, anxious, or irritable. Other patients become agitated and begin hallucinating without apparent change in the underlying medical condition. Waxing and waning of symptoms and perceptual disturbances may reflect the fact that the nondominant cortex is involved.

Common features of delirium include sleep disturbance and either decreased or agitated level of consciousness. Delirium may first present as *sundowning* with daytime drowsiness and nighttime insomnia with confusion. As the patient becomes more ill, disorientation and inattention dominate the clinical picture. Nonetheless, consciousness does not always follow the course of the underlying illness. When the patient's sleep is disturbed and the affect is labile, delirium usually lasts longer. This cluster of symptoms points to involvement of the reticular activating system of the brainstem and ascending pathways in delirium. Symptoms usually resolve quickly when the underlying disorder is treated, but a degree of confusion can last as long as 1 month after the medical condition has resolved, and some patients are even left with a longterm dementia.

C. PSYCHOLOGICAL TESTING

The Mini-Mental Status Exam (MMSE) is often used to quantify cognitive impairment, but only specific items on the MMSE are useful for evaluating delirium. Delirious patients have the most difficulty with calculation, orientation, attention, memory, and writing. The other higher cortical functions and language are usually preserved. The MMSE may be normal in as many as one-third of patients with clinical delirium. More specific delirium scales can be helpful. The Confusion Assessment Method is a rapid test designed to be administered by trained nonpsychiatrists. The Delirium Rating Scale is a 10-item scale for assessment of delirium severity. One study found that patients whose delirious episode improved within 1 week had much lower Delirium Rating Scale scores at the time of psychiatric consultation than did patients whose delirium lasted more than 1 week. The Trail Making Test (Parts A and B) and clock drawing tests are psychomotor tasks that are sensitive and easy to administer. Unfortunately, these tests measure specific cognitive functions that may not be impaired in delirium. For the busy clinician, the MMSE is the most practical tool, however, the clock drawing test also provides useful information in a short time.

D. LABORATORY FINDINGS

The vital signs are often abnormal. Common tests that often reveal the etiology of the delirium include complete blood count, sedimentation rate, electrolytes, blood urea nitrogen, glucose, liver function tests, toxic screen, electrocardiogram (ECG), chest X ray, urinalysis, and others. Blood gases or appropriate cultures may be helpful. A computed tomography (CT) scan is sometimes necessary to diagnose structural damage. Prompt lumbar puncture will confirm the diagnosis of suspected intrathecal infection.

Imaging studies are needed when the neurologic examination suggests a focal process or when initial screening tests have not revealed a treatable cause of the delirium. Even in nonneurological causes of delirium, CT scans often reveal ventricular dilatation, cortical atrophy, and ischemic changes. The right-hemisphere association cortex is often involved when some patients who are not paralyzed become delirious, suggesting a predisposing role for structural brain disease in the elderly with delirium. Subarachnoid hemorrhage, subdural hematoma, or right-hemisphere stroke can cause early mental status changes. Structural neurologic injury is sometimes the sole reason for delirium.

The EEG is useful in the evaluation of delirium when all other studies have been unrevealing. Generalized slowing is the typical pattern. A normal EEG is atypical but does not rule out delirium. Confusion and clouding of consciousness correlate partially with EEG slowing. In mild delirium, the dominant posterior rhythm is slowed. In more severe cases, theta and delta rhythms are present throughout the brain. Quantitative methods of EEG analysis supplement visual assessment in difficult cases. The severity of EEG slowing is correlated with the severity and duration of delirium and with the length of hospital stay. In more severe cases of metabolic or toxic delirium, triphasic waves replace diffuse symmetrical slowing. The appearance of periodic lateralized epileptiform discharges suggests a structural etiology. Rarely, the EEG reveals nonconvulsive status epilepticus as the cause of the delirium. In sedative or alcohol withdrawal, the EEG may show low-voltage fast activity.

Differential Diagnosis (Including Comorbid Conditions)

Distinguishing delirium from dementia can be difficult, because many clinical findings on mental status examination are similar. According to DSM-IV, the most common differential diagnoses are as follows: whether the patient has dementia rather than delirium; whether he or she has a delirium alone; or whether the patient has a delirium superimposed on preexisting dementia. Regardless, the clinical history is the most important tool in the diagnosis. Delirium is an acute illness. Dementia is longstanding. Physical examination and mental status are also important. Tremor, asterixis, restlessness, tachycardia, fever, hypertension, sweating, and other psychomotor and autonomic abnormalities are more common in delirium than dementia. Positive neurobehavioral symptoms such as agitation, delusional thinking, and hallucinations are much more common in delirium than dementia. On the other hand, cortical disorders such as dysphasia (language impairment) or apraxia (motor impairment) are not as common in delirium as in dementia. Clinicians should remember, however, that the two conditions often coexist.

Patients with delirium frequently have altered perceptions. As a result, delirium is sometimes mistaken for a psychosis. It is usually possible to separate delirium from a psychosis because signs of cognitive dysfunction are more common in delirium than in psychotic disorders. Psychotic patients are not normally disoriented, and they can usually perform well on bedside tests of attention and memory. The EEG is normal in psychoses. When the laboratory evidence does not support a medical illness, the clinician should consider the possibility of a psychiatric cause. When a psychiatric illness causes symptoms of delirium, patients are said to have a *pseudodelirium*. A history of past psychiatric illness may help clarify whether a patient has delirium or a psychiatric illness with pseudodelirium (e.g., a dissociative fugue or trauma state).

In some clinical situations, the boundaries are blurred between delirium and purely psychiatric illness. Psychiatric illness causes certain populations to become prone to physical disease. As a result, delirium can be surprisingly prevalent in psychiatric patients. Delirium and depression often coexist in seniors because depressed older patients are prone to become dehydrated and malnourished. Psychiatric patients may misuse prescribed drugs or abuse street drugs. Psychiatrists must be alert for delirium in all psychiatric patients.

Treatment

The correct treatment of delirium entails a search for the underlying causes and an attempt to treat the acute symptoms. Close nursing supervision to protect the patient is essential. Staff should remove all dangerous objects. Brief visits from a familiar person and a supportive environment with television, radio, a calendar, and proper lighting help orient the patient. The physician should review the patient's medications for unnecessary drugs and stop them; he or she should also monitor the patient's electrolyte balance, hydration, and nutrition.

A. HANDLING TREATMENT RESISTANCE

When delirious patients become agitated, they may resist treatment, threaten staff, or place themselves in danger. Of equal importance, these patients have elevated circulating catecholamines, which causes an increase in heart rate, blood pressure, and ventilation. Hospital personnel must protect patient rights and apply the least restrictive intervention when dealing with an agitated patient (see Chapter 34). The use of mechanical restraints increases morbidity, especially if the restraints are applied for more than 4 days. A sitter, although expensive, can sometimes obviate the need for physical restraint. Specially designed beds can also reduce the need for restraints. The Health Care Financing Administration has recently introduced strict guidelines for the use of restraints in psychiatric settings.

When other methods fail to control agitated patients, chemical sedation is usually more effective and less dangerous than physical restraint. According to the practice parameters of the Society of Critical Care Medicine, haloperidol is the preferred agent for the treatment of delirium in the critically ill adult. Many clinicians prefer the atypical antipsychotic agents in elderly patients because of the lower incidence of extrapyramidal side effects. The U.S. Food and Drug Administration (USFDA) has issued a warning because of the risk of cardiac complications and type II diabetes accompanying these agents. Whether or not these warnings are meaningful during the short-term use of these agents in patients with delirium is unknown. One recent study, however, indicated that haloperidol and other high-potency neuroleptics had a higher risk in elderly patients than the atypical antipsychotic agents such as olanzapine or quetiapine. In emergencies, haloperidol should be administered intravenously for a painless, rapid, and reliable onset of action that occurs in about 11 minutes. The dose regimen can be adjusted every 30 minutes until the patient is under control. For mildly agitated patients, 1–2 mg may suffice. Severely agitated patients may do better with an initial dose of 4 mg. Every 30 minutes the dose is doubled until the patient's behavior is contained. About 80% of patients will respond to less than 20 mg per day of intravenous haloperidol. This dose should be minimized in the elderly patient. Although intravenous haloperidol is safe, significant Q-T interval prolongation and "torsades de pointes" (an atypical rapid ventricular tachycardia) are possible complications of high-dose intravenous haloperidol therapy. Droperidol was used in similar fashion in the past, but is no longer available for this purpose because of the high frequency of "torsades de pointes". Hypotension may occur rarely. Acute dystonic reactions occur in less than 1% of patients. Other extrapyramidal side effects, however, such as Parkinsonism and tardive dyskinesia, are very common with this agent.

B. TREATING COMORBID ANXIETY

Patients admitted to the intensive care unit are often anxious and in pain, conditions that make delirium worse. Anxiety and delirium may be difficult to distinguish from one another. The interplay between confusion and anxiety may cause patients to become agitated when they are encouraged to engage in stressful activities such as weaning from mechanical ventilation. Benzodiazepines, if carefully monitored, can help in these situations. If benzodiazepines are given intravenously, they can cause respiratory depression or hypotension, however, this class of drugs can be easily titrated when monitoring is appropriate. As a result, benzodiazepines are effective in the treatment of delirium in many patients. Neuroleptic agents such as haloperidol may act synergistically with benzodiazepines, resulting in control of agitation. The patient's level of consciousness and respiratory drive are usually maintained but should be monitored. Once sedation has been achieved, intermittent administration of a neuroleptic agent in combination with a benzodiazepine can usually maintain control.

C. MANAGING SIDE EFFECTS

Physicians need to be aware of the side effects of benzodiazepines. Even when these medications are used as hypnotics, they may cause a decrease in the patient's MMSE score. Note that benzodiazepines are also employed to produce amnesia for uncomfortable procedures such as colonoscopy or transesophageal echocardiography. A variety of factors, including reduction in hepatic metabolism, modify the pharmacokinetics of many benzodiazepines in elderly patients. Lorazepam and oxazepam may be less affected by hepatic factors and are therefore preferred. Midazolam has been used as an intravenous infusion in intensive care settings because it is safe and has a short half-life.

Barbiturates are highly effective sedatives, but they depress the respiratory and cardiovascular systems. Given the efficacy of benzodiazepines, barbiturates should probably be reserved for agitated patients who have special indications for these drugs. Etomidate and propofol should be avoided for long-term use in agitated patients because of potentially serious side effects.

D. MANAGING PAIN

Pain relief is important. Opiates are the cornerstone of analgesia, but they may also contribute to delirium. In acute settings, opiates with short half-lives are the most efficacious. The Society of Critical Care Medicine recommends morphine, however, the total daily dosage must be monitored carefully in situations in which as-needed dosing is permitted. Naloxone can reverse the effects of a morphine overdose, but the clinician must be aware of the 20-minute half-life of this antagonist. Morphine is contraindicated in patients who have renal failure. Meperidine has been associated with hallucinations and seizures and should not be given to patients with delirium.

E. SPECIAL CONSIDERATIONS

The determination of the effective dosage of sedatives and analgesics in patients who have multiple organ system insufficiency requires careful planning and monitoring. Because the liver and kidney eliminate these drugs, organ system failure usually affects their distributive volume and clearance. The physician must assess the patient's creatinine clearance and liver function. Malnourished patients may have reduced plasma binding. By reducing the size and frequency of doses, the physician can avoid toxic effects. In life-threatening delirium, consultation with the anesthesia service is recommended, and therapeutic paralysis with muscle relaxants and anesthetic agents can be considered.

Prognosis

Patients with delirium have longer hospital stays and higher mortality than lucid patients. About half of all patients with acute encephalopathies improve if they receive proper treatment. Of the remainder, half will die and half will prove to have early signs of dementia. The severity of the underlying illness determines whether the delirious person will live or die, and patients with the poorest cognitive status on admission have the poorest long-term outcome. Ideal management requires awareness of the causes of delirium and active preventive efforts. Very elderly patients and patients with sensory impairment are at highest risk. The alert physician who recognizes systemic illness early and avoids complicated drug regimens can help prevent delirium.

Adams R, Victor M: Delirium and other acute confusional states. In: *Principles of Neurology*, 6th edn. New York: McGraw-Hill, 1996.

Ayd FJ: Intravenous haloperidol-lorazepam therapy for delirium. *Drug Ther Newslett* 1984;19:33.

Bowen BC, et al.: MR signal abnormalities in memory disorder and dementia. *Am J Roentgenol* 1990;154:1285.

Ely EW, Inouye SK, Bernard GR, et al.: Delirium in mechanically ventilated patients. Validity and reliability of the confusion assessment method for the intensive care unit (CAM-ICU). *JAMA* 2001;286:2703–2710.

Ely EW, Shintani A, Truman B, et al.: Delirium as a predictor of mortality in mechanically ventilated patients in the intensive care unit. *JAMA* 2004;291:1753–1762.

Food and Drug Administration. FDA public health advisory: Deaths with antipsychotics in elderly patients with behavioral disturbances. www.fda.gov/cder/drug/advisory/antipsychotics.htm

Inouye SK, Bogardus ST, Charpentier PA, et al.: A multicomponent intervention to prevent delirium in hospitalized older patients. *JAMA* 1999;340:669–676.

Koponen H, et al.: EEG spectral analysis in delirium. *J Neurol Neurosurg Psychiatry* 1989;52:980–985.

Ross CA, et al.: Delirium: Phenomenologic and etiologic subtypes. *Int Psychogeriatr* 1991;3:135.

Trzepacz PT, Dew MA: Further analyses of the Delirium Rating Scale. *Gen Hosp Psychiatry* 1995;17:75.

Wang PS, Schneeweiss S, Avorn J, et al.: Risk of death in elderly users of conventional vs. atypical antipsychotic medications. *N Engl J Med* 2005;353:2335–2341.

■ DEMENTIA

General Considerations

Slow evolution of multiple cognitive deficits characterizes dementia. Usually dementia patients have prominent memory impairment, however, dementia has many presentations. Personality disturbance or impaired information processing may reflect the early stages of a dementing process. Occasionally, language disorders or visuospatial syndromes are the presenting features of dementia. Sometimes the clinical syndrome is specific for a particular underlying pathology, but often the presentation may reflect a variety of possible pathologies. DSM-IV categorizes dementias according to presumed etiology, but this categorization will undoubtedly continue to undergo substantial revision because of the explosion of knowledge emerging from dementia research. In this chapter, DSM-IV criteria are included wherever possible (see "DSM-IV Diagnostic Criteria" sections, where applicable), however, in some cases alternative classifications better express the growing field of knowledge (see "Essentials of Diagnosis" sections, where applicable).

Evaluation

Clinical diagnosis is ultimately an attempt to deduce the neuropathologic basis of the patient's problem. Most dementias are associated with destruction or degeneration of brain structures. The autopsy shows whether the damage is the result of degenerative disease, vascular disease, infection, inflammation, tumors, hydrocephalus, or traumatic brain injury. Multiple causes for dementia are often apparent at an autopsy. Because the autopsy comes too late to help the patient or the family, the clinician must be knowledgeable about the pathology that is most likely to be associated with a given clinical presentation.

Clinical diagnosis is based on the patient's history and mental status and on laboratory examination. Several basic tests are recommended in the evaluation of dementia. These include complete blood count with differential, electrolytes, liver function tests, blood urea nitrogen, creatinine, protein, albumin, glucose, vitamin B_{12}, urinalysis, and thyroid function tests. A brain imaging study, either CT or magnetic resonance imaging (MRI), is virtually always required. CT generally gives less information than MRI. In a significant minority of cases, imaging does not clarify the diagnosis, but nonetheless provides comfort to the family and the clinician that "no stone has been unturned." Imaging studies are recommended in some practice guidelines, including those of the American Academy of Neurology. Optional tests include sedimentation rate, blood gases, folate, HIV screen, syphilis serology, heavy metals screen, positron emission tomography (PET) or single photon emission computed tomography (SPECT) scanning. Genetic testing (for apolipoprotein E), cerebrospinal fluid (CSF) assays of tau, and neural thread protein are available but generally not recommended.

CT and MRI scans are especially important in excluding focal lesions or conditions such as hydrocephalus, subdural hematoma, silent strokes, or brain tumors. The physician must be careful not to over-interpret findings.

EEG was previously used more commonly in the evaluation of dementia, however, EEG slowing is difficult to interpret. Intermittent slowing is not related to MRI change or to decline in neuropsychological function. Runs of intermittent slowing increase in frequency with advancing age, but such episodes are brief and infrequent. Focal slow waves sometimes occur in temporal and frontal areas without significance. When any of these changes become prominent, pathology is usually present. Older people in good health may have an average occipital frequency that is a full cycle slower than young adults, however, they do not show EEG dominant frequencies below 8 hertz.

Occasionally, a dementia evaluation leads to the diagnosis of a treatable illness and permits curative treatment, especially when the dementia has toxic or metabolic etiologies. More commonly the physician establishes a plausible explanation of the clinical findings and suggests palliative care. Because families come to physicians for a diagnosis and a prognosis, the physician's explanation should include statements about what is likely to happen to the patient. The family needs an interpretation of the observed behavior and suggestions about ways to deal with it. The physician gives the family some understanding of what is happening and helps them in planning for future decline in the patient's status. The psychiatrist often manages the troubling behavior that occurs toward the end of many dementing illnesses. The psychiatrist also recognizes the needs of the caregiver and makes suitable suggestions to help the caregiver relinquish part of the burden.

CLINICAL SYNDROMES

DEGENERATIVE DEMENTIAS

Dementia of the Alzheimer's type (AD), frontotemporal dementia (FTD), and diffuse Lewy body disease are primary degenerative processes occurring within the CNS. These syndromes are progressive and lead inevitably to severe disability and death. Other degenerative dementias are associated with diseases that affect other neurological systems; these include Huntington's disease, Parkinson's disease (PD), progressive supranuclear palsy, corticobasal degeneration, and multiple system atrophy.

1. Dementia of the Alzheimer's Type

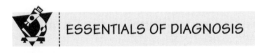

ESSENTIALS OF DIAGNOSIS

The most widely applied criteria for the clinical definition of AD are those of the National Institute of Neuro-logical and Communicative Disorders and Stroke and those of the AD and Related Disorders Association. The diagnosis of probable AD requires the presence of dementia established by clinical examination, documented by standardized mental status assessment, and confirmed by neuropsychological tests. These tests must demonstrate deficits in two or more areas of cognition, with progressive worsening of memory and other cognitive functions in the absence of delirium. The onset must be between ages 40 and 90 years, and there must be no other brain disease that could account for the clinical observations (this implies a work-up, including the blood studies and brain imaging tests discussed above). The disorder must also be progressive and associated with disability in routine activities. Supportive features include family history, specific progressive deficits in cognitive functions, and laboratory data such as PET or SPECT scans. PET ligands that bind to amyloid, such as the Pittsburgh Compound, may provide more accurate AD diagnosis in the future.

General Considerations

AD is the most common form of dementia, accounting for over half of all dementias. Oddly enough, just 25 years ago, many textbooks considered AD to be rare, likely because the disease was confined to "presenile" cases, younger than age 65. We now know that the neuropathology of presenile and senile dementia is the same. There has been a veritable explosion in research in AD.

Although memory problems dominate the early stages of the disorder, AD affects cognition, mood, and behavior. Cognitive impairment affects daily life because patients are unable to perform normal activities of daily living. Behavioral manifestations of the disease such as temper outbursts, screaming, agitation, and severe personality changes are more troubling than the cognitive difficulties. No two patients with AD are exactly alike when it comes to the behavioral manifestations of the disorder. Only recently has this aspect of the disease received substantial attention.

A. EPIDEMIOLOGY

AD is the most common type of progressive dementia. This degenerative disease reaches 20% prevalence in 80-year-olds, as much as 48% prevalence in one study of community-dwelling elderly people over age 85, and afflicts over four million Americans. It is projected to affect 8–14 million by the year 2030. The disease affects women more often than men. The economic impact of AD has been estimated at over $100 billion annually.

B. ETIOLOGY

In general, AD represents an imbalance between neuronal injury and repair. Factors contributing to injury may include free radical formation, vascular insufficiency, inflammation, head trauma, hypoglycemia, and aggregated β-amyloid protein. Factors contributing to ineffective repair may include the presence of the apolipoprotein E (ApoE) E4 gene, altered synthesis of amyloid precursor protein, and hypothyroidism. Some researchers hypothesize that β-amyloid causes chronic inflammation. AD also involves formation of tau-containing neurofibrillary tangles; most researchers feel that the tau protein changes (see below) are a secondary phenomenon in AD, though they may be primary in FTD and other diseases. Ultimately, the deficit of key neurotransmitters, especially acetylcholine, plays a major role in the cognitive symptoms.

Plaques and tangles identify the illness at the microscopic level. Amyloid plaques occur in vast numbers in severe cases. Amyloid plaques were first recognized in 1892. PAS or Congo Red stains identify these structures. β-Amyloid peptide, which is concentrated in senile plaques, has been linked to AD. The β-amyloid protein, in the form of pleated sheets, appears early in the brain and in blood vessels in AD. Some studies suggest that β-amyloid is toxic to mature neurons in the brains of Alzheimer's patients. Neurons in these areas begin to develop neurofibrillary tangles. Amyloid plaques and neurofibrillary tangles gradually accumulate in the frontal, temporal, and parietal lobes. The density of plaques determines postmortem diagnosis. Amyloid binding can now be imaged in PET studies, using the Pittsburgh compound and other ligands. The number of neurons and synapses is reduced. This is particularly true of acetylcholine-cholinergic-containing neurons in the basal nucleus of Meynert, which project to wide areas of the cerebral cortex. PET studies demonstrate a reduction in acetyl cholinesterase and decreased binding of cholinergic ligands. Hirano bodies and granulovacuolar degeneration occur in the hippocampus and represent further degeneration.

Neocortical neurofibrillary tangles are extremely rare in normal individuals, however, neuropil threads and neurofibrillary tangles appear at the onset of dementia. These intracytoplasmic filaments displace the nucleus and the cellular organelles. Neurofibrillary tangles contain an abnormally phosphorylated protein named tau. The abnormal phosphorylation of tau protein probably causes defective construction of microtubules and neurofilaments. The neurofibrillary tangles in brains affected by AD abnormally express Alz-50, a protein antigen commonly found in fetal brain neurons. Neural thread protein is present in the long axonal processes that emerge from the nerve cell body and is found in association with neurofibrillary tangles. This protein may be involved in neural repair and regeneration.

Neurons bearing neurofibrillary tangles often project to brain regions that are rich in senile plaques containing β-amyloid. These plaques are found in areas innervated by cholinergic neurons. Cholinergic neurons in the hippocampus and the basal nucleus of Meynert degenerate early in AD, causing impairment of cortical and hippocampal neurotransmission and cognitive difficulty. The affected cortical areas become anatomically disconnected. One of the earliest areas to be disconnected is the hippocampus, which explains why memory disorder is one of the early manifestations of AD. As time goes on, there is a loss of communication between other cortical zones and subsequent loss of higher cognitive abilities.

These basal forebrain cholinergic projections not only mediate cognitive function but also mediate brain responses to emotionally relevant stimuli. In the late stages of AD, a wide range of behavioral changes occur, including psychosis, agitation, depression, anxiety, sleep disturbance, appetite change, and altered sexual behavior. These changes are mediated by cholinergic degeneration and by degeneration in other neural systems. Serotonergic neurons and noradrenergic neurons degenerate as the disease progresses. Degeneration of these systems also contributes to some of the later cognitive and behavioral manifestations of the disorder. Because dopaminergic neurons are relatively immune to degeneration in AD, the performance of well-learned motor behaviors is preserved well into the late stages of the disease.

C. GENETICS

AD has demonstrated genetic diversity. Chromosome 21 has been implicated for many years because it is well known that patients with Down syndrome are very likely to develop the histological features of AD. Genetic mutations usually cause familial, autosomal dominantly transmitted, early-onset AD. Several mutations of the amyloid precursor protein gene on chromosome 21 have been described. These mutations increase the production of an abnormal amyloid that has been associated with neurotoxicity. Another form of early-onset disease has been localized to a variety of defects on chromosome 14. These mutations are associated with presenilin 1 and account for the majority of familial Alzheimer's cases. A mutation on chromosome 1 is associated with presenilin 2. Both of these mutations also cause increased production of amyloid, in that the presenilins are now known to be secretase enzymes involved in the formation of beta-amyloid peptide, a 40–42 amino acid peptide, from the amyloid precursor protein.

The ApoE E4 allele is associated with the risk of late-onset familial and sporadic forms of AD. ApoE; a plasma protein involved in the transport of cholesterol is encoded by a gene on chromosome 19. Disease risk increases in proportion to the number of ApoE E4 alleles. The population that is positive for ApoE E4 has a lower age at onset. The ApoE E2 allele may offer some protection. Although patients with the ApoE E4 allele may be more likely to have AD, a full diagnostic evaluation including imaging, laboratory tests, and neuropsychological evaluation is still indicated when the clinical situation warrants. It is premature to regard ApoE testing as a screening tool for AD, and it is not recommended for presymptomatic screening in family members of patients with AD. Another gene, SORL1, has recently been described as a marker for sporadic AD.

Clinical Findings

A. SIGNS AND SYMPTOMS

A subjective sense of memory loss appears first, followed by loss of memory detail and temporal relationships. All areas of memory function deteriorate including encoding, retrieval, and consolidation. Patients forget landmarks in their lives less often than other events. Amnesia for names and specific nouns is the earliest language abnormality in AD, and a mild anomic aphasia is often found in patients with early AD. Agnosia (failure to recognize or identify objects), more severe aphasia (language disturbance), apraxia, and visuospatial-topographical impairments such as getting lost while walking or driving occur later in the disease.

In the early stages of AD, a subjective memory deficit is difficult to distinguish from benign forgetfulness. Considerable research has examined patients with impaired memory but otherwise normal cognitive function, a disorder called "mild cognitive impairment." These patients are more likely to develop AD over time than age-matched controls. Deficits in memory, language, concept formation, and visual spatial praxis evolve slowly. Later, patients with AD become passive, coarse, and less spontaneous. Many become depressed, and depression may worsen the patient's cognitive function. Depressed Alzheimer's patients often exhibit degeneration of the locus coeruleus or substantia nigra.

More than half of patients with mild Alzheimer's patients present with at least one psychiatric symptom, and one-third present with two or more symptoms. After the initial stage of the disease, patients enter a stage of global cognitive deterioration. Denial or loss of self-awareness replaces anxiety, and cognitive deficits are noticeable to family and friends. In the final stages, patients become aimless, abulic (unable to make decisions), aphasic, and restless. At this stage, abnormal neurologic reflexes, such as the snout, palmomental, and grasp reflexes, are common.

B. PSYCHOLOGICAL TESTING

The clinical assessment and staging of AD have always been difficult. The MMSE is often used but sometimes seriously underestimates cognitive impairment. The Standardized MMSE has better reliability than the MMSE. The Blessed Dementia Scale uses collateral sources and correlates well with postmortem pathology. The interrater reliability of the Blessed Dementia Scale is low.

The Extended Scale for Dementia is a rating scale designed to distinguish the intellectual function of dementia patients from normal seniors. The Neurobehavioral Cognitive Status Examination (NCSE) is a tool that assesses a patient's cognitive abilities in a short amount of time. This instrument uses independent tests to estimate functioning within five major cognitive ability areas: language, constructions, memory, calculations, and reasoning. The Mattis Dementia Rating Scale (DRS) is useful in staging dementia. Both the NCSE and the DRS are sensitive, but they are more time consuming than the MMSE. In most clinical practices, the MMSE is used for assessment of dementia and for following the patient's progress, and common recommendations for drug therapy are based on the MMSE score.

Comprehensive scales combine clinical judgment, objective data, and specific rating criteria. The Reisberg Brief Cognitive Rating Scale and the Global Deterioration Scale are brief comprehensive scales. The Clinical Dementia Rating Scale (CDR) is a more extensive instrument that includes subject interview, collateral interview, brief neuropsychological assessment, and interview impression. Patients with a CDR score of 0.5 are likely to have "very mild" AD. The CDR has a complicated scoring algorithm and is best reserved for research.

The Alzheimer's disease Assessment: Cognitive (ADAS COG) and the Behavioral Pathology in AD (Behave-AD) instruments are used in clinical drug trials to determine pharmacologic efficacy in cognitive areas or behavioral areas, respectively.

The Consortium to Establish a Registry for Alzheimer's disease Criteria (CERAD) examination includes general physical and neurologic examinations as well as laboratory tests. Specified neuropsychological tests and a depression scale are also administered.

C. LABORATORY FINDINGS AND IMAGING

Although CT scans reveal atrophy in Alzheimer's patients as a group, atrophy alone does not reliably predict AD in individual patients. Atrophy can be quantified using appropriate ratios and progresses on serial evaluation, but this information adds little to the patient's clinical care.

MRI region-of-interest techniques reveal reduced brain volume and higher CSF volume in patients with

AD. AD may be associated with enlarged CSF spaces or atypical signal intensity in the medial temporal lobes. These findings imply that advancing AD is associated with increased brain water, where either the atrophy leads to an increase in CSF spaces, or there are associated ischemic changes in the deep cerebral white matter. Finally, volumetric studies may show hippocampal sclerosis in the brains of Alzheimer's patients. Hippocampal atrophy may be relatively specific to AD and may be useful for early detection and differential diagnosis.

^{31}P–nuclear magnetic resonance (NMR) spectroscopy profiles may be helpful in the evaluation of AD. ^{31}P NMR profiles of AD patients show elevated ratios of phosphomonoesterase to phosphodiesters in the temporoparietal region.

In the early stage of dementia, functional brain imaging (i.e., PET and SPECT scans) is more sensitive than structural brain imaging (i.e., MRI and CT scan). PET scans reveal changes in temporoparietal metabolism that differentiate patients with AD from the normal elderly. PET scans reveal the following abnormalities in AD: (1) reductions in whole-brain metabolism (paralleling dementia severity), (2) hypometabolism in the association cortex exceeding that in the primary sensorimotor cortex, and (3) metabolic asymmetry in suitable cortical areas accompanying neuropsychological deficits. In AD metabolic deficits start in the parietal cortex. Frontal metabolism decreases as dementia progresses. AD spares the primary motor cortex, sensory cortex, and basal ganglia.

SPECT scans can reveal information about regional brain function at a much lower cost and degree of complexity than PET scans, but the spatial resolution is not as good. In more advanced AD cases, SPECT scans reveal decreased perfusion in the bilateral temporoparietal regions.

EEG abnormalities are not common early in AD, but they develop as the disease progresses. Diffuse slow wave abnormalities occur first in the left temporal regions and become more frequent and longer as the disease progresses. EEG abnormalities that occur early in dementia suggest a coexisting delirium. Because dementia often presents first in association with delirium, infectious, toxic, or metabolic disturbances should be considered if the EEG slowing is severe.

Evoked potentials are an EEG technology that average many signals following a specific stimulus. In AD, the auditory P300 amplitude in the posterior parietal regions is suppressed on evoked potential maps. Other studies have not demonstrated clinically useful abnormalities of the P300 component in dementia. Compared to control subjects, AD patients show longer P100 latencies of pattern-reversal visual evoked potentials. The flash P100 distinguishes them only marginally. The long-latency auditory evoked potential helps differentiate between cortical and subcortical dementias. Patients with subcortical dementias exhibit prolonged latencies.

Differential Diagnosis (Including Comorbid Conditions)

Clinicians have traditionally used a battery of laboratory tests to differentiate AD from a variety of medical conditions that cause memory impairment. These tests include complete blood count, comprehensive metabolic panel, thyroid function tests, and vitamin B$_{12}$. In appropriate cases, the erythrocyte sedimentation rate, serological tests for syphilis, and even a lumbar puncture may be indicated. In many cases, a careful history and bedside mental status examination can reliably diagnose presumed AD and distinguish it from other forms of dementia. A detailed drug history is necessary because drugs, especially those with anticholinergic properties, can cause Alzheimer-like symptomatology. A normal neurologic examination is entirely consistent with AD. Neurologic abnormalities are much more common in other dementing illnesses. The relationship between AD and depression is complex and is discussed later in this chapter.

Memory loss is common in nondemented seniors. Many of these patients become terrified that they have AD and seek medical help. Physicians have difficulty distinguishing normal age-associated memory loss, benign forgetfulness, and early AD.

Benign senile forgetfulness is a condition that occurs when effects of aging on memory are greater than expected. Elderly patients with benign forgetfulness forget unimportant details. This contrasts with Alzheimer's patients, who forget events randomly. Seniors who experience benign senile forgetfulness have trouble remembering recent information; typically, Alzheimer's patients have difficulty with recent and remote memory. The most important aspect of the treatment of benign senile forgetfulness is reassurance, but cognitive retraining can sometimes be helpful. When the memory loss is clearly more than normal for age, the diagnosis should be "mild cognitive impairment" (MCI). As mentioned earlier, this condition is not as benign, in that almost half of patients with MCI progress to AD over a 3–4-year period. Drug treatment for patients with MCI is the subject of active research, but no specific recommendation exists, as yet. Treatment should be considered when the cognitive disorder becomes disabling, or by common insurance company guidelines, when the MMSE drops below 24.

Although AD can be diagnosed accurately in clinical settings, inaccuracy of diagnosis continues to plague clinical care. AD is over-diagnosed. Patients with FTD, PD, diffuse Lewy body disease, or even metabolic conditions mistakenly receive the diagnosis of AD. Unfortunately, even patients taking multiple medications and those who have delirium may receive the diagnosis of AD.

Treatment

The aim of pharmacotherapy in AD is as follows: (1) to prevent the disease in asymptomatic individuals, (2) to alter the natural course of the disease in those already diagnosed, and (3) to enhance patients' cognition and memory. As yet, no treatment has been shown to be effective in preventing the disease, though general health measures such as exercise, healthy diet, treatment of hypertension and hyperlipidemia, and avoidance of tobacco and excessive alcohol are all suggested to delay or prevent the disease. Treatment to enhance memory in Alzheimer's patients has focused on improving cholinergic activity. Cholinergic enhancement can occur through the administration of acetylcholine precursors, choline esterase inhibitors, and combinations of AChE with precursors, muscarinic agonists, nicotinic agonists, or drugs facilitating AChE release. To date, only cholinesterase inhibitors have proved effective in clinical trials.

Early attempts to treat dementia with ergoloid mesylates were of limited benefit. In some studies, ergoloid mesylates were more effective than placebo. The dose-response relation suggests that the effective dosage may be higher than currently approved. Unfortunately, the original clinical trial designs were flawed, leaving their benefit unproved.

Attempts to enhance acetylcholine transmission with precursors such as lecithin and choline failed to show benefit in AD. Cholinomimetic substances such as arecoline were more successful but have had limited use because of adverse side effects, short half-life, and narrow dose range. Physostigmine, an acetylcholinesterase inhibitor, has limited benefit because of its short half-life and significant side effects.

The first acetylcholinesterase inhibitor approved for use in mild to moderate AD was tetrahydroaminoacridine (Tacrine). Tacrine frequently causes adverse side effects, particularly gastrointestinal hyperactivity. Elevation of liver transaminase is another significant side effect. Of the patients who take tacrine, 25% will experience elevations (up to three times the normal) in alanine amino transferase levels. For these reasons, tacrine is rarely used currently.

Second-generation cholinesterase inhibitors such as donepezil are more specific for CNS acetylcholinesterase than for peripheral acetylcholinesterase. These drugs do not have the limitations associated with tacrine. Donepezil has the additional advantage of daily dosing. It does not cause significant hepatotoxicity. Donepizil has an orally dissolving tablet form and has been approved for mild, moderate, and severe AD. Rivastigmine is a cholinesterase inhibitor that has a relative specificity for both acetylcholinesterase and butyrylcholinesterase, an effect shared only with tacrine. There is evidence that butyrylcholinesterase is present at high concentrations in the brains of patients with AD, but the relevance of this factor to its clinical effect is unknown. The drug has more gastrointestinal side effects than donepizil. It is given twice daily at doses of 1.5, 3, 4.5, and finally 6 mg, with dose advances made every four weeks. A last cholinesterase agent, galantamine, has similar effects on the acetylcholinesterase enzyme, but may also increase presynaptic release of acetylcholine. This agent is available in both twice daily and extended release preparations. The daily doses are 8, 16, and 24 mg. The gastrointestinal side effects of this agent are intermediate between those of donepizil and rivastigmine, but individual patients may tolerate one better than another.

New delivery mechanisms for the anticholenesterase medications have made them more tolerable. Galantamine is available in an extended release formulation. Rivastigmine will be available in a patch formulation that provided similar efficacy to that achieved at the highest doses of the capsule with three times fewer reports of nausea and vomiting.

Muscarinic M1 receptors are relatively intact in AD, despite the degeneration of presynaptic cholinergic innervation. Several muscarinic agonists have been studied in clinical trials, but none has been approved, to date. Finally, stimulation of nicotinic receptors may have a protective effect in AD.

The newest drug to be USFDA approved for AD is memantine, an antagonist at the NMDA receptor. The exact mechanism of action of this drug is not known; the NMDA effect could represent a neuroprotective effect on "excitotoxicity" of glutamate on surviving neurons, but this drug appears to have other beneficial effects on learning and memory. It has been approved for moderate to advanced AD, that is, patients with MMSE <20.

Treatment of behavioral complications of AD is problematic. Depression should always be treated, usually with an SSRI agent. Anxiety can be helped with trazodone at bedtime, but benzodiazepines tend to worsen the memory loss and may cause paradoxical agitation. Valproic acid has been found helpful in some, but not all studies. Both donepezil and memantine appear to ameliorate behavioral disturbances in patients with AD. The same therapeutic considerations discussed under delirium are relevant in the treatment of psychosis in AD. Atypical antipsychotic agents are not greatly effective and have a black box warning. In general, we recommend low doses of olanzapine, risperidone, aripiprazole or quetiapine, with increases in dosage or shifting to another agent if symptoms persist. In the CATIE trial, the benefit for those taking active drug compared to placebo, was small. While antipsychotic medications were more often associated with distressing adverse effects. Patients and families must be warned of the potential risks of these agents.

Therapeutic strategies intended to slow progression of AD have not been very successful. Early studies suggested that the incidence of AD was reduced in postmenopausal women taking estrogen, but the Women's Health Initiative studies found the opposite: postmenopausal estrogen and progesterone hormone replacement therapy appears associated with a higher incidence of cognitive deficits and dementia. Use of non-steroidal anti-inflammatory drugs has been inversely associated with incidence of dementia in population studies, but a therapeutic use of these agents in AD has not been proved. The Cox II inhibitor refoxicib (Vioxx) was taken off the market because of increased cardiovascular events, and one of the two studies with this finding involved patients with AD. Antioxidants such as vitamin E and selegiline have shown a beneficial effect in some studies, but several recent studies have failed to establish any role for these agents. In particular, a study of mild cognitive impairment showed a limited benefit for donepizil, but none whatsoever for Vitamin E. Nicotine may have protective properties, but the toxic effect of the drug on other body systems currently precludes its use as treatment. Attempts to treat AD with nerve growth factor have been limited by the inability of the substance to cross the blood–brain barrier.

Treatments to reduce the deposition of amyloid protein in the brain have not proved effective as yet, but this field has great promise. A trial of a vaccine against amyloid had to be stopped because of the development of an encephalitis in about 10% of the recipients; one case, studied at autopsy, had little remaining amyloid staining. More selective vaccines and passive immunity with monoclonal antibodies against amyloid are currently in testing. An experimental drug called Alzhemed represents another attempt to reduce amyloid deposition; this clinical trial is still in progress. In general, AD is a very active area of clinical research.

Prognosis

An early-onset form of AD occurs in some people in their 40s, 50s, or 60s. A prolonged, indolent, subtle deterioration in mental function characterizes the clinical course of illness. From the time of clinical diagnosis the course is variable, but survival is possible up to 20 years from clinical recognition. Early-onset cases tend to progress more rapidly. Ultimately, functional performance declines. The patient's ability to drive becomes impaired, and he or she becomes unable to manage personal finances or to produce a complete meal. In general, studies suggest that patients with a MMSE score below 20 are probably not safe drivers. Later, impairment of language and inability to recognize familiar people lead to agitation, restlessness, and wandering. Hallucinations and other disruptive behaviors may make management difficult. In the final stages of the disease, the patient is generally mute and completely devoid of comprehension. Death most often results from a comorbid illness such as pneumonia.

American College of Medical Genetics/American Society of Human Genetics Working Group on ApoE and Alzheimer Disease Consensus Statement: Statement on use of apolipoprotein testing for Alzheimer disease. *J Am Med Assoc* 1995;20:1627.

Chartier-Harlin MC, et al.: Early onset Alzheimer's disease by mutation at codon 17 of the beta-amyloid precursor protein gene. *Nature* 1991;353:844.

Cummings JL, Kaufer D: Neuropsychiatric aspects of Alzheimer's disease: The cholinergic hypothesis revisited. *Neurology* 1996; 47:876.

Cummings JL, Schneider E, Tariot PN, et al.: Behavioral effects of memantine in Alzheimer disease patients receiving donepezil treatment. *Neurology* 2006;67:57–63.

Cummings JL: Alzheimer's disease. *N Engl J Med* 2004;351:56–67.

Farlow MR, Evans RM: Pharmacologic treatment of cognition and Alzheimer's dementia. *Neurology* 1998;51(Suppl 1):S36.

Holmes C, Wilkinson D, Dean C, et al.: The efficacy of donepezil in the treatment of neuropsychiatric symptoms in Alzheimer's disease. *Neurology* 2004;63:214–219.

Kirshner HS (2005). Mild Cognitive Impairment: To Treat or Not to Treat. *Curr Neurol Neurosci Rep*, 5:455–457.

Klunk WE, Engler H, Norberg A, et al.: Imaging brain amyloid in Alzheimer's disease with pittsburgh Compound-B. *Ann Neurol* 2004;55:306–319.

Knopman DS, DeKosky ST, Cummings JL, et al.: Practice parameter: Diagnosis of dementia (an evidence-based review). *Neurology* 2001;56:1143–1153.

Petersen RC, Stevens JC, Ganguli M, et al.: Practice parameter: Early detection of dementia: Mild cognitive impairment (an evidence-based review). *Neurology* 2001;56:1133–1142.

Rogaeva E, Meng Y, Lee JH, et al.: The neuronal sortilin-related receptor SORL1 is genetically associated with Alzheimer disease. *Nat Genet* 2007;39:168–177.

Roses AD: Apolipoprotein E affects the rate of Alzheimer disease expression: β-amyloid burden is a secondary consequence dependent on APO E genotype and duration of disease. *J Neuropathol Exp Neurol* 1994;53:429.

Schneider LS, Olin JT: Overview of clinical trials of hydergine in dementia. *Arch Neurol* 1994;51:787.

Schneider LS, Tariot PN, Dagerman KS, et al.: Effectiveness of atypical antipsychotic drugs in patients with Alzheimer's disease. *N Engl J Med* 2006;355:1528–1538.

Sink KM, Holden KF, Yaffe K: Pharmacological treatment of neuropsychiatric symptoms of dementia. A review of the evidence. *JAMA* 2005;293:596–608.

Small GW, et al.: Diagnosis and treatment of Alzheimer disease and related disorders. Consensus statement of the American Association for geriatric psychiatry, the Alzheimer's association, and the American geriatrics society. *J Am Med Assoc* 1997;278: 1363.

Small GW, Leiter F: Neuroimaging for diagnosis of dementia. *J Clin Psychiatry* 1998;59(Suppl 11):4.

Wang PS, Schneeweiss S, Avorn J, et al.: Risk of death in elderly users of conventional vs. atypical antipsychotic medications. *N Engl J Med* 2005;353:2335–2341.

Winblad B, Kilander L, Eriksson S, et al.: Donepizil in patients with severe Alzheimer's disease: Double-blind, parallel-group, placebo-controlled study. *Lancet* 2006;367:1057–1065.

Wolfe MS. Shutting down Alzheimer's. *Sci Am* 2006;73–79.

Yankner BA, et al.: Neurotoxicity of a fragment of the amyloid precursor associated with Alzheimer's disease. *Science* 1989;245:417.

2. *Frontotemporal Dementia*

 ESSENTIALS OF DIAGNOSIS

- *FTDs represent a cluster of related disorders associated with degeneration of the frontal and temporal lobes. These disorders differ from AD primarily in the presentation with focal symptoms such as frontal lobe dysfunction or aphasia, rather than memory loss. In the frontal lobe variants of this disorder, personality changes usually precede or overshadow the patient's cognitive problems. Many patients become apathetic and stop caring about hygiene or social involvement. Others become disinhibited or impulsive. Sexual inappropriateness is common. Executive functions such as planning and judgment may also be abnormal in some patients. Alternatively, patients may tend to exhibit anger, irritability, and even mania. In rare cases, the Klüver-Bucy syndrome may develop with hyperorality, hypersexuality, and a compulsion to attend to any visual stimulus; this syndrome is associated with bilateral temporal lobe pathology. These patients also have impaired visual object recognition. Many FTD patients present with progressive aphasia. In the U.S., these patients have been referred to under the diagnosis "primary progressive aphasia." The term "FTD" is now considered a more general category, of which primary progressive aphasia is one subtype.*

- *The variety of presentations is the result of the segmental nature of the pathology. Some areas of the frontal lobe may be devastated, whereas adjacent areas may be entirely normal. Therefore, any behavioral syndrome compatible with damage to a specific frontal region is possible.*

General Considerations

FTDs represent about 10% of degenerative dementias. About 40% of patients with these disorders have a family history of dementia, which suggests dominantly inher-

ited illness. Other risk factors include electroconvulsive therapy (ECT) and alcoholism. Pick's disease is historically the most recognized frontal lobe dementia. It is often familial.

Clinical Findings

A. Signs and Symptoms

FTDs are pathologically heterogeneous conditions. Only rare patients with this type of presentation have AD, and those represent primarily patients who present with fluent aphasia. One variant is "semantic dementia," in which patients not only become unable to name objects, but they lose the meaning of words said to them. These patients have either AD or one of the other variants of FTD at autopsy. Most FTD cases have a lobar atrophy pattern involving one or both frontal and temporal lobes. The microscopic pathology is variable. Some have intraneuronal, intracytoplasmic, silver-staining inclusions called Pick bodies; these cases are traditionally diagnosed as "Pick's disease". In some patients, neuropathologic evaluation shows no specific histopathologic changes, other than neuronal loss, microvacuolation of the neuropil, and gliosis. Many of these patients have abnormal tau proteins within neurofibrillary tangles. These disorders are often familial, and several gene mutations involving the tau gene on Chromosome 17 have been described. Some families have been described with features of progressive aphasia, FTD, and Parkinsonism. Other cases are tau-negative, but ubiquitin-positive. In other patients, frontal lobe dementia occurs simultaneously with lower motor neuron disease as in amyotrophic lateral sclerosis. The genetic and molecular biogical characterization of these variants of FTD is an active field of research at present.

Core features of frontal lobe dementias include insidious onset and gradual progression. There is early decline in social interpersonal conduct. Emotional blunting and apathy also occurs early without insight. There's a marked decline in personal hygiene and significant distractibility and motor impersistence (failure to maintain a motor activity). In the types associated with aphasia, language is affected more significantly than personality.

Personality change, lack of insight, and poor judgment dominate the early stages of frontal lobe dementias. Frontal lobe dementias cause patients to be apathetic when medial frontal damage occurs and disinhibited when basal-frontal dysfunction predominates. Social withdrawal and behavioral disinhibition may precede the onset of dementia by several years. Sometimes memory is impaired, but attention, language, and visuospatial skills are spared.

In patients whose frontal lobe dementia primarily affects frontal language, loss of spontaneity of speech is often the first noticeable symptom. Selective language defects may occur in the absence of significant cognitive decline. In these patients, the clinical picture resembles a progressive aphasia.

Most patients with frontal lobe dementias lack drive and motivation. Others are tactless or insensitive in the early stages of the illness. Some patients develop symptoms of Klüver-Bucy syndrome with hypersexuality and hyperorality, going on later to exhibit perseverative speech, apathy, or stereotyped behavior. The memory disorder of frontal lobe dementias is more prominent concerning recently acquired material. Remote memory remains intact until later in the disease. Behavioral symptoms are usually more prominent in frontal lobe dementias, whereas parietal lobe symptoms such as receptive aphasia and agnosia are less common.

B. Psychological Testing

On psychological testing, patients exhibit features consistent with frontal lobe dysfunction. Useful tests include the Wisconsin Card Sorting Test, the Stroop Test, another test in which the subject is asked to list words beginning with the letters F, A, and S (FAS test) and the response is timed, the Trail Making Test, and other tests designed to ferret out frontal lobe dysfunction. Some measures of aphasia should also be included in the neuropsychological test battery.

C. Laboratory Findings and Imaging

In classic cases of Pick's disease, the patient's brain exhibits marked atrophy of the frontal and temporal lobes, resulting in a knife-like appearance of the gyri. MRI may show a dramatic frontal pole or temporal pole atrophy that clearly differentiates Pick's and other frontal lobe dementias from the pattern of temporoparietal atrophy seen in Alzheimer's patients. In frontal lobe dementias, the EEG may remain normal despite severe pathology. PET and SPECT imaging also show the focal, lobar nature of the degeneration.

PET scans in patients with Pick's disease show bilateral frontal hypometabolism without temporoparietal defects. These findings are not always observed in early Pick's disease. In some patients the findings may be unilateral. In cases with progressive aphasia, left frontal and temporal hypometabolism or hypoperfusion are evident.

At a microscopic level, cell loss is particularly marked in the outer layers of the cortex. Degenerating neurons may have Pick's bodies. The structural changes of AD, including amyloid plaques and tangles, are entirely lacking. Frontal lobe dementias are not associated with Lewy bodies, however, areas of spongiform degeneration, similar to those found in Creutzfeldt-Jakob disease, may be observed. The pathology is patchy: Some frontal lobe areas remain normal. From a histopathologic point of view, frontal lobe dementia (Pick's disease) is characterized by gliosis, microvacuolation, neuronal atrophy loss, and 40–50% loss of synapses in three superficial cortical

laminae of the frontal convexity and anterior temporal cortex. The deeper laminae are little changed.

Differential Diagnosis

Other conditions can present with frontal lobe behaviors and dementia, for example, vascular dementias, normal pressure hydrocephalus, Huntington's disease, and mass lesions. Butterfly gliomas are particularly likely to present with pure frontal lobe behaviors and dementia. Frontal lobe dementias can also be confused with personality disorder, mania, and depression. This is particularly true early in the course of the illness when the cognitive involvement is minimal.

Treatment

Treatment of frontal lobe dementias is limited to psychosocial interventions, such as protecting the patient from his or her indiscretions, and symptomatic psychiatric treatment. At times an associated depression occurs. Treatment of this depression with SSRIs may be helpful. Psychostimulants, such as methylphenidate, may help motivate apathetic patients. Carbamazepine may be helpful for Klüver-Bucy syndrome by reducing the frequency of behaviors. Olanzapine may be helpful when extreme disinhibition occurs. In patients with memory disorder, donepezil may be helpful, but no treatment trials have confirmed a benefit of either anticholinesterase medications or memantine in FTDs, and it is not clear that degeneration of the cholinergic system is prominent in this condition.

Prognosis

FTDs often have primarily a presenile onset. Progression is quite variable but, generally speaking, slow. Memory functions may be retained until later in the illness. Patients with frontal lobe dementias can later develop motor neuron disease, although the clinical features of motor neuron disease may accompany or occasionally precede the onset of dementia.

Diehl J, Grimmer T, Drzezga A, et al.: Cerebral metabolic patterns at early stages of frontotemporal dementia and semantic dementia. A PET study. *Neurobiol Aging* 2004;25:1051–1056.

Grossman M, Mickanin J, Onishi K, et al.: Progressive nonfluent aphasia: Language, cognitive, and PET measures contrasted with probable Alzheimer's disease. *J Cog Neurosci* 1996;8:135–154.

Heutink P, Stevens M, Rizzu P, et al.: Hereditary frontotemporal dementia is linked to Chromosome 17q21–q22; a genetic and clinicopathological study of three Dutch families. *Ann Neurol* 1997;41:150–159.

Hodges JR, Davies RR, Xuereb JH, et al.: Clinicopathological correlates in frontotemporal dementia. *Ann Neurol* 2004;56:399–406.

Hodges JR, Patterson K, Oxbury S, Funnell E. Semantic dementia. Progressive fluent aphasia with temporal lobe atrophy. *Brain* 1992;115:1783–1806.

Huey ED, Putnam KT, Grafman J: A systematic review of neurotransmitter deficits and treatments in frontotemporal dementia. *Neurology* 2006;66:17–22.

Kertesz A, Munoz DG: Primary progressive aphasia and pick complex. *J Neurol Sci* 2003;206:97–107.

Kirshner HS, Tanridag O, Thurman L, Whetsell WO, Jr.: Progressive aphasia without dementia: Two cases with focal, spongiform degeneration. *Ann Neurol* 1987;22:527–532.

Lebert F, Stekke W, Hasenbroekx C, et al.: Frontotemporal dementia: A randomized, controlled trial with trazodone. *Dement Geriatr Cogn Disord* 2004;17:355–359.

Mesulam MM: Primary progressive aphasia. *Ann Neurol* 2001;49: 425–432.

Mesulam MM: Primary progressive aphasia—a language-based dementia. *N Engl J Med* 2003;349:1535–1542.

Neary D, et al.: Frontotemporal lobar degeneration: A consensus on clinical diagnostic criteria. *Neurology* 1998;51:1546.

Sonty SP, Mesulam MM, Thompson CK, et al.: Primary progressive aphasia: PPA and the language network. *Ann Neurol* 2003;53: 35–49.

3. Lewy Body Dementia

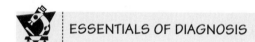 ESSENTIALS OF DIAGNOSIS

Lewy bodies are cytoplasmic inclusions seen in the neurons of the substantia nigra and other pigmented nuclei in patients with PD. In recent years, similar neuronal inclusions have been discovered in cortical neurons in patients with dementia. The term "Lewy body dementia" refers to patients who present with dementia symptoms before or simultaneously with motor disturbances suggestive of PD. Patients with Lewy body disease typically demonstrate fluctuating cognitive impairment, with active confusion and hallucinations, in addition to deterioration of memory and higher cortical functions. This fluctuating, delirium-like presentation distinguishes this disorder from AD. Associated features include visual or auditory hallucinations, mild extrapyramidal signs, or repeated and unexplained falls. Autonomic findings are common, and diffuse Lewy body disease may present as part of the multiple systems atrophy or Shy-Drager syndrome. The illness progresses at a variable rate to an end stage of severe dementia. Vascular dementias and other physical illness must be excluded.

General Considerations

The prevalence of diffuse Lewy body disease may have been underestimated in the past because of the difficulty of making the neuropathologic diagnosis. Lewy bodies may occur in the cortex or in subcortical regions. They may also be intermixed with plaques and tangles. When Lewy bodies occur together with the pathology of AD, the term Lewy body variant of AD is used. This condition is also referred to as the common form of Lewy body disease. The pure form of Lewy body disease lacks Alzheimer's pathologic features. This form is sometimes referred to as diffuse Lewy body disease. Both disorders are included in the more general term Lewy body dementia. Diffuse Lewy body disease may underlie the dementia associated with PD, but many such cases have AD pathology at autopsy.

A. EPIDEMIOLOGY

The disease represents approximately 15% of dementias seen at autopsy. The age at onset is somewhat earlier than Alzheimer's and shows a greater degree of variability. There is substantial overlap with AD, and many patients exhibit mixed pathology. The mean age at onset is 68 and at death is 75 years. Men are affected more often than women.

B. GENETICS

The ApoE E4 allele is over-represented in patients with Lewy body disease. The mutant allele of *CYP2D6B* is a risk factor for both PD and Lewy body disease. This gene encodes an enzyme that is involved in detoxifying environmental toxins. The mutation eliminates the active form of the enzyme.

Clinical Findings

A. SIGNS AND SYMPTOMS

In the early stages of diffuse Lewy body disease, memory loss, inattention, and difficulty in sustaining a train of thought are characteristic. Psychiatric signs are prominent in many patients with diffuse Lewy body disease and may be the first indication of the disorder. Psychiatric symptoms include personality change, depression, hallucinations, or delusions. Weight loss is common. Extrapyramidal signs are less severe in diffuse Lewy body disease than in PD. Bradykinesia is more common than the tremor. Sometimes extrapyramidal signs are limited to the patient's gait. The anatomic location of the Lewy bodies explains some characteristics of the disorder. Diffuse Lewy body disease affects both cholinergic and dopaminergic systems.

B. PSYCHOLOGICAL TESTING

Patients with diffuse Lewy body disease present with both cortical and subcortical neuropsychological findings. The subcortical features distinguish the condition from AD. Although not a pure subcortical dementia, diffuse Lewy body disease has prominent subcortical features.

The primary symptoms of subcortical dementias include forgetfulness, slowed thinking, and apathy. In addition, the patient's ability to manage information efficiently is reduced. Executive functions are also diminished. Memory is more disturbed for free recall than recognition. Patients with subcortical dementias are unable to profit from feedback because of poor concentration and inability to maintain set. They have difficulty sequencing and conceptualizing ideas. Another symptom is perseveration. Memory problems and visual spatial disturbances are also common but are not as severe as in AD. Subcortical dementias differ from AD in that the former are not associated with aphasia, recognition deficits, and denial of illness.

C. Laboratory Findings and Imaging

The hallmark of diffuse Lewy body disease is extensive Lewy body formation in the neocortex. The severity of dementia is related to the density of cortical Lewy bodies. Lewy bodies are usually found in the pigmented neurons of the substantia nigra in PD. Cortical Lewy bodies are much easier to overlook. Staining with anti-ubiquitin antibodies simplifies identification and increases the recognition of diffuse Lewy body disease. In contrast, Alz-50 immunoreactivity is small or nonexistent.

The EEG can be helpful in distinguishing between diffuse Lewy body disease and AD. Diffuse slowing and frontal intermittent delta activity are common in Lewy body disease. Significant slowing and frontal intermittent rhythmic delta are not usually present in early AD, however, slowing of the background EEG does occur in vascular dementias. Vascular dementias, particularly those caused by stroke, are likely to demonstrate focal EEG changes consistent with the underlying structural damage. Focal EEG findings are not consistent with either diffuse Lewy body disease or AD. Even though the EEG may provide useful information, EEG alone cannot reliably differentiate vascular dementias from AD or diffuse Lewy body disease.

Differential Diagnosis

A noninvasive diagnostic test does not exist for Lewy body disease. The most distinctive feature of the disease is the delirium-like episodes with psychotic features that occur and then remit spontaneously. Diffuse Lewy body disease shares some features with progressive supranuclear palsy, FTD, PD, AD, and normal pressure hydrocephalus. The dementia caused by the later stages of small vessel disease may also bear a striking resemblance to Lewy body dementia. Late-life psychosis, delirium, syncope, and drug toxicity must also be considered.

Treatment

Because diffuse Lewy body disease affects neocortical dopamine systems, typical neuroleptic treatment of the psychiatric symptoms is usually not successful and can produce significant extrapyramidal side effects. Severe and often fatal neuroleptic sensitivity may occur in some elderly patients with dementia of the Lewy body type. Neuroleptic sensitivity may be manifested as neuroleptic malignant syndrome. Although the typical neuroleptics are not well tolerated, atypical neuroleptics such as olanzapine, clozapine, or quetiapine may produce significant antipsychotic effect without serious side effects.

The response to L-dopa is less dramatic than in other Parkinson's syndromes. Higher doses of L-dopa often produce or aggravate psychosis, and this is even more true of dopamine agonist drugs such as pramipexole or ropinirole. In contrast, depression is treatable and responds readily to antidepressant agents, often with a corresponding improvement in cognition. Antidepressants that cause orthostasis should be avoided. Some patients may need fludrocortisone to support blood pressure. Anticholinesterase agents may be of benefit for the memory disorder of Lewy body dementia; rivastigmine has recently been approved by the USFDA for the treatment of patients with PD and dementia. Neuroprotective agents such as vitamin E or selegiline may be tried, but there is no proof of their benefit.

Prognosis

Diffuse Lewy body disease has quite a variable course but generally progresses more rapidly than AD. The average time from diagnosis to death is approximately 6 years. The disease often presents as a psychiatric condition because of the strange and complex hallucinations and delusions. The psychiatric symptoms occur much earlier in the course of diffuse Lewy body disease than in AD. Cardinal features of fully developed Lewy body dementia include delirium, hallucinatory-delusional states, disturbed behavior, akinesia, rigidity, and orthostatic hypotension. Aphasia is notably absent. Although the cognitive impairment is progressive, there is marked daily variability. As the disease progresses, parkinsonian signs may become more severe. Involuntary movements, myoclonus, quadriparesis in flexion, and dysphagia (difficulty swallowing) occur in the final stages.

Bonanni L, Thomas A, Onofrj M: Diagnosis and management of dementia with lewy bodies: Third report of the DLB consortium. *Neurology* 2006;66:1455.

Emre M, Aarsland D, Albanese A, et al.: Rivastigmine for dementia associated with Parkinson's disease. *N Engl J Med* 2004; 351:2509–2518.

Filley CM: Neuropsychiatric features of Lewy body disease. *Brain Cogn* 1995;28:229–239.

Karla S, Bergeron C, Lang AE: Lewy body disease and dementia. *Arch Intern Med* 1996;156:487.

McKeith I, et al.: Neuroleptic sensitivity in patients with senile dementia of Lewy body type [see comments]. *Br Med J* 1992;305:673.

McKeith I, Del Ser T, Spano P: Efficacy of rivastigmine in dementia with Lewy bodies: A randomized, double-blind, placebo-controlled international study. *Lancet* 2000;356:2031–2036.

Schmidt ML, et al.: Epitope map of neurofilament protein domains in cortical and peripheral nervous system Lewy bodies. *Am J Pathol* 1991;139:53.

4. *Subcortical Dementias*

 ESSENTIALS OF DIAGNOSIS

Patients with subcortical dementias have a diagnosed disorder of deeper brain structures in the presence of a relatively unaffected cerebral cortex. These patients have problems with arousal, attention, mood, motivation, language, and memory. Subcortical dementias may occur in PD, Huntington's disease, progressive supranuclear palsy, cortical basal ganglia degeneration (now called corticobasal degeneration), Hallervorden-Spatz disease, idiopathic basal ganglia calcification, and the spinocerebellar degenerations. Subcortical dementias have also been identified in inflammatory, infectious, vascular, and demyelinating illness.

General Considerations

The concept of subcortical dementias unifies conceptually those conditions affecting the relationship of deeper structures to the cortex. In subcortical dementias, cerebral cortical functioning is relatively intact, but the basal ganglia are dysfunctional or disconnected. Subcortical dementias are not entirely homogeneous entities, and specific features will depend on the pathologic causes. Thus the features of the cognitive disorder observed in PD are not exactly the same as that seen in Huntington's disease or in progressive supranuclear palsy.

A. EPIDEMIOLOGY

Estimates of the prevalence of dementia in Parkinson's patients depends on the population studied and criteria used. Estimates ranging from 30% to 50% have frequently been reported, but if neuropsychological testing criteria are used, prevalence may reach 90%. The overall prevalence rate of PD with dementia is estimated to be about 40 per 100,000.

The prevalence of Huntington's disease is about six per 100,000. Dementia is a ubiquitous feature of Huntington's disease, but the severity of impairment varies greatly among patients. There are other degenerative diseases of the basal ganglia frontal circuits that lead to subcortical dementia. Progressive supranuclear palsy, the disease in which subcortical dementia was first described, is less common than PD. Striatonigral degeneration and corticobasal degeneration can also cause subcortical dementia, though corticobasal degeneration also affects cortical structures and often presents with language and cognitive deficits. Corticobasal degeneration is associated with tau protein abnormalities and often overlaps with the FTD syndrome. Parkinsonism and apraxia of one upper limb are associated symptoms. These entities are more widely recognized with improved diagnostic techniques.

B. ETIOLOGY

Subcortical dementias involve primarily the thalamus, basal ganglia, and related brainstem nuclei with relative sparing of the cerebral cortex. Patients with basal ganglia disease or with disease affecting basal ganglia frontal circuits develop subcortical dementias. PD is always associated with neuronal loss in the substantia nigra, leading to destruction of dopaminergic connections to the basal ganglia. As a result, subcortico–cortical pathways function defectively. Striatal dopamine depletion disrupts the normal pattern of basal ganglia function in PD and, consequently, interrupts normal transmission of information through frontostriatal circuitry. Dopaminergic transmission, along the nigrostriatal pathway, may be implicated in sustaining various cognitive and motor processes.

In addition, neuronal loss occurs throughout the CNS. Patients with dementia due to PD have significant cell loss in many other CNS structures, particularly in the basal nucleus of Meynert. The depletion of acetylcholine in the cortex is less severe than in AD. There is significant damage to the locus coeruleus, secondary loss of cortical norepinephrine, and cell loss in the raphe nucleus leading to serotonin depletion. This may explain the anxiety and depression so commonly associated with PD.

C. GENETICS

Huntington's disease has an autosomal dominant mode of inheritance. An excess number of CAG trinucleotide repeats in the 5′-translated region of chromosome 4 causes Huntington's disease. A DNA test can detect the gene before symptoms appear. Virtually 100% of patients with more than 40 repeats of the gene will manifest the disease at some point in their lives, however, the age at which the disease manifests itself is quite variable. Huntington's disease exhibits an earlier onset in successive generations of a pedigree, especially when transmitted through the father. There is greater variability of repeat length with paternal transmission, and the gene tends to have everincreasing CAG repeats. The change in repeat length with paternal transmission is correlated significantly with decreasing age at onset between the father and offspring.

The genetics of progressive supranuclear palsy have recently been clarified. Studies suggest that progressive supranuclear palsy is an autosomal recessive condition that maps to a polymorphism in the tau gene. It has been reported that a genetic variant of tau, known as the A0 allele, was represented excessively in patients with progressive supranuclear palsy in comparison to control subjects. A highly significant overrepresentation of the A0/A0 genotype and a decrease in the frequency of the A0/A3 genotype were found in patients with progressive supranuclear palsy. The presence of the tau A0/A0 genotype is a risk factor for developing the disorder, whereas A3 may be protective. PSP, made famous by the comedian and actor Dudley Moore, is also a tauopathy.

Hallervorden-Spatz syndrome is a rare, autosomal recessive neurodegenerative disorder in which iron accumulates in the basal ganglia. Extrapyramidal signs are dominant and include dystonia. Mental deterioration occurs as the disease progresses. MRI reveals marked overall low signal from the globus pallidus.

The genetics of PD are extremely complex and reflect the fact that the disorder has multiple etiologies. Several genes have been discovered in families with more than one member with PD; to date, these genetic types of PD account for less than 10% of the cases. There may be genetic factors influencing susceptibility to PD. In addition, it has long been believed that PD represents an interaction between genetic and environmental factors. A large twin study also suggests that genetic influences are less important in patients with disease beginning after the age of 50 years. In contrast, genetic influences are larger in earlier-onset disease.

Several purely genetic forms of PD have been identified. The *g209a* mutation in the *alpha-synuclein* gene has been associated with autosomal dominant PD in a number of families. Other gene loci have been reported. Different mutations in the microtubule-associated tau protein gene have been identified in several families with hereditary FTD and Parkinsonism (*ftdp-17*) linked to chromosome 17q21–22. Another gene, *Gstp1–1*, expressed in the blood–brain barrier, may influence response to neurotoxins and explain the susceptibility of some people to the parkinsonism-inducing effects of pesticides. The dopamine receptor gene has also been implicated in PD. Autosomal recessive juvenile parkinsonism and early-onset parkinsonism with diurnal fluctuation are other forms of PD with relatively clear genetic causes.

Clinical Findings

In contrast to cortical dementias such as AD, subcortical dementias are relatively circumscribed syndromes. The principal features of subcortical dementias include slowed mentation, impairment of executive function, recall abnormalities, and visuospatial disturbances. Recall is better than in AD, and overall memory impairment is not as severe. At each functional stage, patients with subcortical dementias are less intellectually impaired than are patients with AD. Subcortical dementias do not involve aphasia, agnosia, or apraxia.

Subcortical dementias may constitute a group of partially treatable forms of dementia. Subcortical dementias create a cognitive picture similar to that of major affective disorder. Moreover, if the patient becomes depressed, his or her cognitive abilities are reduced even further. Psychiatric consultation may be obtained to treat depression and apathy. Depression aggravates the memory and language impairments associated with subcortical dementias. Antidepressants may improve cognition in subcortical syndromes. Specific subtypes of cognitive impairment are related directly to the neuropathology of each disease. In progressive supranuclear palsy, behavioral and cognitive changes resemble those associated with lesions of the frontal lobes.

Symptoms of subcortical dementias may respond to psychotropic medication. Mood disorders are extremely common in subcortical dementias and may respond to antidepressants. Sometimes the cognitive deficits improve along with the mood disorder. The response of psychotic symptoms to neuroleptics is more variable. The choice of neuroleptic must be thought out more carefully. Antipsychotics may be required to control psychotic symptoms and agitation, however, many of these patients have associated movement disorders and antipsychotics may affect motor symptoms in either a positive or a negative manner depending on the specific movement disorder.

The dementias associated with PD and Huntington's disease are discussed in detail in the sections that follow. Normal pressure hydrocephalus and AIDS dementia complex also present as subcortical dementias, but will be discussed in later sections.

DEMENTIA DUE TO PD

Clinical Findings

A. SIGNS AND SYMPTOMS

Cognitive changes, particularly mild impairment in memory, executive functions, attention, and information processing, occur early in Parkinson's disease. The time required to make decisions is prolonged. These effects are more noticeable if the primary symptoms are bradykinesia and rigidity. Patients who complain primarily of tremors have fewer cognitive abnormalities.

Some Parkinson's patients have only a subcortical dementia. Others are more seriously mentally impaired, and these patients appear to have either cortical Lewy bodies or plaques and tangles, suggesting AD. These patients also differ from others with the disorder in that they present a more marked severity of the extrapyramidal syndrome with predominant bradykinesia and an earlier deteriorating response to L-dopa treatment. The presence of dysphasia or other cortical deficits early in the course of the illness suggests the presence of coexisting AD. These patients are also more likely to develop a significant depression early in the course of the illness. In the presence of depression, Parkinson's patients are more likely to develop a cognitive disorder that persists even when the depression is treated.

B. PSYCHOLOGICAL TESTING

Very early in the disease course, Parkinson's patients demonstrate mild impairment on tests sensitive to information processing speed, maintaining set, and visuospatial discrimination. Neuropsychological tests suggest that an underlying perceptual motor deficit exists in PD. Personality changes occur early whereas recall abnormalities and apathy tend to occur later. These subtle cognitive difficulties might underlie the mental inflexibility and rigidity associated with PD and could be attributed to destruction of the ascending dopaminergic and mesocorticolimbic pathway.

Parkinson's patients whose disease develops relatively late in life are prone to develop comorbid dementing illness such as AD, diffuse Lewy body disease, or vascular dementia. Neuropsychological testing can help determine whether these patients are developing a mixed syndrome, sometimes referred to as Parkinson's plus.

C. LABORATORY FINDINGS AND IMAGING

PET scans using [18F]fluorodeoxyglucose will often show hypofrontality in nondemented Parkinson's patients or in those with mild subcortical dementia. The presence of bilateral temporoparietal deficits in addition to hypofrontality suggests the coexistence of either Lewy body disease or AD.

PET scans can be used to examine glucose metabolism through the use of [18F] fluorodeoxyglucose and to examine dopamine metabolic patterns through the use of [18F] fluorodopa. [11C] raclopride can be used to examine dopamine D_2 receptor binding; this ligand is not routinely available in clinical practice. These techniques hold promise for future diagnostic clarification.

In Parkinson's patients, SPECT scans demonstrate decreased frontal lobe blood flow that is more significant on the left side than on the right. Basal ganglia decrements are also visible. These changes appear to be particularly accentuated in the early stages of PD with subcortical dementia. SPECT binding studies demonstrate decreased basal ganglia binding in demented Parkinson's patients compared to nondemented Parkinson's patients. Bilateral temporoparietal deficits probably indicate concomitant AD.

NMR spectroscopy indicates an increase in cerebral lactate in patients with PD, especially in those with dementia. Finally, evoked potential studies indicate some difference between Parkinson's patients with and without dementia. Reaction time is prolonged in both groups of patients. The event-related P300 evoked potential is normal in nondemented Parkinson's patients but is prolonged in demented Parkinson's patients. Visual evoked potentials show an increased latency of P100 in demented Parkinson's patients compared to nondemented Parkinson's patients.

Differential Diagnosis

PD with subcortical dementia must be distinguished first from PD with coexisting Alzheimer's or diffuse Lewy body disease. Functional imaging may help. Other conditions to consider include vascular dementias and other parkinsonian syndromes such as progressive supranuclear palsy.

Treatment

Many medications affect cognition in PD patients. As a rule, anticholinergic medication impairs cognition, whereas dopaminergic medication may mildly enhance it. The dosage of dopaminergic medication is important, because at higher dosages patients may become confused or hallucinate. Levodopa–carbidopa or direct dopamine agonists such as pramipexole and ropinirole are the standard initial treatments for PD. Neuroleptics may cause significant rigidity in patients with PD or diffuse Lewy body dementia. Atypical neuroleptics are usually preferred in these patients because standard neuroleptics cause extrapyramidal side effects, tardive dyskinesia, and neuroleptic malignant syndrome. Clozapine or quetiapine may be preferred neuroleptics for patients with subcortical dementias because these atypical agents may improve psychotic symptoms without adverse motor effects.

ECT has been used in the management of psychiatric complications in PD. Not only do affective symptoms respond, but motor symptoms improve. Unfortunately patients with dementia due to PD may develop post-ECT delirium. Nonetheless, ECT remains an occasionally used treatment for intractable depression associated with PD. The dosage of antidepressant or number of ECT treatments should be considered together with anti-parkinsonian therapies. Demented parkinsonian patients often experience side effects after taking anti-parkinsonian medication. As a result, the clinician should be inclined to treat the motor symptoms conservatively in order to minimize cognitive side effects. The use of rivastigmine for dementia associated with PD was discussed above, under Lewy body dementia.

Prognosis

Patients with PD who become demented are older, have a longer duration of disease, and a later age at onset than those who do not become demented. Age is the biggest risk factor. The development of dementia is strongly related to the age at which the patient developed motor manifestations. In some patients, cortical Lewy bodies cause the dementia. Although most patients with PD do not have AD, some Parkinson's patients have dementia that is due to the coexistence of AD. The dual diagnosis of Parkinson's and AD is associated with a particularly poor prognosis.

The cognitive deficits evident in early PD do not progress to dementia in all patients. When dementia does develop, the symptoms are quite heterogeneous. Patients with Parkinson's dementia have a great deal of difficulty with tasks that involve visual and spatial orientation. Intellectual ability begins a global decline in PD with dementia, but memory is more severely impaired than are language and other cortical functions. Episodic memory (i.e., memory for items relating to date and time) is especially distorted. Although the patient can drive an automobile, decline in spatial memory may make following directions difficult and slowed reaction time makes driving dangerous.

The association between depression and PD has been recognized for more than 150 years. Depression affects up to 50% of Parkinson's patients and is more pronounced during the early stages of the illness. Affective disorder aggravates the poor concentration and impaired information processing associated with PD. The treatment of depression tends to improve some of these cognitive deficiencies.

Christine CW, Aminoff MJ: Clinical differentiation of Parkinsonian syndromes: Prognostic and therapeutic relevance. *Am J Med* 2004;117:412–419.

Cummings JL: Depression and Parkinson's disease: A review. *Am J Psychiatry* 1992;149:443.

Eskandar EN, Cosgrove GR, Shinobu SA: Surgical treatment of Parkinson's disease. *JAMA* 2001;286:3056–3059.

Feany MB: New genetic insights into Parkinson's disease. *New Engl J Med* 2004;351:1937–1940.

Freed CR, Greene PE, Breeze RE, et al.: Transplantation of embryonic dopamine neurons for severe Parkinson's disease. *N Engl J Med* 2001;344:710–719.

Lang AE, Lozano AM: Parkinson's disease. First of two parts. *New Engl J Med* 1998;339:1044–1053.

Lang AE, Lozano AM: Parkinson's disease. Second of two parts. *New Engl J Med* 1998;339:1130–1143.

Miyasaki JM, Martin W, Suchowersky O, et al.: Practice parameter: Initiation of treatment for Parkinson's disease: An evidence-based review: Report of the quality standards subcommittee of the American Academy of neurology. *Neurology* 2002;58:11–17.

Nutt JG, Wooten GF: Diagnosis and initial management of Parkinson's disease. *N Engl J Med* 2005;353:1021–1027.

Schapira AH, Olanow CW: Neuroprotection in Parkinson disease. Mysteries, myths, and misconceptions. *JAMA* 2004;291:358–364.

The Deep-Brain Stimulation for Parkinson's Disease Study Group. Deep-brain stimulation of the subthalamic nucleus or the pars interna of the globus pallidus in Parkinson's disease. *New Engl J Med* 2001;345:956–963.

Lewy Body Dementia

Aarsland D, Perry R, Brown A, et al.: Neuropathology of dementia in Parkinson's disease: A prospective, community-based study. *Ann Neurol* 2005;58:773–6.

Cummings JL: Lewy body diseases with dementia: Pathophysiology and treatment. *Brain Cogn* 1995;28:266–280.

Poewe W: Treatment of dementia with Lewy bodies and Parkinson's disease dementia. *Mov Disord* 2005;20(Suppl 12):S77–S82.

Progressive Supranuclear Palsy

Daniel SE, deBruin VM, Lees AJ: The clinical and pathological spectrum of Steele-Richardson-Olszewski syndrome (progressive supranuclear palsy): A reappraisal. *Brain* 1995;118:759–770.

Litvan I, Campbell G, Mangone CA, et al.: Which clinical features differentiate progressive supranuclear palsy (Steele-Richardson-Olszewski syndrome) from related disorders? A clinicopathological study. *Brain* 1997;120:65–74.

Multisystem Atrophy

Mark MH: Lumping and splitting the Parkinson plus syndromes: Dementia with Lewy bodies, multiple system atrophy, progressive supranuclear palsy, and cortical-basal ganglionic degeneration. *Neurol Clin* 2001;19:607–627.

Wenning GK, Colosimo C, Geser F, Poewe W: Multiple system atrophy. *Lancet Neurol* 2004;3:93–103.

Corticobasal Degeneration

Bergeron C, Pollanen MS, Weyer L, et al.: Unusual clinical presentations of cortical-basal ganglionic degeneration. *Ann Neurol* 1996;40:893–900.

Gibb WRG, Luthert PJ, Marsden CD: Corticobasal degeneration. *Brain* 1989;112:1171–1192.

Litvan I, Cummings JL, Mega M: Neuropsychiatric features of corticobasal degeneration. *J Neurol Neurosurg Psychiatry* 1998;65:717–721.

DEMENTIA DUE TO HUNTINGTON'S DISEASE

Clinical Findings

A. SIGNS AND SYMPTOMS

Huntington's disease often has a delayed onset, with a mean age at onset of about 40 years. Progressive cognitive decline is a cardinal feature of Huntington's disease, however, mild deficits in cognitive function are an early finding. Severe mental deterioration is apparent later in the disease. The onset is proportional to the number of cytosine-adenine-guanine (CAG) repeats in the Huntington's disease allele, although the degree of cognitive deficit is not proportional to the number of CAG repeats but rather to chronicity of the illness.

Huntington's disease usually presents with choreiform movements, but it can present as incipient dementia or depression. As the disease progresses, all patients become demented. The cognitive changes are quite varied, even in the late stages of the illness.

The dementia develops slowly and is consistent with damage to pathways linking the frontal areas to the striatum. Prominent complaints are apathy, slow information processing, and problems in maintaining attention. Difficulty with attention and concentration is more pronounced than in PD. Compared to patients with AD, those with Huntington's disease have less memory impairment. Cortical symptoms such as aphasia, agnosia, and apraxia are less common in Huntington's than in AD.

Most patients with Huntington's disease develop prominent psychiatric symptoms. Depression is the most common symptom, but up to 10% of patients have symptoms resembling bipolar disorder. Irritability, personality change, and other behavioral problems are also common. Frontal lobe impairment results in poor judgment that may lead to embarrassing or even illegal activities. A paranoid psychosis is common in Huntington's patients.

B. PSYCHOLOGICAL TESTING

Huntington's patients initially show difficulty with attention tasks. Other early deficits include psychomotor speed and the ability to shift set. Go/no-go tasks are impaired early as are other tasks that require internal cues. Huntington's patients are unable to maintain divided attention and to perform tasks in which multimodal sensory information is provided. When compared to Alzheimer's patients, Huntington's patients demonstrate greater impairment on the initiation/perseveration subscale of the DRS. Alzheimer's patients demonstrate greater impairment on the memory subscale than do Huntington's patients. Constructional praxis becomes apparent at moderate and severe levels of dementia in Huntington's patients but appears relatively early in Alzheimer's patients.

C. LABORATORY FINDINGS AND IMAGING

At autopsy, there is a marked decrease in small cholinergic neurons in the striatum, with low levels of choline acetyl transferase. The disease also damages the small cells containing GABA. Consequently the basal ganglia have decreased concentrations of GABA. Acetylcholine-containing neurons in the basal nucleus of Meynert are preserved. The dopaminergic system is also spared. In Huntington's disease, brain imaging reveals atrophy in the caudate nucleus, reflecting this loss of neurons.

CT scans and MRI show atrophy of the basal ganglia years before the development of symptoms. The putamen is less affected than the caudate. PET scans show striatal hypometabolism in the brains of Huntington's patients early in the course of the disease. Asymptomatic carriers can be identified with 86% sensitivity and 100% specificity. Glucose metabolism decreases at a rate of about 2% per year. Raclopride binding is decreased by about 6% per year and correlates with the number of CAG repeats. The easy availability of the genetic test for Huntington's disease has made brain imaging less crucial in this disease.

Differential Diagnosis

Huntington's disease must be differentiated from other choreiform disorders. The existence of a specific genetic test has aided greatly in diagnosis. The most compelling question of differential diagnosis is whether to perform this test on asymptomatic individuals who have not yet developed the disease; in general, this should be reserved for genetics clinics with counseling readily available.

Treatment

Patients with Huntington's disease may experience an improvement in chorea from neuroleptics but may concurrently experience cognitive decline. Affective disorder is extremely common in HD patients. Mood-stabilizing agents, particularly lithium, can be helpful. Ten percent of patients become psychotic. Clozapine can be used effectively in psychotic Huntington's patients. Other patients show prominent obsessive–compulsive features. Chlorimipramine may be effective for associated obsessive–compulsive disorder. An interesting finding is that psychiatric illness is increased significantly in patients who are at risk for the disease but in whom later genetic testing reveals the absence of the HD gene. This finding emphasizes the need for considerable counseling and social support in this disease.

Prognosis

The prognosis of HD is universally fatal. The later the onset of Huntington's disease the greater the probability that cognitive decline will be minimal, however, 60% of Huntington's patients develop features typical of subcortical dementia. Initially chorea predominates, but later the patient becomes rigid. Striatal damage progresses at a rate that is determined by the length of the CAG repeat. If the patient is affected by psychiatric illness, particularly affective disorder, there is a high prevalence of suicide. The relationship between the severity of chorea and dementia is robust, particularly regarding memory loss. The degree of cognitive disability is ultimately related to the chronicity of the illness but not to the length of the CAG repeat.

Foroud T, et al.: Cognitive scores in carriers of Huntington's disease gene compared to noncarriers. *Ann Neurol* 1995;37:657.

Furtado S, Sucherowsky O. Huntington's disease: Recent advances in diagnosis and management. *Can J Neurol Sci* 1995;22:5–12.

Pillon B, et al.: Severity and specificity of cognitive impairment in Alzheimer's, Huntington's, and Parkinson's diseases and progressive supranuclear palsy. *Neurology* 1991;41:634.

Walling HW, Baldassae JJ, Westfall TC. Molecular aspecits of Huntington's disease. *J Neuroscience Res* 1998;54:301–308.

Wilson's Disease

Brewer GJ, Yuzbasiyan-Gurkan V: Wilson's disease. *Medicine* 1992; 71:139–164.

El-Youssef M: Wilson disease. *Mayo Clin Proc* 2003;78:1126–1136.

VASCULAR DEMENTIA

 ESSENTIALS OF DIAGNOSIS

Vascular dementias are a varied group of disorders. The true incidence of dementia cases that represent pure vascular dementia is unknown. Because of the variety of types of vascular diseases, the diagnosis of this disorder has been problematic. Cases with mixed vascular disease and AD are likely the second most common dementia, after AD itself.

DSM-IV Diagnostic Criteria

A. *The development of multiple cognitive deficits manifested by both*

  (1) memory impairment (impaired ability to learn new information or to recall previously learned information)

  (2) one (or more) of the following cognitive disturbances:

    (a) aphasia (language disturbance)

    (b) apraxia (impaired ability to carry out motor activities despite intact motor function)

    (c) agnosia (failure to recognize or identify objects despite intact sensory function)

    (d) disturbance in executive functioning (i.e., planning, organizing, sequencing, abstracting)

B. *The cognitive deficits in Criteria A1 and A2 each cause significant impairment in social or occupational functioning and represent a significant decline from a previous level of functioning.*

C. *Focal neurological signs and symptoms or laboratory evidence indicative of cerebrovascular disease that are judged to be etiologically related to the disturbance.*

D. *The deficits do not occur exclusively during the course of a delirium.*

(Adapted with permission from Diagnostic and Statistical Manual of Mental Disorders, 4th edn. Copyright 1994 American Psychiatric Association.)

- *Diagnostic subclassifications and the concept of vascular dementia are very much in flux. The Hachinski Scale is used primarily to exclude vascular dementia when studying AD. The criteria from the National Institute of Neurological Disorders and Stroke and from the European Association Internationale pour la Recherche et l'Enseignement en Neurosciences are more specific in regard to etiology and are more flexible.*

General Considerations

Because such a large number of possible etiologic mechanisms exist, the clinical features related to vascular dementia differ from one patient to another. Vascular dementias have many causes: Small vessel disease, multi-infarct dementia, strategic strokes, cerebral hypoperfusion, vasculitis, subarachnoid hemorrhage, genetic causes, and cerebral amyloid angiopathy. Recent neuroimaging studies have revealed that vascular dementias may be more common than previously supposed.

Factors in cerebrovascular disease leading to vascular dementia include (1) volume of lesion (e.g., one large lesion or several small lesions), (2) number of cerebral injuries, (3) location of cerebral injury (e.g., cortical lesions produce a different form of dementia than do subcortical lesions; strokes in strategic locations may produce dementia), (4) white-matter ischemia due to small vessel disease, and (5) co-occurrence of vascular disease and AD or another dementing process.

Vascular dementias may be more amenable to prevention and treatment than is AD. Generally, the risk factors for vascular dementias are the same as those for strokes: Hypertension, diabetes mellitus, advanced age, male sex, smoking, and cardiac disease.

1. Dementia Due to Small Vessel Disease

Small vessel disease can cause a subcortical dementia syndrome. Personality and mood changes are frequent. Psychomotor retardation and poor judgment accompany memory deficits. Binswanger's disease is an extreme form of this condition and is characterized by pseudobulbar signs, abulia, and significant mood and behavior change. Binswanger's disease is associated with multiple small areas of hemispheric softening and demyelination. It occurs mainly in hypertensive males. In most cases, there is not only atherosclerosis of the extracranial arteries but also fibrous and muscular thickening of the small vessels.

Clinical Findings

Small vessel disease can cause cortical and subcortical lesions. Imaging studies can identify these lesions, often referred to as leukoaraiosis, or ischemic deep white-matter disease. Imaging studies identify excessive CNS water caused by damage to the capillaries and postcapillary venules: Collagen is deposited in the media and adventitia and may eventually block the lumen of the arteriole, ultimately affecting the regulation of blood flow in the brain parenchyma. The result is a characteristic pathologic change in the nervous system: rarefaction of the white matter. This finding on MRI scans is extremely common in elderly people, whereas Binswanger's disease is rare in autopsy series. To qualify as a stroke, white matter lesions must be clearly dark on CT or on T1-weighted MRI. Most ischemic changes in the white matter are bright on T2 and Fluid-Attenuated Inversion Recovery (FLAIR) but not clearly dark on T1. The correlates of ischemic white matter changes with behavioral and cognitive measures have been controversial. The presence of these lesions correlates both with age and with vascular risk factors such as hypertension. In some series, cognitive decline has correlated with the degree of white matter ischemic change, but many normal people have some degree of white matter change. Neurologists and psychiatrists spend a great deal of time explaining the significance of "ischemic white matter changes" on MRI to patients and families. Anxiety, depression, and overall severity of neuropsychiatric symptoms are also associated with white-matter ischemia.

The effects of small vessel disease are synergistic with lacunar infarcts. PET research has shown that reduction in cortical metabolism is related to the severity of subcortical pathology. Pathology in the subcortical nuclei greatly influences the metabolism of the frontal cortex.

2. Multi-Infarct Dementia

Lacunar infarcts are small, punctate lesions usually found in the deep white matter, basal ganglia, and brainstem. Multiple lacunar strokes or a few larger strokes can lead to multi-infarct dementia. Hypertension is the greatest risk factor. Previous strokes or myocardial infarction often precede dementia; as compared to AD, most patients have had abrupt, stroke-like events. Previous strokes and cortical atrophy are also correlated with dementia.

Clinical Findings

Multi-infarct dementia advances in stepwise fashion. The clinical signs and symptoms of the disease are associated with changes in MRI, CT scan, and EEG. The Hachinski Scale is a rating scale based on clinical course and illness features that is intended to assess the probability of multi-infarct dementia. Mean Hachinski ischemic scores of 10 predict the presence of infarcts in 93% of patients. Small, localized strokes in brain areas that are functionally important cause well-recognized conditions such as Weber's or Wallenberg's syndromes, however, these lesions may not cause dementia. In patients with multi-infarct dementia, the deep middle cerebral artery territory supplied by the lenticulostriate branches is most likely to be affected. Bilateral infarcts are very common.

A subcortical dementia can sometimes develop in patients with strokes. Paramedial mesencephalic and diencephalic infarcts cause cognitive and affective disorder closely resembling that associated with subcortical degenerative disorders. In these cases, CT scans or MRI sometimes delineate clinical anatomic relationships that account for specific constituents of the syndrome. Dementia resulting from small deep infarctions may involve disease in the same cholinergic projections from the deep frontal nuclei to the cerebral cortex involved in AD. Multiple lesions are thought to have a cumulative effect on mental function.

3. Dementia Due to Strategic Strokes

Strategic single infarcts in specific areas of the brain can cause dementia. Patients who have strokes in the left supramarginal or angular gyrus may develop profound difficulties with comprehension. Strategic strokes in the frontal lobes or in the nondominant parietal lobe can lead to significant reduction in cognitive abilities. Right temporal lesions can be associated with acute confusional states. One or more strategically placed strokes can therefore lead to dementia. The most common single strokes associated with dementia would be major middle cerebral artery strokes on either side, posterior cerebral strokes that affect the hippocampus, and frontal lobe strokes.

Stroke patients are prone to affective disorder that can affect recovery. About 40% of stroke patients develop poststroke depression. In some studies, depression correlates with infarctions in the left hemisphere and frontal more than posterior location. Systemic vascular disease, drug therapy, and psychological reactions to disability contribute to poststroke depression. Subcortical atrophy may predispose to the development of poststroke depression. Patients with ventricular enlargement may be more likely than those without atrophy to develop major depression following a left frontal or left basal ganglia lesion. Whereas left-hemisphere injury leads to early depression, right-hemisphere lesions and preexisting subcortical atrophy predispose to delayed onset of depression, and occasionally to mania.

Clinical Findings

Each brain hemisphere has a different biochemical response to injury. PET scan findings suggest the biochemical response of the two hemispheres to stroke may be different. Right-hemisphere stroke increases serotonin-receptor binding. This does not occur following comparable left-hemisphere stroke. The lower the serotonin binding within the left hemisphere, the more severe the depression is likely to be. This finding suggests that the right, not the left, hemisphere produces biochemical "compensation" for damage by increasing serotonin binding in the noninjured regions. After a stroke, depression may be a result of the failure to up-regulate serotonin receptors. Other factors influencing the differences between hemispheres in poststroke depression undoubtedly include the dominance of the right hemisphere for emotions, such that damage to the right hemisphere causes emotional flatness or apathy, and the presence of neglect of deficit in right hemisphere stroke patients (see below), which often results in a delayed onset of poststroke depression. Nondepressed patients experience less cognitive impairment than do depressed patients. Structural neurologic damage may produce either classic affective disorder or disorders of affective expression and personality that bear little resemblance to classic affective disorder. Stroke patients with depression often respond to antidepressant treatment.

A. RIGHT-HEMISPHERE LESIONS

The expression and understanding of affect are right-hemisphere functions. Evaluation of mood disorders in patients with right-hemisphere damage requires consideration of alterations of affective communication. Depression may be underdiagnosed in patients with right temporoparietal lesions. These patients are often unable to understand nuances of affect. Common cognitive complications of right parietal dysfunction include denial of illness, hemi-inattention (lack of attention to one side of the body), constructional apraxia, and spatial discrimination. Patients with right posterior lesions may not verbally acknowledge depressed feelings. They may appear emotionally flat, or indifferent. A late-onset depression may occur in these patients.

Right frontal lobe damage causes expressive aprosodia (impairment in the normal variations of speech), an inability to express nuances of affect. Affective explosiveness, a temporal lobe function, is preserved. Depressed patients with expressive aprosodia do not appear depressed during a psychiatric interview.

B. LEFT-HEMISPHERE LESIONS

With left-hemisphere lesions, language impairment complicates the diagnosis of affective disorder. Patients with Broca's aphasia exhibit nonfluent speech, impaired writing, defective naming, and (usually) hemiparesis (one-sided paralysis). Verbal acknowledgment of a depressed mood may be difficult to elicit. In spite of diagnostic difficulties, the incidence of depression in patients with unilateral left frontal lobe damage is striking. The putative mechanism is interruption of catecholamine axons to, and arborization in, the cerebral cortex. Comprehension deficits in patients with posterior aphasia make accurate diagnosis of affective disorder difficult. Clinically, posterior aphasia can resemble either dementia or affective disorder. Speech is fluent and associated neurologic deficits often subtle, however, neologisms and paraphasic errors punctuate the speech of patients with Wernicke's aphasia. In addition, Wernicke's patients exhibit impaired reading, writing, naming, repetition, and comprehension. Patients with left posterior lesions display exaggerated affect because the main remaining vehicle of communication is affective expression. When their speech is not understood, they may become angry or even paranoid.

Left parietal dysfunction can mimic AD because it produces ideomotor apraxia, right-left disorientation, finger agnosia, amnestic aphasia, dyslexia (inability to read, spell, and write words), dysgraphia (difficulty in writing), and acalculia (inability to do simple arithmetic calculations). Right parietal dysfunction causes left spatial neglect and "dressing apraxia." These patients do not usually have as great a memory impairment as do AD patients. Some visuospatial disruption attends normal aging. Neuropsychological evaluation distinguishes normal elders from those with parietal disorder or dementia.

Clinical deterioration may occur in brain-disordered patients without a new lesion. Erratic recovery and poor cooperation during rehabilitation suggest affective disorder. Pathologic laughing or crying, depressive propositional language, and perhaps abnormal dexamethasone suppression test suggest depression. Bilateral hemispheric dysfunction may cause excessive crying.

Differential Diagnosis

A. DIFFERENTIATING FRONTAL LOBE DISORDER FROM DEPRESSION

Several characteristics differentiate frontal lobe disorder from depression. Frontal patients are apathetic and not deeply depressed. Frontal personality changes are more dramatic than are those in depression. Frontal lobe systems are responsible for affect modulation. When these systems disconnect from brainstem centers, pseudobulbar affect develops. Patients who feel a fleeting emotion may be unable to inhibit a prolonged affective display such as crying. The phrase "emotionally incontinent" is sometimes applied to these patients because of their inability to inhibit emotional expression. Patients with frontal lobe disease often have impaired insight and judgment. They are perseverative concerning some social responses, yet they may be unable to initiate others. As a result, they can appear bizarre in social settings.

4. Dementia Due to Cerebral Hypoperfusion of Watershed Areas

Hypotension, decreased volume of body fluids, cardiac arrhythmias, and other causes of hypoperfusion can cause ischemia in the watershed areas between the major sources of cerebral arterial supply. Significant watershed strokes can lead to serious disconnection syndromes. Lesions circling Broca's area cause a transcortical motor aphasia. Transcortical motor aphasia displays elements of Broca's aphasia with intact repetition. Patients with transcortical motor aphasia have decreased speech production (abulia). Mild forms of the disorder can be identified by poor performance on the FAS test and on other frontal lobe tests.

Watershed lesions surrounding Wernicke's area cause transcortical sensory aphasia. This syndrome is similar to Wernicke's aphasia, but repetition remains intact. The most severe form of watershed infarct causes isolation of the speech area. In this condition the entire language apparatus is disconnected from other brain structures. Echolalia is the only form of speech of which the patient is capable.

Bilateral strokes in the posterior parts of the hemispheres can result in complex neurobehavioral deficits such as visual agnosia, prosopagnosia (inability to recognize familiar faces), or auditory agnosias. These deficits are often explained by disconnections between sensory input and centers that interpret the information. Unilateral left posterior cerebral artery territory strokes are associated with alexia without agraphia, and severe memory disorder. These cognitive deficits can contribute to vascular dementia.

5. Dementia Due to Cerebral Vasculitis

Autoimmune vasculitis is an uncommon cause of dementia. Systemic vasculitis that affects the CNS occurs most often in conjunction with collagen vascular disease (such as polyarteriitis nodosa). The most common autoimmune disease associated with stroke is systemic lupus erythematosus, but this disease is associated with antineuronal antibodies that cause delirium and antiphospholipid antibodies associated with stroke; a true vasculitis is rare. Antiphospholipid antibodies can also be associated with stroke syndromes in patients who do not have lupus. CNS vasculitis can occur in isolation (e.g., granulomatous angiitis or isolated CNS vasculitis). Infectious diseases such as neurosyphilis and Lyme disease can cause CNS vasculitis, which can be extremely difficult to diagnose but should be considered in the presence of any rapidly progressing dementia.

6. Dementia Due to Subarachnoid Hemorrhage

Subarachnoid hemorrhage causes intense vasospasm, which can lead to significant ischemia. This ischemia can cause a dementing syndrome that persists after the subarachnoid hemorrhage has resolved.

7. Dementia Due to Cerebral Autosomal Dominant Arteriopathy with Subcortical Infarcts & Leukoencephalopathy (CADASIL)

CADASIL is an inherited arterial disease of the brain recently mapped to chromosome 19p13.1. Features of the disorder include recurrent subcortical ischemic events, progressive or stepwise subcortical dementia, pseudobulbar palsy, migraine with aura, and severe depressive episodes. Attacks of migraine with aura occur earlier in life than ischemic events. The diagnosis should be considered in patients with recurrent small subcortical infarcts leading to dementia that also have transient ischemic attacks (TIAs), migraine with aura, and severe depression. Demented patients exhibit frontal, temporal, and basal ganglia deficits on SPECT scans despite the relative absence of focal neurologic findings.

8. Dementia Due to Cerebral Amyloid Angiopathy

Cerebral amyloid **angiopathy** is the term given to a condition in which amyloid is deposited on the walls of small arteries and arterioles, weakening the blood vessels and leading to an increased incidence of intracerebral hemorrhage. Amyloid angiopathy can also interfere with blood flow in small vessels and contribute to deep white-matter ischemic changes. The hemorrhages are lobar, may be recurrent, and often occur in patients without hypertension. Cerebral amyloid angiopathy often occurs within the context of AD and is a cause of mixed vascular-Alzheimer's dementia.

Clinical Findings

A. SIGNS AND SYMPTOMS

See discussions of individual dementias.

B. PSYCHOLOGICAL TESTING

The neuropsychological deficits in vascular dementias tend to be variable and depend on both the underlying pathology and the location of the lesion. Although memory is almost always affected, executive, subcortical, and frontal lobe functions may exhibit significant deterioration. Patients with vascular dementias generally have better language function and better memory than do those with AD (unless the language areas are directly affected by strokes).

Neuropsychological findings in vascular dementias depend heavily on the volume and location of the infarct. Usually multiple forms of vascular pathology contribute concurrently to the overall findings of vascular cognitive impairment.

C. LABORATORY FINDINGS AND IMAGING

A variety of clinical laboratory findings may be indicated in the investigation of vascular dementias. A complete blood count, sedimentation rate, blood glucose, and ECG are obtained routinely. Often a carotid Doppler, transesophageal echocardiography, and Holter monitor (recording ambulatory ECG) add to the investigation. In some cases, coagulation screen, lipid profile, lupus anticoagulant, anticardiolipin antibodies, and autoantibody screens may be necessary. Cerebral angiography may be necessary to diagnose cerebral vasculitis but is not routinely obtained. If an infection or inflammation is suspected, then a spinal tap may be helpful.

MRI is the most helpful radiologic tool in the diagnosis of vascular dementias, but CT scans may be helpful in some cases. Patchy diffuse white-matter lucency on CT scan or hyperintensity on MRI suggests leukoaraiosis. Normal scans may show lesions that are punctate or partially confluent. The aging brain becomes susceptible to an assortment of changes in the periventricular and subcortical white matter. These changes are radiolucent on CT scans and hyperintense on T2-weighted MRI. White-matter changes are common in patients with chronic hypertension. Examination of affected tissues reveals dilated perivascular (Virchow-Robin) spaces, mild demyelination, gliosis, and diffuse neuropil vacuolation. The associated clinical abnormalities are usually not serious, but defects of attention, mental processing speed, and psychomotor control may be evident, although usually only through neuropsychological testing. As a result, significant overlap occurs between the scans of normal patients and those who have clinically significant vascular disease. These changes also appear in early AD, making the interpretation of early disease more difficult. Leukoaraiosis is associated with increased age, hypertension, limb weakness, and extensor-plantar responses. Some patients have extensive deep white-matter brain lesions without detriment to cognitive, behavioral, or neurologic functioning.

Pathology becomes evident when periventricular capping and plaque-like hyperintensities become confluent. When these changes are at their most severe, the diagnosis of Binswanger's disease can be suspected. Lesions that distinguish patients with vascular dementias include definite infarctions, dark on T1 and bright on T2 weighted MRI scans. Irregular periventricular hyperintensities extending into the deep white matter and large confluent areas of deep white-matter hyperintensity likely contribute, but these alone cannot be used to diagnose vascular dementia. These abnormalities are associated with extensive arteriosclerosis, diffuse white-matter rarefication, and even necrosis. In general, the hyperintensities associated with AD are smaller.

A relationship exists between the extent of MRI abnormality and dementia, in population studies, but not in individual patients. MRI white matter abnormalities relate to advanced age, vascular risk factors, and loosely to degree of cognitive impairment. In CADASIL, MRI reveals prominent signal abnormalities in the subcortical white matter and basal ganglia. Cognitive impairment is linked to signal abnormalities and hypoperfusion in the basal ganglia.

^{31}P NMR spectroscopy profiles may be helpful in the evaluation of vascular dementias. Patients with vascular dementias exhibit elevations of the phosphocreatine/inorganic orthophosphate ratio in tempo roparietal and frontal regions.

PET scans may be helpful in diagnosing vascular dementias. They may demonstrate focal areas of hypometabolism that correspond roughly to areas of impairment discovered on neuropsychological testing. Hypometabolism, even without atrophy, is visible on anatomic images. Areas of hypometabolism seen on PET scans conform to cortical high-signal intensity on MRI. In addition, cerebral metabolism is reduced globally because isolated lesions have extensive and distant metabolic effects. The pattern of hypometabolism observed in vascular dementias is distinct from that observed in AD. Vascular dementias are associated with multiple defects in the cortex, deep nuclei, subcortical white matter, and cerebellum. Dementia increases as global and frontal hypometabolism evolve. Consequently, PET scans detect more widespread brain involvement than does structural imaging. In AD, hypometabolism can involve areas that appear structurally normal on MRI, but in vascular dementia the two imaging modalities correlate better. SPECT scans of patients with vascular dementias show varying degrees of irregular uptake in the cerebral cortex, similar to that seen in PET scans. In SPECT studies of individuals affected with CADASIL, cerebral blood flow reduction matched with MRI signal abnormalities.

EEG often shows focal slowing corresponding to areas of cerebral ischemia or infarction. These areas of slowing may be demonstrated visually on EEG brain maps. Computer-analyzed EEGs use mathematical formulas to break the EEG into power distributions across frequencies. This technique reveals decreased alpha power and increased theta power and delta power that parallel the degree of dementia. The ratio of high-frequency to low-frequency electrical activity in the left temporal region is decreased. Compared to AD, vascular dementias are associated with lower EEG frequency and reduced synchronization. Somatosensory evoked potentials show prolonged central conduction time and a reduction of the primary cortical response amplitude in multi-infarct dementia but not in AD.

Treatment

Prevention is important in vascular dementias. Control of hypertension is probably the single most important preventive measure, however, caution must be taken not to lower the blood pressure too much and thus cause hypoperfusion. Control of diabetes, cholesterol and lipid management, and abstinence from cigarettes are also important. Treatment of atrial fibrillation can prevent embolic strokes. Although anticoagulants are highly effective for preventing cardioembolic strokes, their effectiveness in noncardioembolic strokes is uncertain. Antiplatelet agents, including aspirin, clopidogrel, or aspirin and extended release dipyridamole have been shown to reduce the incidence of second strokes. These agents are likely beneficial also in patients with vascular dementia. Diagnosis and surgical or endovascular treatment of carotid disease is also important in patients with TIA and stroke secondary to carotid artery stenosis. Pentoxifylline has been tested but has demonstrated limited efficacy. In cases of either systemic or cerebral vasculitis, high-dose corticosteroids may prevent further cognitive loss. As yet, no specific agent has been approved for vascular dementia itself, though clinical trials have supported efficacy of anticholinesterase medications.

Table 14–1. Hachinski Ischemic Score*

Feature	Score
Abrupt onset	2
Stepwise deterioration	1
Fluctuating course	2
Nocturnal confusion	1
Relative preservation of personality	1
Depression	1
Somatic complaints	1
Emotional incontinence	1
History of hypertension	1
History of strokes	2
Evidence of associated atherosclerosis	1
Focal neurological symptoms	2
Focal neurological signs	2

*Patients with a total score of 7 or more are considered to have multi-infarct dementia; those scoring ≤ 4 have primary degenerative dementia.
(Adapted from Hachinski VC, Iliff LD, Zilkha E, et al.: Cerebral blood flow in dementia. *Arch Neurol* 1975;32: 632–637.)

Prognosis

Vascular dementias shorten life expectancy. Three-year mortality is almost three times greater in the very elderly than in age-matched controls. About one-third of patients die from dementia itself; the others die from cerebral vascular disease, cardiac disease, or other, unrelated conditions (Tables 14–1 and 14–2).

Table 14–2. California Criteria for Ischemic Vascular Dementia (IVD) (Chui et al., Neurology, 1992)

1 Dementia established by clinical examination
2 Progressive worsening of cognitive function
3 Evidence of at least two strokes by clinical or neuroradiological criteria
4 Evidence of at least one hemisphere infarct by CT or MRI (T1-weighted)
5 Diagnosis of definite IVD requires neuropathology

(Adapted from Chui HC, Victoroff JI, Margolin D, et al.: Criteria for the diagnosis of ischemic vascular dementia proposed by the State of California Alzheimer's disease diagnostic and treatment centers. *Neurology* 1992;42: 473–480.)

Chabriat H, et al.: Clinical spectrum of CADASIL: A study of 7 families. Cerebral autosomal dominant arteriopathy with subcortical infarcts and leukoencephalopathy [see comments]. *Lancet* 1995;346:934.

Chui HC, Victoroff JI, Margolin D, et al.: Criteria for the diagnosis of ischemic vascular dementia proposed by the State of California Alzheimer's disease diagnostic and treatment centers. *Neurology* 1992;42:473–480.

Dichgans M, Mayer M, Uttner I, et al.: The phenotypic spectrum of CADASIL: Clinical findings in 102 cases. *Neurology* 1998;44:731–739.

Gorelick PB, Erkinjuntti T, Hofman A, Rocca WA, Skoog I, Winblad B. Prevention of vascular dementia. *Alzheimer Dis Assoc Disord* 1999;13(Suppl 3):S131–S139.

Hachinski VC, Iliff LD, Zilkha E, et al.: Cerebral blood flow in dementia. *Arch Neurol* 1975;32:632–637.

Hachinski VC, Potter P, Merskey H: Leuko-araiosis. *Arch Neurol* 1987;44:21–23.

Kirk A, Kertesz A, Polk MJl: Dementia with leukoencephalopathy in systemic lupus erythematosus. *Can J Neurol Sci* 1991;18:344–348.

Moore PM, Richardson B: Neurology of the vasculitides and connective tissue diseases. *J Neurol Neurosurg Psychiatry* 1998;65:10–22.

Robinson RG, Starkstein SE: Mood disorders following stroke: New findings and future directions. *J Geriatr Psychiatry* 1989;22:1.

Rockwood K, Bowler J, Erkinjuntti T, Hachinski V, Wallin A: Subtypes of vascular dementia. *Alzheimer Dis Assoc Disord* 1999; 13(Suppl 3):S59–S65.

Roman GC, Tatemichi TK, Erkinjuntti T, et al.: Vascular dementia: Diagnostic criteria for research studies. Report of the NINDS-AIREN International Work Group. *Neurology* 1993;43:250–260

Tatemichi TK, Paik M, Bagiella E, et al.: Risk of dementia after stroke in a hospitalized cohort: Results of a longitudinal study. *Neurology* 1994;44:1885–1891.

Verhey FRJ, et al.: Comparison of seven sets of criteria used for the diagnosis of vascular dementia. *Neuroepidemiology* 1996;15:166.

Zhang WW, et al.: Structural and vasoactive factors influencing intracerebral arterioles in cases of vascular dementia and other cerebrovascular disease: A review. Immunohistochemical studies on expression of collagens, basal lamina components and endothelin-1. *Dementia* 1994;5:153.

DEMENTIA DUE TO CEREBRAL INFECTION & INFLAMMATION

 ESSENTIALS OF DIAGNOSIS

Infectious processes can cause a sustained, progressive loss of intellectual function. The diagnosis of dementia due to cerebral infection or inflammation is made when the infectious process can be established as a causal agent of the dementia.

General Considerations

Neurosyphilis is the classic dementia due to an infectious process. More recently, the AIDS dementia complex has become the most common form of infectious dementia. Other viral causes of dementia include herpes simplex, progressive multifocal leuko encephalopathy, and subacute sclerosing panencephalitis. Any severe encephalitis can cause a subsequent dementia. Creutzfeldt-Jakob disease is an uncommon cause of rapidly developing dementia caused by a prion, a novel infectious entity that produces a spongiform encephalopathy.

1. Dementia Due to HIV Disease, Opportunistic Infection, or Multifocal Leukoencephalopathy

Dementia due to HIV disease is often referred to as the AIDS dementia complex, which eventually affects about 15% of AIDS patients.

Clinical Findings

A. SIGNS AND SYMPTOMS

Early in HIV infection, patients are likely to experience an acute encephalitis or aseptic meningitis. In HIV-infected patients, impaired memory and reduced psychomotor speed are more common than is global intellectual deterioration. HIV-induced neuropsychological impairment does not correlate with subjective complaints, neurologic signs, reduced T4 lymphocytes, CSF abnormalities, EEG slowing, atrophy on brain CT scan, or nonspecific hyperintensities on brain MRI. Dementia, cancer of the CNS, and opportunistic infection present later in HIV infection.

AIDS dementia complex is characterized by a clinical triad of progressive cognitive decline, motor dysfunction, and behavioral abnormality. Early symptoms include memory difficulty and psychomotor slowing. Behavioral symptoms include apathy and social withdrawal. It can be difficult to distinguish the AIDS dementia complex from depression, and the pattern of dementia is subcortical. Eventually, cognitive and motor impairment progresses, leading in the final stages to global dementia and paraplegia. Although the AIDS dementia complex may present at any stage of HIV infection, it usually appears relatively late in the course of the disease. The mean survival time in patients with AIDS dementia complex was 7 months before the introduction of protease inhibitors.

B. PSYCHOLOGICAL TESTING

Patients with the AIDS dementia complex have a neuropsychological profile consisting of decreased motor speed, decreased memory, and failure on frontal lobe tasks. The HIV Dementia Scale tests specific abilities including timed motor tasks, frontal lobe function, and memory. The test is easy to administer and may be used to follow the patient's progress and response to treatment. Physical findings in the HIV dementia complex include hyperreflexia and hypertonia.

C. Laboratory Findings and Imaging

In the AIDS dementia complex, HIV probably enters the CNS through macrophages that cross the blood–brain barrier. These macrophages infect microglia. In the AIDS dementia complex, the HIV virus can be detected in macrophage- and glial-activated cells in the white matter and deep gray matter. Activated macrophages and microglia probably cause dementia through the secretion of neurotoxins that cause neuronal depopulation and a loss of dendritic arborization. The most common neuropathologic finding is a diffuse destruction of white matter and subcortical gray matter.

Sixty percent of patients show a slightly elevated spinal fluid protein. There may also be an elevated IgG fraction and oligoclonal bands. CSF lymphocytosis may occur; the CD4/CD8 ratio mirrors that of the peripheral blood. HIV can usually be isolated directly from the CSF.

Brain imaging is essential in the evaluation of patients with the AIDS dementia complex because infection with the human immunodeficiency virus-type 1 (HIV-1) predisposes the individual to a number of opportunistic CNS infections and tumors. In order to diagnose the AIDS dementia complex, the clinician must exclude these opportunistic infections, including progressive multifocal leukoencephalopathy, toxoplasmosis, tuberculosis, and cryptococcosis. On MRI and CT scans, the brains of patients with the AIDS dementia complex demonstrate atrophy. MRI shows scattered white-matter abnormalities.

Differential Diagnosis

Diagnostic uncertainty may exist in severe cases. Progressive multifocal leukoencephalopathy produces focal white-matter abnormalities due to multiple foci of demyelination. PET brain imaging techniques help to distinguish opportunistic infections from intracerebral lymphoma.

Treatment

The most effective therapy is to reduce the number of viruses with antiretroviral agents such as 3′-azido-3′deoxythymidine (AZT). AZT can improve the mental function of HIV-infected patients. If AZT therapy is not initially effective, the dosage can be increased to the patient's ability to tolerate side effects or another antiviral agent can be added. Protease inhibitors have a similar effect, and multidrug regimens are now the standard treatment of HIV. Psychostimulants have been reported to provide symptomatic relief in some patients.

Prognosis

In the early stages of the illness, the AIDS patient experiences forgetfulness, lapses in concentration, and social withdrawal. Cognitive and motor slowing are prominent. The memory problem is mild compared to that observed in AD. Patients retain a relatively good sense of self-awareness and rarely experience the denial of illness that often occurs in other dementias. As the disease progresses patients become unable to perform activities of daily living. Motor function is affected simultaneously. Patients become unable to walk or require a walker and personal assistance. In the final stages of the disease, patients are nearly vegetative.

2. Dementia Due to Other Viruses

Herpes simplex encephalitis damages the temporal lobes. The disease can present initially with confusion or psychiatric symptomatology. Later the patient develops a severe headache, fever, often seizures, and confusion. MRI and CSF examination are helpful for early diagnosis. A specific EEG pattern is associated with the disorder. Early recognition is essential so that antiviral therapy can be initiated. If the disease progresses, the patient may be left with rather severe deficits. Klüver-Bucy syndrome, an amnestic syndrome, or global dementia are common residuals of herpetic encephalitis.

Progressive multifocal leukoencephalopathy generally occurs in older immunocompromised patients. It may also occur in the later stages of AIDS. This disorder proceeds extremely rapidly, and death usually occurs within months. Subacute sclerosing panencephalitis is a rare disease of late childhood caused by measles virus. It has become extremely rare since the measles vaccine was introduced. Sporadic encephalitis is another uncommon cause of dementia.

3. Dementia Due to Neurosyphilis

Neurosyphilis, caused by the spirochaete bacterium *Treponema pallidum,* was historically a major cause of dementia, but it is a rare diagnosis in the current era. Neurosyphilis presents as a vascular occlusive disease. The meninges may appear thickened and inflamed. Neuroimaging may show infarction, arteriitis, cortical lesions, or meningeal enhancement. The basal areas of the brain are preferentially affected, leading to frontal and temporal lobe dysfunction.

Clinical Findings

A. Signs and Symptoms

Neurosyphilis frequently causes psychiatric symptoms such as labile affect, depression, or mania. Patients are usually moderately demented but experience a preponderance of personality disturbances. The Argyll Robertson pupil (the pupil accommodates but does not react to light) is observed occasionally, but many patients become demented without exhibiting this sign. Tabes dorsalis, with posterior column sensory loss and lightening pains, is an associated finding in some patients.

B. LABORATORY FINDINGS

A variety of screening tests are used to establish the possibility of syphilitic infection. Once the infection is suspected, a spinal tap is indicated. The diagnosis of neurosyphilis is made by performing the Venereal Disease Research Laboratory (VDRL) test on the patient's CSF.

Treatment

The principal mode of treatment for neurosyphilis is intravenous penicillin. The decision to retreat a patient who has already had a course of penicillin is difficult to make and is usually based on the patient's clinical response, CSF cell count, and protein concentration. Even after successful treatment of the infection, the patient may continue to have significant deficits. VDRL titer may be an indicator of continued *T. pallidum* activity in patients without obvious clinical deterioration.

Prognosis

Neurosyphilis can occur decades after the original infection. It is not uncommon for an elderly woman to present with this disorder, having been infected many years earlier by her spouse. Early symptoms include fatigue, personality change, and forgetfulness. Neurosyphilis is a great imitator and can produce almost any psychiatric or cognitive disorder. Late in the disease the patient becomes confused and disoriented. Myoclonus, seizures, and dysarthria are common.

4. Dementia Due to Lyme Disease

Lyme disease is a multisystemic illness that can affect the CNS, causing neurologic and psychiatric symptoms. It is caused by the spirochaete *Borrelia burgdorferi,* which enters the host after a bite by a deer tick.

Clinical Findings

Lyme disease may involve either the peripheral or the CNS. Dissemination to the CNS can occur within the first few weeks after skin infection. Like syphilis, Lyme disease may have a latency period of months to years before symptoms of late infection emerge. A broad range of psychiatric reactions have been associated with Lyme disease including dementia, psychosis, and depression.

5. Dementia Due to Creutzfeldt-Jakob Disease

An unusual infectious agent, known as a prion, leads to Creutzfeldt-Jakob disease (CJD), a condition associated with a rapidly progressive dementia. There are three forms of Creutzfeldt-Jakob disease: Infectious, sporadic, and inherited. Until recently, the infectious variety was usually iatrogenic, however, the addition of sheep brain to cow feed in Britain has led to an outbreak of an atypical variant of the disease, bovine spongiform encephalopathy ("mad cow disease") among beefeaters in Britain.

Clinical Findings

A. SIGNS AND SYMPTOMS

The majority of patients with CJD present with myoclonus, exaggerated startle responses, seizures, and pyramidal signs. Although most cases are sporadic, 10–15% are familial. Gerstmann-Straussler syndrome is a rare familial dementia caused by a prion and related to Creutzfeldt-Jakob syndrome. It resembles olivopontocerebellar degeneration. Spongiform encephalopathy accompanies both Gerstmann-Straussler syndrome and CJD. Mutation in the prion protein (PrP) gene occurs in Gerstmann-Straussler syndrome. Fatal familial insomnia is another rare inherited dementia caused by the prion. Patients with this disorder experience a complete lack of sleep in the year or two prior to death. PrP gene analysis is potentially useful for diagnosis and genetic counseling.

B. LABORATORY FINDINGS

Creutzfeldt-Jakob disease is the only dementia that can be distinguished by characteristic electrical patterns. EEG shows triphasic bursts, sometimes correlating with myoclonic jerks. PrP genetic analysis can be helpful in some cases of prion disease. MRI also shows lesions early in the course, often affecting the basal ganglia and cortex; in relatively acute cases, the diffusion weighted MRI shows bright lesions resembling strokes.

Prognosis

Prion disease is uniformly fatal. The time between diagnosis and death is generally less than 2 years. There are no treatments. Because the disease has been transmitted through careless production and processing of meat, primary prevention is possible.

Geraci AP, Di Rocco A, Simpson DM: Neurologic complications of AIDS. *The Neurologist* 2001;7:82–97.

Navia BA, Cho ES, Petito RW: The AIDS dementia complex: II. Neuropathology. *Ann Neurol* 1986;19:517.

Price RW: Management of AIDS dementia complex and HIV-1 brain infection. Clinical-virological correlations. *Ann Neurol* 1995;38:563.

Prusiner SB: Genetic and infectious prion diseases. *Arch Neurol* 1993;50:1129.

Simpson DM, Berger JR. Neurologic manifestations of HIV infection. *Med Clin NA* 1996;80:1363–1394.

DEMENTIA DUE TO OTHER GENERAL MEDICAL CONDITIONS

Metabolic causes of dementia include dialysis dementia, repeated episodes of diabetic hypoglycemia, prolonged hepatic encephalopathy, hypothyroidism, and hypoxia. Many diseases can cause dementia in older people, for example, pernicious anemia, thyroid disorder, systemic infection, collagen disease, brain hypoxia, and toxic exposure.

Vitamin B_{12} deficiency causes subacute combined degeneration. Subacute combined degeneration causes demyelination in the posterior columns and loss of pyramidal cells in the motor strip. Often a peripheral neuropathy is present. Slow information processing, confusion, memory changes, delirium, hallucinations, delusions ("megaloblastic madness"), depression, and psychosis have been observed in patients with vitamin B_{12} deficiency.

Anemia is not necessary for the syndrome to develop. Sometimes a familial pattern occurs. Antiparietal-cell antibodies are often present. Current state-of-the-art testing uses serum cobalamin levels as a screening test and serum or urine homocysteine and methylmalonic acid determinations as confirmatory tests. Homocysteine abnormalities are associated with neurologic deficits and psychiatric symptomatology. A Schilling test follows the patient's vitamin B_{12} level to help determine etiology.

Depression and dementia respond rapidly to the administration of vitamin B_{12} when the condition is diagnosed in its early stages. Vitamin B_{12} deficiency is treatable with monthly injections, daily oral supplements, or an intranasal gel. If the condition is not diagnosed in the early stages, neurologic, psychiatric, and cognitive impairment may persist and become irreversible. The prevalence of low cobalamin levels is significantly increased in AD. Contrary to widely accepted beliefs, subnormal serum vitamin B_{12} levels are a rare cause of reversible dementia.

Older people frequently have mildly decreased thyroid function. This does not cause an irreversible dementia. In some people, hypothyroidism exacerbates a depression. Thyroid deficiency can also hasten a severe melancholic depression that causes a patient to appear demented. Consequently, thyroid function tests (including thyroid stimulating hormone level) should be obtained. On exceedingly rare occasions, hyperthyroidism or hypothyroidism cause a delirium that can be mistaken for dementia. Patients with vascular dementias often have hypothyroidism. The reason for this association is unclear, but thyroid replacement can improve the performance of patients who have this condition.

Patients who are undergoing dialysis may experience impaired mental functioning that can be secondary to a parathyroid hormone abnormality and its effect on calcium metabolism. Patients who have been on dialysis for extended periods may experience a general decline in intellectual function that is usually mild. True dialysis dementia has become rare since aluminum was eliminated from the dialysate.

Many toxins can cause dementia. Organic solvents inhaled in the workplace cause cognitive deficits. Organic solvents can occasionally cause dementia when used as intoxicants. Carbon monoxide and heavy metals are other toxins that affect mental function. Appropriate history, physical examination, and toxicology evaluation are necessary for the diagnosis of toxin-induced dementias.

Dementia can be caused by the direct or indirect effect of cancer. Patients with cancer develop dementia as a result of intracranial tumors, cerebral metastases, carcinomatous meningitis, progressive multifocal leukoencephalitis, opportunistic infections, and paraneoplastic effects ("limbic encephalitis"). Tumors can lead to noncommunicating hydrocephalus by obstructing the outflow of CSF. Some patients develop progressive dementia as a complication of whole-brain radiotherapy.

1. Dementia Due to Normal Pressure Hydrocephalus

 ESSENTIALS OF DIAGNOSIS

Normal pressure hydrocephalus causes a relatively distinct syndrome consisting of gait difficulty, sometimes called gait apraxia, urinary incontinence, and dementia. Normal pressure hydrocephalus may be idiopathic, but it may follow a subarachnoid hemorrhage, meningitis, or other entity that can cause altered spinal fluid dynamics.

General Considerations

A. Epidemiology

Normal pressure hydrocephalus is the most common type of hydrocephalus diagnosed in people over age 60 years.

B. Etiology

Normal pressure hydrocephalus occurs when the CSF pressure inside the ventricles is higher than that in the subarachnoid space, and the ventricles expand.

Clinical Findings

The clinical diagnosis of hydrocephalus as a cause of dementia is confusing because many conditions can cause similar symptoms. Nonetheless, a timely diagnosis is important because dementia caused by normal pressure hydrocephalus can sometimes be reversed if the diagnosis is made early enough.

A. Signs and Symptoms

The patient presents the classic triad of dementia, incontinence, and gait disturbance. The dementia develops at a rapid pace. The patient's gait becomes magnetic in quality, and he or she is likely to experience frequent falls.

B. Psychological Testing

Patients with normal pressure hydrocephalus are impaired on tests designed to detect frontal lobe involvement. The pattern of dementia suggests a subcortical process. Successful ventriculoperitoneal shunt placement improves the patient's cognitive function in 50–67% of cases, in published series.

C. Laboratory Findings and Imaging

The clinical picture associated with vascular dementias can closely resemble that associated with normal pressure hydrocephalus. Unfortunately, MRI findings in patients with normal pressure hydrocephalus overlap those seen in patients who have small vessel disease. Both conditions are associated with increased ventricular size and significant periventricular hyperintensity, as shown on T2-weighted MRI. Normal pressure hydrocephalus differs from small vessel disease in that in the former the MRI can show a large cerebral aqueduct when the pulsation of CSF creates a flow void.

When radioisotope-labeled albumin (RISA) is injected into the lumbar sac (the RISA cisternogram test), it usually diffuses readily over the cerebral convexities. Patients with normal pressure hydrocephalus have abnormal CSF dynamics: Radioactivity appears in the ventricles but is absent over the convexities. Although this test may sometimes be useful, it is not often used today.

Cerebral fluid drainage procedures are sometimes used to help predict whether surgery will be successful. If the patient's gait improves after removal of a large amount of CSF, then the patient is judged to be a better candidate for surgery. Lack of improvement militates against surgery.

Differential Diagnosis

Normal pressure hydrocephalus can be difficult to distinguish from vascular dementias and AD. Although imaging tests help, there is some overlap between the findings of normal pressure hydrocephalus and other forms of dementia. Tests of spinal fluid dynamics help clarify the matter, but ultimately, improvement after shunt placement clarifies the issue. Unfortunately, clinical experience with shunt placement may not be as favorable

as that seen in published reports. Improvement may be more transient.

Treatment

Dementia from normal pressure hydrocephalus may respond to shunting, the treatment of choice, however, shunting is associated with significant morbidity. Thus the procedure should probably be carried out only in cases in which the indications are clear and in which the dementia has not progressed to an irreversible degree.

Prognosis

Patients whose normal pressure hydrocephalus has a defined etiology, such as previous head trauma or subarachnoid hemorrhage, respond more reliably to shunting than patients with idiopathic hydrocephalus. Variables associated with a positive outcome from CSF shunting include CSF pressure, duration of dementia, and gait abnormality preceding dementia.

2. Dementia Due to Traumatic Brain Injury

 ESSENTIALS OF DIAGNOSIS

Dementia due to traumatic brain injury refers to a wide range of alterations in thinking, mood, and behavior resulting from specific neurologic damage associated with brain trauma. The severity of the injury is an important determinant of outcome. Specific vulnerabilities such as age, preexisting neurologic or psychiatric disease, and social support determine the ultimate prognosis.

General Considerations

A. Epidemiology

The annual rate of traumatic brain injury among the general population is about 200 per 100,000 people in the United States. Traumatic brain injuries are most common among young adult males and most often are the result of automobile accidents. Older adults also represent a significant risk group. Falls are the most common cause of injury in children and older adults. Most head injuries are considered to be mild. Older adults are more likely than younger adults to have a severe injury.

B. ETIOLOGY

Head trauma severe enough to cause brief loss of consciousness or posttraumatic amnesia can produce long-lasting cognitive and behavioral changes.

The principal mechanisms underlying traumatic brain injury have been well established. Forces of deceleration and acceleration act within the cranial compartment to produce injury. The swirling movement of brain tissue causes diffuse injury to axons and contusions to cortical areas adjacent to jagged bone. Because the hippocampus is found near the sphenoid ridge, it is especially susceptible to damage when the brain is set in sudden motion. Memory mechanisms fail, and both anterograde and retrograde amnesia follow. The length of posttraumatic amnesia is closely related to the overall severity of diffuse brain damage. The frontal lobes are also susceptible to contracoup injury. Closed head trauma causes both diffuse and focal brain injury. Subarachnoid hemorrhage and subdural hematoma may produce additional damage, and cerebral edema further complicates the picture.

Beyond structural changes, biochemical alterations also develop. For example, free acetylcholine may appear in large quantities in the CSF, or anoxic damage may produce an increase in CSF lactate.

Clinical Findings

A. SIGNS AND SYMPTOMS

Fatigue, headache, and dizziness may occur shortly after a mild head trauma. Later a postconcussive disorder may develop. The most significant features of postconcussive syndrome are slowing of information processing, impaired attention, and poor memory.

More severe head injuries are rated according to the Glasgow coma scale. This is a measure of consciousness that analyzes eye opening response, verbal response, and motor response. Head trauma is categorized on this scale as mild, moderate, or severe. The Glasgow coma scale gives a rough judgment regarding prognosis.

Recovery from moderate and severe head trauma is an extremely long process. Recovery is most rapid during the first year or two, and it can continue for many years. In the initial stages of recovery, progress can be followed with the Rancho Los Amigos scale. In the later stages of recovery, measurement of recovery is based on clinical indicators such as return to work.

Recovery from head trauma is also affected by secondary brain injury. Intracranial hematomas, brain edema, and vasospasm affect prognosis by causing occlusion of intracranial vessels, thus producing secondary strokes. Infection, seizures, or metabolic imbalance may affect the postinjury course. Traumatic brain injury produces physical disability ranging from sensory and mo-

tor deficits to posttraumatic epilepsy. In addition, there is usually some deterioration in cognitive ability. Emotional or behavioral deviation usually produces the most significant disability. Some individuals show personality disturbance characterized by anxiety, depression, or irritability. Others may demonstrate a classic frontotemporal syndrome with memory impairment, apathy, lack of motivation, and indifference to the environment. Physicians must consider these emotional difficulties when providing treatment and rehabilitation to these patients.

B. PSYCHOLOGICAL TESTING

Neuropsychological test data are used to develop treatment strategies tailored for an individual's strengths and deficits. Neuropsychological testing can sometimes reveal subtle changes in information processing in patients who otherwise appear normal. A commonly used test is the paced auditory serial addition task. During this exercise, subjects listen to digits presented at a standard rate and add each digit to the one immediately preceding. Head trauma patients are both slower and less accurate than are normal subjects.

Patients with mild to moderate postconcussive disorder may become irritable or even aggressive, and exhibit blunt affect, apathy, or lack of spontaneity. The effects of mild to moderate head trauma can be subtle, and both patients and practitioners may make light of the cognitive impairment associated with mild head trauma despite sometimes devastating consequences.

In more severe forms of head trauma, neuropsychological testing can be used to measure the extent of secondary injury. To some extent this helps establish the prognosis. Neuropsychological testing can then be used to measure progress. Because cognitive rehabilitation is an important part of recovery, neuropsychological testing can help the psychologist focus on the particular areas of deficit.

C. LABORATORY FINDINGS AND IMAGING

The EEG is sensitive to brain changes following trauma. Local suppression of the alpha rhythm may extend bilaterally. In more severe injury, EEG discharges become progressively slower and delta activity may predominate. The EEG is not a reliable guide to prognosis, and other clinical features must be considered. An EEG that becomes normal early in the course of the illness usually predicts good recovery following head trauma. MRI is invaluable in detecting areas of structural damage.

Treatment

Recovery from head trauma is a dynamic process rather than a static one. As a result, treatment evolves during the course of recovery. In mild head trauma, treatment consists in determining the neuropsychological deficit and giving appropriate counseling. In addition, symptomatic treatment of headaches, dizziness, and mood alteration is useful. Intervention with the patient's employer may help foster understanding and help encourage work conditions that are more conducive to success.

In moderate or severe head trauma, the goals of treatment change as the patient recovers. The early stages of treatment may be oriented to merely suppressing violent outbursts and improving sleep. Later, therapy is tailored to improving memory, impulsiveness, irritability, and affective disorder. Both pharmacotherapy and psychotherapy are useful in this regard. Carbamazepine is generally useful for impulsiveness and may be combined with an atypical neuroleptic. Sleep disturbance may respond to trazodone. The affective disorders respond to SSRIs and other antidepressants. In general, these agents should be started at low doses, with gradual increases. Head trauma patients tend to be sensitive to medication side effects.

Complications/Adverse Outcomes of Treatment

Depression and anxiety are common in outpatients with traumatic brain injuries. These symptoms add to the morbidity of closed head trauma because depressed or anxious patients perceive themselves as more severely disabled. Death by suicide is a risk after head injury.

Alcohol and substance abuse also alter the outcome of traumatic brain injury. Alcohol intoxication is present in up to one-half of patients hospitalized for brain injury. Two-thirds of rehabilitation patients have a history of substance abuse preceding their injuries. Untreated substance abuse adversely affects cognitive status in rehabilitation patients.

Repeated head trauma in boxers produces dementia pugilistica. In its fully developed form, the disorder consists of cerebellar, pyramidal, and extrapyramidal features, along with intellectual deterioration. The syndrome may progress even after the boxer has retired from the sport.

Prognosis

Periods of unconsciousness may last several hours yet still be compatible with complete recovery. The longer the patient is unconscious, the poorer the outcome. As the patient recovers from severe head trauma, a period of confusion may follow lasting from hours to months. Some patients pass through a period of extremely disturbed behavior that poses severe management problems. The patient may be abusive, aggressive, or uncooperative. The patient may appear delirious during this time with vivid audiovisual hallucinations. When head trauma is associated with prolonged unconsciousness, recovery is usually followed by some degree of dementia. Recovery from mild to moderate head trauma is more variable and difficult to predict.

Graff-Radford NR, Godersky JC, Jones MP: Variables predicting surgical outcome in symptomatic hydrocephalus in the elderly. *Neurology* 1989;39:1601.

Levin HS, et al.: Serial MRI and neurobehavioral findings after mild to moderate closed head injury. *J Neurol Neurosurg Psychiatry* 1992;55:255.

DEMENTIA & DEPRESSION

Depressed seniors often deny mood disorder and focus on memory problems, complaining of memory loss disproportionate to their actual decrement in memory functioning. Because depressed seniors commonly exhibit impaired attention, perception, problem solving, or memory, psychometric testing may not distinguish depression from AD. This lack of diagnostic clarity has led to the term **pseudodementia.** This term creates unrealistic expectations for a psychiatric cure for dementia. Cognitive disorder seen during late-life affective disorder is real and not simulated. **Depressive cognitive dysfunction** is a more accurate term. In most cases, depression is a factor worsening dementia rather than the sole cause.

 ESSENTIALS OF DIAGNOSIS

The cognitive decline encountered in depressed older people is more precipitous than in demented patients. The history often reveals previous depression. The combined effects of age and depression produce a pattern of deficits distinct from that found in younger depressed patients and less severe than that in Alzheimer's patients. The actual memory impairment is modest in depressed patients, but the level of subjective complaint is high. In contrast, organically impaired patients have more memory loss and less subjective complaints. The cognitive dysfunction encountered in depressed patients is probably secondary to decreased arousal with associated deficits in motivation and attention. Depressed patients do well on simple tasks but poorly on tasks requiring sustained attention or concentration. Following drug treatment, their performance improves. Patients' cognitive complaints correlate with depressive symptoms rather than with MMSE scores.

Clinical Findings

A. Signs and Symptoms

Patients with depressive dementia often exhibit early morning awakening, anxiety, weight loss, psychomotor retardation, and decreased libido. Patients with dementia present with disorientation, and their daily activities are more seriously impaired. Despite these differences, there is no definitive diagnostic tool. Cognitive decline in depressed older people commonly has a multifactorial etiology. In fact, depression may be the presenting symptom of a degenerative disorder.

B. Laboratory Findings

The dexamethasone suppression test is not useful in discriminating between depression and dementia or between subtypes of dementia. Sleep studies distinguish depression from dementia with about 85% accuracy. Depressed seniors experience shorter rapid eye movement (REM) latency, higher REM sleep percentage, less non-REM sleep disturbance, and early morning awakening. Patients with AD experience less REM sleep. Computerized techniques, including amplitude frequency measures and spectral analyses, permit new approaches to the examination of delta sleep. Many depressed patients show lower delta wave intensity during the first non-REM period than during the second period.

Several studies have shown an association between depressive dementia and degenerative dementia. The longer the follow-up, the more likely that depressive dementia will evolve into degenerative dementia. Elderly depressed patients also display a remarkable increase in prevalence of cortical infarcts and leukoencephalopathy. Depressed patients tend also to have basal ganglia lesions, sulcal atrophy, large cerebral ventricles, and subcortical white-matter lesions. Nevertheless, AD patients have more prominent cortical atrophy compared to those with major depression.

C. Imaging

PET scans distinguish dementia from late-life depression more clearly than does structural imaging (i.e., CT scan and MRI). The temporoparietal pattern observed in patients with primary degenerative dementia is not observed in those with affective disorder. In severely depressed patients, PET scans show left-right prefrontal asymmetry in resting-state cerebral metabolic rates. Successful drug therapy reduces the asymmetry. In depression, the decrease in glucose metabolism is more pronounced in prefrontal areas, and these changes persist despite clinical improvement, suggesting that the abnormality is not state dependent.

Differential Diagnosis

Both mania and depression can present as pseudodelirium. Vegetative signs are not helpful in distinguishing depression from delirium. Laboratory investigations are required. Mania may present with symptoms of dementia, but delirium is more common. About one quarter of manic patients over age 65 years have no history of affective illness. Cognitive changes often persist even after the patient has "switched" into depression.

Treatment

Treatment with lithium, carbamazepine, or valproate resolves both mania and cognitive impairment. Antidepressant medication for affective disorder is usually effective, however, side effects are troublesome in older patients. Previous treatment response should help guide therapy. Unfortunately, one-third of the seniors hospitalized for mania experience a permanent decline in their MMSE scores. This suggests that late-life mania is related to structural changes in the brain.

Because TCAs are likely to cause adverse drug reactions in seniors, SSRI's or SNRI's are generally preferred. Occasionally, monoamine oxidase inhibitors, alprazolam, and bupropion are useful. For mild depression, SSRIs are the first-line agents. Psychostimulants such as methylphenidate and dextroamphetamine present yet another treatment option. These drugs appear to be of particular benefit when used in the short term for the treatment of depression that complicates medical illness.

Lithium is effective in treating bipolar disorder, but its side effect of impairing renal function limits its use. In elderly patients, lithium has a very narrow therapeutic index. Lithium toxicity can occur quickly, damaging already-compromised kidneys. Valproate may be preferred if the patient has a new-onset illness and has not previously been exposed to treatment. If lithium is used, very close monitoring is required. When other therapies have failed, ECT may reverse pseudodementia or pseudodelirium dramatically. ECT is safe and effective, even in patients older than 80 years or in those with poststroke depression. Common complications of ECT in the elderly include severe confusion, falls, and cardiorespiratory problems.

DELUSIONS & BEHAVIORAL DISTURBANCE

As dementia worsens, behavioral problems emerge. Problem behavior often stems from the inability of staff to understand patients' needs. It is important to identify the cause of the dementia before rushing into pharmacologic treatment. Patients can exhibit behavioral disturbances because they are hungry, thirsty, bored, constipated, tired, sexually aroused, or in pain. Patients with dementia, like all of us, need to feel loved, and they benefit from opportunities to develop self-esteem. An initial psychosocial approach to these problematic patients should assess whether these needs are being met.

A multidisciplinary team setting is the most appropriate format for setting treatment goals that are then communicated to the family. It is essential to involve the family in order to educate them and to initiate social interventions. Patients and family members need to believe that a meaningful life is possible despite dementia. This is particularly true if family members are taught to validate the patient's emotional experience. Very little can be gained by approaches aimed at reorientation or enforcing confrontation with reality. Support groups help family members learn not only to cope with the negative outcomes but also to understand their loved one in the context of the illness.

Drug therapy of abnormal behaviors associated with dementia are problematic. First, the anticholinesterase agents and memantine have been demonstrated to improve behavior to some degree. Psychotropic medications must be used cautiously. The Omnibus Reconciliation Act of 1990 introduced specific restrictions on the use of psychotropic medication in the care of nursing home residents. Nonetheless, pharmacotherapy is often essential for treatment of the behavioral disorders that accompany dementia. Psychiatrists are frequently asked to treat agitation in demented patients. Antipsychotics, antidepressants, and sedative-hypnotics are used widely for this purpose, however, data from double-blind clinical trials are limited.

Neuroleptics are effective in some patients with dementia related psychosis. In many other patients they are of absolutely no benefit and may even be harmful. Although atypical agents have a lower incidence of extrapyramidal side effects including tardive dyskinesia, these newer agents all carry a black box warning regarding an increase in death rate in treated patients. A review of 17 placebo-controlled studies involving four of the atypical antipsychotics showed that the death rate for elderly patients with dementia was about 1.6–1.7 times that of placebo.

There is no evidence that atypical agents offer convincing benefits in this population. Despite many millions of dollars spent by pharmaceutical companies on double blind placebo controlled trials, these agents demonstrate limited or no efficacy when compared to placebo. In the Clinical Antipsychotic Trials of Intervention Effectiveness (CATIE) study, a large government study of atypical antipsychotics in AD, about 30% of those taking the active medications improved, compared to 21% of those taking placebo. But atypical antipsychotic medications also were more often associated with troubling side effects, such as sedation, confusion, and weight gain, compared to placebo. All neuroleptics should be used in as low doses as possible and for as short a duration as possible. Neuroleptics should be reduced periodically or discontinued in order to determine ongoing need. Dementia is a progressive and dynamic process. Patients who required therapy at an early stage of the illness may no longer benefit at a later stage.

Short-acting benzodiazepines control agitation and may be used on occasion in the short term to treat agitation or as a hypnotic in severely demented patients. They can be used in conjunction with antipsychotics. Benzodiazepines are effective for only a minority of patients, and they cause drowsiness, paradoxical agitation, memory loss, an increased risk of falling, and potential habituation. Their use should be reserved for the management of short-term crisis situations in which a rapid response is necessary.

Trazodone has been used to control aggression in demented patients on the theory that aggression is related to serotonergic depletion. Patients generally receive a mild benefit with nighttime doses of 50–100 mg/day. Because some elderly patients experience gait disturbances immediately after the nighttime dose, fall precautions must be taken. Buspirone reduces agitation in dementia in dosages of 20–40 mg/day. Some patients respond preferentially to valproic acid. These patients often have manic symptoms associated with agitation, including pressured speech, flight of ideas, and sleeplessness.

There are few placebo-controlled studies of the drugs used to treat agitation in older people, but the use of psychopharmacology is common in patients who have failed conventional treatment. Carbamazepine or valproate may be best for patients with manic symptoms, buspirone for patients with anxiety, and antidepressants for patients who appear depressed. Because these medications often are given to dementia patients for prolonged periods, studies are needed to define their long-term clinical efficacy.

Some behaviors such as wandering, purposeless repetitive activity, stealing, and screaming are not amenable to pharmacologic intervention. These behaviors must be dealt with by environmental design such as the wanderguard system (a wristband alarm system) or appropriate soundproofing. Clinicians can reduce the occurrence of sundowning by promoting daytime activity, preventing daytime napping, and enforcing a regular sleep schedule. The medical treatment of sundowning can be frustrating, however, sedatives are sometimes helpful.

Burke WJ: Neuroleptic drug use in the nursing home: The impact of OBRA. *Am Fam Physician* 1991;43:2125.

Cummings JL, Schneider E, Tariot PN, et al.: Behavioral effects of memantine in Alzheimer disease patients receiving donepezil therapy. *Neurology* 2006;67:57–63.

Flint AJ, van Reekum R: The pharmacologic treatment of Alzheimer's disease: A guide for the general psychiatrist [see comments]. *Can J Psychiatry* 1998;43:689.

Schneider LS, Dagerman KS, Insel P. Risk of death with atypical antipsychotic drug treatment for dementia. Meta-analysis of randomized placebo-controlled trials. *JAMA* 2005;294:1934–1943.

Schneider L, Tariot P, Dagerman K, et al.: Effectiveness of Atypical Antipsychotic Drugs in Patients with Alzheimer's Disease. *N Engl J Med* 2006;355:1525–1538.

Sink KM, Holden KF, Yaffe K: Pharmacological treatment of neuropsychiatric symptoms of dementia. A review of the evidence. *JAMA* 2005;293:596–608.

Wang PS, Schneeweiss S, Avorn J, et al.: Risk of death in elderly users of conventional vs. atypical antipsychotic medications. *N Engl J Med* 2005;353:2335–2341.

■ AMNESTIC DISORDERS

MEMORY FUNCTION

The study of memory is a great challenge because the systems that underlie memory function are complex. Patients are diagnosed with an amnestic disorder when they are unable to learn new information or recall previously learned facts or events, in the absence of a delirium or dementia. An amnestic disorder may be due to a general medical condition or induced by a particular toxin. The physician must report the responsible medical condition as part of the Axis I diagnosis. Amnestic disorders are difficult to categorize and may be difficult to distinguish from mild generalized cognitive impairment.

SHORT-TERM VERSUS LONG-TERM MEMORY

There is much controversy about the nature and measurement of memory. Although some cognitive scientists use the term "short-term memory" to mean immediate attention span and long-term storage for longer retained memories, clinicians generally use the terms "immediate," "short-term," and "long-term" or remote memory. Immediate memory, also called "working memory," consists of registration and attention span, as for 7 digits forwards. Immediate memory is retained for seconds only, unless the subject actively rehearses the information. Immediate memory retains information in reverberating neural circuits involving the frontal lobes. If it is not converted to short-term storage, data is lost. Memories are stored through a process called consolidation. Short-term memories are recalled through the hippocampi and related structures, also the amygdala when emotion or fear are important to the memory. Long-term, or remote memory, is thought to be stored in the cortex and may not require the hippocampus for access. Short-term memory is a biochemical process that depends on protein synthesis and the development of dendritic connections. In the clinical setting, patients who have difficulty learning new material are described as having an anterograde amnesia.

Patients who have difficulty recalling information stored before the onset of an illness or injury have retrograde amnesia. The retention of material in long-term storage depends on that part of the cerebral cortex related to the specific sensory modality involved. Thus if both the occipital and occipital-parietal cortices are involved in an injury, visual memories may be impaired significantly.

IMPLICIT VERSUS EXPLICIT MEMORY

Cognitive neuroscience has provided strong support for the idea that multiple memory systems exist. One system divides memory into explicit and implicit types. **Explicit memory** is synonymous with declarative memory. Declarative memory reflects a conscious recollection of the past. The short-term memory discussed above, **episodic memory** of a person's own conscious experiences, is a form of declarative or explicit memory, but so is the recall of factual information, often called **semantic memory.** Declarative memories are consciously known and are therefore explicit. Explicit memory disorders are well recognized clinically. Lesions in the medial temporal lobes, midline diencephalon, or basal forebrain can impair declarative memory because relationships between sensory modalities are processed through the hippocampal diencephalic system.

Patients with semantic deficits may retain factual autobiographical information. The retention of this information implies that episodic memory is intact. Patients with the classic amnestic syndromes often have impairment of episodic memory. In contrast, patients with AD have significant deficiencies in semantic memory, as well as in episodic memory.

Nondeclarative memory is sometimes called implicit memory. **Implicit memory** implies that a person may be able to know something without being aware of remembering it. Implicit memory is not usually tested clinically. Implicit memory does not involve the conscious recollection of recent experiences for the execution of tasks. Procedural learning (e.g., how to drive a car) is an example of implicit memory. Apraxia can be seen as a deficit in implicit memory. Amnestic patients can learn certain skills or acquire problem-solving abilities, even though they have no memory of having learned the behavior.

The basal ganglia, cerebellum, and frontal lobes have been linked to procedural learning. Procedural learning does not involve the hippocampal diencephalic system.

Procedural learning is most affected in subcortical dementias such as Huntington's and PDs.

Additional examples of implicit learning include classical conditioning (stimulus-response) and operant conditioning (reinforcing behaviors). Even people who do not have amnestic disorders learn by classical conditioning but may not be able to recollect the experience. People who have severe declarative memory disorders are quite capable of learning through stimulus-response and reinforcement paradigms. The cerebellum is heavily involved in this type of memory.

Yet another form of memory is **probabilistic learning,** in which we learn from past experiences to predict the future. This form of memory is also relatively independent of medial temporal lobe functions.

All memories are influenced heavily by emotions. Memory for emotionally arousing events is modulated by an endogenous memory-modulating system consisting of stress hormones and the amygdala. This system is an adaptive method of creating memory strength that is proportional to memory importance. In addition, some memory is state specific so that these memories can be recalled only during emotional states similar to the ones present when they were created.

It is important for the practitioner to realize that memory is highly complex and difficult to quantify at the bedside. It is equally important to recognize that in patients with amnestic syndromes, neuropsychological testing reveals normal perception, language, motor functions, and preserved intellectual skills.

THEORIES OF MEMORY

Recently neural network theories of memory have been proposed. Distinct neural networks mediate different memory modalities. Neural networks are based on the idea that streams of information are combined by forming, strengthening, or pruning connections between neurons to form new representations which can later be retrieved. Evidence for this process comes from the fact that damage to specific areas of the association cortex affects individual sensory memory modalities. Currently, research in functional brain imaging is being combined with these theories to provide a new source of information about how memory systems function.

CLINICAL SYNDROMES

Clinical bedside diagnosis of amnestic disorders is easiest to establish with damage to the medial temporal lobe. The severity of memory impairment depends heavily on the location and extent of damage in these brain structures. The thalamus, basal ganglia, cerebellum, frontal lobe, and other cortical structures also play a role.

The anatomic structures affected in amnestic disorders include the medial temporal lobes, mammillary bodies, fornix, medial dorsal thalamus, and frontal lobes, known as Papez's circuit. Damage to these pathways by neurologic insults or toxins causes clinical memory problems. Injuries and toxic exposures can produce either reversible or irreversible amnestic conditions.

SUBSTANCE-INDUCED PERSISTING AMNESTIC DISORDER

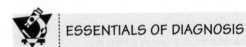

ESSENTIALS OF DIAGNOSIS

DSM-IV Diagnostic Criteria

A. The development of memory impairment as manifested by impairment in the ability to learn new information or the inability to recall previously learned information.

B. The memory disturbance causes significant impairment in social or occupational functioning and represents a significant decline from a previous level of functioning.

C. The memory disturbance does not occur exclusively during the course of a delirium or a dementia and persists beyond the usual duration of substance intoxication or withdrawal.

D. There is evidence from the history, physical examination, or laboratory findings that the memory disturbance is etiologically related to persisting effects of substance use (e.g., a drug of abuse, a medication).

(Reprinted with permission from Diagnostic and Statistical Manual of Mental Disorders, 4th edn. Copyright 1994 American Psychiatric Association.)

1. Korsakoff's Syndrome

Korsakoff's syndrome, now usually referred to as the **Wernicke-Korsakoff syndrome,** is a severe anterograde learning defect associated with confabulations. These patients have difficulty encoding and consolidating explicit memory. Storage is mildly impaired, but retrieval and new learning are severely impaired. When Korsakoff's patients process new material, they forget information at a normal rate, but learning new material is extremely difficult; in severe cases, new learning is impossible. Retrograde memory is also impaired in Korsakoff's syndrome, especially back to the onset of illness and perhaps a period earlier. The most remote memories prior to the onset of illness are spared. As a result, Korsakoff's patients retain more distant memories dramatically more proficiently than they learn new material.

Korsakoff's patients have little impairment in implicit memory, and their ability to perform motor procedures remains intact. They may retain the capacity to complete complex motor tasks. Typically general intelligence, perceptual skills, and language remain relatively normal. The cardinal symptom of Korsakoff's syndrome is confabulation. Although remote memory for events before the neurologic insult is often surprisingly intact, Korsakoff's patients are unable to organize memories in a temporal context. Because they distort the relationships between facts, Korsakoff's patients have remote memory deficits.

Korsakoff's syndrome commonly follows an episode of Wernicke's encephalopathy. This neurologic condition is manifested by confusion, ataxia, and nystagmus; thiamine deficiency is its direct cause. If thiamine is given during the acute stage of Wernicke's encephalopathy, Korsakoff's syndrome can be prevented. The administration of glucose-containing fluid must be avoided, for it will hasten Korsakoff's syndrome unless the patient has been adequately dosed with thiamine and recovery has begun. Alcohol abuse causes the conditions that lead to Korsakoff's syndrome, but malnutrition alone can cause the disorder, for example, in hyperemesis gravidarum or in patients with surgery for morbid obesity. The lesions caused by thiamine deficiency occur in the hippocampus, the mammillary bodies, and the anterior and dorsal nucleus of the thalamus, and disrupt the Papez's circuit, referred to earlier.

2. Amnesia from Drugs & Toxins

Patients prescribed sedatives, hypnotics, and anxiolytics can develop substance-induced amnestic disorders. Amnestic syndromes usually follow intense, continuous use of these drugs, but recovery usually occurs when the patient stops using the offending agent. Toxins can also cause amnestic disorders. Neurotransmitters involved in memory include acetylcholine, catecholamines, GABA, and glutamic acid. Disruption of these transmitter systems by drugs or toxins also disrupts specific memory functions. Drugs having this effect include benzodiazepines, anticonvulsants, and antiarrhythmics. Amnesia is a characteristic of all the benzodiazepines, with the effect depending on the route of administration, dose, and pharmacokinetics of the specific drug. The amnestic effects of benzodiazepines are sometimes used for therapeutic purposes during surgical procedures. Toxins that affect memory include organophosphates, carbon monoxide, and organic solvents. Chronic exposure to these and other neurotoxins may also affect memory. The patient's ability to recover memory functions depends on the substance, the length of exposure, and other comorbidities.

AMNESTIC DISORDER DUE TO A GENERAL MEDICAL CONDITION

 ESSENTIALS OF DIAGNOSIS

DSM-IV Diagnostic Criteria

A. The development of memory impairment as manifested by impairment in the ability to learn new information or the inability to recall previously learned information.

B. The memory disturbance causes significant impairment in social or occupational functioning and represents a significant decline from a previous level of functioning.

C. The memory disturbance does not occur exclusively during the course of a delirium or a dementia.

D. There is evidence from the history, physical examination, or laboratory findings that the disturbance is the direct physiological consequence of a general medical condition (including physical trauma).

Specify if:
Transient: if memory impairment lasts for 1 month or less. When the diagnosis is made within the first month without waiting for recovery, the term "provisional" may be added.

Chronic: If memory impairment lasts for more than 1 month.

(Reprinted with permission from Diagnostic and Statistical Manual of Mental Disorders, 4th edn. Copyright 1994 American Psychiatric Association.)

1. Temporal Lobe Memory Syndromes

The medial temporal lobe system consists of the hippocampus and adjacent, anatomically related entorhinal, perirhinal, and parahippocampal cortices. These structures have widespread and reciprocal connections with the neocortex. Medial temporal structures are essential for consolidating short-term memory for facts and events, however, the function of this system is temporary. As time passes, memory stored in the neocortex becomes independent of the medial temporal lobe. Lesions that involve the medial temporal lobes are the most important clinical cause of the amnestic syndrome. Earlier in this chapter we discussed the Wernicke-Korsakoff syndrome, the prototypic example of an amnestic syndrome. Bilateral strokes in the distribution of the posterior cerebral arteries, bilateral medial temporal lobectomy for epilepsy, or Herpes simplex encephalitis can produce bilateral temporal lobe lesions. Patients with bilateral temporal lobe damage develop an amnestic syndrome with profound deficits in learning and retention. Lesions of the fornix and bilateral paramedial thalamic lesions also disrupt temporal lobe memory circuits, causing patterns of amnesia that resemble the Wernicke-Korsakoff syndrome.

Unilateral damage to the medial temporal lobe produces distinct temporal lobe memory syndromes. These memory deficits are commonly observed in patients with hippocampal sclerosis. Deficits may be selective for verbal material if the lesion is in the left temporal lobe, or for nonverbal material if the right temporal lobe is involved. Patients with these deficits often have complex partial seizures as well as memory problems. When the seizure disorder is highly active, the memory deficit may be more profound. Patients with temporal lobe resections for epilepsy or posterior cerebral artery territory strokes on one side can develop similar syndromes.

Partial amnesia syndromes can also result from temporal lobe damage. Damage to the lateral temporal lobe causes aphasia or loss of long-stored auditory memories. Temporal lobe lesions that disconnect the hippocampus from the association cortex can produce memory disorders specific for a sensory modality such as vision or touch. Temporal lobe damage can result from prolonged seizures, anoxia, trauma, ischemia, or basilar meningitis.

2. Frontal Lobe Memory Syndromes

The frontal lobes, via connections to the striatum and thalamus, is involved in the executive component of working memory, which plays an important role in some forms of sensorimotor skill learning. In patients with frontal lobe damage, memory for procedural steps may be impaired. A phenomenon of frontal lobe memory disorder is "forgetting to remember," such as going to the basement to get a tool and also remembering to get something out of the freezer. Patients with frontal memory problems have difficulty maintaining set. They interpret the world concretely. Not only do they have a tendency to become distracted, they also perseverate. Working mem-

ory deficits correlate with frontal lobe convexity damage, especially on the left side. Patients with left frontal lobe damage have difficulty with rote verbal learning, whereas patients with right frontal lobe damage may have difficulty keeping visuospatial memories preserved for rehearsal and learning of spatial relationships.

3. Transient Global Amnesia

Transient global amnesia is a syndrome of temporary memory loss, called "global" because it affects all types of short-term memory. Consciousness and self-awareness are preserved. Associated behavioral changes include repetitive questioning, with failure to recall the answers to the questions. The syndrome resolves within 24 hours. After the attack the only remaining symptom is a permanent amnestic gap for the duration of the episode, and perhaps a few minutes before the onset of the memory loss. The syndrome is recurrent in a minority of cases. Transient global amnesia was originally thought to have cerebrovascular etiology; although the disorder is associated with conventional risk factors for cerebrovascular disease, it does not appear to carry the same risk of stroke as a TIA, and in general the syndrome carries a benign prognosis. Some patients have been reported to have diffusion-weighted MRI lesions in the hippocampus during Transposition of Great Arteries (TGA) attacks. The etiologies of TGA may be multiple; recurrent attacks are often related to migraine or partial epilepsy.

4. Post-ECT Memory Disorders

Memory loss is a well-known side effect of ECT. Anterograde memory loss for events during the series of treatments is to be expected. Mild retrograde amnesia also occurs. Memory complaints are more common in individuals who receive bilateral ECT. Nondominant unilateral ECT has been shown in a small number of poorly designed studies to improve memory in some depressed patients, however, it is often less efficacious than bilateral ECT.

The long-term memory problems associated with ECT are more troubling to patients than are the short-term ones. ECT creates a persistent storage deficit that results in accelerated forgetting. Capacity for new learning recovers substantially by several months after ECT, but accelerated forgetting can be documented for up to 6 months post-ECT.

5. Amnestic Disorders Due to Head Trauma

Memory deficits are frequent after head trauma. The pattern of memory disorder depends on the nature of the injury. Patients who are severely injured have damage to multiple cortical structures. The variability of the damage is so great that no single pattern of amnestic disorder occurs after head trauma. Mild head trauma produces short-term memory deficits that recover over a few months. More severe damage may cause deficits that prevent the patient from returning to school or to work. In general, the duration of total antegrade amnesia, the length of retrograde amnesia, and the length of loss of consciousness all correlate with the severity of posttraumatic amnesia. Because damage to structures involved in the maintenance of attention interferes with the patient's ability to learn new material, frontal lobe damage can contribute to the memory deficits observed in closed head trauma. Other neurologic damage, emotional difficulties, and psychiatric disorder may contribute significantly to the memory disorder observed in head trauma patients. Finally, head trauma patients are frequently involved in legal action; therefore, some individuals intentionally exaggerate deficits to derive secondary gain.

Retrograde deficits after closed head injury last for variable amounts of time, with a characteristic pattern of greatest deficits immediately after injury and improvement during the 2 years that follow. "Shrinking retrograde amnesia" has been described, in which memories more distant from the injury are recovered first. More recent events are recovered later. A focal retrograde amnesia, in which patients are unable to remember specific events, has also been described. This focal retrograde amnesia has involved autobiographical information in some patients. Posttraumatic amnesia is related both to deficits in information processing speed and to cognitive outcome.

Baddeley A: Working memory. *Science* 1992;255:556–559.

Budson AE, Price BH: Memory dysfunction. *N Engl J Med* 2005; 352:692–699.

Cabeza R, Mangels J, Nyberg L, et al.: Brain regions differentially involved in remembering what and when: A PETstudy. *Neuron* 1997;19:863–870.

Haslam C, et al.: Post-coma disturbance and post-traumatic amnesia as nonlinear predictors of cognitive outcome following severe closed head injury: Findings from the Westmead Head Injury Project. *Brain Inj* 1994;8:519.

Hodges JR, Warlow CP: The aetiology of transient global amnesia. A case-control study of 114 cases with prospective follow-up. *Brain* 1990;113:639.

Kirshner HS: Approaches to intellectual and memory impairments. In: Bradley W, et al.: (ed). *Clinical Practice*, 4th edn. Butterworth Heinemann (Elsevier), 2004, pp. 65–74.

Kopelman MD: The Korsakoff syndrome. *Br J Psychiatry* 1995;166: 154.

Milner B: Some cognitive effects of frontal-lobe lesions in man. *Phil Trans R Soc Lond (Biol)* 1982;298:211.

Polster MR: Drug-induced amnesia: Implications for cognitive neuropsychological investigations of memory. *Psychol Bull* 1993; 114:477.

Ross ED: Sensory-specific and fractional disorders of recent memory in man. II. Unilateral loss of tactile recent memory. *Arch Neurol* 1980;37:267.

Squire LR, Zola SM: Structure and function of declarative and nondeclarative memory systems. *Proc Natl Acad Sci U S A* 1996; 93:13515–13522.

Squire LR, Zola-Morgan S: The medial temporal lobe memory system. *Science* 1991;253:1380–1386.

Strupp M, Bruning R, Wu RH, et al.: Diffusion-weighted MRI in ransient global amnesia: Elevated signal intensity in the left mesial temporal lobe in 7 of 10 patients. *Ann Neurol* 1998; 43:164–170.

Thompson RF, Kim JJ: Memory systems in the brain and localization of a memory. *Proc Natl Acad Sci U S A* 1996;93:13438–13444.

Ungerleider LG, Courtney SM, Haxby JV: A neural system for human visual working memory. *Proc Natl Acad Sci U S A* 1998;95: 883–890.

Wagner AD, Schacter DL, Rotte M, et al.: Building memories: Remembering and forgetting of verbal experiences as predicted by brain activity. *Science* 1998;281:1188–1191.

Squire LR: ECT and memory loss. *Am J Psychiatry* 1977;134:997.

CONCLUSION

The psychiatrist must use the medical model skillfully to participate fully in the care of patients who have delirium, dementia, or other cognitive disorders. The dual diagnosis of neurologic and affective disorders is more the rule than the exception. In many patients, affective state and optimal cognitive functioning are mutually dependent. The diagnostic skills obtained through the practice of general psychiatry have tremendous value. Treatment of affective disorders and other psychiatric conditions contribute significantly to the patient's ultimate cognitive outcome.

In the care of patients who have delirium and dementia, the boundary between neurology and psychiatry is blurred; the specialties of neuropsychiatry and behavioral neurology have evolved to meet the needs of patients with these disorders. Specific neurologic disorders cause specific neurobehavioral disorders and psychiatric symptoms. Although diagnosis does not determine a cure, it does suggest an appropriate clinical treatment plan. The cost-effective treatment of neuropsychiatric disorders requires a basic understanding of the neurological underpinnings to their disorders. The psychiatrist must have a thorough understanding of the effects of normal aging, delirium, and dementia. Eventually research will uncover prevention techniques based on diet, exercise, antioxidants, or other yet undiscovered compounds. Until then, the medical model remains the most useful method for the treatment of these mental disorders.

Substance-Related Disorders[1]

15

Peter R. Martin, MD

ESSENTIALS OF DIAGNOSIS

DSM-IV Diagnostic Criteria

Substance Dependence

A maladaptive pattern of substance use, leading to clinically significant impairment or distress, as manifested by three (or more) of the following, occurring at any time in the same 12-month period:

(1) tolerance

(2) withdrawal

(3) the substance is often taken in larger amounts or over a longer period than was intended

(4) there is a persistent desire or unsuccessful efforts to cut down or control substance use

(5) a great deal of time is spent in activities necessary to obtain the substance, use the substance, or recover from its effects

(6) important social, occupational, or recreational activities are given up or reduced because of substance use

(7) the substance use is continued despite knowledge of having a persistent or recurrent physical or psychological problem that is likely to have been caused or exacerbated by the substance

Substance Abuse

A. A maladaptive pattern of substance use leading to clinically significant impairment or distress, as manifested by one (or more) of the following, occurring within a 12-month period:

    (1) recurrent substance use resulting in failure to fulfill major role obligations at work, school, or home

    (2) recurrent substance use in situations in which it is physically hazardous

    (3) recurrent substance-related legal problems

    (4) continued substance use despite having persistent or recurrent social or interpersonal problems caused or exacerbated by the effects of the substance

B. The symptoms have never met the criteria for substance dependence for this class of substance.

Substance Intoxication

A. The development of a reversible substance-specific syndrome due to recent ingestion of (or exposure to) a substance.

B. Clinically significant maladaptive behavioral or psychological changes that are due to the effect of the substance on the central nervous system.

C. The symptoms are not due to a general medical condition and are not better accounted for by another mental disorder.

Substance Withdrawal

A. The development of a substance-specific syndrome due to the cessation of (or reduction in) substance use that has been heavy and prolonged.

B. The substance-specific syndrome causes clinically significant distress or impairment in social, occupational, or other important areas of functioning.

C. The symptoms are not due to a general medical condition and are not better accounted for by another mental disorder.

(Adapted, with permission, from *Diagnostic and Statistical Manual of Mental Disorders*, 4th edn. Copyright 1994 American Psychiatric Association.)

[1] This work was supported in part by the National Institute on Alcohol Abuse and Alcoholism (RO1 AA014969) and the National Institute on Drug Abuse (RO1 DA015713 and T32 DA021123).

Table 15–1. Substance-Related Disorders as Classified in DSM-IV-TR

Substance-use disorders
Substance dependence
Substance abuse

Substance-induced disorders
Substance-induced intoxication
Substance withdrawal
Substance-induced delirium
Substance-induced persisting dementia
Substance-induced persisting amnestic disorder
Substance-induced psychotic disorder
Substance-induced mood disorder
Substance-induced anxiety disorder
Substance-induced sexual dysfunction
Substance-induced sleep disorder

Classification of Substance-Related Disorders

The substance-related disorders are classified into two categories: (1) substance-use disorders and (2) substance-induced disorders (Table 15–1). The substance-use disorders are (somewhat arbitrarily) dichotomized into substance abuse and substance dependence based on the number of relevant symptoms that the patient exhibits. The *Diagnostic and Statistical Manual of Mental Disorders,* fourth edition (DSM-IV) specifies substance-use disorders that result from the self-administration of several different drugs of abuse (Table 15–2).

The specific criteria for diagnosis of substance-use disorders draw heavily on the concept of the **dependence syndrome.** This important advance in our thinking about these disorders frames the interactions among the pharmacologic actions of the drug, individual psychopathology, and the effects of the environment in a clinically meaningful construct that is generalizable to all drugs of abuse. This concept is derived from the clinical observation that patients may have maladaptive behavior as a result of drug use without the presence of neurophysiologic adaptive changes such as tolerance or withdrawal (also referred to as **neuroadaptation**). Neuroadaptation is not necessarily dysfunctional if there is no concomitant inappropriate desire to continue the use of the drug (**drug seeking**). For example, driving while drunk may have devastating consequences, particularly in the sporadically drinking young driver who has not acquired tolerance to ethanol. In another example, the postsurgical patient who has been receiving morphine

Table 15–2. Classes of Substances of Abuse in DSM-IV-TR

Class	Common Examples
Alcohol	Beer, wine, sherry, whiskey, vodka, gin
Amphetamine and amphetamine-like substances	Amphetamine, dextroamphetamine, methamphetamine, methylphenidate, diet pills, khat
Caffeine	Coffee, tea, soft drinks, analgesics, cold remedies, stimulants, diet pills
Cannabis	Marijuana, hashish, delta-9-tetrahydrocannabinol (THC)
Cocaine	Coca leaves or paste, cocaine hydrochloride, cocaine alkaloid (crack)
Hallucinogens	Lysergic acid diethylamide (LSD), psilocybin, dimethyltryptamine, mescaline
Inhalants	Aliphatic, aromatic, and halogenated hydrocarbons (e.g., gasoline, glue, paint, paint thinners, other volatile compounds)
Nicotine	Cigarettes and other types of tobacco products
Opioids	Heroin, morphine, methadone, codeine, hydromorphone, oxycodone, meperidine, fentanyl, pentazocine, buprenorphine
Phencyclidine and phencyclidine-like substances	Phencyclidine, ketamine
Sedatives, hypnotics, and anxiolytics	Benzodiazepines (e.g., diazepam, oxazepam, chlordiazepoxide, alprazolam, midazolam, clonazepam), barbiturates (e.g., secobarbital, amobarbital, pentobarbital, phenobarbital), nonbarbiturate hypnosedatives (e.g., ethchlorvynol, glutethimide, chloral hydrate, methaqualone)
Other	Anabolic steroids, nitrite inhalants, nitrous oxide, and various over-the-counter and prescription drugs that do not readily fall into the other categories

for pain relief clearly exhibits neuroadaptation but is not likely to develop the dependence syndrome.

Fundamental to the concept of the dependence syndrome is the priority of drug seeking over other behaviors in the maintenance of dysfunctional drug use. Lesser weight is attributed to the presence of tolerance or withdrawal. In general, three (or more) individual symptoms from among the following three symptom clusters need to be part of the clinical presentation for the diagnosis of substance dependence: (1) loss of control (i.e., the substance is taken in larger amounts or over a longer period than intended, or there are unsuccessful efforts to reduce use); (2) salience to the behavioral repertoire (i.e., a great deal of time is spent in substance-related activities at the expense of important social, occupational, or recreational activities that are reduced or given up, or there is continued substance use despite knowledge of having a persistent or recurrent physical or psychological problem likely to have been caused or exacerbated by the substance); and (3) neuroadaptation (i.e., the presence of tolerance or withdrawal).

Diagnosis of a substance-use disorder by the presence of a given number of symptoms provides at best an incomplete picture of various clinically important features of the illness, such as severity, course, and prognosis, as well as indicated treatment for this heterogeneous patient population. The issue of illness severity is addressed in DSM-IV primarily by a distinction between substance abuse and dependence. The importance of diagnostic criteria for drug abuse is evident: They identify the substantial minority of individuals who have a history of maladaptive substance use but do not progress to dependence despite continuing substance abuse and developing certain associated problems. However, the distinction between drug abuse and dependence may not be practical, or possible, if substance-use disorders are considered in terms of continuities rather than categorically. As a result, substance abuse is a residual category, applied only to individuals who do not meet criteria for substance dependence (for the given class of substance) but still experience clinically significant impairment or distress in life functioning as a result of substance use. In order to augment diagnostic sensitivity and also maintain the primacy of drug-seeking behavior, a person can be diagnosed as substance dependent without ever having exhibited tolerance or withdrawal. In DSM-IV, dependence is formally subtyped according to whether or not there is physiologic dependence (i.e., the presence of tolerance or withdrawal). Finally, to better characterize individual patients, certain descriptive terms, or **course specifiers,** have been added to distinguish among different clinical courses of the dependence syndrome. For example, a dependent patient may be in remission (which may be early or sustained, full or partial), on agonist therapy (e.g., methadone or, more recently, buprenorphine, a mixed μ-opioid receptor agonist–antagonist, that is now

used for maintenance treatment much as methadone), or in a controlled environment (e.g., locked hospital ward).

It may be exceedingly difficult to establish whether psychopathology in a given individual who has a substance-use disorder is a consequence of drug use or is due to an additional psychiatric diagnosis. Table 15–3 indicates the broad overlap between substance-induced disorders and other psychiatric syndromes considered in this book. For example, diverse psychiatric signs and symptoms, including those of delirium (see Chapter 14), psychotic disorders (see Chapters 16 and 17), mood disorders (see Chapter 18), anxiety disorders (see Chapter 19), sexual dysfunction (see Chapter 25), and sleep disorders (see Chapter 27), can have their onset during intoxication or withdrawal. Dementia, amnestic disorder, and flashbacks (recurrences of the intoxicating effects of the drug that may occur years after use) associated with hallucinogen use may persist long after the acute effects of intoxication and withdrawal have abated. Accordingly, it is helpful to determine, preferably by longitudinal observation or by history, the timing of the onset of psychopathology with respect to the initiation of drug use, and whether it is still present when drug use has ceased, recognizing that the duration of abstinence can be a determining variable.

Pharmacotherapy of a complicating psychiatric disorder is currently considered appropriate if it is an independent (i.e., a primary) disorder, but not if it is a consequence (i.e., a secondary disorder) of a substance-use disorder. The distinction between whether a complicating psychiatric disorder is primary or secondary to substance dependence is not easily made, particularly if both disorders started early in life or are historically closely intertwined. Nevertheless, the use of medications with dependence liability per se (e.g., benzodiazepines, methylphenidate, barbiturates, anticholinergics) for the treatment of a coexisting psychiatric disorder may be severely detrimental to the patient. Moreover, treatment of a secondary disorder is unlikely to be successful if the co-occurring substance dependence is not adequately addressed.

Integration via a multiaxial diagnostic classification system of the physical, psychological, and social domains of each patient's clinical presentation is an important feature of DSM-IV. However, this classification approach is not always adequate to describe fully how the dependence syndrome may be modified by diverse factors such as complex drug-use patterns (i.e., more than one drug via different routes of administration), disabilities resulting from drug-use (e.g., mood disorders, brain dysfunction, medical complications), or various personality disorders and the sociocultural context of drug use. Physicians cannot ignore these more difficult issues as they communicate with each other and with other health care professionals or as they serve as legal consultants,

Table 15–3. Substance-Induced Psychiatric Syndromes Associated with Psychoactive Substances

Psychiatric Syndrome	Psychoactive Substance*
Delirium	Depressants (I/W), stimulants (I), opioids (I), cannabinoids (I), hallucinogens (I), arylcyclohexylamines (I), inhalants (I)
Dementia	Depressants (P), inhalants (P)
Amnestic disorder	Depressants (P)
Psychotic disorders	Depressants (I/W), stimulants (I), opioids (I), cannabinoids (I), hallucinogens (I/P), arylcyclohexylamines (I), inhalants (I)
Mood disorders	Depressants (I/W), stimulants (I/W), opioids (I), hallucinogens (I), arylcyclohexylamines (I), inhalants (I)
Anxiety disorders	Depressants (I/W), stimulants (I/W), caffeine (I), cannabinoids (I), hallucinogens (I), arylcyclohexylamines (I), inhalants (I)
Sexual dysfunction	Depressants (I), stimulants (I), opioids (I)
Sleep disorders	Depressants (I/W), stimulants (I/W), opioids (I/W), caffeine (I)

*Letters in parentheses denote that the disorder has its onset during intoxication (I), withdrawal (W), intoxication or withdrawal (I/W), or the disturbance persists (P) long after the acute effects of intoxication or withdrawal. Depressants include alcohol, sedatives, hypnotics, and anxiolytics; stimulants include cocaine and amphetamine and amphetamine-like substances.

Adapted, with permission, from American Psychiatric Association: *Diagnostic and Statistical Manual of Mental Disorders*, 4th edn. American Psychiatric Association, 1994.

perform disability assessments, and help develop health care policy.

Use of Psychoactive Substances

Throughout history, members of almost every society have used indigenous psychoactive substances (e.g., opium, stimulants, cannabis, tobacco) for widely accepted medical, religious, or recreational purposes. In more recent times, a wide range of substances (e.g., central nervous system [CNS] depressants and stimulants, hallucinogens, and dissociative anesthetics), synthesized de novo or structurally modified from naturally occurring psychoactive compounds, have also become available for self-administration.

Descriptors of the magnitude and context of psychoactive drug use (e.g., excessive use, abuse, misuse, addiction) represent difficult value judgments. Even if such terms are defined explicitly, they are not likely to be readily generalizable from one society (or group within the society) to another. To demonstrate the arbitrary nature of these terms one needs only to examine the changes in perceptions of drug use in the United States since the 1960s.

Maladaptive Patterns of Drug Use

Maladaptive patterns of use involve the self-administration of psychoactive agents to alter one's subjective state and experience of the environment, under inappropriate circumstances or in greater amounts than generally considered acceptable within the social constraints of one's culture. Medical diagnosis of substance-related disorders requires meaningful diagnostic criteria that are generalizable across cultures and drugs of abuse. Definition of maladaptive patterns of use in terms of their consequences, presumably less influenced by value judgments, has provided the conceptual basis for DSM-IV diagnostic criteria. Accordingly, considerable weight is placed on behavioral factors rather than on purely medical complications of use or physiologic effects. This conceptual advance, theoretically consistent with the biopsychosocial model of health care, is readily amenable to prevention and has important implications for treatment. The diagnostic focus has shifted from the drug per se to the interactions of drug, individual, and societal factors. Such a perspective is quite different from the traditional medical model of considering drug use as merely a bad "habit" until organ damage is diagnosable, or the social model in which even use sufficient to cause physical complications is not considered an illness.

General Considerations

A. EPIDEMIOLOGY

Surveys conducted by various government agencies at fixed intervals since the 1960s have monitored changes in population attitudes, the prevalences of different types of drug use, health consequences, estimated costs to society, and treatment outcome. Cross-sectional epidemiologic studies are valuable to the clinician, because knowledge of the prevalence of drug-related problems suggests the likelihood with which these problems will be encountered in the patient population. For example, a physician may be assisted in the management of an overdose or other drug-related emergency by knowing "what's on the street" at that point in time. Longitudinal population studies of cohorts of drug users are particularly informative with respect to understanding antecedents of substance-use disorders, dose-response relationships for consequences of use, and determinants of effective treatment outcome.

1. Prevalence of drug use—Patterns of drug use change over time, and contemporaneous prevalence rates can vary according to the epidemiologic survey quoted. Epidemiologic surveys in the United States documented epidemics of marijuana abuse in the 1960s, heroin in the 1970s, and cocaine in the 1980s. While no single drug captured society's imagination in the 1990s, opioid dependence has been on the rise, and methamphetamine is perceived to have reached "epidemic" proportions at the onset of the new millennium. Furthermore, epidemiologic studies have documented an upward trend in the usage of all drugs and alcohol during the 1970s, followed by a downward trend in the 1980s; this trend reversed and then stabilized in the 1990s and beyond. Knowledge about the prevalence of **drug use** is highly predictive of the proportion of the population that will develop **abuse** or **dependence** (see below).

Although Americans use alcohol more often than they do any other drug, younger individuals tend to combine alcohol with multiple illicit drugs. Older cohorts (age 35 years and older) frequently use alcohol alone, or with prescribed drugs of abuse. According to the 2004 National Survey on Drug Use and Health (Table 15–4), 121 million Americans (50.3% of the population aged 12 years and older) reported being current drinkers of alcohol (at least one drink in the past month). An estimated 55 million (22.8%) were binge drinkers (5 or more drinks at the same time or within a couple of hours of each other at least once in the past 30 days), and 17 million (6.9%) were heavy drinkers (5 or more drinks on the same occasion on at least 5 different days in the past 30 days). An estimated 70.3 million persons (29.2%) reported use of the other legal drug, tobacco.

An estimated 19.1 million (7.9% of the U.S. population aged 12 or older) used an illicit drug during the month prior to the survey. Marijuana is the most prevalent illicit drug by far, used by 14.6 million in the past month. An estimated 8.2 million people (3.4%) were current users of illicit drugs other than marijuana. Most (6 million) used psychotherapeutic drugs nonmedically. An estimated 4.4 million used pain relievers, 1.6 million used tranquilizers, 1.2 million used stimulants (including 583,000 methamphetamine users), and 300,000 used

Table 15–4. Prevalence of Substance Use in Last Month (Per 100 Persons Aged 12 Years or Older)

Drug	Prevalence (%)
Alcohol	50.3
● Binge drinker	22.8
● Heavy drinker	6.9
Tobacco	29.2
An illicit drug	7.9
● Marijuana	6.1
● Cocaine	0.8
— Crack	0.2
● Methamphetamine	0.3
● Hallucinogens	0.4
● Ecstasy	0.2
● Heroin	0.1
Nonmedical use of psychotherapeutic drugs	2.5
● Pain relievers	1.8
● Tranquillizers	0.7
● Stimulants	0.5
● Sedatives	0.1

Adapted from Substance Abuse and Mental Health Services Administration: *Overview of Findings from the 2004 National Survey on Drug Use and Health* (Office of Applied Studies, NSDUH Series H-27, DHHS Publication No. SMA 05-4061) Rockville, MD, 2005.)

sedatives. An estimated 2 million persons were current cocaine users (467,000 used crack); hallucinogens were used by 929,000 persons; 166,000 were current heroin users; and 450,000 were current Ecstasy users. National data have consistently shown that substance use, abuse, and dependence are most prevalent among the young (age 18–34 years) and that the highest rates are observed in young men.

2. Prevalence of substance-use disorders—According to the National Comorbidity Survey, the first survey to be administered in the early 1990s using a structured psychiatric interview (Composite International Diagnostic Interview) to a nationally representative household sample of over 8,000 respondents, the lifetime prevalence rate of a substance-use disorder (except for use of nicotine or caffeine) was 19.5 per 100 persons 18 years and older. Drugs covered by this survey included alcohol, tobacco, sedatives, stimulants, tranquilizers, analgesics, inhalants, marijuana/hashish, cocaine, hallucinogens, heroin, nonmedical use of prescription drugs, and polysubstance use. Alcohol abuse or dependence was identified in 13.2% of the population during their lifetime, and drug abuse or dependence in 8% of the population. According to the 2004 National Survey on Drug Use and Health, an

Table 15–5. Prevalence of Substance-Use Disorders During the Previous Year (Per 100 Persons Aged 12 Years or Older)

Substance-Use Disorder	Prevalence (%)
Any substance-use disorder	9.4
• Alcohol abuse or dependence, no illicit drug-use disorder	6.4
• Illicit drug abuse or dependence, no alcohol use disorder	1.6
• Alcohol and illicit drug abuse or dependence	1.4
—Marijuana abuse or dependence	1.9
—Cocaine abuse or dependence	0.7
—Opioid abuse or dependence	0.6

Adapted from Substance Abuse and Mental Health Services Administration: *Overview of Findings from the 2004 National Survey on Drug Use and Health* (Office of Applied Studies, NSDUH Series H-27, DHHS Publication No. SMA 05-4061) Rockville, MD, 2005.)

estimated 22.5 million persons (9.4% of persons 12 years and older) were classified as having substance dependence or abuse in the past year (Table 15–5). Of these, 3.4 million were dependent on, or abused, both alcohol and illicit drugs; 3.9 million were dependent on, or abused, only illicit drugs; and 15.2 million were dependent on, or abused, only alcohol. Of the 7.3 million persons classified as being dependent on, or abusing, illicit drugs; 4.5 million were dependent on, or abused, marijuana; 1.6 million were dependent on, or abused, cocaine; and 1.4 million were dependent on, or abused, pain relievers. The majority of other illicit drugs were used in combination with alcohol, marijuana, cocaine, or opioids and by a relatively small proportion of the population who met criteria for substance-use disorder.

3. Risk of co-occurring psychiatric diagnoses—According to the National Institute of Mental Health Epidemiologic Catchment Area Survey, in which 20,291 persons representative of the US community and institutional population were interviewed, the odds of having a mental disorder were 2.7 times greater if one also had substance abuse or dependence (excluding nicotine or caffeine) in comparison with no drug-use disorder. Drug-use disorders occurred at higher rates in individuals who had alcohol abuse or dependence (21.5%) than in those who did not (3.7%). Alcohol use disorders were more prevalent among those who met criteria for drug abuse or dependence (47.3%) than among those who did not (11.3%). Specific psychiatric diagnoses, such as major depressive disorder, bipolar affective disorder, schizophrenia, anxiety disorders, and antisocial personality disorder, have been associated with substance-use

disorders in epidemiologic studies, leading to theories of common pathogenesis. For example, according to the 2004 National Survey on Drug Use and Health, persons with a major depressive episode (MDE) in the previous year were twice as likely (28.8% vs. 13.8%) as those without MDE to have used an illicit drug in the past year. Similar patterns were observed for specific illicit drugs in the previous year, such as marijuana, cocaine, heroin, hallucinogens, inhalants, and the nonmedically used psychopharmacologic agents. Also, persons with MDE in the past year were 1.3 times as likely (9.2% vs. 6.9%) than those without MDE to be heavy alcohol users. The rate of daily cigarette use was 1.7 times greater in those who had MDE in the last year.

Persons with MDE were more likely than those without MDE to be dependent on, or abuse illicit drugs (9.6% vs. 2.7%) and alcohol (16.8% vs. 7.1%). Among persons with substance dependence or abuse, 18.5% had at least one MDE in the past year compared with 7% among those who did not have substance dependence or abuse.

Such associations suggest that the clinician should have a high index of suspicion for substance-use disorders when dealing with clinical populations diagnosed with mental disorders. The clinician should also be circumspect about prescribing psychoactive medications with dependence liability to these patients.

B. Etiology

The etiology of substance-use disorders has been conceptualized in terms of an integration of biological, psychological, and social theories. A recent advance has been recognition of shared clinical features, similar biopsychosocial underpinnings, and frequent co-occurrence of substance-use disorders and so-called "behavioral addictions," such as pathological gambling, problematic hypersexuality, and obesity or other eating disorders.

1. Individual vulnerabilities—The major goal of any etiologic theory is to explain why, in the face of widespread availability of drugs and alcohol, certain individuals develop a substance-use disorder, and others do not. This is a gargantuan task because these are complex and multifaceted disorders. Substance abuse and dependence are heterogeneous disorders that represent the final common pathway for a variety of behavioral difficulties in diverse sociocultural contexts. Also, circumstances that lead to these complex and multifaceted disorders differ among individuals. Equally difficult to understand is why in some patients substance-use disorders continue inexorably to death in spite of treatment, whereas in other patients drug use can be decreased or stopped (either spontaneously or with treatment). Therefore, substance-use disorders are perhaps most usefully conceptualized in terms of multiple simultaneous variables interacting over time.

The fact that not all individuals who self-administer psychoactive agents, during given developmental stages or life circumstances, progress to repeated problematic use, has led to the search for factors that determine individual vulnerability. Biological factors that may contribute to the development of substance-use disorders include interindividual differences in (1) susceptibility to acute psychopharmacologic effects of a given drug; (2) metabolism of the drug; (3) cellular adaptation within the CNS to chronic exposure to the drug; (4) predisposing personality characteristics (e.g., sensation seeking, poor impulse control, difficulty delaying gratification, or antisocial traits); and (5) susceptibility to medical and neuropsychiatric complications of chronic drug self-administration. Psychological factors—such as the presence of co-occurring psychopathology (e.g., depression, anxiety, attention-deficit/hyperactivity disorder, psychosis, pathological gambling, eating disorders, or problematic hypersexuality); medical illnesses (e.g., chronic pain, essential tremor); or past or present severe stress (e.g., resulting from crime, battle exposure, sexual trauma, or economic difficulties)—have received considerable attention as potential causes for "self-medication." The possibility exists that susceptibility to psychological stressors and substance-use disorders may have similar etiologies. For example, some of the etiologic factors that predispose an individual to depression following major losses (e.g., dysregulation of noradrenergic neurotransmission or the hypothalamic-pituitary-adrenal axis) may also contribute to the development of substance-use disorders. Similarly, prefrontal cortical dysfunction manifested by impulsiveness or poor decision making is observed in individuals diagnosed with either pathological gambling or cocaine dependence. Finally, social factors also contribute to the initiation of drug use and progression of substance-use disorders. Such social factors include peer group attitudes toward, and shared expectations of the benefits of, drug use (such as enhanced pleasurable activities with drug use); the availability of competing reinforcers in the form of educational, recreational, and occupational alternatives to substance use; and the availability of drugs during particular developmental stages.

The fact that individuals often use more than one drug simultaneously, or give a history of having used different drugs at different times during their lifetime, has led to an emphasis on the similarities rather than the differences among abused substances with respect to the ontogeny of drug-use behaviors. Further, the stepwise development of different substance-use disorders over time suggests common mechanisms of susceptibility and generalizable diagnostic criteria and treatment strategies. Likewise, the co-occurrence and parallel life courses of substance-use disorders and other out-of-control and self-destructive behaviors, such as pathological gambling, problematic hypersexuality, and over-eating have pointed to shared abnormalities of fundamental brain reward (drive) mechanisms that may be generalized beyond drug self-administration.

i. Drug-seeking behavior—Conceptualization of substance-use disorders in terms of the biopsychosocial model, rather than as simply the physiologic consequences of chronic drug use, has led to recognition of the central role of conditioning and learning in drug dependence. The behavioral perspective provides a framework for understanding the entire spectrum of psychoactive substance use, from its initiation to its progression to compulsive drug use, as well as the acquisition of tolerance and physical dependence; it also explains how co-occurring psychopathology so frequently influences the clinical course of substance-use disorders. Psychopharmacologic processes that initiate, maintain, and regulate drug-seeking behavior include (1) the positive reinforcing and discriminative effects of drugs, (2) the environmental stimuli associated with drug effects (which facilitate drug seeking), and (3) the aversive effects of drugs (which extinguish drug seeking). These processes are modulated by social, environmental, and genetic factors such as the individual's personal history, the presence of psychopathology (e.g., anxiety, depression, thought disorders), and the individual's previous exposure to (expectancy of) psychoactive drugs (Figure 15–1). The neural mechanisms and behavioral factors that influence psychoactive drug use are amenable to detailed analysis using drug self-administration models in laboratory animals, in which the neuropharmacology and neuroanatomy of the brain systems that mediate reward can be explored.

ii. Drug intoxication—Individual factors that affect the quality and magnitude of intoxication also influence drug reinforcement, and ultimately, the development of substance-use disorders. Among these are variables such as initial tolerance, previous experience with the drug, the social context of administration, and presence of disorders that affect CNS responses to the drug or disorders of other organs that determine the brain concentration of the drug. Direct adverse consequences of acute intoxication are predictable from the pharmacologic actions of the drug. For example, CNS depressants have a spectrum of dose-related effects from initial disinhibition at low doses to stupor and coma at higher doses. Similarly, CNS stimulants enhance arousal, attention, and performance at low doses but can lead to psychomotor agitation, psychotic disorganization, and convulsions at higher doses. Often the most serious consequences of these agents are indirect effects, namely, impaired performance or judgment, which can cause automobile or work-related accidents, drug-related violence, or unprotected sexual

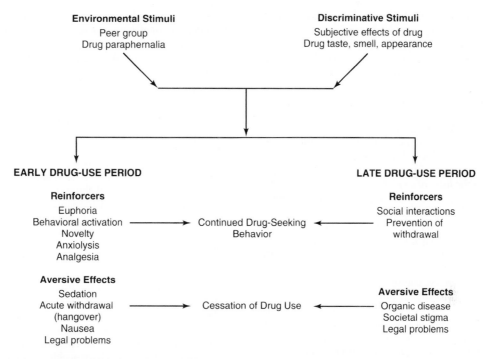

Figure 15–1. Factors contributing to drug-seeking behavior. (Adapted, with permission, from Martin PR, Lovinger DM, Breese GR: Alcohol and other abused substances. In: Munson P, Mueller RA, Breese GR (eds). *Principles of Pharmacology: Basic Concepts and Clinical Applications.* Chapman & Hall, 1995, pp. 417–452.)

activity. Finally, the route of drug administration can greatly influence intoxication. For example, both intravenous administration and smoking result in rapid entry of the drug into the brain with intense but relatively short-lived euphoria; for highly reinforcing drugs (e.g., cocaine, opioids), this can result in compulsive, binge-like use. Nasal insufflation, subcutaneous administration (so-called "skin popping"), and oral ingestion result in relatively slower access to the drug's site of action in the brain, with greater variability in drug bioavailability and less reinforcement.

iii. Neural mechanisms—Investigation of the neural pathways that mediate the powerful (positive) reinforcing effects of drugs of abuse have implicated dopamine, opioid, glutamate and gamma-amino butyric acid (GABA) systems within a midbrain-forebrain-extrapyramidal reward circuit with its focus in the nucleus accumbens. The connections of the ventral midbrain and forebrain, commonly called the medial forebrain bundle, are a major conduit for hypothalamic afferents and efferents and also support (more than any other brain region) the repeated self-administration of current through electrodes (an intracranial self-stimulation model of addiction). This system modulates, or filters, signals from the limbic system that mediate basic biological drives and motivational variables, convert emotion into motivated action and movement via the extrapyramidal system, and may also be the neuronal substrate for the rewarding effects of drugs of abuse. It has been hypothesized that the mesocorticolimbic dopamine system may be critical in motor arousal associated with anticipation of reward, and that all addictive drugs have a psychostimulant (dopaminergic) action as a common underlying mechanism that contributes to reinforcement. Therefore, drugs of abuse activate neural pathways evolved to guide an organism through the challenges of the environment by reinforcing behavior essential for the survival of the species. If drugs of abuse are repeatedly administered, these reward circuits may cease to shape survival behavior effectively.

iv. Behavioral mechanisms—The effects of drugs that mediate their positive reinforcing influence are desirable changes in mood (euphoria), alleviation of negative affective states (e.g., anxiety, depression), functional enhancement (e.g., improved psychomotor or cognitive performance), and alleviation of withdrawal. It is difficult to understand why certain psychoactive drugs with profound aversive effects can nonetheless maintain drug-seeking behavior and have dependence liability. Aversive effects of drugs counteract the tendency toward self-administration and may limit drug use if they result in dose-dependent toxicity. For example, initial exposure to nicotine in the form of cigarettes often results in distressing symptoms, such as coughing, nausea, and lightheadedness, which may terminate smoking. Similarly, severe gastritis in the chronic alcoholic patient may result in attempts to cut down drinking or limit continued alcohol ingestion. It is now recognized that the stimulus properties of most drugs of abuse, a major determinant of drug-seeking behavior, are complex and multifaceted. Specifically, their pharmacologic profiles include both positive reinforcing and aversive components, and their effects are modified readily by associated environmental stimuli and individual differences among drug users.

If a drug is repeatedly administered under given circumstances (situation, time, place), environmental stimuli can become associated with effects of the drug by means of classical (Pavlovian) conditioning. Subsequently, the circumstances under which the drug was administered (without actual presentation of the drug) comprise certain environmental (conditioned) stimuli that can modify drug-seeking behavior, subjective state, or psychophysiologic responses (conditioned reinforcement). For example, patients who have abstained from intravenous heroin for many years can experience a desire to use heroin when they return to the location where they previously used or when they view a film that portrays others who are injecting drugs intravenously. Using positron emission tomography (PET), researchers have shown that in dependent patients, dopaminergic activation accompanies the presentation of relevant cues from the environment or the anticipation of drug (without its administration). Moreover, similar patterns of brain activation are demonstrable using functional magnetic resonance imaging (fMRI) when a subject is presented cues related to highly rewarding behaviors that do not involve drug self-administration, such as gambling, sexual activity, and food. The importance of conditioned stimuli in the response to drugs is also demonstrated readily in laboratory animals by tolerance after a drug is tested in an environment in which it was administered previously that is greater than in a distinctly different environment.

2. Neuroadaptation—Neuroadaptation refers to the neuronal changes and consequent clinical signs and symptoms that result from repeated drug administration independent of drug-seeking behavior or use-related organ damage. It encompasses the biological substrata of tolerance and physical (as opposed to psychological) dependence.

i. Tolerance—After repeated exposure to many psychopharmacologic agents, individuals require a larger dose to produce intoxication of the magnitude that was experienced when the drug was first administered. Conversely, a smaller degree of intoxication results from doses of the drug that were used initially. This phenomenon, called tolerance, is a pharmacologic characteristic shared by many of the substances of abuse considered in DSM-IV (particularly the CNS depressants and the opioids). Tolerance allows and may encourage progressively greater doses to be self-administered. (After repeated exposure to CNS stimulants, reverse tolerance, or a greater pharmacologic effect, may be observed.) Tolerance is an adaptive physiologic response of the intact organism that opposes the pharmacologic effects of the drug. The mechanistic underpinnings reside in molecular changes at the cellular level and in interactions between the organ systems of the body. The components of tolerance include (1) increased capacity for clearance of a drug by metabolizing enzymes in the liver (pharmacokinetic or metabolic tolerance), (2) reduced response from the same drug concentration (functional or pharmacodynamic tolerance), and (3) accommodation to drug effects through learning (behavioral or learned tolerance). Tolerance to one CNS depressant usually results in some cross-tolerance to other (sometimes chemically unrelated) CNS depressants. Tolerance accelerates dose-related complications of drug use.

Acquired tolerance should be distinguished from sensitivity to a given drug on first administration and from acute tolerance that develops over the course of a single exposure to the drug. Differences in the population in initial or acute tolerance to a given drug are innate characteristics of the CNS that may influence individual vulnerability to the development of psychoactive substance-use disorders.

ii. Dependence—Traditionally, dependence refers to the neuronal changes that develop after repeated exposure to a given agent, the clinical syndrome characterized by out-of-control drug use, and the serious biopsychosocial consequences that accompany these neuronal changes. At present, dependence can be defined only indirectly in terms of (1) the presence of tolerance or the emergence of a withdrawal syndrome (immediate and protracted) upon drug discontinuation (physical dependence) and (2) the craving or drug-seeking behavior manifested as a result of conditioned stimuli (psychological dependence). The dependence syndrome represents the elements of psychological dependence, including drug seeking and psychosocial consequences of drug use. Physical dependence usually develops in concert with tolerance, and controversy remains over whether physical dependence and tolerance are simply different manifestations of the same neuronal changes. The reacquisition of both tolerance and physical dependence are accelerated following repeated cycles of drug administration and withdrawal, suggesting certain similarities between these phenomena and learning and memory. Furthermore, the reinforcing and aversive affects of drugs may differ considerably at different stages in the course of a substance-use disorder (see Figure 15–1).

iii. Withdrawal—Upon discontinuation of chronic administration of many psychoactive agents (or administration of a specific antagonist), a withdrawal (abstinence) syndrome emerges as drug concentrations (or receptor occupancy) at the pharmacologic sites of action decline. This syndrome is characterized by a spectrum of signs and symptoms that are generally opposite to those of intoxication and whose severity is related to the cumulative dose (dosage and duration of administration). For example, withdrawal from CNS depressants results in CNS hyper excitability, whereas withdrawal from psychostimulants causes CNS depression. For most drugs of abuse, the withdrawal syndrome also involves homeostatic responses. These represent reversal of the neuroadaptive changes that occurred with long-term drug administration, resulting in significant activation of the autonomic nervous system.

iv. Cellular & molecular mechanisms of neuroadaptation—Advances in neuroscience, such as the development of specific receptor antagonists, electrophysiological and brain imaging techniques, and molecular methods to measure subtle cellular alterations, have enhanced our fundamental understanding of neuroadaptation. Neuroadaptation can be conceptualized not only in terms of the intact organism (of particular relevance to understanding the clinical signs and symptoms of withdrawal), but also at the level of neuronal signal transduction, which can be studied in vitro. Changes in synaptic membrane composition, receptor function, and postreceptor intracellular events have all been proposed as the basis of neuroadaptation to psychoactive drugs of abuse. For example, acute alcohol exposure fluidizes cell membranes, but chronic alcohol exposure results in alterations in the lipid composition that render synaptic membranes more rigid. The inhibition by cocaine of dopamine reuptake leads to increased intrasynaptic dopamine, subsequent depletion of presynaptic dopamine due to reduced synthesis of the neurotransmitter, and eventual upregulation (enhanced sensitivity) of postsynaptic dopamine receptors. Finally, in rats, chronic morphine administration increases G proteins, cyclic adenosine monophosphate–dependent protein kinase, and the phosphorylation of a number of proteins, including transcription factors. Emerging evidence points to similar functional changes on reward pathways following administration of many of the drugs of abuse, as well as natural reinforcers. Such a common pathway of responses might be akin to the molecular-level alterations that occur during learning and memory. Keys to molecular changes during acute drug administration and during neuroadaptation have clear implications for the pharmacotherapy of dependence and withdrawal.

C. GENETICS

The clinical features and course of alcohol dependence have been studied more extensively than have those of other substance-use disorders. Alcohol dependence is a heuristically useful paradigm for understanding the genetic factors that contribute to the development of most substance-use disorders. In fact, recent studies show shared genetic factors associated with alcohol and other drug-use disorders. As discussed earlier in this chapter, individual vulnerabilities to substance-use disorders span biological, psychological, and social domains. These domains are tightly interrelated and can influence one another, such that it may be difficult to unravel the role(s) of single variables. Furthermore, substance abuse or dependence in family members disrupts family life in countless ways, thereby affecting developmental processes in children within the family. It is not surprising, therefore, that higher than normal rates of alcohol or drug dependence, as well as of other forms of psychopathology, exist among children of these families. In addition to these environmental factors, genetic factors also play a role in the familial predisposition to substance-use disorders. However, it is recognized that **interactions** of the genetic and environmental factors associated with drug-use disorders may be more important than either of these factors alone.

1. Inheritance of alcohol dependence—Findings from twin and adoption studies demonstrate the relative contributions of genetic and environmental factors in predisposition to alcohol dependence. For example, the concordance rate for alcohol dependence is substantially higher in monozygotic (0.70) than dizygotic (0.33) twins, whereas concordance rates are no different for less severe forms of the disorder, such as alcohol abuse (0.8 for both monozygotic and dizygotic twins). Adoption studies show that adopted-away men with alcoholic biological parents have an increased likelihood of developing alcoholism regardless of whether they are raised in an alcoholic or nonalcoholic environment. In general, the severity of parental alcoholism tends to influence the prevalence of alcoholism in adopted-away sons; patients with the most severe alcoholism have the highest rates of alcohol dependence in their offspring. These studies suggest that the relative contributions of environmental and genetic factors in development of alcoholism may vary with the severity or type of alcohol dependence.

2. Heterogeneity of alcohol dependence—As discussed earlier in this chapter, groups of alcohol-dependent patients are heterogeneous. The challenge in genetic studies of alcoholism has been to identify homogenous subgroups of alcohol-dependent patients. Clearly defined phenotypes in patients (and their families) could then be studied in depth to identify predictors of etiology, longitudinal course, and response to treatment. One heuristically useful classification is based predominantly on age at onset of alcohol dependence: onset after age 25 (type 1) and onset before age 25 (type 2). Reliably different clusters of alcohol-related problems and personality traits tend to occur with these two subtypes of alcohol dependence. In general, patients with type 2 alcoholism are characterized by thrill seeking, impulsiveness, and aggressiveness, whereas those with type 1 alcoholism have a greater tendency to become anxious and depressed as a result of their drinking. Type 2 alcoholism tends to be more recalcitrant to treatment than is type 1 alcoholism.

Both genetic predisposition and an alcoholic rearing environment were required for adopted-away sons of fathers with type 1 alcoholism to express type 1 alcoholism. In contrast, adopted-away sons of fathers with type 2 alcoholism were significantly more likely to manifest this type of alcohol dependence than were the offspring of fathers without type 2 alcoholism, whether or not they were raised in an alcoholic family. This observation indicates that the genetic loading for alcohol dependence is influenced profoundly by the environment in the case of late-onset alcohol dependence, whereas environmental background is relatively less important for early-onset alcohol dependence.

3. Women & addiction—There are distinct differences between the genders in the inheritance, clinical presentation, and longitudinal course of alcohol dependence. It is particularly important to understand alcohol use disorders in women because of the adverse effects of drinking on the developing fetus, and the disruptive effects of alcohol use or dependence on the mother–child relationship. Both of these consequences of alcohol consumption in women can perpetuate the transmission of alcohol use and other psychiatric disorders from one generation to the next via nongenetic means.

Women have lower rates of alcohol dependence compared to men, although these rates are rising at a disquieting pace. Lower rates of alcohol dependence result in part from the smaller amounts of alcohol consumed by women in general, for a number of psychosocial and biological reasons. Even though women start drinking later than men, they tend to develop, at about the same age as men, more serious physical complications. These observations suggest greater intrinsic toxicity of ethanol to the liver, brain, and possibly other organ systems of women compared to men. Established gender-related differences in predisposition to co-occurring psychopathology (e.g., depression and somatic anxiety) may complicate and exacerbate alcohol dependence. Daughters of fathers with type 1 alcoholism are at increased risk for alcoholism but not for other psychopathology; daughters of fathers with type 2 alcoholism are at higher risk only for somatization disorder.

4. Genetic factors in development of alcoholism—Although genetic studies suggest that genetic factors are important contributors to the development of alcohol dependence, the mechanisms involved are only now beginning to be elucidated. This is an exciting area of research, but its clinical relevance is not yet apparent. Because there is likely a complex cascade of events between the genetic underpinnings of alcohol dependence and the eventual manifestation of symptoms, this clinical diagnosis is probably not the best phenotype for use in genetic analyses. A preferable phenotype for genetic analyses might be an intermediary measure of the neuropsychiatric functioning involved in the pathway between genotype and the outcome of interest (endophenotype). For example, it has been suggested that children of alcoholic fathers are less sensitive to the intoxicating effects of ethanol than are children of nonalcoholic fathers. Presumably, these children would have to drink more than would children of nonalcoholic fathers in order to become intoxicated and, thus, be more likely to become alcohol dependent. The abilities of researchers to match subjects retrospectively in terms of lifetime exposure to, and experience with, alcohol are important limitations of these studies. Such limitations can be overcome only by carefully conducted longitudinal investigations beginning in childhood. Early notions that differences in innate tolerance to ethanol or susceptibility to alcohol dependence were based on differences in ethanol metabolism have not been firmly established. More recently, researchers have focused on molecular underpinnings of interindividual differences in, for example, the $GABA_A$ receptor genotype or brain biogenic amine metabolism as predisposing to development of alcohol dependence. Specifically, considerable preclinical and human data implicate low brain serotonergic activity in stimulating alcohol consumption and in producing the aggressive and impulsive behavior often associated with type 2 alcoholism. In addition, an impaired ability to allocate significance to targeted stimuli, as manifested by reduced amplitude of the late positive component of event-related electroencephalographic (EEG) potential, has been identified in children of fathers with type 2 alcoholism, and is considered a genetic factor predisposing to alcohol dependence. Early onset alcoholics may be more prone to develop brain damage as a result of alcohol consumption. They may be cognitively impaired prior to beginning drinking, especially with respect to attention and motor control. This line of reasoning is supported by relationships found between adult alcohol dependence and early delays in motor development, suggesting that fronto-cerebellar deficits play a causal role.

5. Inheritance of substance-use disorders other than alcohol dependence—It is unknown whether the genetic mechanisms that predispose individuals to alcohol dependence also influence the development of other substance-use disorders. Common causality is suggested (though difficult to prove) because many (particularly younger) individuals tend to combine alcohol and other drugs of abuse, often indiscriminately.

The twin and adoption studies described earlier in this chapter provide guidelines for how to study this question in patients with drug abuse or dependence. For example, in one adoption study of genetic and environmental factors in drug abuse, drug abuse in adult adoptees was associated in equivalent proportions with (1) antisocial personality in the adoptees, related to a biological background of antisocial personality; (2) no antisocial personality in the adoptees but with a biological background of alcoholism; and (3) neither antisocial personality nor alcoholism in either the adoptee or the biological background but psychosocial factors such as divorce and psychiatric illness in the adopting family environment. Such studies show that interactions between genetic and environmental factors are as important in the development of other substance-use disorders as they are for alcohol dependence. A shared underlying mechanism seems most likely to involve endophenotypes related to attention, impulse control, executive functioning, related abnormalities of brain functioning, or the presence of, or vulnerability to, depression, anxiety, or related psychopathology.

Koob GF, Le Moal M: Plasticity of reward neurocircuitry and the 'dark side' of drug addiction. *Nat Neurosci* 2005;8:1442–1444.

Martin PR, Petry NM: Are nonsubstance-related addictions really addictions? *Am J Addict* 2005;14:1–7.

McLellan AT, Lewis DC, O'Brien CP, Kleber HD: Drug dependence, a chronic medical illness: Implications for treatment, insurance, and outcomes evaluation. *JAMA* 2000;284:1689–1695.

Nestler EJ: Is there a common molecular pathway for addiction? *Nat Neurosci* 2005;8:1445–1449.

Clinical Findings

A. SIGNS & SYMPTOMS

1. Alcohol & other CNS depressants—

i. Intoxication—Alcohol and other CNS depressant intoxication proceeds in stages that depend on dosage and time following administration. Apparent CNS stimulation, which occurs early in alcohol or CNS depressant intoxication or at low dosages, results from depression of inhibitory control mechanisms. The most sensitive parts of the brain are the polysynaptic structures of the reticular activating system and the cortex, depression of which causes euphoria and dulling of performance that depends on training and previous experience. Excitation resulting from intoxication is characterized by increased activity, verbal communication, and often aggression (Table 15–6). Euphoric feelings or calming effects are typically the expressed reason for drug self-administration. Higher blood concentrations of alcohol or other CNS depressants cause mild impairment of motor skills and slowing of reaction time, followed by sedation, decreased motor coordination, impaired judgment, diminished memory and other cognitive deficits, and eventually diminished psychomotor activity and sleep. At still higher concentrations, alcohol and most CNS depressants can induce stupor, and ultimately coma and death, by progressive depression of midbrain functions and interference with spinal reflexes, temperature

Table 15–6. Signs and Symptoms of CNS Depressant Intoxication and Withdrawal

Intoxication	Withdrawal
Disinhibition (e.g., inappropriate sexual or aggressive behavior, impaired judgment, mood lability)	Anxiety or psychomotor agitation
Somnolence, stupor, or coma	Tremor
Impaired attention or memory	Craving
Slurred speech	Autonomic hyperactivity (e.g., tachycardia, hypertension, sweating, hyperthermia, arrhythmia)
Incoordination	Insomnia
Unsteady gait	Sensory distortions or hallucinations (e.g., transient visual, tactile, or auditory)
Nystagmus	Nausea or vomiting
	Seizures
	Delirium

regulation, and the medullary centers controlling cardiorespiratory functions. Death due to benzodiazepine overdose is very unlikely unless combined with alcohol or other CNS depressants.

The dose–response curve of ethanol has been studied in greater depth than has any other CNS depressant. Sensitivity to alcohol intoxication varies widely within the population as a whole. For example, at blood ethanol concentrations of 50, 100–150, and 200 mg/100 mL, it is estimated that approximately 10%, 64%, and almost all of the general population, respectively, would be overtly intoxicated. In contrast, at a blood ethanol concentration of 300 mg/100 mL, some alcoholic individuals may appear only mildly intoxicated even though their psychomotor performance and judgment are impaired significantly. According to the Council of Scientific Affairs of the American Medical Association, blood alcohol concentrations of 60, 100, and 150 mg/100 mL increase an individual's relative probability of causing an automobile accident 2-, 6-, and 25-fold, respectively. Legal limits of blood ethanol concentration for automobile drivers are 100 mg/100 mL (the term in common use is 0.10) for most states in the United States, 80 mg/100 mL for most countries in Western Europe, and between 0 and 50 mg/100 mL for Scandinavian and Eastern European countries.

ii. Drug-seeking behavior—The classic sedative–hypnotic actions of ethanol, barbiturates, and benzodiazepines correlate well with their shared ability to modulate GABA-induced chloride anion fluxes in vitro. These drugs can also act as anxiolytics; however, benzodiazepines are unique among CNS depressants because of their ability to reduce anxiety while causing relatively little sedation. It is believed that the reinforcing actions and abuse potential of CNS depressants reside primarily in their anxiolytic and tension-reducing properties mediated by activation of GABA$_A$ receptors. Furthermore, in animal models, established GABA efferents from the nucleus accumbens to the substantia innominata-ventral pallidum can influence the expression of cocaine- or opioid-induced behavioral stimulation. This may explain why alcohol and other CNS depressants are often used by addicted individuals along with cocaine or opioids.

iii. Neuroadaptation—Adaptive neuronal changes resulting from the continued presence of alcohol or other CNS depressants involve a decrease in inhibitory functions of the nervous system. Although the molecular basis of such neuronal adaptation has not been elucidated fully, the clinical consequences are well characterized and include the development of tolerance and dependence, which usually proceed in parallel. Although pharmacokinetic differences among CNS depressants may alter the duration of time the agent is present at its site of pharmacologic action, and subtle molecular differences may influence the precise interactions of the different agents with their binding site(s) and the neuronal receptors occupied, the neuroadaptive changes that eventually result from chronic ingestion of alcohol, benzodiazepines, barbiturates, or nonbarbiturate hypnosedatives are for practical purposes much the same.

The development of tolerance to, and dependence on, CNS depressants can occur after only a few days of repeated ingestion. As with all drugs, tolerance and dependence are determined by dosage and frequency of use. For example, a drug dosage that initially caused sedation and anxiolysis may in time be insufficient to induce sleep or reduce anxiety; thus, higher dosages are needed to attain these therapeutic goals. Tolerance may not develop at the same rate to all actions of a CNS depressant. For example, whereas sedation usually diminishes after the first few days of treatment with most benzodiazepines, anxiolytic effects may persist for months without a need to increase the dosage. Euphoric effects may not be as predictable, which can cause rapid increases in dosage if the drug is being self-administered for this purpose. In general, for alcohol and other CNS depressants there is no marked elevation of the lethal dosage with repeated use, and respiratory depression may be superimposed on chronic consumption after a severe, acute overdose.

iv. Withdrawal—Cessation of alcohol or CNS depressant intake after prolonged use is associated with a syndrome of neuronal hyperexcitability with increased noradrenergic and adrenocortical activity. This syndrome is initially characterized by anxiety, apprehension, restlessness, irritability, and insomnia with clinically apparent tremor and hyperreflexia (see Table 15–6). Moderately severe cases progress to signs of autonomic hyperactivity with tachycardia, hypertension, diaphoresis, hyperthermia, and muscle fasciculations. Often patients experience anorexia, nausea, or vomiting with subsequent dehydration and electrolyte disturbances. Paroxysmal EEG discharges may precede generalized tonic–clonic seizure activity. The most severe cases develop delirium (agitation, disorientation, fluctuating level of consciousness, visual and auditory hallucinations, and intense autonomic arousal).

Among the CNS depressants, the most severe and potentially dangerous withdrawal syndrome results from barbiturates and nonbarbiturate hypnosedatives; alcohol withdrawal is of intermediate severity; and withdrawal from benzodiazepines poses the least risk. The onset, severity, and duration of the withdrawal syndrome in a given class of CNS depressants are determined by the rate of elimination of the drug and its metabolites from the body. In the alcohol withdrawal syndrome, generalized tonic–clonic seizures typically occur 12–48 hours after the last drink, and delirium tremens begins at 48–72 hours. The signs of acute alcohol withdrawal typically

Table 15–7. Signs and Symptoms of Psychostimulant Intoxication and Withdrawal

Intoxication	Withdrawal
Stimulation (euphoria, hypervigilance, anxiety, tension, anger, impaired judgment)	Depression (dysphoria)
Psychomotor agitation (stereotyped behaviors, dyskinesias, dystonias)	Psychomotor retardation
Energy (decreased need for sleep)	Fatigue (increased need for sleep)
Anorexia (nausea or vomiting, weight loss)	Increased appetite
Autonomic arousal (tachycardia, hypertension, pupillary dilation, perspiration, or chills)	Craving
Chest pain, cardiac arrhythmias, respiratory depression	
Confusion	
Seizures	

abate by 3–5 days after the last drink, but subtle brain abnormalities may persist for an undetermined period. Among the barbiturates, nonbarbiturate hypnosedatives, and benzodiazepines, withdrawal usually begins within 12 hours and is most severe for rapidly eliminated compounds (e.g., amobarbital, methyprylon, triazolam). For slowly metabolized compounds (e.g., phenobarbital, diazepam, clonazepam), the syndrome may be delayed for several days after drug discontinuation. More protracted effects of withdrawal from CNS depressants have not been well studied, but residual problems related to cognitive impairment, anxiety and depressive symptoms, and insomnia may result.

2. Psychostimulants: cocaine & amphetamines—

i. Intoxication—The main clinically relevant pharmacologic action of cocaine and amphetamine-related stimulants is the blockade of reuptake of the catecholamine neurotransmitters norepinephrine and dopamine. The consequences of noradrenergic reuptake blockade include tachycardia, hypertension, vasoconstriction, mydriasis, diaphoresis, and tremor. The effects of dopamine reuptake blockade include self-stimulation, anorexia, stereotyped movements, hyperactivity, and sexual excitement. As a result, many of the signs and symptoms of cocaine and amphetamine intoxication are similar (Table 15–7). CNS stimulation and a subjective "high" are accompanied by an increased sense of energy, psychomotor agitation, and autonomic arousal.

The psychoactive effects of most amphetamine-like substances last longer than those of cocaine. Furthermore, because cocaine has local anesthetic actions, the risk of its causing severe medical complications such as cardiac arrhythmia and seizures is greater than for amphetamine-like stimulants. Amphetamine-related compounds therefore remain popular in the stimulant-abusing population.

ii. Drug-seeking behavior—The most striking pharmacologic characteristic of cocaine is its tremendous reinforcing effect. Women who are cocaine dependent have higher rates of primary major depression than do cocaine-dependent men, consistent with drug use as a form of self-medication. Men with cocaine dependence have higher rates of co-occurring antisocial personality disorder than do cocaine-dependent women. Studies in animal models have shown that animals will self-administer cocaine in preference to food, leading to emaciation and death (in contrast to other highly reinforcing agents such as opioids). Dopamine seems to be the main neurotransmitter involved in the positive reinforcement of cocaine.

iii. Neuroadaptation—Although not well-understood, neuroadaptation appears to occur in response to chronic psychostimulant use. Users develop acute tolerance to the subjective effects of cocaine, which can play a major role in dose escalation and subsequent toxicity. Sensitization appears to play a role in cocaine-induced panic attacks, paranoia, and lethality.

iv. Withdrawal—In humans, discontinuation of cocaine leads to dysphoria (a so-called "crash"). Hypersomnolence and anergia are also common (see Table 15–7). In rats, termination of repeated cocaine administration produces interoceptive stimuli that are similar to the discriminative stimulus effects of pentetrazole, a drug that is anxiogenic in humans. As a result, the typical cycle of use consists of binges, each followed by a "crash" (lasting 9 hours to 4 days), followed by withdrawal (lasting 1–10 weeks), during which craving and relapse is common.

3. Opioids—

i. Intoxication—The characteristic pharmacologic action of opioids is analgesia. Centrally, opioids are activating at low dosages and sedating at higher dosages.

Table 15–8. Signs and Symptoms of Opioid Intoxication and Withdrawal

Intoxication	Withdrawal
Activation or "rush" (early or with low dosages) and sedation/apathy or "nod" (late or with high dosages)	Depressed mood and anxiety Dysphoria
Euphoria or dysphoria	Craving
Feelings of warmth, facial flushing, or itching	Piloerection ("goose flesh") Lacrimation or rhinorrhea
Impaired judgment, attention, or memory	
Analgesia	Hyperalgia, joint and muscle aches
Constipation	Diarrhea and gastrointestinal cramping, nausea, or vomiting
Pupillary constriction	Pupillary dilation and photophobia
Drowsiness	Insomnia
Respiratory depression, areflexia, hypotension, tachycardia	Autonomic hyperactivity (e.g., tachypnea, hyperreflexia, tachycardia, hypertension, sweating, hyperthermia)
Apnea, cyanosis, coma	Yawning

Other major features of intoxication are feelings of euphoria or dysphoria, feelings of warmth, facial flushing, itchy face, dry mouth, and pupil constriction (Table 15–8). Intravenous use can cause lower abdominal sensations described as an orgasm-like "rush." This is followed by a feeling of sedation (called the "nod") and dreaming. Severe intoxication may cause respiratory suppression, areflexia, hypotension, tachycardia, apnea, cyanosis, and death.

ii. Drug-seeking behavior—Addiction to opioids (particularly heroin) can be severe and often leads individuals to dysfunctional behavior to support their habit. Animals tend to repeat opioid self-administration and prolong its effects.

Self-administered opioid compounds affect the endogenous opioid systems of the body. Endogenous opioid peptides are distributed throughout the brain and form three major functional systems defined by their precursor molecules: β-endorphin from pro-opiomelanocortin, enkephalins from proenkephalin, and dynorphin from prodynorphin. Endogenous opioids modulate nociceptive responses to painful stimuli, stressors, reward, and homeostatic adaptive functions (hunger, thirst, and temperature regulation). Rats will self-administer opioid peptides into the ventral tegmental area and nucleus accumbens, suggesting that these regions may be responsible, at least in part, for the reinforcing properties of opioids (and cocaine). Other regions supporting rewarding effects for opioids are the hippocampus and hypothalamus. Endogenous opioid tone contributes to the maintenance of normal mood and a nondopaminergic system of opioid reward.

There are three main types of opioid receptor: μ, δ, and κ. These G protein-coupled proteins inhibit adenylcyclases in various tissues and cause their pharmacologic actions by reducing cyclic adenosine monophosphate levels. The μ-opioid receptor appears to be important for the reinforcing actions of opioids, whereas the δ-opioid receptor may play a role in the opioid motor stimulation that is dopamine (D_1 receptor) dependent. Like other substances of abuse, opioids can increase dopamine release in the nucleus accumbens as measured by in vivo microdialysis in awake, freely moving animals; but the reinforcing effect of opioids in the nucleus accumbens can be independent of dopamine release. The reinforcing actions of opioids may involve both a dopamine-dependent (i.e., ventral tegmental area) and a dopamine-independent (nucleus accumbens) mechanism.

iii. Neuroadaptation—Neuroadaptation occurs in response to regular opioid use. For example, when chronically abused by humans, heroin rapidly loses its aversive properties and increases its reinforcing ones. The tolerance that develops when opioids are administered repeatedly appears to be receptor selective. It has been theorized that μ receptors couple less well to G proteins in rat locus coeruleus neurons that have been chronically treated with morphine. Tolerance occurs both to specific opioid effects such as analgesia and motor inhibition and to the generally depressant properties of opioids, whereas the psychomotor effects are potentiated.

iv. Withdrawal—Withdrawal of opioids is characterized by hyperalgesia, photophobia, goose flesh, diarrhea, tachycardia, increased blood pressure, gastrointestinal cramps, joint and muscle aches, and anxiety and depressed mood (see Table 15–8). Spontaneous withdrawal results in intense craving because of the reduction of dopamine release in the nucleus accumbens, but the degree of physical dependence does not predict the severity of craving. The motivational (affective) properties of withdrawal are independent of the intensity and pattern of the physical symptoms. Because opioids can counteract withdrawal dysphoria and the reduction of dopaminergic transmission, these changes may contribute to maintenance of opioid addiction.

4. Cannabinoids—

i. Intoxication—The subjective effect of marijuana intoxication varies from individual to individual. It is determined in part by highly variable pharmacokinetics, dosage, route of administration, setting, experience and expectation, and individual vulnerability to certain psychotoxic effects. Typically, intoxication is characterized by an initial period of "high" that has been described as a sense of well-being and happiness (Table 15–9). This euphoria is followed frequently by a period of drowsiness or sedation. The perception of time is altered and hearing and vision distorted. The subjective effects of intoxication often include dissociative reactions. Impaired functioning occurs in a variety of cognitive and performance tasks, including memory, reaction time, concept formation, learning, perception, motor coordination, attention, and signal detection. At dosages equivalent to one or two "joints" (marijuana cigarettes), processes involved in the operation of motor vehicles or airplanes are impaired. The impairment persists for 4–8 hours, long after the user perceives the subjective effects of the drug. The impairment produced by alcohol is additive to that produced by marijuana. Tolerant individuals may exhibit somewhat less performance decrement.

Physically, dilation of conjunctival blood vessels and tachycardia may be noted. Blood pressure remains relatively unchanged unless high dosages are used, in which case orthostatic hypotension ensues. Increased appetite is often attributed to marijuana but has not been observed consistently in controlled studies. At higher dosages, acute panic reactions, paranoia, hallucinations, illusions, thought disorganization, and agitation have been observed. With extremely high dosages, an acute toxic psychosis is accompanied by depersonalization and loss of insight.

ii. Drug-seeking behavior—In chronic cannabinoid users, dependence and degree of drug-seeking behaviors are controversial. In some patients, drug-seeking behavior appears to be manifested primarily as drug craving. The psychological and physiologic mechanisms underpinning this craving are not understood. Laboratory animals do not self-administer the drug. The recognition and characterization of the endogenous cannabinoid system has led to important advances in our understanding of cannabinoid abuse and dependence. Moreover, there is a growing body of evidence that the endogenous cannabinoid system might participate in the motivational and dopamine-releasing effects of several drugs of abuse other than cannabinoids.

iii. Neuroadaptation—Neuroadaptation in response to cannabinoid use has been more difficult to document than in some of the other drugs of abuse. Tolerance to cannabinoids appears to develop in animals and in humans, although it does not seem to be as profound as with some other drugs. It occurs mostly with heavy use. Chronic abuse of exogenous cannabinoids activates the same receptors as do endogenous cannabinoids, the CB1 and CB2 cannabinoid receptors. These G protein-coupled receptors play an important role in many processes, including metabolic regulation, craving, pain, anxiety, bone growth, and immune function. The functioning of cannabinoid receptors can now be studied directly by the use of agonists or antagonists, or indirectly by manipulating endocannabinoid metabolism and this will likely help elucidate processes of neuroadaptation.

iv. Withdrawal—Cannabinoid withdrawal does not produce well-characterized withdrawal symptoms, perhaps because cannabinoids are so lipophilic that they are very slowly eliminated from the body. The DSM-IV does not include cannabis withdrawal, but there is an impetus to include the condition in future versions of DSM. Converging evidence from basic laboratory and clinical studies indicates that a withdrawal syndrome consistently follows discontinuation of chronic heavy use of cannabis, or treatment with cannabinoid receptor antagonists. Some patients report insomnia, irritability, dysphoria, anorexia, weight loss, hand tremor, mild fever, or slight nausea with discontinuation of use. These symptoms occur primarily in patients who smoke very potent preparations.

Table 15–9. Signs and Symptoms of Cannabis Intoxication

Euphoria, drowsiness, or sedation
Sensation of slowed time
Auditory or visual distortions, dissociation
Impaired judgment, motor coordination, attention, or memory
Slowed reaction time
Conjunctival injection
Tachycardia
Increased appetite
Anxiety, acute panic reactions, paranoia, illusions, or agitation

5. Nicotine & tobacco—

i. Intoxication—Nicotine intoxication is not a DSM-IV diagnosis. However, nicotine intake has multiple effects. For example, many users report improved mood, skeletal muscle relaxation, and diminished anxiety and appetite. In addition, cognitive effects including enhanced attention, problem solving, learning, and memory have been reported.

ii. Drug-seeking behavior—Users of tobacco products frequently exhibit substance-seeking behavior. Smokers often describe strong cravings for tobacco, especially in particular situations such as after eating or while experiencing stress. The degree of craving differs among individuals, and the ability to discontinue tobacco products varies greatly.

iii. Neuroadaptation—Nicotine is thought to be the chief substance in tobacco that causes neuroadaptation. Tolerance to nicotine has been shown in both laboratory animals and humans. Dependence is indicated by the difficulty of discontinuing use of nicotine products despite a desire to quit.

The primary pharmacologic actions of nicotine appear to occur via nicotine binding to acetylcholine receptors in the brain and autonomic ganglia. Several subtypes of nicotinic cholinergic receptors are found in the CNS. Activation of these receptors appears to cause the reinforcing effects and diminished appetite associated with nicotine. Some of the reinforcing actions of nicotine may be due to the effects of nicotine on dopamine pathways projecting from the ventral tegmental area to the limbic system and the cerebral cortex. Stimulation of peripheral nicotine receptors causes many of the autonomic effects associated with nicotine use. Short-term use of tobacco appears to increase cerebral blood flow, whereas long-term use has the opposite effect. Aspects of neuroadaptation to nicotine may also be secondary to release of hormones such as β-endorphin, adrenocorticotropic hormone, cortisol, epinephrine, norepinephrine, endocannabinoids, and vasopressin.

iv. Withdrawal—Withdrawal symptoms often occur with abrupt discontinuation of nicotine intake: craving, anxiety, depression, irritability, headaches, poor concentration, sleep disturbances, enhanced blood pressure, and increased heart rate. In some cases, craving lasts for years under appropriate circumstances. Management of withdrawal symptoms has been one strategy to prevent relapse in those trying to quit smoking.

6. Hallucinogens & volatile inhalants—

i. Intoxication—Intoxication with hallucinogens causes effects that vary greatly and may last 8–12 hours. Flashbacks are possible after termination of use (Table 15–10). The cardinal features of hallucinogen intoxication include visual hallucinations and disturbance of

Table 15–10. Signs and Symptoms of Hallucinogen Intoxication

Marked anxiety or depression
Perceptual changes (e.g., intense perceptions, depersonalization, derealization, illusions, hallucinations, synesthesias)
Thought disorders (e.g., ideas of reference, paranoia, impaired reality testing)
Impaired judgment
Autonomic arousal (e.g., pupillary dilation, tachycardia, sweating, palpitations, blurring of vision, tremors, incoordination)

thoughts and perception in multiple sensory modalities. These features can lead to devastating consequences if they occur in dangerous situations (e.g., when driving or standing in precarious areas such as on a balcony). Other features include sensory changes (e.g., colors, shapes), synesthesia (the perception in one modality when a different modality has been stimulated), delusions, paranoia, derealization, depersonalization, cognitive impairment, coordination problems, behavioral changes, euphoria (or dysphoria), nausea, tremors, time distortion, dizziness, weakness, and giddiness. A "bad trip" involves striking dysphoria. Visual hallucinations with perception of various light patterns, and incorrect movement perception or object recognition have been reported. Augmented sensory perception (particularly tactile), which can be pleasurable (thus the term "ecstasy" for MDMA), often occurs with methamphetamine use. Other symptoms such as ataxia, dizziness, nausea, perspiration, and bruxism can occur with use. Many complications are related to hallucinogen use (e.g., panic reactions, seizures, exacerbation of psychiatric illnesses). Suicidal or homicidal tendencies may be enhanced.

Anticholinergic drugs of abuse include antihistamines and the belladonna alkaloids such as scopolamine and atropine. Anticholinergic drugs are characterized by "dream-like" states, feelings of euphoria, heightened social interaction, and sedation. At high dosages, disorientation or paranoia may occur. These substances are sometimes used with mild opioids (called "Juice and Beans" or "T's and Blues" on the streets) to enhance the euphoric effect.

Arylcyclohexylamines, such as PCP (phencyclidine), act as dissociative anesthetics. Behavioral alterations include paranoia, mood shift, agitation, catalepsy, and violence. PCP may be smoked, snorted, or injected. It causes reddening of the skin, pupillary changes, dissociation, delusions, amnesia, dry skin, dizziness, poor coordination, excitement, and nystagmus. Increased blood pressure and tachycardia may also occur.

Intoxication by volatile inhalants generally lasts only several minutes. Confusion, sedation, and euphoria may often result from use. Physical effects include analgesia, respiratory depression, hypotension, and ataxia. Nitrous oxide is associated with euphoria and laughter ("laughing gas").

ii. Drug-seeking behavior—Psychedelic substances produce little or no dependence, and regular use is not common. Animals generally do not self-administer these drugs (except for MDMA-like compounds), and frequent users generally do not report craving. Tolerance to LSD occurs after only days of use; however, the intoxicating effects return after a few days without use. Other indolamines are cross-tolerant with LSD, but the phenylethylamine hallucinogens are not. Tolerance to anticholinergic drugs can also occur but usually requires prolonged use.

iii. Neuroadaptation—Little is known about neuroadaptation to the actions of hallucinogens. Phenylalkylamines and indolamines are serotonin receptor agonists, which probably relates to their clinical effects. Phosphatidylinositol hydrolysis is stimulated after receptor binding and leads to enhanced excitability of certain neurons in the limbic system, cerebral cortex, and brainstem.

The phenylisopropylamines inhibit reuptake of catecholamine and indolamine neurotransmitters and may be transported into serotonin neurons. It is hypothesized that the serotonergic action of these drugs accounts for their hallucinogenic effects (as with other hallucinogens), while the effect on catecholamines causes arousal.

Anticholinergic drugs such as scopolamine and atropine act as antagonists of muscarinic receptors. These receptors are found in the cerebral cortex, and several subtypes have been reported. Stimulation may excite or inhibit neuronal activity including effects on serotonin receptors.

Arylcyclohexylamines, such as PCP, act as antagonists to the N-methyl-D-aspartate class of glutamate receptors, which are themselves ion channels. PCP also binds to σ-type opioid receptors and inhibits catecholamine reuptake.

iv. Withdrawal—Withdrawal symptoms are not common with these drugs; however, the anticholinergic substances may cause tachycardia, sweating, depression, anxiety, or psychomotor agitation after use has been discontinued.

B. PSYCHOLOGICAL TESTING

Alcohol and other substances of abuse can cause both transient and enduring damage to the brain. Neuropsychological testing is important in the overall assessment of some patients with substance-related disorders. Most of these tests are readily available, noninvasive, and inexpensive. They require the full participation of the patient; therefore, they may not be as objective as blood chemistries or radiologic procedures. Neuropsychological tests are preferably conducted at least 3 weeks after the most recent substance use so that lasting brain dysfunction can be detected. Although these tests are useful, many factors influence them, including medication, co-occurring medical conditions or psychiatric disorder, and compliance with testing.

Intelligence tests such as the Wechsler Adult Intelligence Scale (WAIS) are useful in determining the patient's global behavioral and adaptive potential. The WAIS is predictive of the patient's likely success in activities such as work and school. Other intelligence tests may be more appropriate for specific patient populations. Different aspects of cognition may be evaluated by specific tests. For example, the Wechsler Memory Scale is useful for patients who have possible substance-induced memory impairment.

Neuropsychological batteries such as the Halstead-Reitan Neuropsychological Test Battery and the Luria-Nebraska Neuropsychological Battery can provide comprehensive information about many aspects of brain functioning. In alcoholic patients, the Halstead-Reitan Battery frequently reveals impairment on many of the individual tests such as Tactual Performance, Categories (visual–spatial abstracting), Trails B (perceptual motor speed), and Tactual Performance Test-Location (incidental memory for spatial relationships).

Some assessment tools have been developed for evaluation of substance abuse itself (as opposed to possible causes or consequences thereof). One of the major difficulties in using such measures is in distinguishing use from abuse. The four-question CAGE assessment is used to screen patients for alcoholism. CAGE stands for an acronym reflecting (1) the subjective need to **cut down**, (2) being **annoyed** at other people when they comment on one's drinking, (3) feelings of **guilt** over use, and (4) the need for an "**eye opener**." Generally, two out of four yes answers are considered positive. Sensitivity and specificity are high for most populations. The more complex Michigan Alcoholism Screening Test (MAST) is often used in the assessment of alcohol intake and the consequences of consumption. It has 25 differentially weighted items in a true–false format. Sensitivity, specificity, and validity testing have all been favorable. Shorter 10- and 13-item forms are available with reasonably good validity. A reliable test of the consumption and consequences of drug abuse is the Drug Abuse Screening Test. It has 28 items (unlike the MAST, not differentially weighted), in a true–false format. Another useful instrument is the Alcohol Dependence Scale. This scale has 25 multiple-choice items and is concerned primarily with the loss of ability to control drinking.

Because co-occurring psychiatric illnesses and social difficulties are common in substance abusers, other psychological tests may be of value in certain patients. For example, the Addiction Severity Index (ASI), a semistructured interview designed to address seven problem areas in substance-abusing patients: medical status, employment and support, drug use, alcohol use, legal status, family/social status, and psychiatric status. The ASI provides an overview of recent (past 30 days) and lifetime problems related to substance use. The Minnesota Multiphasic Personality Inventory, a commonly used assessment tool with over 500 items (with results formatted into 10 clinical scales and 3 validity scales), provides typical personality profiles for substance-dependent patients. (See also Chapter 6, *Psychological and Neuropsychological Assessment*.)

C. LABORATORY FINDINGS

A number of laboratory findings are of use in the evaluation and care of substance abuse patients. Urine drug screens and blood alcohol levels provide objective information as to what drugs are in the patient's system, at what concentration. The relative degree of intoxication or withdrawal at specific drug levels can provide clues as to the patient's level of tolerance and dependence. A complete evaluation considers whether particular drugs are detectable in urine and the length of time that they are detectable. This will vary according to many factors, including dosage, duration of use, and individual metabolic and renal clearance rates. Average upper limits on urine detection times are provided in Table 15–11.

Many other blood chemistries are useful. The toxic effects of alcohol on the liver are evaluated with liver function tests, such as SGOT (serum glutamic oxaloacetic transaminase) and SGPT (serum glutamic pyruvic transaminase). GGT (γ-glutamyl transpeptidase) is perhaps the most sensitive monitor of alcohol consumption. Alcohol-induced hepatitis classically presents with

Table 15–11. The Upper Limit of Urine Detection

Drug	Limit
Alcohol	12 h
Amphetamine	2 d
Cannabis	4 wk
Cocaine	8 h (4 d for metabolites)
Opioids	3 d
Phencyclidine (PCP)	8 d
Benzodiazepines	3 d
Barbiturates	1 d (short-acting); 3 wk (long-acting)
Codeine	2 d

a SGOT:SGPT ratio of about 2:1. Viral hepatitis screens can help differentiate causes of abnormalities in hepatic function. Serum amylase is valuable in the detection of pancreatitis. A complete blood cell count can monitor bone marrow functioning: mild, macrocytic anemia is often observed in alcohol-abusing patients. Low potassium and bicarbonate are consistent with drug-related diarrhea. Chloride deficiencies are associated with chronic vomiting. Although total body stores of magnesium may be difficult to assess, alcohol-induced magnesium wasting can lead to detectable extracellular deficiencies. Protein, albumin, potassium, and phosphorus are helpful indicators of nutritional status.

D. NEUROIMAGING

Intellectual impairment is perhaps the earliest complication of chronic alcoholism. It is difficult to determine whether subtle neuropsychological impairments are consequences of chronic alcohol consumption. Computed tomography or magnetic resonance imaging studies of patients with 2–36 weeks of abstinence have shown that a large proportion of alcoholic patients have detectable cerebral and cerebellar atrophy and ventricular dilation. Recently, functional measures of brain activity have corroborated these neuroanatomic findings.

E. COURSE OF ILLNESS

1. Alcohol & other CNS depressants—The CNS depressants include brewed or distilled alcoholic beverages and various pharmaceutical agents prescribed for the treatment of insomnia, anxiety, depression, and, less frequently, for seizure control or as muscle relaxants (see Table 15–2). No CNS depressant (e.g., alprazolam, zolpidem, eszopiclone, zaleplon) has been developed that is totally free of abuse liability and the potential for a withdrawal syndrome, problems shared with alcoholic beverages.

Alcoholic beverages are readily available at affordable cost with minimal legal restrictions. Accordingly, there is widespread use of alcohol in diverse recreational and work-related circumstances, and traumatic injuries sustained while under the influence of elevated blood alcohol are among the most common public health problems today. Youngsters with little experience with drinking are particularly vulnerable as they first begin to participate in high-risk activities such as sports, sexuality, and driving. Heavy drinkers, who often have blood alcohol concentrations that impair judgment and motor skills or who use other drugs in combination with alcohol, are particularly at risk for alcohol-related violence, traumatic injury, and death.

The benzodiazepines are currently (as barbiturates were previously) among the most widely prescribed medications and the most commonly misused or abused type of prescription drug. With continued use, individuals develop tolerance and need higher doses to achieve symptomatic relief. If the physician does not educate the patient and provide careful prescription monitoring, the patient may eventually receive high doses of these medications with attendant side effects such as mood disorder, cognitive dysfunction, social difficulties, impaired work performance, and traumatic injury due to falls or vehicular accidents. In order to maintain symptomatic relief in the face of tighter controls by the prescribing physician, the patient may combine alcohol, medications, or illicit drugs (e.g., marijuana, opioids) with the prescribed dose of CNS depressant, seeking other physicians to provide additional prescriptions (so-called doctor shopping), or engaging in illegal activities such as forging prescriptions. The combination of alcohol with other CNS depressants greatly increases the risk associated with its use and is the most common clinical cause of severe drug overdose. Cessation of drug use leads to undesirable, and potentially harmful, withdrawal symptoms (such as seizures). Thus, drug-seeking behavior and repeated drug use is often continued in order to prevent these effects. Fulminant withdrawal occasionally occurs in patients who discontinue CNS depressant use because of illness or other unforeseen circumstances such as hospitalization for a motor vehicle accident.

2. Psychostimulants: cocaine & amphetamines—The alkaloid cocaine is derived from *Erythroxylon coca,* a plant indigenous to South America, where since time immemorial its leaves have been chewed for their stimulating effects. Because the only contemporary medical use for cocaine is as a local anesthetic, the drug is almost always purchased illegally by users. Amphetamine and amphetamine-like stimulants may be obtained by prescription for the treatment of obesity, attention-deficit/hyperactivity disorder, and narcolepsy. As a result, prescribed stimulants are commonly diverted into the illegal market (see Table 15–2). An epidemic of cocaine use started in the late 1970s, preceded by a period in which it was thought not to be particularly dangerous. Cocaine's significant dependence liability came to be recognized later, resulting in a diminution in use of the drug in the late 1980s. Abuse of amphetamine-like compounds has continued unabated because of their widespread availability and relatively low cost. Recently, use of illegally manufactured methamphetamine derivatives has reached epidemic proportions, reminiscent of the cocaine epidemic of the 1980s. Methamphetamine, including a crystallized, smokable form called "ice," is representative of a group of "designer drugs". These ring-substituted derivatives of amphetamine and methamphetamine, synthesized in clandestine laboratories, derive their popularity from their mixed stimulant and hallucinogenic effects.

Cocaine and other stimulants are almost always used with other psychoactive substances, most commonly alcohol but also other CNS depressants or opioids. Alcohol is considered a gateway drug for cocaine and other stimulant use. It can accentuate the "high" obtained from stimulants, alleviate some of the adverse effects (e.g., "wired" feelings), and is a readily available (i.e., legal) substitute. Heroin (sometimes called "speedball") is another drug that is commonly combined with cocaine and is reported to increase cocaine euphoria.

Methods of use include inhalation via the nostrils ("snorting"), subcutaneous or intravenous injection, and smoking ("free basing"). Nasal insufflation is the most common and least dangerous method, but it does not provide the ecstatic sensation associated with smoking or injection. These latter routes of administration give the drug rapid access to the brain, thereby increasing its reinforcing effect and toxicity.

3. Opioids—Opioid use and addiction has occurred for centuries, and many opioid compounds are abused throughout the world (see Table 15–2). Opioid abuse may start with initially appropriate use for medical analgesia. Some drugs such as codeine and pentazocine can be found in nonprescription medications such as cough syrup and abused when more potent illicit drugs are not readily available. The use of long acting oral forms (e.g., morphine sulfate, MS Contin and oxycodone, OxyContin) has surpassed that of illicit heroin or morphine in most Western countries. Urban dwellers in the northeast are the most frequent abusers of heroin, whereas in rural regions, oral formulations of morphine and oxycodone have become the primary opioids of abuse. Medical professionals with easy access to opioids are at increased risk. In Asia, opium use is still widespread.

Unrefined opium is often smoked using a water pipe. Intravenous heroin (mainlining) and morphine are popular because of the sudden (less than a minute) "rush" produced. Subcutaneous injection is sometimes used, especially if veins have become unusable because of frequent injections. Refined opioids can also be nasal insufflation, a method often preferred by new users. Long-acting oral opioid preparations are typically used with medical prescription or ground up and injected. Although the euphoric state of opioid intake is short, its sedative and analgesic effects can continue for hours. Street drugs are frequently "cut" (mixed or combined) with other substances, such as caffeine, powdered milk, quinine, and strychnine, to dilute the concentration of the active ingredient. These other substances can lead to altered clinical effects and medical difficulties beyond those associated with the opioid; however, the unpredictable potency of these street preparations can often lead to accidental overdose.

4. Cannabinoids—Marijuana is the common name for the plant *Cannabis sativa.* Other names for the plant or its products include hemp, hashish, chasra, bhang, ganja, and daga. The highest concentrations of the psychoactive cannabinoids are found in the flowering tops of both male and female plants. Most commonly the plant is cut, dried, chopped, and then incorporated into cigarettes. The primary psychoactive constituent of marijuana is delta-9-tetrahydrocannabinol, although many other active cannabinoids are known. The hemp plant synthesizes at least 400 of these chemicals.

Since the 1960s, marijuana has been the most commonly used illicit substance. It is a leading candidate for legalization for medical purposes. Marijuana is often the first illicit drug, other than alcohol, used by youngsters. For the first time in history, the use rate in females appears to be higher than in males. The likelihood of having used cocaine and other illicit drugs increases with the extent of marijuana use in all age groups. The epidemiology of marijuana use, therefore, can be viewed as a predictor of illicit drug-related problems in a given population.

5. Nicotine & tobacco—Tobacco is a substance commonly used in many countries and across age groups, from early teens to the elderly. Cigarette smoking is the most common method of use, although cigar smoking, pipe smoking, and smokeless tobacco (snuff) use each have had varying levels of popularity at different times and among different groups. Primarily because of educational programs, the use of tobacco products has declined over the past 30 years in North America. Nevertheless, the use of tobacco products continues to be a significant public health problem and has increased recently in some subpopulations, such as teenage girls.

According to studies that alter the nicotine and tar content of cigarettes, user satisfaction appears to be related to nicotine content, suggesting that this agent is responsible for the reinforcing effects. Heated debate, litigation, changes in laws, and greater enforcement of existing laws regulating the cigarette industry have evolved as the adverse public health effects of smoking have become more widely appreciated.

6. Hallucinogens & volatile inhalants—Hallucinogens are subdivided into two major categories: the indoalkylamines (such as D-lysergic acid diethylamide [LSD], dimethyltryptamine [DMT], psilocin, psilocybin, diethyltryptamine [DET]), the phenylethylamines (such as trimethoxyphenyl ethylamine [mescaline], 3,4-methylenedioxy methamphetamine [MDMA; called "ecstasy" on the streets], 2,5-dimethoxytryptamine [DOM, STP], and 3,4-methylenedioxy amphetamine [MDA]). Other hallucinogens include peyote (mescaline, from Mexican cactus), *Myristica fragrans* (nutmeg), and morning-glory seeds (similar in effect to LSD). Arylcyclohexylamines include phencyclidine (PCP; called "angel dust," "crystal," "weed," and "hog" on the streets) and ketamine. Ketamine is most commonly used as an anesthetic in veterinary medicine; PCP has no current medical uses.

Volatile inhalants include aromatic, aliphatic, and halogenated hydrocarbon compounds such as gasoline, industrial solvents (e.g., acetone, toluene), paints, glues, refrigerants (e.g., Freon), and paint thinners (e.g., turpentine). Nitrous oxide (an anesthetic) and amyl nitrite (a vasodilator; called "poppers" on the streets) are included.

Native Americans used psychedelic drugs such as mushrooms (psilocybin and psilocin) and peyote before the Spanish exploration of Mexico. Hoffman described the hallucinogenic effects of LSD in 1943. Scopolamine (and other belladonna alkaloids), mescaline (a plant product), and amphetamine designer drugs have similar effects. Hallucinogens in the United States were most popular in the 1960s and early 1970s, with a dramatic decline shortly afterward. The use of these drugs has continued, however, at a fairly constant level since the late 1970s. An increase of use, particularly of the designer drugs, has been noted among teens and young adults. A recent disturbing trend involves the use of several of these drugs by large numbers of youngsters during all-night dance parties ("raves"). Some Native Americans and other groups continue to use plant hallucinogens in their mystic ceremonies. PCP is used most commonly in urban areas.

Users of volatile inhalants are most often in their preteen and teenage years. Professionals, such as dentists, who have easy access to substances such as nitrous oxide, are also at increased risk of use. The use of volatile inhalants was perhaps greatest in the late 1970s and early 1980s.

Budney AJ, Hughes JR, Moore BA, Vandrey R: Review of the validity and significance of cannabis withdrawal syndrome. *Am J Psychiatry* 2004;161:1967–1977.

Dani JA, Harris RA: Nicotine addiction and comorbidity with alcohol abuse and mental illness. *Nat Neurosci* 2005;8:1465–1470.

Volkow ND, Fowler JS, Wang GJ: The addicted human brain viewed in the light of imaging studies: Brain circuits and treatment strategies. *Neuropharmacology* 2004;47:3–13.

Differential Diagnosis

Patients are unlikely to present to physicians complaining of difficulties with the use of psychoactive substances. Rather, they present for treatment of the complications of substance use. Such patients are unlikely to offer information that they use psychoactive agents, much less admit to problematic drug use. They may deny that they have a drug problem when questioned. The nonspecificity and wide variety of symptoms that accompany these psychoactive substances, as well as the unreliability of patient reports, make the diagnosis of these disorders difficult. The physician must approach, with a high index of suspicion, patients who exhibit signs and symptoms consistent with a substance-use disorder. Only if the physician is open to the diagnosis will it be made appropriately.

Because of the many clinical manifestations of substance-use disorder, the physician must consider it in the differential diagnosis of myriad medical and psychiatric illnesses. For example, a withdrawal-induced delirium must be differentiated from the many other causes of delirium, ranging from CNS infection and metabolic disturbance, to medication toxicity. Similarly, numerous medical problems must be eliminated before a physician can assume that all the signs and symptoms exhibited by a drug-abusing patient are the result of a substance of abuse (even if one or more drugs have been used). For example, an intoxicated substance abuser may have fallen and incurred a closed head injury or be in diabetic ketoacidosis.

Numerous similar presentations can be cited. For example, patients with hyperthyroidism or bipolar affective disorder may have similar initial clinical features to those on stimulants, and vice versa. Patients with psychosis (e.g., schizophrenia, bipolar affective disorder, or major depressive disorder with psychotic features) may exhibit signs and symptoms similar to those of a person withdrawing from CNS depressants, or vice versa.

A common problem is the differential diagnosis of the anxious or depressed alcoholic patient. The physician must determine whether the patient has a primary mood or anxiety disorder with subsequent substance-abuse or a substance-induced mood disorder. In such circumstances, the only way the physician can differentiate the cause(s) of the depressed mood or anxiety is by taking a careful history or by observing the patient's response to treatment. On the other hand, the correct diagnosis may require discussion with others who have known the patient over time.

In the differential diagnosis of substance abuse, the physician must be aware that the patient could be in denial, in which case the reported history may be intentionally or unintentionally inaccurate or incomplete. Denial may be followed by unexpected medical or psychiatric problems or concomitant drug abuse.

Lukens TW, Wolf SJ, Edlow JA, et al.: Clinical policy: Critical issues in the diagnosis and management of the adult psychiatric patient in the emergency department. *Ann Emerg Med* 2006;47:79–99.

Ziedonis DM, Smelson D, Rosenthal RN, et al.: Improving the care of individuals with schizophrenia and substance use disorders: Consensus recommendations. *J Psychiatr Pract* 2005;11:315–339.

Treatment

A. OTHER INTERVENTIONS

The treatment of substance-use disorders is perhaps influenced more by the widely held societal attributions of responsibility for causation of the problem than by an understanding of etiology. Such attributions can lead to a broad range of responses, the most extreme being to view the addict as either a patient or a criminal, and as moral or immoral, innocent or guilty, victim or perpetrator.

A corollary of this viewpoint is to regard rehabilitation from substance use as belonging either in the realm of medicine or in the criminal justice system. However, the social control mechanisms used for prevention or deterrence are not so easily dichotomized. There are distinct inconsistencies and tensions between the medical (i.e., prevention) and legal (i.e., deterrence) systems as evidenced by the lack of a straightforward relationship between the pharmacologic properties and health risks of a drug, and whether it is considered legal or illegal (the term "illicit" is often used) within criminal law. Drugs such as alcohol and nicotine (as smoked in tobacco)—which cause the greatest expense by far for the health care system—are freely available. Whether other drugs that present societal problems should be legally controlled is heatedly debated. In general, the more alternatives available to the law for controlling dysfunctional drug use, the less legal regulation is required. Attitudinal changes in society have contributed to the reemergence over time of "epidemics" of drug use. This is currently the case with respect to methamphetamine, but it has been observed in the past century for most other psychoactive drugs. For example, there are historical examples of failed attempts at prohibition of caffeine and nicotine; the chief focus of legal suppression during the twentieth century has been, in turn, alcohol, heroin, cannabis, cocaine, and methamphetamine.

The treatment of substance abuse is a multistage process. Generally, patients must go through detoxification, rehabilitation, and relapse prevention (aftercare). Emphasis is currently on similarities (e.g., common neurochemical mechanisms of drug-seeking behavior and underlying psychopathology) rather than differences (as was the case in the past) among substances of abuse. Thus, patients who abuse different drugs can receive treatment in the same programs, and abstinence from all substances of abuse is promoted. In addition, the treatment of co-occurring psychiatric and medical problems is begun simultaneously with treatment of the substance-use disorder. One problem affects the other. This has resulted in the emergence of so-called "dual diagnosis" treatment units, which provide general psychiatric care for those who have both addiction and a co-occurring disorder. The pharmacologic treatment of concomitant psychiatric disorder requires careful diagnosis and the avoidance of potentially addicting psychoactive substances (e.g., treatment of panic attacks with alprazolam).

The biopsychosocial model is a useful guide to the treatment of substance-use disorder. As a result, both pharmacologic and psychosocial approaches, combined

Table 15–12. Nonpharmacologic Modalities of Substance-Abuse Treatment

---

Education
12-Step support program facilitation (e.g., Alcoholics
 Anonymous, Narcotics Anonymous, Cocaine
 Anonymous)
Enhancement of coping strategies
Relaxation training
Family therapy
Lifestyle change (avoiding drug use trigger situations)
Psychotherapy (usually cognitive, relational, or
 supportive, in a group or individual setting)
Vocational and physical rehabilitation
Recreational therapy
Sexual education
Health and nutritional counseling
Spiritual growth
Aftercare

---

in a so-called pharmacopsychosocial strategy, are implemented.

B. PSYCHOTHERAPEUTIC INTERVENTIONS

Whereas detoxification (treatment of withdrawal) differs among individual drugs of abuse because of differing pharmacologic profiles, long-term management is more similar than different for the numerous substances of abuse (Table 15–12).

The quality of outside social support and the reliability and stability of the patient's social circumstances are the chief determinants of whether inpatient or outpatient treatment is indicated. After initial detoxification (usually inpatient, but outpatient if appropriate), a rehabilitation program is initiated. Substance abuse education (of the patient and family) is very helpful and can be achieved in formal or informal settings. Coping skills and relaxation training are of great value to many patients who have clinical anxiety. Inpatient and outpatient treatment should include appropriately selected psychotherapy (e.g., social/milieu, insight-oriented, behavioral, individual, cognitive, and group, in various combinations). Patients should participate in self-support groups.

Health maintenance issues must be addressed with an emphasis on smoking cessation, hygiene, exercise, diet, sex education (e.g., preventing the transmission of HIV and other sexually transmitted diseases). Nonaddictive medications for conditions such as chronic pain should be used. Physicians should coordinate the care of each patient. An examination of spirituality should be encouraged if appropriate for the needs of the patient.

Aftercare is at least as important as the initial treatment program. Participation in organized aftercare groups following formal treatment keeps patients engaged with the professionals and peer groups with whom care was initiated, and allows them to monitor their relative progress. Individuals with a disorganized family situation or no outside support benefit from structured living facilities such as halfway houses. Lifestyle changes may be needed, the patient removing himself or herself from people and circumstances that promote drug use or stimulate craving. Vocational rehabilitation can be valuable. Twelve-step programs (e.g., Alcoholics Anonymous and Narcotics Anonymous) and other mutual support groups are helpful.

The psychiatric treatment of co-occurring conditions, such as depression, anxiety disorder, bipolar affective disorder, and chronic pain disorder, is essential in preventing relapse, for example, if the patient has been using addictive drugs as misguided self-medication. Appropriate pharmacologic and psychosocial therapies should be prescribed, but potentially addicting medication avoided. It is important that the physician recognizes it may be counterproductive to treat comorbid psychiatric symptoms that will disappear or diminish with abstinence. Education should be provided about commonly used medications that are mood altering and can lead to relapse (e.g., anxiolytics or opioid analgesics).

C. PSYCHOPHARMACOLOGIC INTERVENTIONS

The following sections describe some of the well-accepted pharmacologic approaches for the treatment of withdrawal from drugs of abuse (Table 15–13). Pharmacologic strategies for the long-term treatment of substance-use disorder, independent of co-occurring psychopathology, is an exciting new field of research. Its clinical utility remains adjunctive to psychosocial approaches and will not be discussed in detail here (Table 15–14). The physician must not treat psychopathology before being sure that it is not a complication of drug use. Inappropriate treatment is very unlikely to be effective and may actually harm the patient.

1. Alcohol & other CNS depressants—Cross-tolerance and cross-dependence among alcohol and other CNS depressants indicates shared cellular and molecular mechanisms of action and provides the rationale for pharmacologic treatment of CNS depressant withdrawal. Once the obvious clinical signs of withdrawal are apparent, the strategy is to administer a CNS depressant that has a longer elimination half-life than the drug from which the patient is being withdrawn. A long-acting benzodiazepine such as diazepam (or chlordiazepoxide) is the treatment of choice for alcohol withdrawal. The slowly eliminated barbiturate phenobarbital is optimal for other CNS depressants (see Table 15–13). Hourly doses are administered until withdrawal symptoms are eliminated (for treatment of alcohol withdrawal) or until the patient manifests signs of mild intoxication (for other forms of

Table 15–13. Pharmacological Treatment of Withdrawal Syndromes from Substances of Abuse

Substance	Agent and Dosage	Other Treatment
Alcohol	Diazepam, 10–20 mg/1–2 hours (typical dosage required, 60 mg)	Thiamine, 100 mg intramuscularly or 50 mg twice daily by mouth, and multivitamin tablets for 3 days
Other CNS depressants	Phenobarbital, 120 mg/hour (typical dosage, 900–1500 mg)	
Stimulants	Not usually needed	Anxiolytics or neuroleptics acutely for agitation or toxic psychosis
Opioids	3–5 days of clonidine 0.1–0.3 mg every 4–6 hours (check BP prior to each dose, hold for BP ≤90/60) Alternatively, methadone dosed at 10–20 mg by mouth every 12 hours initially, or buprenorphine dosed at 4–12 mg under tongue daily initially, both taper over a 5–10-day period to reduce withdrawal symptoms (1 mg buprenorphine is equivalent to 5 mg methadone, 5 mg of heroin, 15 mg of morphine, 100 mg of meperidine)	Ibuprofen for muscle cramps, loperamide for loose stools, and promethazine for nausea or vomiting
Nicotine and tobacco	Nicotine patch started at 7–21 mg per day based on addiction severity with slow taper over 3 months Nicotine gum started at 2–4 mg every 1–3 hours based on addiction severity with slow taper over 3 months Varenicline by mouth at 1 mg twice per day for 12 weeks	Clonidine acutely can minimize withdrawal discomfort
Cannabinoids	Not usually needed	Anxiolytics or neuroleptics acutely for agitation or severe anxiety
Hallucinogens	Not usually needed	Anxiolytics or neuroleptics acutely for toxic psychosis

Table 15–14. Pharmacological Maintenance Strategies for Substance Dependence After Detoxification Completed

Substance	Agent and Dosage
Alcohol	Disulfiram 125–500 mg daily Naltrexone 25–100 mg daily Acamprosate 666 mg three times per day Topiramate 25–150 mg twice per day (not FDA approved)
Other CNS depressants	None approved or recommended
Stimulants	None approved or recommended
Opioids	Methadone by mouth at 30–140 mg per day Buprenorphine 4–32 mg under the tongue (available as buprenorphine/naloxone [4/1] to prevent diversion)
Nicotine and tobacco	Antidepressants often used
Cannabinoids	None approved or recommended
Hallucinogens	None approved or recommended

CNS depressant withdrawal). Physicians sometimes use a tapering dose of the abused benzodiazepine for detoxification; however, the phenobarbital loading-dose strategy appears to be the better treatment option. Alprazolam tapers are generally very slow (about 10% per week) because of the risk of significant withdrawal reactions and are often associated with poor compliance or an exacerbation of dependence.

All drugs currently used for the treatment of CNS depressant withdrawal are liable to reactivate dependence. When prescribing these medications, careful patient education is needed concerning risks and benefits, and particularly with regard to the potential for dependence. Problems can occur if patients are not monitored carefully, or if they take the medication(s) in excess of that prescribed. The treating physician may not be aware that the patient is obtaining prescriptions of the same (or similar) drug(s). A major challenge for pharmacologists is to develop agents that ease CNS depressant withdrawal without risking abuse and dependence.

Patients in alcohol detoxification should be prescribed thiamin and other vitamins to prevent the neurologic, hematopoietic, and cognitive effects of chronic drinking. The ultimate goal is to institute a nutritional diet. The FDA has approved the administration of naltrexone to prevent alcohol craving and relapse (Table 15–14). Aversion therapy with disulfiram has also been used; however, its long-term effectiveness has not been established, and patients must be carefully educated and monitored because of the potential for serious reactions if disulfiram is combined with alcohol (see section "Adverse Outcomes of Treatment"). Randomized placebo-controlled studies have shown that acamprosate and topiramate are efficacious in treatment of alcohol dependence. Acamprosate is now FDA approved for the long-term treatment of relapse in alcohol dependent patients. However, there is little research to help the physician select one or another of these medications.

2. Psychostimulants: cocaine & amphetamines— The treatment of stimulant intoxication is usually supportive. Anxiolytics or neuroleptics may be needed for agitation. Psychostimulants can be highly addictive, and chronic users must understand the causes of relapse and design strategies for relapse prevention. Pharmacologic agents such as anticonvulsants (e.g., carbamazepine) and antidepressants can help prevent relapse, but controlled studies have been inconclusive. In animal models, environmental manipulation such as inflicting punishment, increasing the amount of effort required to obtain the drug, or offering alternative reinforcers decrease its self-administration. Such behavioral observations have guided clinical treatment approaches, such as contingency management. Only if the patient can maintain abstinence beyond the withdrawal period can extinction

and ultimate abstinence follow. Therefore, treatment should address the conditions that lead to relapse, reducing the effects of conditioned cues that trigger craving. Such conditions involve the persons with whom, or situations in which, the individual has used cocaine, together with the availability of cocaine in the neighborhood. Rewards should be provided contingent on abstinence.

After stimulant overdose, further treatment may be needed. In the case of amphetamines, the patient's urine can be acidified with ammonium chloride to increase excretion of the substance. An α-adrenergic antagonist can be used to decrease elevated blood pressure, and antipsychotic medication may be needed to alleviate CNS overstimulation.

Cocaine overdoses are more complicated because of the greater potential for cardiac arrhythmia, respiratory failure, and seizures. Chlorpromazine can be useful in reducing CNS and cardiovascular problems (as it has some α-adrenergic–antagonist action). Artificial respiration or cardiac life support may be needed. Severe anhedonia and depression is associated with damage to brain-reward pathways (e.g., after methamphetamine use) and can necessitate antidepressant treatment.

3. Opioids—Opioid withdrawal can be treated in several ways, depending on whether the ultimate goal is abstinence or maintenance treatment with methadone or buprenorphine. Often, a slow taper of methadone (a long-acting opioid agonist that requires special licensure for use in opioid maintenance treatment) is used for gradual detoxification over weeks to months. In other circumstances, the abused opioid is discontinued abruptly and clonidine, methadone, or buprenorphine used short term to reduce withdrawal symptoms. Clonidine has the advantage of not being an opioid and not having addicting properties, but it may not provide as smooth a withdrawal. Baseline readings of blood pressure and regular monitoring are advised. Methadone, a pure μ-opioid agonist, or buprenorphine, a mixed μ-opioid agonist–antagonist, alleviate the symptoms of withdrawal, but each has significant dependence liability. Proper hydration and supportive care can be combined with other agents, such as ibuprofen for muscle cramps, loperamide for loose stools, and promethazine for nausea.

Methadone maintenance programs (1–2 years or longer) are used in some locations to reduce the risk of reverting to the drug and promoting crime cultures (Table 15–14). Some patients on methadone maintenance use other drugs such as alcohol and cocaine, and sell the methadone they receive to support their drug use. Other pharmacologic means of relapse prevention currently being investigated include buprenorphine and naltrexone. Buprenorphine was approved for the office-based treatment of opioid dependence by trained physicians through the Drug Abuse Treatment Act of

2000. In the treatment of chronic pain, nonaddicting medication (e.g., gabapentin and certain antidepressants) and other treatments (e.g., physical therapy, nerve blocks) should be used when appropriate to minimize the likelihood of relapse.

4. Cannabinoids—The treatment of cannabinoid intoxication usually requires no more than a safe, calm environment. Anxiolytic medication is used only in cases of severe agitation or anxiety. Educational programs are important for prevention, particularly among younger people.

5. Nicotine & tobacco—Nonpharmacologic approaches are frequently used to help tobacco users quit smoking. Weight gain and mood lability may need to be addressed. Strategies may need to be developed to help users endure the day without tobacco use. Clonidine can help reduce withdrawal symptoms. Nicotine-containing products such as dermal patches and gum can be used to taper smokers from nicotine. Antidepressants have been helpful in some patients. A significant recent addition to the treatment of nicotine dependence is verenicline (Table 15–14).

6. Hallucinogens & volatile inhalants—Detoxification from low dosages of hallucinogens can often be achieved in a safe, structured environment with emotional support. Anxiolytics and possibly neuroleptics (such as haloperidol, but not phenothiazines because of possible side effects) may be needed. If respiratory suppression occurs, emergency oxygen may be required. The primary treatment for arylcyclohexylamine overdose is removal from sensory stimulation, and possibly treatment with benzodiazepines or neuroleptics.

Co-Occurring Disorders

Psychoactive substance abuse can contribute to or result from various forms of psychopathology. Physicians are most likely to encounter patients with substance-use disorders when they present for the treatment of a complicating or associated physical or emotional illness. Medical and psychiatric complications of drug use are attributable to either the direct pharmacologic actions of the substance (e.g., overdose, organ toxicity, metabolic consequences) or to the indirect effects of drug self-administration on lifestyle. The indirect effects include use of other than the primary drug of abuse (including tobacco), inappropriate use of prescribed medications such as analgesics or anxiolytics, malnutrition, trauma, infection, neglect, or lack of compliance with the medical regimen for coexistent illnesses. The treatment of severe medical complications takes precedence if the illness is life threatening or incapacitating. However, if the underlying substance-use disorder and emotional concomitants

are not recognized and addressed, treatment may be for naught.

Martin PR, Weinberg BA, Bealer BK: *Healing Addiction: An Integrated Pharmacopsychosocial Approach to Treatment.* Hoboken, New Jersey: John Wiley & Sons, 2007.

Nunes EV, Levin FR: Treatment of depression in patients with alcohol or other drug dependence: A Meta-analysis. *JAMA* 2004;291:1887–1896.

O'Brien CP: Anticraving medications for relapse prevention: A possible new class of psychoactive medications. *Am J Psychiatry* 2005;162:1423–1431.

Complications

A. Alcohol

The medical complications of chronic alcoholism derive from the pharmacologic effects of ethanol, the changes in intermediary metabolism resulting from its biotransformation to acetaldehyde in the liver, and the toxic effects of this metabolite in various body tissues (Table 15–15). Moreover, poor nutrition, which is frequently associated with chronic alcohol consumption can complicate those related to alcohol alone.

Ethanol metabolism leads to conversion of pyruvate to lactate and to the formation of acetoacetate, acetone, and β-hydroxybutyrate. These chemicals can interfere with the renal tubular secretion of uric acid, causing increases in blood urate and exacerbating gout.

Heavy drinking after a period of not eating can cause severe, sometimes fatal, hypoglycemia. This is the result of the combination of low hepatic glycogen stores and inhibition by ethanol of gluconeogenesis. Fatty liver can be caused by single episodes of ethanol binging. Chronic fatty liver, probably in combination with nutritional deficiencies, progresses to alcoholic hepatitis and finally cirrhosis. Ethanol can induce an isozyme of cytochrome P450 to convert some chemicals to hepatotoxic metabolites. Alcoholic cirrhosis continues as a major preventable cause of death among individuals aged 24–44 years in large urban areas.

The diuresis associated with drinking alcoholic beverages is caused primarily by inhibition of ADH release from the posterior pituitary. Alcohol also increases the release of adrenocorticotropic hormone, glucocorticoids, and catecholamines. The synthesis of testosterone is inhibited, and its hepatic metabolism increased. Men with chronic alcoholism often have signs of hypogonadism and feminization (e.g., gynecomastia).

Ethanol stimulates the secretion of gastric and pancreatic juices. This effect on gastric juices and the direct irritant action of concentrated solutions of ethanol help to explain why one of every three heavy drinkers has chronic gastritis. High dosages of ethanol can cause vomiting independent of any local irritation. Alcohol

Table 15–15. Medical Complications of Alcoholism

Metabolic and malnutrition
  Gout
  Hyperlipidemia and fatty liver
  Hypoglycemia
  Weight loss or obesity
  Immune compromise (opportunistic infections)
  Impaired protein synthesis
  Mineral and electrolyte imbalances
  Vitamin deficiencies
  Decreased blood clotting

Gastrointestinal
  Esophagitis
  Gastritis or ulcer
  Pancreatitis
  Liver disease (alcoholic hepatitis, cirrhosis)
  Malabsorption
  Altered drug and carcinogen metabolism
  Increased cancer incidence

Endocrine
  Pancreatic insufficiency (glucose intolerance)
  Increased ACTH, glucocorticoid, or catecholamine
    release
  Inhibited testosterone synthesis (male
    hypogonadism)
  Inhibition of ADH, oxytocin release

Neurologic
  Dementia
  Amnesia
  Cerebellar degeneration
  Fetal alcohol effects
  Neuropathy

Cardiovascular
  Hypertension
  Stroke
  Arrhythmias
  Coronary heart disease

Table 15–16. Medical Complications of Psychostimulant Abuse

General health
  Chronic fatigue
  Sleep problems
  Nasal congestion, ulceration, or bleeding
  Chronic cough or sore throat
  Nausea or vomiting
  Sexual disinterest
  Intravenously or sexually transmitted hepatitis
    or HIV
  Traumatic injuries and overdose

Neurologic
  Selzure
  Cerebrovascular accident
  Hyperpyrexia and rhabdomyolysis
  Headaches
  Dystonias
  Cerebrovasculitis

Cardiovascular
  Arrhythmia
  Angina pectoris
  Myocardial infarction
  Syncope
  Pulmonary edema
  Aortic dissection

---

abuse is associated with acute and chronic pancreatitis and esophagitis. An increased incidence of carcinoma of the pharynx, larynx, and esophagus has been found among heavy users of alcoholic beverages. Nutritional problems are common among alcoholic patients and are manifested by weight loss or obesity, impaired protein synthesis, altered amino acid metabolism, immune incompetence, mineral and electrolyte imbalance, and vitamin deficiencies.

B. PSYCHOSTIMULANTS: COCAINE & AMPHETAMINES

Physical consequences of stimulant abuse include sleep problems, chronic fatigue, severe headaches, and, depending on the route of administration, nasal sores and bleeding, severe dental caries, chronic cough and sore throat, nausea, and vomiting (Table 15–16).

Stimulant abuse can lead to seizures, cerebrovascular accidents, cerebrovasculitis, hyperpyrexia with rhabdomyolysis, and dystonia. Possible mechanisms for neuropsychiatric complications include cerebrovascular vasoconstriction, neurotransmitter depletion, and a reduction of the limbic seizure threshold by repeated subconvulsant stimulation.

Cocaine abuse is particularly dangerous because of the devastating cardiovascular effects that can occur in healthy and young individuals: angina pectoris, myocardial infarction, syncope, aortic dissection, pulmonary edema, and sudden arrhythmic death. Similar cardiovascular morbidity has been observed for amphetamine-related drugs.

C. OPIOIDS

Opioid abuse can lead to many serious medical complications in addition to dependence (Table 15–17). For example, injuries can result from sedation, especially if an individual drives or uses dangerous machinery while taking opioid medication. The analgesic effect can block natural mechanisms that alert the user of physical injury. Decreased respiratory drive, vomiting, and death (from respiratory suppression) can occur

Table 15–17. Medical Complications of Opioid Abuse

General health
Chronic fatigue
Sleep problems
Nausea or vomiting
Sexual disinterest
Traumatic injuries

Pulmonary
Pulmonary edema
Overdose
Respiratory depression
Death

Infectious diseases
Intravenously or sexually transmitted hepatitis
or HIV
Thrombophlebitis
Pulmonary emboli or abscess

with overdose. Shared needle use in intravenous users increases the risk of HIV infection, hepatitis, brain abscess, thrombophlebitis, pulmonary emboli, pulmonary infection, acute endocarditis, septic arthritis, and other infectious diseases. Substances added to opioid street preparations (e.g., strychnine) can lead to peripheral neuropathy, myelopathy, and amblyopia. It has been estimated that over 25% of street opioid addicts are dead within 10–20 years of abuse.

D. CANNABINOIDS

A controversial amotivational syndrome has been described in the literature, wherein chronic marijuana users have been noted to exhibit apathy; dullness; impairment of judgment, concentration, and memory; and loss of interest in personal appearance and conventional goals. Well-controlled clinical studies have not provided strong evidence that an amotivational syndrome is a direct consequence of marijuana use; however, such symptoms would be of particular concern to school-aged adolescents. There is evidence of alterations in heart rate; blood pressure; and reproductive, immunological, and pulmonary function. Cannabinoid-induced testosterone suppression is an issue of concern. It has become apparent that chronic marijuana use has widespread physiological consequences.

E. NICOTINE & TOBACCO

Much has been written and debated about the adverse effects of tobacco use. It is generally accepted that users have significantly increased risk of many serious illnesses: pulmonary disease (e.g., emphysema, lung cancer); cardiovascular disease (e.g., coronary artery disease); peripheral vascular disease, particularly with chronic use;

dental disease (e.g., oral cancer, especially with smokeless tobacco); nicotine stomatitis and stained teeth; and diminished birth weight in the babies of mothers who smoke. Some researchers have estimated that as many as 25% of deaths in the United States are associated with tobacco use. Exposure to high doses of nicotine, as is found in some insecticides, can cause diarrhea, nausea, vomiting, irritability, headache, convulsions, tachypnea, coma, or death.

F. HALLUCINOGENS & VOLATILE INHALANTS

The acute effects of hallucinogens include sympathomimetic actions such as high blood pressure and seizures, particularly with use of phenylisopropylamine compounds. Anticholinergic substances can cause amnesia, hallucinations, dry mouth, constipation, bronchodilation, tachycardia, urinary retention, diminished penile erection, photophobia, increased intraocular pressure, and blurred vision (from dilated pupils). Long-term complications include flashbacks that seem to be stimulated by stress and fatigue.

PCP use can lead to paranoid hallucinations, violent behavior, and self injury. Medical effects include hypersalivation, catalepsy, perspiration, rigidity, myoclonus, stereotyped movements, hyperreflexia, cardiac arrhythmia, hypertension, and convulsions.

Intoxication with volatile inhalants can be associated with dizziness and syncope. Cardiac arrhythmia, pulmonary edema, liver damage, asphyxiation, and renal dysfunction can occur. Neurotoxic effects can lead to severe dementia in young adults.

Lieber CS: Relationships between nutrition, alcohol use, and liver disease. *Alcohol Res Health* 2003;27:220–231.

Naimi TS, Brewer RD, Mokdad A, Denny C, Serdula MK, Marks JS: Binge drinking among us adults. *JAMA* 2003;289:70–75.

Marzuk PM: Fatal injuries after cocaine use as a leading cause of death among young adults in New York City. *N Engl J Med* 1995;332:1753.

Adverse Outcomes of Treatment

A. UNRECOGNIZED OR UNTREATED MEDICAL COMPLICATIONS

Patients with alcohol and drug dependence are often inappropriately triaged to treatment facilities lacking the medical expertise needed to manage medical complications. This may be because intoxicated patients cannot provide adequate histories or because of hostile attitudes among treating professionals. All substance-dependent patients deserve a meticulous history, physical examination, and appropriate laboratory examination to rule out common medical complications. Medical and surgical consultation and joint management are often necessary for more complex cases. In addition, it is important to recognize addictive disorders in patients who have the medical disorders typically complicating alcohol or drug abuse and diagnose correctly patients who are recalcitrant to usually effective treatments. These points are discussed in greater detail in the section "Differential Diagnosis."

B. UNRECOGNIZED OR UNTREATED OTHER PSYCHIATRIC DISORDERS

It can be disastrous if a treatable psychiatric disorder is overlooked in a substance-abusing patient. Many jurisdictions artificially separate the psychiatric care of patients with addictions from those with other psychiatric disorders. Some 12-step support groups proscribe the use of all psychopharmacologic agents, even if they have no known abuse liability and are potentially beneficial. This is to some degree the result of a mistrust of psychiatrists, who until recently believed that the care of patients with substance-use disorders was outside their bailiwick. It is now commonly accepted that all psychiatrists should develop the expertise needed for the diagnosis and appropriate treatment or referral of substance-dependent patients and should seek collaborative relationships with community resources such as 12-step programs.

Drug Interactions

Disulfiram inhibits aldehyde dehydrogenase (involved in alcohol metabolism), and its effects in the drinker are largely if not entirely due to accumulation of acetaldehyde. Taken alone, disulfiram causes little or no effects. With alcohol, it causes intense flushing of the face and neck, tachycardia, hypotension, nausea, and vomiting. It has caused death. Disulfiram also significantly inhibits microsomal drug-metabolizing enzymes and increases the elimination half-life of many drugs such as phenytoin, warfarin, thiopental, and caffeine. In treating alcoholism, physicians must use disulfiram with caution and combine it with psychosocial treatment.

Although alcohol can alter absorption of some drugs (e.g., it increases the absorption of diazepam), the basis for most pharmacokinetic ethanol-drug interactions involves the alcohol dehydrogenase pathway and/or liver microsomal enzymes. Microsomal drug metabolism (cytochrome P450) is inhibited in the presence of high concentrations of ethanol. Therefore, when ethanol and prescribed drugs are taken together, the drug's effect may be augmented (in the case of phenytoin and warfarin) or the effect of alcohol prolonged (in the case of chloral hydrate, chlorpromazine, or cimetidine). Microsomal induction after long-term alcohol consumption contributes to accelerated ethanol metabolism at high blood ethanol concentrations. Increased drug metabolism and activation of xenobiotics (e.g., carcinogens) following microsomal induction results in lower-than-therapeutic blood levels (in the case of barbiturates, phenytoin,

isoniazid, meprobamate, methadone, and warfarin) or increased production of toxic metabolites (in the case of acetaminophen). Although most recently launched drugs have been developed by the pharmaceutical industry so as to minimize drug interactions via microsomal enzyme metabolism, pharmacodynamic interactions are still widespread. Common mechanisms for pharmacodynamic ethanol-drug interactions include increased drug effects when an individual is intoxicated with ethanol, because of additive CNS depression (in the case of antihistamines, other CNS depressants, opioids, antipsychotics, and antidepressants); or diminished drug effects when the individual has not been drinking, because of the presence of cross-tolerance to other CNS depressants.

Metabolism of methadone can be altered by the coadministration of medications that induce cytochrome P450 (e.g., rifampin, phenytoin, barbiturates, carbamazepine), thereby complicating dosing during methadone maintenance.

Prognosis

The prognosis and course of illness in substance abuse disorders depends on numerous factors involving a complex interaction of biological, psychological, and environmental elements. The specific substance(s) used, the duration and dosage of substance use, co-occurring psychiatric and medical disorders, coping skills, developmental history, socioeconomic status, social support, genetic predispositions, treatment choices, and other aspects are all important. The prognosis for individuals who abuse drugs other than alcohol is complicated by an antisocial lifestyle. In addition, the intravenous use of those drugs (as well as sex-for-drugs transactions) increases the risk and spread of life-threatening illnesses such as AIDS and hepatitis.

The outcome of substance-related problems is enhanced by relapse prevention using nonpharmacologic approaches involving psychotherapy and self-help groups (such as Alcoholics Anonymous). Appropriate adjunctive pharmacologic treatments can be effectively combined with psychosocial treatments to prevent relapse.

It is important to treat co-occurring psychiatric illnesses. Most alcoholic patients have another psychiatric illness, particularly affective, anxiety, and personality disorders, which can worsen prognosis if not addressed. Co-occurrence of psychiatric disorders is also prevalent among the other substance-use disorders. Complete psychiatric evaluation and treatment is therefore essential in patients with substance and related disorders.

A. ALCOHOL & OTHER CNS DEPRESSANTS

Naltrexone and acamprosate are the only medications approved by the FDA to prevent alcohol relapse. Naltrexone is a μ-opioid receptor antagonist. Acamprosate (calcium bisacetylhomotaurinate), a chemical analog of L-glutamic acid, affects GABAergic and glutamatergic neurotransmission. Both naltrexone and acamprosate reduce relapse by approximately half that of placebo control subjects over a 2- to 3-month period (down to a rate of about 20–25%). Moreover, the type of psychotherapy used with naltrexone appears to influence treatment outcome as lower rates of relapse were reported in patients using supportive therapy compared to coping skills therapy.

More recently investigators have studied whether combining these medications improves alcoholism treatment outcome. Naltrexone or acamprosate as well as the combination of the two were significantly more effective than placebo in one study. Naltrexone treatment tended to be superior to acamprosate regarding time to first drink and time to relapse in this study. Naltrexone/acamprosate combined was most effective with significantly lower relapse rates than placebo and acamprosate alone; but the combination was not significantly better than naltrexone alone. In spite of some demonstrated benefits from these medications they should always be used in conjunction with psychosocial therapies.

B. Psychostimulants: Cocaine & Amphetamines

Users of stimulants such as cocaine and amphetamines tend to use the drug nearly daily (in low or high dosages) or intermittently (e.g., weekend binges). Binge use of psychostimulants often leads to dependence. Daily users often increase rapidly the dosage taken. Intravenous use or smoking of cocaine can lead to dependence in a matter of weeks or months. Dependence takes longer to develop in individuals who nasally insufflate the drug. Preliminary studies indicate that cognitive–behavioral therapy is more effective than interpersonal psychotherapy in preventing relapse in cocaine-dependent patients (with abstinence rates over a 3-week period of 60% and 33%, respectively). Behavioral treatment (contracting, counseling, community reinforcement) increases abstinence to about 40% in a 3- to 4-month period compared to 5% in those who participate in drug counseling only. In addition, preliminary trials suggest that some patients with cocaine dependence benefit from antidepressants and anticonvulsants (e.g., carbamazepine).

C. Opioids

Opioid dependence is often characterized by short periods of abstinence followed by relapse. Even after years of forced abstinence by incarceration, many subjects relapse after being released from jail. Relapse often occurs when patients fail to inform their physician about their addictions and opioids are prescribed for medical ailments. Psychosocial therapies for opioid dependence are often helpful. Agonist substitution with methadone is well established to benefit the most severely addicted patient

population when provided in methadone maintenance programs. Buprenorphine, recently approved for administration by appropriately trained physicians in office-based practice, provides an alternative to methadone in treatment of opioid dependence. However, it is not yet established for which patients methadone or buprenorphine is the preferred treatment modality. On the other hand, similar benefits have been found for standard outpatient counseling or psychotherapy in patients on methadone maintenance (for opioid dependence) compared to those in therapeutic communities. Subjects who remain in combined treatment have lower relapse rates than do those who drop out. Psychodynamic therapy and cognitive therapy have been of greater benefit than standard drug counseling alone. Interestingly, limited monthly interactions with a psychotherapist, when combined with methadone maintenance, appear to be as effective as more intensive and frequent interpersonal psychotherapy.

D. Cannabinoids

Cannabis dependence occurs slowly in those who develop patterns of increasing dosage and frequency of use. The pleasurable effects of cannabis often diminish with regular heavy use. In patients with marijuana dependence, manual-guided individual treatment and group therapy appear to have similar beneficial effects. Marijuana use drops about 50% in response to these treatment modalities.

E. Nicotine & Tobacco

Tobacco smokers usually start in their early teen years, often in social settings. Children are at increased risk if their parents or close friends smoke. Since the 1970s, smoking has decreased in the U.S. population but less in females than in males. The greatest prevalence rate of smoking is in the psychiatric population, especially among patients with schizophrenia or depression. Smoking is very reinforcing, and although some people can stop smoking "cold turkey," overall failure rates of treatment are high (over 70% at 1 year).

F. Hallucinogens & Volatile Inhalants

The onset of hallucinogen use depends on availability, social and cultural setting, and expectations. Use is often experimental and intermittent, but chronic or heavy use can lead to long-term consequences such as flashbacks, mood lability, personality disturbances, and dementia.

Kessler RC: The epidemiology of dual diagnosis. *Biol Psychiatry* 2004;56:730–737.

Vaillant GE: A long-term follow-up of male alcohol abuse. *Arch Gen Psychiatry* 1996;53:243.

CONCLUSION

The substance-related disorders exact an immense toll on the mental and physical well-being of many individuals. Consequently, they jeopardize the integrity of the family and other social forces represented by the health-care system, the law, and the economy. Because of the prevalence of substance-related disorders, and because they can masquerade as diverse medical and other psychiatric disorders, their recognition and initial treatment are relevant to all physicians, in particular, to psychiatrists. Substance-related disorders are heterogeneous in terms of the interactions between the manifest psychopathology of the individual patient and the psychopharmacologic actions of a given drug, within the relevant sociocultural context. This perspective is useful in seeking an etiologic understanding of these disorders, conducting a clinical assessment, planning for the initial treatment of the direct consequences of drug use, and developing and implementing a comprehensive treatment strategy for patients. Recent perspectives of addictive disorders have broadened to include other out-of-control, self-destructive, so-called behavioral addictions, which for many individuals seem to be woven into the fabric of substance-use and co-occurring psychiatric disorders.

Future directions in substance abuse treatment research are likely to focus on understanding issues of co-occurring psychiatric conditions, developing new psychopharmacologic treatment options, and combining pharmacotherapy and psychotherapy in the management of these disorders. Agents that can help reduce drug craving and relapse are of particular interest as are genetically based interindividual differences in these disorders. Overall, considerably more research is needed on the optimal combination of treatment modalities to prevent relapse in substance-dependent patients and improve prognosis.

Schizophrenia

Herbert Y. Meltzer, MD, William V. Bobo, MD, Stephan H. Heckers, MD, &
Hossein S. Fatemi, MD, PhD

ESSENTIAL OF DIAGNOSIS

DSM-IV-TR Diagnostic Criteria for Schizophrenia

A. Characteristic symptoms: *Two (or more) of the following, each present for a significant portion of time during a 1-month period (or less if successfully treated):*

(1) *delusions*

(2) *hallucinations*

(3) *disorganized speech (e.g., frequent derailment or incoherence)*

(4) *grossly disorganized or catatonic behavior*

(5) *negative symptoms, i.e., affective flattening, alogia, or avolition*

Note: *Only one Criterion A symptom is required if delusions are bizarre or hallucinations consist of a voice keeping up a running commentary on the person's behavior or thoughts, or two or more voices conversing with each other.*

B. Social/occupational dysfunction: *For a significant portion of the time since the onset of the disturbance, one or more major areas of functioning such as work, interpersonal relations, or self-care are markedly below the level achieved prior to the onset (or when the onset is in childhood or adolescence, failure to achieve expected level of interpersonal, academic, or occupational achievement).*

C. Duration: *Continuous signs of the disturbance persist for at least 6 months. This 6-month period must include at least 1 month of symptoms (or less if successfully treated) that meet Criterion A (i.e., active-phase symptoms) and may include periods of prodromal or residual symptoms. During these prodromal or residual periods, the signs of the disturbance may be manifested by only negative symptoms or two or more symptoms listed in Criterion A present in an attenuated form (e.g., odd beliefs, unusual perceptual experiences).*

D. Schizoaffective and mood disorder exclusion: *Schizoaffective disorder and mood disorder with psychotic features have been ruled out because either (1) no major depressive, manic, or mixed episodes have occurred concurrently with the active-phase symptoms; or (2) if mood episodes have occurred during active-phase symptoms, their total duration has been brief relative to the duration of the active and residual periods.*

E. Substance/general medical condition exclusion: *The disturbance is not due to the direct physiological effects of a substance (e.g., a drug of abuse, a medication) or a general medical condition.*

F. Relationship to a pervasive developmental disorder: *If there is a history of autistic disorder or another pervasive developmental disorder, the additional diagnosis of schizophrenia is made only if prominent delusions or hallucinations are also present for at least a month (or less if successfully treated).*

(Adapted, with permission, from *Diagnostic and Statistical Manual of Mental Disorders*, 4th edn., Text Revision. Washington, DC: American Psychiatric Association, 2000.)

- **Diagnostic criteria** met, as specified in the box above. Note that these criteria allow the diagnosis in absence of prominent hallucinations or delusions (e.g., there is instead some combination of negative symptoms, disorganized speech, and/or disorganized or catatonic behavior).
- **Duration of active psychotic symptoms** for at least 1 month, or for a shorter duration if active treatment was initiated.
- **Total duration of illness for at least 6 months,** including prodrome, acute phase, and residual symptoms.

- **Cognitive impairment**, characterized by disorganized, illogical, loosely associated or bizarre **speech**, or by inappropriate or bizarre **behaviors**.
- **The above symptoms are idiopathic in nature.**
- **Dysfunction in one or more life domains** as a result of the above signs or symptoms.

Other common features:

- **Lack of insight** that symptoms and difficulties that stem from them are products of a mental illness that requires treatment.
- **Deterioration in personal appearance and hygiene.**
- **Depressive and anxiety-based symptoms,** including **suicidal thinking.**
- **Abnormal motor activity,** including rocking, pacing, grimacing, maintaining uncomfortable postures, stereotypies, and odd mannerisms.
- **Poor compliance** with treatment.
- Comorbid **drug** (including nicotine) and **alcohol use disorders,** and chronic **physical health problems.**

General Considerations

Schizophrenia is a clinical syndrome historically characterized by a heterogeneous mixture of clinical features referred to as **psychosis**. These clinical features include hallucinations, delusions, abnormal emotions, cognitive problems, and abnormal behaviors. The clinical diagnosis of schizophrenia is currently made on the basis of these characteristic signs and symptoms, their time course, their adverse impact on functional capacity, and their idiopathic nature (e.g., they are not the psychiatric manifestations of general medical conditions or effects of substances, and are not better accounted for by other diagnoses that feature psychotic symptoms or severe functional or cognitive incapacity).

Even after excluding the secondary causes of psychotic symptoms, the diagnosis of schizophrenia and related disorders remains challenging. For one, the etiology and the neuropathophysiology of schizophrenia is unknown. Second, no single sign or symptom is pathognomonic to schizophrenia. Finally, there is no clinically reliable biological marker, including functional or structural neuroimaging or pattern of genetic heritability.

The concept of schizophrenia as a diagnostic entity is still evolving even though the diagnostic criteria in use today have been unchanged for over two decades. Although it is likely that the schizophrenic syndrome has been described in one form or another since ancient times, the twentieth-century observations of Emil Kraepelin, Eugen Bleuler and Kurt Schneider have contributed most to our current classification of the disorder. Kraepelin was credited with distinguishing manic–depressive illness

(now called bipolar disorder) from **dementia praecox** (the forerunner of schizophrenia) based on relative age of onset (younger in the case of manic–depressive illness), symptom course (episodic for manic–depressive illness, chronic for dementia praecox), vocational/social outcome (better for manic–depressive illness) and level of cognitive impairment (more severe in dementia praecox). Bleuler coined the term "schizophrenia" based on his observation that long-term outcome was quite variable among patients with dementia praecox and on the hypothesis that a split between thought and affect was the central feature of the illness. Bleuler specifically identified four components (also known as Bleuler's "four A's") as the essence of the syndrome: **Autism** (i.e., a disconnect from reality), **Ambivalence** (of affect and will), **Affectivity** (in Bleuler's words: an "indifference to everything"), and **Association** (in Bleuler's words: "the associations lose their continuity").

Schneider contributed the concept of **first-rank symptoms** (e.g., thought insertion, thought withdrawal, thought broadcast, voices arguing or discussing, delusions of control, etc.), which he believed were pathognomonic of schizophrenia and became the forerunner of the notion of positive signs and symptoms. Schneider's first-rank symptoms are now known not to be specific for schizophrenia, for they may also occur in mania, drug induced states, and other disorders. Nonetheless, these and other signs and symptoms together have undergone extensive empirical testing to be criteria with sufficient diagnostic specificity, reliability, and validity for use in clinical practice

Lieberman JA, Stroup TS, Perkins DO (eds): *Textbook of Schizophrenia.* Washington, DC: American Psychiatric Publishing, 2006.

Mueser KT, McGurk SR: Schizophrenia. *Lancet* 2004;363:147.

A. EPIDEMIOLOGY

1. Incidence & prevalence—The **incidence** of schizophrenia ranges from 10 to 40 new cases per 100,000 population, while the age-corrected median **point prevalence** and **lifetime prevalence** estimates of the disorder are 4.6 and 4.0 cases per 1000 population, respectively. This figure for lifetime prevalence estimate is lower than the often reported range of 0.5% to 1.0%, which is believed to be an overestimate. Differences between site estimates of incidence and prevalence may be due to a variety of factors, including sex, urbanicity, migrant status, month of birth, recovery, suicide, and other forms of early mortality.

2. Life expectancy, drug use, & physical health problems—The life expectancy in schizophrenia is lower by about 20% relative to the general population. Increased early mortality among schizophrenics is attributed to increased rates of **suicide** (10–13% lifetime risk of completed suicide, 18–55% risk for attempted suicide), accidents, and poor physical health. At baseline, schizophrenics appear to be at higher risk for a host of metabolic and cardiovascular disorders, including obesity, diabetes, dyslipidemia, and coronary artery and cerebrovascular disease. Other contributors to the medical morbidity of schizophrenia include unhealthy lifestyle, alcohol and drug abuse, and high rates (70–80%) of chronic heavy smoking. High rates of substance abuse alone contribute to poor physical health, infrequent medical and psychiatric follow up, and poor compliance with medical and psychiatric treatment. In addition, several of the most efficacious treatments for schizophrenia may elevate cardiovascular risk as a result of weight gain, dyslipidemia and glucose elevation.

In spite of the health concerns that accompany schizophrenia, there is a disproportionately low rate of health service utilization among this population. Cognitive dysfunction, paranoid symptoms, apathy, comorbid disorders, poverty and illness-associated stigma may all impede utilization of necessary medical services. Concrete recommendations for health screening and monitoring are provided later (see section "Treatment").

B. Demographics

1. Gender—Schizophrenia is slightly more common in males than in females (male:female risk ratio is 1.4); however, as noted above, the average age of onset of schizophrenia for women is at least 5 years later than for men. Others have found no statistically significant differences in prevalence estimates between males and females. Differences in **sex distribution** for new-onset cases are especially apparent after the age of 45, where there is a 2:1 sex ratio in favor of women. Compared with men, women with schizophrenia tend to have better premorbid functioning, fewer negative symptoms, more prominent mood symptoms, more complete recovery from episodes, better clinical response to antipsychotic medication, milder long-term course, better social functioning, less comorbid substance abuse and less potential for suicide. Symptoms in females may worsen after menopause.

2. Age—The age of onset for men appears to be earlier (age 18–25 years) than for women (age 25–35 years). For men, there is a second but much smaller incidence peak between age 30 and 35 years. Onset prior to the age of 10 is considered rare, though when it does occur, symptoms are typically very severe. Onset after the age of 45 (**late onset**) is also uncommon, and very uncommon after the age of 65 (**very late onset**). Patients with poor outcome, as indicated by poor response to currently available therapies, have an earlier age at onset than do those who are more responsive to treatment. The average age at onset of neuroleptic-resistant schizophrenia in female patients may be 4–5 years lower than in female patients with neuroleptic-responsive schizophrenia, but male and female patients with neuroleptic-resistant schizophrenia have similar ages at onset: 20–21 years, on average, according to one study.

3. Social status—The prevalence rates of schizophrenia are higher in densely populated urban areas, as well as in industrialized nations. The prevalence of schizophrenia is lower in developing countries compared with developed nations. Patients in developing countries have a more benign illness course than those in developed countries. Especially in Western societies, individuals with schizophrenia are at higher risk for poverty, unemployment, homelessness or inadequate housing, ill health, and poor access to health care. It has been theorized that the limitations posed by the symptoms of schizophrenia result in a **downward drift** in socioeconomic status, or prevent upward social mobility, or both.

Individuals in lower socioeconomic classes have higher rates of schizophrenia because of the markedly impaired work function of patients with this illness. Lower income is to be expected in the families of schizophrenics because 10% of the parents of schizophrenic patients have schizophrenia themselves, and other parents may have subclinical forms of the illness, including cognitive impairments and Axis II pathology, impairing their earning capacity.

4. Social support—Individuals with schizophrenia are more likely to be single (never married), divorced, or separated relative to age-matched controls. Individuals with schizophrenia who are unmarried tend to have earlier onset of psychosis, poorer premorbid functioning, and more severe illness, relative to those who have married. Conversely, adequate social support in any form and avoidance of high "**expressed emotion**" environments (overcritical or over-protective) both predict better long-term course.

5. Ethnicity—Schizophrenia affects individuals from all racial and ethnic groups. While schizophrenia was once believed to be more prevalent among nonimmigrant minority groups in the United States, especially African Americans, recent studies have shown that such groups do not appear to be at greater risk for schizophrenia compared with the general population. There is conflicting evidence as to the influence of immigration status on overall risk of developing schizophrenia. The disproportionately high prevalence of schizophrenia observed among first-generation immigrants in Western countries appears to normalize in subsequent generations.

6. Other factors—Epidemiologic data consistently show that schizophrenic patients have an increased likelihood of having been born in the **late winter and spring months**. The seasonal effect has been linked to epidemics of influenza or viral infections that occur more frequently during winter months. A number of epidemiologic studies have attributed the increased rate of schizophrenic births to maternal influenza or other viral infections during the second trimester. Maternal influenza during the second trimester may impair fetal growth and predispose to obstetric complications and lower birth weight in about 2% of individuals destined to develop schizophrenia. Recent epidemiologic evidence based on 2669 cases of schizophrenia in a population cohort of 1.75 million showed significant relative risks of developing schizophrenia with increased urbanization and season of birth. The highest association was for births in the months of February and March, presumably due to the increased risk of viral infection during pregnancy. Other complicating factors such as maternal malnutrition and Rh incompatibility during gestation have been associated with increased vulnerability to schizophrenia.

C. ETIOLOGY

Kraepelin conjectured that schizophrenia was caused by a biological abnormality, even though the attempts to identify an abnormality (including neuropathological studies by Alois Alzheimer) were unsuccessful. In the middle of the twentieth century, the view that schizophrenia was the result of specific disturbances in child-rearing received considerable attention. In particular, communication deviance between parents and the child who was diagnosed with schizophrenia was considered by some clinicians to be a sufficient cause of schizophrenia. Although communication deviance in families with a schizophrenic child has been demonstrated in a number of studies, evidence that this feature was specific for schizophrenia or causative was unconvincing. Nevertheless, this line of research led to a continual interest in how family (and other caregiver) interactions can contribute to or diminish the stress and coping skills of patients with schizophrenia and, thus, modulate the course of the illness.

The view that schizophrenia is a brain disease now prevails, based on evidence from studies of neurotransmitter systems, histological, and neuroimaging studies of brain structure, and studies of brain function.

Neurochemical Abnormalities

A. DOPAMINE HYPOTHESIS

The most widely accepted original hypothesis of the etiology of schizophrenia and of the action of antipsychotic drugs implicates the neurotransmitter dopamine (DA). Dopaminergic neurons arise from two midbrain nuclei: (1) the **nigrostriatal tract** originates in the substantia nigra, terminates in the striatum, and is involved in modulation of motoric behavior, cognition, and sensory gating; and (2) the **mesolimbic** and **mesocortical tracts** originate in the ventral tegmental area and terminate in limbic and cortical structures, respectively, affecting cognitive, motivational, and reward systems. The dopamine 1 (D_1) receptor family, which includes D_1 and D_5 receptors, is present in high concentration in the cortex and striatum. The dopamine 2 (D_2) receptor family consists of D_2, D_3, and D_4 receptors and is concentrated in the limbic and striatal regions. Presynaptic DA receptors (i.e., D_2 and D_3) can consist of either somatodendritic autoreceptors localized to cell bodies in the substantia nigra and ventral tegmental area or terminal autoreceptors limited to axons of these DA cells. The somatodendritic and terminal autoreceptors affect the firing of DA cells and the synthesis and release of DA, respectively.

1. Positive symptoms—The DA hypothesis of schizophrenia, as originally postulated, proposed that schizophrenia is due to an excess of DA activity in limbic brain areas, especially the nucleus accumbens, as well as the stria terminalis, lateral septum, and olfactory tubercle (e.g., **mesolimbic dopamine hyperactivity**). This hypothesis was based on evidence that chronic administration of the stimulant D-amphetamine produced a psychosis that resembles paranoid schizophrenia. D-Amphetamine increases the release of DA and norepinephrine (NE) and inhibits their reuptake. Isomers of D-amphetamine with different effects on the availability of NE and DA in rodents were used to show that increased locomotor activity, which correlates best with psychosis in humans, is due to an increased release of DA rather than NE.

The second line of evidence relating DA to schizophrenia is that antipsychotic drugs decrease DA activity by receptor depletion (reserpine) and blockade (neuroleptics). The most compelling evidence that linked DA to the positive symptoms of schizophrenia was the finding that chlorpromazine was an effective antipsychotic drug and that it blocked DA receptors in vivo, inhibiting the effect of D-amphetamine on locomotor activity. The discovery that a number of different chemical classes of DA-receptor antagonists are effective as antipsychotic drugs and that there is a high correlation between the drug's average daily dosage and its affinity for the D_2-receptor family led to the view that increased stimulation of these receptors caused schizophrenia.

2. Negative symptoms and cognitive dysfunction—Decreased dopamine activity in the prefrontal cortex (**mesocortical dopamine deficit**) may mediate the negative symptoms and cognitive dysfunction associated with schizophrenia.

The concept of increased DA activity as the core deficit in schizophrenia was developed at the time when delusions and hallucinations were central to the diagnosis of schizophrenia, whereas negative symptoms, affective symptoms, and cognitive dysfunction were relegated to a secondary role. The latter aspects of schizophrenia have never been associated with excessive DA activity. As mentioned earlier in this chapter, researchers have proposed that decreased DA activity may lead to cognitive impairment and depression. There is little evidence that blockade of D_2 or D_4 receptors induces depression or cognitive impairment. Recent studies in primates have implicated the D_1-receptor family in the control of working memory, a cognitive function impaired in schizophrenia.

3. Limitations of the dopamine hypotheses—Clinically, factors that challenge the primacy of dopamine imbalance at the expense of other transmitter systems stem from at least two observations. First, drugs that act on other transmitter systems, such as hallucinogens (e.g., lysergic acid, psilocybin) and dissociative anesthetics (e.g., phencyclidine, ketamine), also cause psychotic symptoms. Phencyclidine exposure results in a psychotic syndrome that models schizophrenic psychosis more accurately than amphetamine does (see below). Second, while D_2-receptor blockade occurs very quickly after antipsychotic dosing, clinical antipsychotic effects typically require several weeks to ensue.

Furthermore, postmortem studies of patients with schizophrenia have not found consistent abnormalities in the density of any of the five DA receptors or changes in their affinities for DA, with the possible exception of the D_3 receptor, which may have an abnormal form. Several research groups have also reported a link between D_3 polymorphisms and schizophrenia. There is no reliable evidence, from either postmortem studies or positron emission tomography (PET) studies, for an increase in the density of D_2 receptors in schizophrenia. Recent PET studies of the release of DA in the striatum of patients with schizophrenia suggest that the extracellular concentration of DA in this region is increased compared to that in normal subjects. Plasma and cerebrospinal fluid (CSF) levels of homovanillic acid, the major metabolite of DA, are not elevated in patients who have schizophrenia. Some researchers have suggested that DA-receptor sensitization occurs in schizophrenia, but only indirect evidence supports this hypothesis.

Abi-Dargham A, Gil R, Krystal J, et al.: Increased striatal dopamine transmission in schizophrenia: Confirmation in a second cohort. *Am J Psychiatry* 1998;155:761–767.

Capuano B, Crosby IT, Lloyd EJ: Schizophrenia: Genesis, receptorology and current therapeutics. *Curr Med Chem* 2002;9:521.

Charney DS, Nestler EJ (eds): *Neurobiology of Mental Illness*, 2nd edn. New York, NY: Oxford, 2004.

Heinz A, Romero B, Gallinat J, Juckel G, Weinberger DR: Molecular brain imaging and the neurobiology and genetics of schizophrenia. *Pharmacopsychiatry* 2003;36(suppl 3):S152.

Jaskiw GE, Weinberger DR: Dopamine and schizophrenia: A cortically correct perspective. *Semin Neurosci* 1992;4:179.

Laruelle M: Imaging dopamine transmission in schizophrenia. A review and meta analysis. *Q J Nucl Med* 1998;42:211–221.

Voruganti LP, Awad AG: Brain imaging research on subjective responses to psychotropic drugs. *Acta Psychiatr Scand Suppl* 2005;427:22.

B. SEROTONIN HYPOTHESIS

Serotonin (5-HT) neurons originate in the midbrain dorsal and median raphe nuclei, which project to the cortex, striatum, hippocampus, and other limbic regions. There are at least 15 types of 5-HT receptors; of these, the most relevant to schizophrenia are the 5-HT_1, 5-HT_{1D}, 5-HT_2, 5-HT_3, 5-HT_6, and 5-HT_7 receptors. Somatodendritic autoreceptors (of the 5-HT_{1A} type) are present on the cell bodies of 5-HT raphe neurons and inhibit firing of serotonergic neurons. Terminal autoreceptors (5-HT_{1D} in humans) regulate the synthesis and release of 5-HT. 5-HT_3 receptors stimulate DA release. Postsynaptic 5-HT_{2A} receptors are localized on pyramidal neurons in mesocortical areas. The complex interaction between 5-HT and DA varies by brain region and by types of 5-HT and DA receptor.

An early theory of the etiology of schizophrenia was that it is due to an excess of brain serotonergic activity. This theory was based on the belief that the psychotomimetic properties of lysergic acid diethyl amide (LSD), an indole compound, are due to its 5-HT agonist properties. This led to a search for endogenous indole hallucinogens in the brain, blood, and urine of schizophrenic patients. The enzymes that synthesize and catabolize indoles, of which 5-HT is the most important, were also studied in detail; however, none of the putative abnormalities was confirmed by subsequent careful study.

The notion that the effects of LSD and other indole hallucinogens, such as psilocybin and *N,N*-dimethyltryptamine, provide an adequate model of schizophrenia was also rejected because the primary effect of these drugs is to cause visual hallucinations. The potency of these agents as hallucinogens is highly correlated with their 5-HT_{2A}-receptor affinity. The thought disorder, auditory hallucinations, and bizarre behavior usually present in schizophrenia are generally absent in normal individuals given these agents. However, ingestion of these agents can cause an exacerbation of positive symptoms in schizophrenic patients.

Neuroleptic drugs are not particularly useful in decreasing the effects of the indole hallucinogens. Newer antipsychotic drugs such as clozapine, olanzapine, risperidone, quetiapine, and sertindole are potent antagonists of the 5-HT_{2A} receptor. Some of the advantages of these drugs may result from their greater potency as 5-HT_{2A}-receptor antagonists, relative to D_2-receptor blockade. The most likely advantages of these drugs, related to their higher affinity to 5-HT_{2A} versus DA receptors, are their low D_2-induced extrapyramidal symptoms (EPS) profile and their ability to improve negative symptoms. Increased stimulation of 5-HT_{2A} receptors may be important in the etiology of negative symptoms and EPS. Although this concept of the role of 5-HT in schizophrenia is no longer considered viable, alternative theories of the role of 5-HT are of interest and are discussed in subsequent sections.

Abi-DarghamA, Laruelle M, Aghajanian GK, Charney D, Krystal J: The role of serotonin in the pathophysiology and treatment of schizophrenia. *J Neuropsychiatry Clin Neurosci* 1997;9:1.

Capuano B, Crosby IT, Lloyd EJ: Schiozphrenia: Genesis, receptorology and current therapeutics. *Curr Med Chem* 2002;9:521.

Meltzer HY, Fatemi SH: The role of serotonin in schizophrenia and the mechanisms of action of antipsychotic drugs. In: Kane JM, Möller HJ, Awouters F (eds). *Serotonin in Antipsychotic Treatment: Mechanisms and Clinical Practice.* Marcel Dekker, New York, NY 1996, pp. 77–107.

C. GLUTAMATE HYPOTHESIS

Clinical and experimental evidence has supported a complex role for glutamate in the etiology of schizophrenia. The original evidence for an abnormality of the glutamatergic system was a decreased level of glutamate in the CSF of patients with schizophrenia. Subsequent studies have revealed decreased expression of glutamatergic receptors, such as the *N*-methyl-D-aspartate (NMDA) and AMPA/Kainate receptors. Evidence indicates that decreased glutamatergic activity is the result of decreased levels of glutamate receptors of the NMDA subtype. Consistent with the role of glutamate in schizophrenia, three noncompetitive antagonists of NMDA receptors (phencyclidine [PCP], ketamine, and MK-801), and three competitive antagonists (CPP, CPP-ene, and CGS 19,755), can produce a range of positive and negative symptoms and cognitive dysfunction in normal control subjects closely mimicking the clinical signs and symptoms of schizophrenia. Exposing schizophrenic patients to these agents results in marked intensification of core schizophrenic symptoms.

Neuroleptics can block some of the clinical effects of PCP. The ability of the 5-HT$_{2A}$- and D$_2$-receptor antagonists, such as clozapine and olanzapine, to block the clinical effects of these NMDA-receptor antagonists is unknown. However, the preclinical effects of PCP, such as disruption of sensory gating, can be blocked by selective 5-HT$_{2A}$-receptor antagonists, such as MDL100,907, and by clozapine. Several compounds that enhance NMDA receptor function (e.g., glycine, D-serine, D-cycloserine) have been reported to alleviate negative and positive symptoms in patients with schizophrenia when administered in conjunction with typical neuroleptic drugs. It has also been suggested that increased levels of glutamate can have neurotoxic effects on various neurons; however, there is no conclusive evidence for neurodegenerative change in schizophrenia.

Coyle JT: Glutamate and schizophrenia: Beyond the dopamine hypothesis. *Cell Mol Neurobiol* 2006; 26: 365–384.

Goff DC, Coyle JT: The emerging role of glutamate in the pathophysiology and treatment of schizophrenia. *Am J Psychiatry* 2001;158:1367.

Olney JW, Farber NB: Glutamate receptor dysfunction and schizophrenia. *Arch Gen Psychiatry* 1995;52:998.

D. GAMMA-AMINOBUTYRIC ACID

The major inhibitory neurotransmitter gamma-aminobutyric acid (GABA) has been implicated in the pathophysiology of schizophrenia. After initial reports of decreased GABA levels in CSF, recent postmortem studies have implicated a decreased function of GABAergic neurons in schizophrenia. The most replicated finding is a decreased expression of the messenger RNA for glutamic acid decarboxylase (GAD), the enzyme necessary for the synthesis of GABA. The 67 kDa isoform of GAD has been reported as decreased in the cerebral cortex and hippocampus of schizophrenic subjects. Subsequent studies have identified gene and protein expression changes in specific subsets of GABAergic neurons in the cerebral cortex, such as parvalbumin-positive GABAergic neurons in the prefrontal cortex, which play a crucial role in the modulation of pyramidal cell firing and the synchronization of cortical activity.

Benes FM, Berretta S: Gabaergic interneurons: Implications for understanding schizophrenia and bipolar disorder. *Neuropsychopharmacology* 2001;25:1–27.

Lewis DA, Hashimoto T, Volk DW: Cortical inhibitory neurons and schizophrenia. *Nat Rev Neurosci* 2005;6:312–324.

Structural Brain Abnormalities

The neuropathological exploration of schizophrenia is experiencing a renaissance and has been complemented recently by neuroimaging studies of the cortical gray and white matter, and subcortical regions.

A. CORTEX AND HIPPOCAMPUS

The study of the cerebral cortex remains at the center of schizophrenia research. Ever since Kraepelin's original conceptualizations of dementia praecox as a disorder of uniquely human qualities (such as volition and insight), most studies of brain structure have focused on the prefrontal cortex, primarily its dorsolateral aspects (i.e., dorsolateral prefrontal cortex [DLPFC]). Recently, the medial temporal lobe, especially the hippocampus, has attracted significant interest, originally because of the reports of psychotic symptoms in patients with medial temporal lobe lesions. Other regions of interest include the anterior cingulate cortex and the superior temporal gyrus. Improved neuroimaging methods allow for the in vivo measurement of regional brain volumes, the estimation of cortical thickness, and the shape analysis of cortical and subcortical structures. Two important morphometric findings have been replicated, with achieve significant effect sizes in meta-analyses. First, the lateral and third ventricles are enlarged. Second, the volumes of several cortical regions are decreased in the medial temporal lobe.

At the cellular level of cortical organization, abnormalities of cell number, protein expression, and gene expression have been reported. The well-established finding of decreased cortical volume in schizophrenia is not mirrored, as in most neurological disorders, by reports of marked neuronal loss. Some investigators have interpreted the lack of marked cell loss and the lack of an associated increase in the number of glial cells as evidence against a neurodegenerative and in favor of a neurodevelopmental abnormality.

Some studies provide evidence of a decreased prominence of dendrites and axons (referred to, in aggregate, as neuropil), resulting in an increased density of cortical neurons. This is complemented by emerging evidence for decreased oligodendrocyte functioning, i.e., of the glial cells crucial for the myelination of fiber pathways.

The application of sophisticated methods of protein and gene expression in postmortem brain tissue has provided researchers with the opportunity to study subtle abnormalities of cellular architecture, not detected by the standard neuropathological examination of brain tissue. Such studies have demonstrated deficits in cortical and hippocampal neurons, such as subtypes of GABAergic neurons in the prefrontal cortex.

Longitudinal neuroimaging studies have shown convincingly that the changes in cortical structure are visible at the time of the first episode of schizophrenia, and not simply the effect of longstanding illness or treatment. Furthermore, some studies provide evidence that abnormalities of brain structure can be found in individuals who are at high risk of developing schizophrenia, but have not yet become symptomatic. Finally, neuroimaging studies reveal that some of the abnormalities found in schizophrenia are present also in unaffected first-degree relatives. Taken together, there is a compelling evidence for structural abnormalities of the cortex and hippocampus in schizophrenia.

B. Subcortical Regions

Initial reports indicated a significant decrease of mediodorsal thalamic nucleus volume and neuronal population. Some reports specifically implicated those neurons of the mediodorsal thalamic nucleus that establish strong reciprocal connections with the DLPFC. Recent rigorous, larger studies, however, have not been able to replicate the finding of thalamic neuronal loss.

The basal ganglia have been studied extensively in schizophrenia, as they are a projection site of dopaminergic fibers from the substantia nigra. While several studies have demonstrated an increased release of dopamine into the striatum (especially during periods of acute psychosis), there is little evidence for an abnormality in basal ganglia volume, cell number, or protein and gene expression.

C. White Matter

Recent studies reveal abnormalities of glial cells and myelinated fiber pathways in schizophrenia. The cellular abnormalities include a decreased number of oligodendroglia and a decreased expression of myelin-related genes. Either abnormality could lead to a disturbance of myelinated fiber pathways in the brain. Neuroimaging studies of fractional aniostropy, a measure of the alignment and organization of fiber bundles in the brain, have indeed revealed such patterns of cortical disconnection. They appear to affect regions in the prefrontal cortex as well as several large-scale networks of brain regions, such as the frontal and temporo-parietal brain regions subserving language function.

Functional Brain Abnormalities

There is little doubt that the core features of schizophrenia (i.e., the positive and negative symptoms and the significant decline in social functioning) are caused by abnormalities of brain function. The extensive literature on neuropsychological deficits in schizophrenia is supported by more recent reports of the neural basis of such deficits.

A. Neuropsychological Studies

Most patients with schizophrenia show significant deficits on standard neuropsychological tests. While some investigators have proposed that such deficits are selective (e.g., for verbal memory or attention), meta-analyses reveal abnormalities in most aspects of cognition in schizophrenia. The deficits of cognition are present in the early stages of the illness. Cohort studies of subjects, who later develop schizophrenia reveal significant cognitive deficits before the onset of the illness. While schizophrenia as a whole is characterized by cognitive deficits, their severity varies and predicts the level of functioning in the community.

B. Prefrontal Cortex Function

Behavioral, neuroimaging, and electrophysiological studies have shown convincingly that several functions of the prefrontal cortex are impaired in schizophrenia. These include abnormal DLPFC function during the storage of information as well as the retrieval of information from working memory. Abnormal anterior cingulate cortex function is found when inhibiting responses to sensory stimuli. Functional neuroimaging studies using PET and functional magnetic resonance imaging (fMRI) reveal a complex pattern of abnormal DLPFC activation in schizophrenia. While patients show a decreased activation of the DLPFC compared to healthy control subjects (referred to as hypofrontality) during some cognitive tasks, they show normal or increased DLPFC activation on other tasks. Task performance, which is typically lower in schizophrenia, explains some of the variable patterns. When the performance on tasks of DLPFC function is equilibrated between subjects, subjects with schizophrenia typically show an increased pattern activation. This has been interpreted as a sign of decreased cortical efficiency, since greater DLPFC activation (i.e., more activity in the same number of cortical neurons or the same degree of activity in a larger number of neurons) is required for the same level of task performance. Some have speculated that such patterns could be the result of abnormal dopaminergic modulation of cortical neurons, while others have proposed decreased cortical inhibition and impaired cortical synchronization as the cause.

C. HIPPOCAMPAL FUNCTION

Some aspects of hippocampal function during the encoding and retrieval of memory are abnormal in schizophrenia. There are patterns of increased hippocampal activity at baseline and during passive viewing of stimuli, and a decreased ability to modulate hippocampal responses during the retrieval of previously stored information. The impairment of hippocampal function appears to be particularly pronounced when the relationship between previously learned items has to be recalled.

D. SENSORY FUNCTIONS

The reception and integration of sensory information is abnormal in schizophrenia. An extensive electrophysiological literature has documented abnormalities in early sensory processing. These abnormalities involve the thalamic nuclei, the primary sensory cortices, and the multimodal cortices.

E. OTHER FUNCTIONS

Several other brain regions, including thalamus, basal ganglia, and cerebellum have been shown to be impaired during the performance of cognitive tasks in schizophrenia.

Davis KL, Stewart DG, Friedman JI, et al.: White matter changes in schizophrenia: Evidence for myelin-related dysfunction. *Arch Gen Psychiatry* 2003;60:443–456.

Lewis DA, Lieberman JA: Catching up on schizophrenia: Natural history and neurobiology. *Neuron* 2000;28:325–334.

Sim K, Cullen T, Ongur D, Heckers S: Testing models of thalamic dysfunction in schizophrenia using neuroimaging. *J Neural Transm* 2006;113:907–928.

Wright IC, Rabe-Hesketh S, Woodruff PW, David AS, Murray RM, Bullmore ET: Meta-analysis of regional brain volumes in schizophrenia. *Am J Psychiatry* 2000;157:16–25.

Table 16–1. Lifetime Expectancy (Morbid Risk) Estimates of Schizophrenia

	Lifetime Expectancy (%)
If no relative has schizophrenia	1
If the following relative has schizophrenia:	
One Parent	10
Both Parents	46
Sibling	10
Child	6
For twin if cotwin has schizophrenia:	Proband-wise concordance (%)
Dizygotic twin	14
Monozygotic twin	46

Genetic Hypothesis

It has been known for many years that the risk of schizophrenia is increased if another family member is affected (Table 16–1). Family, twin, and adoption studies of schizophrenia have revealed a high degree of heritability, approximately 80%. Heritability is the proportion of phenotypic variance accounted for by genetic effects. It refers to variance in the population and does not translate into a straightforward risk assessment for an individual. Furthermore, high heritability does not exclude a role for nongenetic factors. This is evidenced by the fact that, despite the high heritability of schizophrenia, the concordance rate in monozygotic twins is only 50%, pointing to the importance of environmental factors. Taken together, there is convincing evidence that a combination of risk genes contributes to the development of schizophrenia. However, it is also apparent that schizophrenia is not completely determined by genes (as in an autosomal dominant condition with full penetrance, such as Huntington disease).

The exact genetic mechanism of schizophrenia remains elusive. The introduction of molecular biological techniques has resulted in many reports of linkages between the diagnosis of schizophrenia and polymorphisms in the human genome. However, linkage to particular chromosomal regions has been hard to confirm in independent replication studies, most likely due to a combination of small genetic effects, inadequate sample sizes, and the use of marker maps of insufficient density. Two recent meta-analyses have attempted to overcome the issue of limited power in individual studies. Both analyses provided support for the existence of susceptibility genes

Table 16–2. Risk Genes for Schizophrenia

Gene	Abbreviation	Locus
Neuregulin	NRG1	NRG1-p21
Dysbindin	DTNBP1	6p22
G72	G72	13q34
D-Amino acid oxidase	DAAO	12q24
RGS4	RGS4	1q21–22
Catechol-O-methyl transferase	COMT	22q11
Proline dehydrogenase	PRODH	22q11

on chromosomes 8p and 22q, but they differed with regard to specific regions on chromosomes 1q, 3p, 5q, 6p, 11q, 13q, 14p, and 20q.

Recently, the detailed mapping of chromosomal regions has led to the identification of several genes that are being examined (Table 16–2). Several genes code for proteins known to affect pathways relevant to schizophrenia. For example, the newly found protein neuregulin 1 (NRG1), which is coded for by gene G72 on chromosome 13q34, and the enzyme D-amino acid oxidase (DAAO) are all in a position to affect glutamatergic neurotransmission. On the other hand, a mutation in the gene coding for catechol-O-methyl transferase (COMT), the catabolic enzyme of dopamine, is associated with impaired brain function in schizophrenia. Thus, there is now compelling evidence for specific risk genes for schizophrenia. This could lead to a better understanding of disease mechanisms and the identification of targets for drug development.

Owen MJ, Craddock N, O'Donovan MC: Schizophrenia: Genes at last? *Trends Genet* 2005;21:518–525.

A. GENETICS

There is clear evidence that genetic factors influence the risk of developing schizophrenia.

The concordance rate in monozygotic twins, about 48%, is nearly three times that in dizygotic twins. Higher estimates of disease heritability range from 60% to 85%. The concordance rate for children of two schizophrenic parents is nearly that for monozygotic twins (Table 16–1), and the odds of being diagnosed with schizophrenia decline precipitously the greater the distance from a proband case. A more detailed discussion of genetic factors is provided later (see section "Etiology").

Genetic profile is responsible, on the other hand, for only about 50–70% of the risk for developing schizophrenia; thus, environmental (nongenetic) factors are involved in the development of the disorder. The **stress–diathesis model** posits that a biological predisposition toward developing schizophrenia is inherited genetically, and that this vulnerability interacts with environmental challenges, which, together, lead to development of the full syndrome. Several nongenetic factors have been explored, including obstetric, birth and early childhood complications, season of birth (e.g., during spring and early winter months), exposure to infection, drug use, stressful life events and societal modernization. The precise contribution of these and other factors to the overall risk of developing schizophrenia is difficult to assess, given the heterogeneity of the disorder, its course, and the wide variety of exposures that individuals with the disorder encounter.

Bromet EJ, Fennig S: Epidemiology and natural history of schizophrenia. *Biol Psychiatry* 1999;46:871.

Brown S, Inskip H, Barraclough B: Causes of excess mortality of schizophrenia. *Br J Psychiatry* 2000;177:212.

Haefner H, An der Heiden W: Epidemiology of schizophrenia. *Can J Psychiatry* 1997;42:139.

Jablensky A: Epidemiology of schizophrenia: A global burden of disease and disability. *Eur Arch Psychiatry Clin Neurosci* 2000;250:274.

Jones P, Cannon M: The new epidemiology of schizophrenia. *Psychiatr Clin North Am* 1998;21:1.

McGrath JJ: Myths and plain truths about schizophrenia epidemiology: The NAPE lecture 2004. *Acta Psychiatr Scand* 2005;111:4–11.

Mortensen PB, et al.: Effects of family history and place and season of birth on the risk of schizophrenia. *N Engl J Med* 1999;340:603.

Saha S, et al.: A systematic review of the prevalence of schizophrenia. *PLoS Med* 2005;2:413.

Tsuang MT, Tohen M (eds): *Textbook in Psychiatric Epidemiology,* 2nd edn. New York, NY: Wiley-Liss, 2002.

Clinical Findings

The *Diagnostic and Statistical Manual of Mental Disorders,* fourth edn, Text Revision (DSM-IV-TR) (see "DSM-IV-TR Diagnostic Criteria for Schizophrenia" box) requires at least two of five types of positive and negative symptoms (Criterion A). The four positive symptoms (Criteria A1–A4)—delusions, hallucinations, disorganized speech, and grossly disorganized or catatonic behavior—are considered psychotic symptoms, in that these behaviors, beliefs, and precepts are not considered consistent with normal human experience.

A. SIGNS & SYMPTOMS

1. Delusions—Delusions are defined by the DSM-IV-TR as "fixed, false beliefs that are not widely held within the context of the individual's cultural or religious group," that persist despite contradictory evidence or dysfunction clearly linked to the belief. Most often, delusions have the

Table 16–3. Common Types of Delusions

Delusions of control: Belief that one's thoughts, feelings, or actions are being controlled or actively manipulated by outside forces or agencies.
Delusions of grandiosity: Belief that one has extraordinary powers, gifts, or abilities that are clearly exaggerated and often bizarre.
Delusions of guilt: Belief that one has committed a terrible act or crime. Often, there is also the belief that transgressions will lead to impossibly terrible outcomes, and that they are deserving of punishment.
Delusions of reference: Belief that actions or remarks of others, or external events, have a significant personal and often private meaning for the patient.
Persecutory delusions: Belief that one is being conspired against or threatened by others, including but not limited to individuals, organizations (such as the FBI), religious figures, or extraterrestrials.
Somatic delusions: Belief that one is carrying a severe disease or other malfunction not supported by medical evidence, and are often bizarre and attributed to outside forces.
Thought insertion, withdrawal, or broadcasting: Belief that one's own thoughts have been implanted by an outside agency (insertion), that one's thoughts have been taken out of their mind (withdrawal) or can be read or heard by others via telepathy or other passive means (broadcasting).

form of distorted and highly illogical misinterpretations of actual events or experiences (**errors of inference**). In the clinical setting, it can sometimes be difficult to determine if a patient's conviction is so distorted, illogical and impermeable as to be considered delusional. It is helpful to garner as much detail as possible from the patient about their belief(s) in order to uncover errors of inference. Suggesting rational explanations for a patient's belief may elicit a willingness to consider alternatives (less consistent with delusional thought). On the other hand, it may demonstrate that the patient is unwilling or incapable of doing so (more consistent with delusional thought, especially if the belief clearly leads to dysfunctional behavior). Common delusional themes are exemplified in Table 16–3.

2. Hallucinations—Hallucinations are typically prominent, occurring several times a day. They usually appear in the form of one or more voices that keep a running commentary on the patient's everyday activities. They occasionally are unfriendly, insulting, or accusatory. Hallucinations are usually associated with delusions and are consistent with delusional themes. On occasion, voices command patients to perform acts that could result in harm to themselves or others (**command auditory hallucinations**). Only rarely do patients carry out the commands; however, command auditory hallucinations increase risk of suicidal and violent behaviors. Although patients with schizophrenia can experience visual, olfactory, gustatory, somatosensory, viscerosensory, or tactile hallucinations, these types of hallucinatory activity should raise the suspicion of a general medical cause (Table 16–4). The same may generally be said for single auditory hallucinations that

occur in the context of cognitive dysfunction and altered sensorium, or in the absence of delusion.

3. Disorganized speech & behavior—Examples of **disorganized speech** (Criterion A3) **and behavior** (Criterion A4) are many, as summarized in Table 16–5. In general, disorganized speech is believed to reflect an underlying impairment in thought processes—that is, the inability to process stimuli accurately and link thoughts or ideas in a coherent and logical manner. Alternatively referred to as **thought disorder**, these clinical signs are believed by many to be the cardinal feature of schizophrenia, and to be more closely associated with functional disability than positive symptoms are. As is the case with speech, for a behavior to be considered disorganized, it must result in significant impairment and be obvious to casual observers. Organized behaviors that occur in response to delusions are not considered to be "disorganized." **Catatonic behaviors** (Table 16–6) are found in other mental disorders, medical conditions, and drug toxicity. They warrant immediate medical evaluation if new in onset.

4. Negative symptoms—The fifth group of symptoms (Criterion A5) are referred to as **negative symptoms** because they represent deficits of normal function and are not psychotic, per se (Table 16–7). It is generally accepted that there are **primary and secondary negative symptoms**, the former of which represent longstanding illness features that persist between psychotic episodes and may even predate the onset of psychotic symptoms. Primary negative symptoms tend to respond less well to drug treatment and cause more dysfunction than positive symptoms. Secondary negative symptoms are believed to stem from side effects of medication, depression or

Table 16–4. Characteristics of Psychiatric Presentations that Raise Suspicion of Organic Etiology*

Atypical age at first symptom onset

Atypical symptom presentation (e.g., does not conform to descriptive diagnostic criteria)

Fluctuations in sensorium

Rapid onset cognitive impairment

Abnormal vital signs

History of chronic general medical problems of use of substances that cause psychotic symptoms

Recent deterioration or change in physical health status coincident with onset of psychotic symptoms

History of significant polypharmacy, including use of over-the-counter preparations

Abnormal body habitus, neurological examination

Absence of personal or family history of psychiatric illness

Atypical or absence of response to established treatment(s)

*No single factor alone can establish an organic cause for psychiatric symptoms. A thorough evaluation taking into account history from the patient and collateral informants, available medical records, physical and neurological examination, appropriate laboratory and neurodiagnostics, and clinical observation is required.

Table 16–5. Disorganized/Catatonic Speech and Behavior

SPEECH

Circumstantiality: Speech that is goal directed but excessive in unneeded detail. Questions are eventually answered; however, direct answers are difficult to come by.

Tangentiality: Speech that begins in a goal directed manner, but deviates gradually and consistently such that answers to questions are not reached. New topics arise from the topic previously under discussion, so an association between thoughts can be appreciated.

Derailment: Speech that begins in a goal directed manner, but topics shift rapidly between sentences with no logical connection to the topic previously under discussion.

Illogicality: Speech that is goal directed but gives illogical responses to logical questions, or bases assertions on premises that have no logical or coherent basis.

Concrete speech: Speech that reflects an inability to use abstract thinking, which may bring about literal interpretations of proverbs during mental status examination, or a pattern of speech that conveys little to no information due to use of excessively vague or meaningless phrases (**verbigeration**).

Incoherence: Incomprehensible speech due to loss of logical connections between words, phrases and sentences, the extreme form of which is termed **word salad.**

Clanging: Words are used based on how they sound rather than what they mean.

Neologism: Use of nonsensical words, often as a combination of parts of two or more different words.

Thought blocking: Sudden and involuntary interruption in the progress of speech or thought.

BEHAVIOR

Unprovoked outbursts of laughter or other emotions

Unprovoked outbursts of hyperactive, agitated, or violent behavior

Inappropriate social behaviors

Severe neglect of hygiene or bizarreness of choice in clothing and general appearance

Table 16–6. Selected Catatonic Signs

Psychomotor Signs
Excitement: Extreme but purposeless hyperactivity
Stupor: Extreme hypoactivity or immobility with little if any responsiveness to external stimuli
Staring
Maintaining postures for long periods without reacting
Maintaining odd facial expressions (several seconds to several minutes)
Echopraxia
Stereotypies: Repetitive but purposeless (non-goal-directed) activity
Rigidity
Mannerisms: Purposeful movements executed in an odd or exaggerated manner
Negativism: Purposeless resistance to instructions or efforts at being moved
Waxy flexibility
Refusal to eat, drink, and/or make eye contact
Sudden and inappropriate behaviors, with no apparent provocation (including combativeness)
Perseveration: Repeatedly returns to same movement or motor activity
Speech
Mutism: Absent or minimal verbal responses
Echolalia
Verbigeration: Aimless repetition of phrases or sentences
Perseveration: Repeatedly returns to same topic
Other
Primitive reflexes
Autonomic hyperactivity

demoralization associated with the illness, or as a reaction to psychotic symptoms. Secondary negative symptoms may not persist and can respond to treatment of the underlying cause.

5. Diagnostic threshold—While the diagnostic threshold put forth by the DSM-IV-TR generally calls for two or more symptoms from Criteria A1–A5, there are three exceptions. The diagnosis of schizophrenia can be made on the basis of presence of only **bizarre delusions** (i.e., completely implausible beliefs), or the auditory hallucination of a voice keeping a running commentary on the subject's daily activities, or two or more voices conversing with each other.

Table 16–7. Negative Symptoms of Schizophrenia

Affective flattening: Absence of outward emotional reaction to stimuli. There is a decrease in or absence of spontaneous movement, expressive gestures, eye contact, shifts in vocal inflections
Avolition: Lack of motivation for initiating or completing tasks, reflective of a loss of drive and of interest in one's surroundings
Alogia: Decrease in the production and fluency of spontaneous speech (but not refusal to speak), which is believed to reflect poverty of thought. Abnormalities may also include prolonged pauses before answering questions
Anhedonia: Diminished or absent capacity to experience pleasure
Attention deficits: Inability to maintain engagement in a goal directed activity or task
Social withdrawal, diminished capacity to feel close to others

Table 16–8. DSM-IV-TR Subtypes of Schizophrenia

Subtype	
Paranoid	Prominent persecutory or grandiose delusions or auditory hallucinations. Cognition remains relatively well intact. Negative symptoms, disorganized speech/behavior, and catatonic symptoms are absent relative to hallucinations or delusions. The most common form of the illness, and has a more favorable prognosis than catatonic, undifferentiated and disorganized types.
Disorganized	Disorganized speech, disorganized behavior, and flat or inappropriate affect are all present, and are the most prominent features of the illness. Absence of systematized delusions. Criteria for catatonic subtype are not met.
Catatonic	A minimum of two of the following groups of symptoms: (a) Catalepsy, waxy flexibility, or catatonic stupor; (b) Catatonic excitement; (c) Extreme negativism, or mutism; (d) Catatonic posturing, stereotypies, odd mannerisms or grimacing; (c) Echolalia or echopraxia. Considered rare. Prognosis nearly as good as for paranoid subtype.
Undifferentiated	Second most common of the illness. Symptoms that meet Criterion A are present, but do not satisfy criteria for paranoid, disorganized, or catatonic subtypes. Intermediate prognosis (better than disorganized subtype, but less favorable than paranoid or catatonic subtypes).
Residual	Some attenuated but persisting symptoms left after partial or near resolution of hallucinations, delusions, disorganized speech, or grossly disorganized or catatonic behavior.

Even though the above symptoms are not necessarily present in all schizophrenic patients, many patients express all of these symptoms at one time or another. The clinical manifestations of the illness as described above can vary greatly in intensity over time in a particular patient. The DSM-IV-TR requires that the symptoms result in significant **functional impairment** in work, relationships, self-care, or other life domains. The symptoms must be present in one form or another (e.g., prodromal or residual symptoms) for a period of 6 months or greater, but with at least 1 month of fully expressed, active symptoms as described in Criterion A. The signs and symptoms should not be better accounted for by another psychiatric disorder, general medical illnesses or the effects of substances (see section "Differential diagnosis" below).

6. Subtyping in schizophrenia—Considerable effort has been made to sort through the heterogeneous clinical presentations of schizophrenia and identify homogenous groups that share characteristic symptoms, course, prognosis, and patterns of response to treatment. The DSM-IV-TR describes five such subtypes (Table 16–8). These subtypes were intended for use as a hierarchical system based on the most recent examination of the patient. Under this scheme, the **catatonic type** is considered first and is diagnosed as long as the criteria in Table 16–6 are met,

even in the presence of prominent positive symptoms. If these criteria are unmet, the **disorganized type** is considered next, and is diagnosed if all three criteria in Table 16–6 are met, again regardless of positive-symptom load. Therefore, the **paranoid type** can be diagnosed only if the criteria for the first two are not met. The **undifferentiated type** is left for cases that manifest disorganization in combination with delusions and/or hallucinations but do not fit neatly into one of the above categories, while the **residual type** is reserved for cases in which delusions, hallucinations, disorganization and/or catatonic behaviors are no longer prominent, but persist in an attenuated or less severe form.

7. Other clinical features—Mild neurologic deficits are often present in schizophrenia: Abnormal body movements, gait, mannerisms, or reflexes; increased or decreased muscle tone; abnormal rapid eye movements (saccades); frequent blinking; dysdiadochokinesia; astereognosis; and poor right–left discrimination.

Cognitive dysfunction is a cardinal feature of schizophrenia. On average, the intelligence quotient (IQ) of schizophrenic patients, when first diagnosed with the disorder, is 10 points lower than comparison groups, including unaffected siblings or co-twins. Children at risk of schizophrenia have lower IQs than do control subjects with abnormalities in attention and concentration.

Patients in their first episode of schizophrenia exhibit impairments in attention, working memory, visual–spatial memory, semantic memory, recall memory, and executive function.

The diverse nature of the cognitive disturbance in schizophrenia suggests that the disturbance is based on diffuse rather than localized brain disease. With treatment, that impairment might improve slightly, but there is little evidence that antipsychotic drugs, with the exception of clozapine, have a significant effect on the cognitive disturbance in schizophrenia. Cognitive impairment is often independent of positive and negative symptoms and even of disorganization. Over the course of the illness, a small percentage of schizophrenic patients experience a great deterioration in cognition and reach the levels of impairment of patients with senile psychosis, such as Alzheimer's disease. The majority of schizophrenic patients do not exhibit such marked dilapidation of cognitive function. Cognitive disturbance plays a major role in limiting the social life and occupational performance of schizophrenic patients. For this reason, therapies that reverse cognitive disturbance in schizophrenia will be of immense value.

American Psychiatric Association: *Diagnostic and Statistical Manual of Mental Disorders*, 4th edn, Washington, DC: Text Revision (DSM-IV-TR). American Psychiatric Association, 2000.

Frances A, First MB, Pincus HA (eds): *DSM-IV Guidebook*. Washington, DC: American Psychiatric Press, 1995.

B. PSYCHOLOGICAL TESTING

The presence of significant cognitive abnormalities in schizophrenic patients warrants the use of **neuropsychological testing** to establish evidence of brain disorder early during the diagnosis of the disease, or to establish a cognitive pretreatment baseline. Formal neuropsychological assessment using objective tests, such as the Halstead-Reitan Battery, the Luria-Nebraska Battery, the Wechsler Adult Intelligence Scale, the Wechsler Intelligence Scale for Children, and the Wisconsin Card Sorting Test (WCST), can identify various abnormalities involving the frontotemporal areas of the brain. The usefulness of **projective** and **personality tests** in the diagnosis of schizophrenia may be limited because, although these tests identify bizarre ideations and abnormal personality traits, respectively, they are prone to unreliable, subjective interpretation.

Lesak MD, Howieson DB, Loring DW (eds): *Neuropsychological Assessment*. Oxford, 2004.

C. LABORATORY & NEUROIMAGING FINDINGS

No laboratory or neuroimaging findings are considered pathognomonic for schizophrenia. The utility of these investigations is therefore limited to the ruling out of nonpsychiatric etiologies for psychotic presentations (discussed later). Some findings have been replicated and have shed light on neuropathological processes that may eventually be found to characterize schizophrenia.

1. Cerebral ventricular enlargement—Despite the large body of supportive imaging studies, ventricular enlargement is not present in all patients with schizophrenia and is not specific for schizophrenia. For example, ventricular enlargement and increased sulcal prominence can also be observed in patients with mood disorders.

2. Structural and functional brain abnormalities—A number of brain abnormalities have been identified with neuroimaging (reviewed above). However, none of the findings reported so far have achieved the status of a diagnostic test. There is an emerging literature on the longitudinal aspects of brain changes in schizophrenia. Such studies will be helpful to better understand the differences in disease outcome and treatment response.

Course of Illness

A. ONSET & NATURAL COURSE

1. Onset—The **onset** of the disorder is quite variable. Classically, the onset is gradual, with a **prodromal** phase of varying duration that predates the first psychotic break. The prodromal phase is generally considered the first of **three phases** of schizophrenia (prodromal, active, and residual phases). During this time, patients may evidence gradually increasing social withdrawal, poor motivation, restricted affective range, cognitive difficulties, and increasingly odd behavior. These changes are subthreshold for a diagnosis of schizophrenia. For others, the onset can be quite rapid, evolving over a period of weeks.

2. Course—**Active phase** symptoms emerge following the prodrome (referred to as a "first psychotic break") often in the context of significant life stress or substance use. Treatment may begin after a variable period of time, referred to as the **duration of untreated psychosis**. There is considerable evidence that the longer the duration of untreated psychosis, the poorer the response to treatment, though not all studies are in agreement. After initiation of treatment, pooled data analysis suggests that about one third of patients with first-break schizophrenia have a benign **illness course** (i.e., they fully or nearly fully recover, with minimal or no impairment), while the remainder have either an intermediate or poor outcome.

The **residual phase** is characterized by persisting schizophrenic symptoms. Of the two thirds of patients who do not achieve full or nearly full recovery during active phase treatment, approximately half experience a stable course without further deterioration, but significant residual deficits remain. The remaining group of patients with poor treatment outcome often exhibit progressive deterioration. Thus, the level of psychopathology and impairment during the residual phase can vary considerably. In general, the more incomplete the symptom recovery, the more likely the patient is to function poorly and relapse in the future. Relative to positive symptoms, negative symptoms are less responsive to medication.

3. Late- and very-late-onset disease—Most older patients with schizophrenia have had an onset of illness during early adulthood (**early-onset** schizophrenia); however, about 20% of patients manifest psychotic symptoms for the first time during middle (**late-onset,** after age 45 years) or old age (**very-late-onset,** after age 65 years). In general, the clinical symptoms of early- and late-onset schizophrenia are similar, though some important differences characterize late-onset illness. These include higher prevalence among women, less severe negative symptoms and cognitive impairment, the predominance of paranoid delusions, and lower dose requirement for antipsychotic medication.

Hafner H, an der Heiden W: Epidemiology of schizophrenia. *Can J Psychiatry* 1997;42:139.

Harrison G, Hopper K, Craig T, et al.: Recovery from psychotic illness: A 15- and 25-year international follow-up study. *Br J Psychiatry* 2001;178:506.

Howard R, Rabins PV, Seeman MV, et al.: Late-onset schizophrenia and very-late-onset schizophrenia-like psychosis: An international consensus. *Am J Psychiatry* 2000;157:172.

Perkins DO, Gu H, Boteva K, Lieberman JA: Relationship between duration of untreated psychosis and outcome in first-episode schizophrenia: A critical review and meta-analysis. *Am J Psychiatry* 2005;162:1785.

Differential Diagnosis

A detailed workup, often in the context of the safety and structure afforded by psychiatric hospitalization, is necessary, especially at the first onset of psychotic symptoms. Serial patient interviews and additional history from collateral sources (e.g., prior medical records, collateral informants) are required.

A. ORGANIC ETIOLOGIES OF PSYCHOTIC SYMPTOMS

Most reversible secondary causes of psychosis (Table 16–9) can be ruled out on the basis of a meticulous history, mental status examination, physical and neurological examination and appropriate laboratory and neurodiagnostic testing (Table 16–10). Some general clinical guidelines can be applied to the raising of suspicion of an organic etiology for psychotic symptoms (Table 16–11). They must always be followed by adequate clinical assessment.

Table 16–9. Selected Secondary Causes of Psychotic Symptoms

CNS infections
Viral
Herpes, Mumps, Mononucleosis
Bacteria
Syphilis
Parasitic
Schistosomiasis, trypanosomiasis
Substance related
Medications
Anticholinergic drugs
Prodopaminergic agents
Antimalarials
Antiparkinson drugs
Antihypertensives
Antituberculous agents
Over-the-counter stimulants (ephedrine, phenylephrine, pseudoephedrine)
Methylphenidate, psychostimulants
Corticosteroids
Certain antiarrhythmics (digitalis, procainamide)
Agents of abuse
Hallucinogens
Cannabis
Psychostimulants
Dissociative anesthetics (phencyclidine, ketamine, dextromethorphan)
Withdrawal states (alcohol, sedative–hypnotic, psychostimulant)
Acute cardiovascular
Anoxia, any cause
Metabolic
Hypoglycemia, hyponatremia, hypercalcemia
Hepatic or uremic encephalopathy, postdialysis state
Porphyria
Postoperative state
Traumatic brain injury
Other CNS pathology
Demyelinating (e.g., multiple sclerosis)

Table 16–9. (continued)

Primary dementing disorders
Alzheimer disease, Pick disease,
Dementia with Lewy bodies
Epilepsy
Cerebrovascular disease
Space occupying lesions
Malignancy, abscesses
Endocrine
Hypo- or hyperthyroidism
Hypo- or hyperadrenalism
Hypo- or hyperparathyroidism
Postpartum psychosis
Connective tissue disorders
Systemic lupus erythematosus, temporal arteritis Sarcoidosis
Toxicological (drug overdose, heavy metal poisoning)
Nutritional
Deficiency in thiamine, vitamin B12, folate, niacin

Table 16–10. Suggested Diagnostic Workup for First-Break Psychotic Symptoms

Serial (repeated) histories from patient and collateral informants
Thorough review of all available medical records
Complete physical and neurological examinations
Routine laboratory tests
Electrolytes, blood urea nitrogen (BUN), creatinine
Glucose
Complete blood count, with differential
Thyroid panel
Liver function tests
Syphilis screening (VDRL, etc.)
Vitamin B12, folate levels
HIV screen (if indicated)
Urine drug/toxicology screen, blood alcohol level
Routine urinalysis
Other laboratory tests to consider
Pregnancy test
Serum drug levels
Lumbar puncture for CSF analysis
Coagulation studies
Radiographic tests to consider
Indications for cranial CT or MRI
Previously unevaluated psychotic symptoms
New onset cognitive deficits
Atypical psychotic presentation
Nonauditory hallucinations
Rapid onset
Onset age > 50 years
Altered/fluctuating sensorium
Focal neurological deficits or soft signs
History of recent head injury
Electroconvulsive therapy being considered
Chest X-ray (geriatric patients)
Electroencephalogram (as clinical situation warrants)

B. PSYCHIATRIC DISORDERS THAT PRESENT WITH PSYCHOTIC (OR PSYCHOTIC-LIKE) SYMPTOMS

1. Other psychotic disorders—In differentiating between schizophrenia and other psychotic disorders, the duration of symptoms must be accurately assessed. **Schizophreniform disorder** involves prodromal, active-phase and residual symptoms identical to schizophrenia, but the total duration of illness is less than 6 months before full recovery. It should be noted, however, that while about one third of patients fully recover within 6 months and retain a diagnosis of schizophreniform disorder, two thirds eventually progress to schizophrenia or schizoaffective disorder. With **brief psychotic disorder**, psychotic symptoms endure for less than 1 month before full recovery. **Delusional disorder** is distinguished by its later age of onset (35–50 years) and the persistence of nonbizarre delusions in absence of hallucinations, disorganized thoughts or behaviors, and negative symptoms. Patients with delusional disorder do not typically manifest the degree of functional incapacity observed among patients with schizophrenia, and do not experience significant changes in cognition. Therefore, delusional disorder is a very difficult diagnosis to recognize in the clinical setting.

2. Mood disorders with psychotic features—In distinguishing between **mood disorders (bipolar I disorder and major depression)** with psychotic features, **schizoaffective disorders (bipolar or depressed subtype)** and schizophrenia, it is helpful to determine whether the mood and psychotic symptoms occurred simultaneously, whether the psychotic symptoms

Table 16–11. Drugs Used in the Treatment of Schizophrenia

Generic Name	Recommended Dose Range (mg/d)	Chlorpromazine Equivalents (mg/d)	Adverse Effects EPS	Tardive Dyskinesia	Prolactin Elevation	Sedation	Weight Gain	Orthostasis	Anticholinergic	Diabetes Exacerbation and Dyslipidemia
TYPICAL ANTIPSYCHOTIC DRUGS										
Chlorpromazine	300–1000	100	Some (for low-potency drugs) – +++ (for high-potency drugs)	++ – +++	++ – +++ (risk higher for high-potency drugs)	Some (for high-potency drugs) – +++ (for low-potency drugs); possibly least for molindone	Some (for high-potency drugs) – +++ (for low-potency drugs); possibly least for molindone	Some (for high-potency drugs) – +++ (for low-potency drugs)	Some (for high-potency drugs) – +++ (for low-potency drugs)	+ – ++
Fluphenazine*	5–20	2								
Haloperidol*	5–20	2								
Loxapine	30–100	10								
Mesoridazine	150–400	50								
Molindone	30–100	10								
Perphenazine	16–64	10								
Thioridazine	300–800	100								
Thiothixene	15–50	5								
Trifluoperazine	15–50	5								
ATYPICAL ANTIPSYCHOTIC DRUGS										
Aripiprazole	10–30		0 – +	0 – +	0	0 – +	0 – +	+ – ++	0	0
Clozapine	150–600		0	0	Transient	+++	+++	+++	+++	+++
Olanzapine	10–30		0 – + (if >10 mg/d)	Rare	+ (if >20 mg/d)	++	+++	+	+	+++
Quetiapine	300–800		0	Rare	0	++	+ – ++	++	0 – +	++
Risperidone*	2–8		+ (less if >4 mg/d)	Rare	+++	+	+ – ++	++	0	+
Ziprasidone	120–200		0 – +	Rare	0 – +	0 – ++	0	+ – ++	0	0

*Also available in long-acting injectable preparations.

Adapted with permission from the International Psychopharmacology Algorithm Project (IPAP) algorithm for the treatment of schizophrenia, available at www.ipap.org.

277

persisted at any point independent of mood symptoms, and whether the mood symptoms were brief relative to the total period of the disturbance. In mood disorder with psychotic features and schizoaffective disorder, psychotic symptoms occur at the same time as mood symptoms; however, in schizoaffective disorder, psychotic symptoms exist independently of mood changes for at least 2 weeks (and often longer). For mood disorders with psychotic features, psychotic symptoms do not persist apart from mood dysfunction. Another important distinction between mood disorder and schizophrenia is that, after resolution of acute mood and psychotic symptoms, there is a return to normal functioning. Schizophrenic patients rarely return to baseline functioning, and each subsequent psychotic relapse may result in progressive dilapidation.

3. Personality disorders—Individuals with personality disorders may be suspicious and hypervigilant (**paranoid personality disorder**), with marked eccentricities of appearance and behavior, perceptual distortions and diminished capacity for close relationships (**schizotypal personality disorder**). They may evidence an incapacity for relationships of any kind and extreme isolativeness (**schizoid personality disorder**). Individuals with cluster-disorders and those with **borderline personality disorder** are prone to severe stress-induced paranoia, which may be difficult to distinguish from a primary psychotic disturbance on the basis of only one clinical encounter. However, personality disorders have mild relative symptoms compared to those observed among schizophrenics, and the symptoms have been present throughout the patient's lifetime. None with personality disorder present with prominent hallucinations or frank delusions. They also lack chronic negative symptoms or disorganization.

4. Anxiety disorders—Patients with **posttraumatic stress disorder (PTSD)** are prone to severe hallucinatory-like symptoms and fearful (paranoid) behavior; however, patients with PTSD usually retain insight in to the nature of their disturbances, which are inextricably linked to exposure to past traumatic event(s). Insight is typically preserved in **obsessive–compulsive disorder (OCD)**, even though uncontrollable intrusive thoughts and compulsive mental or physical rituals can mimic psychosis. A rare subtype of OCD is characterized by poor insight; however, these disorders do not feature negative or disorganization symptoms and are not associated with the same degree of functional incapacity as the typical patient with schizophrenia.

5. Other disorders—Patients with **hypochondriasis** or **body dysmorphic disorder** are convinced of the presence of an occult disease or bodily defect in absence of objective evidence to support their belief(s).

The absence of hallucinations and disorganization symptoms, and exclusively somatically circumscribed preoccupations, quickly distinguish these disorders from schizophrenia.

C. Differential Diagnosis of Negative Symptoms

The workup of a patient who presents with prominent negative symptoms must be especially thorough. Many conditions, some very serious, can mimic the negative symptoms of schizophrenia. These include malignant catatonia, delirium, frontal lobe injury, intracranial space occupying lesions (e.g., tumors, etc.), substance abuse, hypothyroidism, severe depression, bipolar mania (catatonic presentation), parkinsonism (idiopathic or neuroleptic-induced), and neuroleptic-induced akinesia.

American Psychiatric Association: *Diagnostic and Statistical Manual of Mental Disorders*, 4th edn. Washington, DC: Text Revision (DSM-IV-TR). American Psychiatric Association, 2000.

Goff DC, Freudenreich O, Henderson DC: Psychotic patients. In: Stern TA, Fricchione GL, Cassem NH, Jellinek MS, Rosenbaum JL (eds). *Handbook of General Hospital Psychiatry*. Philadelphia, PA: Mosby, 2004, pp. 37–48.

Marsh CM: Psychiatric presentations of medical illness. *Psychiatr Clin North Am* 1997;20:181.

Whiteford HA, Peabody CA: The differential diagnosis of negative symptoms in chronic schizophrenia. *Aust N Z J Psychiatry* 1989;23:491.

Schooler NR: Deficit symptoms in schizophrenia: Negative symptoms versus neuroleptic-induced deficits. *Acta Psychiatr Scand Suppl* 1994;380:21.

Siris SG: Depression in schizophrenia: Perspective in the era of "Atypical" antipsychotic agents. *Am J Psychiatry* 2000;157:1379.

Treatment

The modern treatment of schizophrenia has as its **goals** the reduction of symptomatology and the maximization of functioning. To achieve this, a number of **treatment targets** have been identified, including (1) positive symptoms, (2) negative symptoms, (3) conceptual disorganization, (4) neurocognitive deficits, and (5) anxious/depressive symptoms and suicidality. The situation is more complicated in cases of comorbid substance abuse or severe physical morbidity, both of which are common in community mental health settings. A number of treatment modalities—both pharmacological and nonpharmacological—must therefore be utilized.

As a general rule, **positive symptoms** such as hallucinations and delusions, as well as **disorganized speech and behavior** and psychotic **agitation**, all respond very well to antipsychotic drug treatment. Though dramatic in appearance and distressing and potentially dangerous to the patient and others, the severity of positive symptoms does not appear to correlate significantly with long-term functioning.

By contrast, **negative symptoms** such as anhedonia, affective flattening, alogia, avolition, and social withdrawal are far more difficult to treat pharmacologically, and are robust predictors of long-term functional incapacity. Older generation ("typical") neuroleptic medications, such as haloperidol and perphenazine, have little impact on these devastating symptoms. On the other hand, the efficacy profile of atypical antipsychotic drugs in treating negative symptoms is more encouraging.

Cognitive function is severely impaired in schizophrenia. Patients demonstrate neuropsychological deficits in a broad array of domains; however, impairments in executive skills, working memory, verbal skills, and learning and memory are especially severe. Cognitive impairment has important consequences for the everyday functioning, and is a critical determinant of capacity for work, social functioning, and independent living. Not surprisingly, cognitive impairment has become an important therapeutic target, based on the rationale that improvements in cognitive function will lead to subsequent improvement in functional status.

An underappreciated phenomenon is the severity and pervasiveness of **depression and anxiety** symptoms associated with schizophrenia. Depression in schizophrenia is very common; however, mood symptoms have only been recently recognized as a core feature of the illness. Depressive symptoms frequently emerge during acute psychotic episodes or shortly after their resolution (i.e., **postpsychotic depression**). Over time, they tend to occur and persist independently of positive symptoms, and may occur at any stage of the illness. By the same token, **suicidal behavior**, though common among schizophrenic patients, has only recently become an independent treatment target.

A. Psychopharmacologic Interventions

Antipsychotic drugs are the treatment of choice for virtually all patients with schizophrenia. There are two broad classes of antipsychotic drugs: The **typical** (a.k.a., "first-generation" or "conventional") antipsychotic drugs and the **atypical** (a.k.a., "second-generation" or "novel") antipsychotics (Table 16–11). What follows is a description of each of these broad classes, followed by guidelines for choosing antipsychotic medications and for their clinical use in treating schizophrenia during the acute phase and long-term treatment.

1. Typical antipsychotic drugs—The discovery of chlorpromazine in 1950 revolutionized the treatment of schizophrenia. It and the other typical drugs have a simple **mechanism of action**: They are direct-acting dopamine D_2-receptor antagonists. Thus, they occupy D_2 receptors in each of the relevant dopamine pathways, including the mesolimbic tract (where excessive dopamine transmission is believed to underlie positive symptoms), mesocortical tract (where deficits in dopamine transmission are thought to cause cognitive dysfunction and negative symptoms), nigrostriatal tract (where D_2 blockade results in extrapyramidal adverse effects, as will be discussed shortly), and the tuberoinfundibular tract (where activation pf D_2 receptors controls pituitary prolactin release). By this one mechanism, typical neuroleptics remedy positive symptoms but coincidentally result in troublesome antidopaminergic adverse effects (EPS, hyperprolactinemia) and either fail to address adequately or even worsen negative symptoms and cognitive dysfunction. This class of agents does not have a useful impact on work capacity and social functioning.

i. Clinical use—In terms of **treatment response**, about 70% of patients with schizophrenia who manifest delusions or hallucinations during some phase of their illness will have a good response of those symptoms to these agents. The **therapeutic lag time** is about 4–6 weeks. For many, an antipsychotic response will be observed sooner, sometimes within the first week of treatment. The other 30% will have moderate to severe positive symptoms despite adequate doses of these agents for at least 6 weeks, which is considered the minimum, adequate **therapeutic trial length**. Evidence suggests that lower **dosages** of typical antipsychotics can bring relief to patients as rapidly and effectively as higher doses and with fewer side effects. For instance, daily dosages of 5–10 mg of haloperidol, or its equivalent (Table 16–11), may be adequate for many, if not most, patients with acute psychosis. First-episode and recent-onset patients almost always respond to lower dosages. Ordinarily, higher dosages should not be tried until at least 4–6 weeks of treatment at the starting dose have been tried. Then, if positive symptoms persist, the dosage may be increased. Plasma levels of antipsychotics and their metabolites vary greatly between patients. The only typical agent with a possible therapeutic window is haloperidol. For haloperidol, a steady-state plasma range of 12–17 ng/L has been associated with optimal antipsychotic action.

ii. Adverse effects—The term **neuroleptic** refers to the neurologic side effects of the typical antipsychotics, such as catalepsy in rodents and **EPS** in humans. These effects occur in the same dosage range as is associated with an antipsychotic effect; therefore, for typical antipsychotics, treatment emergent EPS is a common and significant treatment-limiting factor. The EPS may be divided into acute and delayed effects. The predominant acute effects are **parkinsonism** (coarse resting tremor, bradykinesia, hypertonia, unstable gait), **akathisia** (subjective restlessness and psychomotor agitation), and **dystonic reactions** (sudden-onset, sustained, intense and often painful muscular contraction). The late occurring

Table 16–12. Common Causes of Suboptimal Response to Antipsychotic Treatment in Schizophrenia

Misdiagnosis of schizophrenia
Diagnosis of schizophrenia should be reconfirmed in every instance of suboptimal treatment response
Undiagnosed psychiatric comorbidity
Comorbid substance use disorder(s)
Poor compliance with treatment
Can confirm using plasma levels for haloperidol and clozapine
Inadequate drug dose (see Table 16–10)
400–600 mg/d chlorpromazine equivalents for all typical agents
Target serum level of $\geq$350 ng/L for clozapine
Inadequate trial length
$\geq$4–6 weeks is usually necessary
Possibly longer for clozapine treatment or history of refractory disease
Possibly longer for any agent where negative symptoms are prominent
Intolerable side effects, especially:
EPS, including akathisia and parkinsonism
Sedation
Cognitive dulling (with traditional neuroleptics)
Worsening affective symptoms (with traditional neuroleptics)
Intolerable drug–drug interactions
Poor social support

side effects are **tardive dyskinesia** and **tardive dystonia**. The late occurring effects are sometimes irreversible and, rarely, life threatening. No one with tardive dyskinesia should be treated with a typical neuroleptic now that the atypical antipsychotics are readily available.

As mentioned beforehand, the antipsychotic action and motor side effects of neuroleptics are secondary to their ability to decrease dopaminergic activity due to blockade of D_2 receptors in the mesolimbic and nigrostriatal pathways of the brain, respectively. The affinities that antipsychotic agents have for D_2, 5-HT_{2A}, and muscarinic receptors are key determinants of their liability to cause EPS. These drugs also have variable affinities for other neurotransmitter receptors which have predictable effects on antipsychotic profile (Table 16–12).

These receptors include histamine 1 (H1, antagonism of which may result in sedation and weight gain), alpha-1 (α-1) adrenergic (antagonism of which may result in sedation, orthostatic hypotension, and reflex tachycardia), muscarinic-1 (M1) cholinergic (antagonism of which may result in blurring of vision, dry mouth, urinary retention, constipation, and cognitive dulling) receptors. Hematologic effects, jaundice, cardiac effects (e.g., electrocardiographic changes such as QTc interval prolongation, especially for thioridazine, pimozide, and droperidol), photosensitivity, and retinitis pigmentosa (associated especially with the use of higher doses of thioridazine, which may result in blindness) result from toxic effects on specific target tissues.

iii. Choice of agent:—The choice of typical neuroleptic drug is based on a variety of initial considerations, which include the following:

- side-effect profile,
- past response(s) to antipsychotic drugs,
- the availability of long-acting preparations (e.g., fluphenazine and haloperidol decanoate) required for patients who frequently relapse due to poor medication compliance. In chronically noncompliant patients who are unwilling to take oral medication, biweekly or monthly injections of fluphenazine decanoate or haloperidol decanoate (given at clinics or by visiting nurses) often decrease relapse rates significantly.
- the availability of short-acting injectable or intravenous formulations for use in acute situations (to control agitation and combative behavior) where oral dosing is not feasible, or when the oral route is not available.

Other considerations are based on the side-effect profile. Differences in side-effect profile between low- and high-potency typical neuroleptics are predicted to a great degree by their receptor-binding profiles. For instance, low-potency drugs (e.g., chlorpromazine, thioridazine, mesoridazine), so named because of their relatively lower affinity for D_2 receptors and therefore higher dose requirement for antipsychotic potency (300 mg/d or greater), may result in lower EPS or hyperprolactinemic liability compared to high-potency agents (e.g., haloperidol, fluphenazine). However, low-potency drugs result in more sedation, weight gain, orthostasis, and antimuscarinic effects than high-potency agents do because of their higher affinities for H1, α-1 and M1 receptors. The latter agents produce more EPS than do the low-potency agents (see Table 16–11).

If the patient's history of drug response does not indicate an unusual sensitivity to EPS, high-potency agents such as haloperidol and fluphenazine are preferred to low-potency agents. Thioridazine is believed to have more risk of causing a ventricular arrhythmia than other typical antipsychotic drugs. If EPS develop, anticholinergic agents such as benztropine, diphenhydramine, biperiden, or trihexyphenidyl can be used as a pharmacological adjunct, or the patient can be switched from a high-potency agent to a medium-potency drug (e.g., trifluoperazine) or to a low-potency drug (e.g., thioridazine). A more important strategy for the minimization of EPS is to keep the dose as low as possible (e.g., no more than 5–10 mg/d of haloperidol equivalents), assuming there is a reason why an atypical antipsychotic drug could not be substituted. Persistent EPS, especially akathisia, can contribute to noncompliance or lead to increased agitation or even suicide risk. Thus, in cases of apparently increased agitation and disorganized behavior in the face of ongoing treatment especially with typical antipsychotics, screening for akathisia should always be considered.

2. Atypical antipsychotic drugs—The "atypical" antipsychotic drugs were given this name because they were able to produce an antipsychotic effect at doses which produced little or no EPS (and very few cases of tardive dyskinesia). The prototypical atypical is clozapine, a dibenzodiazepine, which was first identified in 1959. After the hypothesis was advanced that its atypicality was due to a weak D_2-receptor blockade coupled to potent serotonin (5-HT_{2A}) antagonism (**mechanism of action**), a number of other atypical antipsychotic drugs were discovered which shared this mechanism: Risperidone, olanzapine, quetiapine, ziprasidone, and aripiprazole. The latter differs from the others in substituting partial D_2-receptor blockade for D_2-receptor antagonism. Other atypical antipsychotics including asenapine, Iloperidone, laurisdione, paliperidone, and perospirone are in development, and have mechanisms of action similar to clozapine. Bifeprunox has a mechanism similar to that of aripiprazole (partial dopamine D_2-receptor agonism). Besides being a partial D_2 agonist, aripiprazole is also a 5-HT_{2A} antagonist (like most other atypicals) and a 5-HT_{1A}-partial agonist (similar to clozapine, quetiapine and ziprasidone). Bifeprunox is a 5-HT_{1A}-partial agonist and has weak 5-HT_{2A}-antagonist properties.

i. Clozapine—Clozapine was the first antipsychotic drug shown in controlled clinical trials to alleviate both positive and negative symptoms in patients who had failed to respond to adequate trials of typical neuroleptic drugs. In this treatment-resistant group, clozapine treatment results in a clinical response in 30–60% of cases. It produces almost no EPS, akathisia, tardive dyskinesia, or hyperprolactinemia. The onset of a significant response to clozapine in treatment-resistant patients may be delayed for up to 6 months. Primary negative symptoms tend to improve more slowly than do other types of symptoms. The response to clozapine is usually only partial,

but for patients whose symptoms have been virtually nonresponsive to all other therapies, the change can be highly significant.

The remarkable advantages of clozapine (described later in this section) must be balanced against its ability to cause **agranulocytosis**, in 1% of patients. As a result, clozapine has been approved in the United States only for patients with schizophrenia who have failed to respond adequately to typical neuroleptic drugs (**treatment-resistant schizophrenia**) or who are intolerant of typical neuroleptic drugs because of EPS or tardive dyskinesia, or who are at high risk for **suicide**. Poor work function or moderate-to-severe residual negative symptoms are considered a poor response, even if only mild positive symptoms are present.

Clozapine has been shown to reduce depression and suicidality. The latter effect leads to a major decrease in the overall mortality rate associated with schizophrenia, despite the slight increase due to agranulocytosis. Numerous studies have reported that clozapine can improve some aspects of cognitive function, especially verbal fluency, attention, and recall memory. This effect appears to be unrelated to the drug's lack of adverse effect on motor function.

About 40% of patients have positive symptoms that fail to respond adequately to clozapine monotherapy. As previously mentioned, it often takes 6 months and sometimes longer for positive symptoms to be controlled in very treatment-resistant patients. Patience is required. Polypharmacy with other antipsychotic drugs should be avoided, if possible. Only ECT has sometimes been found to be effective as an adjunctive treatment. The effectiveness of adding of mood stabilizers and antidepressants when mood instability or depression is inadequately treated with clozapine has not been studied in a controlled manner. On clinical grounds, trials with various mood stabilizers may be attempted. There is some evidence that lamotrigine and valproate are useful.

Agranulocytosis during clozapine treatment generally occurs within 4–18 weeks after treatment begins, but it can occur rarely at later times. In the United States, white blood cell and absolute neutrophil count (ANC) must be monitored weekly for 6 months, then every 2 weeks for months 7–12, followed by monthly monitoring on an indefinite basis. When the white blood cell count falls below 3000 cells per mm^3, or the ANC below 1500 cells per mm^3, clozapine should be stopped and not restarted. If agranulocytosis has developed, granulocyte colony stimulating factor (G-CSF) or other growth factors can be used to hasten the recovery process. Recovery generally takes 7–14 days. Hospitalization to prevent or treat sepsis is essential. To date, the death rate from clozapine due to agranulocytosis is about 1 per 10,000.

Clozapine can also cause **leukocytosis** and **eosinophilia** in the early stages of treatment. The development of these disorders does not predict later development of agranulocytosis. Other side effects of clozapine include sedation, weight gain, type II diabetes, hyperlipidemia and atherosclerotic heart disease, major motor **seizures**, obsessive–compulsive symptoms or treatment-emergent obsessive–compulsive disorder, hypersalivation, tachycardia, hypotension, hypertension, stuttering, neuroleptic malignant syndrome, urinary incontinence, myocarditis, and constipation. Many of these side effects diminish over time or are responsive to pharmacologic agents and decreased dosage.

The dosage of clozapine ranges from 100 to 900 mg/d for most patients. It must be titrated slowly because of tachycardia and hypotensive side effects, with a starting dosage of 25 mg/d. The average dosage is 400–500 mg/d, usually given twice daily. Plasma levels of 350–400 ng/L are more likely to be associated with clinical response than are lower levels.

Clozapine has a very complex pharmacologic profile. It has a high affinity for serotonergic ($5-HT_{2A,2C,6,7}$), adrenergic ($a_{1,2}$), muscarinic, and histaminergic receptors. Clozapine and related drugs are inverse agonists at $5-HT_{2A}$ and $5-HT_{2C}$ receptors, meaning they can block the constitutive activity of these receptors, (i.e., activation of the receptor that is independent of 5-HT stimulation). The major metabolite of clozapine, *N*-desmethylclozapine is a M1 muscarinic agonist. This mechanism may improve cognitive function and reduce psychosis. No other atypical or a metabolite thereof has M1 muscarinic properties.

ii. Other D_2 and $5-HT_{2A}$ Antagonists—This group of drugs includes **quetiapine, olanzapine, risperidone, and ziprasidone**. As a class, these agents are as effective as the typical antipsychotic drugs with regard to the control of positive symptoms. The recent CATIE study suggested that olanzapine is superior with regard to some outcome measures; however, CATIE permitted olanzapine to be dosed at a higher than the approved dose range which probably enabled it to be more effective in the subset of patients who were treatment resistant. At clinically equivalent doses, there is no reliable evidence that any of these drugs is significantly more efficacious than the others. Anecdotal evidence suggests that ziprasidone causes an activation syndrome earlier and at lower doses than other treatments do. However, controlled clinical trials do not support this. It may be that patients vulnerable to this type of activation are underrepresented in clinical trials.

These drugs differ in side-effect profiles (Table 16–11). Olanzapine, like clozapine, has the greatest likelihood of causing metabolic side effects. Both drugs show relatively high-affinity binding to H1, α-1 and M1 receptors and thus are associated with corresponding adverse effects. Metabolic effects include weight gain and abnormalities in indices of insulin resistance, including increased fasting blood sugar and an atherogenic lipid profile. Some patients develop type II diabetes or diabetic ketoacidosis. In rank order, the other drugs likely to produce these effects are quetiapine and risperidone (moderate risk), and ziprasidone and aripiprazole (lower risk). Both risperidone and ziprasidone are mild, overall, in this regard. Nevertheless, some patients treated with any of these drugs will gain weight or have glucose and lipid changes. Despite the fact that many patients who develop insulin resistance also experience significant weight gain, these two factors are not highly correlated in many patients. Patients who do not gain weight may therefore show other facets of the insulin resistance syndrome and vice versa. Patients should be monitored for increased lipids and fasting blood sugar after the first 3 and 6 months of treatment, and every 6 months thereafter.

Relative to typical neuroleptics, atypical antipsychotic drugs have less treatment-emergent antidopaminergic side effects than typical neuroleptics do. At higher doses (e.g., above 6 mg/d), dose-dependent EPS and hyperprolactinemic effects can be observed with risperidone, however.

The dose of these drugs should be kept as low as possible in non–treatment-resistant patients. First-episode patients and those within the first 5 years of illness usually require the low end of the dose range. All atypical drugs, with the exception of quetiapine, which has a very short half-life, can be given once a day, generally prior to sleep, to minimize daytime sedation, for example, olanzapine, 10–20 mg/d; quetiapine, 200–1000 mg/d; and risperidone, 2–8 mg/d. Polypharmacy with two antipsychotic drugs should be avoided. If control of positive symptoms is inadequate at these dosages after 6 weeks, it might be useful to increase the dose. However, a switch to clozapine, where the dose can be relatively high with minimal EPS, is often a better strategy, especially after the failure of two adequate antipsychotic trials (e.g., 6 or more weeks at an adequate dose). As with clozapine, augmentation with mood stabilizers, antidepressant drugs or ECT can be attempted on clinical grounds.

Currently, only risperidone is available in a long-acting form. It must be given every 2 weeks and takes 6 weeks before steady state plasma levels are achieved. Therefore, oral risperidone must be continued for at least 3 weeks after the first long-acting risperidone injection, or even longer in some cases. The typical dose of long-acting injectable risperidone is between 35–50 mg every 2 weeks.

iii. Partial D_2 agonists—**Aripiprazole** is the first partial dopamine agonist which has been approved for the treatment of schizophrenia. The basis of partial

dopamine agonism as a block to dopaminergic blockade is that aripiprazole occupies the receptor, but causes significantly less activation of the receptor than the full agonist, dopamine does. The efficacy of aripiprazole is no doubt dependent, in addition, on its serotonergic properties. It is a 5-HT$_{2A}$ antagonist and a 5-HT$_{1A}$-partial agonist, both of which effects would be expected to minimize EPS. Aripiprazole is generally given once daily, at a dose of 15 mg/d. Sometimes, doses of 20–30 mg are required. Combination with a typical neuroleptic should be avoided as that could interfere with the partial dopamine agonist properties. Aripiprazole produces mild metabolic side effects, comparable to those of risperidone and ziprasidone. It may also be associated with activation when first administered, and can cause nausea.

The management of schizophrenia is often conceived of as occurring in three phases of treatment (acute, continuation, and maintenance).

1. Acute phase treatment—The acute phase of schizophrenia is characterized by fully expressed psychotic symptoms. The acuity of symptoms is often such that hospitalization is necessary for control of acute, life-threatening agitation and combativeness. In order to avoid use of physical restraints, oral antipsychotic medication may be offered; however, oral medication is often refused or, more commonly, cannot be safely administered in an acute situation. For patients who are acutely agitated or likely to harm themselves or others, short-acting injectable antipsychotics, benzodiazepines, alone or in combination, may be considered. Currently, the only atypical antipsychotics available in an acute injectable form are ziprasidone and olanzapine. Several typical neuroleptics are available in this form (haloperidol, 5 mg IM), and are often administered alone or in combination with an injectable benzodiazepine (e.g., lorazepam) and/or an anticholinergic drug (e.g., benztropine or diphenhydramine). It is necessary to isolate such patients in a quiet room, with as much supervision as possible. Parenteral haloperidol may be repeated, as needed, every 2–4 hours. Rarely, ECT will be needed.

Once agitation has been controlled or if injectable medication is not indicated, treatment with an orally administered antipsychotic may be initiated. Ordinarily, the first antipsychotic administered should be chosen from aripiprazole, quetiapine, risperidone, and ziprasidone in a never-treated or medication-free patient who has a history of response to antipsychotic drug treatment (Figure 16–1). Olanzapine, because of its higher burden of metabolic side effects, might be kept in reserve. However, not all patients treated with olanzapine develop metabolic side effects. For patients on one of these drugs for whom a switch is indicated to another of the same class, there is no accepted preferred way to do this. Stopping the current drug as the new drug is introduced may be as safe and effective as rapid or slow cross-titration.

In choosing among the various first-line options, no convincing data suggest superior efficacy in target symptom domains for a particular agent. The clinical decision about which agent to use is based on other factors: side-effect profile, past therapeutic response to agent(s), and patient/caregiver preference. The issue of tolerability due to side-effect burden is no small one, since relapse into acute phase illness is often preceded by unilateral discontinuation of medication.

If circumstances are such that a patient requires treatment with a typical neuroleptic (i.e., prior treatment response to typical rather than atypical drugs in absence of significant EPS, limited formularies, cost considerations, or patient/caregiver preference), treatment is best commenced with an oral drug at low dosage (i.e., 10 mg/d haloperidol equivalent). The dose should not be increased for 4–6 weeks unless psychotic or aggressive symptoms or sleeplessness are severe. Rapid dose increases aggravate the risk of EPS and secondary negative symptoms without added antipsychotic benefit. Routine use of short-acting parenteral medication for newly hospitalized patients is to be avoided unless absolutely necessary.

Long-acting (depot) medication should not be given initially except to those patients noncompliant with other forms of treatment. On the other hand, acute-phase symptoms due to illness relapse in the setting of poor compliance call specifically for consideration of long-acting injectable antipsychotic medication. As previously discussed, long-acting risperidone is the only atypical drug available for such use, whereas haloperidol and fluphenazine are available among the typical drugs. Because of its atypical profile, long-acting risperidone should be the first choice.

2. Continuation phase treatment—Psychotic symptoms respond, usually partially, within the first several days of treatment, or even on the first day in some patients. However, most patients do not achieve a full response at a given dose for 2–6 weeks, and remain vulnerable to early relapse. The purpose of continuation-phase treatment is to monitor patient compliance, therapeutic response, and treatment tolerance. In addition, because a significant lag time may be required to full therapeutic effect at a given dose of drug, it is inadvisable to discontinue a drug prematurely and substitute a different class of neuroleptic agent before the optimal 4–6 weeks of therapy has passed, unless significant side effects develop that are not amenable to treatment. After initial stabilization, continuation treatment ranges in duration up to 6–8 weeks, depending upon treatment response.

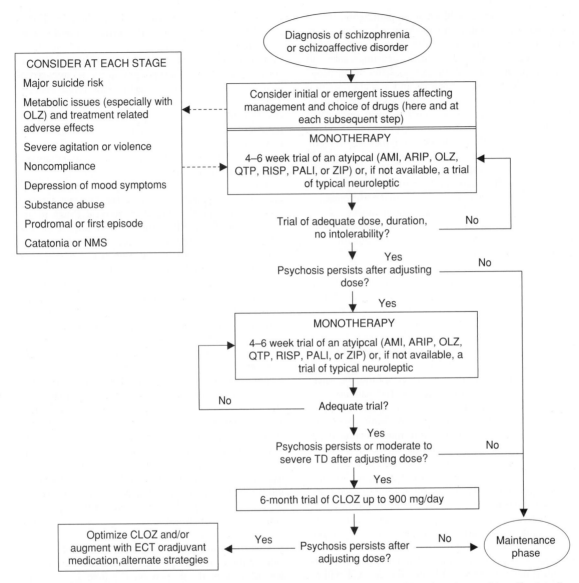

Figure 16–1. Algorithm for the pharmacological treatment of patients with schizophrenia or schizoaffective disorder. First-line options include amisulpiride (AMI, not available in the United States), aripiprazole (ARIP), olanzapine (OLZ), quetiapine (QTP), risperidone (RISP), paliperidone (PALI), or ziprasidone (ZIP). An adequate trial of medication is 4–6 weeks at an adequate dosage before trying a different agent. Clozapine should be considered if a patient does not respond to two or more adequate medication trials. Patients should receive 6 months of clozapine treatment before adequacy of treatment response is judged. If response is inadequate, a number of less well-studied options may be considered. At first assessment and at each initial visits, there are a number of clinical considerations and other important areas that should be assessed, as indicated in the box in the upper left hand corner of the figure. Adapted from the International Psychopharmacology Algorithm Project (IPAP) schizophrenia treatment algorithm, available online at www.ipap.org.

In general, the same medication dosage that resulted in control of acute phase symptoms is appropriate for the continuation phase, though the dose may be "fine tuned" during this time in order to minimize adverse effects or bring about a more adequate clinical response. Although some evidence supports intermittent dosing of antipsychotic medication, this strategy has been associated with increased rates of relapse. Continuous dosing is preferred.

The use of several neuroleptics at the same time should be avoided. There is no justification for the concomitant use of two classes of typical neuroleptic drugs (e.g., a parenteral and an oral antipsychotic) unless the patient's route of treatment is being converted from intramuscular to oral. In some instances, particularly when a neuroleptic does not adequately control anxiety and agitation, the adjunctive use of benzodiazepines may be helpful.

3. Maintenance treatment—The primary goals of maintenance treatment are prevention of relapse and optimization of psychosocial functioning. Long-term illness management also calls for monitoring and treating medical comorbidities (including the effects of antipsychotic treatment), addressing comorbid psychiatric and substance use disorders, and addressing the important issue of medication compliance.

As is the case with continuation-phase treatment, the dosage used to achieve clinical response in the acute phase is often continued, but may be subject to "fine tuning" for the reasons specified above. Continuous dosing is preferred. Ongoing monitoring of medication compliance must be paramount, as this is still the most common reason for relapse. Noncompliance stems from a number of factors: Denial of illness (poor insight); intolerable side effects; suboptimal management of clinical symptoms; cognitive deficits; and other reasons. Weight gain, EPS (especially akathisia), and sedation can also be distressing to patients. Because many of the adverse effects of medication are dose dependent, problems with compliance may be managed by lowering the dosage, or switching to agents that result in fewer side effects. Pharmacological adjuncts may be required to counter particular adverse effects if dosage adjustment or switching are not clinically feasible. For most patients, treatment with antipsychotic medications will be of indefinite duration.

In spite of recent advances in antipsychotic treatment, a significant proportion of patients are left with persisting symptoms, especially negative and neurocognitive symptoms. Even under the best of circumstances, however, positive symptoms frequently persist, though in a less acute form. Incompletely treated symptoms are associated with significant psychiatric and physical health-related morbidity, and with an increased risk of relapse and rehospitalization. Thus, management during maintenance phase must endeavor to achieve as optimal a treatment response as possible. If at least a partial response to a well-executed antipsychotic trial has been achieved, remaining options include watchful waiting (since some treatment effects may take longer to appear), upwardly adjusting the drug dosage, using adjunctive medication, or switching to another medication, assuming that other factors that contribute to suboptimal treatment response have been ruled out (Table 16–12). For typical neuroleptics, clinical evidence indicates that the dose–response profiles eventually either plateau, or the side-effect liability begins to outweigh therapeutic benefit as doses are increased. For atypical antipsychotics, the dose–response interactions have been less well studied, though there is some evidence in favor of high-dose strategies for olanzapine and other atypicals.

The evidence for augmenting nonclozapine atypical antipsychotics is generally lacking. Serial trials of antipsychotic monotherapy are preferred. For treatment-refractory patients, a trial of clozapine monotherapy is clearly indicated (discussed later). However, when dosages of antipsychotic medication cannot be raised, when the risk of losing the partial response already achieved outweighs the potential benefit of switching medication, or when no other options are feasible, augmentation may be considered for specific target symptoms or psychiatric comorbidities that antipsychotic monotherapy cannot address. When an adjunct is being considered, great care must be taken to review all medications, in order to anticipate unwanted drug interactions and other risks of combining medications. Specific clinical subgroups for whom adjuncts have at least some support include patients with aggressive behavior (valproate, benzodiazepines), anxiety (benzodiazepines, antidepressants), substance use problems (naltrexone), prominent affective symptoms (valproate, lithium, antidepressants), positive symptoms (benzodiazepines), negative symptoms (antidepressants) and cognitive difficulties (antidepressants, buspirone). These strategies, again, are based on anecdotal reporting and, in cases where the evidence is stronger, clinical responses can be highly variable or even worse, especially in the case of benzodiazepines.

4. Treatment-refractory schizophrenia—Treatment-resistant schizophrenia is variously defined. Failure of two well-carried-out therapeutic trials of antipsychotic from any pharmacological class is a generally accepted definition. The atypical antipsychotic, clozapine, is the only drug with proven efficacy for treatment-resistant patients. It remains the gold standard in this subgroup. Approximately 30–60% of all schizophrenic patients who fail to respond to typical antipsychotics respond to clozapine. Data concerning the usefulness of other atypical antipsychotics at conventional doses are not convincing, though higher-than-usual doses of other atypical antipsychotics may be of benefit. As was previously discussed in regard to other atypicals, there are several potentially useful adjuncts for addressing a partial antipsychotic response to clozapine, though none have a particularly strong empirical basis. To date, the most evidence is for ECT. While the rationale for the use of augmenting therapies would be the strongest for clozapine, given its status as a treatment of last resort, the potential for dangerous adverse effects with certain drug combinations is considerable. Thus, the need for caution may be even greater when augmenting clozapine partial response than for other agents.

Casey DE: Neuroleptic drug-induced extrapyramidal syndromes and tardive dyskinesia. *Schizophr Res* 1991;4:109–120.

Christison GW, Kirch DG, Wyatt RJ: When symptoms persist: Choosing among alternative somatic treatments for schizophrenia. *Schizophr Bull* 1991;17:217–245.

Conley RR, Buchanan RW: Evaluation of treatment-resistant schizophrenia. *Schizophr Bull* 1997;23:663–674.

Dolder CR, Lacro JP, Leckband S, Jeste DV: Interventions to improve antipsychotic medication adherence: Review of recent literature. *J Clin Psychopharmacology* 2003;23:389–399.

Goldman LS: Medical illness in patients with schizophrenia. *J Clin Psychiatry* 1999;60:10–15.

Jin H, Meyer JM, Jeste DV: Atypical antipsychotics and glucose dysregulation: A systematic review. *Schizophr Res* 2004;71:195–212.

Keith SJ, Kane JM: Partial compliance and patient consequences in schizophrenia: Our patients can do better. *J Clin Psychiatry* 2003;64:1308–1315.

Kinon BJ, Ahl J, Stauffer VL, Hill AL, Buckley PF: Dose response and atypical antipsychotics in schizophrenia. *CNS Drugs* 2004;18:597–616.

Kontaxakis VP, Ferentinos PP, Havaki-Kontaxaki BJ, Roukas DK: Randomized controlled augmentation trials in clozapine-resistant schizophrenic patients: A critical review. *Eur Psychiatry* 2005;20:409–415.

Lehman AF, Kreyenbuhl J, Buchanan RW, et al.: The Schizophrenia Patient Outcomes Research Team (PORT): Updated treatment recommendations 2003. *Schizophr Bull* 2004;30:193–217.

Newcomer JW: Second-generation (atypical) antipsychotics and metabolic effects: A comprehensive literature review. *CNS Drugs* 2005;19(suppl 1):1–93.

Richelson E, Souder T: Binding of antipsychotic drugs to human brain receptors: Focus on newer generation compounds. *Life Sci* 2000;68:29–39.

Schatzberg AF, Nemeroff CB (eds): *Textbook of Psychopharmacology*, 3rd edn. Washington, DC: American Psychiatric Publishing, 2004.

B. Psychotherapeutic Interventions

Although antipsychotic drugs are the mainstay of treatment of schizophrenia, significant residual symptoms often remain, even with optimal management. Furthermore, the rate of nonadherence to pharmacological treatment is high. Both of these facts make it imperative for every clinician to explore nonpharmacological modalities of treatment. Such treatments are aimed at improving compliance with drug therapy, supporting the patient, fostering independent living skills, improving psychosocial and work functioning, and reducing caretaker burden.

The major forms of psychotherapeutic interventions for schizophrenia are cognitive–behavioral therapy (CBT), personal therapy, compliance therapy, acceptance and commitment therapy, and supportive psychotherapy. The CBT, originally developed for the treatment of depression and anxiety, has been modified for the treatment of schizophrenia. The goals of CBT in the treatment of schizophrenia include belief modification, reattribution, and normalizing of psychotic experiences. A recent meta-analysis of CBT trials in schizophrenia reported a modest effect size (0.37) for the reduction of positive symptoms. A variation of CBT is acceptance and commitment therapy, which does not aim to change thoughts and feelings, but to "just notice" and accept them. Personal therapy focuses on affective dysregulation and aims to achieve recovery in several stages of decreasing acuity, making it a long-term therapeutic effort. Compliance therapy is short term and uses motivational interviewing to improve medication adherence in the acute stage of the illness (often at the time of hospitalization).

Other psychosocial approaches include illness education, cognitive remediation, and social skills training. Providing education and support to family members is a crucial component of comprehensive treatment. Family treatment that ameliorates expressed emotion reduces the likelihood of relapse, especially if the patient's response to antipsychotic medication is less than optimal.

In most mental health systems, case management has been developed to provide low-cost support for patients living in the community, many of whom were formerly institutionalized. Case managers help patients find housing; manage financial resources; get access to psychiatric clinics, rehabilitation services, and crisis intervention; and comply with medication regimens. Such assistance enables patients to live in settings with no or minimal mental health worker provided supervision. Some mental health systems assign patients at especially high risk of rehospitalization to a multidisciplinary team that is available around-the-clock, an approach termed "assertive community treatment."

Finally, many communities offer supported employment programs, whereby patients are assessed for skills and are matched with an appropriate job with on-site support and training from a work coach familiar with the special needs of patients with schizophrenia. The goal of supported employment is similar to that of sheltered work programs—assisting patients to obtain employment.

Garety PA, Fowler D, Kuipers E: Congitive-behavioral therapy for medication-resistant symptoms. *Schizophr Bull* 2000;26:73–86.

Heinssen RK, Libwerman RP, Kopelowicz A: Psychosocial skills training for schizophrenia: Lessons from the laboratory. *Schizophr Bull* 2000;26:21–46.

Lenroot R, Bustillo JR, Lauriello J, Keith SJ: Integrated treatment of schizophrenia. *Psychiatr Serv* 2003;54:1499–1507.

Penn DL, Mueser KT, Tarrier N, et al.: Supportive therapy for schizophrenia: Possible mechanisms and implications for adjunctive psychosocial treatments. *Schizophr Bull* 2004;30:101–112.

Prognosis

As indicated above, the course of schizophrenia is highly variable; however, the typical pattern is of relative remissions with residual symptoms and dysfunction, punctuated by periodic symptom exacerbation. About 10% of patients eventually recover, while an additional 20% have a good outcome. One third of treated patients have a stable but only intermediate outcome, while the remaining one third have a deteriorating course.

Thus, a significant proportion of treated patients (about 40%) continue to manifest psychotic symptoms. Even low-grade residual symptoms can be enough to impede functional capacity (e.g., to work, sustain meaningful relationships, maintain adequate self-care, and live independently). Therefore, in spite of advances in the treatment of the disorder, more is needed before patients with schizophrenia can enjoy a quality of life comparable to that of the general population.

Table 16–13. Predictors of Course and Outcome in Schizophrenia

Factor	Better Outcome	Poorer Outcome
Age at onset*	About 20–25	Below 20
CT/MRI studies*	Normal morphology	Dilated ventricles, brain atrophy
Initial clinical symptoms*,[†]	Catatonia, paranoia, depression, schizoaffective diagnosis, atypical symptoms, confusion	Negative symptoms (e.g., flat affect, poverty of thought, apathy, asociality); obsessive–compulsive symptoms
Occupational record*	Stable	Irregular
Onset*	Acute, late	Insidious
Rate of progression*	Rapid	Slow
Sex*	Possibly females	Possibly males
Length of episode prior to assessment[†]	Months or less	Years
Being in a developing country[‡]	Present	Absent
Cannabis use[‡]	Absent	Present
Optimal prenatal care[‡]	Present	Absent
Precipitating factors[‡]	Present	Absent
Socioeconomic status[‡]	Middle, high	Low
Substance abuse[‡]	Absent	Present
Stressful life[‡]	Absent	Present
Early treatment with medications[§]	Present	Absent
Long-term drug maintenance[§]	Present	Absent
Response to medications initially[§]	Present	Absent
Family history of mental illness[¶]	Affective	Schizophrenia
Other adverse social factors[¶]	Absent	Present
Prenatal adverse events[¶]	None	Present
Presence of certain gene polymorphism, e.g., COMT. NMDA2A[¶]	Absent	Present

*Clinical; [†]diagnosis; [‡]environment; [§]treatment; [¶]genetic.

A. PREDICTORS OF BETTER LONG-TERM COURSE

Predictors of better long-term course are summarized in Table 16–13. Even under these circumstances, return to a full premorbid level of functioning is rarely observed, and milder residual deficits persist as indicated above. The long-term prognosis for independent living is unfavorable.

B. PREDICTORS OF POORER LONG-TERM COURSE

Predictors of poorer long-term course are summarized in Table 16–13. Taking into account the different syndromal domains of schizophrenia, negative symptoms, and cognitive dysfunction are more closely tied than positive symptoms to functional disability and problems with independent living. This is probably due to the combination of illness-specific factors and the limitations of available treatment, the latter of which may successfully address combativeness, agitation, neurovegetative problems and other positive symptoms but provide less benefit for negative symptoms, social dysfunction, impeded cognition, and poor insight. On the other hand, negative symptoms and cognitive dysfunction are more responsive to the atypical antipsychotic drugs than to the typical neuroleptics.

More than half of patients with schizophrenia have poor insight. Many are unaware that their symptoms are attributable to mental illness. Even if appropriate treatment is initiated, the rates of relapse are high, especially in the context of poor treatment compliance, the most common form of which is "partial" noncompliance rather than outright treatment refusal or discontinuation.

C. EARLY MORTALITY

Early mortality is frequently encountered among schizophrenic patients, roughly 1.5–2.0 times more often than in the general population. Excess mortality is attributed not only to illness-related psychopathological symptoms and cognitive dysfunction, but also to medical comorbidity, accidents, and suicide. The standardized mortality ratios for "natural causes," accidents, and suicide among patients with schizophrenia are approximately 1.1, 2.2, and 8.4, respectively. The lifetime risk for suicide among patients with schizophrenia is 10–13%. At some point during their lifetime, 18–55% of patients attempt suicide.

Successful treatment of the disorder, therefore, requires attention not only to psychopathological domains such as positive and negative symptoms, but also to cognition, functional capacity, treatment compliance, affective/anxiety symptoms, psychosocial support, comorbid conditions (psychiatric and substance related) and general medical care. Advances in pharmacological and psychosocial treatment, and increased attention to medical problems and the other special needs of schizophrenic patients, offer hope to many.

Davidson L, McGlashan TH: The varied outcomes of schizophrenia. *Can J Psychiatry* 1997;42:34.

Jobe TH, Harrow M: Long-term outcome of patients with schizophrenia: A review. *Can J Psychiatry* 2005;50:892.

Tsuang MT, Tohen M (eds): *Textbook in Psychiatric Epidemiology*, 2nd edn. New York, NY: Wiley-Liss, 2002.

Other Psychotic Disorders

17

Richard C. Shelton, MD

■ SCHIZOPHRENIFORM DISORDER

 ESSENTIALS OF DIAGNOSIS

DSM-IV-TR Diagnostic Criteria

A. Criteria A, D, and E of schizophrenia must be met.

B. An episode of the disorder (including prodromal, active, and residual phases) lasts at least 1 month but less than 6 months. When the diagnosis must be made without waiting for recovery, it should be qualified as "provisional."

Specify if:
Without good prognostic features
With good prognostic features: as evidenced by two (or more) of the following:

(1) onset of prominent psychotic symptoms within 4 weeks of the first noticeable change in usual behavior or functioning

(2) confusion or perplexity at the height of the psychotic episode

(3) good premorbid social and occupational functioning

(4) absence of blunted or flat affect

(Reprinted, with permission, from the *Diagnostic and Statistical Manual of Mental Disorders*, 4th edn. Text Revision. Washington, DC: American Psychiatric Association, 2000)

General Considerations

A. EPIDEMIOLOGY

Diagnostically, schizophreniform disorder is "positioned" in time between brief psychotic disorder (discussed later in this chapter), which lasts 1 month or less, and schizophrenia (see Chapter 16), which by definition continues beyond 6 months. Although many patients eventually will be shown to have schizophrenia, a small but significant number of patients with persisting psychotic disorders will show complete recovery of their illness. The proportion of recovery is likely to be small, although the exact percentage is unknown. Those who do show recovery typically exhibit characteristics known to predict better outcome in other diagnostic categories (e.g., acute onset, brief prodrome, lack of psychosocial deterioration, and prominent mood symptoms).

B. ETIOLOGY

Schizophreniform disorder is a heterogeneous category; therefore, in all likelihood, it has several distinct etiologies. Because most patients with this disorder will proceed on to meet diagnostic criteria for schizophrenia, the etiologies will be the same as for that condition, discussed in detail in Chapter 16. Some patients with this disorder appear to recover significantly and thus represent a manifestation that is distinct from typical schizophrenia.

C. GENETICS

Because schizophreniform disorder is likely to be an etiologically heterogeneous disorder, genetic relationships are unclear. Those persons who proceed on to manifest typical schizophrenia show genetic predispositions that are similar to this condition. Those who recover completely may have increased family histories of both psychotic and affective disorders, especially bipolar disorder.

Clinical Findings

A. SIGNS & SYMPTOMS

Patients with schizophreniform disorder exhibit symptoms consistent with Criterion A of schizophrenia (i.e., typically hallucinations; delusions; negative symptoms; disorganization of thought, speech, and behavior) that last between 1 and 6 months. Patients with these symptoms may proceed on to a typical pattern of schizophrenia and should be diagnosed as such if the symptoms are present for more than 6 months. However, others may proceed to complete or near-complete resolution of their symptoms. These patients generally have good premorbid function, acute onset (often after a stressor), and complete resolution without residual deficits in psychosocial function. In addition, mood symptoms tend to be more prominent and a family history of mood disorder is common in these patients.

B. PSYCHOLOGICAL TESTING

Psychological testing will reveal a pattern of symptoms more typical of schizophrenia (see Chapter 16). These findings will include the common symptoms of thought disorganization, hallucinations, and delusions. However, overt cognitive impairment (including memory problems) is uncommon, and prominent mood symptoms may occur. Persons with schizophreniform disorder may demonstrate frontal cortical regional deficits such as impaired performance on the Wisconsin Card Sorting Test.

C. LABORATORY FINDINGS & NEUROIMAGING

Brain imaging studies may show the same results as those reported for schizophrenia. However, the differences often are less prominent, owing to the shorter duration of the condition. Alternatively, many patients do not show differences from normal controls, which may be associated with recovery. However, diagnostic imaging studies are not indicated.

A relative activation deficit in the inferior prefrontal region during performing the Wisconsin Card Sorting Test has been reported in both patients with schizophrenic and patients with schizophreniform disorder.

Course of Illness

Schizophreniform disorder often follows a course typical of schizophrenia. If symptoms are present for more than 6 months, psychological and social deterioration typically associated with schizophrenia may occur. First generation antipsychotics such as haloperidol reduce the symptoms of the illness but will not prevent deterioration if the symptoms are present for more than 6 months. The potential beneficial effects of newer, atypical antipsychotics (e.g., clozapine, risperidone, olanzapine, quetiapine) in preventing psychosocial deterioration or cognitive impairment has been hypothesized but not conclusively established.

Differential Diagnosis (Including Comorbid Conditions)

Although the major differential diagnoses are brief psychotic disorder and schizophrenia, the rapid onset of acute psychosis may be the most important diagnostic point. Attention should focus on the prior 6 months, the pattern of onset, and the presence of mood changes, alcohol and substance abuse, and other illness and prescriptive medications.

Treatment

The treatment of schizophreniform disorder is similar to that of schizophrenia (see Chapter 16).

Hospitalization is usually required in the acute stages of overt psychotic symptoms.

A. PSYCHOPHARMACOLOGIC INTERVENTIONS

Antipsychotic drugs represent the mainstay of symptomatic management, and resolution of psychosis often is fairly rapid. It has been shown that patients with schizophreniform disorder respond to antipsychotic treatment much more rapidly than do patients with schizophrenia. Sedative agents, especially benzodiazepines, may be needed to manage acute agitation. Electroconvulsive therapy may be indicated for some patients.

B. PSYCHOTHERAPEUTIC INTERVENTIONS

Psychotherapy is usually needed to help patients integrate the psychotic experience. Psychosocial support and rehabilitation is critical with these patients to help reduce the deterioration in function more typical of schizophrenia. Therefore, rapid treatment of symptoms and social reintegration of the patient is important.

C. OTHER INTERVENTIONS

After the resolution of acute symptoms, psychological, social, and occupational or educational treatment becomes the main focus of treatment. An acute schizophreniform psychotic episode represents a catastrophic event in the life of the patient, and psychotherapy is needed to help the patient understand the event and gain a sense of control over future episodes. A variety of issues should be discussed with the patient and his or her family or significant other: (1) the fundamental biological nature of the disorder; (2) the role of medication in controlling current and future symptoms, particularly the possible effect of symptom management on the evolution of the disorder; (3) the early-warning signs that indicate a return of psychosis; (4) the impact of the disturbance on the person's life and that of the family; (5) the need for gradual reintegration into work or school; and (6) the importance of future psychosocial management, including intensive case management or occupational or educational rehabilitation.

Prognosis

Most individuals with schizophreniform disorder are simply in the early stages of the development of more typical schizophrenia. The 6-month cutoff for the diagnosis of schizophreniform disorder acknowledges that although patients with typical schizophrenia symptoms sometimes show complete resolution, this seldom occurs when the symptoms have been present for 6 months or more. Almost all patients will then proceed to a course more consistent with schizophrenia, with persistent deterioration and impairment in psychosocial functioning. Exceptions to this rule are very rare.

Strakowski SM: Diagnostic validity of schizophreniform disorder. *Am J Psychiatry* 1994;151:815.

■ SCHIZOAFFECTIVE DISORDER

 ESSENTIALS OF DIAGNOSIS

DSM-IV-TR Diagnostic Criteria

A. *An uninterrupted period of illness during which, at some time, there is either a major depressive disorder, a manic episode, or a mixed episode concurrent with symptoms that meet Criterion A for schizophrenia.*

Note: *The major depressive episode must include Criterion A1: depressed mood.*

B. *During the same period of illness, there have been delusions or hallucinations for at least 2 weeks in the absence of prominent mood symptoms.*

C. *Symptoms that meet criteria for a mood episode are present for a substantial portion of the total duration of the active and residual periods of the illness.*

D. *The disturbance is not due to the direct physiological effects of a substance (e.g., a drug of abuse, a medication) or a general medical condition.*

Specify *type:*
Bipolar type: *if the disturbance includes a manic or a mixed episode (or a manic or a mixed episode and major depressive episodes)*
Depressive type: *if the disturbance only includes major depressive episodes*

(Reprinted, with permission, from the *Diagnostic and Statistical Manual of Mental Disorders.* 4th edn. Text Revision. Washington, DC: American Psychiatric Association, 2000)

General Considerations

A. EPIDEMIOLOGY

The lifetime prevalence of schizoaffective disorder is less than 1%. Schizoaffective disorder is characterized by prominent mood symptoms (mania or depression) occurring during the course of a chronic psychotic disorder. Phenomenologically, schizoaffective disorder holds the middle ground between mood disorders, especially psychotic mood disorders, and chronic psychotic conditions such as schizophrenia. The debate continues over whether schizoaffective disorder "belongs" to the spectrum of either schizophrenia or affective disorders, or represents a distinct category. Schizoaffective disorder likely represents a heterogeneous disorder with multiple distinct etiologies.

B. ETIOLOGY

Recent research indicates that there appear to be distinct etiologies and outcomes depending on whether the course of schizoaffective disorder is typified by episodes of bipolar-type cycling or simple depressive episodes in the absence of mania.

C. GENETICS

In the bipolar variant, there is an increased proportion of family history of bipolar disorder (but not schizophrenia) and a better overall outcome. Although a family history of affective disorder is observed in the depressive variant, a history of psychotic disorder seems to be more common and outcome is poorer than in the bipolar form. Both variants usually have a better prognosis than does schizophrenia without prominent mood symptoms.

Clinical Findings

A. SIGNS & SYMPTOMS

Patients with schizoaffective disorder exhibit symptoms consistent with DSM-IV-TR diagnostic Criterion A for schizophrenia. However, during the course of illness, there are superimposed episodes of depressive or manic symptoms. These patients would be diagnosed as having schizoaffective disorder, depressed or manic types, respectively. However, psychotic symptoms consistent with schizophrenia must be present for at least 2 weeks independently of the mania or depression syndromes.

Schizoaffective disorder, bipolar type, usually involves cycling of mania, depression, or mixed states in a way that is consistent with bipolar disorder. Similarly, patients with schizoaffective disorder, depressive type, may have repeated episodes of major depression, as in major depressive disorder. However, unlike depressive or bipolar disorders, there are consistent symptoms of schizophrenia in the absence of overt mood disorder. In schizoaffective disorder, depressive type, depressive episodes in which the patient meets full diagnostic criteria for major depression must be distinguished from the mood and negative symptoms associated with schizophrenia. For example, DSM-IV-TR criteria require the presence of persisting depressed mood for this diagnosis. Similarly, care should be taken to avoid misdiagnosing as mania agitation, hostility, insomnia, and other symptoms of an acute exacerbation of schizophrenia.

B. PSYCHOLOGICAL TESTING

The results of psychological tests depend on the state of illness of a given patient. That is, although the typical results of schizophrenia usually are present (see Chapters 6, 16), characteristics of mood disorders also may be present. For example, psychological testing results will be consistent with depression or mania during corresponding episodes of illness. However, schizoaffective disorder, bipolar type, may be associated with less psychosocial and cognitive impairments than are schizophrenia or schizoaffective disorder, depressive type.

Course of Illness

Generally, persons with schizoaffective disorder have a course of illness that is intermediate between the mood disorders (with a relatively better prognosis) and schizophrenia (with marked residual psychosocial deterioration). However, distinctions also can be made for patients within the schizoaffective spectrum. Patients with schizoaffective disorder, bipolar type (i.e., those with a history of manic or mixed bipolar episode), have a course of illness that is more similar to bipolar disorder. These patients often have better functioning between acute episodes of illness than patients with either schizophrenia or schizoaffective disorder, depressive type. Patients with schizoaffective disorder, depressive type, tend to exhibit more typical schizophrenic symptoms and course, although when the disorder is managed properly, the prognosis may be better than typical schizophrenia without comorbid depression.

Differential Diagnosis (Including Comorbid Conditions)

Persons with schizophrenia are not immune to the occurrence of mood symptoms. When these features meet the diagnostic criteria for a mood disorder concurrently with features of schizophrenia, the diagnosis of schizoaffective disorder may be made. However, great care must be exercised in the evaluation in order to provide appropriate management of the disorder. For example, depressive symptoms not meeting full diagnostic criteria for a major depressive episode are common in schizophrenia and do not warrant a diagnosis of schizoaffective disorder per se. In fact, treatment of schizophrenia, especially management with atypical antipsychotics, may reduce these symptoms in many patients without reliance on antidepressants. Alternatively, the negative symptoms of schizophrenia (e.g., apathy, withdrawal, avolition, blunted affect) may be confused with the symptoms of depression. Again, these symptoms generally are treated more effectively with atypical antipsychotics. Finally, the agitation, insomnia, and grandiose delusions of an acutely psychotic patient with schizophrenia sometimes can be confused with mania. However, a careful examination of the course of illness, prodromal symptoms, and acute presentation can be helpful in making the correct diagnosis. For example, the acutely agitated patient who presents for treatment after a period of progressive withdrawal, isolation, and bizarre behavior is unlikely to have mania. A good diagnostic rule of thumb is to evaluate the patient for the presence of current or past mood disorder by excluding the symptoms of schizophrenia, prior to confirming the diagnosis of schizoaffective disorder.

Psychotic mood disorders also may present with a confusing picture. DSM-IV-TR diagnostic criteria are written to aid the clinician in making this distinction. The presence of mood symptoms concurrent with psychosis, even symptoms that otherwise appear to be more like typical schizophrenia (i.e., bizarre behavior or disorganized speech) are not adequate to make the diagnosis of schizoaffective disorder. This condition is understood as representing a mood disorder superimposed on a course of schizophrenia. Therefore, the criteria require the symptoms of schizophrenia to be present for at least 2 weeks in the absence of prominent mood symptoms meeting diagnostic criteria for major depression, mania, or mixed state. A course consistent with dysthymia concurrent with schizophrenia does not constitute a diagnosis of schizophrenia.

Treatment

A. PSYCHOPHARMACOLOGIC INTERVENTIONS

Once a definite diagnosis of schizoaffective disorder is made, treatment must take into consideration the necessity of managing both mood symptoms and psychotic symptoms (Table 17–1). Antipsychotics are required for the management of the psychotic features (see Chapter 17) and are typically used in these patients in acute manic states. Atypical antipsychotics are the first

---

Table 17–1. Principles of Management of Schizoaffective Disorder

- Acute and chronic antipsychotic drug therapies usually are required.
- Atypical antipsychotics may be more effective in managing psychotic and mood symptoms.
- Additional mood stabilizers may be needed for patients with a history of mania.
- Antidepressants will sometimes be required for both depressive and bipolar types; however, exposure to antidepressant medications should be minimized for patients with a history of mania.
- Psychological, social, educational, and occupational support and rehabilitation usually are needed as with schizophrenia.

treatments of choice for several reasons. They can reduce both psychotic and more purely manic symptoms. They also exhibit mood stabilizing effects which are needed if cycling is present. Antidepressant drugs should be used as required in a manner similar to that discussed in Chapter 18 for the treatment of major depression. Alternatively, mood-stabilizing agents such as lithium, carbamazepine, or divalproex may be required adjunctively for the treatment of mood cycling. The effectiveness of lamotrigine as an adjunctive antidepressant or mood stabilizer in this population is largely unknown. Finally, psychosocial management often is needed in much the same fashion as with schizophrenia or schizophreniform disorder to aid in social reintegration.

B. Psychotherapeutic Interventions

No single specific psychotherapeutic intervention has been recommended for schizoaffective disorder. However, patients may benefit from a combination of family therapy, social skills training, and cognitive rehabilitation.

Prognosis

Regardless of the diagnostic category (i.e., bipolar or depressive type), certain factors are associated with a poor outcome. They include insidious onset prior to the first psychotic episode; early onset of illness; poor or deteriorating premorbid functioning; the absence of a clear precipitating stressor; prominent negative symptoms in the prodromal, acute, or residual phases of illness; and a family history of schizophrenia. These factors are also associated with a poorer outcome in persons with schizophrenia without prominent mood symptoms.

Keck PE, Jr., McElroy SL, Strakowski SM: New developments in the pharmacologic treatment of schizoaffective disorder. *J Clin Psychiatry* 1996;57(Suppl 9):41.

Marneros A: The schizoaffective phenomenon: The state of the art. *Acta Psychiatr Scand Suppl* 2003;418:29–33.

■ DELUSIONAL DISORDER

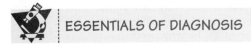

ESSENTIALS OF DIAGNOSIS

DSM-IV-TR Diagnostic Criteria

A. *Nonbizarre delusions (i.e., involving situations that occur in real life, such as being followed, poisoned, infected, loved at a distance, or deceived by spouse or lover, or having a disease) of at least 1 month's duration.*

B. *Criterion A for schizophrenia has never been met.*
Note: *Tactile and olfactory hallucinations may be present in delusional disorder if they are related to the delusional theme.*

C. *Apart from the impact of the delusion(s) or its ramifications, functioning is not markedly impaired and behavior is not obviously odd or bizarre.*

D. *If mood episodes have occurred concurrently with delusions, their total duration has been brief relative to the duration of the delusional periods.*

E. *The disturbance is not due to the direct physiological effects of a substance (e.g., a drug of abuse, a medication) or a general medical condition.*

Specify *type (the following types are assigned based on the predominant delusional theme):*

Erotomanic type: *delusions that another person, usually of higher status, is in love with the individual*

Grandiose type: *delusions of inflated worth, power, knowledge, identity, or special relationship to a deity or famous person*

Jealous type: *delusions that the individual's sexual partner is unfaithful*

Persecutory type: *delusions that the person (or someone to whom the person is close) is being malevolently treated in some way*

Somatic type: *delusions that the person has some physical defect or general medical condition*

Mixed type: *delusions characteristic of more than one of the above types but no one theme predominates*

(Reprinted, with permission, from the *Diagnostic and Statistical Manual of Mental Disorders.* 4th edn. Text Revision. Washington, DC: American Psychiatric Association, 2000)

General Considerations

A. Epidemiology

The cause of delusional disorder is unknown. A very small proportion of the population (roughly 0.03%) experience persistent, relatively fixed delusions in the absence of the characteristic features of other psychotic disorders like schizophrenia.

B. Etiology

Etiologic theories about the development of delusional disorder abound, but systematic study is sparse. Early concepts of etiology focused on the denial and projection of unacceptable impulses. Hence, as examples, homosexual attraction would be reformulated unconsciously to homosexual delusions or a belief in a love relationship with a famous person. Other theories focus on projection of unacceptable sexual and aggressive drives, leading to paranoid fears of others. These and other psychodynamic theories have certain heuristic appeal, but little systematic study has been done to support these conjectures.

C. GENETICS

Little is known about the genetics of delusional disorder. Family studies have suggested a decided lack of increased family history of psychotic or mood disorder.

Clinical Findings

A. SIGNS & SYMPTOMS

Delusional disorder is characterized by nonbizarre delusions. Most often the delusional content appears possible, albeit far-fetched. For example, people with this condition may have fixed delusions that they are in an unrequited love relationship with a famous person or that they are being watched by the CIA, but not that their movements are being controlled by an external force. Persons with this condition may appear otherwise quite normal. They often hold jobs and may be married. The oddness and eccentricity of their beliefs and behavior may manifest itself only around the topic of the delusion.

The diagnosis of delusional disorder depends on the presence of nonbizarre delusions in the absence of meeting Criterion A for schizophrenia (see Chapter 16). Specifically, there should not be significant hallucinatory experiences, marked thought disorder, prominent negative symptoms, or psychosocial deterioration. Except for the behaviors associated with the delusions (e.g., delusional accusations of unfaithfulness in the spouse), the actions of the individual are not otherwise impaired. Although people with delusional disorder may have comorbid major depression or bipolar disorder, the delusions should be present at times when a mood disorder is not present and not just concurrently with an episode of depression or mania. Under these circumstances, however, care must be taken to distinguish this condition from schizoaffective disorder. Specifically, the symptoms must not meet criterion A of the schizophrenia diagnostic criteria.

Specific types of delusional disorder have distinguishing features. The most familiar is the so-called **persecutory type**, in which patients experience fixed (and often focal) paranoid delusions that other persons are intending to harm them in some way. These patients may believe that they are being watched or followed, or that malevolent parties are engaging in other persecutory or threatening behavior. The affected person will act in a way that is consistent with the content of the persecutory delusion but will otherwise be normal.

Another common variant is the **jealous type**. These patients exhibit delusional beliefs that their significant other is being unfaithful. As with the persecutory type, the plausible nature of the belief system may make it difficult to distinguish delusional beliefs from normal fears or real experiences. Patients with delusional disorder, jealous type, either have beliefs that cross the threshold of credibility or refuse to accept reasonable reassurances. For example, a 90-year-old man who believes that his 88-year-old wife is having sex regularly with young men may be suffering from delusional disorder.

In delusional disorder, **erotomanic type** (also referred to as de Clerambault syndrome), the delusion is that another person, usually someone who is famous or of higher social status, is in love with the affected individual. These beliefs may be highly elaborate, although plausibility is maintained. For example, a young woman with delusional disorder, erotomanic type, may travel around the country to attend the concerts of a famous performer. She may believe that the performer gives her secret signals during his concert that indicate his love. However, she also may believe that there is some external reason that he cannot express his love more directly, for example, because he is married, or has an ill mother, or some other reason. Persons with this condition seldom make direct contact with their paramour, although they may, occasionally, engage in more aggressive stalking behavior. Whenever the disorder occurs, it typically becomes the central focus of the person's life.

In the **grandiose type** of the disorder, the person experiences fixed, false beliefs of power (e.g., being the owner of a major corporation), money, identity (e.g., being the Prince of England), a special relationship with God (e.g., being Jesus Christ) or famous people, or some other distinguishing characteristic. These patients may be quietly psychotic but may come to treatment as a result of a contact with a government agency or other organization. For example, a person who believes that he is the President of the United States may be picked up trying to enter the grounds of the White House.

The **somatic type** of delusional disorder involves a fixed belief of some physical abnormality or characteristic. Distinguishing this disorder from simple hypochondriasis may be difficult and generally depends of the content of the belief and the degree to which the belief is held in spite of evidence to the contrary. People with somatoform disorders such as hypochondriasis or body dysmorphic disorder may have a fixed belief regarding a specific, serious, but plausible physical illness, such as cancer or AIDS. In hypochondriasis, these beliefs often relate to specific symptoms, such as pain, stiffness, or swelling. Patients with delusional disorder, somatic type, may have beliefs about other, more unusual conditions. These delusions may involve beliefs about contamination with toxic substances, infestations of insects or other vermin, foul body odors, malfunctions of specific body parts such as the liver or intestines, or other unusual content.

Finally, the **mixed type** of delusional disorder involves more than one of the types described above, without one taking prominence, and the **unspecified type** involves delusions that do not fall into one of the other categories. For example, the delusion of Capgras Syndrome is the belief that a familiar person has been replaced by an imposter.

B. PSYCHOLOGICAL TESTING

Psychological testing will reveal the presence of the delusional psychotic material in these patients but, most often, little else. The cognitive impairments or social deterioration seen in schizophrenia are absent; if such impairments are present, the diagnosis of schizophrenia should be considered. Similarly, prominent mood symptoms might suggest a diagnosis of a psychotic mood disorder.

C. LABORATORY FINDINGS & IMAGING

Neuroimaging data on delusional disorder are rare. Limited evidence indicates that persons with delusional disorder show reduced cortical gray matter and increased ventricular and sulcal size similar to that seen in schizophrenia. However, there has been little systemic study of this condition.

Course of Illness

Occasionally, patients with delusional disorder will go on to develop schizophrenia. This is an exception, though; most patients maintain the delusional diagnosis. About half of patients recover fully and about one-third improve significantly. Only about 20% maintain the delusion indefinitely.

Differential Diagnosis (Including Comorbid Conditions)

The differential diagnosis of delusional disorder encompasses broad categories of disorders. For example, delusional thinking may occur in patients with other psychotic disorders such as schizophrenia, schizoaffective disorder, mood disorders (bipolar disorder, manic or depressed type or major depression) with psychotic features, psychotic disorders due to a general medical condition, or substance-induced psychotic disorder. In delusional disorder, however, important features of those conditions will be absent. For example, the prominent hallucinations, negative symptoms, thought disorder, or social deterioration consistent with schizophrenia are not present. Similarly, mood symptoms, if present, are not prominent. The delusional thinking should not be accounted for by the presence of a medical condition or substance, including substances of abuse. For example, a young patient with a history of stimulant abuse who exhibits paranoid ideation after a recent cocaine binge would not necessarily have delusional disorder.

A delusional diagnosis also may be easily confused with the obsessions of obsessive-compulsive disorder (OCD; see Chapter 21); however, in OCD the patient almost always has at least some insight into the exaggerated nature of the thoughts. Further, obsessions associated with OCD most often involve an inappropriate or exaggerated appraisal of a real threat. This could include a fear of contamination, loss of control of impulses, loss of important documents, and similar threats. When delusional disorder involves a fear of a specific threat, the fears are more typically paranoid or persecutory in nature.

Somatoform disorders such as hypochondriasis or somatization disorder are easily confused with delusional disorder, somatic type (see Chapter 22). As noted earlier, delusional disorder, somatic type, generally differs in both degree and type of belief. That is, in delusional disorder the beliefs are held tenaciously, and often will involve implausible content. Alternatively, people with body dysmorphic disorder often hold tenaciously to their preoccupation with a specific body part and are not easily dissuaded from the belief. In this case, the belief may seem like a delusion. The distinction is that the problem is perceptual, – i.e., is fixed on the appearance of a body part, and does not extend to other types of delusional beliefs.

Paranoid personality disorder also may be confused with delusional disorder (see Chapter 30). Two significant characteristics distinguish these disorders. In paranoid personality disorder, the hostility and paranoid thinking most often are generalized and affect multiple areas of the person's life. For example, the patient may be jealous of the spouse but also will exhibit hypersensitivity at work and in other areas. By contrast, the psychotic thoughts of delusional disorder usually are focused in a single area with remarkable preservation of other areas of thinking and functioning. Another feature distinguishing the disorders is the tenacity of the delusional belief. Persons with delusional disorder most often will maintain a stable but false belief system for long periods. Alternatively, the threatening beliefs of the person with paranoid personality disorder do not reach delusional proportions and often wax and wane in intensity.

Treatment

A. PSYCHOPHARMACOLOGIC INTERVENTIONS

The treatment of delusional disorder relies heavily on the use of antipsychotic drugs, particularly the atypical antipsychotics; however, little systematic study has examined the effectiveness of this approach. Pharmacotherapy should be undertaken with caution: Patients with delusional disorder are convinced of the delusional beliefs and will usually resist medication management. Drug treatment should only be undertaken in the context of an ongoing therapeutic relationship in which there has been an effort to establish rapport, collaboration, and shared goals. For example, it is of little use to try to convince patients who have persecutory delusions that medicine will help them by changing how they think about the feared situation. Patients may be willing to take a drug that will calm the anxiety that has resulted from the persecution. Pimozide has been recommended for this condition; however, systematic study of this approach is lacking.

B. PSYCHOTHERAPEUTIC INTERVENTIONS

Individual supportive psychotherapy as well as family therapy may also be required.

Complications/Adverse Outcomes of Treatment

The main complication of delusional disorder has to do with whether the affected person acts on the delusion in some way. Most people with this disorder lead quiet, uneventful lives otherwise. However, a sudden, unexpected event may intervene, such as the stalking of a famous person. These events may lead to incarceration or involuntary hospitalization, which may surprise friends and coworkers. These actions are consistent with the content of the delusion. Unfortunately, treatment, at least in the short term, often is ineffective, leading to a repetition of the behaviors related to the false beliefs.

Prognosis

The prognosis of delusional disorder is good in most cases. About two third of patients recover or improve significantly; however, in about 20% of patients delusional symptoms persist and are usually treatment-resistant.

Manschreck TC: Delusional disorder: The recognition and management of paranoia. *J Clin Psychiatry* 1996;57(Suppl 3):32–49.

Manschreck TC, Khan NL: Recent advances in the treatment of delusional disorder. *Can J Psychiatry* 2006;51:114.

■ BRIEF PSYCHOTIC DISORDER

 ESSENTIALS OF DIAGNOSIS

DSM-IV-TR Diagnostic Criteria

A. *Presence of one or more of the following symptoms:*
   (1) delusions
   (2) hallucinations
   (3) disorganized speech (e.g., frequent derailment or incoherence)
   (4) grossly disorganized or catatonic behavior

Note: *Do not include a symptom if it is a culturally sanctioned response pattern.*

B. *Duration of an episode of the disturbance is at least 1 day but less than 1 month, with eventual full return to premorbid level of functioning.*

C. *The disturbance is not better accounted for by a mood disorder with psychotic features, schizoaffective disorder, or schizophrenia and is not due to the direct physiological effects of a substance (e.g., a drug of abuse, a medication) or a general medical condition.*

Specify *if*:

With marked stressor(s) (brief reactive psychosis): *if symptoms occur shortly after and apparently in response to events that, singly or together, would be markedly stressful to almost anyone in similar circumstances in the person's culture*

Without marked stressor(s): *if psychotic symptoms do not occur shortly after, or are not apparently in response to events that, singly or together, would be markedly stressful to almost anyone in similar circumstances in the person's culture.*

With postpartum onset: *if onset within 4 weeks postpartum*

(Reprinted, with permission, from the *Diagnostic and Statistical Manual of Mental Disorders.* 4th edn. Text Revision. Washington, DC: American Psychiatric Association, 2000)

General Considerations

The emergence of transient psychotic symptoms, particularly after a severe psychological or social stressor such as a move or loss of a loved one, is not rare. Brief psychotic symptoms in the absence of a clear stressor are less common but also may occur. This disorder is generally associated with very acute onset and florid symptoms that decline rapidly even in the absence of the use of antipsychotic drugs. A diagnosis of brief psychotic disorder should be considered if a psychotic patient has a history of good premorbid functioning and an acute onset that resolves rapidly and completely in response to antipsychotic therapy.

A. EPIDEMIOLOGY

Reliable estimates of the frequency of this disorder are not available; however, an increased frequency is observed in populations that have experienced significant life stresses (e.g., immigrants, refugees, military recruits, and persons who have experienced a disaster such as an earthquake or hurricane). Therefore the frequency is going to depend on the population under study. Predisposing variables include comorbidity of personality disorder, substance use disorder, or dementia, or low socioeconomic status. Socioeconomic status may be associated with brief psychotic disorder in part because persons of lower social class may be at increased risk for major life stresses.

B. Etiology

A variety of stressors may occur prior to the onset of brief psychotic disorder. If the onset occurs within 4 weeks of giving birth, the specifier *with postpartum onset* is used. Many other stressors may predispose to the occurrence of this condition. For example, the disorder may occur after the death of a loved one, after a move to a new country (culture shock), during a natural disaster, or during combat or other military activity. A variety of factors are associated with the occurrence of brief psychotic disorder. They can be associated either with an increased likelihood of experiencing a stressor (e.g., lower socioeconomic status, refugee or immigrant status, presence in a war zone) or limitations in coping skills (e.g., persons with personality disorders, children or adolescents). However, the problem may also occur in people experiencing mild or no stressor and without predisposing characteristics.

C. Genetics

Family history relationships are unclear; however, there may be an increased risk of psychotic disorder (including brief psychotic episodes) or affective disorder in relatives of persons with this condition.

Clinical Findings

A. Signs & Symptoms

Psychotic symptoms occurring for 1 month or less with complete resolution constitute brief psychotic disorder. This condition occurs most often after a significant external stressor, although DSM-IV-TR allows the diagnosis without an obvious stress. The presentation is usually particularly florid. Patients can exhibit confusion, marked agitation or catatonia, emotional lability, and psychotic symptoms such as hallucinations or delusions. The symptoms may be so severe as to mimic the appearance of delirium.

B. Psychological Testing

Psychological testing has not been shown to be useful in adding to the diagnosis of brief psychotic disorder.

C. Laboratory Findings

There are no laboratory findings suggestive or supportive of brief psychotic disorder.

Course of Illness

Though by definition symptoms are brief and time-limited, recurrence of psychotic events often occurs, especially in the face of ongoing stressors or comorbid conditions such as personality disorder. When recurrence is frequent, long-term management with an antipsychotic (usually an atypical antipsychotic agent) may be indicated.

Differential Diagnosis (Including Comorbid Conditions)

The diagnosis of brief psychotic disorder is often difficult to make, and corroborative information from a family member or friend may be required to distinguish this problem from another psychotic disorder or cognitive disorder such as delirium.

A variety of disorders should be considered in the differential, including schizophrenia spectrum disorders (i.e., schizophreniform disorder, schizophrenia, or schizoaffective disorder), psychotic affective disorder, delusional disorder, personality disorder, substance use disorder (including withdrawal), delirium, psychotic disorder due to medical condition, or substance-induced psychotic disorder. Schizophrenia and related disorders (including delusional disorder) are distinguished by the duration of psychotic symptoms and impairments. Persons with brief psychotic disorder show complete resolution of their psychotic symptoms and impairments within the 30 days allotted for the diagnosis. The symptoms of persons with delusional disorder are more confined to the delusional content and are not as pervasive as that usually seen in brief psychotic disorder.

A diagnosis of psychotic affective disorder should be made in the presence of prominent mood symptoms meeting diagnostic criteria for mania or depression. This distinction may be difficult to make, especially in highly agitated or otherwise distressed patients. The mood, psychotic, and behavioral symptoms of affective psychosis rarely resolve completely within 30 days of initiation of treatment; therefore, if patients show complete return of baseline function within this time frame, a diagnosis of brief psychotic disorder should be considered, especially in the absence of a history of mood disorder.

Patients with personality disorder may present transient episodes of psychosis. This is particularly true of borderline personality disorder but may be seen in other disorders, including histrionic, schizotypal, or obsessive-compulsive personality. These events almost always follow a significant stressor, especially an interpersonal

Table 17–2. Principles of Management of Brief Psychotic Disorder

- Hospitalization usually is indicated.
- Undertake a thorough psychiatric and medical evaluation and laboratory testing to rule out other major psychiatric, medical, or substance use disorders.
- Attempt to identify and eliminate or modify significant stressors.
- Antipsychotic and sedative drugs (such as benzodiazepines) often are indicated in acute management; however, long-term treatment with these medicines should be avoided when the diagnosis of brief psychotic disorder is clear and the patient experiences complete resolution of symptoms.
- Long-term treatment should focus on several major elements:
  Improving coping skills
  Eliminating or stabilizing ongoing psychological or social stressors
  Establishing a network of social support
  Managing comorbid conditions, including personality disorders
  Reintegrating the patient into the social, educational, or occupational milieu
  Helping the patient and social network to understand the condition and to recognize early prodromal symptoms of impending psychosis, especially sleeplessness
  Facilitating sleep, nutrition, and hygiene

stressful event. These occurrences may be very brief (i.e., less than 1 day) and would be included in the category of psychotic disorder not otherwise classified. However, if they occur for more than 1 day but less than 1 month, the patient should be given a diagnosis of brief psychotic disorder along with the personality disorder diagnosis. Finally, if the psychotic symptoms seem related to substance use or withdrawal or to a medical condition, the alternatives of substance use disorder (including substance-induced psychotic disorder) or psychotic disorder due to medical condition should be given diagnostic primacy.

Treatment

Treatment proceeds as with any other form of psychosis (Table 17–2). Hospitalization is usually required, and a reduction in sensory stimulation is helpful.

A. PSYCHOPHARMACOLOGIC INTERVENTIONS

Antipsychotics and sedatives help to ameliorate the symptoms, especially by inducing sleep. Response to antipsychotic drug treatment is often rapid and complete. If complete resolution of psychotic symptoms occurs, the duration of treatment can be relatively brief i.e., one to three months. If brief psychotic disorder is recurrent, then longer-term treatment with an atypical antipsychotic should be considered.

B. PSYCHOTHERAPEUTIC INTERVENTIONS

Subsequent psychotherapeutic management should be aimed at three goals. The first goal of treatment is to help the person understand the nature of the problem, especially as it relates to the reaction to a specific stressor (if any). An acute onset of a major psychotic episode is a highly disruptive and disturbing event. Any person so affected needs to make sense of the experience. The second goal is rapid reintegration into the environment.

C. OTHER INTERVENTIONS

Third, longer-term goals include the development of coping skills to help prevent subsequent episodes of illness. Because the problem may recur, it is important to help the patient and family recognize early prodromal signs (e.g., sleeplessness) of an impending episode.

Complications/Adverse Outcomes of Treatment

The principal complications of brief psychotic disorder have to do with the disruptions of social function, including employment, that may occur. As a result, rapid but stepwise reintegration is indicated in most patients. Careful attention should be paid to predisposing variables, including ongoing stressors (e.g., relationship stress, especially abuse) and comorbid disorders (e.g., comorbid personality or substance use disorders or medical conditions). Longer-term adverse outcomes may be more related to the outcome of these predisposing variables (especially personality disorder) than to the brief psychotic disorder per se. Some patients will never experience another psychotic event, whereas others will experience recurrences.

Prognosis

By definition, the short-term outcome of this disorder is good, though recurrence of symptoms is common, especially in the face of stressors or comorbid conditions. Long-term antipsychotic management may be indicated in some cases. Table 17–3 summarizes the favorable prognostic indicators of brief psychotic disorder.

Correll CU, Lencz T, Smith CW, et al.: Prospective study of adolescents with subsyndromal psychosis: Characteristics and outcome. *J Child Adolesc Psychopharmacol* 2005;15:418.

Jorgensen P, Bennedsen B, Christensen J, Hyllested A: Acute and transient psychotic disorder: Comorbidity with personality disorder. *Acta Psychiatr Scand* 1996;94:460.

Table 17–3. Favorable Prognostic Indicators of Brief Psychotic Disorder

Good premorbid adjustment
Few premorbid schizoid traits
Severe precipitating stressors
Sudden onset of symptoms
Affective symptoms
Confusion and perplexity during psychosis
Little affective blunting
Short duration of symptoms
Absence of schizophrenic relatives

■ SHARED PSYCHOTIC DISORDER

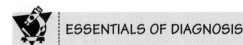 ESSENTIALS OF DIAGNOSIS

DSM-IV-TR Diagnostic Criteria

A. *A delusion develops in the context of a close relationship with another person(s), who has an already-established delusion.*

B. *The delusion is similar in content to that of the person who already has the established delusion.*

C. *The disturbance is not better accounted for by another psychotic disorder (e.g., schizophrenia) or a mood disorder with psychotic features and is not due to the direct physiological effects of a substance (e.g., a drug of abuse, a medication) or a general medical condition.*

(Reprinted, with permission, from the *Diagnostic and Statistical Manual of Mental Disorders*. 4th edn. Text Revision. Washington, DC: American Psychiatric Association, 2000)

General Considerations

A. Epidemiology

The exact frequency of shared psychotic disorder is not known. It may occur with greater frequency in certain groups or situations, especially with social isolation of the involved parties.

B. Etiology

The etiology of shared psychotic disorder is generally thought to be psychological. The dominant, psychotic person simply imposes the delusional belief on the submissive party.

C. Genetics

A genetic predisposition to idiopathic psychoses has been suggested as a possible risk factor for shared psychotic disorder.

Clinical Findings

A. Signs & Symptoms

Shared psychotic disorder, commonly referred to as *folie à deux,* occurs when a delusion develops in a person who has a close relationship with another person who already has a fixed delusion in the context of another psychotic illness such as schizophrenia or delusional disorder. Most often the person experiencing shared psychotic disorder is in a dependent or submissive position. This would include, as examples, the position of a dependent spouse or child of a psychotic person. Most cases involve members of a family, although it may occur in other situations (e.g., religious cults). Moreover, other factors such as old age, social isolation, low intelligence, sensory deprivation, cerebrovascular disease, and alcohol abuse are associated with shared psychotic disorder.

Course of Illness

In shared psychotic disorder, the patients must be separated for treatment purposes. In general, the healthier of the two will give up the delusional belief. The sicker of the two will maintain the false fixed belief.

Differential Diagnosis (Including Comorbid Conditions)

Differential diagnosis should consider the following: Delirium and dementia; alcohol-induced psychotic disorder; intoxications with sympathomimetics (incl. amphetamine, marijuana, L-Dopa); mood disorders; schizophrenia, and malingering and factitious disorders.

Treatment

A. Psychotherapeutic Interventions

In the most common situation, simple separation results in resolution of the delusional belief in the submissive member *(folie imposée)*. Less commonly, the delusion fails to remit in either of the parties at separation *(folie simultanée)*. In the rarest form, the dominant person induces a delusion in a second person, but that person goes on to develop his or her own additional delusional ideation *(folie communiquée)*.

Table 17–4. Principles of Management of Shared Psychotic Disorder

Separate the involved persons. Make an effort to maintain separation if possible.
Hospitalization or alternative community residence (such as respite care) may be needed.
Avoid the use of medications if possible.
Provide ongoing psychological and social support after acute treatment.
Ongoing psychological treatment should focus on the development of coping skills and social independence.
Social monitoring and intervention (including family therapy) are indicated if the patient is going to return to the same environment.

In the latter two conditions, antipsychotic drug therapy may be required to help reduce the psychosis of the submissive person. Table 17–4 summarizes the treatment options.

Mentjox R, van Houten CA, Kooiman CG: Induced psychotic disorder: Clinical aspects, theoretical considerations, and some guidelines for treatment. *Compr Psychiatry* 1993;34:120.

Silveira JM, Seeman MV: Shared psychotic disorder: a critical review of the literature. *Can J Psychiatry* 1995;40:389

■ PSYCHOTIC DISORDER DUE TO A GENERAL MEDICAL CONDITION & SUBSTANCE-INDUCED PSYCHOTIC DISORDER

ESSENTIALS OF DIAGNOSIS

DSM-IV-TR Diagnostic Criteria
Psychotic Disorder Due to a General Medical Condition

A. *Prominent hallucinations or delusions.*

B. *There is evidence from the history, physical examination, or laboratory findings that the disturbance is the direct physiological consequence of a general medical condition.*

C. *The disturbance is not better accounted for by another mental disorder.*

D. *The disturbance does not occur exclusively during the course of a delirium.*

Substance-Induced Psychotic Disorder

A. *Prominent hallucinations or delusions.*

Note: *Do not include hallucinations if the person has insight that they are substance induced.*

B. *There is evidence from the history, physical examination, or laboratory findings of either (1) or (2):*

(1) the symptoms in Criterion A developed during, or within a month of, substance intoxication or withdrawal

(2) medication use is etiologically related to the disturbance

C. *The disturbance is not better accounted for by a psychotic disorder that is not substance induced. Evidence that the symptoms are better accounted for by a psychotic disorder that is not substance induced might include the following: the symptoms precede the onset of the use (or medication use); the symptoms persist for a substantial period of time (e.g., about a month) after the cessation of acute withdrawal or severe intoxication, or are substantially in excess of what would be expected given the duration of use; or there is other evidence that suggests the existence of an independent non-substance-induced psychotic disorder (e.g., a history of recurrent non-substance-related episodes).*

D. *The disturbance does not occur exclusively during the course of delirium.*

(Reprinted, with permission, from the *Diagnostic and Statistical Manual of Mental Disorders*. 4th edn. Text Revision. Washington, DC: American Psychiatric Association, 2000)

General Considerations

Many medical illnesses (Table 17–5) and drugs (Table 17–6) can induce psychotic symptoms. Other medical conditions, toxins, and drugs should be considered with any patient presenting with psychosis or with an exacerbation of a preexisting psychotic disorder. Psychotic conditions related to medical conditions are very common, especially in the hospital setting. Clinicians should be prepared to treat these conditions vigorously.

Clinical Findings

SIGNS & SYMPTOMS

Hallucinations and delusions are common; however, the hallucinations of illness-related psychosis tend to be fairly specific to the underlying illness. For example, olfactory (smell) and gustatory (taste) hallucinations are

Table 17–5. Medical Conditions Associated with Psychotic Symptoms

Brain neoplasm
Cerebrovascular accident
Creutzfeldt–Jakob disease
Encephalitis
Deficiency states (vitamin B12, folate, thiamin, niacin)
Dementias (e.g., Alzheimer disease, Pick disease)
Fabry disease
Fahr disease
Hallervorden–Spatz disease
Heavy metal poisoning
Herpes encephalitis
HIV/AIDS
Huntington disease
Lewy body disease
Metachromatic leukodystrophy
Neurosyphilis
Parkinson disease
Porphyria
Seizure disorder (complex partial seizures)
Systemic lupus erythematosus
Wilson disease

Table 17–6. Drugs Associated with the Induction of Psychosis

Anticholinergics (atropine)
Antidepressants
Dopamine agonists (L-dopa, bromocriptine, pramipexole)
Hallucinogens (D-lysergic acid diethylamide, phencyclidine, cannabis, mescaline)
Histamine-2 antagonists (cimetidine)
Inhalants (toluene)
Psychostimulants (cocaine, amphetamine, sympathomimetics)
Sedative-hypnotic, alcohol, or anxiolytic withdrawal
Sympathomimetics (pseudoephedrine)

associated with basal lesions of the brain or seizure disorders involving the temporal lobe or hippocampus. Alcohol or other sedative withdrawal may result in tactile (touch) hallucinations. Visual hallucinations may be reported in psychotic states induced by dopamine agonists,

Table 17–7. Management of Psychotic Disorder Due to Medical Condition and Substance-Induced Psychotic Disorder

Evaluate all acutely psychotic patients for medical or substance-induced causes, even those with chronic psychotic conditions.
Identify and vigorously treat the underlying medical or substance use disorder (including withdrawal).
Minimize exposure to all drugs.
Judiciously use antipsychotics or sedatives (including benzodiazepines).
Drug management may include low-dose typical (e.g., haloperidol 0.5–2 mg/d) or atypical (e.g., risperidone 0.5–2 mg/d, olanzapine 2.5–5 mg/d) antipsychotics or low-dose, short-acting benzodiazepines (e.g., alprazolam, lorazepam 0.25–1 mg/d).
Lower the dose or discontinue psychotropic medications as soon as possible.
Longer-term management should focus on the vigorous treatment of the underlying condition. In addition, special attention should be paid to sleep hygiene.

sympathomimetics, anticholinergics, or hallucinogenic drugs.

Treatment

A. PSYCHOTHERAPEUTIC INTERVENTIONS

The management of these disorders requires identification and aggressive management of the underlying illness or drug that has induced the psychosis (Table 17–7).

B. PSYCHOPHARMACOLOGIC INTERVENTIONS

In addition, antipsychotics may be required to treat the psychotic symptoms acutely. Generally, elimination of the offending illness or drug will resolve the psychotic state. Drug treatment should be conservative and targeted to the offending symptoms, such as psychosis, insomnia, or agitation.

PROGNOSIS

The long-term prognosis of these conditions relates to the course of the underlying illness. Psychosis in the face of medical conditions does not portend a favorable outcome in many patients, and may be seen in parallel with delirium, a poor prognostic feature. In addition, psychosis may recur if the fundamental medical disorder recurs.

Fricchione GL, Carbone L, Bennett WI: Psychotic disorder caused by a general medical condition, with delusions. Secondary "organic" delusional syndromes. *Psychiatr Clin North Am* 1995;18:363

PSYCHOTIC DISORDER NOT OTHERWISE SPECIFIED (NOS)

Certain psychotic states cannot be classified into one of the foregoing categories of psychoses and are referred to as psychotic disorder NOS.

 ESSENTIALS OF DIAGNOSIS

DSM-IV-TR Diagnostic Criteria
This category includes psychotic symptomatology (i.e., delusions, hallucinations, disorganized speech, grossly disorganized or catatonic behavior) about which there is inadequate information to make a specific diagnosis or about which there is contradictory information, or disorders with psychotic symptoms that do not meet the criteria for any specific psychotic disorder. Examples include:

(1) Postpartum psychosis that does not meet criteria for mood disorder with psychotic features, brief psychotic disorder, psychotic disorder due to a general disorder

(2) Psychotic symptoms that have lasted for less than 1 month but that have not yet remitted, so that the criteria for brief psychotic disorder are not met

(3) Persistent auditory hallucinations in the absence of any other features

(4) Persistent nonbizarre delusions with periods of overlapping mood episodes that have been present for a substantial portion of the delusional disturbance

(5) Situations in which the clinician has concluded that a psychotic disorder is present, but is unable to determine whether it is primary, due to a general medical condition, or substance induced

(Reprinted, with permission, from the *Diagnostic and Statistical Manual of Mental Disorders*. 4th edn. Text Revision. Washington, DC: American Psychiatric Association, 2000)

Kendler KS, Walsh D: Schizophreniform disorder, delusional disorder and psychotic disorder not otherwise specified: Clinical features, outcome and familial psychopathology. *Acta Psychiatr Scand* 1995;91:370.

OTHER SPECIFIED OR CULTURE-BOUND PSYCHOTIC DISORDERS

Several psychotic disorders have specific presentations or are contained within certain demographic groups. These disorders are widely recognized but are not accorded formal diagnostic status in DSM-IV-TR.

1. Capgras Syndrome (delusion of doubles)

This disorder represents a fixed belief that familiar persons have been replaced by identical imposters who behave identically to the original person.

2. Lycanthropy

This is a delusion that the person is a werewolf or other animal.

3. Frégoli Phenomenon

In this delusion, a persecutor (who usually is following the person) changes faces or makeup to avoid detection.

4. Cotard Syndrome (délire de négation)

A false perception of having lost everything, including money, status, strength, health, but also internal organs. This may be seen in schizophrenia or psychotic depression and responds to treatment of the underlying condition.

5. Autoscopic Psychosis

The main symptom is a visual hallucination of a transparent phantom of one's own body.

6. Koro

This disorder in males is characterized by a sudden belief that the penis is shrinking and may disappear into the abdomen. An associated feature may be the belief that when this occurs the person will die. A similar condition may be seen in women with fears of the loss of the genitals or breasts. Although this problem is seen more commonly in Asia, presentations in Western countries occur occasionally.

7. Amok

The amok syndrome consists of an abrupt onset of unprovoked and uncontrolled rage in which the affected person may run about savagely attacking and even killing people and animals in his or her way. It is seen most often in Malayan natives but has been reported in other cultures. In some circumstances, this problem is observed in individuals with preexisting psychotic disorders.

8. Piblokto (Arctic hysteria)

This disorder occurs among the Eskimos and is characterized by a sudden onset of screaming, crying, and tearing off of clothes. The affected person may then run or roll about in the snow. It usually resolves rapidly, and the person will usually have no memory of the event.

9. Windigo (Witigo)

Specific North American Indian tribes, including the Cree and Ojibwa, manifest this rare psychotic state.

People affected may believe that they are possessed by a demon or monster that murders and eats human flesh. Trivial symptoms including hunger or nausea may induce intense agitation because of a fear of transformation into the demon.

Bernstein RL, Gaw AC: Koro: Proposed classification for DSM-IV. *Am J Psychiatry* 1990;147:1670.

Berrios GE, Luque R: Cotard's syndrome: Analysis of 100 cases. *Acta Psychiatr Scand* 1995;91:185.

Koehler K, Ebel H, Vartzopoulos D: Lycanthropy and demonomania: Some psychopathological issues. *Psychol Med* 1990;20: 629.

Kon Y: Amok. *Br J Psychiatry* 1994;165:685.

Mojtabai R: Fregoli syndrome. *Aust N Z J Psychiatry* 1994;28: 458.

Mood Disorders

18

Peter T. Loosen, MD, PhD, & Richard C. Shelton, MD

■ MAJOR DEPRESSIVE DISORDER

ESSENTIALS OF DIAGNOSIS

DSM-IV-TR Diagnostic Criteria
Major Depressive Episode

A. *Five (or more) of the following symptoms have been present during the same 2-week period and represent a change from previous functioning; at least one of the symptoms is either (1) depressed mood or (2) loss of interest or pleasure.*

Note: *Do not include symptoms that are clearly due to a general medical condition, or mood-incongruent delusions and hallucinations.*

(1) depressed mood
(2) markedly diminished interest or pleasure
(3) significant weight loss when not dieting or weight gain, or decrease or increase in appetite
(4) insomnia or hypersomnia
(5) psychomotor agitation or retardation
(6) fatigue or loss of energy
(7) feelings of worthlessness or excessive or inappropriate guilt
(8) diminished ability to think or concentrate, or indecisiveness
(9) recurrent thoughts of death or suicide

B. *The symptoms do not meet criteria for a Mixed Episode.*

C. *The symptoms cause significant distress or impairment in social, occupational, or other important areas of functioning.*

D. *The symptoms are not due to the direct physiological effects of a substance (e.g., a drug of abuse, a medication) or a general medical condition (e.g., hypothyroidism).*

E. *The symptoms are not better accounted for by Bereavement, i.e., after the loss of a loved one, the symptoms persist for longer than 2 months and are characterized by marked functional impairment, morbid preoccupation with worthlessness, suicidal ideation, psychotic symptoms, or psychomotor retardation.*

(Adapted, with permission, from *the Diagnostic and Statistical Manual of Mental Disorders,* 4th edn., Text Revision. Washington DC: American Psychiatric Association, 2000.)

General Considerations

A. EPIDEMIOLOGY

The separation into bipolar and non-bipolar disorder has proved clinically and diagnostically useful. It is supported by family studies, twin studies, and biological studies. It is supported further by differential clinical responses to treatment and differential disease onsets and outcomes. To these factors, we can add the epidemiologic risk factors detailed in Table 18–1.

Symptoms and disorders of the depression spectrum are rather common. Lifetime prevalence rates for significant depressive symptoms are 13–20% and for major depressive disorder 3.7–6.7%. Major depressive disorder is about two to three times as common in adolescent and adult females as in adolescent and adult males. In prepubertal children, boys and girls are affected equally. Rates in women and men are highest in the 25–44-year-old age group.

Boyd JH, Weissman MM: Epidemiology. In: Paykel ES (ed). *Handbook of Affective Disorders.* New York: Guilford Press, 1982, pp. 109–125.
Weissman MN, Livingston Bruce M, Leaf PJ, Florio LP, Holzer C: Affective Disorders. In: Robins LN, Regier DA (eds). *Psychiatric Disorders in America.* New York: Free Press, 1991, pp. 53–80.

B. ETIOLOGY

Despite intensive attempts to establish its etiologic or pathophysiologic basis, the precise cause of major

Table 18–1. Risk Factors for Major Depressive Disorder

Family history	High risk in families with history of depression (7%) or alcoholism (8%)
Social class	No relationship
Race	May be less common in African Americans
Life events	Recent negative life events may precede episode
Personality	Insecure, worried, introverted, stress sensitive, obsessive, unassertive, dependent
Childhood experience	Early childhood trauma (e.g., significant loss, disruptive, hostile, negative environment)
Postpartum	Depressive episodes common
Menopause	No relationship
Social network	Relative lack of interpersonal relationships

depressive disorder is not known. There is consensus that multiple etiologic factors—genetic, biochemical, psychodynamic, and socioenvironmental—may interact in complex ways and that the modern-day understanding of depressive disorder requires an understanding of the interrelationships among these factors.

1. Life events—Recent evidence confirms that crucial life events, particularly the death or loss of a loved one, can precede the onset of depression. However, such losses precede only a small (though substantial) number of cases of depression. Fewer than 20% of individuals experiencing losses become clinically depressed. Although other major life events may occur prior to the onset of depression, many patients become depressed with little or no apparent provocation. These observations argue strongly for a predisposing factor, probably genetic, developmental, or temperamental in nature.

2. Biological theories

i. Neurotransmitters—Associations between mood and monoamines (i.e., norepinephrine, serotonin, and dopamine) were first indicated serendipitously by the mood-altering effects of isoniazid (used initially for the treatment of tuberculosis) and later by reports that isoniazid (a monoamine oxidase inhibitor [MAOI]) affects monoamine concentrations in the brains of laboratory animals. We now know that all clinically-effective antidepressants affect postsynaptic signaling of serotonin, norepinephrine, or both at the postsynaptic membrane. This action has led to the hypothesis that depression is caused by a neurotransmitter deficiency and that antidepressants exert their clinical effect by treating this imbalance.

In the late 1970s, emphasis shifted from acute presynaptic to delayed postsynaptic receptor—mediated events after it was shown that most chronic antidepressant treatments (including pharmacotherapy and electroconvulsive therapy [ECT]) cause subsensitivity of the norepinephrine receptor—coupled adenylate cyclase system in brain. This desensitization of norepinephrine receptor systems was linked to a decrease in the density of β–adrenoceptors. More importantly, it paralleled the delayed onset of action common to all antidepressants. More recent concepts have evolved from the original deficiency hypotheses, emphasizing the integration of multiple intracellular signals that regulate neuronal response (i.e., changes in G protein, cyclic adenosine monophosphate, or protein kinase and the induction of gene transcription). These cellular mechanisms are thought to ultimately affect the expression of specific genes. Therefore, abnormalities of intracellular signal transduction and/or gene expression are now thought to underlie the physiology of depression. Other neurotransmitters (e.g., acetylcholine, gamma amino butyric acid, melatonin, glycine, histamine), hormones (e.g., thyroid and adrenal hormones), and neuropeptides (e.g., corticotropin-releasing hormone, endorphins, enkephalins, vasopressin, cholecystokinin, substance P) may play significant roles in the modulation of mood.

ii. Neuroendocrine factors—Emotional trauma sometimes immediately precedes the onset of depression. Emotional trauma can also precede the onset of endocrine disorders such as hyperthyroidism and Cushing's disease, both of which are commonly associated with psychological disturbance, most commonly in mood and cognition. When endocrine changes are associated with psychological disturbance it is often unclear whether such changes are precipitants, perpetuating influences, or secondary effects.

The two endocrine systems most extensively studied in psychiatry are the hypothalamic-pituitary-adrenal (HPA) axis and the hypothalamic-pituitary-thyroid (HPT) axis. About half of patients with major depression exhibit cortisol hypersecretion that returns to normal once the depression is cured. The evidence of cortisol hypersecretion includes increased adrenocorticotropin (ACTH) secretion, increased plasma concentration and urinary excretion of cortisol and its metabolites, alterations in the normal circadian rhythm of cortisol secretion, relative resistance to glucocorticoid negative feedback inhibition of ACTH secretion, and blunted ACTH responses to corticotropin-releasing hormone. However, not all depressed patients exhibit evidence of significant hypercortisolism. Several studies have attempted to document the psychological effects of manipulating plasma glucocorticoid concentrations in depressed patients. They reported antidepressant effects in some depressed patients after administration of such antiglucorticoid medications as aminoglutethimide, metyrapone, and ketokonazole.

Human studies have also demonstrated a profound effect of thyroid hormones on brain development, maturation, and connectivity. The effects of thyroid hormones on mature brain function, as they pertain to mood, are less marked. The most common effects are as follows: (1) Depression and cognitive decline are the most frequently observed psychiatric symptoms in patients who have adult hypothyroidism, (2) A small dose of thyroid hormone, preferably triiodothyronine (T_3), will accelerate the therapeutic effect of various antidepressants, particularly in women, and can convert antidepressant nonresponders into responders in both sexes, (3) Most longitudinal studies have revealed dynamic reductions in serum thyroxine (T_4) concentrations in depressed patients during a wide range of somatic treatments, including various antidepressants, lithium, sleep deprivation, and ECT, (4) Administration of thyrotropin-releasing hormone (TRH) may induce an increased sense of well-being and relaxation in normal subjects and in patients with neurologic and psychiatric disease, especially depression, and (5) Although overt thyroid disease is rare in major depression, subtle forms of thyroid dysfunction are common—for example, absence or flattening of the diurnal thyroid-stimulating hormone (TSH) curve, often caused by a reduction in the nocturnal TSH surge; a blunted TSH response after administration of TRH (discussed in greater detail later in this section); and subclinical hypothyroidism or positive antithyroid antibodies.

iii. Early Life Stress—In recent years, an increasing number of studies have evaluated both the immediate and long-term neurobiological effects of early childhood trauma (e.g., physical or emotional abuse, neglect, or parental loss). Studies of traumatized persons or animal models of early life stress suggest long-lasting effects on neuroendocrine, psychophysiological, and neurochemical systems. Together, these effects may present the biological basis of an enhanced risk for psychopathology, including depression. In addition to having added childhood trauma to the existing list of risk factors for depression, these studies have created a burgeoning awareness and consensus that the high number of children who are exposed in our society to early trauma is unacceptable. Hopefully, further studies may elucidate the many factors that determine individual vulnerability or resilience to the neurobiological effects of early trauma and help to prevent their deleterious neurobiological and psychopathological consequences.

Ahmed N, Loosen PT: Thyroid hormones in major depressive and bipolar disorders. In: Casper R (ed). *Women's Health*

and Emotion. England: Cambridge University Press, 1997, pp. 83–108.

Goodwin FK, Jamison KR: *Manic Depressive Illness.* New York: Oxford University Press, 1990.

Heim C, Nemeroff CB: Neurobiology of early life stress: Clinical studies. *Semin Clin Neuropsych* 2002;7:147.

Loosen PT: Hormones of the hypothalamic-pituitary-thyroid axis: A psychoneuroendocrine perspective. *Pharmacopsychiatry* 1986;19:401.

Flores BH, Musselman DL, DeBattista C, Garlow SJ, Schatzberg AF, Nemeroff CB: Biology of mood disorders. In: Schatzberg AF, Nemeroff CB (eds). *Textbook of Psychopharmacology,* 3rd edn. Washington, DC: American Psychiatric Press, 2004, pp. 717–763.

Nemeroff CB, Loosen PT (eds): *Handbook of Clinical Psychoneuroendocrinology.* New York: Guilford Press: 1987, pp. 384–396.

Pearson Murphy BE: Steroids and depression. *J Steroid Biochem Mol Biol* 1991;38:537.

Wolkowitz OM, Reus VI: Treatment of depression with antiglucocortoid drugs. *Psychosom Med* 1999;61:698.

Wolkowitz OM, Rothschild AJ (eds): *Psychoneuroendocrinology.* Arlington, VA: American Psychiatric Publishing, 2003.

3. Psychosocial theories

i. Psychoanalytic and psychodynamic models—In the early 20th century, psychoanalytic interpretations of mental illness were prominent. Karl Abraham (1911) wrote the first important psychoanalytic paper on depression, stating that depression is unconsciously motivated and the result of repressed sexual and aggressive drives. Concurrent writings of Sigmund Freud suggested that depression and, to a lesser extent, mania were understood as precipitated by loss and manifested by regressions to anal and oral phases of libidinal development. These regressions in adult life resulted from an unfortunate combination of predisposition (constitutional overaccentuation of oral eroticism) and critical childhood disappointments. Armed with Freud's concepts on the role of introjection in normal mourning and in melancholia, Abraham wrote of the "severe conflict of ambivalent feelings from which [the patient] can only escape by turning against himself the hostility he originally felt towards his object."

The precepts that depression is the result of a loss and that it symptomatically represents "anger turned against the self" are part of the enduring legacy of classic psychoanalytic thinking. Freud believed that the real, threatened, or imagined loss of a narcissistic object choice (meaning that the individual's love of the object was equivalent to love of the self) would trigger a withdrawal of libido away from the object and back into the self through introjection of the ambivalently cathected object. The patient then would attack himself (depressive symptoms) as though for misdeeds that were the doing of the lost object. In other words, the depressed patient experiences a loss as a narcissistic wound; suicide becomes an unconscious attempt to destroy the now hated object that dwells in the patient's ego by means of introjection. Like Abraham, Freud also emphasized the importance of somatic factors in predisposing the individual to depression and in the clinical picture itself. Diurnal variation of mood, for example, was beyond psychological explanation. Later psychoanalytic writers (e.g., M. Klein, D. W. Winicott, E. Bibring) sought to expand on Freud's thinking, incorporating further developments in ego-psychology, object relations theory, and self-psychology. Although widely held, traditional psychodynamic theories have not held up to careful study. Moreover, psychoanalysis or most forms of psychodynamic therapy either have not been formally tested or have not been shown to be more effective than simple interpersonal contact.

ii. Behavioral models—In the mid-1900s, three models based on behavioral theory emerged (see Chapter 10). Peter Lewinsohn showed that depression can be caused by inadequate or insufficient positive reinforcement. In everyday life, this can occur in two main ways: (1) if an environment lacks positive reinforcement (e.g., through individual or mass unemployment) or (2) if the person is not able to take advantage of reinforcement (e.g., through isolation induced by poor social skills). Inadequate positive reinforcement may lead to a self-perpetuating cycle consisting of dysphoria, a reduction in behaviors that would normally obtain the reinforcement, lowered self-esteem and increased hopelessness, and increased isolation.

Martin Seligman developed the theory of learned helplessness as he was searching for an animal model of depression. Laboratory animals given random shocks from which they cannot escape develop apathy to any stimulus. Generalizing this observation to humans, Seligman's theory suggests that depression can result from situations in which a person has lost (actual or imagined) control over negative life events.

The cognitive-behavioral model of depression developed by Aaron Beck suggests that depression develops when the patient cognitively misinterprets life events. The conceptual core of this model consists of the cognitive triad of depression: (1) a negative self-view (i.e., "things are bad because I am bad"), (2) a negative interpretation of experience (i.e., "everything has always been bad"), and (3) a negative view of the future (i.e., "everything will always be bad"). It is a basic tenet of this theory that a depressed person interprets the world through depressive schemata that distort experiences in a negative direction. Typical cognitive distortions include arbitrary inference (in which the person assumes a negative event was caused by himself or herself), selective abstraction (in which the person focuses on the negative element in an otherwise positive set of information), magnification and minimization (in which the person overemphasizes

negatives and underemphasizes positives), and inexact labeling (in which the person gives a distorted label to an event and then reacts to the label rather than to the event).

Beck AT: Cognitive therapy. A 30 year retrospective. *Am Psychol* 1991;46:368.

Freud S: Mourning and melancholia (1917). In Strachey J (ed & trans). *Standard Edition of the Complete Psychological Works of Sigmund Freud,* Vol 14. London: Hogarth, 1957, pp. 237–260.

Roose S: Depression. In Nersessian E, Kopff R (eds). *Textbook of Psychoanalysis.* Washington, DC: American Psychiatric Press, 1996, pp. 301–318.

C. GENETICS

Mood disorders are familial, but the exact mode of transmission is not understood (see Chapter 3).

Clinical Findings

A. SIGNS & SYMPTOMS

1. Major depressive episode—The cardinal feature of a major depressive episode is a depressed mood or the loss of interest or pleasure (see items *i* and *ii* below) that predominates for at least 2 weeks and causes significant distress or impairment in the individual's social, occupational, or other important areas of functioning. During this time, the individual must also exhibit at least four additional symptoms (i.e., other than depressed mood or anhedonia), drawn from the following common features of depression:

i. Depressed mood—Depressed mood is the most characteristic symptom, occurring in over 90% of patients. The patient usually describes himself or herself as feeling sad, low, empty, hopeless, gloomy, or down in the dumps. The quality of mood is likely to be portrayed as different from a normal sense of sadness or grief. The physician often observes changes in the patient's posture, speech, facies (e.g., a melancholic expression known as facies melancholica), dress, and grooming consistent with the patient's self-report. Many depressed patients state that they are unable to cry, whereas others report frequent weeping spells that occur without significant precipitants.

A small percentage of patients do not report a depressed mood, sometimes referred to as **masked depression**. These patients are usually brought to their physician by the family members/coworkers who have noticed the patients' social withdrawal or decreased activity. Patients may associate depression with feelings of sadness. However, depression as often involves emotional numbness or lack of positive reactivity. Similarly, some children and adolescents do not exhibit a sad demeanor, presenting instead as irritable.

ii. Anhedonia—An inability to enjoy usual activities is almost universal among depressed patients. The patient or his or her family may report markedly diminished interest in all, or almost all, activities previously enjoyed such as sex, hobbies, and daily routines.

iii. Change in appetite—About 70% of patients observe a reduction in appetite with accompanying weight loss; only a minority of patients experience an increase in appetite, often associated with cravings for particular foods such as sweets.

iv. Change in sleep—About 80% of depressed patients complain of some type of sleep disturbance, the most common being insomnia. Insomnia is usually classified as initial (i.e., problems in falling asleep), middle (i.e., problems of staying asleep with frequent awakenings throughout the night), or late (i.e., early morning awakening). The most common and unpleasant form of sleep disturbance in major depressive disorder is late insomnia, with awakenings in the early morning (usually around 4–5 AM) and significant worsening of depressive symptoms in the first part of the day. In contrast, initial insomnia is especially common in those with significant comorbid anxiety. Some patients complain of hypersomnia rather than insomnia; hypersomnia is common in atypical depression and seasonal affective disorder (SAD) and is often associated with hyperphagia.

v. Change in body activity—About one-half of depressed patients develop a slowing, or retardation, of their normal level of activity. They may exhibit a slowness in thinking, speaking, or body movement or a decrease in volume or content of speech, with long pauses before answering. In about 75% of depressed women and 50% of depressed men, anxiety is expressed in the form of psychomotor agitation, with pacing, an inability to sit still, and hand-wringing.

vi. Loss of energy—Almost all depressed patients report a significant loss of energy (anergia), unusual fatigue or tiredness, and a general lack of efficiency even in small or elementary tasks.

vii. Feelings of worthlessness and excessive or inappropriate guilt—A depressed individual may experience a marked (and often unrealistic) decrease in self-esteem. In European cultures, well over half of depressed patients exhibit some guilt, ranging from a vague feeling that their current condition is the result of something they have done, to frank delusions and hallucinations of poverty or of having committed an unpardonable sin. In other cultures, shame or humiliation is experienced.

viii. Indecisiveness or decreased concentration—About one-half of depressed patients complain of or exhibit a slowing of thought. They may feel that they are not able to think as well as before, that they cannot concentrate, or that they are easily distracted. Frequently they will doubt their ability to make good judgments and find themselves unable to make even small decisions. On formal psychological testing, the patient's accuracy is usually retained, but speed and performance are slow. In severe forms, called **pseudodementia**, particularly among the elderly, memory deficits may be mistaken for early signs of dementia. In contrast to dementia, pseudodementia usually reverses after treatment of the underlying depression. However, when cognitive symptoms are comorbid with depression, they may represent an emerging dementia that can still be present after the depression has resolved.

ix. Suicidal ideation—Many depressed individuals experience recurrent thoughts of death, ranging from transient feelings that others would be better off without them, to the actual planning and implementing of suicide.

Suicide is the eighth leading cause of death in the United States, accounting for more than 30,000 deaths each year. Major depression accounts for roughly 50% of suicides, and 15% of patients with depression eventually die by suicide. The risk of suicide is present throughout a depressive episode but is probably highest immediately after initiation of treatment and during the 6–9-month period following symptomatic recovery. Table 18–2 lists common predictors of suicide risk.

Alcohol and drug dependence account for roughly 25% of suicides, and psychosis is present in 10% of suicides. For each person who completes suicide, 8–10 people attempt suicide, and for every completed suicide, 18–20 attempts are made. Patients with a history of suicide attempts account for 50% of completed suicides. Medical illnesses are associated with as many as 35–40%

Table 18–2. Factors Associated with Elevated Risk of Suicide

Older than 45 yr, male, white (i.e., risk is greater in males, especially white males, where it appears to increase with age)
Prior suicide attempt or history of other self-injury
Family history of suicide or psychiatric illness
Recent severe loss
Present or anticipated poor health
Detailed plan
Inability to accept help
Lack of available support from society (e.g., living alone, unemployment)
Psychotic symptoms
Comorbid alcoholism or drug abuse

of suicides, and with as many as 70% of suicides occurring in those over the age of 60 years. As much as 10% of general medical admissions result from failed suicide attempts.

2. Melancholic subtype—The diagnosis of major depression with melancholic features is made when the patient has either loss of pleasure in all, or almost all, activities, or lack of reactivity to usually pleasurable stimuli, along with three or more of the following: (1) distinct quality of depressed mood (i.e., the mood is different than that experienced after the loss of a loved one); (2) depression regularly worse in the morning, (3) early morning awakening (at least 2 hours prior to the usual time of awakening), (4) marked psychomotor retardation or agitation, (5) significant anorexia or weight loss, and (6) excessive or inappropriate guilt. Other characteristics sometimes associated with melancholia include the absence of personality disturbance before first episode, the occurrence of one or more previous episodes followed by complete remission, and prior good response to specific and adequate somatic antidepressant therapy (e.g., ECT, tricyclic antidepressants [TCAs], MAOIs, lithium).

3. Atypical depression—Although the term depression often calls to mind the pattern of symptoms associated with melancholia (especially insomnia and loss of appetite), some patients experience a reversed pattern – that is, symptoms that are opposite to those seen in melancholia. The *Diagnostic and Statistical Manual of Mental Disorders*, fourth edition (DSM-IV) diagnostic criteria for major depression with atypical features include mood reactivity (that is, mood that brightens in response to a positive event) along with two or more of the following: (1) significant weight gain or increase in appetite, (2) hypersomnia, (3) leaden paralysis (i.e., heavy, leaden feelings in arms or legs), (4) a long-standing pattern of sensitivity to real or perceived interpersonal rejection (that are not limited to episodes of mood disturbance) that results in significant social or occupational impairment. In the case of rejection sensitivity, emotional reactions may occur after imagined, anticipated, or real rejection by others and may be extreme at times. This diagnostic subcategory was derived in the 1960's by British psychiatrists based on differential responses to TCAs and MAOIs. They posited that melancholic depression responded preferentially to the former, while atypical depression to the latter. Subsequent research has confirmed that persons with atypical features respond better to MAOIs than to tricyclics.

4. Seasonal affective disorder—Occasionally patients experience depressive episodes at characteristic times of the year. Most commonly the episodes of SAD begin in fall or winter and remit in spring, but occasionally they can also be observed in summer. SAD with prevalence during the winter months (winter depression) appears to vary with latitude, age, and sex. SAD is more common in higher latitudes (i.e., closer to the north or south poles) and among younger people, particularly in females. SAD is characterized clinically by hypersomnia, anergia, and a craving for sweets. SAD responds particularly well to light therapy and typically to serotonergic agents (i.e., selective serotonin reuptake inhibitors [SSRIs]).

The seasonal pattern specifier is given if all of the following are true: (1) there has been a regular temporal relationship between the onset of major depressive episodes in bipolar I or bipolar II disorder or major depressive disorder, recurrent, and a particular time of the year (e.g., fall or spring), (2) full remissions (or a change from depression to mania or hypomania) also occur at a characteristic time of the year.

B. PSYCHOLOGICAL TESTING

Psychological testing has not been found useful in aiding the diagnosis of major depressive disorder.

C. LABORATORY FINDINGS & IMAGING

No laboratory findings are diagnostic of a major depressive episode; however, several laboratory findings are abnormal in some patients with major depression, compared to the general population. It appears that most laboratory abnormalities are state dependent (i.e., they occur while patients are depressed), but some findings may precede the onset of an episode or persist after its remission.

1. HPA axis

i. Dexamethasone suppression test—Although the dexamethasone suppression test (DST) has little use as a clinical marker for depression, it is worth mentioning some of the more pertinent DST findings: (1) The overall sensitivity (i.e., positive DST outcome) was 44% among all patients with major depression given 1 mg dexamethasone; sensitivity was significantly higher (65%) in elderly depressed patients but dropped to 31% in a smaller group of patients who received 2 mg of dexamethasone, (2) Within the depression spectrum, the rates of DST nonsuppression increased strikingly from grief reactions (10%) and dysthymic disorders (23%), to major depressive disorders (44%), major depressive disorders with melancholia (50%), psychotic affective disorders (69%), and depression with serious suicidality (78%), (3) In some depressed patients, the DST allowed researchers to predict or monitor long-term treatment outcome, (4) DST-positive patients appeared to respond more favorably to biological interventions such as antidepressants or ECT, (5) Among depressed patients, abnormal DST results correlated mostly with initial insomnia, weight loss, loss of sexual interest, ruminative thinking, and psychomotor retardation or agitation, and (6) HPA axis dysregulation contributed to cognitive dysfunction, although it is not known whether hypercortisolemia and cognitive impairment in depression are related indirectly or causally.

A hyperactive HPA axis has been observed in stroke patients with major depression; in pain patients with major depression; and in patients with anorexia nervosa, bulimia nervosa, alcoholism, obsessive–compulsive disorder, or anxiety disorders. It has not been observed in schizophrenic patients.

ii. Corticotropin-releasing hormone test—A blunted adrenocorticotropic hormone response after corticotropin-releasing hormone administration is another HPA axis abnormality commonly observed in major depression.

2. HPT axis

i. T4 concentrations—Most depressed patients appear to be euthyroid; however, longitudinal studies consistently found significant serum T_4 reductions during a wide range of somatic treatments, including various antidepressants, lithium, sleep deprivation, or ECT. Evidence indicates that the T_4 reduction was greater in treatment responders than in nonresponders. It is not known whether the initial T_4 increase in depression is part of the pathophysiology of the illness, or whether it is a compensatory mechanism by which the organism delivers thyroid hormone to the brain.

ii. Subclinical hypothyroidism—Subtle thyroid dysfunctions are common in depression. Between 1% and 4% of patients show evidence of overt hypothyroidism, and between 4% and 40% show evidence of subclinical hypothyroidism. Comorbid subclinical hypothyroidism can be associated with cognitive dysfunction or with a diminished response to standard psychiatric treatments. Some depressed patients with subclinical hypothyroidism may respond behaviorally to thyroid hormone substitution.

iii. TRH test—The TRH test (i.e., measurement of serum TSH following TRH administration) has been used widely in psychiatry. More than 3000 patients have been studied, the majority of whom had major depressive disorder. Approximately 30% of patients had a blunted TSH response during depression, and a smaller number showed TSH blunting during remission; however, definitions of TSH blunting have varied among studies, different assays have been used, and a standard amount of TRH has not always been injected.

There appears to be no association between the TRH-induced TSH response and (1) the patient's body surface or age, (2) serum thyroid hormone or cortisol concentrations, (3) severity of depression, or (4) previous intake of antidepressant drugs (excluding long-term lithium administration). Further, the TRH test does not aid in the distinction between primary and secondary depression or between unipolar and bipolar subgroups. Preliminary evidence suggests that TSH blunting may be associated with a more prolonged course of depression and with a history of violent suicidal behavior.

Within psychiatric disorders, TSH blunting can also occur in some patients who have borderline personality disorder, anorexia nervosa, panic disorder, primary degenerative dementia, chronic pain, premenstrual syndrome, or alcoholism, both during acute withdrawal and after prolonged abstinence. The absence of TSH blunting in both schizophrenic patients and phobic patients during exposure therapy suggests that the abnormality is not a mere correlate of mental distress.

3. Sleep electroencephalogram—Most depressed patients have insomnia. Sleep problems commonly reported include interruptions throughout the night, early morning awakenings, and less frequently, difficulty falling asleep. Sleep electroencephalogram (EEG) recordings reveal the following: (1) a shortened rapid eye movement (REM) latency (i.e., a shorter than normal interval between sleep onset and first REM period), more common in elderly depressed patients and often associated with unipolar depression; (2) a shift of slow-wave sleep (i.e., sleep stages 3 and 4), normally occurring during the first non-REM period, into the second non-REM period; and (3) an increased REM density (i.e., more frequent REM episodes) during the first few hours of sleep.

Because most of these sleep EEG abnormalities can be found in other illnesses, and some accompany normal aging, there is no agreement as to whether these abnormalities constitute diagnostic markers of depression or whether they reflect abnormal functioning in sleep-related processes but lack diagnostic specificity (see Chapter 27). There is evidence that EEG sleep variables are normal in depressed patients 6 months after an acute episode.

4. Brain imaging—The rapidly increasing sophistication of neuroimaging techniques has improved our understanding of the neural substrates of emotion and its disorders. Neuroimaging studies have been particularly useful in characterizing the circuitry underlying emotional disorders.

Mood disorders may be associated with global and regional changes in cerebral blood flow and metabolism. Global cerebral blood flow and glucose metabolism appear normal, but may be decreased in late life depression. Decreased prefrontal cortex (PFC), especially left PFC, blood flow and metabolism in depressed unipolar patients are the most consistently replicated findings; there is preliminary evidence that they may correlate with severity of illness and cognitive impairment. Basal ganglia abnormalities have also been found in depressed unipolar patients, involving decreased blood flow and metabolism. Increased activity of amygdala is also observed. Other neuroimaging studies in major depression point to abnormalities in the hippocampus, cingulate, and related parts of the striatum and thalamus. These data suggest a neural model in which dysfunction of limbic, striatal, and PFC structures impair the modulation of the amygdala/hippocampus complex, leading to abnormal processing of emotional stimuli.

In unipolar depression, little is known about the state or trait characteristics of these findings, as the exact relationships between functional neuroimaging findings and clinical course has not been systematically investigated. Depression also tends to be associated with lesions in the left frontotemporal or right parieto-occipital regions. This concept is consistent with neuroanatomical and behavioral findings in stroke patients. Patients with dominant anterior or nondominant posterior strokes are especially vulnerable to secondary depressions, whereas patients with nondominant anterior or dominant posterior strokes are especially vulnerable to mania or hypomania.

D. COURSE OF ILLNESS

Major depressive disorder may be preceded by dysthymic disorder (10% in community samples, and 15–25% in clinical samples). Table 18–14 summarizes the course and prognosis of both non-bipolar disorders and bipolar disorders.

Major depressive disorder may begin at any age, with an average age at onset in the mid-teens to late 20s. Symptoms typically develop over days to weeks, and prodromal symptoms and preexisting comorbid conditions (e.g., generalized anxiety, panic attacks, phobias) are common. Although some patients have only a single episode, with full return to premorbid functioning, approximately 50% of patients with such episodes will eventually have another episode, at which time they will meet criteria for recurrent depression.

The course of recurrent depression is variable. Some patients have a few isolated episodes separated by stable intervals (years) of normal functioning. Others have clusters of episodes, and still others have increasingly frequent episodes with shortening of the interepisode interval and generally increased disease severity. Some patients experience a major depression without full remission before the next; this is referred to as major depression without interepisode recovery. About 50% of patients with one depressive episode will have a recurrence, and about 90% of patients who have had three episodes can be expected to have a fourth. Thus the number of past episodes can serve as a predictor of the future (i.e., as the number of recurrences increases, the episodes lengthen in duration and increase in both frequency and intensity). The average number of lifetime episodes is around five. About 5–10% of patients with an initial diagnosis of major depressive disorder subsequently develop a manic episode.

Depressive episodes may remit completely, partially, or not at all. The patient's functioning usually returns to the premorbid level between episodes, but 20–35% of patients show persistent residual symptoms and social or occupational impairment. Data from the prepsychopharmacology era (i.e., before 1960) suggest that, if untreated, a depressive episode may last about 12 months. Relapse is common. Almost 25% of patients relapse within the first 6 months of remission, especially if they have discontinued their antidepressant medications; 30–50% relapse in the first 2 years; and 50–75% relapse within the first 5 years. The risk of relapse during early remission can be reduced significantly by maintaining patients on antidepressants for at least 6 months—a regimen now generally viewed as important in managing the recurring nature of the illness.

A major depressive episode often follows acute psychosocial stressors, such as death, loss of a loved one, divorce, or acute medical illness. There is evidence that psychosocial stressors are more important in triggering or facilitating the first two depressive episodes and that their influence becomes less important in subsequent episodes.

Ahmed N, Loosen PT: Thyroid hormones in major depressive and bipolar disorders. In: Casper R (ed). *Women's Health and Emotion.* England: Cambridge University Press, 1997, pp. 83–108.

Beyer JL, Krishnan KR: Volumetric brain imaging findings in mood disorders. *Bipolar Disord* 2002;4:89–104.

Drevets WC: Functional anatomical abnormalities in limbic and prefrontal cortical structures in major depression. *Prog Brain Res* 2000;126:413–431.

Goodwin FK, Jamison KR: *Manic Depressive Illness.* New York: Oxford University Press, 1990.

Loosen PT: Hormones of the hypothalamic-pituitary-thyroid axis: A psychoneuroendocrine perspective. *Pharmacopsychiatry* 1986;19:401.

Nemeroff CB, Loosen PT (eds): *Handbook of Clinical Psychoneuroendocrinology.* New York: Guilford Press, 1987.

Soares JC, Mann JJ: The functional neuroanatomy of mood disorders. *J Psychiat Res* 1997;31(4):393–432.

Wolkowitz OM, Rothschild AJ (eds): *Psychoneuroendocrinology.* Arlington, VA: American Psychiatric Publishing, 2003.

Differential Diagnosis

A diagnosis of depression is made if the individual is significantly impaired by the depressive symptoms outlined in the preceding section, and if three exclusion criteria are met: (1) the illness is not due to the effects of a substance (e.g., drug of abuse or medication) or a general medical condition, (2) the illness is not part of a mixed episode (see section on Bipolar Disorders later in this chapter), and (3) the symptoms are not better accounted for by bereavement.

A. MEDICAL CONDITIONS

Most patients with depression will initially present not to a psychiatrist but to their general medical practitioner and often with a somatic complaint (i.e., "I can't sleep," or "I have no energy") rather than a psychiatric complaint (i.e., "I'm depressed"). This is especially true for elderly patients. It is also true that many medications and medical disorders commonly produce symptoms of depression (Table 18–3). Most of these sources of depression can be detected by a thorough review of a patient's history, a complete physical and neurologic examination, and standard laboratory tests. If an etiologic relationship exists between one of these causes and a mood disturbance, the diagnosis will be mood disorder due to a general medical condition (see section on Mood Disorder Due to a General Medical Condition later in this chapter).

B. Other Psychiatric Disorders

Depression can be a feature of almost all other psychiatric disorders; however, the diagnosis should not be made if the episode is part of a bipolar disorder or schizoaffective disorder.

C. Uncomplicated Bereavement

Bereavement generally refers to the grief symptoms experienced after the loss of a loved one. Bereavement is not considered a mental disorder even though it may have symptoms characteristic of a major depressive episode (e.g., sadness, insomnia, loss of appetite, weight loss, feelings of guilt or hopelessness). Data indicate that almost 25% of bereaved individuals meet criteria for major depression at 2 months and again at 7 months and that many of these people continue to do so at 13 months. Patients with more prolonged symptoms tend to be younger and tend to have a history of major depression. Antidepressant treatment is justified in bereavement when the behavioral symptoms are prolonged or if they are associated with continued functional impairment.

Treatment

An important aspect of the treatment of depression is for the physician to discuss with patients and their families the illness, its symptoms and course, and particularly its recurrent nature. Patients should recognize that the illness may recur; they—and their close family members—should be cognizant of the premonitory signs and symptoms of an impending episode (i.e., insomnia, especially early morning awakening, loss of energy, loss of appetite and libido, and diurnal changes in well-being); and they should be told to return to their physician as soon as they have noticed any combination of the premonitory signs for, say, longer than 1 week. This, of course, is best achieved if patients are followed up closely in and out of episodes, if the communication between the physician and the patient or patient's family is open and

Table 18–3. Organic Causes of Depression

Medications
Analgesics (e.g., indomethacin, opiates)
Antibiotics/anti-infectives (e.g., interferon)
Antihypertensive agents with catecholamine effects (e.g., propranolol, reserpine, α-methyldopa, clonidine)
Antineoplastic agents (e.g., cycloserine, vincristine, vinblastine, amphotericin B, Procarbazine, Interferon)
Gastrointestinal motility drugs (e.g., metoclopramide)
Histamine$_2$ receptor antagonists (Cimetidine, Ranitidine) Heavy metals (mercury, lead)
L-Dopa
Insecticides (e.g., organophosphates)
Oral contraceptives
Sedative-hypnotics (e.g., barbiturates, benzodiazepines, chloral hydrate)
Corticosteroids
Substances of Abuse
Alcohol
Cocaine
Opiates
Amphetamine or cocaine withdrawal
Neurologic Disease
Chronic subdural hematoma
Dementias
Huntington's disease
Migraine headaches
Multiple sclerosis
Normal pressure hydrocephalus
Parkinson's disease
Strokes
Temporal lobe epilepsy
Wilson's disease
Infectious Disease
Brucellosis
Encephalitis
HIV
Infectious hepatitis
Influenza
Lyme disease
Mononucleosis

Table 18–3. (Continued)

Subacute bacterial endocarditis
Syphilis
Tuberculosis
Neoplasms
Bronchogenic carcinoma
CNS tumors
Disseminated carcinomatosis
Lymphoma
Pancreatic cancer
Metabolic and Endocrine Disorders
Addison's disease
Anemia
Apathetic hyperthyroidism
Cushing's disease
Diabetes
Hepatic disease
Hypokalemia
Hyponatremia
Hypoparathyroidism
Hypopituitarism (Sheehan's disease)
Hypothyroidism
Pellagra
Pernicious anemia
Porphyria
Thiamine, B_{12}, and folate deficiencies
Uremia
Collagen-Vascular Conditions
Giant cell arteriitis
Rheumatoid arthritis
Systemic lupus erythematosus
Cardiovascular Conditions
Chronic heart failure
Hypoxia
Mitral valve prolapse
Postmyocardial infarction or coronary artery bypass graft
Miscellaneous
Chronic pyelonephritis
Pancreatitis
Postpartum depression

continuous, and if all parties are thoroughly aware that the nature of the illness necessitates both close, continuous observation of its course and early, decisive intervention to prevent relapse. It is also important to recognize that clinical features often have significant treatment implications. A summary of these features and their suggested solutions is provided in Table 18–4.

A. PSYCHOPHARMACOLOGIC INTERVENTIONS

1. Clinical pharmacology

i. Principles of use—The following general principles provide a useful framework for the clinical use of antidepressants in major depressive disorder: (1) diagnose properly; (2) avoid treatment of symptoms (e.g., agitation, insomnia, memory disturbances) if possible, because most symptoms fit into specific diagnostic entities; and (3) be aware of the cycling course of the disease, because it necessitates different treatment approaches: Acute treatment for florid symptoms; continuation therapy to prevent early relapse; and maintenance therapy to make relapse (i.e., recurrence) less likely or, if it occurs, less severe.

ii. Indications—Antidepressant drugs are used successfully to treat a variety of psychiatric and other conditions (19.1–4). In mood disorders, they are used most widely in the treatment of major depressive disorder, but they also have some (albeit reduced) therapeutic activity in treating dysthymic disorder and bipolar disorder (see sections on Dysthymic Disorders and Bipolar Disorders later in this chapter).

The effectiveness of antidepressants in young patients remains controversial, because some controlled clinical trials failed to show consistent beneficial effects in children and adolescents. Even though mitigating factors such as different study designs, medication compliance, and the impact of exogenous factors (e.g., family discord) on symptom manifestation limit the interpretation of these studies, antidepressant drugs are used widely in depressed children and adolescents. Moreover, antidepressants may increase risk of self-injury transiently. However, the best data suggest that the overall risk of suicide in children and adolescents is reduced by antidepressant treatment.

In contrast, antidepressants are very useful in elderly depressed patients, in whom daily dosage requirements are normally reduced because of pharmacokinetic changes associated with aging (i.e., reductions in both hepatic clearance and protein binding).

Antidepressants are usually initiated at a low dosage and increased over a 7–10-day period to achieve the initial target dosage. The dosage may have to be increased further in some patients in order to achieve the best results. With suicidal patients, the physician must take extra care early in the treatment because behavioral activation can

Table 18–4. Clinical Features Influencing Treatment and Their Solutions

Features	Treatment Considerations
Severity	Even mild depression, if unresponsive to nonsomatic treatment, should be considered for antidepressants.
Recurrent depression	Consider for maintenance therapy.
Prior mania or hypomania	Somatic treatments may provoke (hypo)manic episodes in approximately 5–20% of patients (most have a history of bipolar disorder). Such treatments may also precipitate rapid-cycling bipolar disorder. The treatments of choice are lithium alone or in combination with a MAOI or buproprion.
Depression with psychotic features	Carries a higher risk of suicide and recurrent depression. Combine a neuroleptic with an antidepressant or use amoxapine.
Depression with catatonic features	If intravenous injections of lorazepam or amobarbital are not immediately helpful, consider ECT.
Depression with atypical features	Features include anxiety, reverse polarity (e.g., hypersomnia, hyperphagia, marked mood reactivity), and a sense of severe fatigue. TCAs are useful in only 35–50% of patients; in contrast, MAOIs yield response rates of 55–75%.
Depression with alcohol and/or substance abuse	A patient who has major depression with comorbid addiction is more likely to require hospitalization, more likely to attempt suicide, and less likely to comply with treatment than is a patient without such comorbidity. Advisable to detoxify the patient before initiating antidepressant treatment.
Depression with panic and/or anxiety disorder	Panic disorder complicates major depression in 15–30% of cases. Good response to non-MAOI antidepressants, especially imipramine.
Pseudodementia	Lacks the signs of cortical dysfunction seen in true dementia (e.g., aphasia, apraxia, agnosia); treat early and aggressively.
Postpsychotic depression	Depressive symptoms complicate the course of schizophrenia in 25% of cases. Add antidepressant to neuroleptic regimen.
Depression during or after pregnancy	Carefully assess the benefit-risk ratio, especially if treatment is prescribed during the first trimester. If possible, avoid pharmacologic treatment in nursing mothers. Be aware of the possible teratogenic effects of benzodiazepines (i.e., cleft lip and palate) and lithium (i.e., cardiac malformations). Consider ECT as alternative treatment.
Depression superimposed on dysthymia	Antidepressant treatment may resolve both major depression and underlying dysthymia. SSRIs and MAOIs may be the most helpful.
Depression superimposed on personality disorder	Frequently associated with atypical features; more likely to respond to MAOIs or SSRIs. Patients usually show less satisfactory treatment response in regard to both social functioning and residual depressive symptoms.

(Modified after American Psychiatric Association: Practice guidelines for major depressive disorder in adults. *Am J Psychiatry* 1993;150(Suppl):4.)

precede observable mood effects, providing patients with sufficient energy to act on suicidal impulses.

Response to treatment should be evaluated every 3–4 weeks. If the patient is not fully recovered, and if there are no dose-limiting side effects, the dosage should be increased to the next incremental level. This plan should be followed until remission is achieved, dose-limiting side effects occur, or the upper end of the therapeutic range is reached. Absent full remission, the treatment should then be switched to a drug of a different therapeutic class. Augmentation or combination therapy should be considered if there is only partial response.

Once a therapeutic effect is achieved, the antidepressant medication should be continued through the period of high vulnerability for relapse (i.e., at least 6 months for continuation therapy). Because more than 60% of depressed patients will eventually relapse, especially if unprotected by medication, and because future episodes are more severe, it has been proposed that some depressed patients be placed on long-term treatment. Such maintenance therapy for extended periods of time (even years) should be considered if (1) the patient is older than 40 years and had two or more prior episodes of illness, (2) the first episode occurred at age 50 years or older, (3) the

Table 18–5. Common Clinical Uses of
Antidepressants

Major Indications	Secondary Indications
Major depressive disorder	Obsessive-compulsive disorder *
Dysthymia	Generalized anxiety disorder
Bipolar disorder, depressed type	Social phobia
Panic disorder (with or without agoraphobia)	Bulimia nervosa
	Attention-deficit/ hyperactivity disorder* Diabetic polyneuropathy[†] Chronic pain syndromes* Sleep disorders Enuresis[‡]

*Mainly serotonergic antidepressants.
[†]Especially TCAs such as imipramine and desipramine.
[‡]Specific for the use of imipramine in children.

patient has a history of three or more depressive episodes, or (4) the patient has been depressed or dysthymic for 2 or more years before treatment.

Slow tapering of the antidepressant medication can be considered after at least 5 years of treatment if the patient is completely asymptomatic and is not experiencing or anticipating significant stressors. Some patients prefer lifetime treatment rather than risking a return of depression.

2. Adverse effects—Table 18–5 lists common adverse effects associated with antidepressant drugs, their possible mechanisms, and their management. Table 18–6 indicates the relative potency of antidepressants at producing these effects (Table 18–7).

i. Monoamine oxidase inhibitors—Common side effects of MAOIs include those associated with α_1-adrenergic or muscarinic/cholinergic antagonism (see Table 18–5). They are generally manageable by slowing the dose titration or by adjusting the maximum dosage. Less common reactions include ataxia, color blindness, hepatotoxicity, or induction of mania in bipolar patients. Withdrawal reactions—including anxiety, restlessness, insomnia, nausea, agitation, myoclonus, and in extreme cases, the induction of mania—may occur after abrupt discontinuation.

The most serious side effect associated with MAOI use is the development of an acute hypertensive crisis. The metabolism of certain dietary amino acids, especially tyramine, is blocked by MAOIs. The resulting increase in neurotransmitter availability can lead to an acute hypertensive crisis, with patients complaining about pounding headaches and presenting with flushing and blood vessel

distention. The reaction must be considered a medical emergency to be treated with slow intravenous administration of the α-adrenergic antagonist phentolamine, 5 mg (which may be repeated hourly as needed).

MAOIs may also produce acute toxicity by interfering with the metabolic clearance of other drugs, including general anesthetics, barbiturates and other sedatives, antihistamines, alcohol, narcotics (particularly meperidine), anticholinergic agents, TCAs, and sympathomimetic amines (e.g., pseudoephedrine used commonly in decongestants).

Coadministration of MAOIs with either SSRIs or L-tryptophan can provoke a central serotonin syndrome, characterized by acute mental status changes (e.g., confusion, hypomania), restlessness, myoclonus, diaphoresis, tremor, diarrhea, hyperreflexia, and occasionally, seizures, coma, and death. The syndrome is usually mild in nature and resolves within 24 hours after drug discontinuation. MAOIs should therefore not be started within 2 weeks of discontinuation of most SSRIs (5 weeks in the case of fluoxetine, because of its long half-life time [HLT] [see next section]).

Coadministration of TCAs and MAOIs (used occasionally for the management of treatment-refractory depression) can produce serious side effects, including delirium and hypertension. It is therefore advisable to wait at least 2 weeks after discontinuing TCAs before initiating treatment with MAOIs. Table 18–8 lists foods and drugs that can produce serious adverse effects. Patients should be given a copy of this list before beginning treatment with MAOIs.

ii. TCAs & related antidepressants—Tricyclic-induced side effects are the result of their binding to both specific (e.g., norepinephrine or serotonin) and nonspecific (e.g., histamine, muscarinic) sites. Table 18–6 summarizes these actions and their consequences.

The tertiary amine TCAs—amitriptyline, imipramine, and doxepin—tend to be more potent at binding sites unrelated to the mechanism of action and, therefore, tend to produce more severe side effects than the secondary amine TCAs nortriptyline and desipramine (see Tables 18–6 and 18–7).

TCAs and trazodone can affect the heart in the same way as the class 1 antiarrhythmics quinidine or procainamide, inducing atrioventricular (A-V) conduction delays. Special care should be taken with patients who have a first-degree A-V block (a relative contraindication) or a second-degree A-V block (an absolute contraindication) (see Table 18–6). As type 1 antiarrhythmics, these antidepressants may pose greater long-term risk than previously thought. The primary antiarrhythmics can increase the risk of sudden death from a presumed arrhythmic source. This may explain the long-standing observation of increased risk of sudden death in patients treated chronically with TCAs.

Table 18–6. Mechanisms and Management of Common Antidepressant Side Effects of Antidepressants

Mechanism	Side Effects	Management	Drug Examples
Muscarinic/cholinergic blockade	Dry mouth, blurred vision, constipation, urinary retention, mild sinus tachycardia, memory problems.	*Dry mouth*: Candy, sugarless gum. *Constipation*: Hydration, bulk laxatives. *Urinary retention*: Bethanechol, 30–200mg/day. Use bupropion, sertraline, or trazodone.	TCAs, MAOIs
α–adrenergic antagonism	Orthostatic hypotension, dizziness, reflex tachycardia, flushing, diaphoresis, potentiation of the antihypertensive effect of prazosin.	*Orthostatic hypotension*: Increase dosage slowly, use safer agents such as nortriptyline, desipramine, bupropion, or SSRIs. Exert especial caution in elderly patients who are susceptible to falls and fractures.	TCAs, MAOIs, trazodone, nefazodone
Histaminic (H) antagonism	Somnolence, weight gain, hypotension, and potentiation of CNS depressants.	*Weight gain*: Bupropion, fluoxetine, sertraline, and trazodone are alternatives; bupropion and fluoxetine may reduce weight.	TCAs
NE reuptake blockade	Tremor, tachycardia, insomnia, anxiety, erectile and orgasmic dysfunction, blockade of the antihypertensive effect of guanethidine and guanadrel.		TCAs, most heterocyclics
5-HT reuptake blockade	Nausea, diarrhea, anorexia, anxiety, headache, insomnia, sexual dysfunction (loss of erectile or ejaculatory function in men, loss of libido and anorgasmia in women).	*Sexual dysfunction:* Neostigmine, 7.5–15.0 mg taken 30 min before intercourse will enhance libido and reverse delayed ejaculation. Cyproheptadine, 4 mg/day orally may reverse anorgasmia.	SSRIs, clomipramine, venlafaxine, MAOIs
DA reuptake blockade	Psychomotor activation, insomnia, anxiety, aggravation of psychosis, potentiation of antiparkinsonian agents.	NA	TCAs (weak), bupropion
DA receptor blockade	Parkinsonian (i.e., extrapyramidal) effects, elevation of prolactin with gynecomastia and galactorrhea.	NA	Amoxapine, TCAs (weak)
5-HT receptor antagonism	Hypotension, somnolence.	NA	Trazodone, nefazodone, amitriptyline
	Neurologic side effects: Seizures, mild myoclonus, toxic confusional state.	*Seizures*: Fluoxetine, sertraline, trazodone, and MAOIs carry a lower risk to induce seizures. *Myoclonus*: Clonazepam, 0.25 mg three times daily. *Toxic confusional state*: Seen at higher dose and blood levels, responds to lowering the dose.	TCAs
Effects like those of class I antiarrhythmic agents	Cardiovascular effects: TCAs may induce symptomatic conduction defects and orthostatic hypotension	Monitor those patients carefully who take already another class I antiarrhythmic agent.	TCAs, trazodone

Table 18–6. (Continued)

Mechanism	Side Effects	Management	Drug Examples
	among patients with preexisting but asymptomatic conduction defects. TCAs may also provoke arrhythmia in patients with subclinical sinus node dysfunction.	Evaluate patients for preexisting but asymptomatic conduction defects such as interventricular conduction delay and bundle branch block. Be aware that patients with prolonged QT intervals, whether preexisting or drug-induced, are predisposed to the development of ventricular tachycardia. Obtain ECG in all patients older than 40 yr before initiating treatment.	TCAs, trazodone
	Insomnia and anxiety.	Minimize anxiety by starting at a low dose. Manage insomnia by adding trazodone, 100 mg at bedtime (be aware that trazodone can induce priapism in some patients).	Fluoxetine (anxiety and insomnia); desipramine and bupropion (anxiety)

NE: norepinephrine; 5-HT: Serotonin; DA: dopamine; CNS: central nervous system; TCAs: tricyclic antidepressants; SSRIs: selective serotonin reuptake inhibitors; MAOIs: monoamine oxidase inhibitors; ECG: electrocardiogram.

(Modified after American Psychiatric Association: Practice guidelines for major depressive disorder in adults. *Am J Psychiatry* 1993;150(Suppl):4.)

Maprotiline is associated with an increased risk for seizures at higher dosages and plasma levels and has never gained wide use in the United States. Venlafaxine, a mixed norepinephrine and serotonin reuptake inhibitor, can produce mild hypertensive reactions, especially at dosages greater than 300 mg/day. Risk factors for hypertension, such as age, race, or preexisting renal or hypertensive disorder, are usually not associated with this effect.

iii. Selective serotonin reuptake inhibitors—SSRIs potently and selectively block the uptake of serotonin, thereby producing characteristic side effects such as nausea, diarrhea, anorexia, anxiety, headache, insomnia, and orgasmic dysfunction (see Table 18–6). Sexual dysfunction is troublesome and can be persistent. It can be managed by reducing the dosage or by switching to bupropion or nefazodone. Cyproheptadine, yohimbine, or methylphenidate are also occasionally useful in reversing these effects. Finally, sildenafil has been shown in controlled trials to be beneficial in both men and women.

3. Pharmacokinetics

i. Absorption—All antidepressant drugs are highly lipophilic and are absorbed readily from the gastrointestinal tract. Plasma peaks typically occur within 30–60 minutes and remain unbound for 30 minutes.

ii. Distribution—Most (80–90%) antidepressants are highly protein bound, although individual differences in binding can produce a fourfold variation in the amount of free drug. Tissue distribution and demethylation, the first step in metabolism of tertiary heterocyclics, occur rapidly. All antidepressants can be displaced by other drugs with similar protein-binding characteristics. Similarly, antidepressants will displace other compounds that are highly protein bound (e.g., the anticoagulant warfarin); this can increase the free fraction of these drugs and, therefore, both its therapeutic and its adverse effects.

iii. Metabolism—Antidepressants are metabolized mainly in the liver. Metabolism includes demethylation, hydroxylation, and glucuronide conjugation. Individual differences in a patient's microsomal enzyme activity produce steady-state plasma concentrations (bound and unbound) that may vary as much as 40-fold. During the first pass through the liver, about 80% of the drug is degraded (the so-called **first-pass effect**). The first demethylation of imipramine and amitriptyline produces (the clinically highly active) desipramine and nortriptyline, respectively; these and other drugs have active metabolites that significantly prolong their biological half-lives. Glucuronide conjugation occurs after hydroxylation and makes the derivative water soluble; approximately 65% of the drug is eventually eliminated in the urine. Plasma clearance is slow.

Impairment of hepatic or renal function will reduce plasma clearance of antidepressants and thus potentiate their effects. Antipsychotics, by competing for

Table 18–7. Clinical Characteristics of Antidepressants

Drug	Dose Range (mg)	Central Action[†]	Side Effects[‡]				
			Ach	A1	H1	S2	Quin
Tricyclics							
Amitriptyline	100–300	NE (5-HT)	VH	VH	H	M	+
Nortriptyline	50–200	NE (5-HT)	M	M	M	M	+
Imipramine	100–300	NE (5-HT)	H	M	M	L	+
Desipramine	100–300	NE	M	L	L	L	+
Protriptyline	20–60	NE	VH	L	M	L	+
Doxepin	100–300	NE (5-HT)	H	VH	VH	M	+
Trimipramine	75–300	NE (5-HT)	H	VH	VH	M	+
Clomipramine[§]	100–250	5-HT (NE)	VH	M	M	M	+
Heterocyclics							
Maprotiline	100–225	NE	L	M	H	L	+
Amoxapine	100–400	NE	L	M	M	VH	+
Trazodone	150–400	5-HT$_2$ antagonism (NE, 5-HT)	L	H	L	H	+
Bupropion	300–450	DA(?)	VL	VL	VL	VL	—
Venlafaxine	75–375	5-HT	VL	VL	VL	VL	—
Nefazodone	100–500	5-HT$_2$ antagonism (NE, 5-HT)	H	VL	H	VL	—
SSRIs							
Fluoxetine[§]	20–80	5-HT	L	VL	VL	VL	—
Fluvoxamine[§]	100–300	5-HT	VL	VL	M	VL	—
Paroxetine	20–80	5-HT	L	VL	VL	VL	—
Sertraline	50–200	5-HT	VL	VL	VL	VL	—
MAOIs							
Phenelzine	30–90	MAO inhibition	L	M	H	(?)	—
Tranylcypromine	10–40	MAO inhibition	L	M	H	(?)	—

NE: norepinephrine; 5-HT: 5-hydroxytryptamine (serotonin); DA: dopamine; MAO: monoamine oxidase; Ach: acetylcholine; A1: α_1-adrenergic; H1: histamine-1; S2: 5-HT$_2$; Quin: quinidine-like effect; HTN: hypertensive; H: high; VH: very high; M: medium; L low; VL: very low.
[†]Reuptake inhibition, except as otherwise indicated. Less significant clinical effects are shown in parentheses.
[‡]Side effects are listed on mg/kg basis; always multiply by the total dose to get the true clinical side effect profile.
[§]Established benefit in obsessive-compulsive disorder.

(Modified after American Psychiatric Association: Practice guidelines for major depressive disorder in adults. Am J Psychiatry 1993;150(Suppl):4; Baldessarini RJ: Drugs and the treatment of psychiatric disorders, depression and mania. In Hardman JG, Limbird LE (eds). *The Pharmacological Basis of Therapeutics.* New York: McGraw-Hill, 1996, pp. 431–459.)

Table 18–8. Dietary and Drug Restrictions Associated with MAOI Antidepressants

Danger Level	Foods	Drugs
Very dangerous (must be avoided under all circumstances)	All cheese (cottage cheese, cream cheese, and yogurt are safe) Sauerkraut	Amphetamines Asthma inhalants (*pure* steroid inhalants are safe) Cyclopentamine Decongestants, cold, and sinus medications Ephedrine Meperidine Metaraminol Methylphenidate Phenylephrine Phenylpropamolamine Pseudoephedrine Serotonin-active antidepressants (e.g., clomipramine, fluoxetine, sertraline, paroxetine, fluvoxamine)
Moderately dangerous (should be avoided)	All fermented or aged foods (e.g., aged corned beef, salami, fermented sausage, pepperoni, summer sausage, pickled herring) Fermented alcohol beverages (e.g., red wine, sherry, vermouth, cognac, beer, and ale) (clear alcoholic drinks are permitted in true moderation) Broad bean pods (e.g., English broad beans, Chinese pea pods) Liver (chicken, beef or pork) or liverwurst Meat or yeast extracts Spoiled fruit (e.g., spoiled bananas, pineapples, avocados, figs, raisins)	Antihistamines Dopamine L-Dopa Local anesthetics with epinephrine (safe without epinephrine—e.g., carbocaine) Narcotics (codeine is safe) TCAs (e.g., imipramine, amitriptyline, nortriptyline, desipramine, doxepin)
Minimal danger (rarely associated with hypertensive episodes and can be eaten in small amounts)	Anchovies Beets Caviar Chocolate Coffee Colas Curry powder Figs Junket Licorice Mushrooms Rhubarb Snails Soy sauce Worcestershire sauce	

Note: Diabetics taking insulin may have increased hypoglycemia, requiring adjustment in dose of insulin (otherwise safe); patients taking hypotensive agents for high blood pressure may have more hypotension, also requiring adjustment (but also otherwise safe).

metabolism, can have a similar effect. Conversely carbamazepine and barbiturates, by inducing metabolism, can reduce their therapeutic efficacy.

iv. Half-life times—After a single oral dose, distribution is most important in regard to clinical efficacy; after chronic dosing, HLT becomes more important. The HLTs of the most commonly used antidepressants are given in Table 18–9.

4. Predicting treatment response & managing treatment failure—Several factors are useful in predicting a patient's clinical response (positive and negative) to an antidepressant (Table 18–10).

Table 18–9. HLTs of Common Antidepressants

Drug	HLT (h)
Trazodone	5
Imipramine	16
Amitriptyline	16
Paroxetine	20
Desipramine	22
Nortriptyline	24
Amoxapine	30
Citalopram	33
Maprotiline	47
Fluoxetine	24–72
Clomipramine	54–77
Protriptyline	126

Between 60% and 70% of persons with major depressive disorder respond to an adequate antidepressant drug trial. However, only about one-third of patients fully recover. The reasons for treatment failure include inadequate dose and/or serum level, inadequate duration of treatment (minimum 6 weeks), prominent side effects, noncompliance, and incorrect diagnosis.

Table 18–10. Predictors of Antidepressant Response

Positive Predictors	Negative Predictors
Vegetative symptoms (anorexia, weight loss, middle and late insomnia)	Coexistence of other significant psychiatric disturbances (particularly with hysterical or externalizing features)
Diurnal mood variation	
Psychomotor agitation or retardation	
Autonomous and pervasive symptoms	Chronic symptoms
Acute onset	Psychotic features
Family history of depression	Hypochondriacal concerns or predominant somatic features
Dose of imipramine (or equivalent dose of another heterocyclic) above 125–150 mg/day	
Blood levels of desipramine (or imipramine and desipramine) above 200 ng/ml, and nortryptiline between 50 and 150 ng/ml	Previous drug trial failure(s)
	History of sensitivity to adverse reactions

Table 18–11. Therapeutic Plasma Levels of Antidepressants

Drug	Plasma Concentration (ng/ml)
Amitriptyline (plus nortriptyline)	150–250
Nortriptyline	50–150*
Imipramine (plus desipramine)	150–250
Desipramine	50–150
Doxepin (plus desmethyldoxepin)	>100

*Therapeutic window.

Because single doses of antidepressants can produce widely varying drug serum levels, the patient's plasma levels should be measured in order to ensure optimal dosing when available. Unfortunately, only plasma levels of tricyclics are widely available. Associations between plasma levels and clinical response are known for several antidepressants (Table 18–11). The monitoring of the plasma level of nortriptyline is particularly important because there appears to be a therapeutic window in which the drug is most effective. Plasma levels can also be assessed for other antidepressants, including fluoxetine, but the relationship between plasma levels and clinical response is less well understood for these agents. Indications for monitoring drug levels of antidepressants are (1) failure to respond to a presumably adequate trial in terms of dose and duration; (2) concurrent physical illness, especially cardiovascular disease; (3) use of higher than usual doses (i.e., greater than 300 mg/day of imipramine); (4) treatment in the very young or old (or in any patient with decreased protein binding); (5) the presence of side effects uncertainly related to drug treatment; and (6) drug overdose.

When a true treatment failure has occurred, the physician needs to consider an alternative approach. This may involve trying another treatment approach (e.g., ECT or combining TCAs with an MAOI) or using one of several augmentation strategies (Table 18–12). A large body of evidence supports these strategies, and particularly in tertiary care centers (to which most nonresponders normally are referred) they are widely and safely used.

Lithium carbonate, thyroid hormone (preferably T_3), or sleep deprivation are effective in augmenting the therapeutic effects of TCAs. Among these strategies, sleep deprivation is the least invasive and most easily conducted technique. Its antidepressant effects, observed in about 65% of patients after only one night of wakefulness, are immediate; it is entirely free of side effects; and patients

Table 18–12. Alternative Therapies for Treatment-Resistant Depression

Augmentation of TCAs or MAOIs with
Sleep deprivation*
Lithium*
Thyroid hormone[†]
L-Tryptophan[‡]
Psychostimulants (amphetamine, methylphenidate—in combination with TCAs only)[‡]
Carbamazepine[†]
TCA/MAOI combination (use with extreme care)[†]
ECT (reserved primarily for severe intractable depression or when the patient is acutely suicidal)*
Phototherapy or light therapy[†]
Psychostimulants alone (reserved largely for treatment in elderly depressed patients)[‡]
Psychotherapy (cognitive-behavioral and interpersonal psychotherapy) alone or in combination with TCAs[†]

*Recommended with substantial clinical confidence.
[†]Recommended with moderate clinical confidence.
[‡]Options that may be recommended on the basis of individual circumstances.

(Modified after American Psychiatric Association: Practice guidelines for major depressive disorder in adults. Am J Psychiatry 1993;150(Suppl):1–26. For 2nd guideline edition see Am J Psychiatry 2000;157(Suppl 4):1–45.)

can repeat it easily and safely even after they have been discharged from the hospital. Care must be taken, however, since patients may relapse quickly after recovery sleep. Lithium can be titrated to standard serum levels and T_3 started at 25 µg/day; both augmentation strategies should be maintained for a minimum of 3 weeks in the absence of therapeutic response. About half of patients who have not responded to the standard antidepressants will experience sudden clinical improvement. It is not known whether lithium or T_3 should be continued after a clinical response has occurred. T_3 appears to be effective in the augmentation of SSRI's and related newer medications. However, the effectiveness of lithium has been called into question.

Alternative methods for treating refractory depression include the use of a combination of a noradrenergic antidepressant such as desipramine or bupropion with a serotonergic one such as fluoxetine. If TCA's are used, care must be taken to measure the plasma level since SSRIs are competitive inhibitors of metabolism by liver cytochrome enzymes, especially CYP2D6. This can lead to a dangerous increase in plasma levels. Hence TCA plasma levels should be measured with concomitant use. Psychostimulants such as amphetamine or methylphenidate may be useful in some patients but in a more limited way.

The addition of cognitive–behavioral psychotherapy (CBT) to antidepressant treatment also appears to be beneficial in many patients. In particular, a version of CBT specifically designed to aid in chronic depression,

referred to as cognitive behavioral analysis system of psychotherapy (CBASP) has been shown to be effective in one large scale clinical trial. The effects of other psychotherapies have not been established.

If these techniques are ineffective, two other options remain. The first is to use a TCA and an MAOI together, but this strategy bears some risk of acute and potentially serious side effects. As well, the data supporting the effectiveness of this combination is very limited. Imipramine and phenelzine are commonly employed. Typically, the MAOI is started first. Once a stable dose is achieved, a tricyclic may be started at low dose. Patients must be cautioned regarding potential negative consequences, including hypertensive reactions. ECT is another available treatment that can be used in the face of nonresponse. A more extensive discussion of ECT is found below.

American Psychiatric Association: Practice guidelines for the treatment of patients with major depressive disorder in adults. *Am J Psychiatry* 2000;157(Suppl 4):1–45.

Baldessarini RJ: Drugs and the treatment of psychiatric disorders, depression and mania. In: Hardman JG, Limbird LE (eds). *The Pharmacological Basis of Therapeutics.* New York: McGraw-Hill, 1996, pp. 431–459.

Charney DS, Berman RM, Miller HL: Treatment of depression. In: Schatzberg AF, Nemeroff CB (eds). *Textbook of Psychopharmacology*, 2nd edn. Washington, DC: American Psychiatric Press, 1998.

Glassman AH, Roose SP, Bigger JT, Jr.: The safety of tricyclic antidepressants in cardiac patients: Risk-benefit reconsidered. *J Am Med Assoc* 1993;269:2673.

Goodwin FK, Jamison KR: *Manic Depressive Illness.* New York: Oxford University Press, 1990.

Schatzberg AF, Nemeroff CB (eds): *Textbook of Psychopharmacology,* 2nd edn. Washington, DC: American Psychiatric Press, 1998.

Keller MB, McCullough JP, Klein DN, et al.: A comparison of nefazodone, the cognitive behavioral-analysis system of psychotherapy, and their combination for the treatment of chronic depression. *N Engl J Med* 2000;342:1462–1470.

B. OTHER INTERVENTIONS

1. Electroconvulsive therapy—Between 80% and 90% of all ECT treatments in the United States are performed for the treatment of major depressive disorder. Although ECT appears to be most effective in the most severely depressed patients, attempts to use clinical symptoms, patient history, demographics, or other factors as predictors of clinical response have been largely unsuccessful.

ECT has shown efficacy in all types of major depressive disorder. Recent evidence suggests that it is less useful in patients whose depressive episodes occur in the context of a concurrent mental or medical disease (i.e., secondary depression) or in the treatment of depression that has been refractory to medications during the present episode.

i. When to use ECT—The decision to refer a patient for treatment with ECT is made only after careful considerations of its risks and benefits. ECT is used as primary treatment when (1) an urgent need (either psychiatrically or medically) for a rapid response exists, (2) there is less risk with ECT than with other treatment alternatives, (3) there is a patient history of better response to ECT, or (4) there is a strong patient preference for its use. A majority of patients referred for ECT do not meet these criteria. ECT is used as a secondary treatment when (1) the patient has responded poorly to or is intolerant of alternative treatments or (2) the patient has deteriorated to the point at which a rapid response is needed urgently.

ii. Contraindications—There are no absolute contraindications to the use of ECT, but some conditions are relative contraindications (Table 18–13). If treatment with ECT becomes necessary on a life- saving basis, these

Table 18–13. Relative Contraindications to ECT

Space-occupying intracerebral lesions (except for small, slow growing tumors without edema or other mass effect)
Conditions with increased intracranial pressure
Unstable vascular aneurysms or malformations
Intracerebral hemorrhage
Pheochromocytoma
Recent myocardial infarction

risks can generally be minimized to some extent using appropriate pharmacologic interventions. With appropriate preparation, ECT can be used effectively and safely in both pregnant and elderly patients.

iii. Adverse outcomes of treatment

i. Mortality— The overall mortality rate of ECT is extremely low; it approximates that of brief general anesthesia. Estimates range between 1 in 10,000 (0.01%) and 1 in 1000 (0.1%) patients.

ii. Cognitive changes— There is no relationship between ECT and brain damage; however, temporary cognitive changes do occur and are often the most notable and most distressing side effects. Three types of cognitive change may be observed:

Postictal confusion. Because ECT induces seizure activity, all patients experience some transient confusion, lasting from a few minutes to a few hours, after they awaken from the ECT treatment. Most patients usually will not remember the immediate postictal period and will not experience the cognitive changes following a seizure as a significant disturbance. Reassurance, support, and avoidance of cognitive demands during the acute postictal period are typically all that is necessary for treatment. Postictal sedation with a short-acting benzodiazepine such as midazolam may be necessary if the patient becomes agitated.

Interictal confusion. Occasionally postictal confusion may not disappear fully, and when severe, it may develop into an interictal confusional state or delirium. This phenomenon, which is uncommon, may be cumulative over the ECT course but disappears rapidly over a period of days after the conclusion of treatments.

Memory impairment. Amnesia often occurs with ECT and varies considerably in both severity and persistence. Memory disturbances consist of both retrograde amnesia (i.e., difficulty in recalling information learned prior to the ECT course) and anterograde amnesia (i.e., difficulty in retaining newly learned information). When present, anterograde and retrograde amnesia disappear rapidly over a period of days to weeks after completion of the ECT course.

A small group of patients report that their memory never returned to normal after ECT. The etiology for this phenomenon is unclear, and objective memory testing generally does not substantiate the subjective complaint. Possible explanations for this phenomenon may include (1) patients incorrectly attribute memory problems associated with depression to prior ECT, (2) anesthetic misadventure (e.g., hypoxia), or (3) other, occult memory impairment (e.g., evolving dementia).

iii. Cardiovascular complications— During the seizure and acute postictal period, the sympathetic and parasympathetic autonomic systems are stimulated sequentially. Activation of the sympathetic system increases heart rate, blood pressure, and myocardial oxygen consumption, placing an increased demand on the cardiovascular system. Activation of the parasympathetic system causes a transient reduction in cardiac rate. These changes in heart rate and cardiac output challenge the cardiovascular system, occasionally giving rise to transient arrhythmias and, in susceptible individuals, transient ischemic changes. Most cardiovascular changes are minor, and the risk of complications can be diminished greatly by the use of oxygen and appropriate medications in susceptible patients.

iv. Other adverse effects— General somatic complaints (i.e., headaches, nausea, muscle soreness) are common after ECT. Analgesics may be given prophylactically prior to ECT to patients who routinely have post-ECT headaches. The dosage of muscle relaxant should be increased if muscle soreness and headaches are due to inadequate relaxation.

About 7% of depressed bipolar patients switch into a manic or mixed state after ECT. This state can be managed by either continuing ECT or stopping ECT and administering an antimanic agent.

2. Course of treatment

i. Number of treatments—A typical ECT course involves 6–12 treatments, but the number required may be as low as 3 or as high as 20. Alterations in the ECT course should be considered for nonresponders or for patients whose clinical progress is minimal after approximately six treatments. Alterations may include changing from unilateral to bilateral electrode placement, increasing stimulus intensity, or potentiating the seizure pharmacologically. If there is still no response after three or four additional treatments, or if the patient's response has reached a plateau below a full level of remission, the ECT course should be terminated.

ii. Multiple monitored ECT—Multiple monitored electroconvulsive therapy (MMECT) was developed in an attempt to decrease the average length of the treatment course by inducing multiple seizures (usually 2–10) during a single treatment. MMECT appears to be associated with a more rapid clinical response, but the total number of seizures required is greater. There is also evidence that MMECT is associated with a higher frequency of prolonged seizure activity, exaggerated cardiovascular responses, and increased cognitive side effects.

iii. Frequency of treatments—In the United States, most ECT treatments are given three times a week (e.g., Monday, Wednesday, and Friday). An increase in the frequency is associated with a more rapid response but also increased cognitive side effects.

iv. Continuation treatment—Most psychiatrists agree that after the remission of a depressive or manic episode, ECT treatment should be continued for at least 6–12 months. After the conclusion of a course of ECT, there are three options for continued treatment:

(1) administration of appropriate psychotropic medications (e.g., antidepressants); (2) continuation of ECT; or (3) psychotherapy, combined with pharmacotherapy or ECT.

v. Maintenance treatment—Because of the severity and chronicity of some patients' illnesses, many practitioners now prophylactically continue pharmacotherapy or ECT for longer time periods, particularly when attempts to discontinue treatment have resulted in a recurrence of the illness. Maintenance ECT treatments may be given monthly, although some individuals require more frequent administration (e.g., weekly). There is no lifetime maximum number of treatments that a patient may have. Cumulative amnestic effects are not usually seen.

American Psychiatric Association: *The Practice of ECT: Recommendations for Treatment, Training, and Privileging*. Washington, DC, American Psychiatric Press, 1990.

Weiner RD, Coffey CE: Electroconvulsive therapy in the medical and neurologic patient. In: Stoudemire A, Fogel BS (eds). *Psychiatric Care of the Medical Patient*. New York: Oxford University Press, 1993, pp. 207–224.

3. Vagus nerve stimulation—A number of clinical studies have shown that vagus nerve stimulation (VNS) has antidepressant effects in patients with depression resistant to four or more treatments. Improvement with VNS result in enhanced neurocognitive function in many patients. VNS appears to be most effective in patients with low to moderate antidepressant resistance. Response rates usually range from 30–40%, and long-term VNS treatment appears to be associated with sustained symptomatic improvement. VNS is also known to improve mood in depressed patients with epilepsy.

4. Transcranial magnetic stimulation—Repetitive transcranial magnetic stimulation (rTMS) is a noninvasive and easily tolerated method of altering cortical physiology. Clinical studies support an antidepressant effect of high-frequency rTMS administered to the left PFC; however, antidepressive efficacy is not consistent, and where efficacy is demonstrated, degree of clinical improvement appears to be small. The absence of psychosis, and younger age may be predictors of treatment success. Low frequency TMS to the right PFC also has shown promise. Repetitive TMS may be useful in augmenting or hastening the response of antidepressant drugs in patients with major depressive disorder.

C. PSYCHOTHERAPEUTIC INTERVENTIONS

The establishment and maintenance of a supportive therapeutic relationship, wherein the therapist gains the patient's confidence and is available in times of crisis, is crucial in the treatment of depression. Beyond pure psychotherapeutic management the therapeutic relationship contains other important factors. These include observing emerging destructive impulses toward self or others; providing ongoing education, knowledge, and feedback about the patient's illness, its prognosis, and treatment; discouraging the patient from making major life changes while he or she is depressed; setting realistic, attainable, and tangible goals; and enlisting the support of others in the patient's social network.

Depression is often treated with psychotherapy, either alone or in combination with antidepressants. This is particularly true for unipolar depression. The psychosocial interventions that have fared well in controlled trials relative to antidepressants include interpersonal psychotherapy, cognitive–behavioral therapy, and some of the marital and family interventions. Traditional dynamic psychotherapy has not proved effective but may not have been evaluated adequately.

1. Interpersonal psychotherapy—Interpersonal psychotherapy seeks to recognize and explore depressive precipitants that involve interpersonal losses, role disputes and transitions, social isolation, or deficits in social skills. It focuses on current interpersonal problems and deemphasizes childhood antecedents or extensive attention to transference in the therapeutic relationship. Interpersonal psychotherapy can be effective in reducing depressive symptoms in the acute phase of nonmelancholic major depression of lesser severity. It seems to produce a greater change in social functioning than antidepressants; this change may not appear until after several months of treatment (or until several months after treatment is over).

2. Cognitive–behavioral therapy—Cognitive–behavioral therapy is based on the premise that helping patients recognize and correct erroneous beliefs and maladaptive behaviors can relieve their affective distress. It also can be effective in reducing depressive symptoms in the acute phase of major depression. Cognitive–behavioral therapy may have an enduring effect that protects the patient against subsequent relapse following treatment termination. A recent large-scale clinical trial has shown that CBT is about as effective as the antidepressant paroxetine in moderate to severe major depression. Moreover, CBT reduced the likelihood of relapse over continuation placebo or medication over the subsequent year. Comorbid generalized anxiety disorder favored treatment with paroxetine. In the treatment of very severe depression in outpatients neither interpersonal therapy nor cognitive–behavioral therapy are quite as effective as antidepressant drugs.

A recent multi-center trial of patients with chronic depression compared the antidepressant effects of an antidepressant (Nefazodone), Cognitive Behavioral Analysis System of Psychopathology (CBASP), a psychotherapy method designed for chronic depression, or the combination. Overall, the effects of the antidepressant alone and psychotherapy alone were equal and significantly less effective than combination treatment. Among those with a history of early childhood trauma or abuse, psychotherapy alone was superior to antidepressant monotherapy, suggesting an important role of psychotherapy in the management of patients with chronic forms of major depression and a history of childhood trauma.

3. Marital therapy & family therapy—Marital and family problems are common in the course of mood disorders. They may be a consequence of depression but may also increase the patient's vulnerability to depression and in some instances retard recovery. Research suggests that marital therapy and family therapy may reduce depressive symptoms and the risk of relapse in patients with marital or family problems.

4. Selection of specific therapies—Patient preference plays a large role in the selection of a particular form of psychotherapy. In choosing the most appropriate form, the psychiatrist should consider that an interpersonal approach may be more useful for patients who are in the midst of conflicts with significant others and for those having difficulty adjusting to an altered career or social role or other life transition. A cognitive approach can be helpful for patients who seek and are able to tolerate explicit, structured guidance from another party.

Berman RM, Narasimhan M, Sanacora G, et al.: A randomized clinical trial of repetitive transcranial magnetic stimulation in the treatment of major depression. *Biol Psych* 2000;47:332.

DeRubeis RJ, Hollon SD, Amsterdam JD, et al.: Cognitive therapy vs. antidepressant medications in the treatment of moderate to severe major depressive disorder: Response to short-term treatment. *Arch Gen Psychiatry* 2005;62:409.

Fitzgerald PB, Brown TL, Marston NA, Daskalakis ZJ, Kulkarni J: Transcranial magnetic stimulation in the treatment of depression: A double-blind, placebo-controlled trial. *Arch Gen Psych* 2003;60:1002.

Gershon AA, Dannon PN, Grunhaus L: Transcranial magnetic stimulation in the treatment of depression. *Am J Psych* 2003;160:835.

Hollon SD, DeRubeis RJ, Shelton RC, et al.: Prevention of relapse following cognitive therapy versus medications in moderate to severe depression. *Arch Gen Psychiatry* 2005;62:417.

Holtzheimer PE, Russo J, Avery DH: A meta-analysis of repetitive transcranial stimulation in the treatment of depression. *Pyschopharm Bull* 2001;35:149.

Jarrett RB, Rush AJ: Short-term psychotherapy of depressive disorders: Current status and future directions. *Psychiatry* 1994;57:115.

Loo CK, Mitchell PB: A review of the efficacy of transcranial magnetic stimulation treatment for depression, and current and future strategies to optimize efficacy. *J Aff Dis* 2005;88:255.

Marangell LB, Rush AJ, George MS, et al.: Vagus nerve stimulation for major depressive episodes: One year outcomes. *Biol Psych* 2002;51:280.

Nemeroff CB, Heim CM, Thase ME, et al.: Differential responses to psychotherapy versus pharmacotherapy in patients with chronic forms of major depression and childhood trauma. *Proc Natl Acad Sci U S A* 2003;100:14293.

Rush AJ, George MS, Sackeim HA, et al.: Vagus nerve stimulation for treatment-resistant depressions: A multicenter study. *Biol Psych* 2000;47:276.

Sackeim HA, Rush AJ, George MS, et al.: Vagus nerve stimulation for treatment-resistant depression: Efficacy, side effects, and predictors of outcome. *Neuropsychopharm* 2001;25:713.

Weissman MM, Markowitz JC: Interpersonal psychotherapy: Current status. *Arch Gen Psychiatry* 1994;51:599.

Complications/Adverse Outcomes of Treatment

Major depressive disorder is associated with considerable morbidity, disability, and risk for suicide. Up to 15% of patients with severe major depressive disorder commit suicide (among patients with recurrent depression, death by suicide occurs at the rate of about 1% per year). Among patients with major depressive disorder who are older than 55 years, the death rate is increased fourfold. Compared to nondepressive subjects, patients with major depressive disorder admitted to a nursing home are more likely to die within the first 5 years. Among patients in general medical settings, physically ill patients with depression have increased pain and physical illness and decreased social and role functioning. In fact, deterioration of functioning associated with depression or depressive symptoms can be equal to or worse than that associated with severe medical conditions. The combination of advanced coronary artery disease (CAD) and depressive symptoms was associated with roughly twice the reduction in social functioning as with either condition alone, suggesting that the effects of depressive symptoms and chronic medical conditions on functioning can be additive.

Major depression and depressive symptoms, although commonly observed in medical populations, are often underdiagnosed and undertreated. This is particularly relevant in cardiovascular disease where depression and its associated symptoms have been shown to be a major risk factor for both development of cardiovascular disease and death after myocardial infarction. In patients with cardiovascular disease, treatment of depression may thus stabilize mood imbalance, improve quality of life, and perhaps positively affect such outcome measures as longevity.

Major depressive disorder exacts a large toll on patients, family members, and society, because of its high level of morbidity and mortality. It may account for more bed days than any other physical disorder except cardiovascular disease, and it may be more costly to the economy than chronic respiratory illness, diabetes, arthritis, or hypertension. It has been estimated that depression and other mood disorders account for $43.7 billion in direct costs (i.e., treatment) and indirect costs (i.e., lost productivity through illness, absenteeism, or suicide). Before modern treatments, depressed patients typically spent one-fourth of their adult lives in the hospital and fully one-half of their lives disabled.

Goodwin FK, Jamison KR: *Manic Depressive Illness.* New York: Oxford University Press, 1990.

Musselman DL, Evans DL, Nemeroff CB: The relationship of depression to cardiovascular disease: Epidemiology, biology, and treatment. *Arch Gen Psychiatry* 1998;55:580.

Prognosis

Table 18–14 summarizes the relevant prognosis factors. Major depressive disorder is not a benign condition, but careful management, including early, aggressive therapeutic intervention can largely improve its otherwise poor prognosis. Although the literature on long-term outcome has produced variable results because of study design (i.e., short duration of observation, focus on hospitalized episodes, exclusion of episodes preceding the index episode, and retrospective rather than prospective analysis) and different case definitions, the IOWA 500 study, involving 35 years of retrospective follow-up of patients initially presenting with a manic episode, found that outcome was good in 64% of patients, fair in 14%, and poor in 22%. Compared to well-matched patients with minor surgery or schizophrenia, the depressed

Table 18–14. Course and Prognosis of Mood Disorders

	Bipolar Disorders	Non-Bipolar Disorders
Age at onset	28–33 yr	38–45 yr
Duration of episode	Before 1960: 7–13 months; after 1960: 2–4 months	Before 1960: 24% develop episodes > 1 yr; after 1960: 18% develop episodes > 1 yr
Recovery	5–10% do not recover from index episode	Similar
Long-term outcome	More chronic course, more episodes, length of cycle shortens with more frequent episodes	More benign in one-third of patients, length of cycle shortens with more frequent episodes
Mortality and suicide	Completed suicide occurs in 10–15% of patients with bipolar I disorder	Up to 15% commit suicide

Note: Non-bipolar disorders refers to the clinical category under which major depressive disorders is classified.

patients' outcome was intermediate (i.e., better than that of schizophrenic patients but worse than that of surgery patients).

Positive prognostic indicators include an absence of psychotic symptoms, a short hospitalization or duration of depression, and good family functioning. Poor prognostic indicators include a comorbid psychiatric disorder, substance abuse, early age at onset, long duration of the index episode, and inpatient hospitalization. A patient who has major depression with comorbid addiction is more likely to require hospitalization, more likely to attempt suicide, and less likely to comply with treatment than is a patient with depression of similar severity not complicated by comorbid addiction.

Clinicians have noted substantially increased mortality rates in major depressive disorder and bipolar disorder for more than 60 years. They recognized suicide as the most significant factor contributing to mortality, although other factors (e.g., malnutrition, comorbid medical illness) are likely to contribute. Early studies reported up to six times the mortality rates expected for a normal population of the same age, but later studies found a less striking yet still significant increase in mortality, averaging about two times the expected rates.

■ DYSTHYMIC DISORDER

 ## ESSENTIALS OF DIAGNOSIS

DSM-IV-TR Diagnostic Criteria

A. *Depressed mood for most of the day, for more days than not, as indicated either by subjective account or observation made by others, for at least 2 years.*
   Note: *In children and adolescents, mood can be irritable and duration must be at least 1 year.*

B. *Presence, while depressed, of two (or more) of the following:*
   (1) poor appetite or overeating
   (2) insomnia or hypersomnia
   (3) low energy or fatigue
   (4) low self-esteem
   (5) poor concentration or difficulty making decisions
   (6) feelings of hopelessness

C. *During the 2-year period (1 year for children or adolescents) of the disturbance, the person has never been without the symptoms in Criteria A and B for more than 2 months at a time.*

D. *No major depressive episode has been present during the first 2 years of the disturbance (1 year for children and adolescents); i.e., the disturbance is not better accounted for by chronic major depressive disorder, or major depressive disorder, in partial remission.*
   Note: *There may have been a previous major depressive episode provided there was a full remission (no significant signs or symptoms for 2 months) before development of the dysthymic disorder. In addition, after the initial 2 years (1 year in children and adolescents) of dysthymic disorder, there may be superimposed episodes of major depressive disorder, in which case both diagnoses may be given when the criteria are met for a major depressive episode.*

E. *There has never been a manic episode, a mixed episode, or a hypomanic episode, and criteria have never been met for cyclothymic disorder.*

F. *The disturbance does not occur exclusively during the course of a chronic psychotic disorder, such as schizophrenia or delusional disorder.*

G. *The symptoms are not due to the direct physiologic effects of a substance (e.g., a drug of abuse, a medication) or a general medical condition (e.g., hypothyroidism).*

H. *The symptoms cause clinically significant distress or impairment in social, occupational, or other important areas of functioning.*

Specify if:

Early Onset: if onset is before age 21 years
Late Onset: if onset is age 21 years or older
Specify (for most recent 2 years of Dysthymic Disorder With Atypical Features)

(Reprinted, with permission, from *the Diagnostic and Statistical Manual of Mental Disorders*, 4th edn., Text Revision. Washington DC: American Psychiatric Association, 2000.)

General Considerations

The term **dysthymia** is derived from the Greek word *thymos*, and its literal meaning is "disordered mood." The classic dysthymic patient has been described by Akiskal as "ill-humored ... (having the) ... disposition to low-grade dysphoria ... habitually brooding, overcontentious, incapable of fun, and preoccupied with personal inadequacy" (1995, p. 1073). The term **dysthymic disorder** was first used in the *Diagnostic and Statistical Manual of Mental Disorders*, third edition (DSM-III), which attempted to create a diagnostic concept under which a heterogeneous group of disorders previously referred to as depressive neurosis could be subsumed. The creation of this diagnostic entity as separate from major depressive disorder has been an impetus for increased research activity.

Despite our improved understanding of this condition, dysthymic disorder, as Max Hamilton stated just before his death in 1989, "lies on the border between the normal and pathological." Because patients with dysthymic disorder experience symptoms that are of a lower intensity than those associated with major depression, the term **subsyndromal mood disorder** has been applied. In a rural primary care population, 3.8–6.0% of patients were classified as having low-grade or intermittent depressions according to research diagnostic criteria (which were used mainly for research purposes and preceded the development of the DSM-III), and almost twice as many patients (11.2%) had a psychiatric disorder with significant depressive symptomatology that did not fit into a specific depressive disorder category. (The diagnosis of intermittent depression using research diagnostic criteria can be seen as the precursor of the diagnosis of dysthymic disorder in DSM-III.) The data suggest that dysthymic disorder is the tip of a very large iceberg of subsyndromal mood states.

A. Epidemiology

Table 18–15 summarizes the relevant risk factors. The lifetime prevalence of dysthymic disorder in the general population (3.2%) is exceeded only by that for major depression (4.9%). Even more dramatic are the 1-month point prevalence rate estimates from the Epidemiologic Catchment Area (ECA) survey, which at 3.3% rank dysthymic disorder second only to phobia and more common than alcoholism and all other mental disorders assessed. The protracted course of dysthymic disorder makes it the most commonly encountered form of mood disorder. It affects women more often than men, with a ratio of nearly 2–1. Dysthymic disorder usually sets in

Table 18–15. Risk Factors for Dysthymic Disorder

Familial pattern	Dysthymia is more common among first-degree relatives of people with major depression than among the general population.
Age at onset	Disease onset is usually before age 45, but a sizeable subgroup of patients develop the disorder in late life (45% after age 45, and 19% after age 65).
Social class	No relationship.
Race	Possibly low occurrence in African Americans (2.5% vs. 3.3% in whites).

before the age of 45 years. Although dysthymic disorder appears to be the least common among African Americans (2.5%), the ECA survey noted the largest number of depressive and dysthymic symptoms in that population. This finding may imply either denial of illness by some respondents or a higher rate of subsyndromal mood disorder (currently diagnosed as depressive disorder not otherwise specified or the proposed depressive personality disorder).

B. Etiology

1. Life events—Personality features may be involved in the pathogenesis of dysthymic disorder. Psychoanalytic theorists have stressed the concept of inordinate interpersonal dependency, in which the patient's self-esteem is excessively reliant on approval, reassurance, attention, and love from others. Thus when such interpersonal concern from others wanes or terminates, depression ensues.

Cognitive theorists ascribe the symptoms of depression to disordered basic cognitive schema, or dysfunctional thoughts, that are developed early in life. The learned helplessness model holds that after repeated, inescapable shock, experimental animals will not initiate avoidance from aversive stimuli, even when avenues of escape are readily available. Even when faced with major traumatic events and losses, most people do not progress from grief to pathologic depression, suggesting that adverse life events and an underlying vulnerability interact to produce symptoms of chronic depression. It is also true that mood disorders create adverse conditions, such as separation, divorce, and suicide. When such conditions occur in parents, an already predisposed child is exposed to environmentally determined object losses that might precipitate more severe illness or earlier onset of depressive episodes.

2. Biological theories—Family studies demonstrate that patients with dysthymic disorder and patients with major depression exhibit similar rates of mood disorders in first-degree relatives. Patients with dysthymic disorder also exhibit shortened REM latency during sleep onset, as do patients with major depression. Thus there may be a biological or familial relationship between these two disorders.

Personality inventories of patients with dysthymic disorder often reveal a disturbed personality structure; dependent, avoidant, borderline, and narcissistic personality disorders are the most common. Little is known about the exact biological determinants of dysthymic disorder. Many dysthymic individuals respond well to antidepressants, although the percentage of those who respond and the magnitude of their response are generally less than that observed in patients with major depression.

C. Genetics

Family studies support a genetic link between dysthymic disorder and major depression. Twin studies have not corroborated a strong relationship between dysthymic disorder and other personality disorders, with the exception of the depressive personality disorder. Depressive personality disorder is a construct noted in the DSM-IV, in which individuals demonstrate a pervasive pattern of depressive cognitions and behaviors beginning in early adulthood but do not develop dysthymic disorder or major depressive episodes. Depressive personality disorder may be a condition that subsumes the persistent trait-like qualities of the depressive disorders. Preliminary evidence from family studies indicates that this disorder is related to the major mood disorders such as dysthymic disorder. Thus far, research has not identified any specific gene or set of genes associated with dysthymic disorder.

Akiskal HS: Mood disorders: Introduction and overview. In: Kaplan HI, Sadock BJ (eds). *Comprehensive Textbook of Psychiatry*, Vol 1, 6th edn. Baltimore, MD: Williams & Wilkins, 1995.

Barrett JE, Barrett JA, Oxman TE, Gerber PD: The prevalence of psychiatric disorders in a primary care practice. *Arch Gen Psychiatry* 1988;45:1100.

Hamilton M: Foreword. In: Burton SW, Akiskal HS (eds). *Dysthymic Disorder*. London: Royal College of Psychiatrists, 1990.

Kessler RC: Dysthymia in the community and its comorbidity with psychiatric and substance use disorders. NIMH Sponsored Workshop: Subsyndromal Mood Disorders: Dysthymia and Cyclothymia. Bethesda, MD, April 26, 1993.

Regier DA, Boyd JH, Birk JD, et al.: One-month prevalence of mental disorders in the United States. *Arch Gen Psychiatry* 1988;45:977.

Weissman MN, Livingston Bruce M, Leaf PJ, Florio LP, Holzer C: Affective Disorders. In: Robins LN, Regier DA (eds). *Psychiatric Disorders in America*. New York: Free Press, 1991, pp. 53–80.

Clinical Findings

A. SIGNS & SYMPTOMS

Although there has been some controversy concerning the symptoms that best define dysthymic disorder, recent studies suggest that the symptoms most commonly encountered in dysthymic disorder may be those found in the alternative DSM-IV research criterion B for dysthymic disorder (Table 18–16).

In children, dysthymic disorder often results in impaired social interaction and school performance. Children and adolescents with dysthymic disorder are usually irritable, pessimistic, cranky, and depressed and have low self-esteem and poor social skills.

B. PSYCHOLOGICAL TESTING

Patients with dysthymic disorder have increased scores for neuroticism and introversion on the Maudsley Personality Inventory; these abnormalities persist even after recovery.

Table 18–16. Symptoms Most Commonly Encountered in Dysthymic Disorder

Low self-esteem or self-confidence, or feelings of inadequacy
Feelings of pessimism, despair, or hopelessness
Generalized loss of interest or pleasure
Social withdrawal
Chronic fatigue or tiredness
Feelings of guilt, brooding about past
Subjective feelings of irritability or excessive anger
Decreased activity, effectiveness, or productivity
Difficulty in thinking, reflected by poor concentration, poor memory, or indecisiveness

(Modified after *Diagnostic and Statistical Manual of Mental Disorders*, 4th edn. [DSM-IV].)

C. LABORATORY FINDINGS & NEUROIMAGING

About 25–50% of adults with dysthymic disorder have EEG abnormalities similar to those found in major depressive disorder (e.g., reduced REM latency, increased REM density, reduced slow-wave sleep, impaired sleep continuity). Dysthymic patients with these abnormalities have a positive family history for major depressive disorder more often than do patients without these abnormalities; they also appear to respond better to antidepressant medications. It is not clear whether EEG abnormalities can also be observed in patients with pure dysthymic disorder (i.e., in those with no history of major depressive episodes). An abnormal DST is not common in dysthymic disorder, unless criteria are also met for a major depressive episode.

Differential Diagnosis

Major depressive disorder usually consists of one or more discrete episodes of depression that can be distinguished, by both onset and duration, from the person's usual functioning. During these episodes, vegetative symptoms such as insomnia, loss of appetite, loss of libido, weight loss, and psychomotor symptoms are common. In contrast, dysthymic disorder is characterized by chronic, less severe depressive symptoms that can persist for 2 or more years; vegetative symptoms are less common in dysthymic disorder than in major depressive disorder.

Depressive symptoms may be associated with chronic psychotic disorders and are not considered to indicate dysthymic disorder if they occur only during the course of the psychotic disorder (including residual phases). If mood disturbance is judged to be the direct physiologic consequence of a specific, usually chronic, general

Table 18–17. Treatment of Dysthymic Disorder

Treatment Approach	Primary Method	Secondary Methods
Behavioral	Interpersonal psychotherapy, cognitive–behavioral therapy	
Pharmacologic	SSRIs* (e.g., fluoxetine, paroxetine, sertraline, venlafaxine)	TCAs* (e.g., desipramine, nortriptyline), MAOIs (e.g., phenelzine)

* Table 18.6 provides the range for normal dosage.

medical condition (e.g., multiple sclerosis), then the diagnosis is mood disorder due to a general medical condition. Similarly, substance-induced mood disorder is diagnosed when the depressive symptoms are thought to result from the ingestion of a drug of abuse or a medication or from exposure to a toxin.

Treatment

A. Psychopharmacologic Interventions

Substantial evidence from controlled treatment trials indicates that antidepressants are useful in the treatment of dysthymic disorder, with or without comorbid major depression (Table 18–17). TCAs, MAOIs, and SSRIs all appear to be effective treatments. Rates of response have varied, and there is currently no information assessing the rates of response to a second antidepressant if the first trial was unsuccessful. Controlled maintenance treatment studies are under way. Most dysthymic patients, if they respond to an antidepressant, require continued treatment for at least 6–12 months.

Because dysthymic patients with mild symptoms are not likely to tolerate side effects, the clinician should initiate treatment with an SSRI, because it produces less anticholinergic and sedating side effects and less weight gain. This is particularly important in women receiving long-term treatment. SSRIs can produce a number of mild and time-limited side effects, including gastrointestinal symptoms, insomnia, nervousness, sweating, tremor, dizziness, occasional somnolence, and sexual dysfunction. In patients who do not respond to SSRIs, nortriptyline and desipramine are effective. Among nonselective MAOIs, phenelzine is particularly beneficial for those with atypical reversed vegetative symptoms (e.g., hypersomnia, hyperphagia).

Many of the controlled medication trials reported only partial responses in some subjects with dysthymic disorder. Such patients might benefit from augmentation with a second antidepressant, lithium, thyroid hormone, or combined treatment with psychotherapy. However, there have been controlled studies neither of pharmacologic augmentation strategies, nor of combined pharmacotherapy and psychotherapy approaches.

B. Psychotherapeutic Interventions

Although antidepressants are effective in treating dysthymic disorder, a substantial proportion of patients either fail to respond or are unable to tolerate the side effects. Psychotherapy should be used to address impairments in social and occupational functioning, chronic pessimism and hopelessness, and lack of assertiveness (see Table 18–17). Interpersonal psychotherapy and cognitive–behavioral therapy are useful in treating major depression. Recent modifications of these approaches for dysthymic disorder have been investigated in small naturalistic studies, with successful results. Both therapies are typically time-limited (i.e., lasting less than 6 months).

Interpersonal psychotherapy emphasizes the interaction between the individual and his or her psychosocial environment. Interpersonal psychotherapy has the dual therapeutic goals of reducing depressive symptoms and developing more effective strategies for dealing with social and interpersonal relations. As applied to dysthymic disorder, interpersonal psychotherapy has a major focus on the therapeutic relationship, which is used as a model for other interpersonal interactions. The therapist encourages the patient to engage in occupational and social activities and helps the patient to identify personal needs, to assert those needs, and to set limits.

Cognitive–behavioral therapy is based on the assertion that depression is associated with negative thought patterns, cognitive errors, and faulty information processing that can be altered by specific psychotherapeutic strategies. These strategies help the patient to identify and test negative cognitions and to replace them with alternative, more flexible schemata, which are subsequently rehearsed and studied. As applied to dysthymic disorder, chronic beliefs of helplessness and lack of control are challenged and modified by the experience of mastery in producing desired outcomes, especially in the area of interactions with others.

C. Other Interventions

Interventions based on other than psychopharmacological or psychotherapeutic strategies have not been shown to be of value in the management of dysthymic disorder.

Charney DS, Berman RM, Miller HL: Treatment of depression. In: Schatzberg AF, Nemeroff CB (eds). *Textbook of Psychopharmacology*, 2nd edn. Washington, DC: American Psychiatric Press, 1998.

Harrison WA, Stewart JW: Pharmacotherapy of dysthymia. *Psychiatr Ann* 1993;23:638.

Hirschfeld RMA, Shea MT: Mood disorders: Psychosocial treatments. In: Kaplan HI, Sadock BJ (eds). *Comprehensive Textbook of Psychiatry*, 6th edn. Williams & Wilkins, 1995, pp. 1178–1187.

Complications/Adverse Outcomes of Treatment

Pure dysthymic disorder without prior major depressive disorder is a risk factor for developing major depressive disorder. Ten percent of patients with pure dysthymic disorder will develop major depressive disorder over the ensuing year. In clinical settings, individuals with dysthymic disorder frequently have superimposed major depressive disorder, which is often the reason for seeking treatment.

The condition that co-occurs most frequently with dysthymic disorder is major depressive disorder. The ECA survey estimated that 3.5% of the population had major depression only, 1.8% had dysthymic disorder only, and 1.4% of the population had both disorders, or double depression, at some point in their lives. Moreover, major depressive disorder occurred in 42% of patients with dysthymic disorder, and dysthymic disorders occurred in 28% of patients with major depressive disorder.

The National Comorbidity Survey (NCS) has confirmed that patients with dysthymic disorder have high rates of coexisting psychopathology. In that sample, only 8% of dysthymic patients were unaffected by another Axis I disorder. Besides major depression, the NCS revealed high rates of social phobia, posttraumatic stress disorder, and generalized anxiety disorder. Eating disorders, especially bulimia nervosa, are also associated with nonendogenous depression of only moderate severity. Furthermore, subjective observations and objective investigations have found that depressive symptoms in bulimia are highly reactive, unstable, short lived, and temporally related to bingeing and purging episodes.

Chronic mood symptoms can contribute to interpersonal problems or be associated with distorted self-perception. Thus the assessment of features of a personality disorder is difficult in such individuals. Nevertheless, concomitant personality disorders—especially cluster C personality diagnosis (i.e., avoidant, obsessive-compulsive, and dependent)—can complicate dysthymic disorder. The disorder can also be associated with the cluster B personality diagnoses (i.e., borderline, histrionic, and narcissistic).

Other chronic Axis I disorders (e.g., substance dependence) or chronic psychosocial stressors can be associated with dysthymic disorder in adults. In children, dysthymic disorder can be comorbid with attention-deficit/hyperactivity disorder (ADHD), conduct disorder, anxiety disorders, learning disorders, and mental retardation.

Kessler RC: Dysthymia in the community and its comorbidity with psychiatric and substance use disorders. NIMH Sponsored Workshop: Subsyndromal Mood Disorders: Dysthymia and Cyclothymia. Bethesda, MD, April 26, 1993.

Weissman MN, Livingston Bruce M, Leaf PJ, Florio LP, Holzer C: Affective Disorders. In: Robins LN, Regier DA (eds). *Psychiatric Disorders in America*. New York: Free Press, 1991, pp. 53–80.

Prognosis

Dysthymic disorder often has an early and insidious onset (i.e., in childhood, adolescence, or early adult life) and a chronic course. Disease onset is usually before age 45, but a sizable subgroup of patients develop the disorder in late life (45% after age 45, and 19% after age 65). If dysthymic disorder precedes the onset of major depressive disorder, there is less probability that there will be spontaneous full recovery between major depressive episodes and a greater likelihood of having more frequent subsequent major depressive episodes.

The outcome literature of dysthymic disorder is not encouraging: Of dysthymic inpatients, only about 40% recovered after 2 years of follow-up, and only about 30% after 5 years of follow-up. Thus one can conclude that the available treatments for dysthymic disorder, as currently delivered, are only modestly effective and that relapse is quite common.

■ BIPOLAR DISORDERS

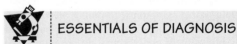 ESSENTIALS OF DIAGNOSIS

DSM-IV-TR Diagnostic Criteria
Manic Episode

A. *A distinct period of abnormally and persistently elevated, expansive, or irritable mood lasting at least 1 week (or any duration if hospitalization is necessary).*

B. *During the period of mood disturbance, three (or more) of the following symptoms have persisted (four if the mood is only irritable) and have been present to a significant degree:*

(1) *inflated self-esteem or grandiosity*

(2) *decreased need for sleep (e.g., feels rested after only 3 hours of sleep)*

(3) *more talkative than usual or pressure to keep talking*

(4) *flight of ideas or subjective experience that thoughts are racing*

(5) *distractibility (i.e., attention too easily drawn to unimportant or irrelevant external stimuli)*

(6) *increase in goal-directed activity (either socially, at work or school, or sexually) or psychomotor agitation*

(7) *excessive involvement in pleasurable activities that have a high potential for painful consequences (e.g., engaging in unrestrained buying sprees, sexual indiscretions, or foolish business investments)*

C. *The symptoms do not meet the criteria for a mixed episode.*

D. *The mood disturbance is sufficiently severe to cause marked impairment in occupational functioning or in usual social activities or relationships with others, or to necessitate hospitalization to prevent harm to self or others, or there are psychotic features.*

E. *The symptoms are not due to the direct physiological effects of a substance (e.g., a drug of abuse, a medication, or other treatment) or a general medical condition (e.g., hyperthyroidism).*

Note: *Manic-like episodes that are clearly caused by somatic antidepressant treatment (e.g., medication, electroconvulsive treatment, light therapy) should not count toward a diagnosis of bipolar I disorder.*

(Reprinted, with permission, from the *Diagnostic and Statistical Manual of Mental Disorders*, 4th edn., Text Revision. Washington DC: American Psychiatric Association, 2000.)

General Considerations

Bipolar disorders can be conceptualized into three distinct entities: **Bipolar I disorder**, consisting of episodes of mania cycling with depressive episodes; **bipolar II disorder**, consisting of episodes of hypomania cycling with depressive episodes; and **cyclothymic disorder**, consisting of hypomania and less severe episodes of depression (see section on Cyclothymic Disorder later in this chapter). Very few patients have only manic episodes.

A. Epidemiology

Table 18–18 summarizes the relevant risk factors. Among the key risk factors for bipolar disorder are being female, having a family history of bipolar disorder, and coming from an upper socioeconomic class. Data also suggest that people under age 50 years are at higher risk of a first attack of bipolar disorder, whereas someone who already has the disorder faces an increasing risk of a recurrent manic or depressive episode, as he or she grows older.

ECA studies support a lifetime prevalence of bipolar disorder ranging from 0.6% to 1.1% (between 0.8% and 1.1% in men, and between 0.5% and 1.3% in women). Estimates from community samples range from 0.4% to 1.6%, suggesting that the disorder affects over 3 million persons in the United States. Bipolar disorder accounts for one quarter of all mood disorders. Prevalence rates of bipolar disorders are usually underestimated, because of problems in identifying manic and, more so, hypomanic episodes.

Bipolar disorders are about equally distributed among males and females, but there are more females with serious bipolar disorder, especially rapid-cycling bipolar disorder. Higher rates of hypothyroidism, greater use of antidepressant medication, and changes in reproductive status and gonadal steroids may account for

Table 18–18. Risk Factors for Bipolar Disorder

Age	People under the age of 50 are at higher risk of a first episode, whereas those who already have the disorder face an increasing risk of a recurrent episode as they age.
Social class	Found more frequently in the upper socioeconomic class.
Race	No relationship.
Life events	No relationship.
Personality	No relationship.
Childhood experience	No relationship.
Marital status	Data not uniform.
Family history	Bipolar patients have both bipolar and unipolar first-degree relatives in roughly equal proportions.

(Modified after Boyd JH, Weissman MM: Epidemiology. In: Paykel ES (ed). *Handbook of Affective Disorders*. New York: Guilford Press, 1982, pp. 109–125; Robins LN, Regier DA (eds). *Psychiatric Disorders in America*. New York: Free Press, 1991, pp. 53–80.)

the greater prevalence of rapid-cycling bipolar disorder among women.

Approximately 10–15% of adolescents with the diagnosis of recurrent major depression will later develop bipolar I disorder. Mixed episodes are more likely in adolescents and young adults than in older adults. The first occurrence of a manic episode after the age of 50 years should alert the clinician to the possibility that the episode may be due either to a general medical condition or to substance use. Bipolar disorder is often misdiagnosed in adolescents (e.g., as ADHD). Patients with early-onset bipolar disorder are more likely to display psychotic symptoms and to have a poorer prognosis in terms of lifetime outcome.

Mood disorders often have seasonal patterns. Acute episodes of depression are common in spring and fall, whereas mania appears to cluster in the summer months. Corresponding data on suicides also show a peak in the spring and a (smaller) peak in the late fall.

B. Etiology

Despite intensive attempts to establish its etiologic or pathophysiologic basis, the precise cause of bipolar disorder is not known. As in major depressive disorder, there is consensus that multiple etiologic factors—genetic, biochemical, and socioenvironmental—may interact in complex ways. Bipolar disorder has a fairly strong genetic association, two-thirds or more of patients showing family history. Association studies have demonstrated linkage at several loci, most consistently at 18p/q and 21q, with others demonstrated as well (5p, 6p, 10q, 12q, 16p, 22p).

1. Life events—Although psychosocial stressors can occasionally precede the onset of bipolar disorder, there is no clear association between life events and the onset of manic or hypomanic episodes. In fact, given the disruptive nature of mood cycling, bipolar disorder may be more likely to induce negative life events. For example, poor judgment during a manic episode may expose people to greater risk for trauma, sexual abuse, or debt.

2. Biological theories

i. Neurotransmitters—Neurotransmitter theories initially conceptualized that depression and mania are on the opposite ends of the same continuum. For example, the norepinephrine hypothesis of affective illness centered around the availability of norepinephrine at synaptic sites, with less norepinephrine being available in depression, and more in mania. This theory, and later modifications of it, especially as they pertain to the separation of unipolar and bipolar disorders, are discussed earlier in this chapter. Simple models of variable transmitter levels have given way to more complex conceptualizations of the illness.

ii. Neuroendocrine factors—Abnormalities in the HPA axis and, more so, in the HPT axis are common in bipolar disorder; they are discussed later in this section.

3. Psychosocial theories—Psychosocial theories pertaining to the etiology of bipolar disorders are the same as those described for major depressive disorder (see section on Major Depressive Disorder earlier in this chapter).

Environmental conditions contribute more to the timing of a bipolar episode than to the patient's inherent underlying vulnerability. In other words, more stressful life events appear to precede early episodes than later ones, and there is a pattern of increased frequency over time. It is possible that early precipitating events merely activate preexisting vulnerability, thereby making an individual more vulnerable for future episodes.

This clinical observation is supported conceptually by the **kindling model**. In laboratory animals, repeated electrical stimulation of the hippocampus will lead to the development of a spontaneous seizure disorder, in which seizures occur without external stimulation. Applied to bipolar disorder, this model provides a better understanding of several phenomena inherent in the illness, including the above-mentioned effects of repeated episodes on disease severity and outcome (e.g., rapid-cycling bipolar disorder usually develops late in the course of the illness) and the acute and prophylactic treatment effects of ECT and anticonvulsants such as carbamazepine and valproic acid. Because these therapies inhibit kindling in laboratory animals, their therapeutic effect in bipolar disorder may involve interruption of kindling.

The kindling model also has enormous treatment implications. Because it suggests that preventing or treating early episodes will favorably affect outcome, it stresses the need for early identification and intervention techniques. This pertains particularly to younger patients, because the risk of kindling is highest during adolescence.

C. Genetics

Twin and family studies provide strong evidence for a genetic component in bipolar disorder, but the precise mechanisms of inheritance are not known. In monozygotic twins, the concordance rate is higher for bipolar disorder (80%) than for unipolar disorder (54%). In dizygotic twins, concordance rates are 24% for bipolar disorder and 19% for unipolar disorder. Adoption studies have shown that the biological children of affected parents have an increased risk for developing a mood disorder, even when reared by unaffected parents, although the data are not uniform. Finally, first-degree biological relatives of bipolar I patients have elevated rates of bipolar I disorder (4–20%), bipolar II disorder (1–5%), and major depressive disorder (4–24%).

Ahmed N, Loosen PT: Thyroid hormones in major depressive and bipolar disorders. In: Casper R (ed). *Women's Health and Emotion.* England: Cambridge University Press, 1997, pp. 83–108.

Arana GW, Baldessarini RJ, Ornsteen M: The dexamethasone suppression test for diagnosis and prognosis in psychiatry. Commentary and review. *Arch Gen Psychiatry* 1985;42:1193.

Boyd JH, Weissman MM: Epidemiology. In: Paykel ES (ed). *Handbook of Affective Disorders.* New York: Guilford Press, 1982, pp. 109–125.

Flores BH, Musselman DL, DeBattista C, Garlow SJ, Schatzberg AF, Nemeroff CB: Biology of mood disorders. In: Schatzberg AF, Nemeroff CB (eds). *Textbook of Psychopharmacology,* 3rd edn. Washington, DC: American Psychiatric Press, 2004, pp. 717–763.

Goodwin FK, Jamison KR: *Manic Depressive Illness.* New York: Oxford University Press, 1990.

Weissman MN, Livingston Bruce M, Leaf PJ, Florio LP, Holzer C: Affective Disorders. In: Robins LN, Regier DA (eds). *Psychiatric Disorders in America.* New York: Free Press, 1991, pp. 53–80.

Clinical Findings

A. Signs & Symptoms

Bipolar disorders can be subdivided into two diagnostic entities: Bipolar I disorder (recurrent major depressive episodes with manic episodes) and bipolar II disorder (recurrent major depressive episodes with hypomanic episodes). The symptoms of both bipolar disorders involve changes in mood, cognition, and behavior (Table 18–19).

1. Bipolar I disorder—Episodes typically begin relatively quickly, with a rapid escalation through the stages summarized in Table 18–19. In 50–60% of cases, a depressive episode immediately precedes or follows a manic episode. Mania without history of depression is very rare. The hallmark of a manic episode is abnormally and persistently elevated, expansive, or irritable mood. The elevated mood can be described as euphoric, cheerful, and with indiscriminate enthusiasm and optimism; therefore, others often perceive it as infectious. Although the patient's mood may be predominantly elevated, it may quickly become irritable, especially after demands are not satisfied.

i. Somatic features—The sleep of bipolar patients varies with their clinical state. When depressed, bipolar patients may sleep too much; when manic, they sleep little or not at all and typically report feeling fully rested nevertheless. As the manic episode intensifies, patients may go without sleep for nights, their insomnia further intensifying the manic syndrome. There is speculation as to whether the insomnia precedes, and perhaps triggers or fuels, the manic episode. It is difficult to control an acute manic episode clinically if one cannot control the associated insomnia. Conversely, some bipolar patients may experience a manic or hypomanic episode after a single night of sleep deprivation.

ii. Behavioral features—Bipolar patients are initially social, outgoing, self-confident, and talkative and can be difficult to interrupt. Their speech is full of puns, jokes, and irrelevancies. Patients are often hypersexual, promiscuous, disinhibited, and seductive; they may present to an emergency room setting dressed in colorful, flamboyant, and inappropriate clothing. As the manic episode intensifies, their speech becomes loud, intrusive, rapid, and difficult to follow, and they can become irritable, assaultive, and threatening.

Table 18–19. Stages of Mania

	Stage I	**Stage II**	**Stage III**
Mood	Labile affect; euphoria predominates; irritability if demands not satisfied	Increased dysphoria and depression; open hostility and anger	Very dysphoric; panic-stricken; hopeless
Cognition	Expansive, grandiose, overconfident; thoughts coherent but occasionally tangential; sexual and religious preoccupations; racing thoughts	Flight of ideas; disorganization of cognition; delusions	Incoherent, definite loosening of associations; bizarre and idiosyncratic delusions; hallucinations in one-third of patients; disorientation to time and place; occasional ideas of reference
Behavior	Increased psychomotor activity; increased rate of speech; increased spending, smoking, telephone use	Increased psychomotor activity; pressured speech; occasional assaultive behavior	Frenzied, frequently bizarre psychomotor activity

(Adapted from Goodwin FK, Jamison KR: *Manic Depressive Illness.* New York: Oxford University Press, 1990.)

iii. **Cognitive features**—Manic patients are easily distracted. Their thought processes are difficult to follow because of racing thoughts and flight of ideas. They appear to have an unrestrained and accelerated flow of thoughts and ideas, which are often unrelated. Patients can be overly self-confident and become preoccupied with political, personal, religious, and sexual themes. They may exhibit an inappropriate increase in self-esteem and may have grandiose beliefs (e.g., of brilliance, success, wealth, etc.). Their judgment is impaired significantly, resulting in buying sprees, sexual indiscretions, and unwise business investments. Psychotic features such as paranoia, delusions, and hallucinations are sometimes present, not unlike those seen in patients with schizophrenia.

iv. **Risk of suicide**—Bipolar patients are at a substantial risk for suicide, with a mortality rate estimated to be 2–3 times higher than that of the general population. There is burgeoning evidence that lithium maintenance treatment attenuates the risk of suicide attempts and completions. When 16,800 bipolar patients were followed for a 2-year period, the annual risk of suicide or suicide attempts was 0.26–0.4 in patients taking lithium, and 1.68–1.5 in patients not taking lithium. Risk factors for suicide in bipolar patients include a history of previous suicide attempts, a history of rapid-cycling bipolar disorder, comorbid substance abuse, a mixed episode, and a current depressive episode.

2. Bipolar II disorder—Characterized by recurrent episodes of major depression and hypomania, bipolar II disorder has been identified as a distinct disorder only in DSM-IV. Hypomanic symptoms are similar to manic symptoms but do not reach the same level of symptom severity or social impairment (i.e., the patient's capacity to function vocationally is seldom compromised). Hypomania, though associated with elated mood and increased self-assuredness, does not present with psychotic symptoms, or may not show severe racing thoughts, or marked psychomotor agitation. Hypomanic patients thus do not perceive themselves as being ill and are likely to minimize their symptoms and to resist treatment.

3. Rapid-cycling bipolar disorder—By definition, patients with rapid-cycling bipolar disorder experience four or more affective episodes per year. Approximately 10–15% of bipolar patients experience rapid cycling. Although similar to other bipolar patients nosologically and demographically, patients with rapid-cycling bipolar disorder tend to have a longer duration and a more refractory course of the illness. Women are represented disproportionately, making up 80–95% of rapid-cycling patients, compared to about 50% of non-rapid-cycling patients. A variety of factors may predispose bipolar illness to a rapid-cycling course, including treatment with antidepressants. The development of clinical or subclinical hypothyroidism (spontaneously or during lithium treatment) in a manic patient predisposes to a more rapidly cycling course.

B. PSYCHOLOGICAL TESTING

Psychological testing has not been shown to be of value in the management of bipolar disorder.

C. LABORATORY FINDINGS & NEUROIMAGING

No laboratory findings are diagnostic of a bipolar disorder or of a manic or hypomanic episode; however, several laboratory findings have been noted to be abnormal in groups of individuals with bipolar disorder. Compared to the wealth of findings in major depressive disorder, research findings in bipolar disorder are in general scarce and inconclusive. For one thing, bipolar disorder is not as common as major depressive disorder. Beyond that, patients with acute manic states are not as likely to collaborate in research studies; they experience lack of insight, agitation, irritability, and racing thoughts, among other symptoms; and they are normally in need of rapid containment of symptoms.

1. HPA axis—The few available cross-sectional and longitudinal studies reveal increased plasma cortisol levels in some depressed bipolar patients. Abnormalities in the DST have also been noted. DST nonsuppression occurs more frequently in the mixed phase of the illness (78%), but also occurs in bipolar depression (38%) and mania (49%). Both hypercortisolemia and DST results normalize after the acute episode subsides, suggesting that these abnormalities are state and not trait dependent. Although these abnormalities are not specific for bipolar disorder or even major depression, their pathophysiology is suggestive of central (i.e., hypothalamic) rather than peripheral dysregulation of cortisol.

2. HPT axis—HPT axis abnormalities are rather common in bipolar disorder, especially in rapid-cycling bipolar disorder, but the precise relationship of these abnormalities with the illness and its various clinical presentations is not known. Among these abnormalities are an attenuated nocturnal TSH peak, a blunted TSH response to TRH administration, and a high prevalence of various degrees of hypothyroidism.

There are intriguing associations among thyroid function, bipolar disorder, and gender. Hypothyroidism is very common in patients with bipolar disorder; it is especially common in female patients who present with a rapid-cycling course. Treatment with hypermetabolic doses of T_4 has shown some promise in that it may reduce acute symptoms, number of relapses, and duration of hospitalizations.

Two main conclusions can be drawn from these observations. Clinically, comorbid hypothyroidism seems to negatively affect disease outcome by predisposing the individual patient to a rapid-cycling course. Substitution with T_4 has proven useful in some patients, but often, high doses are necessary to induce clinical response. Conceptually these findings support the hypothesis that a relative central thyroid hormone deficit may predispose to the marked and frequent mood swings that characterize rapid-cycling bipolar disorder. We may ask whether the central thyroid hormone deficit serves only as a risk factor for the development of rapid cycling in a known bipolar patient, or whether it can predispose most affectively ill patients to any major behavioral change (i.e., the switch from depression into recovery, from recovery into depression, or from depression into mania).

3. Sleep EEG—Sleep EEG recordings have revealed normal results in acutely ill bipolar patients, including normal REM latencies, but not all studies agree. These data, of course, are in stark contrast to those reported in major depressive disorder, in which shortened REM latencies are common. However, bipolar patients in full clinical remission can exhibit an increased density and percentage of REM and a sleep architecture more sensitive to arecoline (an acetylcholine agonist known to produce a shortened REM latency). The discrepancies between unipolar and bipolar patients are thought to be the result of different levels of clinical severity, variable proportions of bipolar I and bipolar II patients, and age differences.

4. Brain imaging—The most consistent neuroimaging findings in depressed (unipolar and) bipolar patients are decreased PFC blood flow and metabolism. Basal ganglia abnormalities have also been found in depressed bipolar patients, involving decreased blood flow and metabolism. In bipolar disorders, structural imaging studies suggest an increased number of white matter hyperintensities, which may be unique to bipolar disorder and its treatment, or related to cardiovascular factors. Metabolic and blood flow studies provide evidence for decreased activity of the PFC in depressed bipolar patients. It is presently not known whether these findings are state or trait related.

D. COURSE OF ILLNESS

The natural course of bipolar disorders is variable. Patients usually experience their first manic episode in their early 20s, but bipolar disorders sometimes start in adolescence or after age 40 years. Manic episodes typically begin suddenly, with a rapid escalation of symptoms over a few days, often, they are triggered by psychosocial stressors. In about 50% of patients a depressive episode immediately precedes a manic episode.

Although medications are effective in treating acute episodes and in maintaining patients in remission, they are not completely effective in preventing future episodes. Studies have shown that patients maintained with lithium levels of 0.8–1.0 ng/mL are less likely

to have a recurrence than are patients maintained on lower lithium levels (0.4–0.6 ng/mL). Combinations of lithium and anticonvulsants have shown promise in maintaining euthymia and increasing cycle intervals.

Ahmed N, Loosen PT: Thyroid hormones in major depressive and bipolar disorders. In: Casper R (ed). *Women's Health and Emotion.* England: Cambridge University Press, 1997, pp. 83–108.

Arana GW, Baldessarini RJ, Ornsteen M: The dexamethasone suppression test for diagnosis and prognosis in psychiatry; commentary and review. *Arch Gen Psychiatry* 1985;42:1193.

Bauer MS, Whybrow PC: Thyroid hormones and the central nervous system in affective illness: Interactions that may have clinical significance. *Integr Psychiatry* 1988;6:75.

Beyer JL, Krishnan KR: Volumetric brain imaging findings in mood disorders. *Bipolar Disord* 2002;4:89.

Flores BH, Musselman DL, DeBattista C, Garlow SJ, Schatzberg AF, Nemeroff CB: Biology of mood disorders. In: Schatzberg AF, Nemeroff CB (eds). *Textbook of Psychopharmacology*, 3rd edn. Wahington, DC: American Psychiatric Press, 2004, pp. 717–763.

Goodwin FK, Jamison KR: *Manic Depressive Illness.* New York: Oxford University Press, 1990.

Soares JC, Mann JJ: The functional neuroanatomy of mood disorders. *J Psychiat Res* 1997;31:393.

Stoll AL, Renshaw PF, Yurgelun-Todd DA, Cohen BM: Neuroimaging in bipolar disorder: What have we learned? *Biol Psych* 2000;48:505.

Differential Diagnosis

A. MEDICAL DISORDERS

Numerous medical disorders and medications can induce or mimic the clinical picture of bipolar disorder, exacerbate its course and severity, or complicate its treatment. It has been widely noted that psychopharmacologic interventions are less successful if the bipolar disorder is due to a primary medical condition; whenever possible, it is advisable to attempt to correct the underlying medical disorder before beginning psychopharmacologic treatment.

DSM-IV criteria specify that to make a diagnosis of bipolar disorder, the symptoms cannot be the direct result of a substance or a general medical condition. A late onset of the first manic episode (over age 50) should prompt the clinician to carefully exclude a possible medical cause. Table 18–20 lists the many organic causes of mania and hypomania.

B. PSYCHIATRIC DISORDERS

The Axis I and Axis II disorders associated with hypomanic or manic symptoms need to be included in the differential diagnosis of bipolar disorders (Table 18–21). First, the psychotic features associated with schizophrenia or schizoaffective disorder are often indistinguishable from those associated with acute mania. Second, major depressive episodes may be associated prominently with

Table 18–20. Organic Causes of Mania and Hypomania

Medications	Dialysis
Isoniazid	Hyperthyroidism
Procarbazine	**Neurologic Disorders**
L-Dopa	Right temporal lobe seizures
Bromide	Multiple sclerosis
Decongestants	Right hemisphere damage
Bronchodilators	Seizure disorders
Procyclidine	Huntington's disease
Calcium replacement	Poststroke
Phencyclidine	**Infectious Diseases**
Metoclopramide	Neurosyphilis
Corticosteroids and ACTH	Herpes simplex encephalitis
Hallucinogens	Q fever
Cimetidine	HIV infection, influenza
Sympathomimetic amines	**Neoplasms**
Disulfiram	Diencephalic glioma
Barbiturates	Suprasellar craniopharyngioma
Anticonvulsants	Parasagittal meningioma
Benzodiazepines	Right intraventricular meningioma
Cocaine	Right temperoparietal occipital metastases
TCAs	Tumor of floor of the fourth ventricle
Metabolic Disturbances	**Other Conditions**
Postoperative states	Postisolation syndrome
Hemodialysis	Posttraumatic confusion
Vitamin B_{12}	Post-ECT
Addison's disease	Delirium
Iatrogenic Cushing's disease	Serotonin syndrome
Postinfection states	Right temporal lobectomy

(Modified from Goodwin FK, Jamison KR: *Manic Depressive Illness.* New York: Oxford University Press, 1990.)

irritable mood and may thus be difficult to distinguish from a mixed bipolar episode. Third, in children and adolescents, ADHD and mania are both characterized by overactivity, impulsive behavior, poor judgment and academic performance, and psychological denial. Fourth, patients with certain personality disorders (e.g., borderline or histrionic personality disorders) can exhibit impulsivity, affective instability, and paranoid ideations, as do manic patients.

Finally, substance abuse is exceedingly common in patients with bipolar disorder. As many as 41% of bipolar patients abuse or are dependent on drugs, 46% abuse or are dependent on alcohol, and as many as 61% abuse or are dependent on any substance. Careful etiologic evaluation and a drug-free washout period after intoxication are often necessary to distinguish whether the mood disturbance is the consequence of substance abuse or whether the substance abuse is the consequence of a mood disturbance. Such differentiation is important because psychiatric comorbidity complicates the acute manic state and negatively affects disease outcome. The mood disorders complicated by substance abuse are therefore

Table 18–21. Axis I and Axis II Disorders that May be Associated with Manic or Hypomanic Symptoms

Axis I
Delirium
Dementia
Substance-related disorders
Schizophrenia
Schizoaffective disorder
Delusional disorders
Psychotic disorder not otherwise specified
Cyclothymic disorder
Factitious disorder
Malingering
Attention-deficit/hyperactivity disorder
Conduct disorder
Axis II
Borderline personality disorder
Histrionic personality disorder

treated in units especially designed to treat aspects of dual diagnosis.

Treatment

A. Psychopharmacologic Interventions

The clinical management of bipolar disorder involves treatment of the acute episodes and maintenance therapy. Acute bipolar episodes usually demand immediate symptom containment, which is achieved most easily using pharmacologic means (Table 18–22). TCAs typically should be avoided in depressive episodes, because of the potential for the induction of mania, mixed state, or rapid cycling. This appears to occur with other antidepressants as well. A limited amount of data suggests that lamotrigine may be effective in bipolar depression, in doses in the range of 200–400 mg/day. It also has mood-stabilizing effects, making it a reasonable medication to use during depressive episodes.

All atypical antipsychotics appear to have acute antimanic effects, and most have been shown to be effective as maintenance treatment. One drug, quetiapine, recently received US Food and Drug Administration (USFDA) approval for bipolar depression as a monotherapy agent. Olanzapine also has been shown to reduce depressive symptoms, although this appears primarily to be vegetative symptoms such as sleep and appetite disturbance, more than so-called "core" depressive symptoms such as down mood or negative thinking. However, the combination of olanzapine with the SSRI fluoxetine has been shown to be quite efficacious, and appears to produce its effects very rapidly. This combination treatment has received approval by the USFDA. However, the use of the combination has been limited. In part, this may be the result of significant issues with weight gain and the potential for metabolic syndrome associated with olanzapine.Acute manic episodes can be managed with lithium, divalproex, or an atypical antipsychotic. If delusional symptoms and agitation are present, antipsychotics (particularly atypical antipsychotics such as olanzapine or risperidone) or benzodiazepines (e.g., clonazepam) need to be added.

After the resolution of depressive or manic episodes, the maintenance treatment phase is aimed at prevention of future episodes. Drugs shown to be effective for maintenance management include lithium, divalproex, lamotrigine, or atypical antipsychotics. Often, treatments will

Table 18–22. Treatment of Bipolar Disorder

Condition	Primary Method	Secondary Methods
Acute depressive episode	SSRI, bupropion	ECT, MAOIs, TCAs
Acute manic episode	Lithium (not useful in mixed episode); valproic acid or carbamazepine, with or without antipsychotic (e.g., haloperidol) or benzodiazepines (e.g., clonazepam)*	Verapamil, ECT
Maintenance treatment	Lithium, valproic acid, or carbamazepine; in difficult cases, lithium plus valproic acid or carbamazepine	Educational and structured psychosocial support

*Lithium should be initiated at 300 mg twice daily and titrated with frequent blood-level monitoring to achieve levels between 0.8 and 1.2 nmol/L acutely (0.6–0.8 nmol/L during maintenance). Carbamazepine should be started at 200 mg twice daily with a gradual increase to plasma levels of 3–14 mg/mL. Valproic acid should be started in the 500–750 mg/day range and titrated in 250-mg increments to achieve plasma levels of 40–110 mg/ml, a range therapeutically effective yet well tolerated.

need to be combined for optimal stabilization. (see Table 18–22).

Mood charting, though cumbersome and time consuming, allows careful delineation of the frequency and severity of episodes and of the drug's efficacy, including evidence of partial response patterns or loss of efficacy. Benzodiazepines (e.g., clonazepam or lorazepam) are often useful in relieving the insomnia and agitation associated with acute illness. Clinicians agree that control of insomnia is paramount in treating acute bipolar illness, and there is speculation that continued insomnia may fuel the illness. Finally, agents with the propensity to destabilize mood (e.g., antidepressants, steroids, alcohol) need to be identified and discontinued if possible (although continuation antidepressant treatment may be needed).

1. Lithium

i. Indications—There are two main indications for lithium in patients with bipolar disorder: (1) for the management of the acute manic or hypomanic episode, and (2) for the prevention of further episodes of both mania and depression. Lithium is also useful in potentiating or augmenting the effects of antidepressants (mainly in refractory depression, as noted earlier in this chapter); in managing impulse-control disorders (especially episodic violence); in the long-term prophylactic treatment of cluster headaches; and in treating schizophrenia in a limited number of patients, particularly if they experience prominent affective symptoms (in which case a neuroleptic is also needed to treat the intrinsic schizophrenic symptoms).

a. Acute management of (hypo)mania— Lithium is useful in acute manic episodes. Approximately 80% of manic patients show at least a partial response to lithium monotherapy. Lithium also has some acute antidepressant effects, but these actions tend to be incomplete and require 3–4 weeks of treatment to achieve maximal effect. Often antidepressants are needed to effectively treat or prevent depressive episodes, but their use is always associated with the risk of precipitating (hypo)manic episodes or of destabilizing the illness course. Bupropion or SSRIs are less likely to produce these unwanted side effects relative to TCAs. In acute manic states, lithium monotherapy can be beneficial in a matter of days, but usually there is a 5–10-day latency of response. Because of this delayed response lithium has not become the sole agent in everyday clinical practice for acute mania. Most clinicians now use antipsychotics or benzodiazepines in addition to lithium in the acute phase of mania to control psychosis, hyperactivity, insomnia, and agitation. Antipsychotics appear to be superior to lithium only in the initial management of the acute state (i.e., in the first few days of treatment).

Patients are often concerned about continuation of treatment indefinitely. The clinician should carefully explain to the patient that he or she may have a chronic condition, that a manic or depressive episode is likely to recur in the future, that it is necessary to be cognizant of the early symptoms of a developing episode (e.g., insomnia, elation or depression of mood, increased or decreased activity), and that treatment should be sought as soon as such symptoms occur. It is also important to point out, ideally to both the patient and family members, that patients are not likely to seek treatment in the early hypomanic states because the associated self-assuredness, mood elation, and boundless energy are generally perceived as pleasant. If lithium is withdrawn abruptly, approximately 50% of patients relapse within 5 months.

b. Prevention of relapse— The efficacy of lithium in the long-term prophylactic treatment of bipolar disorder has been well documented; it appears to involve a reduction in both the number of episodes and their intensity. The preventive effects of lithium are most robust when there is evidence that the interval between episodes has shortened, that is, when the course of bipolar disorder has intensified in both severity of symptoms and frequency of episodes.

c. Management of breakthrough depression— A depressive episode sometimes "breaks through" lithium maintenance treatment. If this occurs, the following steps should be taken: (1) Increase lithium dose; (2) maximize thyroid function; (3) add an SSRI (the drug of choice), bupropion, or an MAOI; (4) consider treatment alternatives (e.g., valproic acid, carbamazepine); and (5) consider sleep deprivation or ECT for severe depression. Because acute side effects and toxicity are common with lithium treatment, a thorough pretreatment and follow-up evaluation are necessary (Table 18–23).

In healthy patients, lithium carbonate can be initiated at 300 mg twice daily and titrated with frequent blood level monitoring. The blood level should be adjusted and maintained in a range of 0.6–1.2 mmol/L. This will require widely varying doses (600–1800 mg/day). However, most patients are maintained effectively at 900–1200 mg/day.

Occasionally treatment calls for the use of medication in liquid form. Lithium citrate, a suspension form of the drug is available. Not only does this preparation allow for finer gradations of titration, but it reduces the likelihood of nausea and vomiting, which are associated with lithium treatment.

ii. Adverse effects—Lithium is well tolerated by most patients. However, careful management of lithium plasma concentrations is required because of its narrow therapeutic window and because of the close association between plasma levels and toxicity (Table 18–24). Within the normal range of lithium plasma levels, one can

Table 18–23. Medical Monitoring of Healthy Patients On Maintenance Lithium

Minimum Recommendations	Frequency
Plasma lithium	4–8 weeks*
T4, free T4, TSH	6 months
Creatinine	12 months
Urinalysis	12 months
Optional recommendations	Frequency
24-h urine volume	6–12 months
Creatinine clearance	6–12 months
Urine osmolality	6–12 months
Complete blood count	6–12 months
EKG (over age 50 yr)	6–12 months

Special circumstances that can alter dose/blood-level relationships

Medical illness, especially with diarrhea, vomiting, or anorexia
Surgery
Crash dieting, sodium restriction diet
Strenuous exercise
Very hot climate
Advanced age
Pregnancy and delivery

*This frequency can be reduced over time, especially with reliable patients.

(Modified after Goodwin FK, Jamison KR: Manic Depressive Illness. New York: Oxford University Press, 1990.)

Table 18–24. Associations Between Lithium Plasma Levels and Toxicity

Lithium Level (mmol/L)	Side Effects
1.0–1.5	Fine tremor, nausea
1.5–2.0	Cogwheeling tremor, nausea and vomiting, somnolence
2.0–2.5	Ataxia, confusion
2.5–3.0	Dysarthria, gross tremor
> 3.0	Delirium, seizures, coma, death

commonly observe persistent but benign side effects, including increased thirst or urination, fine tremor, weight gain, and edema. Above the normal range of lithium plasma levels, serious side effects can occur rapidly; they include (with increasing plasma concentrations and symptom severity) nausea, vomiting, diarrhea, drowsiness and mental dullness, slurred speech, confusion, coarse tremor and twitching, muscle weakness, and above levels of 3.0 mmol/L, seizures, coma and death.

The major side effects of lithium affect the endocrine, renal, hematologic, cardiovascular, cutaneous gastrointestinal, ocular, and nervous systems (Table 18–25). Side effects are usually dosage dependent and transient in nature. Lithium has teratogenic effects, particularly when taken during the first trimester of pregnancy, it has been linked to the serious cardiac birth defect Ebstein's Anomaly and should be avoided in pregnant women. The risk factors predisposing to lithium side effects and toxicity include renal disease or reduced renal clearance with age; organic brain disorder; dehydration after vomiting, diarrhea, increased perspiration, and strenuous exercise; low sodium intake or high sodium excretion; prolonged dieting, especially salt-restriction diets; and early pregnancy.

a. Management of lithium side effects— Because most side effects are dosage dependent, reduction of lithium intake will quickly ameliorate the acute symptoms, but this may increase the risk of relapse (see Table 18–25). Nausea, vomiting, and diarrhea can be reduced in some patients by switching from the carbonate to the citrate salt of lithium. Polydipsia and polyuria can be managed by giving the entire daily dosage of lithium at bedtime. Tremor is often responsive to β-blockers such as atenolol or propranolol. These and other common side effects (i.e., memory problems, weight gain, and tremor)—although not immediately harmful and dangerous—can be quite troublesome, may be intolerable to patients, and often negatively affect compliance. Goodwin and Jamison (1990), pooling percentages from 12 studies including 1094 patients, showed that subjective complaints were common. Among the most frequent were thirst (36%), polyuria (30%), memory problems (28%), tremor (27%), weight gain (19%), drowsiness (12%), and diarrhea (9%). Only 26% of patients had no complaints. Memory problems were most likely to cause noncompliance, followed by weight gain, tremor, polyuria, and drowsiness.

Thyroid dysfunction can be associated with lithium treatment. A small proportion of patients receiving chronic lithium treatment will develop thyroid enlargement with elevations in plasma TSH concentrations. Few patients, however, develop frank hypothyroidism. When this occurs, lithium may be discontinued, if possible, or thyroid hormone supplementation may be initiated.

The most common renal problems in patients taking lithium are polydipsia and polyuria, both of which are

Table 18–25. Common Side Effects of Lithium

Affected System	Side Effect	Comments
Endocrine	Thyroid dysfunction	Lithium inhibits iodine uptake by the thyroid gland, iodination of tyrosine, release of T4 and T3, the peripheral degradation of thyroid hormones, and the stimulating effects of TSH. Approximately 5% of patients taking lithium develop signs of hypothyroidism; another 3% have elevated TSH levels or abnormal clinical signs and symptoms.
	Diabetes mellitus	Lithium may alter glucose tolerance, leading to mild diabetes status in some patients.
Renal	Polydipsia and polyuria	Lithium causes polydipsia and polyuria in about 60% of patients; it persists in 20–25%. Usually these symptoms appear early in treatment and may reappear after several months. This adverse reaction is likely to be the result of an inhibition of the interaction between ADH and adenylate cyclase in the renal tubule and collecting duct system; it is usually reversible.
	Diabetes insipidus	Occasionally a nephrogenic diabetes-insipidus-like syndrome develops in which the patient cannot concentrate urine. Excretion of urine is greater than 3 L/day, and patients must drink comparable amounts of water to avoid dehydration. This condition is almost always reversible.
	Structural kidney damage	This chronic tubulointerstitial nephropathy, perhaps the most worrisome adverse reaction occurring after long-term lithium administration, may be characterized by focal glomerular atrophy, interstitial fibrosis, and significant impairment of tubular functioning. Damage correlates roughly with the length of exposure to lithium. Persistent polyuria may be an early warning sign, but because many patients develop polyuria during maintenance treatment, the physician is often faced with a difficult problem.
	Other kidney effects	Lithium and sodium are managed similarly by the kidney. Perspiration, diarrhea, vomiting, thiazide diuretics, and salt-free diets may thus produce a significant increase in the lithium level, necessitating careful monitoring.
Hematologic	White blood cell count elevation	Because this effect involves a true proliferative response of the bone marrow, lithium can be useful in conditions associated with neutropenia (i.e., radio- or chemotherapy)
Cardiovascular	Significant effects on the heart (e.g., T-wave flattening, U-waves)	Adverse reactions are rare. Several types of conduction problems have appeared, including first degree A-V block, irregular or slowed sinus node rhythms, and increased numbers of ventricular premature contractions.
Cutaneous	Pruritic, maculopapular rash	May appear during first month of treatment.
Gastrointestinal	Gastric irritation, anorexia, abdominal cramps, nausea, vomiting, diarrhea	Common.
CNS and neuromuscular	Mental dullness, decreased memory and concentration, headaches, fatigue and lethargy, muscle weakness, and tremor	Frequent at therapeutic dosages. A fine hand tremor of irregular rhythm and frequency occurs in about 50% of patients; worsened by caffeine, anxiety, and muscle tension; decreases over time. If it persists, propranolol, 20–160 mg/day, may help.
Ocular	Tearing, itching, burning, or blurring of vision	Rare. May occur during first week of treatment.

Table 18–25. (Continued)

Affected System	Side Effect	Comments
Other effects	Weight gain	Between 20% and 60% of patients are said to gain more than 20 pounds during treatment. Etiology unknown.
Pregnancy	Various congenital abnormalities, particularly of the heart and great vessels (Epstein's anomaly)	May occur in babies exposed to lithium in utero during the first trimester. The risk of major congenital malformations with first trimester lithium use is 4–12%; prenatal diagnosis by fetal echocardiogram and high-resolution ultrasound examination at 16–18 weeks' gestation is suggested. The alternatives to lithium—carbamazepine or sodium valproate—are associated with a marked increase in spina bifida. These agents should be avoided during pregnancy. If this is not possible, a thorough risk-benefit analysis is necessary before prescribing any of these drugs during pregnancy.

usually reversible. Rarely, patients can develop diabetes insipidus or an interstitial nephritis-like syndrome (see Table 18–25), both of which require regular monitoring of kidney functioning (see Table 18–23). We now use lower plasma concentrations during maintenance therapy (i.e., 0.6–0.8 nmol/L) than, say, two decades ago; this reduction in lithium dosing has resulted in a lower side-effect profile, especially of renal side effects.

Serious cardiac side effects are uncommon (see Table 18–25). T-wave flattening or inversion occur often and are not associated with negative treatment outcome. Some patients taking lithium over the long-term may experience sudden death of presumed cardiac origin. In particular, sinoatrial node dysfunction (sick sinus syndrome) can occur with increased frequency in these patients. Routine monitoring of the patient's electrocardiogram and pulse is necessary in order to minimize cardiac risk.

The use of lithium during pregnancy is controversial (see Table 18–25). Mild transient hypothyroidism and somnolence are common in newborns exposed in utero. The concentration of lithium in breast milk may also adversely affect nursing infants. The possibility of cardiovascular abnormalities in some infants exposed to lithium during the first trimester in utero necessitates both a careful initial risk-benefit analysis and close monitoring.

b. Contraindications to lithium— Relative or absolute contraindications to lithium are severe renal disease, acute myocardial infarction (in which complications may occur owing to arrhythmias, use of diuretics and digoxin, reduced fluid or salt intake, cardiac failure, and reduced renal function), myasthenia gravis (in which lithium interferes with the release of acetylcholine and the depolarization and repolarization of the motor endplate), first trimester of pregnancy, and breast-feeding mothers. As well, nonsteroidal anti-inflammatory drugs can markedly elevate plasma levels of lithium and should be avoided.

iii. Management of lithium treatment failure— About 60% of bipolar patients respond to lithium treatment alone, although breakthrough of mania or depression is common. If patients do not respond to lithium treatment, the clinician has several alternative options. The first is to change the medication to divalproex. Carbamazepine also has been used as a mood stabilizer, although there are very limited controlled clinical trial data. Lamotrigine also has been shown to have some mood-stabilizing effects and is approved for maintenance use in bipolar disorder. These can be administered with or without continuing lithium. Table 18–26 summarizes other, less common options.

Table 18–26. Alternative or Adjunctive Treatments for Patients who Respond Poorly to Lithium

Assessment of present treatment:
Evaluate possible cycle-inducing effect of adjunctive antidepressant or antimanic medication
Evaluate contribution of drug or alcohol abuse
Change of pharmacological strategy:
Anticonvulsants (e.g., carbamazepine or valproate)
MAOI (e.g., clorgiline) T (hypermetabolic doses)
L-Tryptophan
Calcium channel blockers (e.g., verapamil and others) Magnesium aspartate
Other approaches:
Maintenance ECT
Periodic sleep deprivation

Table 18–27. Pretreatment and Posttreatment Evaluation for Carbamazepine

Complete blood count, including platelets, white blood count, reticulocyte, and serum iron*
Liver function tests[†]
Electrolytes
Thyroid functions: T4, T3, and TSH
Complete urinalysis and blood urea nitrogen
Rule out history of cardiac, hepatic, or renal damage
Rule out history of adverse hematologic response to other drugs

*Repeat at 2 and 4 weeks, and quarterly thereafter.
[†]Repeat at 1, 3, 6, and 12 months, and biannually thereafter.

Preliminary evidence indicates that maintenance treatment with anticonvulsants may carry a higher risk of suicide than maintenance treatment with lithium, but no firm conclusions can be drawn yet. The following are predictors of a good response to anticonvulsants: Rapid-cycling course of the illness, mixed episode, previous poor response to lithium, secondary mania, and recurrent substance abuse.

a. Carbamazepine — Of the two anticonvulsants, carbamazepine has been used clinically for a longer period of time. Doses are typically started at 200–400 mg/day and titrated to achieve a plasma concentration of 3–14 μg/mL. Common side effects include somnolence, dizziness, nausea and vomiting, and mild ataxia; these effects can be managed effectively with dosage reduction or slow dosage titration. Mild elevations of liver enzymes and mildly reduced white blood counts are also common. These problems typically improve or resolve with time. Finally, rash is common and usually requires discontinuation.

Two potentially serious adverse reactions associated with carbamazepine treatment require close and regular monitoring during treatment (Table 18–27). Carbamazepine can acutely damage the liver, resulting in marked increases in liver enzymes and sometimes frank jaundice. Hepatic failure, however, is rare.

Blood dyscrasias, including granulocytopenia, agranulocytosis, or aplastic anemia, pose a second category of problems. Although rare (the incidence of agranulocytosis is approximately six per million population per year, whereas aplastic anemia occurs in two per million per year), the possibility of these adverse reactions necessitates that the patient have a complete blood count taken regularly (see Table 18–27). If the patient's absolute neutrophil count falls below 2000, the count should be monitored at least weekly until a rebound is observed. At below 1500, the carbamazepine dosage should be lowered quickly to about 50% of previous dosage and the count monitored weekly until it rebounds. If the count falls below 1000, carbamazepine should be discontinued and the patient monitored under hospital conditions until the count rebounds.

The teratogenic effects of carbamazepine are well known. Carbamazepine appears to induce neural tube defects such as spina bifida at high rates (about 1% of exposures); therefore, it should not be used in pregnant women. Human chorionic gonadotropin testing is indicated in women of childbearing potential who are to be started on this agent.

b. Valproic acid (divalproex sodium) — Clinical trials have established the effectiveness of valproic acid in the acute management of mania, but long-term maintenance research is lacking. The agent is available as regular sodium valproate or as a dimer molecule divalproex sodium, which is most commonly used. The latter dissociates in the gastrointestinal tract to form free valproate, which is then absorbed. This slower release reduces gastrointestinal side effects that are common with valproic acid.

Divalproex is started in the 500–750 mg/day range and titrated in 250 mg increments to achieve an adequate plasma level. The therapeutic plasma-level range is 50–125 μg/mL. The higher end of the plasma-level range is indicated for patients whose illness is poorly controlled on lower levels.

Common side effects associated with sodium valproate include nausea and vomiting, diarrhea or constipation, mild elevations of liver enzymes, mild drowsiness or fatigue, and skin rash. More serious reactions are rare. Severe hepatitis that can result in hepatic failure has been reported and has resulted in fatalities; it is especially prevalent in young children. Liver function studies are required at baseline and within the first month of treatment. They should be repeated at 3 and 6 months, then at least annually thereafter. Mild elevations of liver enzymes are an indication for more frequent monitoring. Clotting abnormalities also have been reported. Finally, like carbamazepine, valproate may produce spina bifida in infants exposed in utero. Use in pregnancy must be avoided.

c. Atypical antipsychotics — All of the currently available atypical antipsychotics (except for clozapine and the recently approved drug paliperidone) have been described to have acute anti-manic effects. Several appear beneficial in relapse prevention, although only olanzapine has a maintenance indication approved by the USFDA. Nonetheless, all atypicals are used for both acute and maintenance treatment. Side effects of atypicals include extrapyramidal effects, akathisia, somnolence, activation (particularly for ziprasidone and aripiprazole), and weight gain with a risk for the metabolic syndrome. The latter issue is a particular problem for olanzapine, while ziprasidone and aripiprazole produce little weight gain. One concern with the use of antipsychotics of any type (with the possible exception of clozapine) is tardive dyskinesia (TD). TD is a syndrome of abnormal involuntary movements typically involving the face (grimacing), tongue (writhing movements and protrusion), and lips (including lip smacking), but which can involve the trunk and extremities as well. The latter symptoms are typically choreiform in nature. TD may be permanent, so clinicians need to monitor patients for the emergence of symptoms carefully. The risk of TD is much lower with the atypical antipsychotics than with older, typical agents such as haloperidol, with rates under 1% in longer-term use. However, vigilance is needed and other treatments should be used first before considering atypicals. One exception to this rule is the presence of psychotic mania or depression.

B. Psychotherapeutic Interventions

Little is known about the role of psychotherapy in the treatment of bipolar disorder. Efforts are currently under way to evaluate whether treatments such as interpersonal psychotherapy or cognitive therapy work as well in bipolar patients as they do in unipolar patients. Preliminary evidence indicates that family education may reduce the risk for relapse and that cognitive therapy may enhance compliance with medications. On the whole, some of the newer psychosocial interventions appear to represent a viable alternative or valuable adjunct to pharmacotherapy in mild to moderate unipolar disorder. Whether those advantages apply to more severely depressed unipolar patients or to patients with bipolar disorders remains to be determined.

C. Other Interventions

The management of bipolar disorders heavily depends on the utilization of psychopharmacological agents and, if necessary, ECT. Other strategies have not been shown to be therapeutically useful.

1. Electroconvulsive Therapy—Approximately 80% of manic patients show substantial improvement after ECT, but the widespread (and successful) use of lithium and other antimanic agents, often in combination with antipsychotic medications, has limited ECT to patients who are intolerant of medications or whose illness is refractory to medications. ECT has proven especially useful for those manic patients who did not respond to medication and for those in mixed states who present with a high risk for suicide and are thus in need of acute symptom containment.

Baldessarini RJ: Drugs and the treatment of psychiatric disorders, depression and mania. In Hardman JG, Limbird LE (eds). *The Pharmacological Basis of Therapeutics.* New York: McGraw-Hill, 1996, pp. 431–459.

Bowden C: Treatment of bipolar disorder. In: Schatzberg AF, Nemeroff CB (eds). *Textbook of Psychopharmacology*, 2nd edn. Washington, DC: American Psychiatric Press, 1998.

Keck PE, McElroy SL: Antiepileptic drugs. In: Schatzberg AF, Nemeroff CB (eds). *Textbook of Psychopharmacology*, 2nd edn. Washington, DC: American Psychiatric Press, 1998.

Lenox RH, Manji HK: Lithium. In: Schatzberg AF, Nemeroff CB (eds). *Textbook of Psychopharmacology*, 2nd edn. Washington, DC: American Psychiatric Press, 1998.

Complications/Adverse Oucomes of Treatment

Complications and adverse outcomes related to the various biological interventions have been detailed in the above paragraphs where emphasis was given to complications specific to the various therapeutic intervention strategies.

Prognosis

It appears that the availability of treatment for bipolar disorder has significantly affected the length of an average episode. Before 1960 (i.e., before the introduction of psychopharmacologic medications such as lithium), episode length averaged 7–13 months; thereafter, it averaged 2–4 months. With the emergence of early intervention and successful treatment of the illness, the effects of kindling on outcome (described earlier in this section) may have been interrupted, resulting in fewer episodes over time and reduced cycle length. Early disease onset suggests poor prognosis; patients who experience their initial episode in their late teens are likely to have a less favorable outcome than patients who experience their initial episode in their early 30s. Patients with early-onset bipolar disorder should be quickly identified and targeted for aggressive treatment intervention.

As discussed earlier in this section, somatic interventions can have a marked effect on the prognosis of bipolar disorder. Comorbidity with substance abuse, antisocial behavior, and personality disorders often complicates the clinical outcome. Substantial psychosocial morbidity can affect marriage, children, occupation, and other aspects of the patient's life. Divorce rates are two to three times higher in bipolar patients than in the general population, and occupational status is twice as likely to deteriorate. Completed suicide rates approximate 15% in untreated bipolar patients and is usually associated with a depressive or mixed episode.

CYCLOTHYMIC DISORDER

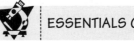 ESSENTIALS OF DIAGNOSIS

DSM-IV-TR Diagnostic Criteria

A. *For at least 2 years, the presence of numerous periods with hypomanic symptoms and numerous* periods with depressive symptoms that do not meet criteria for a major depressive episode. **Note:** In children and adolescents, the duration must be at least 1 year.

B. During the above 2-year period (1 year in children and adolescents), the person has not been without the symptoms in Criterion A for more than 2 months at a time.

C. No major depressive episode, manic episode, or mixed episode has been present during the first 2 years of the disturbance. **Note:** After the initial 2 years (1 year in children and adolescents) of cyclothymic disorder, there may be superimposed manic or mixed episodes (in which case both bipolar I disorder and cyclothymic disorder may be diagnosed) or major depressive episodes (in which case both bipolar II disorder and cyclothymic disorder may be diagnosed).

D. The symptoms in Criterion A are not better accounted for by schizoaffective disorder, and are not superimposed on schizophrenia, schizophreniform disorder, delusional disorder, or psychotic disorder not otherwise specified.

E. The symptoms are not due to the direct physiological effects of a substance (e.g., drugs of abuse, a medication) or a general medical condition (e.g., hyperthyroidism).

F. The symptoms cause clinically significant distress or impairment in social, occupational, or other important areas of functioning.

(Reprinted, with permission, from the Diagnostic and Statistical Manual of Mental Disorders, 4th edn., Text Revision. Washington DC: American Psychiatric Association, 2000.)

General Considerations

A. Epidemiology

Cyclothymic disorder often begins early in life. Lifetime prevalence rates for this disorder range between 0.4% and 1.0% in the general population, and between 3% and 5% in mood disorder clinics. In community samples, cyclothymic disorder is equally common in men and women, but women are more prevalent in clinical settings (in a ratio of approximately 3–2).

B. Etiology

Cyclothymic individuals alternate between the extremes of dysthymia (gloomy and depressed) and hyperthymia (cheerful and uninhibited). They can be moody, impul-

sive, erratic, and volatile but usually do not meet the full syndromal criteria for bipolar disorder. Repeated romantic or conjugal failures occurring in the context of interpersonal and social disturbances are common. Cyclothymia first received an operational definition in the *Diagnostic and Statistical Manual of Mental Disorders*, third edition.

There is still considerable controversy concerning the association between cyclothymic disorder and both other mood disorders and cluster B personality disorders. However, current research favors the conceptualization of cyclothymic disorder as a bona fide mood disorder.

C. Genetics

Among first-degree relatives of cyclothymic patients, the diagnoses of major depressive disorder and bipolar I and II disorders are more common than in the general population (Table 18–28). There may also be an increased familial risk of substance-related disorders.

Akiskal HS: Depression in cyclothymic and related temperaments: Clinical and pharmacologic considerations. *J Clin Psychiatry Monogr* 1992;10:37.

Weissman MN, Livingston Bruce M, Leaf PJ, Florio LP, Holzer C: Affective disorders. In: Robins LN, Regier DA (eds). *Psychiatric Disorders in America*. New York: Free Press, 1991, pp. 53–80.

Clinical Findings

A. Signs and Symptoms

Cyclothymic disorder is characterized by periods of depression alternating with periods of hypomania, which are generally of less severity or shorter duration than those associated with bipolar I disorder. The changes in mood tend to be irregular and abrupt, sometimes occurring within hours of each other. Approximately 50% of patients with cyclothymic disorder are predominantly depressed; a minority has primarily hypomanic symptoms and is unlikely to consult a mental health practitioner.

Table 18–28. Risk Factors for Cyclothymic Disorder

Familial pattern	Approximately 30% of cyclothymic patients have first-degree relatives with bipolar I disorder (a rate similar to that for bipolar I patients). Cyclothymic disorder also occurs more frequently in relatives of bipolar I disorder patients than in relatives of other psychiatrically ill patients.
Age	Often begins early in life
Social class	Not known
Race	Not known

Almost all individuals with cyclothymic disorder have periods of mixed symptoms with marked irritability, leading to unprovoked disagreements with friends, family, and coworkers. Cyclothymic individuals may have a history of multiple geographical moves, involvement in religious cults, or inability to maintain a career pathway.

B. PSYCHOLOGICAL TESTING

Psychological testing has not been shown to be useful in aiding the diagnosis of cyclothymic disorder.

C. LABORATORY FINDINGS

There are no laboratory findings suggesting or supporting the diagnosis of cyclothymic disorder.

D. NEUROIMAGING

There are no neuroimaging findings specific for cyclothymic disorder.

E. COURSE OF ILLNESS

Hypomania can be triggered by interpersonal stressors or by losses. Although most individuals with cyclothymic disorder seek psychiatric help for depression, their problems are often related to the interpersonal and behavioral crises (e.g., romantic failures) caused by their hypomanic episodes. The unpredictable nature of the mood changes causes a great deal of stress, and patients will often feel as if their moods are out of control. Patients will also present with disorganization and work productivity problems following hypomanic episodes.

Howland RH, Thase ME: A comprehensive review of cyclothymic disorder. *J Nerv Ment Dis* 1993;181:485.

Differential Diagnosis

When the mood disturbance is judged to be the direct physiologic consequence of a specific, usually chronic general medical condition (e.g., hypothyroidism), then the diagnosis should be mood disorder due to a general medical condition (see below). If substances, such as stimulants, are judged to be etiologically related to the mood disturbance, then a substance-induced mood disorder should be diagnosed. The mood swings suggestive of substance-induced mood disorder usually dissipate following cessation of drug use.

Although cyclothymic disorder may resemble bipolar I or II disorders with rapid cycling, the mood states in cyclothymic disorder do not meet the criteria for a manic, major depressive, or mixed episode. Borderline personality disorder is frequently confused with cyclothymic disorder, because of its strong affective component with marked shifts in mood. If criteria are met for each disorder, both may be diagnosed. In children and adolescents, ADHD can be clinically difficult to differentiate from cyclothymic disorder, but a pharmacologic trial of stimulants might be diagnostic, as stimulants tend to improve the symptoms of ADHD but may worsen the mood swings of cyclothymic disorder.

Treatment

A. PSYCHOPHARMACOLOGIC INTERVENTIONS

There are no systematic data on the treatment of cyclothymic disorder. Lithium has been used to suppress the hypomanic cycles, but most patients seek treatment for their labile, irritable moods and their anxious, dysphoric depressions. Some of these patients may shift into acute manic states or may develop rapid cycling if their depressions are treated solely with TCAs. In this case, bupropion, MAOIs, and low-dose SSRIs, in conjunction with lithium or other mood stabilizers, may be appropriate.

B. PSYCHOTHERAPEUTIC INTERVENTIONS

Although traditional insight-oriented psychotherapeutic approaches have been used to treat the so-called temperamental and Axis II comorbid features of cyclothymic disorder, experts now also advocate psychoeducational and interpersonal strategies as adjuncts to pharmacotherapy directed at the affective instability.

C. OTHER INTERVENTIONS

Interventions based on other than psychopharmacological or psychotherapeutic strategies have not been shown to be of value in the management of cyclothymic disorder.

Akiskal HS: Dysthymic and cyclothymic depressions: Therapeutic considerations. *J Clin Psychiatry* 1994;55(Suppl):46.

Howland RH, Thase ME: A comprehensive review of cyclothymic disorder. *J Nerv Ment Dis* 1993;181:485.

Complications/Adverse Outcomes of Treatment

There are several sources of comorbidity for cyclothymic disorder. For example, mood disorders, especially major depressive disorder and bipolar II disorder, may follow the onset of cyclothymic disorder. Other comorbid disorders include personality disorders, especially borderline personality disorder (in 10–20% of patients), impulse-control disorders such as intermittent explosive disorder, and substance- related disorders (in 5–10% of patients). Patients may use substances such as alcohol and sedatives to self-medicate the fluctuating moods, or they may ingest stimulants in order to achieve even further stimulation. Sleep disorders (such as problems initiating and maintaining sleep) are occasionally present.

Prognosis

Cyclothymic disorder usually appears in adolescence or early adult life; its onset is insidious and its course chronic. The disorder is considered by some to reflect a temperamental predisposition to other mood disorders, and there is a 15–50% risk that a bipolar I or II disorder will develop subsequently.

MOOD DISORDER DUE TO A GENERAL MEDICAL CONDITION

 ESSENTIALS OF DIAGNOSIS

DSM-IV-TR Diagnostic Criteria

A. A prominent and persistent disturbance in mood predominates in the clinical picture and is characterized by either (or both) of the following:
  (1) depressed mood or markedly diminished interest or pleasure in all, or almost all, activities
  (2) elevated, expansive, or irritable mood

B. There is evidence from the history, physical examination, or laboratory findings that the disturbance is the direct physiological consequence of a general medical condition.

C. The disturbance is not better accounted for by another mental disorder (e.g., adjustment disorder with depressed mood in response to the stress of having a general medical condition).

D. The disturbance does not occur exclusively during the course of a delirium.

E. The symptoms cause clinically significant distress or impairment in social, occupational, or other important areas of functioning.

Specify type:

With depressive features: if the predominant mood is depressed but the full criteria are not met for a Major Depressive Episode

With major depressive-like episode: if the full criteria are met (except Criterion D) for a major depressive episode

With manic features: if the predominant mood is elevated, euphoric, or irritable

With mixed features: if the symptoms of both mania and depression are present but neither predominates

Coding note: Include the name of the general medical condition on Axis I, e.g., mood disorder due to hypothyroidism, with depressive features

Coding note: If depressive symptoms occur as part of a preexisting vascular dementia, indicate the depressive symptoms by coding the appropriate subtype, i.e., vascular dementia, with depressed mood

(Reprinted, with permission, from the Diagnostic and Statistical Manual of Mental Disorders, 4th edn., Text Revision. Washington DC: American Psychiatric Association, 2000.)

General Considerations

A. EPIDEMIOLOGY

Table 18–29 summarizes the prevalence rates of major depression in a variety of medical conditions. As shown

Table 18–29. Likelihood of Developing Major Depression Following Diagnosis of Specific Medical Conditions

Condition	Prevalence (%)
Hemodialysis	7
Coronary artery disease	16–19
Cancer	20–38
Chronic pain	21–32
Neurological disorders	
Stroke	27
Parkinson's disease	21
Multiple sclerosis	6–57
Epilepsy	55
Huntington's disease	41
Dementia	11
Endocrine disorders	
Hyperthyroidism	31
Diabetes Mellitus	24
Cushing's syndrome	67
Hypothyroidism	40
HIV	30
Chronic fatigue	17–47

(Modified after Rouchell AM, Pounds R, Tierney JG: Depression. In Rundell JR, Wise MG (eds). Textbook of Consultation-Liaison Psychiatry. Washington, DC: American Psychiatric Press, 1996, pp. 310–345.)

there, depression is particularly common in certain neurological disorders, endocrine disorders, and cardiovascular disorders. Approximately 27–57% of patients with certain neurologic conditions (e.g., Parkinson's disease, multiple sclerosis, Huntington's disease, and epilepsy) develop symptoms of severe depression at some point during their illness. For medical conditions that do not directly affect the brain, prevalence rates appear to be more variable, ranging from less than 8% (for chronic renal disease), to 19% (for coronary artery disease [CAD]), to 40% (for primary hypothyroidism).

B. ETIOLOGY

Diagnostic criteria require that the disturbance—based on history, physical examination, or laboratory findings—(i) is the direct physiological consequence of a general medical condition, (ii) is not accounted for by another mental disorder, and (iii) does not occur exclusively during the course of a delirium.

C. GENETICS

Little is presently known about the genetics of mood disorders due to a general medical condition.

D. UNDERDIAGNOSIS

Although symptoms of depression are rather common in medically ill patients, depression is usually underdiagnosed and undertreated in medicine clinics or primary care settings. It has been estimated that fewer than 50% of all depressed patients are identified and adequately treated in primary care settings. The primary focus on physical signs and symptoms may only partly explain this problem.

The problem of underdiagnosis appears especially problematic in patients with cancer or cardiovascular disease where treatment of depression can improve quality of life, and perhaps contribute to rising life expectancy.

E. MORBIDITY AND MORTALITY

There is a burgeoning body of evidence suggesting that depression co-occuring with specific medical disorders can negatively affect morbidity and mortality. For example, the presence of either major or minor depression has been shown to (a) predict myocardial infarction, angioplasty and death during the 12 months following catheterization, (b) be a risk factor for mortality in patients with myocardial infarction at 6-month follow-up, (c) increase the risk for death 3.4 times in stroke patients during a 10-year period following the stroke (patients with poststroke depression and few social contacts are especially vulnerable—about 90% died), (d) increase—when co-occurring with a life-threatening illness—the risk for death or further life-threatening illnesses, and (e) increase the likelihood of death in patients with cancer. Although the precise factors that mediate the increased

Table 18–30. Characteristics of Depression Secondary to Medical Illness Compared with Primary Major Depression

Older age at onset
More likely to respond to ECT
More likely to show 'organic' features
More likely to have much lower incidence of family history of alcoholism and depression (19% of medically ill versus 36% of psychiatrically ill)
Less likely to have suicidal thoughts and commit suicide (10% death by suicide in medically ill sample versus 45% in psychiatrically ill group)

Modified after Rouchell AM, Pounds R, Tierney JG: Depression. In Rundell JR, Wise MG (eds). *Textbook of Consultation-Liaison Psychiatry*. Washington, DC: American Psychiatric Press, 1996, pp. 310–345.

risk for morbidity and mortality in medically ill depressed patients remain obscure, there is preliminary evidence that changes in the neuroendocrine and/or immune system may play a critical role.

F. DEPRESSION AS INITIAL MANIFESTATION OF PHYSICAL ILLNESS

Depression may precede the clinical signs and symptoms of some medical illnesses by months and sometimes years. Depressive symptoms are particularly common in the early stages of cancer of the pancreas, cancer of the breast, Huntington disease, or such endocrine disorders as Cushing's disease, Addison's disease, and hypothyroidism. In the endocrine conditions depression can sometimes be seen even before the classic signs and symptoms are present.

G. CHARACTERISTICS OF DEPRESSION SECONDARY TO MEDICAL ILLNESS

Table 18–30 details some of the characteristic differences between major depression and depression secondary to medical illness.

Clinical Findings

A. SIGNS AND SYMPTOMS

The diagnostic criteria for mood disorder due to a general medical condition are less vigorous than those for the primarily psychiatric mood disorders and require only the presence of depressed mood/diminished enjoyment or elevated, expansive, or irritable mood (manic symptoms). Regarding the medical illness, the required signs, symptoms, and laboratory findings are simply those that, in conjunction with the clinical history, yield the medical diagnosis. Furthermore, history, physical examination, or laboratory results must suggest that the mood disturbance is a physiologic consequence of the medical illness. Causality is usually established if the clinician demonstrates the presence of a medical condition known to cause depression and if the symptoms improve as the medical condition is treated. The many medical conditions and medications that are associated with or can cause mood problems are delineated in Tables 18–29 and 18–30.

B. SPECIFIC MEDICAL CONDITIONS ASSOCIATED WITH DEPRESSION

1. Cardiovascular disorders—Depression is common in CAD (Table 18–29). It has been shown that 18% of patients with coronary angiograms that proved CAD met criteria for major depression. Similarly, 16–19% of patients with acute myocardial infarction met criteria for major depression. In CAD, the depressed group was characterized by a positive history of depression, female gender, large infarcts, and poor social relationships.

Comorbid depression in cardiac disease cannot be considered a benign condition, as depression and its associated symptoms have been shown to be a major risk factor for both development of cardiovascular disease and death after myocardial infarction. In patients with cardiovascular disease, depression needs to be identified early and treated aggressively; such treatment may improve quality of life by stabilizing mood imbalance, and perhaps positively affect longevity.

2. Neurological disorders—Among neurological disorders, depression following stroke is the most extensively studied. Among poststroke patients, prevalence rates for depression range from 30% to 50%; these rates include major depression (26%) as well as minor depression (20%). Six months following the stroke, 34% still fulfilled criteria for major depression, and 26% for minor depression. There is evidence that patients with left hemisphere lesions show a higher frequency and severity of depression than patients with right hemisphere lesions; the highest frequency of major depression was seen following left anterior lesions. Psychopharmacologic management using nortriptyline or trazodone has proved beneficial. The high period for developing depression extends to about two years after the stroke.

Other neurological disorder with high prevalence rates for depression are epilepsy, multiple sclerosis, Parkinson's disease, and Huntington's disease (Table 18–29).

3. Endocrine disorder—Endocrine diseases commonly associated with depression are Cushing's disease, primary hypothyroidism (occuring in 1–6% of middle-aged females), diabetes mellitus, and Addison's disease (Table 18–29).

Depression may be among the earliest symptoms of endogenous Cushing's disease, sometimes preceding its final diagnosis by years. Patients with endogenous Cushing's disease usually present with depression (prevalence rates are as high as 65%), whereas patients with iatrogenic Cushing's disease (e.g., resulting after high doses of glucocorticoids for allergic or autoimmune conditions) are more likely to present with mood elevation. It is noteworthy that depressive symptoms not always remit when cortisol levels normalize, suggesting that in Cushing's disease psychological remission does not necessarily parallel endocrine remission or cure. The same phenomenon has been observed in patients whose primary hypothyroidism was treated with thyroid hormone substitution.

About one quarter of patients with diabetes mellitus complain about symptoms of depression. For long period of time, it has been known by primary care physicians and endocrinologists that depression can complicate both course and treatment of diabetes mellitus. During episodes of depression, it may be difficult to appropriately control the endocrine aspects of diabetes mellitus. A burgeoning number of clinical studies shows that comorbid depression can be associated with a less predictable course and wider fluctuations of blood glucose levels, often necessitating a more intensive treatment approach.

C. MEDICATIONS AND SUBSTANCES ASSOCIATED WITH DEPRESSION

Table 18–3 details the list of drugs that are known to cause or exacerbate depressive symptoms. Among them, the most common are analgesics (indomethacin, opiates), antihypertensives (propranol, reserpin, methyl-dopa, clonidine), and steroids.

D. PSYCHOLOGICAL TESTING

Psychological testing has not been shown to be useful in aiding the diagnosis of mood disorder due to a general medical condition.

E. LABORATORY FINDINGS

There are no laboratory findings characteristic of, or specific for, mood disorders due to a general medical condition; this, of course, excepts the laboratory findings characteristic for the primary medical condition.

F. NEUROIMAGING

Little is known about neuroimaging findings in mood disorders due to a general medical condition.

G. COURSE OF ILLNESSS

In most cases, successful treatment of the (primary) medical condition will beneficially affect the (secondary) mood disorder. However, behavioral remission does not always parallel medical remission. For example, patients with Cushing's syndrome who have been cured by surgical removal of the pituitary microadenoma, may continue to fulfill criteria for depression for several months after successful surgery.

Differential Diagnosis

The differential diagnosis of a mood disorder due to a general medical condition must include delirium (a separate diagnosis of mood disorder due to a general medical condition is not given if the mood disturbance is part of a delirium), dementia of the Alzheimer's type, vascular dementia, substance- induced mood disorder, and the other major mood disorders. Table 18–30 compares the characteristics of depression secondary to medical illness with those of (primary) major depression.

Treatment

Treatment approaches are directed primarily at the medical condition. It is noteworthy that particularly in endocrine disorders behavioral remission often does not parallel medical remission, that is, patients may continue to be depressed even after they have been cured endocrinologically. It is possible that in some patients (i.e., in those with a genetic vulnerability for developing depression) the mood disorder was simply triggered by the general medical condition, whereas in others it was more causally linked.

A. PSYCHOPHARMACOLOGIC INTERVENTIONS

The psychopharmacologic treatment of comorbid mood disorders in medically ill patients requires a careful risk-benefit assessment. The considerations necessary for such assessment include the following: (1) side effects of psychotropic agents that may complicate existing medical illness (examples include the use of TCAs in patients with hypothyroidism, orthostatic hypotension, chronic heart disease including myocardial infarction and congestive heart failure, prostatic hypertrophy, or narrow-angle glaucoma); (2) potential interactions of psychotropic agents (e.g., antidepressants) with drugs used to treat medical disorders; and (3) the effects of impaired renal, hepatic, or gastrointestinal functioning on psychotropic drug absorption and metabolism. Medically ill patients are often older and more sensitive to drugs, they require lower dosages, and they metabolize drugs slower than do younger individuals. Therefore, when treating mood disorders in elderly, medically ill patients, clinicians should use low dosages of antidepressants at the beginning of treatment and raise the dosages gradually depending on the patient's toleration of side effects and response to treatment. The following sections summarize the management of comorbid depression in specific medical conditions:

1. Asthma—MAOIs should be administered with caution to patients who have asthma because of interactions with sympathomimetic bronchodilators. Other antidepressants appear to be safe.

2. Cardiac disease—Because of their quinidine-like effects, the TCAs have antiarrhythmic properties and prolong the Q-T interval. A prolonged Q-T interval (i.e., >0.440 seconds) presents a relative contraindication for the use of TCAs. Among patients with preexisting but asymptomatic conduction defects, TCAs may induce symptomatic conduction defects and orthostatic hypotension. TCAs may also provoke arrhythmia in patients with subclinical sinus node dysfunction. SSRIs, trazodone, and bupropion present safer alternatives for treating depression in patients with cardiac disease. It is also advisable to monitor carefully those patients who already take another class I antiarrhythmic agent; to evaluate patients for preexisting but asymptomatic conduction defects such as interventricular conduction delay and bundle branch block; to be aware that patients with prolonged Q-T intervals, whether preexisting or drug induced, are predisposed to the development of ventricular tachycardia; and to obtain an EKG for all patients over age 40 years before initiating treatment.

3. Dementia—Patients with dementia are particularly sensitive to the negative effects of anticholinergic agents on memory and attention. Antidepressants with low anticholinergic profiles are the drugs of choice (e.g., SSRIs, bupropion, trazodone, desipramine, nortriptyline). Stimulants can be useful occasionally. ECT can be used if medications are either contraindicated or not tolerated, and if immediate resolution of depressive symptoms is medically indicated.

4. Hypertension—Antihypertensive medications and antidepressants may interact in various ways, either intensifying or weakening the effects of the antihypertensive therapy. The antihypertensive effect of prazosin is intensified by TCAs, because both block the α-receptors. In contrast, TCAs antagonize the therapeutic actions of guanethidine, clonidine, or α-methyldopa. Orthostatic hypotension can occur when antihypertensives, especially diuretics, are combined with TCAs, trazodone, or MAOIs. β-Blockers, especially propranolol, are known to cause depression in some individuals; the situation is remedied by changing to another antihypertensive medication.

5. Narrow-angle glaucoma—The anticholinergic side effects of TCAs can acutely exacerbate narrow-angle glaucoma in susceptible individuals (i.e., in those with shallow anterior chambers). Patients who receive miotics for their glaucoma may take antidepressants, including those with strong anticholinergic effects, provided that their intraocular pressure is monitored; SSRIs, trazodone, and bupropion present safer alternatives. Trazodone, however, can produce priapism in some patients (about 1 in 7000 men treated); priapism may necessitate surgical intervention, which is often associated with impotence or erectile problems.

6. Obstructive uropathy—Prostate enlargement and other forms of bladder outlet obstruction present relative contraindications to the use of antidepressants with strong anticholinergic effects. Benzodiazepines, trazodone, and MAOIs may also retard bladder emptying. The drugs of choice in this case are SSRIs, bupropion, and desipramine.

7. Orthostatic hypotension—A common side effect of TCAs is orthostatic hypotension, particularly in elderly patients or in patients with preexisting hypotension, impaired left ventricular function, or bundle branch block. Good treatment alternatives are SSRIs and bupropion. They have little affinity for histaminic, muscarinic, and α-adrenergic receptors and are thus not likely to significantly affect pulse rate or blood pressure. Clinicians should advise elderly patients of the potential serious risk of acute orthostatic hypotension (e.g., femur neck fractures) and discuss with them possible ways of avoiding such risk (e.g., not changing positions too rapidly; sitting up in bed before standing up, particularly at night when patients awake because of the need to urinate).

8. Parkinson's disease—Depression is common in patients with Parkinson's disease; 40–50% of patients are so afflicted. The management of depression in this condition often presents great difficulty, and there is no evidence that any particular antidepressant is more efficacious than others. Amoxapine and lithium should be avoided because both can exacerbate neurologic symptoms. MAOIs may adversely interact with L-dopa. The beneficial effects of anticholinergic agents are offset by their induction of memory impairment. ECT may be of transient benefit.

9. Seizure disorders—The effects of antidepressants on the seizure threshold are not completely understood. Two antidepressants, maprotiline and bupropion, are associated with an increased risk for seizures, especially if administered in high dosages. In patients receiving treatment for seizure disorder, fluoxetine may dramatically increase the plasma levels of carbamazepine, whereas TCAs may lower the levels. The plasma levels of TCAs can be increased by valproic acid. ECT can be safely used in patients with seizure disorder.

B. Psychotherapeutic Interventions

There is no evidence that psychotherapeutic interventions are useful as primary treatment strategies in mood disorders due to a general medical condition.

C. Other Interventions

Successful management of the primary medical disorder remains the most important treatment strategy in these conditions. However, if depressive symptoms persist for several months after the medical condition has been treated or cured, or if the medical condition shows a rather chronic course, psychotherapeutic and/or psychopharmacological strategies are useful to assuage depression.

Complications/Adverse Outcomes of Treatment

The complications associated with the management of mood disorders due to a general medical conditions have been detailed in the paragraphs above where emphasis was given to several medical conditions that are known to be associated with specific therapeutic risks.

Prognosis

Comorbid depression is not a clinically benign condition. In diabetes mellitus, comorbid depression can significantly complicate the acute treatment of the illness or negatively affect its outcome. Among patients in a general medical setting, those with comorbid depression report increased pain, more severe physical illness, decreased social functioning, and increased mortality. The deterioration of functioning associated with depression or depressive symptoms may be equal to or worse than that associated with severe medical conditions. Evidence indicates that the combination of current advanced CAD and depressive symptoms can be associated with roughly twice the reduction in social functioning as with either condition alone, suggesting that the effects of depressive symptoms and chronic medical conditions on functioning can be additive. In chronic heart disease, the diagnosis of comorbid depression may be associated with an increased likelihood of medical complications, a more protracted course, and sudden death. It is important to identify such comorbidity early and to treat it aggressively.

Cassem NH, Stern TA, Rosenbaum JF (eds): *Massachusetts General Hospital Handbook of General Hospital Psychiatry.* St. Louis, MO: Mosby, 1997.

Goodwin FK, Jamison KR: *Manic Depressive Illness.* New York: Oxford University Press, 1990.

Loosen PT: Psychiatric manifestations of cushing's syndrome. In: Blevins LS (ed). *Cushing's Syndrome.* Boston: Kluwer Academic Publishers, 2002, pp. 45–64.

Nemeroff CB, Loosen PT (eds): *Handbook of Clinical Psychoneuroendocrinology.* New York: Guilford Press, 1987.

Rouchell AM, Pounds R, Tierney JG: Depression. In: Rundell JR, Wise MG (eds). *Textbook of Consultation-Liaison Psychiatry.* Washington, DC: American Psychiatric Press, 1996, pp. 310–345.

Stoudemire A, Fogel BS: *Principles of Medical Psychiatry.* New York: Grune & Stratton, 1987.

Wolkowitz OM, Rothschild AJ (eds): *Pyschoneuroendocrinology.* Washington, DC: American Psychiatric Publishing, 2003.

Anxiety Disorders

19

Richard C. Shelton, MD

 ESSENTIALS OF DIAGNOSIS

Anxiety disorders range in severity from common, mild phobias (e.g., fear of insects, heights, or storms) to chronic, disabling conditions such as panic disorder or obsessive–compulsive disorder (OCD). Anxiety diagnoses are made according to the specific symptomatic manifestation of each disorder. Table 19–1 lists the anxiety disorder diagnoses included in the Diagnostic and Statistical Manual of Mental Disorders, *fourth edition, Text Revision (DSM-IV-TR). Posttraumatic stress disorder and acute stress disorder are covered in Chapter 20, and OCD is covered in Chapter 21.*

Anxiety is characterized by heightened arousal (i.e., physical symptoms such as tension, tachycardia, tachypnea, tremor) accompanied by apprehension, fear, obsessions, or the like. Anxiety disorders are different from normal fears, although the symptoms can be similar. Generally speaking, normal fears represent emotional reactions to real, external threats, and the emotional response is appropriately related to the actual danger. In contrast, the symptoms of anxiety disorders occur either without obvious external threat or when the response to the threat is excessive. When an extreme or inappropriate fear or worry is present and is coupled with some degree of life impairment, the diagnosis of anxiety disorder should be considered.

General Considerations

A. EPIDEMIOLOGY

Anxiety disorders are among the most common of psychiatric disorders, affecting up to 15% of the general population at any time. Individual anxiety disorders occur frequently. Phobic disorders (i.e., specific or social phobia) may affect as much as 8–10% of the population, generalized anxiety disorder (GAD) about 5%, and OCD and panic disorder each about 1–3%. Although posttraumatic stress disorder appears common, its specific frequency is unknown (see Chapter 20). The comorbid-

ity of anxiety disorders with other psychiatric disorders is high. For example, about 40% of patients with primary anxiety disorders will have a lifetime history of a DSM-IV-TR depressive disorder. Further, in patients who have other psychiatric disorders, significant anxiety symptoms often are associated with those disorders. Therefore, clinically significant anxiety symptoms will occur frequently in patients seen in clinical practice.

B. ETIOLOGY

1. Psychodynamic theory—Traditional psychoanalytic theory describes anxiety disorders as being rooted in unconscious conflict. Freud originally used the term "Angst" (literally, "fear") to describe the simple intrapsychic response to either internal or external threat. He later derived the concept of the pleasure principle, which describes the tendency of the psychic apparatus to seek immediate discharge of impulses. In his earliest organized theory of anxiety, Freud postulated that conflicts or inhibitions result in the failure to dissipate libidinal (i.e., sexual) drives. These restrictions on sexual expression could occur because of external threat and would subsequently result in a fear of the loss of control of the drive. The damming-up of the impulses, along with the fear of loss of control, would result in anxiety.

Freud soon began to see the limitations of this theory and later proposed that anxiety was central to the concept of neurosis. He acknowledged that anxiety was a natural, biologically derived response mechanism required for survival. He abandoned the concept of the transformation of sexual drive (energy) into anxiety and accepted the prevailing notion of the time: anxiety was a result of threat. He recognized two sources of such threat. The first, termed **traumatic situations,** involved stimuli that were too severe for the person to manage effectively and could be considered the common or natural fear response. The second, called **danger situations,** resulted from the recognition or anticipation of upcoming trauma, whether internal (by loss of control of drives) or external. The response to these threats resulted in what was called **signal anxiety,** which was an attenuated and therefore more manageable anxiety response not directly related to trauma. Signal anxiety could be

Table 19–1. DSM-IV-TR Anxiety Disorders

Panic disorder (with or without agoraphobia)
Specific phobia
Social phobia
Generalized anxiety disorder
Obsessive–compulsive disorder
Acute stress disorder
Posttraumatic stress disorder
Anxiety disorder due to medical condition
Substance-induced anxiety disorder

seen as anxiety that resulted from the avoidance of threat.

The structural hypothesis of mental function—which includes the id as the seat of drives, the superego as the location of inhibitions, and the ego as the apparatus for managing drives and inhibitions—evolved during this time period. Central to this hypothesis is the concept of **defense mechanisms.** Psychological defenses are thought to be primarily a function of the ego, which uses these defenses to manage id impulses and superego demands. **Repression** is formulated as the primary defense mechanism, in which unacceptable drive states are maintained largely outside of awareness. Failure of repression could result in anxiety and the use of secondary mechanisms to maintain intrapsychic stability.

The concept of the primacy of the defense mechanism to both generate and manage the anxiety has remained central to psychoanalysis for much of its history. Further, psychoanalytic treatment has focused on the need to uncover childhood trauma, releasing unnecessary defensive inhibitions and developing psychological competence. A number of schools of thought have been elaborated from classical Freudian psychoanalysis, including ego psychology, object relations theory, and self psychology (see Chapter 11).

2. Learning theory—The basic principles of learning theory as they relate to human development are rooted in the work of developmental psychologists, especially Jean Piaget (see Chapter 8). Piaget's observations of children led to an understanding of the progress of development through a series of predictable stages, referred to as epigenesis. Developmental milestones represent an interaction between the maturing brain substrate and environmental influences. Hence children learn according to both the capacity of the brain to manage incoming stimuli and the nature of the stimuli themselves. Appropriate environmental responses facilitate a normal learning process, and aberrant reactions produce problems in development.

As stimuli are assimilated and processed, learning takes place. Learning theory proposes two forms of learning: classical conditioning and operant conditioning (see Chapter 8). The classical conditioning model depends on the pairing of a stimulus that evokes a response (the unconditioned stimulus) with a neutral environmental object or event (the conditioned stimulus). The repeated pairing of the two stimuli would lead to the ability of the conditioned stimulus to elicit the same response as the unconditioned stimulus (the conditioned response).

Whereas classical conditioning views the organism as a relatively passive participant in the learning process, operant conditioning views stimuli as a series of either positive or negative events that influence subsequent behavior. Positive reinforcement occurs when a particular behavior results in a reward. Alternatively, negative reinforcement results when a specific behavior leads to the successful avoidance of an aversive event (i.e., punishment). Positive or negative reinforcements would then enhance the likelihood that the behavior would be repeated. Reinforcements of behaviors, whether they are achievements of rewards or avoidance of pain, underlie learning.

According to learning theory, an anxiety disorder develops when environmental cues become associated with anxiety-producing events during development. Within the construct of GAD, for example, worry and fear become conditioned and are repeated in order to avoid intermittent negative reinforcement. Hence the periodic successful avoidance of a negative outcome reinforces the behavior. For example, an individual's fear (and subsequent avoidance) of air travel would be enhanced by reading about occasional air disasters.

Traditional behavioral therapy of anxiety involves the uncoupling of the unconditioned response from the associated stimulus. Wolpe postulated that actions that inhibited anxiety (i.e., relaxation) in the face of the conditioned stimulus would reduce symptoms. Behavioral treatment of anxiety uses **systematic desensitization** (progressive exposure to an anxiety-evoking stimulus). This type of treatment has been used successfully to treat anxiety disorders such as phobias and OCD, but it has had limited systematic study in other anxiety disorders.

3. Cognitive theory—In a subsequent elaboration of learning theory, a cognitive theory of the etiology of depressive and anxiety disorders has evolved (see Chapter 8, 10). Although several theories have been advanced, Beck's concept of the cognitive triad has gained the broadest acceptance and application. In this view, abnormal emotional states, such as anxiety and depression, are a result of distorted beliefs about the self, the world, and the future. Anxiety disorders, therefore, involve incorrect beliefs that interpret events in an exaggeratedly dangerous or threatening manner. These fundamental belief systems, or schema, result in automatic thought responses to external or internal cues that trigger anxiety. As such, anxiety disorders consistently involve abnormalities of information processing that result in symptom formation.

Cognitive–behavioral therapy involves elements of classical behavioral approaches such as systematic desensitization; however, treatment is extended to the discovery and correction of distorted cognitive schema. The absence of exaggerated misinterpretations of cues leads to a reduction in symptom formation. Cognitive–behavioral psychotherapy has been used successfully to treat a variety of anxiety disorders, including panic disorder, phobias, and OCD.

4. Biological theories—From a biological standpoint, anxiety and fear have high adaptive value in all animals by increasing the animal's capacity for survival. The emotion of anxiety drives a number of highly adaptive behaviors, including escape from threat. The normal brain functions that underlie the anxiety response have been elucidated gradually over the past 50 years. The current understanding of the biological nature of anxiety has been prompted in part by an elucidation of the actions of drugs that reduce the symptoms of anxiety disorders. These observations can be divided into three broad areas: the gamma amino butyric acid (GABA) receptor/benzodiazepine receptor/chloride channel complex; the noradrenergic nucleus locus coeruleus and related brain stem nuclei; and the serotonin system, especially the raphe nuclei and their projections. Abnormalities in the functioning of these areas have been associated with various anxiety disorders.

Gray and colleagues have developed a general theory of a **neural behavioral-inhibition system** that mediates anxiety. The purpose of this system is to evaluate stimuli—consistent with punishment, non-reward, novelty, or fear—that simultaneously produce behavioral inhibition and increase arousal and attention. Antianxiety drugs inhibit responses in these areas. Using pharmacologic and lesioning studies, researchers have related anxiety to several interconnected anatomical areas. Sensory stimuli activate the hippocampus, especially the entorhinal cortex, which secondarily produces habituation by actions on the lateral and medial septal areas. Behavioral inhibition is achieved by projections to the cingulate gyrus. These areas are then influenced by noradrenergic activity of the locus coeruleus and are modulated both by serotonergic innervations from

the raphe and by $GABA_A$-receptor activity. Antianxiety drugs work via mechanisms that influence these areas and receptors. These mechanisms include noradrenergic activation (e.g., tricyclic antidepressants), serotonergic activity (e.g., selective serotonin reuptake inhibitors or buspirone), or benzodiazepine interactions with GABA receptors.

Acute threat results in fear, activating the "fight or flight" response. This, in turn, is mediated by brain regions such as the locus coeruleus and the amygdala. The amygdala participate in the encoding of fearful memory and aversive conditioning; they are therefore involved in both acute fear and negative anticipatory expectation (i.e., anxiety).

Acute fear activates the sympathetic nervous system via the locus coeruleus, resulting in physical symptoms such as tachycardia, tremor, and diaphoresis. Awareness of fear occurs in the cortex, especially the frontal cortex that registers fear and responds with adaptive survival behaviors. The cingulate gyrus is also involved in the mediation of information between cortical and subcortical structures.

C. GENETICS

Controlled family studies of the major subtypes of anxiety disorders including panic disorder, phobic disorders, GAD, and OCD reveal that all of these anxiety subtypes are familial, and twin studies suggest that the familial aggregation is attributable in part to genetic factors. Panic disorder and its spectrum show the strongest genetic determinants; half or more of persons with panic disorder have a family history of the disorder. Although there has been a plethora of studies designed to identify genes underlying these conditions, to date, no specific genetic loci have been identified and replicated in independent samples.

Clinical Findings

A. SIGNS & SYMPTOMS

Anxiety is a normal emotion, a common reaction to the stresses of everyday life. At what point does anxiety become pathologic? In order to make this distinction, one must define the key characteristics of the disorders and recognize that in pathologic anxiety normal psychological adaptive processes have been overwhelmed to the point that daily functioning has been impaired. Anxiety disorders begin at the point of impairment. For example, everyone worries occasionally. When this worry begins to preoccupy a person's thoughts to the point that psychosocial functioning is impeded, an anxiety disorder may be diagnosed.

Anxiety is commonly associated with other medical or psychiatric conditions. Other conditions that give rise to anxiety have their own diagnostic categories: anxiety disorder due to medical condition and substance-induced anxiety disorder.

B. PSYCHOLOGICAL TESTING

Psychological testing has not been shown to be useful in aiding the diagnosis of anxiety disorders.

C. LABORATORY FINDINGS

There are no laboratory findings suggesting or supporting the diagnosis of anxiety disorders, though there is evidence that a family or personal history of panic disorder may convey a liability to experience anxiety with carbon dioxide (CO_2) exposure.

D. NEUROIMAGING

Functional neuroimaging studies in patients with anxiety disorders have shown neurophysiological abnormalities during symptom provocation tests, implicating limbic, paralimbic and sensory association regions.

Course of Illness

The often-chronic course of anxiety disorders, and its frequent comorbidity with other psychiatric conditions, especially mood disorders, are delineated in more detail (i.e., as they pertain to specific subtypes of anxiety disorders) in the paragraphs below.

Differential Diagnosis (Including Comorbid Conditions)

These differential diagnoses, along with other psychiatric disorders that can manifest significant anxiety, are listed in Table 19–2.

■ PANIC DISORDER WITH OR WITHOUT AGORAPHOBIA

ESSENTIALS OF DIAGNOSIS

DSM-IV-TR Diagnostic Criteria

A. Both (1) and (2):

    (1) recurrent, unexpected panic attacks (see below)

    (2) at least one of the attacks has been followed by 1 month (or more) of one (or more) of the following:

        (a) persistent concern about having additional attacks

        (b) worry about the implications of the attack or its consequences (e.g., losing control, having a heart attack, "going crazy")

        (c) A significant change in behavior related to the attacks

B. The presence or absence of agoraphobia (see below).

C. The panic attacks are not due to the direct physiological effects of a substance or a general medical condition.

D. The panic attacks are not better accounted for by another mental disorder, such as social phobia, specific phobia, obsessive-compulsive disorder, posttraumatic stress disorder, or separation anxiety disorder.

Criteria for Panic Attack (not a separate diagnostic category)

A discrete period of intense fear or discomfort, in which four (or more) of the following symptoms developed abruptly and reached a peak within 10 minutes:

    (1) palpitations, pounding heart, or accelerated heart rate

    (2) sweating

    (3) trembling or shaking

    (4) sensations of shortness of breath or smothering

    (5) feeling of choking

    (6) chest pain or discomfort

    (7) nausea or abdominal distress

    (8) feeling dizzy, unsteady, lightheaded, or faint

    (9) derealization or depersonalization

    (10) fear of losing control or going crazy

    (11) fear of dying

    (12) paresthesias (numbness or tingling)

    (13) chills or hot flashes

Criteria for Agoraphobia (not a separate diagnostic category)

A. Anxiety about being in places or situations from which escape might be difficult (or embarrassing) or in which help may not be available in the event of having an unexpected or situationally predisposed panic attack or panic-like symptoms. Agoraphobic fears typically involve characteristic clusters of situations that include being outside the home alone; being in a crowd or standing in

Table 19–2. Differential Diagnosis of Anxiety Disorders

MEDICAL ILLNESSES	*Pulmonary*
Cardiac	Asthma
Angina	Embolism
Arrhythmias	Obstruction
Congestive failure	Obstructive pulmonary disease
Infarction	*Other*
Mitral valve prolapse	Porphyria
Supraventricular tachycardia	**PSYCHIATRIC DISORDERS**
Endocrinologic	Major depression
Hyperthyroidism	Developmental disorders (e.g., Autism, Williams Syndrome)
Cushing disease	Dissociative disorders
Hyperparathyroidism	Personality disorders
Hypoglycemia	Somatoform disorders
Premenstrual dysphoric disorder	Schizophrenia (and other psychotic disorders)
Neoplastic	**SUBSTANCE USE/ABUSE**
Carcinoid	Alcohol/sedative withdrawal
Insulinoma	Antidepressants
Pheochromocytoma	Caffeine
Neurologic	Hallucinogen
Huntington disease	Psychostimulants (e.g., methylphenidate, amphetamine)
Meniere disease	Steroids (corticosteroids, anabolic steroids)
Migraine	Stimulant abuse (e.g., cocaine)
Multiple sclerosis	Sympathomimetics (e.g., pseudoephedrine
Seizure disorder	
Transient ischemic attack	
Vertigo	
Wilson disease	

a line; being on a bridge; and traveling on a bus, train, or automobile.

B. The situations are avoided or endured with marked distress or with anxiety about having a panic attack or panic-like symptoms, or require the presence of a companion.

C. The anxiety of phobic avoidance is not better accounted for by another mental disorder, such as social phobia, specific phobia, obsessive-compulsive disorder, posttraumatic stress disorder, or separation anxiety disorder.

(Adapted, with permission, from the *Diagnostic and Statistical Manual of Mental Disorders*. 4th edn. Text Revision. Washington, DC: American Psychiatric Association, 2000)

General Considerations

A. EPIDEMIOLOGY

Panic disorder occurs in 1–3% of the population and is about twice as common in women as men. Panic-related phenomena, such as isolated panic attacks or limited-symptom attacks, are much more common. Panic may develop at any time in the life span, although the median age at onset is in the mid-twenties. Panic disorder in childhood may be underrecognized or misdiagnosed as conduct disorder or school avoidance. Children with panic disorder often exhibit considerable avoidance behavior with associated educational disability. Panic disorder may flare up in childhood, become quiescent in the teenage years and early adult life, only to reemerge later.

B. ETIOLOGY

Although there have been many theories about the genesis of panic, two dominant (and not mutually exclusive) frameworks have been proposed. There is strong evidence to support a biological foundation. For example, some antidepressant and antianxiety drugs can block the attacks. Further, specific substances known as "panicogens" (e.g., intravenous sodium lactate or inhalation of 5–35% CO_2) can induce panic attacks in persons with panic disorder while sparing those without such a history. These agents collectively activate brain stem nuclei such as the locus coeruleus. Klein and colleagues have postulated that panic attacks are a result of a misperception of suffocation, referred to as a false suffocation response.

There also is support for a cognitive theory of the disorder. Persons with panic disorder often exhibit common cognitive characteristics, with a strong sensitivity to, and misinterpretation of, physical sensations. Cognitive theory suggests that mild physical symptoms are misinterpreted as dangerous. Cognitive–behavioral psychotherapy, with its emphasis on recognizing and correcting catastrophic thoughts, reduces both agoraphobic avoidance and the panic attacks themselves.

C. GENETICS

Of all the major subtypes of anxiety disorders, panic disorder and its spectrum have the strongest familial clustering and genetic underpinnings; half or more of persons with panic disorder have a family history of the disorder. In contrast, the frequency of family history in OCD is low, though family members of OCD patients have a higher than expected rate of tic disorders, indicating a possible genetic linkage between OCD and complex tic disorders. This relationship is further supported by the observation of an increased frequency of tic disorders in OCD patients and vice versa.

Clinical Findings

A. SIGNS & SYMPTOMS

Although the symptoms of panic disorder have been described for over a century, and effective treatment has been available for more than 30 years, the disorder has been recognized widely for only about the last 25 years. Panic disorder is characterized by recurring, spontaneous, unexpected anxiety attacks with rapid onset and short duration. Because of the physical symptoms of the attacks, patients are likely to fear that they are experiencing a heart attack, stroke, or the like. Occasionally patients will think that they are going "crazy" or are "out of control." Patients with panic disorder typically fear further attacks, worry about the implications of the attacks (e.g., that the attacks indicate a serious undiagnosed physical illness), and change their behavior as a result.

Panic attacks involve severe anxiety symptoms of rapid onset. These symptoms climb to maximum severity within 10 minutes, but can peak within a few seconds. Typical symptoms include shortness of breath, tachypnea, tachycardia, tremor, dizziness, hot or cold sensations, chest discomfort, and feelings of depersonalization or derealization. A minimum of four symptoms is required to meet the diagnosis of panic attack. The symptoms usually last for less than 1 hour and most commonly diminish within 30 minutes.

People who experience a panic attack will usually seek help, often at a hospital emergency room. Although this condition is readily diagnosable by clinical signs and symptoms, most cases are not diagnosed initially. This is unfortunate because early detection and treatment can usually prevent disability.

Left untreated, the panic attacks will likely continue. Repeated visits to physicians (of various specialties) and emergency rooms are common. Patients often seek help from many professionals, counselors, therapists, and others. If the diagnosis is not made and treatment is not started, the disorder usually progresses. Patients begin to avoid settings in which panic attacks have happened in the past, particularly social settings such as theaters, malls, grocery stores, churches, and other places where escape might be difficult or embarrassing; such extensive phobic avoidance is referred to as **agoraphobia.**

Agoraphobia is intimately linked with the development of panic disorder. Panic disorder can occur without any significant agoraphobia. This is seen when the panic attacks are relatively mild or are truly spontaneous in nature. However, most people with panic disorder find that particular situations stimulate panic; therefore, they avoid these situations. Most patients find that the likelihood of having an attack is reduced in "safe places" (e.g., at home) or with "safe people" (e.g., a spouse or parent) who will help in the event of an attack. Phobic avoidance is promoted further by anticipatory anxiety, which occurs when patients envision going into a situation in which an attack might occur.

Agoraphobia rarely occurs without a history of frank panic attacks. When it does occur, it is most often accompanied by so-called **limited-symptom attacks** (panic-like attacks that do not meet the full four-symptom criteria for panic attack). Recurrent limited-symptom attacks often predate full panic attacks in many people with panic disorder.

B. LABORATORY FINDINGS

A number of studies have shown that patients with panic disorder have greater anxiety responses to the inhalation of enhanced CO_2 mixtures than do controls or patients with other psychiatric illnesses. There is also evidence that well subjects at high risk for panic disorder (i.e., subjects with a family but no personal history of panic disorder) experience more anxiety following CO_2 exposure than do subjects without such history.

C. NEUROIMAGING

There is emerging evidence that $5-HT_{1A}$-receptor binding is reduced in some patients with panic disorder.

Course of Illness

Though the course of panic disorder is usually chronic, long-term prognosis is good. It is important that panic disorder is treated as early as possible, and that close attention is given to comorbid disorders, especially depression, as they are known to negatively affect outcome.

Differential Diagnosis (Including Comorbid Conditions)

Panic disorder and agoraphobia share features with other mental disorders. Persons with OCD, specific and social phobias, posttraumatic stress disorder, major depression, psychotic disorders, and some personality disorders (e.g., avoidant, paranoid, dependent, schizoid) exhibit social avoidance. These disorders, however, do not share the features of spontaneous panic attacks. The absence of spontaneous panic attacks also distinguishes other disorders with somatic fears including obsessive–compulsive spectrum disorders (e.g., somatic obsessions and body dysmorphic disorder), GAD, and somatization disorders. Although persons with specific and social phobias may have situationally bound panic attacks, recurring unexpected panic attacks do not occur.

Although the diagnosis is usually straightforward, many patients with panic disorder undergo extensive, unnecessary medical evaluation. Some differential diagnostic possibilities for panic attacks include paroxysmal atrial tachycardia, pulmonary embolus, seizure disorder, Meniere disease, transient ischemic attack, carcinoid syndrome, Cushing disease, hyperthyroidism, true hypoglycemia, and pheochromocytoma. Extensive medical evaluation for these disorders is indicated only when other features suggest physical disease (Table 19–2).

Treatment

A. PSYCHOPHARMACOLOGIC INTERVENTIONS

Panic in mildly ill patients often requires no medication and can be managed with psychotherapy alone. Behavioral or cognitive–behavioral therapy is the treatment of choice (see also Chapter 10). Medications in combination with psychotherapy should be reserved for more severely ill patients.

Medication should be considered if the panic disorder impairs functioning, e.g., (1) if agoraphobia is present or developing, (2) if major depression (currently or by history) or a personality disorder is present, (3) if the patient reports significant suicidal ideation, or (4) if the patient voices a strong preference for medication management. The last option is intended to strengthen therapeutic alliance and to encourage the patient's involvement in therapy. Many patients with panic disorder fear behavioral therapy because of the need for exposure to the phobic stimuli.

Tricyclic antidepressants are effective for panic. However, the side effect profile is such that they are rarely used. The physician must warn patients about the potential for the development of transient anxiety, along with other side effects (Table 19–3). The dosage should start low and be titrated upward slowly. High plasma levels appear to worsen outcome.

Imipramine, amitriptyline, and clomipramine have reasonable empirical support for their effectiveness. Other drugs such as nortriptyline or doxepin have limited support. There is some evidence that other antidepressants, such as desipramine, maprotiline, and bupropion, are less effective than imipramine.

The monoamine oxidase inhibitors, especially phenelzine, have relatively strong empirical support. Like tricyclics, phenelzine reduces the frequency and intensity of panic attacks. It also appears to have a substantial antianxiety and antiphobic effect. Unfortunately, the effectiveness of phenelzine is limited by its side effects and safety problems. Besides the side effects listed in Table 19–3, hypertensive reactions can occur when the patient's diet has a high tyramine content. Further, toxicity can be produced when this drug is taken with other agents, such as meperidine or sympathomimetic amines. Although such toxic effects can generally be avoided, patients with panic disorder are especially fearful of them.

Research data support the effectiveness of selective serotonin reuptake inhibitor (SSRI) antidepressants,

Table 19–3. Drugs used for the Treatment of Panic Disorder

Drug	Starting Dosage	Dosing Range	Common Side Effects
Imipramine (or other tricyclic antidepressants)	25 mg at bedtime	50–150 mg	Dry mouth, blurred vision, constipation, urinary hesitancy, orthostasis, somnolence, anxiety, sexual dysfunction
Phenelzine	15 mg twice daily	30–90 mg	Dry mouth, drowsiness, nausea, anxiety/nervousness, orthostatic hypotension, myoclonus, hypertensive reactions
Paroxetine	10 mg	20–40 mg	Nausea, diarrhea, anxiety/nervousness, sexual dysfunction, somnolence
Sertraline	25 mg	25–150 mg	Nausea, diarrhea, anxiety/nervousness, sexual dysfunction
Alprazolam	0.25–0.5 mg	1.5–4.0 mg three times daily	Somnolence, ataxia, memory problems, physical dependence, withdrawal reactions
Clonazepam	0.25–0.5 mg	1.5–4.0 mg twice daily	Somnolence, ataxia, memory problems, physical dependence, withdrawal reactions
Venlafaxine	37.5 mg	37.5–225 mg	Diarrhea, anxiety/nervousness, sexual dysfunction, withdrawal reactions

including paroxetine, sertraline, and the selective norepinephrine reuptake inhibitor (SNRI) venlafaxine extended release, in the treatment of panic disorder. These drugs have become the standard for pharmacological management and have supplanted other antidepressants and benzodiazepines in the treatment of panic disorder; however, in standard antidepressant dosages, these drugs may not be tolerated because of increased anxiety. Dosages should be started low and titrated upward slowly.

Low-dose benzodiazepine management can be used on an as-needed basis to reduce anticipatory anxiety and to facilitate exposure activities. Though virtually any benzodiazepine can be used successfully in this way, the high-potency benzodiazepines alprazolam and clonazepam have specific antipanic effects. Within the usual dosing range, most patients with panic experience a substantial reduction in both panic attacks and in anticipatory anxiety.

Although the likelihood of benzodiazepine abuse is relatively low if the drug is administered acutely in carefully selected patients, benzodiazepines should be avoided in patients with a history of alcohol or drug abuse. However, nearly all patients eventually develop some degree of physical dependency in the case of continuous use. On taper or discontinuation, classical withdrawal effects can occur, such as a rebound return of panic symptoms. Many patients find it very difficult to withdraw completely. As many as 60% of patients with panic disorder will stay on these medications indefinitely. Moderate- to high-dose benzodiazepine therapy should

be reserved for patients who require pharmacotherapy and who have failed on antidepressant treatment, for those who are unable to tolerate antidepressants, or for those for whom antidepressant medications are otherwise inappropriate.

The medications discussed in this section generally reduce the intensity and frequency of panic symptoms as long as they are taken. After discontinuation, most patients relapse. Relapse often occurs during dosage tapering, even with benzodiazepines. As a result, behavioral or cognitive–behavioral therapy with exposure should be combined with pharmacotherapy.

B. PSYCHOTHERAPEUTIC INTERVENTIONS

A variety of therapies have been used to treat panic disorder. Only traditional behavioral treatments and cognitive–behavioral psychotherapy have significant empirical evidence to support their effectiveness. Considerable evidence supports the effectiveness of cognitive–behavioral therapy for treatment of panic disorder. This approach helps patients to recognize the relationships between specific thoughts (i.e., cognitions) and the anxiety that they produce. These thoughts represent misinterpretations of external, or more commonly internal, cues as being threatening. For example, feeling mildly short of breath, slightly tremulous, or having a small increase in heart rate can be misinterpreted as an indication that a catastrophic physical event (e.g., heart attack) is occurring. Successful treatment, then, would help the patient to discover the true relationship between specific internal or external cues and their anxiety, and to correctly interpret the cues as benign.

C. OTHER INTERVENTIONS

An elaboration of cognitive–behavioral therapy includes **interoceptive exposure** as part of the treatment. This method uses experimental manipulations of physical sensations to induce symptoms that are commonly misinterpreted. Exposure techniques may include spinning in place, hyperventilating voluntarily, or ingesting large amounts of caffeine in order to simulate the physical cues that stimulate anxiety. This technique helps the therapist to uncover the catastrophic cognitions and help the client to interpret them correctly.

The last component of cognitive–behavioral therapy of panic disorder involves more traditional relaxation and exposure activities, in which patients gradually and systematically expose themselves to situations that induce anxiety, thereby desensitizing themselves.

Complications/Adverse Outcomes of Treatment

Complications and adverse outcomes related to the various biological interventions have been detailed in the above paragraphs where emphasis was given to complications specific to various therapeutic intervention strategies.

Prognosis

Overall, the long-term prognosis for panic disorder is good, although a significant proportion of patients is likely to develop disability if the condition is not treated soon after the occurrence of the first attack. Major depression occurs in about 40% of patients. Although both depression and panic symptoms respond to antidepressant drugs, comorbid depression worsens the outcome of panic disorder and increases the rate of suicide. About 7% of patients with panic disorder commit suicide, and more than 20% of patients with panic disorder and comorbid psychiatric disorders will eventually commit suicide. Substance abuse, especially alcoholism, also occurs at an increased frequency in panic disorder relative to the general population.

Bakker A, van Balkom AJ, Stein DJ: Evidence-based pharmacotherapy of panic disorder. *Int J Neuropsychopharmacol* 2005;8:473.

Coryell W, Pine D, Fyer A, Klein D: Anxiety responses to CO_2 inhalation in subjects at high-risk for panic disorder. *J Affect Disord* 2006;92:63–70.

Hirschfeld RM: Panic disorder: Diagnosis, epidemiology, and clinical course. *J Clin Psychiatry* 1996;57(Suppl 10):3.

Katon W: Panic disorder: Relationship to high medical utilization, unexplained physical symptoms, and medical costs. *J Clin Psychiatry* 1996;57(Suppl 10):11.

Merikangas KR, Low NC: Genetic epidemiology of anxiety disorders. *Handb Exp Pharmacol* 2005;169:163–179

Pollack MH, Otto MW: Long-term course and outcome of panic disorder. *J Clin Psychiatry* 1997;58(Suppl 2):57.

Rosenbaum JF et al.: Integrated treatment of panic disorder. *Bull Menninger Clin* 1995;59(2 Suppl A):A54.

■ PHOBIC DISORDERS: SPECIFIC PHOBIA & SOCIAL PHOBIA

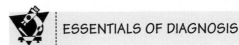 ESSENTIALS OF DIAGNOSIS

DSM-IV-TR Diagnostic Criteria
Specific Phobia

A. *A marked and persistent fear that is excessive or unreasonable, cued by the presence or anticipation of a specific object or situation.*

B. *Exposure to the phobic stimulus almost invariably provokes an immediate anxiety response, which may take the form of a situationally bound or situationally predisposed panic attack.*
Note: In children, the anxiety may be expressed by crying, tantrums, freezing, or clinging.

C. *The person recognizes that the fear is excessive or unreasonable.*
Note: In children, this feature may be absent.

D. *The object or situation is avoided or else is endured with intense anxiety or distress.*

E. *The avoidance, anxious anticipation, or distress in the feared situation(s) interferes significantly with the person's normal routine, occupational (or academic) functioning, or social activities or relationships, or there is marked distress about having the phobia.*

F. *In individuals under age 18 years, the duration is at least 6 months.*

G. *The anxiety, panic attacks, or phobic avoidance associated with the specific object or situation are not better accounted for by another mental disorder, such as obsessive-compulsive disorder, posttraumatic stress disorder, separation anxiety disorder, social phobia, panic disorder with agoraphobia, or agoraphobia without history of panic disorder.*

Specify *type:*

Animal type: *if the fear is cued by animals or insects. This subtype generally has a childhood onset.*

Natural environment type: *if the fear is cued by objects in the natural environment, such as storms, heights, or water. This subtype generally has a childhood onset.*

Blood-injection-injury type: *if the fear is cued by seeing blood or an injury or by receiving an injection or other invasive medical procedure. This subtype is highly familial and is often characterized by a strong vasovagal response.*

Situational type: *if the fear is cued by a specific situation such as public transportation, tunnels, bridges, elevators, flying, driving, or enclosed places. This subtype has a bimodal age-at-onset distribution, with one peak in childhood and another peak in the mid-20s. This subtype appears to be similar to panic disorder with agoraphobia in its characteristic sex ratios, familial aggregation pattern, and age at onset.*

Other type: *if the fear is cued by other stimuli. These stimuli might include the fear or avoidance of situations that might lead to choking, vomiting, or contracting an illness; "space" phobia (i.e., the individual is afraid of falling down if away from walls or other means of physical support); and children's fears of loud sounds or costumed characters.*

Social Phobia

A. *A marked and persistent fear of one or more social or performance situations in which the person is exposed to unfamiliar people or to possible scrutiny by others. The individual fears that he or she will act in a way (or show anxiety symptoms) that will be humiliating or embarrassing.*
   Note: *In children, there must be evidence of the capacity for age-appropriate social relationships with familiar people and the anxiety must occur in peer settings, not just in interactions with adults.*

B. *Exposure to the feared social situation almost invariably provokes anxiety, which may take the form of a situationally bound or situationally predisposed panic attack.*
   Note: *In children, the anxiety may be expressed by crying, tantrums, freezing, or shrinking from social situations with unfamiliar people.*

C. *The person recognizes that the fear is excessive or unreasonable.*
   Note: *In children, this feature may be absent.*

D. *The social or performance situation is avoided or else is endured with intense anxiety or distress.*

E. *The avoidance, anxious anticipation, or distress in the feared social or performance situation(s) interferes significantly with the person's normal routine, occupational (or academic) functioning, or social activities or relationships, or there is marked distress about having the phobia.*

F. *In individuals under age 18 years, the duration is at least 6 months.*

G. *The fear or avoidance is not due to the direct physiological effects of a substance or a general medical condition and is not better accounted for by another mental disorder.*

H. *If a general medical condition or another mental disorder is present, the fear in Criterion A is unrelated to it, e.g., the fear is not of stuttering, trembling in Parkinson's disease, or exhibiting abnormal eating behavior in anorexia nervosa or bulimia nervosa.*

Specify if:

Generalized: *if the fears include most social situations.*
Note: *Also consider the additional diagnosis of avoidant personality disorder.*

(Adapted, with permission, from the *Diagnostic and Statistical Manual of Mental Disorders.* 4th edn. Text Revision. Washington, DC: American Psychiatric Association, 2000)

General Considerations

A. EPIDEMIOLOGY

Phobic disorders are among the most common of all psychiatric disorders. Specific phobia affects 5–10% of the general population, and social phobia (also referred to as social anxiety disorder) affects about 3%. The onset is typically in childhood or early adult life, and the condition is usually chronic. Many people with specific phobia learn to "live around" the feared stimulus. Social phobia is often more disabling.

B. ETIOLOGY

Phobic disorders may develop because of a pairing of anxiety with specific environmental events or experiences. For example, emotional trauma accompanying experiences such as riding in a car or speaking in public may produce a phobia. The majority of individuals with these problems, however, do not report that particular events have led to the disorder. Under these circumstances, the etiology is unknown.

Clinical Findings

A. SIGNS & SYMPTOMS

A specific phobia is an intense, irrational fear or aversion to a particular object or situation, other than a social situation. Typical specific phobias are fears of animals (especially insects or spiders); the natural environment (e.g., storms); blood, injection, or injury; or situations (e.g., heights, closed places, elevators, airplane travel). Most people deal with this problem by simply avoiding the feared stimulus, although this is not always possible. For example, people who have a fear of insects or spiders may avoid basements, attics, or closets; however, the emotional reactions or avoidance behavior may cause more serious problems. People who have a fear of flying may be unable to perform certain kinds of work. People who have a blood-injection-injury phobia may experience vasodilation, bradycardia, orthostatic hypotension, or fainting on exposure.

Social phobia is characterized by an extreme anxiety response in situations in which the affected person may be observed by others. People with social phobia usually fear that they will act in an embarrassing or humiliating manner. As with a specific phobia, social situations are avoided or endured with severe anxiety. Common phobic situations include speaking in public, eating in public, using public restrooms, writing while others are observing, and performing publicly. Rarely, people with this condition suffer from generalized social phobia, in which most or all social situations are avoided.

Neuroimaging

Functional neuroimaging studies have shown that cognitive behavioral therapy (CBT) in patients with phobic disorders resulted in decreased activity in limbic and paralimbic areas; it is noteworthy that similar effects were observed after successful intervention with SSRIs.

Course of Illness

Relatively little is known about the long-term course of phobic disorders; however, untreated phobic disorders often are chronic conditions.

Differential Diagnosis (Including Comorbid Conditions)

DSM-IV-TR diagnostic criteria allow the inclusion of a situationally confined panic attack in the category of phobic disorders. Therefore, panic disorder (with or without accompanying agoraphobia) must be distinguished from phobic disorders. In phobic disorders, anxiety or fear is restricted to a particular object or situation. Panic disorder, by definition, is characterized by severe, unexpected anxiety attacks during at least some phase of the disorder. Agoraphobia is distinguished by its association with panic disorder. This condition is differentiated by anxiety that occurs in situations in which help might not be available in case of a panic attack.

Avoidant personality disorder shares many features—and is often comorbid—with social phobia. The generalized form of social phobia is especially difficult to distinguish from avoidant personality. Avoidant personality disorder is in many ways equivalent to pathologic shyness, it is characterized in DSM-IV-TR by "a pervasive pattern of social inhibition, feelings of inadequacy, and hypersensitivity to negative evaluation." Like social phobia, avoidant personality disorder is usually associated with a fear of being shamed or ridiculed; however, in social phobia the fear is often confined to performance situations, with a relative sparing of other social interactions. For example, a person with social phobia may find it quite impossible to speak or write in public, whereas he or she could conduct a casual conversation without difficulty. This would not be true of someone with avoidant personality disorder.

People with psychotic disorders may experience abnormal fears and avoid others, but these are characterized by delusional beliefs. Patients with somatoform disorders (e.g., hypochondriasis) may exhibit anxiety and avoidance that can be confused with phobic disorders. However, unlike patients with somatoform disorder, those with specific or social phobias retain insight into the irrationality of their condition. In major depression, social avoidance is common, but not related to performance anxiety. Persons with OCD may also avoid situation to prevent stimulation of obsessions and compulsions. However, compulsive behaviors typically do not occur in phobic disorders.

Treatment

A. PSYCHOPHARMACOLOGIC INTERVENTIONS

Although treatments for phobic disorders typically are psychotherapeutic, some drug treatments have been used (Table 19–4). Benzodiazepines are sometimes used to reduce the anxiety associated with specific and social phobias. β-Blockers such as propranolol have been used with success to reduce the autonomic hyperarousal and tremor associated with performance situations. β-Blockers can also be helpful in blood-injection-injury phobia. These medications all have attendant side effects and are often unnecessary because behavioral treatments are so effective. Controlled clinical trials have shown antidepressants, particularly the SSRIs, to be beneficial in treating social phobia.

B. PSYCHOTHERAPEUTIC INTERVENTIONS

Behavioral or cognitive–behavioral psychotherapies are the treatments of choice. A typical treatment regimen

Table 19–4. Pharmacologic Treatment of Social Phobia

Drug	Starting Dosage	Dosing Range	Common Side Effects
Paroxetine	20 mg	20–40 mg	Nausea, diarrhea, anxiety/nervousness, sexual dysfunction, somnolence
Sertraline	50 mg	50–150 mg	Nausea, diarrhea, anxiety/nervousness, sexual dysfunction

involves relaxation training, usually coupled with visualization of the phobic stimulus, followed by progressive desensitization through repeated controlled exposure to the phobic cue. This regimen is generally followed by extinction of the anxiety response. A cognitive–behavioral approach adds the dimension of managing the catastrophic thoughts associated with exposure to the situation.

Complications/Adverse Outcomes of Treatment

Specific and social phobias are common and relatively benign conditions in contrast to panic disorder. Many people experience specific fears but learn to live around them. That is, most people with phobias simply avoid situations in which they may be exposed to a phobic stimulus. Phobias occasionally have a disabling effect. For example, a business executive with a fear of public speaking or flying may find that the phobia restricts his or her ability to benefit from career advancement. Although behavioral treatments may be anxiety provoking, they often produce significant results. Some individuals use substances of abuse, especially alcohol, to endure their anxiety; therefore, a careful alcohol and drug history is important in the evaluation of patients with phobic disorders.

Prognosis

Relatively little is known about the long-term course of phobic disorders; however, untreated, phobias often are chronic conditions.

Curtis GC et al.: Specific fears and phobias. Epidemiology and classification. *Br J Psychiatry* 1998;173:212.

Blanco C, Raza MS, Schneier FR, Liebowitz MR: The evidence-based pharmacological treatment of social anxiety disorder. *Int J Neuropsychopharmacol* 2003;6:427.

Marks I: Blood-injury phobia: A review. *Am J Psychiatry* 1988;145:1207.

Rapaport MH, Paniccia G, Judd LL: A review of social phobia. *Psychopharmacol Bull* 1995;31:125.

■ GENERALIZED ANXIETY DISORDER

 ESSENTIALS OF DIAGNOSIS

DSM-IV-TR Diagnostic Criteria

A. *Excessive anxiety and worry (apprehensive expectation), occurring more days than not for at least 6 months about a number of events or activities (such as work or school performance).*

B. *The person finds it difficult to control the worry.*

C. *The anxiety and worry are associated with three (or more) of the following six symptoms (with at least some symptoms present for more days than not for the past 6 months).*
   Note: *Only one item is required in children.*
   (1) *restlessness or feeling keyed up—-on edge*
   (2) *easily fatigued*
   (3) *difficulty concentrating or mind going blank*
   (4) *irritability*
   (5) *muscle tension*
   (6) *sleep disturbance*

D. *The focus of the anxiety and worry is not confined to features of an Axis I disorder, e.g., the anxiety or worry is not about having a panic attack (as in panic disorder), being contaminated (as in obsessive-compulsive disorder), being away from home or close relatives (as in separation anxiety disorder), gaining weight (as in anorexia nervosa), having multiple physical complaints (as in somatization disorder), or having a serious illness (as in hypochondriasis), and the anxiety and worry do not occur exclusively during posttraumatic stress disorder.*

  E. *The anxiety, worry, or physical symptoms cause clinically significant distress or impairment in social, occupational, or other important areas of functioning.*

  F. *The disturbance is not due to the direct physiological effects of a substance (e.g., a drug of abuse, a medication) or medical condition (e.g., hypothyroidism) and does not occur exclusively during a mood disorder, a psychotic disorder, or a pervasive developmental disorder.*

(Reprinted, with permission, from the *Diagnostic and Statistical Manual of Mental Disorders*. 4th edn. Text Revision. Washington, DC: American Psychiatric Association, 2000)

General Considerations

A. EPIDEMIOLOGY

GAD typically begins in early adult life, is slightly more common in women, and is usually chronic. Although GAD is rather common, it is seen more often in general medical practice than in psychiatry practice. Patients with GAD typically experience persistent worry of variable severity across time that often leads them to their primary care clinician. Continuity of care across time is critical to the recognition and treatment of this disorder. Further, patients with GAD have a high rate of comorbidity with major depression. GAD comes closest to the classic concept of the anxiety neurosis. GAD may be associated with an emotionally reactive temperament (traditionally referred to as neuroticism). In fact, the emotionally reactive temperament appears to have a significant genetic component, and may predispose to a variety of anxiety or depressive disorders.

B. GENETICS

There is emerging evidence from family studies that GAD exhibits a mild to moderate familial aggregation; this appears to hold if subjects are self-selected, or are recruited from a clinical or community setting. Twin studies also indicate that GAD is moderately heritable.

Clinical Findings

A. SIGNS & SYMPTOMS

GAD is a syndrome of persistent worry coupled with symptoms of hyperarousal. Often, patients with GAD do not recognize themselves as having a psychiatric disorder, even though the symptoms can be quite disabling. These patients are much more likely to present in a general medical setting than in a psychiatrist's office. For this reason, primary care clinicians must be particularly sensitive to patients' emotional needs.

B. NEUROIMAGING

A study using proton magnetic resonance spectroscopy has demonstrated that GAD can be associated with asymmetric increases in the N-acetylaspartate–creatine ratio, a suggested marker of neuronal viability, in the (right dorsolateral) prefrontal cortex.

Differential Diagnosis (Including Comorbid Conditions)

Persistent hyperarousal coupled with obsessive thoughts are common to other psychiatric disorders (e.g., major depression). In some ways, GAD could be considered to be major depression without persistently depressed mood or anhedonia (see Chapter 18). In fact, GAD often responds well to treatment with tricyclic antidepressants, as discussed later in this chapter. If the patient worries chronically, depression should always be considered in the differential diagnosis. Other psychiatric disorders with obsessive thinking (e.g., OCD; panic disorder; somatoform disorders; psychotic disorders, especially paranoid subtypes; eating disorders, particularly anorexia nervosa; and many personality disorders) are associated with persistent fear, apprehension, or worry that can be confused with GAD. The focus of the worry should not be related primarily to one of these conditions. For example, if a patient fears the occurrence of a panic attack, the obvious cause of the problem is panic disorder, even if other associated worries (e.g., personal health or well-being of a significant other) are present. Similarly, if the central concern is physical health, without panic attacks, then somatoform disorder is likely to be the primary diagnosis.

Treatment

The management of GAD should consider the long-standing nature of the problem. Treatment should deal with the underlying causes of the condition, such as persistently distorted cognitions. Unfortunately, several factors work against treatment. GAD tends to be under-recognized. Even when it is identified, the problem is often not taken as seriously as the degree of disability associated with the condition would suggest. If treatment is provided, it is likely to be brief. Finally, insurance coverage tends to discriminate against the treatment of GAD. Together, these factors conspire to ensure that most patients with GAD do not get appropriate treatment.

A. PSYCHOPHARMACOLOGIC INTERVENTIONS

Patients with GAD are likely to receive benzodiazepines, even though psychotherapies and other

Table 19–5. Pharmacologic Treatment of Generalized Anxiety Disorder

Drug	Starting Dosage	Dosing Range	Common Side Effects
Buspirone	5 mg three times	15–40 mg daily	Anxiety/nervousness, headache, nausea
Imipramine	25 mg at bedtime	25–150 mg	Dry mouth, blurred vision, constipation, urinary hesitancy, orthostasis, somnolence, anxiety
Venlafaxine	37.5 mg daily	37.5–225 mg daily	Anxiety/nervousness, diarrhea, sexual dysfunction, withdrawal reactions
Benzodiazepines	—	—	Somnolence, ataxia, memory (various) problems, nausea, physical dependence, withdrawal reactions

medications are clearly beneficial. Although benzodiazepines reduce symptoms, GAD is a chronic condition and benzodiazepines are not curative. If benzodiazepines alone are used, long-term management is required to prevent symptoms from returning. Benzodiazepines generally should not be used alone to treat GAD, but they can be helpful adjuncts to treatment, particularly when the symptoms are severe. Short-term, low-to-moderate dosages of benzodiazepines can facilitate psychotherapy. Benzodiazepines can also be used to reduce symptoms and to return the patient to normal functioning. After a few weeks, the benzodiazepine should be reduced and eventually discontinued.

Most clinicians worry about the potential for benzodiazepine abuse. Epidemiologic studies, however, demonstrate that legitimate clinical use far outweighs any abuse. True abuse is relatively uncommon. Benzodiazepine abuse is seen most often when they are used to (1) counteract the adverse effects of psychostimulants such as cocaine; (2) augment the euphoric effects of other sedative drugs such as alcohol; or (3) self-medicate alcohol or other sedative withdrawal.

Benzodiazepines should not be given to patients who have a personal history or strong first-degree family history of drug or alcohol abuse. Even though the primary abuse of benzodiazepines is uncommon, some patients develop psychological and physiologic dependence. Physiologic dependence becomes an increasing problem when benzodiazepines have been given continuously for 3 months or more, although mild withdrawal reactions can occur after shorter treatment periods. Clinicians who are considering treating GAD with benzodiazepines should first weigh the alternatives (described later in this section). In general, brief, interrupted courses of benzodiazepine treatment should be given as psychotherapeutic management is being initiated; prescription refills should be monitored carefully; and the drug should then be tapered if continuous use exceeds 1 month. Problems can generally be avoided under these circumstances.

Benzodiazepines can produce other adverse effects, such as daytime sedation, ataxia (which can cause dangerous falls in the elderly), accident proneness (e.g., motor vehicle accidents), headaches, memory problems (ranging from short-term memory problems to brief periods of profound memory loss), and occasionally, paradoxical excitement or anxiety. These problems are especially prominent in the elderly, in whom due to reduced metabolism drug metabolites can accumulate resulting in high plasma levels.

The anxiolytic buspirone, a serotonin$_{1A}$ receptor partial agonist, is an alternative to benzodiazepines (Table 19–5). Buspirone has several advantages. It produces no motor, memory, or concentration impairments. It has no abuse potential, and it does not cause dependency or withdrawal, even after long periods of exposure. It does not produce drug interactions. It appears to be an almost ideal anxiolytic; however, it has some disadvantages. In contrast to the benzodiazepines, which are often experienced by patients as having an immediate effect, buspirone requires at least 3 weeks to mitigate anxiety. Patients with severe anxiety, especially those who previously received benzodiazepines, may have a reduced level of response. Further, buspirone stimulates the locus coeruleus, which may be associated with a paradoxical increase in anxiety in some patients. Despite these disadvantages, buspirone should be considered a practical alternative to benzodiazepines.

The tricyclic antidepressant imipramine and the heterocyclic antidepressant venlafaxine have demonstrated significant benefit in the treatment of GAD. Like buspirone, the therapeutic effect is delayed, but severely anxious patients appear to improve. Other tricyclic antidepressants or SSRIs may be helpful but have not been tested adequately. β-Blockers and clonidine have been reported to be helpful in treating GAD. Although these drugs can reduce anxiety, side effects of hypotension and depression are prominent. Antipsychotic drugs, such as chlorpromazine or haloperidol, reduce anxiety, but the risk of tardive dyskinesia outweighs the potential benefit.

B. Psychotherapeutic Interventions

Two psychotherapeutic approaches are helpful in treating GAD. Behavioral therapy can teach patients progressive deep muscle relaxation while they imagine anxiety-inducing stimuli. If the patient avoids situations that generate significant anxiety, progressive desensitization can be helpful.

An alternative is cognitive–behavioral therapy. This treatment adds a cognitive component to basic behavioral therapy on the assumption that the anxiety associated with GAD is a result of persistent distortions about the self, other people, and the future. Misinterpretations, especially catastrophic misperceptions of threat or danger, contribute significantly to anxiety. Cognitive–behavioral therapy helps patients to recognize the relationships between specific situations and pathogenic distortions of thinking. Further, the treatment helps to elucidate the faulty fundamental belief systems that underlie the distorted thinking. Patients learn to recognize and counter the distortions with alternative thoughts that eventually become automatic.

C. Other Interventions

Other interventions may be needed, such as marital, family, or occupational therapy. Other primary therapies (e.g., psychodynamic, client-centered, or interpersonal therapy) have little or no empirical support.

Complications/Adverse Outcomes of Treatment

GAD is a highly comorbid condition. The most common comorbid diagnosis is major depression. As noted earlier in this chapter, diagnostic primacy may shift frequently across the patient's lifetime in a more chronic neurotic pattern between the more typical depressive and anxious symptoms. GAD may be comorbid with other conditions, including personality disorders (e.g., obsessive–compulsive, schizoid, histrionic, avoidant) or other anxiety disorders (e.g., OCD, panic disorder). The diagnosis of GAD should be given only if the diagnosis is clearly independent of other Axis I or Axis II disorders. For example, the diagnosis would not be given to a patient who has a history of persistent anxiety or worry occurring only in the context of major depression. Similarly, the diagnosis is excluded if the worries or fears are clearly related to the pattern of OCD, social phobia, or panic disorder. However, the diagnosis can be given if the symptoms of GAD predate the onset of these other conditions or are otherwise definitely temporally independent.

Because the frequency of comorbidity is high, the existence of comorbid disorders should be examined whenever the diagnosis of GAD is considered.

Prognosis

DSM-IV-TR diagnostic criteria require the characteristic features of GAD to be present for at least 6 months before the diagnosis can be made. However, most patients are chronically ill, often for decades. Untreated, GAD typically follows a chronic pattern, with waxing and waning severity. Comorbid conditions may contribute to chronicity. Pharmacologic treatments will relieve symptoms, but the syndrome usually reemerges after treatment has been discontinued. Psychotherapeutic management (with or without symptomatic treatment with medications) often is helpful in reducing the chronicity associated with GAD.

Barlow DH, Wincze J: DSM-IV and beyond: What is generalized anxiety disorder? *Acta Psychiatr Scand* 1998;393(Suppl):23.

Chambless DL, Gillis: Cognitive therapy of anxiety disorders. *J Consult Clin Psychol* 1993;61:248.

Charney DS: Neuroanatomical circuits modulating fear and anxiety behaviors. *Acta Psychiatr Scand Suppl* 2003;417:38–50

Erickson TM, Newman MG: Cognitive behavioral psychotherapy for generalized anxiety disorder: A primer. *Expert Rev Neurother* 2005;5:247.

Gelenberg AJ, Lydiard RB, Rudolph RL, Aguiar L, Haskins JT, Salinas E: Efficacy of venlafaxine extended-release capsules in nondepressed outpatients with generalized anxiety disorder: A 6-month randomized controlled trial. *JAMA* 2000;283:3082.

Hettema JM, Neale MC, Myers JM, Prescott CA, Kendler KS: A population-based twin study of the relationship between neuroticism and internalizing disorders. *Am J Psychiatry* 2006;163:857.

Mackintosh MA, Gatz M, Wetherell JL, Pedersen NL: A twin study of lifetime Generalized Anxiety Disorder (GAD) in older adults: Genetic and environmental influences shared by neuroticism and GAD. *Twin Res Hum Genet* 2006;9:30–37.

Mathew SJ, Mao X, Coplan JD, et al.: Dorsolateral prefrontal cortical pathology in generalized anxiety disorder: A proton magnetic resonance spectroscopic imaging study. *Am J Psychiatry* 2004;161:1119–1121.

Mitte K, Noack P, Steil R, Hautzinger M: A meta-analytic review of the efficacy of drug treatment in generalized anxiety disorder. *J Clin Psychopharmacol* 2005;25:141.

Newman SC, Bland RC: A population based family study of DSM-III generalized anxiety disorder. *Psychol Med* 2006;36:1275–1281.

Rickels K, Downing R, Schweizer E, Hassman H, et al.: Antidepressants for the treatment of generalized anxiety disorder. *Arch Gen Psychiatry* 1993;50:884.

Sellers EM et al.: Alprazolam and benzodiazepine dependence. *J Clin Psychiatry* 1993;54(Suppl):64.

Posttraumatic Stress Disorder and Acute Stress Disorder

20

Douglas C. Johnson, PhD, John H. Krystal, MD, & Steven M. Southwick, MD

■ POSTTRAUMATIC STRESS DISORDER

 ESSENTIALS OF DIAGNOSIS

DSM-IV-TR Diagnostic Criteria

A. The person has been exposed to a traumatic event in which both of the following were present:

   (1) The person experienced, witnessed, or was confronted with an event or events that involved actual or threatened death or serious injury, or a threat to the physical integrity of self or others

   (2) The person's response involved intense fear, helplessness, or horror
   Note: In children, this may be expressed instead by disorganized or agitated behavior.

B. The traumatic event is persistently re-experienced in one (or more) of the following ways:

   (1) Recurrent and intrusive distressing recollections of the event, including images, thoughts, or perceptions
   Note: In young children, repetitive play may occur in which themes or aspects of the trauma are expressed.

   (2) Recurrent distressing dreams of the event
   Note: In children, there may be frightening dreams without recognizable content.

   (3) Acting or feeling as if the traumatic event were recurring (includes a sense of reliving the experience, illusions, hallucinations, and dissociative flashback episodes, including those that occur on awakening or when intoxicated)

Note: In young children, trauma-specific reenactment may occur.

   (4) Intense psychological distress at exposure to internal or external cues that symbolize or resemble an aspect of the traumatic event

   (5) Physiological reactivity on exposure to internal or external cues that symbolize or resemble an aspect of the traumatic event

C. Persistent avoidance of stimuli associated with the trauma and numbing of general responsiveness (not present before the trauma), as indicated by three (or more) of the following:

   (1) Efforts to avoid thoughts, feelings, or conversations associated with the trauma

   (2) Efforts to avoid activities, places, or people that arouse recollections of the trauma

   (3) Inability to recall an important aspect of the trauma

   (4) Markedly diminished interest or participation in significant activities

   (5) Feeling of detachment or estrangement from others

   (6) Restricted range of affect (e.g., unable to have loving feelings)

   (7) Sense of foreshortened future (e.g., does not expect to have a career, marriage, children, or a normal life span)

D. Persistent symptoms of increased arousal (not present before the trauma), as indicated by two (or more) of the following:

   (1) Difficulty falling or staying asleep

   (2) Irritability or outbursts of anger

   (3) Difficulty concentrating

   (4) Hypervigilance

   (5) Exaggerated startle response

E. Duration of the disturbance (symptoms in Criteria B, C, and D) is more than 1 month.

F. The disturbance causes clinically significant distress or impairment in social, occupational, or other important areas of functioning.

(Reprinted, with permission, from *Diagnostic and Statistical Manual of Mental Disorders*, 4th edn., Text Revision. Washington DC: American Psychiatric Association, 2000.)

General Considerations

Despite abundant evidence for persisting and sometimes disabling psychological sequelae of exposure to extreme stressors, the evolution of posttraumatic stress disorder (PTSD) as a modern diagnosis was relatively recent. PTSD-like disorders were described in the U.S. Civil War (DaCosta's Syndrome, Irritable Heart of Soldiers), associated with railroad accidents in the late nineteenth century (Railway Spine), following World Wars I and II (Shell Shock, Traumatic Neurosis, Neurasthenia, Survivor Syndrome).

In the 1950s and 1960s, debate revolved around the issue of whether there was anything unique about the psychiatric symptoms that emerged following extreme stress relative to psychiatric symptoms that were expressed in the context of the stresses of everyday life. Thus, the diagnosis of Gross Stress Reaction appeared in the initial *Diagnostic and Statistical Manual of Mental Disorders* (*DSM*), but was excluded from DSM-II. In 1980, in the wake of the collection of a compelling body of clinical research on soldiers of the Vietnam War, studies of victims of physical and sexual assault, and victims of natural disasters, the American Psychiatric Association introduced PTSD diagnostic criteria in a form that is fundamentally similar to current diagnostic schema. Unlike other anxiety disorders, PTSD is predicated on the occurrence of at least one discrete external event, namely a precipitating trauma. DSM-III defined a trauma as "experiencing an event that is outside the range of usual human experience." However, subsequent epidemiologic studies found that traumatic events are common, that greater than half of the population experienced trauma sometime during their life, and that even witnessing trauma could be predictive of PTSD. The DSM-IV-TR now stipulates two sub-criteria—one objective, one subjective—to meet formal diagnosis of PTSD: (A1) the person experienced, witnessed, or was confronted with an event or events that involved actual or threatened death or serious injury, or a threat to physical integrity of self or others; *and* (A2) the person's response involved fear, helplessness, or horror. The change in the definition of a traumatic event from DSM-III to DSM-IV resulted in higher rates of PTSD in a number of epidemiologic studies. The fiscal year 2005 report from the Veterans Benefits Administration indicated that PTSD was the costliest diagnosis for the VA, and the third most frequently claimed disability, comprising 4.2% of all claims.

A. EPIDEMIOLOGY

1. Extreme stress exposure—Data from the largest mental health epidemiological study to date indicate a majority of Americans have had exposure to at least one potentially traumatic (Criterion A) event. The National Comorbidity Study (NCS) surveyed 5877 Americans (2812 men and 3065 women) aged 15–54 years, and reported that 60.7% of men and 51.2% of women reported experiencing at least one extremely stressful event in their lifetime. Of those who had experienced at least one of these events, the majority of men (56.3%) and a significant percentage of women (48.6%) reported experiencing multiple extremely stressful events.

The prevalence of exposure to extreme stress has also been examined within specific populations such as inner-city residents, women, and combat veterans. For example, in a sample of 4008 American women, 69% of respondents had experienced at least one of these events in their life. Other studies have found extreme stress exposure rates as high as 92.2% for men and 87.1% for women living in inner-city metropolitan areas.

The prevalence of exposure to extreme stressors has recently received increased attention in the United States in the wake of terrorist attacks on civilians and military combat operations in Iraq and Afghanistan. When 3671 U.S. Army and Marine Corps personnel were surveyed 3–4 months after their return from Iraq or Afghanistan, prevalence of life-threatening combat engagement was significantly higher for troops deployed to Iraq compared to Afghanistan: 30% of soldiers from Afghanistan reported "seeing dead or seriously injured or killed Americans," whereas 70% of Iraq veterans endorsed having these experiences; 12% of veterans from Afghanistan reported "handling or uncovering human remains," while over half of all Iraq veterans surveyed (54%) had firsthand experience with war dead.

2. Prevalence rates of PTSD—Despite the ubiquity of extremely stressful life events, only a minority of survivors develop PTSD. For example, the National Vietnam Veterans Readjustment Study (NVVRS) compiled data from 3016 subjects, comprising 1632 Vietnam theater veterans, 716 veterans from the Vietnam era who did not serve in-theater, and a civilian (*n* = 668) cohort (Kulka, Schlenger, Fairbank, Hough, Jordan, Marmar, and Weiss, 1990). Lifetime prevalence for PTSD was 31% for males, and 27% for female veterans; incidence rates 20–25 years after the war were 15%

and 9%, respectively. Overall, these findings indicate that a majority of Vietnam veterans did *not* suffer from chronic maladjustment or PTSD even though most combat-experienced soldiers in this study endured repeated and sustained extreme stress. Recent reanalysis of the NVVRS has adjusted original prevalence rates of PTSD in Vietnam veterans from 30.9% to 18.7% lifetime, and 15.2–9.1% current (Dohrenwend et al., 2006). In comparison, lifetime prevalence of PTSD among adult Americans in the NCS was 7.8%, despite a 60.6% exposure rate for men and 51.2% for women. Among current active-duty combat veterans rates of PTSD were concordant with the difference in combat exposure, with 12.5% of Iraq veterans, and 6.2% of Afghanistan veterans meeting PTSD criteria.

Rates of PTSD vary depending on the nature of trauma. For example, rape results in high rates of PTSD in both men (65%) and women (46%), while automobile accidents have been associated with lower rates of PTSD (men, 25%; women, 13.8%). Prevalence rates for PTSD have been as disparate as 20% for wounded combat veterans and 3% for veterans who were not wounded.

B. Etiology

Multiple psychological, biological, and environmental factors appear to be involved in the etiology of PTSD. In attempting to understand neural and behavioral mechanisms that contribute to the etiology of PTSD, investigators have highlighted four features of PTSD.

1. Fear conditioning and learning—The *Two-Factor* model (Mowrer, 1947) is a combination of classical (Pavlovian) and operant (reinforcement) conditioning. Classical conditioning is the process of pairing together, or associating, two stimuli: the traumatic event (unconditioned stimulus, UCS) and associated sensory stimuli (conditioned stimuli, CS). As a result of this pairing, the formerly neutral CS now elicits the same fear response (conditioned response, CR) (and autonomic arousal) as the UCS.

In cases of PTSD, there may be modality specific (i.e., classical conditioning), as well as polymodal (i.e., contextual conditioning), stimuli paired with the CR. Moreover, behavioral neuroscience research has shown that classical and contextual conditioning are partially mediated by different brain regions. Classical conditioning is known to involve thalamo–amygdala pathways, whereas contextual conditioning occurs via input to the hippocampus and amygdala from higher cortical areas. In the case of contextual conditioning, multiple and often complex environmental stimuli that are present during exposure to the feared stimulus (UCS) become associated. For example, after exposure to a roadside Improvised Explosive Device (IED) in Iraq, a veteran while driving in the United States may experience fear and au-

tonomic arousal when exposed to modality specific (e.g., a loud muffler backfire) or contextual (e.g., hot dirt road, trash in the median, and smell of diesel fuel) stimuli, each of which were previously neutral.

According to the classical conditioning model, a learned CR in PTSD should become extinct over time in the absence of exposure to the original trauma (UCS). However, avoidance or escape thoughts and behaviors often produce a welcome mitigation in anxious arousal, thereby creating a powerful reinforcement (operant conditioning) of continued avoidance. The unintended consequence for the sufferer of PTSD is that new learning (extinction of fear-based arousal) is inhibited.

2. Information processing—Although a stimulus (S) → response (R) model sufficiently explains the acquisition of fear-based conditioning, it is inadequate in that a stimulus does not always produce the same response. For example, the S → R model does not account for the fact that two people can experience the same exact trauma, yet have different reactions. To account for the variability in responses to a stimulus, the S → R model has been modified to the S → O → R model (Eysenck, 1967), where response to a given stimulus is dependent on the nature of the organism. A major component in an information processing model is the appraisal of trauma-related information. Appraisal of a trauma comprises multiple information processing domains including perceived predictability of the event, controllability of the trauma, intensity of emotions, valence of emotions, and personal meaning assigned to the experience. For example, individuals who assign greater positive meaning to stressful events typically exhibit more adaptive responses.

The processing of trauma-related emotions is particularly relevant to avoidance and intrusive memories. According to the Emotion Processing Theory (Foa and Kozack, 1986), memories of traumatic events are stored, along with associated (i.e., conditioned) cues, in information networks called "*fear structures.*" The individual with PTSD avoids encountering or thinking about the trauma, or its cues, in an attempt to avoid activation of the associative network of trauma-related memories. Intrusive memories are believed to occur as a result of implicit exposure to one or more cues that activate the fear structure.

3. Neurobiological systems—A number of neurobiological models have been proposed as an attempt to explain PTSD or specific aspects of PTSD. Prominent among these models are those involving genetic polymorphisms related to stress vulnerability (e.g., polymorphisms of the serotonin transporter gene). Additionally, several models involve detrimental changes to fear, learning, and memory circuits. For example, mammalian learning is known to be optimized by a high degree of neuroplasticity in excitatory inputs to the amygdala from the medial PFC, hippocampus, and thalamus. However, these circuits are also vulnerable to maladaptive alterations secondary to chronic or acute stress, further changing neuromodulation of learning and memory circuits. Such alterations then result in heightened sensitization to stress, enhanced encoding and consolidation of emotional memory, increased fear conditionability, cortical inhibition of limbic activity, and reduced capacity for extinction. Neurobiological vulnerabilities may also be responsible for certain structural abnormalities (e.g., reduced hippocampal volume); although it is uncertain whether these abnormalities are the cause or consequence of PTSD.

C. RISK

Several factors have been identified with increased risk for PTSD. Individual risk factors for PTSD include gender (female), history of prior trauma (i.e., childhood sexual abuse), and a family history of anxiety disorders. For example, data indicate women are twice as likely as men to develop PTSD. However, although several studies do in fact reveal higher rates of PTSD for women, it is necessary to interpret these results within the context of differences in types of trauma to which men and women are most commonly exposed. A review of PTSD research conducted since 1991 did find distinctions in exposure to trauma and PTSD between men and women (Hidalgo and Davidson, 2000). Results suggest that although men are at higher risk of exposure to traumatic events, women are more at risk for developing PTSD. Moreover, men experienced more physical assault and life-threatening traumas, whereas women experienced more sexual assault and childhood parental neglect.

Certain dimensions of personality are also implicated as risk factors for PTSD. In particular, individuals with a stable and consistent pattern of experiencing *negative emotionality* (NEM) may be more vulnerable to PTSD following exposure to an extreme stressor. NEM is a disposition characterized by anxiety, emotional lability, poor interpersonal interactions, and overall negative mood. A related personality construct is neuroticism, which is defined by a high degree of negative affect, and increased acquisition of fear through conditioning. Longitudinal studies of combat veterans pre- and postdeployment have revealed NEM as a significant predictor of both PTSD development and severity. Conversely, positive emotionality (PEM) is hypothesized as a personality factor that moderates the relationship between NEM and PTSD.

Aspects of the trauma and the way it was experienced are also risk factors for PTSD; in general, the greater the intensity of the trauma, the greater the CR and prevalence of PTSD. Factors that contribute to the intensity of the traumatic response and PTSD include duration of the trauma, predictability and controllability of the event, failed attempts to avoid injury, perceived sense of failure, actual loss, proximity to the traumatic event and degree of peritraumatic arousal and dissociation. A survey of 1008 adult survivors of the September 11 World Trade Center attacks found that 7.5% reported symptoms consistent with a diagnosis of PTSD; however, higher rates of PTSD (20%) were found within the larger sample for those living closer to the World Trade Center (Galea, Ahern, Resnick, Kilpatrick, Bucuvalas, Gold, and Vlahov, 2002).

D. RESILIENCE

Given that not all individuals exposed to the same traumatic event will develop PTSD, it becomes vital to understand what it is about those individuals who do well under stress and are able to recover from trauma? In contrast to traditional investigations that seek to determine the causes and catalysts for psychopathology, resilience research, particularly within the field of trauma studies, attempts to explain why some individuals are relatively resistant to the negative impact of trauma, recover rapidly after traumatic exposure, or experience positive growth in response to trauma. Resilience to stress has been investigated from neurobiological (Charney, 2004) and psychosocial perspectives (Southwick, Vythilingam, and Charney, 2005).

1. Neurobiological resilience factors—Numerous genetic factors, developmental influences, brain regions, endocrine and neurotransmitter systems appear to be associated with resilience to stress. Among the neurobiological factors that recently have received attention are: sympathetic nervous system activity that responds robustly to stress but that returns to baseline rapidly perhaps secondary to regulation by neuropeptide Y (NPY) and galanin; capacity to contain the corticotrophin-releasing factor (CRF) response to stress perhaps in association with DHEA, NPY and a host of other regulators; a durable dopamine-mediated reward system that might allow traumatized individuals to remain optimistic and hopeful even in the context of extreme or chronic stress; amygdalae that do not overreact to the environment; hippocampi that provide sufficient inhibition to the hypothalamic-pituitary-adrenal axis (HPA axis); and ample cortical executive and inhibitory capacity.

Elevated levels of plasma NPY have been found in humans following extreme stressors such as military survival training. Moreover, higher levels of NPY have been correlated with better performance during simulated prisoner of war training with Special Forces soldiers. Lower baseline and yohimbine-stimulated levels of NPY have been found in combat veterans with a current diagnosis of PTSD, but other studies of combat-related PTSD and female victims of sexual assault (Seedat, Stein, Kennedy, and Hauger, 2003) have yielded mixed results, suggesting that low levels of NPY are not associated with PTSD, but rather exposure to trauma.

Other neurophysiological factors associated with improved performance under extreme stress and the ability to physically and mentally recover following trauma are low vagal tone and increased heart rate variability (Morgan, Aikins, Steffian, Hazlett, and Southwick, 2007).

A traditional view of resilience is that people who have a stronger constitution are more functional under all circumstances. An alternative view is that people are biased by their genotypes to function best at certain levels of arousal, e.g., COMT gene polymorphism. Under resting conditions, the less functional variant (higher dopamine in PFC) functions better with respect to PFC-related cognitive function, but with stress, the less functional variant is overstimulated and functions more poorly than the other group. The people with higher functioning COMT (less dopamine) are "sluggish" under normal conditions but function more optimally relative to their peers under conditions of high stress.

2. Psychosocial Resilience factors—Resilience to stress has been correlated with *optimism, humor, social support*, and an *active* instead of avoidant *coping-style*. Research has also identified *openness-to-change* and *extroversion* as positive predictors of growth following traumatic experiences. Two closely related constructs associated with resilience are *cognitive flexibility* and *emotion regulation*. *Cognitive flexibility*, marked by the ability to reframe problems and extract personal meaning from stressful situations, has been associated with reappraisal of events as less threatening and a greater sense of self-efficacy in the face of challenge. Moreover, there is some evidence to suggest that resilience is not a static or stable dimension, but is responsive to therapeutic and pharmacological augmentation.

Clearly, resilience to stress is associated with a complex set of interactions between neurobiological and psychosocial factors. For example, Kaufman et al. (2004) studied the effects of social support networks in children who were at risk genetically (s/s allele of the 5-HTTLPR serotonin transporter gene promoter polymorphism) and environmentally (documented history of maltreatment) revealed that strength of social support networks and positive social relationships moderated the risk for depression above and beyond genetic vulnerabilities and early exposure to overwhelming stress.

E. Genetics

A study of 4042 Vietnam era twin pairs indicates that vulnerability to PTSD has a significant genetic component. After controlling for variability in combat exposure, genetic concordance accounted for 13–30% of the variance in reexperiencing symptoms (Cluster B), 30–34% of the variance in avoidance symptoms (Cluster C), and 28–32% of the variance in the (Cluster D) hyperarousal symptoms.

Studies of probands with anxiety disorders and other twin studies indicate that PTSD symptoms are moderately heritable. Increasingly, evidence suggests that PTSD is caused by a complex interaction between genetic vulnerabilities to stress and the nature of the stressor. Given the inherent difficulty in isolating environmental stressors, experimentally controlling for extraneous variables during traumatic events, and the unlikelihood of identifying a single PTSD gene, there is growing interest in endophenotypes.

In monozygotic twins discordant for service in Vietnam, premorbid NSS scores can predict PTSD when coupled with exposure to the stress of combat (Gurvits et al., 2006). However, a longitudinal study, also of co-twins discordant for combat exposure in Vietnam, found that degree of combat stress, not a genetic vulnerability, was the strongest predictor of persistence of PTSD symptoms 30 years after exposure (Roy-Byrne, Arguelles, Vitek, Goldberg, Keane, True, and Pitman, 2004). Results from psychophysiological research similarly suggest that not all PTSD symptoms are genetically determined. For example, a study of ($n = 50$) monozygotic twin pairs discordant for combat exposure in Vietnam showed that the noncombat exposed co-twin failed to demonstrate increased heart rate in response to startling tones. The fact an increased heart rate response to startling tones was evident in the combat exposed group, but not their co-twins, suggests that some aspect of autonomic reactivity is not related to genetic factors.

Clinical Findings

A. Signs and Symptoms

PTSD is characterized by a constellation of reexperiencing, avoidance, and hyperarousal symptoms. Most pathognomonic among these three symptom clusters are episodes of reexperiencing (i.e., flashbacks, nightmares, and intrusive memories). Such memories are rarely, if ever, wanted, and intrude against the will, sometimes for years or even a lifetime. Individuals with PTSD typically try to avoid these memories, both cognitively and behaviorally, and often rearrange their lives around avoiding potential reminders of the trauma that trigger remembrance.

In addition to cognitive and behavioral avoidance, PTSD is marked by significant avoidance of emotional arousal (i.e., emotional numbing); indeed, of the three symptom clusters, avoidance and emotional numbing are most predictive of a PTSD diagnosis and can have debilitating effects on psychosocial function. For instance, evaluation of survivors of the Oklahoma city bombing has shown that Cluster C (avoidance and numbing) symptoms were pivotal to the diagnosis of PTSD, whereas Clusters B (re-experiencing) and D (arousal) were not significantly associated with diagnosis. Of the survivors who met diagnostic criteria for Cluster C, 96% had a diagnosis of PTSD; however, of those who met Cluster B or Cluster D criteria, only 40% and 39% were diagnosed with PTSD, respectively. Conversely, for those individuals who did not receive a diagnosis of PTSD, only 2% met Cluster C criteria, whereas 70% and 73% met criteria for Clusters B and D, respectively.

Some individuals with PTSD experience amnesia for aspects of the traumatic event. This inability to recall certain trauma-related memories, despite hyperaccessibility of other trauma memories, may be explained in part by selective attention, dissociation, or extreme arousal, which can compromise encoding and consolidation of memory at the time of trauma. Likewise, degree of dissociation has been found to be highly predictive of PTSD following life-threatening trauma. Emotional numbing can be difficult to identify clinically since it is not necessarily manifest as flat affect, but rather as a restricted range of affect, and marked detachment from others. In this regard, collateral reporting sources (e.g., family members, significant others) are often integral to an accurate diagnostic assessment. Moreover, emotional numbing can often appear as indifference toward future plans and general apathy about setting goals such as getting married, owning a home, need for a healthy lifestyle, or career advancement.

Insomnia is a major problem for many trauma survivors with PTSD. They often describe difficulty falling asleep and staying asleep secondary to hypervigilance and/or fear of having nightmares. It is not uncommon for vivid nightmares to violently awaken survivors from their sleep.

B. LABORATORY FINDINGS

1. Physiological—A number of psychophysiological findings, characteristic of autonomic reactivity, help to differentiate individuals with current PTSD from those with a past diagnosis of PTSD or no history of PTSD. Increased heart rate reactivity to trauma-related stimuli (e.g., imagery, narratives) has been found in individuals with PTSD. Such cardiac-reactivity appears to be relatively specific to PTSD, as comparison studies including veterans with anxiety disorders other than PTSD have not shown similar increases in heart-rate. Moreover, cardiac reactivity in PTSD does not appear to be a generalized autonomic response to indiscriminate stressors, but rather is associated with trauma specific cues (Orr, Metzger, and Pitman, 2002). PTSD has also been identified by exaggerated startle response, as measured by EMG "eyeblink," increased skin conductance (SC) magnitudes (e.g., galvanic skin response) and slower SC habituation, and increased conditionability to aversive (laboratory shock) stimuli.

2. Cognitive—Information processing biases in PTSD have been studied using various cognitive paradigms. Although some trends in information processing bias have emerged, conclusive results in PTSD have been elusive. For example, individuals with PTSD have demonstrated an attentional bias for threat-related words during the color-naming portion of the Stroop task. Namely, compared to control samples, individuals show an increased latency in naming trauma or emotion words. While this is a robust finding, it is not clear how such results should be interpreted. It remains unclear whether an increased latency for naming trauma words is due to more rapid encoding in individuals with PTSD. Alternatively, those with PTSD may attempt to inhibit (i.e., avoidance) processing of emotionally aversive stimuli.

There is tentative support for biases in judgment showing that individuals with PTSD interpret ambiguous sentences and words (e.g., homographs) as threatening. Memory biases in PTSD have been less consistently demonstrated. In particular, there is some evidence for a mood-congruent memory effect in PTSD, to wit, individuals with PTSD demonstrate a memory advantage for trauma-related information. However, it remains unclear whether this explicit memory bias is the result of recall advantages inherent in personally salient information, or whether the advantages are due to true mood congruency between internal affective state and emotional valence assigned to the remembered material. Support for implicit memory biases in PTSD, based on implicit priming (i.e., below perceptual awareness threshold) and word stem completion task paradigms, is also limited.

Biases in forgetting, in particular thought suppression and cognitive avoidance, have been explored as an explanation for the inconsistent memory findings in PTSD. It has been hypothesized that individuals with PTSD will attempt to suppress or avoid recall of trauma-related memories. In fact, some studies have indicated a bias away from anxiety-provoking information, suggesting there is an implicit or strategic effort to avoid aversive thoughts and memories. However, evidence that individuals with PTSD engage in cognitive avoidance strategies or thought suppression during recall of trauma-related information is tentative.

3. Neuropsychological—Individuals with PTSD demonstrate a range of cognitive abnormalities, particularly in the areas of attention, concentration, learning, and memory (Vasterling and Brewin, 2005). Additionally, PTSD is associated with lower full-scale IQ; however, reliance on estimates of premorbid intellectual functioning makes causal inferences difficult. Individuals with PTSD show deficits in working memory and sustained attention, but not on tasks of executive set switching. Of note, cognitive deficits in these domains occur with threat-neutral, nontrauma-related stimuli.

Similarly, PTSD research with emotionally neutral list-learning tasks has revealed retrieval deficits for newly learned information. That deficits occurred for free recall of recently learned information, but not during recognition trials, suggests that such impairments are not due to encoding impairments, but rather indicate a problem with consolidation of new information into long-term storage. Neuropsychological domains that predominantly remain intact include visuospatial functioning, language, and psychomotor performance.

4. Psychobiological—Multiple neurobiological alterations or abnormalities have been associated with PTSD. The most extensively studied alterations have involved the HPA axis and the sympathetic nervous system. Alterations in the HPA axis in PTSD include (i) elevated resting cerebrospinal fluid levels of CRF; (ii) alterations in 24-hour urine excretion of cortisol, 24-hour plasma cortisol levels, lymphocyte glucocorticoid receptor number, cortisol response to dexamethasone, adrenocorticotropic hormone (ACTH) response to CRF, b-endorphin and ACTH response to metryapone; and (iii) adrenal androgen abnormalities.

Alterations in sympathetic nervous system reactivity include exaggerated increases in heart rate, blood pressure, norepinephrine, and epinephrine in response to traumatic reminders administered in the laboratory; elevated 24-hour plasma norepinephrine; elevated 24-hour urine excretion of norepinephrine and epinephrine, reduced platelet adrenergic receptor number; increased subjective, behavioral, physiological, and biochemical (increased plasma methoxyhydroxyphenylglycol) responses to intravenous yohimbine (an α2-adrenoreceptor antagonist); blunted response to clonidine; and altered yohimbine-induced cerebral blood flow. Alterations in sympathetic nervous system reactivity may contribute to symptoms of reexperiencing and hyperarousal. Neurocognitive and brain imaging studies comparing individuals with PTSD and individuals without psychiatric disorders have reported that subjects with PTSD show biased attention to negative and potentially dangerous information, reductions in hippocampal volume and function, exaggerated amygdala responses to stressful cues, and stress-induced reduction in PFC metabolism.

C. NEUROIMAGING

Positron Emission Tomography (PET) of individuals with PTSD has shown increased activity of the right hemisphere amygdaloid complex during rehearsals of the precipitant trauma. Other research has indicated bilateral hippocampal volume reduction in PTSD, hypothesized to be secondary to the deteriorating effects of glucocorticoids on pyramidal cells in the CA1 and CA2 regions. Moreover, functional magnetic resonance imaging (fMRI) studies of PTSD have shown a positive correlation between symptom severity and reduced hippocampal activity during tests of learning and memory (See Etiology).

D. COURSE OF ILLNESS

PTSD can occur from very early childhood to late in life. Onset of PTSD symptoms most commonly occurs within 3 months following trauma exposure, although symptom manifestation has been known to be delayed for years after the trauma. The course of PTSD is variable, with distinctions sometimes made among chronic, intermittent, residual, and reactivated types. Despite variation in course, epidemiologic studies suggest that the majority of symptoms do attenuate with time. For example, the NCS indicated that PTSD resolve in 6 years for approximately 60% of cases. Follow-up research on 2752 New York city residents 6 months after the terrorist attacks revealed a marked decline in the rates of PTSD from 7.5% to 0.6% (Galea, Vlahov, Resnick, Ahern, Susser, Gold, Bucuvalas and Kilpatrick, 2003). However, it may be that some symptoms are more likely to decrease than others over time. A study of Israeli military personnel over a 2-year period found that symptoms of reexperiencing and intrusive memories decreased, but avoidance and emotional numbing symptoms increased. Although recovery occurs within 3 months in approximately half of those diagnosed with PTSD, for those who do not recover within 3 months PTSD is often chronic and markedly detrimental to physical, social, occupational, and interpersonal functioning.

Moreover, PTSD can be complicated by recurrent exposure to trauma or trauma-associated cues that trigger reactivation of symptoms.

E. PSYCHOLOGICAL TESTING

A variety of rating scales have been developed for the assessment of PTSD, the nature of certain traumas, and specific responses to trauma. Many of these measures have been validated for use in diagnostic and treatment settings.

1. Self-report measures

i. Combat Experiences Scale (CES)—The CES is an assessment of exposure to stereotypical warfare experiences such as firing a weapon, being fired on (by enemy or friendly fire), witnessing injury and death, and going on special missions and patrols that involve such experiences. The CES, standardized in a Persian Gulf War sample, was developed as contemporary version of the Vietnam era Combat Exposure Scale.

ii. Posttraumatic stress checklist (PCL)—The PCL is a 17-item assessment of PTSD symptom severity developed by the National Center for PTSD. The military version of the PCL is keyed to stressful military experiences, and corresponds to 17 items directly adapted from the DSM-IV PTSD criteria. Psychometric data were obtained from veterans of the Vietnam War as well as the Persian Gulf War.

iii. Posttraumatic Diagnostic Scale (PDS)—The PDS is a 49-item measure of PTSD symptom severity and frequency according to the DSM-IV criteria. Symptom severity is anchored to an individual's 'most upsetting traumatic event.' The PDS is distinct from other PTSD assessments in that it also assesses features Criteria A (trauma) and Criteria F (functioning).

2. Clinician administered Scales

i. Clinician administered PTSD scale (CAPS)—The CAPS is a structured clinical interview measuring the frequency and intensity of the 17 DSM-IV symptoms of PTSD and 8 associated symptoms. The CAPS also contains five global rating questions regarding the impact of symptoms on social and occupational functioning, improvement since previous assessment, and overall validity and severity of reported symptoms.

ii. Structured Clinical Interview for DSM Disorders (SCID)—The SCID is a clinician-based structured interview designed to assess the majority of Axis I and Axis II disorders. The PTSD portion of the SCID is found in Module F—Anxiety Disorders. Several versions of the SCID are available for use dependent on the setting (e.g. research, clinical, and nonpatient populations). The SCID is also available in several different languages.

iii. Mississippi scale for PTSD—The scale consists of 39 self-report items derived from the Diagnostic and Statistical Manual of Mental Disorders III-R criteria for PTSD. The first version of the Mississippi Scale contained 35 items, based on the unrevised DSM-III criteria for PTSD. The four added items (items 36–39) assess reexperiencing, psychogenic amnesia, hypervigilance, and increased arousal symptomatology.

iv. Impact of events scale (IES)—The IES is a 22-item self-report measure of reaction to stressful events. The IES was created for the study of bereaved individuals, and was then adopted for studying the psychological impact of trauma.

v. Trauma symptom inventory (TSI)—The TSI is a 100-item evaluation of acute and chronic symptomatology from a wide variety of traumas, including rape, combat experiences, major accidents, natural disasters, as well as childhood abuse. The various scales of the TSI assess a wide range of psychological impacts. These include not only symptoms typically associated with PTSD or acute stress disorder (ASD), but also those intra- and interpersonal difficulties often associated with more chronic psychological trauma. The TSI does not generate DSM-IV diagnoses; instead, it is intended to evaluate the relative level of various forms of posttraumatic distress.

Differential Diagnosis (Including Comorbid Conditions)

1. Adjustment disorder (AD)—Symptoms that arise from an event that is stressful, but not of the life-threatening nature and intensity of Criterion A events for PTSD, fall under the rubric of AD.

2. Acute stress disorder (ASD)—ASD is differentiated from PTSD on two criteria. The first is that ASD symptoms must occur within 4 weeks of the traumatic event, whereas PTSD may have a delayed onset. The second distinction is that ASD symptoms must remit within 4 weeks of their initial presentation; symptoms that last beyond 4 weeks may indicate PTSD.

3. Obsessive-compulsive disorder (OCD)—OCD and PTSD have overlapping symptoms of intrusive thoughts. However, unwanted thoughts in PTSD are distinct in that they are circumscribed to trauma-related events and memories. Although intrusive thoughts in OCD are often distressing, they are not specific to a traumatic event.

4. Psychotic disorders—Delusions and hallucinations, characteristic of psychotic episodes, are distinct from those that occur during PTSD flashbacks. According to diagnostic criteria, persistent reexperiencing of the trauma may include hallucinations and illusions about specific life-threatening events. Such flashbacks may seem, at the time, real to the individual with PTSD. However, conclusion of the PTSD flashback is frequently followed by an acknowledgment that the event was not really reoccurring although it felt like it at the time. In contrast, by their nature, delusions and hallucinations are indistinguishable from reality for the person experiencing psychosis.

5. Personality disorders—An emerging literature on the comorbidity of Axis II disorders with anxiety spectrum disorders requires an understanding of personality disorders that frequently co-occur with PTSD. Both retrospective and longitudinal research have identified significant correlations between PTSD and some Axis II disorders. In particular, there is a close relationship between PTSD and borderline personality disorder (BPD). Longitudinal research documented that a diagnosis of PTSD, rather than a history of mere trauma exposure, was the strongest predictor of features of BPD. Among the Axis II features most closely associated with PTSD: Frantic efforts to avoid abandonment; rejection of help; inappropriate anger; general impulsiveness.

6. Malingering—PTSD diagnostic evaluations rely predominantly, if not exclusively, on self-report measures.

An accurate diagnosis of PTSD can be complicated by the fact that, by definition, it requires an identifiable (Criterion A1) event. As such, issues of secondary gain and remuneration for personal damages make PTSD especially open to legal scrutiny of potential malingering. Thus, ruling out feigned symptoms through collateral reporting sources and psychometrically sound measures is a fundamental component of differential diagnosis for PTSD.

7. Comorbidity—Epidemiological studies indicate that PTSD is rarely a sole diagnosis. In both the NCS and the NVVRS, 50–88% of individuals with a diagnosis of PTSD also had at least one concomitant disorder. In the NVVRS, 99% of those who received a diagnosis of PTSD had at least one other comorbid diagnosis in their lifetime. The most prevalent comorbid diagnoses with PTSD are major depressive disorder (MDD) and alcohol abuse. Although MDD tends to occur equally in males and females as a comorbid diagnosis, alcohol abuse is more frequently found among males with PTSD. Anxiety spectrum disorders such as specific phobias, social phobia, generalized anxiety disorder (GAD), and agoraphobia frequently co-occur with PTSD. Results from the NCS also revealed high comorbidity rates for anti-social personality disorder (43% male and 15% female). Other studies of Axis II disorders and PTSD have been limited by sample size, but reveal notable trends. Among these studies, high PTSD comorbidity rates have been found in BPD and paranoid personality disorder.

Treatment

Empirically validated interventions specifically for PTSD are in their nascency, and have evolved from treatments showing success in the larger set of anxiety spectrum disorders. Prominent among current treatment modalities are cognitive–behavioral therapy (CBT) and selective serotonin reuptake inhibitors (SSRIs). Additionally, treatment combining medication and therapy is often optimal.

A. Psychopharmacologic Interventions

1. Selective serotonin reuptake inhibitors (SSRIs)—Serotonin is implicated in PTSD, as well as a variety of other mood and anxiety disorders that are frequently comorbid with PTSD (e.g., depression, anxiety, impulsivity, substance abuse). Several selective serotonin reuptake inhibitors (SSRIs) have been studied in the treatment of PTSD (Friedman, 2002): sertraline, paroxetine, fluoxetine, and fluvoxamine. Randomized clinical trials (RCTs) have shown SSRIs to be efficacious in treating symptoms in all three PTSD clusters (i.e., reexperiencing, avoidance and numbing, hyperarousal), as well as in treating symptoms associated with PTSD

such as impulsivity, depression, suicidal thoughts, obsessive thinking, and substance abuse. To date, sertraline and paroxetine are the only two medications approved by the U.S. Food and Drug Administration for the treatment of PTSD.

2. Monoamine oxidase inhibitors (MAOIs)—MAOIs have been found especially effective in reducing PTSD symptoms of reexperiencing and sleep disturbance; however, avoidance and hyperarousal symptoms have been largely unaffected. Moreover, RCTs involving MAOIs have been limited because of potential side effects, particularly in patients with comorbid substance abuse disorders.

3. Tricyclic antidepressants (TCAs)—Imipramine, amitriptyline, and desipramine, among the most effective TCAs for depression and other anxiety disorders, have not received sufficient study in the treatment of PTSD. In the relatively few trials that have been conducted, TCAs have appeared to be most helpful for re-experiencing symptoms.

4. Antiadrenergic agents—Similar to MAOIs, antiadrenergic agents (e.g., clonidine, guanfacine, and propranolol) reduce reexperiencing and hyperarousal symptoms in PTSD. A pilot study (Pitman et al., 2002) suggests propanolol may alter consolidation of trauma memories, thereby inhibiting trauma conditioning immediately following acute exposure. However, replication of this finding is pending in several RCTs.

5. Benzodiazepines—As with other anxiety disorders, the long-term risks of prescribing benzodiazepines for PTSD may outweigh their immediate anxiolytic benefits. The short half-life of some benzodiazepines can facilitate medication tolerance and dependence, and also serve as a powerful reinforcement for avoidance and numbing coping mechanisms. Moreover, benzodiazepines often become a safety signal and a significant obstacle to exposure treatments, therein prohibiting extinction learning in CBT. Despite their widespread use for many anxiety disorders, benzodiazepines have not been found efficacious in treating PTSD.

B. Psychotherapeutic Interventions

1. Cognitive–behavioral therapy (CBT)—Although cognitive–behavioral approaches were developed specifically for PTSD, CBT has become the preferred treatment modality given growing treatment outcome data demonstrating its success with other anxiety disorders. CBT comprises several variations, all of which have a goal of fear extinction and improved coping through conditioning and modifying thoughts.

   i. Exposure therapy—Exposure therapy involves re-exposing the traumatized individual to sensory stimuli associated with the traumatic event. Exposure can take the form of mental imagery, pictures, role playing, virtual reality, or reinstatement of physiological arousal cues through interoceptive exercises (i.e., sweating, hyperventilation, increased heart and respiratory rates, etc.). The duration of exposure varies, and can be as short as a few seconds, or as long as 90 minutes (e.g., Prolonged Exposure [PE] therapy). In hierarchical reexposure, trauma cues are introduced systematically, starting with the least threatening stimuli, gradually increasing to exercises of greater intensity as desensitization is achieved. *Systematic desensitization (SD)* occurs over a period of several weeks, though some approaches immediately escalate to the most extreme stressors (e.g., flooding therapy). In either approach, the key to successful exposure therapy is controlling avoidance behaviors, and ensuring a positive outcome at the conclusion of each exposure trial. A positive outcome is imperative for each exposure to facilitate extinction of the original feared cue through learning new associations (i.e., cue = positive or tolerable outcome).

ii. Stress inoculation training (SIT)—The principle goal of SIT is to reduce fear reactions that foster operant avoidance and prohibit extinction learning. This goal is accomplished through a three-stage process involving psychoeducation (conditioning theory and psychobiology of fear), cognitive skills training (reframing and relaxation techniques), and application (scenarios, roleplaying, or in vivo exposures).

iii. Cognitive therapy (CT)—CT for PTSD focuses on thoughts and beliefs about the trauma and its associated cues. Targeted thoughts include "the likelihood the trauma will reoccur," "how the individual has responded to trauma," and "what certain reactions to trauma exposure might mean." Individuals are encouraged to identify assumptions and automatic beliefs about the traumatic event (e.g., "I can't handle this," "I'm going crazy," or "PTSD will ruin my life forever"). Individuals then learn to challenge those assumptions through alternative hypothesis generation and reality testing. Other cognitive skills involve learning how to change perspectives (i.e., cognitive reframing or restructuring), decatastrophizing, and relaxation techniques.

iv. Cognitive processing therapy (CPT)—CPT was developed to address the broader range of emotions other than fear that frequently accompany PTSD in victims of rape and crime: anger, guilt, sadness, and shame (Resick and Schnike, 1992). CPT focuses on memories of the traumatic event, exploring associated intense emotions. Trauma memories are explored through use of diaries and narrative scripts about their trauma, and individuals are encouraged to articulate personal meaning of the traumatic event. Memories of the trauma are reconstructed in narrative format, incorporating as much

sensory stimuli into the description as possible. These narratives are then to be read on a daily basis for several weeks. Therapy sessions involve discussion of the trauma narrative, and examination of irrational thoughts and unpleasant emotions evoked by remembering. Support for CPT continues to grow, due in part to recent comparison studies that highlight larger treatment effect sizes compared to medication. For example, following a 12-session course of CPT in Vietnam combat veterans, 40% of the intention to treat sample no longer met diagnostic criteria for PTSD, a result that was independent of service-connected disability status (Monson et al., 2007).

2. Eye-movement desensitization and reprocessing (EMDR)—EMDR is a controversial technique, not regarding its efficacy, but rather its theoretical underpinnings. EMDR was unintentionally discovered when its originator (Shapiro, 1995) noticed that focusing visual attention on wave movements of tree leaves in the wind provided relief from unpleasant rumination. From this observation, EMDR has evolved as a repetitive lateral eye-movement exercise that facilitates cognitive processing of trauma-related thoughts. EMDR is conducted by the therapist waving the tip of the index finger rapidly back-and-forth in front of the patient's eyes. The finger tip is held 30–35 cm from the patient's face at a rate of 2 waves per second, for a total of 24 waves. Following each eye-movement trial, the patient is instructed first to attempt to block out the memory, take a relaxing breath, and then return to the memory. Each sequence of EMDR is followed by subjective appraisals of distress precipitated by the memory; the sequence is repeated until subject distress decreases to zero.

Complications/Adverse Outcomes of Treatment

The primary complication to psychotherapy for PTSD, especially for cognitive–behavioral-based approaches, is avoidance. Behavioral avoidance can take the form of missed therapy appointments, incomplete treatment homework, or failure to engage trauma cues during in-vivo exposures. Cognitive avoidance can also complicate treatment if it is persistent. Sometimes individuals who appear to engage exposure exercises behaviorally, may be covertly dissociating from the experience in an effort to attenuate arousal and full exposure to the trauma cue. Avoidance may also take the form of self-medication through the use of alcohol and substance abuse. A complication that has received limited attention is the potential impediment that benzodiazepines present to exposure therapies. The short half-life (i.e., fast-acting) of some benzodiazepines is a powerful reinforcement to individuals with PTSD who are averse to autonomic arousal. A heavy reliance on benzodiazepines or alcohol prevents new learning (i.e., extinction conditioning) that is pivotal for extinguishing maladaptive associations with trauma cues. Additional impediments to treatment include sleep irregularities that make new learning more difficult, as well as psychosocial dysfunction that often accompanies chronic, untreated PTSD.

Prognosis

The fact that most individuals with PTSD get better over time does not lessen its psychosocial and functional impact, as subclinical symptom levels can have profound negative consequences. However, the evolution of several promising therapies for PTSD (see Treatment) suggests that even the most difficult cases are treatable. As such, prognosis is best for those who have strong support networks, fewer comorbid diagnoses, and fully engage empirically validated treatments. In contrast, individuals with complex PTSD resulting from multiple childhood traumas, poor interpersonal support networks, Axis II diagnoses, comorbid substance abuse, and diminished cognitive resources are less likely to recover.

American Psychiatric Association: *Diagnostic and Statistical Manual of Mental Disorders*, 4th edn, Text Revision. Washington, DC: American Psychiatric Association, 2000.

American Psychiatric Association: *Diagnostic and Statistical Manual of Mental Disorders*, 4th edn. Washington, DC: American Psychiatric Association, 1994.

Baker DG, Ekhator NN, Kasckow JW, et al.: Higher levels of basal serial CSF cortisol in combat veterans with posttraumatic stress disorder. *Am J Psychiatry* 2005;162:992–994.

Brewin CR, Andrews B, Valentine JD: Meta-analysis of risk factors for posttraumatic stress disorder in trauma exposed adults. *J Consult Clin Psychol* 2000;68:748–766.

Charney DS: Psychobiological mechanisms of resilience and vulnerability: Implications for successful adaptation to extreme stress. *Am J Psychiatry* 2004;161:195–216.

Dohrenwend BP, Turner JB, Turse NA, et al.: The psychological risks of Vietnam for US veterans: A revisit with new data and methods. *Science* 2006;313:979–982.

Eysenck HJ: *The Biological Basis of Personality*. Springfield, IL: Thomas, 1967.

Foa EB, Kozack MJ: Emotional processing of fear: Exposure to corrective information. *Psychol Bull* 1986;99:20–35.

Friedman MJ: Future pharmacotherapy for post-traumatic stress disorder: Prevention and treatment. *Psychiatr Clin North Am* 2002;25:427–441.

Galea S, Ahern J, Resnick H, et al.: Psychological sequelae of the September 11 terrorist attacks in New York City. *N Engl J Med* 2002;346:982–987.

Galea S, Vlahov D, Resnick H, et al.: Trends of probably post-traumatic stress disorder in New York City after the September 11 terrorist attacks. *Am J Epidemiol* 2003;158: 514–524.

Gurvits TV, Metzger LJ, Lasko NB, et al.: Subtle neurologic compromise as a vulnerability factor for combat-related posttraumatic stress disorder: Results of a twin study. *Arch Gen Psychiatry* 2006;63:571–576.

Hoge CW, Castro CA, Messer SC, et al.: Combat duty in Iraq and Afghanistan, mental health problems, and barriers to care. *N Engl J Med* 2004;351:13–22.

Hidalgo RB, Davidson JRT: Posttraumatic stress disorder: Epidemiology and health-related considerations. *J Clin Psychiatry* 2000;61(suppl 7):5–13.

Kaufman J, Yang BZ, Douglas-Palumberi H, et al.: Social supports and serotonin transporter gene moderate depression in maltreated children. *PNAS* 2004;101(49):17316–17321.

Kim JJ, Fanselow MS: Modality specific retrograde amnesia of fear. *Science* 1992;256:675–677.

Kulka RA, Schlenger WE, Fairbank JA, et al.: *Trauma and the Vietnam War Generation: Report of Findings from the National Vietnam Veterans Readjustmetn Study*. New York, NY: Brunner/Mazel, 1990.

Monson CM, Schnurr PP, Resick PA, Friedman MJ, Young-Xu Y, Stevens SP: Cognitive processing therapy for veterans with military-related posttraumatic stress disorder. *J Consult Clin Psychol* 2007;74(5):898–907.

Morgan CA, Aikins DE, Steffian G, et al.: Relation between cardiac vagal tone and performance in male military personnel exposed to high stress: Three prospective studies. *Psychophysiology* 2007;44;120–127.

Mowrer OH: On the dual nature of learning: A re-interpretation of "conditioning" and "problem-solving." *Harv Educ Rev* 1947;17:102–148.

North CE, Pfefferbaum B, Tivis L, Kawasaki A, Chandrashekar R, Spitznagel E: The course of posttraumatic stress disorder in a follow-up study of survivors of the Oklahoma City bombing. *Ann Clin Psychiatry* 2004;16:209–215.

Orr SP, Metzger LJ, Pitman RK: Psychophysiology of post-traumatic stress disorder. *Psychiatr Clin N Am* 2002;25:271–293.

Phillips RG, LeDoux JE: Differential contribution of amygdala and hippocampus cued to contextual fear conditioning. *Behav Neurosci* 1992;106:274–285.

Resnick HS, Kilpatrick DF, Peterson EL, et al.: Prevalence of civilian trauma and posttraumatic stress disorder in a representational national sample of women. *J Consult Clin Psychol* 1993;61:984–991.

Roy-Byrne P, Arguelles L, Vitek ME, et al.: Persistance and change of PTSD symptatology: A longitudinal co-twin analysis of the Vietnam Era Twin Registry. *Soc Psychiatry Psychiatr Epidemiol* 2004;39:681–685.

Seedat S, Stein MB, Kennedy CM, Hauger RL: Plasma cortisol and neuropeptide Y in female victims of intimate partner violence. *Psychoneuroendocrinology* 2003;28;796–808.

Southwick, SM, Vythilingam M, Charney DS: The psychobiology of depression and resilie to stress: Implications for prevention and treatment. *Annu Rev Clin Psychol* 2005;1:255–291.

True WR, Rice J, Eisen SA, et al.: A twin study of genetic and environmental contributions to liability for posttraumatic stress symptoms. *Arch Gen Psychiatry* 1993;50(4):257–265.

Vasterling JJ, Brewin CR: *Neuropsychology of PTSD: Biological, Cognitive, and Clinical Perspectives*. New York, NY: Guilford, 2005.

■ ACUTE STRESS DISORDER

 ESSENTIALS OF DIAGNOSIS

DSM-IV-TR Diagnostic Criteria
Acute Stress Disorder

A. The person has been exposed to a traumatic event in which both of the following were present:

 (1) The person experienced, witnessed, or was confronted with an event or events that involved actual or threatened death or serious injury, or a threat to the physical integrity of self or others

 (2) The person's response involved fear, helplessness, or horror

B. Either while experiencing or after experiencing the distressing event, the individual has three (or more) of the following dissociative symptoms:

 (1) A subjective sense of numbing, detachment, or absence of emotional responsiveness

 (2) A reduction in awareness of his or her surroundings (e.g., "being in a daze")

 (3) Derealization

 (4) Depersonalization

 (5) Dissociative amnesia (i.e. inability to recall an important aspect of the trauma

C. The traumatic event is persistently re-experienced in at least one of the following ways: Recurrent images, thoughts, dreams, illusions, flashback episodes, or a sense of reliving the experience; or distress on exposure to reminders of the traumatic event.

D. Marked avoidance of stimuli that arouse recollections of the trauma.

E. Marked symptoms of anxiety or increased arousal (e.g., difficulty sleeping, irritability, poor concentration, hypervigilance, exaggerated startle response, motor restlessness).

F. The disturbance causes clinically significant distress or impairment in social, occupational, or important areas of functioning.

G. The disturbance lasts for a minimum of 2 days and a maximum of 4 weeks and occurs within 4 weeks of the traumatic event.

H. The disturbance is not due to the direct physiological effects of a substance or a general medical condition, is not merely an exacerbation of a preexisting Axis I or Axis II disorder.

(Adapted, with permission, from *Diagnostic and Statistical Manual of Mental Disorders*, 4th edn. Text Revision. Washington DC: American Psychiatric Association, 2000.)

General Considerations

ASD was first introduced in DSM-IV. The validity of ASD as a disorder distinct form PTSD has been questioned from its inception, and has generated much debate. ASD evolved from an effort to account for symptoms exhibited in the early period following trauma exposure. As such, the primary distinction between ASD and PTSD is the duration of symptoms, with ASD being limited to between 2 days and 4 weeks. Additionally, because ASD is circumscribed to 4 weeks following the traumatic event, diagnostic criteria emphasize dissociative symptoms during, or shortly after, exposure. In addition to at least one symptom from each of the three (reexperiencing, avoidance, and arousal) symptom categories required for a diagnosis of PTSD, ASD requires at least three distinct dissociative symptoms: subjective sense of numbing, detachment, or absence of emotional responsiveness; a reduction in awareness of surroundings; derealization; depersonalization; dissociative amnesia. The presence of dissociative symptoms during or shortly after trauma (i.e., peritraumatic dissociation) has also been a source of contention regarding the validity of ASD, namely the assertion that ASD may pathologize adaptive responses to trauma. While the majority of individuals who meet criteria for ASD do go on to develop PTSD, some individuals with PTSD do not initially meet criteria for ASD (i.e., delayed onset PTSD).

Clinical Findings

In contrast to a vast literature on PTSD, empirical studies of ASD are few. The dearth of research on ASD may be due to its relatively recent introduction into the DSM-IV and because its inclusion was primarily based on theoretical, rather than an empirical considerations. To date, there are three psychometrically valid metrics for assessing ASD: (1) The Stanford Acute Stress Reaction Questionnaire (SASRQ); (2) The Acute Stress Disorder Interview (ASDI); and (3) The Acute Stress Disorder Scale (ASDS).

 ASD is a strong predictor of PTSD. Prospective studies have found that between 72% and 83% of individuals with ASD have gone on to develop PTSD at 6-months posttrauma and that between 63% and 80% of those with ASD meet criteria for PTSD 2 years following trauma.

Differential Diagnosis

Differential diagnosis can be complicated, as a number of seemingly comorbid disorders are mutually exclusive to a diagnosis of ASD. Further complicating the diagnosis of ASD is our increased understanding of the normal range of reactions to human trauma, many of which are also symptoms of ASD and PTSD. Therefore, as with many other disorders, diagnosis is often predicated on duration of the symptoms and functional impairment. In the case of ASD, symptoms must be present for at least 2 days following trauma exposure, and produce significant occupational, social, or functional impairment. If symptoms persist for longer than 30 days, then a diagnosis of PTSD is given.

ASD is also differentiated from disorders that associated with exposure to trauma, namely substance induced disorder and disorder due to a general medical condition such as traumatic brain injury (TBI) suffered from motor vehicle accidents (MVAs) or combat trauma. Individuals who do not meet full criteria for ASD, but have impairment of functioning following a trauma or stressor should be given a diagnosis of adjustment disorder instead.

Treatment and Complications/Adverse Outcomes of Treatment

See section in PTSD.

Prognosis

Extant research shows that the vast majority of individuals who meet criteria for ASD following trauma, go on to develop PTSD. Of note however, is that the majority of PTSD cases resolve over time. In this respect, the prognosis for individuals with ASD is parallel to that of PTSD.

Obsessive–Compulsive Disorder

William A. Hewlett, PhD, MD

 ## ESSENTIALS OF DIAGNOSIS

DSM-IV-TR Diagnostic Criteria

A. Either obsessions or compulsions:

Obsessions as defined by (1), (2), (3), and (4):

(1) recurrent and persistent thoughts, impulses, or images that are experienced, at some time during the disturbance, as intrusive and inappropriate and that cause marked anxiety or distress

(2) the thoughts, impulses, or images are not simply excessive worries about real-life problems

(3) the person attempts to ignore or suppress such thoughts, impulses, or images or neutralize them with some other thought or action

(4) the person recognizes that the thoughts, impulses, or images are a product of his or her own mind (not imposed from without as in thought insertion)

Compulsions as defined by (1) and (2):

(1) repetitive behaviors (e.g., hand washing, ordering, checking) or mental acts (e.g., praying, counting, repeating works silently) that the person feels driven to perform in response to an obsession, or according to rules that must be applied rigidly

(2) the behavior or mental acts are aimed at preventing or reducing distress or preventing some dreaded event or situation; however, these behaviors or mental acts either are not connected in a realistic way with what they are designed to neutralize or prevent or are clearly excessive

B. At some point during the course of the disorder, the person has recognized that the obsessions or compulsions are excessive or unreasonable.

Note: This does not apply to children.

C. The obsessions or compulsions cause marked distress, are time consuming (takes more than 1 hour/day) or significantly interfere with the person's normal routine, occupation (or academic functioning), or usual social activities or relationships.

D. If another Axis I disorder is present, the content of the obsessions or compulsions is not restricted to it.

E. The disturbance is not due to the direct physiological effects of a substance (e.g., a drug of abuse, a medication) or a general medical condition.

Specify *if*:

With poor insight: *if, for most of the time during the current episode, the person does not recognize that the obsessions and compulsions are excessive or unreasonable.*

(Reprinted, with permission, from *Diagnostic and Statistical Manual of Mental Disorders*, 4th edn. Copyright. 1994. Washington DC: American Psychiatric Association, 2000.)

General Considerations

Obsessions are unwanted aversive cognitive experiences usually associated with feelings of dread, loathing, or a disturbing sense that something is not right. The individual recognizes (at some point in time) that these concerns are inappropriate in relation to reality and will generally attempt to ignore or suppress them. Compulsions are overt behaviors or covert mental acts performed to reduce the intensity of the aversive obsessions. They may occur as behaviors that are governed by rigid, but often irrelevant, internal specifications. They are inappropriate in nature or intensity in relation to the external circumstances that provoked them.

A. EPIDEMIOLOGY

1. Population frequencies—Lifetime prevalence rates of obsessive–compulsive disorder (OCD) in the United States range between 2% and 3%, but may be slightly lower in certain ethnic subgroups, including African Americans and possibly Hispanics. Lifetime prevalence rates are similar (approximately 2%) in Europe, Africa, Canada, and the Middle East, but appear to be lower (0.5–0.9%) in certain Asian countries (i.e., India and Taiwan). Lower prevalence rates in selected U.S. and other national populations could be related to cultural factors resulting in underreporting of symptoms, or be related to such biological factors as increased resistance to basal ganglia disease. Although OCD is thought to be a lifetime illness, lifetime prevalence rates in young adults are over twice those seen in the elderly. It is unclear whether this observation represents a reporting bias, a waning of symptoms with advancing age, a shorter life expectancy in patients with OCD, or a changing environmental factor relating to the etiology of the illness.

OCD is usually first seen in childhood or early adulthood: 65% of patients have their onset prior to age 25 years, 15% after the age of 35 years, and 30% in childhood or early adolescence. In the latter population, there is a 2:1 preponderance of males; in contrast, OCD in the adult population is slightly more predominant in women. The frequency of OCD in psychiatric practice may be significantly lower than in the general population. Indeed, the incidence of OCD was previously thought to be as low as 0.05% based on psychiatric samples. Low frequency estimates may be related to the intense shame and secrecy associated with this illness and the patients' reluctance to divulge their symptomatology.

The frequency of specific obsessions and compulsions is fairly constant across populations. Contamination fears are present in approximately 50% of OCD patients, unwarranted fears that something is wrong (called pathologic doubt) in 40%, and other obsessions, including needs for symmetry, fears of harm to self or others, and unwanted sexual concerns, in 25–30%. Checking and decontamination rituals are the predominant rituals in OCD (50–60%). Other rituals, such as arranging, counting, repeating, and repetitive superstitious acts, occur less frequently (30–35%). Most patients with OCD (60%) have multiple obsessions or compulsions.

2. Population subtypes—The only subtype recognized in the *Diagnostic and Statistical Manual of Mental Disorders,* fourth edition, Text Revision (DSM-IV-TR) is OCD with poor insight. Adults given this diagnosis were previously aware that they were symptomatic but became convinced of the validity of their fears and the necessity of their compulsions as their illness progressed. Children with this diagnosis have not yet developed insight regarding their symptoms.

It has not proved helpful to classify OCD according to a symptom dyad (e.g., contamination-washing) as a means of predicting course of the illness, therapeutic outcome, or other relevant measures. Indeed, most individuals have multiple obsessions and compulsions, and symptom clusters can change over time (e.g., a compulsive hand-washer will lose fear of contamination and develop fears of harming others). It has been more useful to classify subtypes of patients according to their underlying experiences. Patients with OCD can be divided into two subgroups based on experiences of (1) pathologic doubt (e.g., dread and uncertainty) or (2) incompletion, or "not-just-right" perceptions. Individuals within these two subgroups appear to share common symptom clusters, co-morbidities, and treatment prognoses.

OCD can also be classified on the basis of the presence or absence of tics. Patients with tics may respond to a different treatment regimen than do those who do not have tics. Because of the relationship between Tourette syndrome and OCD, these patients may also have other symptoms found in the families of Tourette syndrome patients, such as urges to carry out maladaptive acts and problems with impulse control.

Finally, a subset of OCD patients with schizotypal personality disorder has been characterized. These patients are sometimes mistakenly diagnosed as having schizophrenia (though they lack true category A symptoms), are more likely to have poor insight and poor social functioning, may require a different treatment regimen, and are often refractory to treatment.

B. ETIOLOGY

Theories of etiology have invoked psychoanalytic (i.e., relating to early childhood experiences), cognitive, posttraumatic, epileptic, traumatic (i.e., brain injury), genetic, and postinfectious processes. The psychoanalytic view has fallen into disfavor in recent years. Likewise, it is no longer thought that symptoms of OCD are a consequence of psychic trauma. In cases where psychic trauma is associated with the onset of symptoms, the experience is thought to potentiate a propensity for developing OCD symptoms in susceptible individuals and does not create the pathology itself.

OCD can result from pathologic processes affecting cerebral functioning. For example, severe head trauma and epilepsy have been associated with obsessive–compulsive symptoms. Disorders affecting the functioning of the basal ganglia have also been associated with OCD, and a postinfectious autoimmune-related form of OCD has been described in children. OCD symptoms in these children frequently occur after an infection with type A β-hemolytic *Streptococcus* bacteria, with or without classical symptoms of rheumatic fever. In the acute phase of this illness, antibodies directed at streptococcal M-protein react with specific brain proteins located primarily in the basal ganglia and may induce Sydenham chorea (also called St. Vitus' dance). Obsessions, compulsions, or vocal and motor tics indistinguishable from those seen in Tourette syndrome can be prominent when the chorea is present, although the child may not speak of them if not directly questioned. Sydenham chorea is associated with swelling of the head of the caudate nucleus on magnetic resonance imaging (MRI).

Poststreptococcal antineuronal antibodies have also been detected in cases of abrupt-onset OCD that do not exhibit the symptoms of Sydenham chorea nor any other manifestation of rheumatic fever. OCD symptoms appear in conjunction with increasing antibody titers and remit as titers fall. Autoimmune-related OCD has been described only in children. Adults with OCD, however, may have reduced volume in the caudate region of the basal ganglia. It is conceivable that neuropathologic processes, such as repeated autoimmune inflammation, could irreversibly damage central nervous system (CNS) tissue and result in a chronic form of OCD in adults. It is also possible that certain cases of familial OCD or Tourette syndrome could be related to heritable proteins involved in the autoimmune process.

C. Genetics

OCD occurs with greater frequency in family members of OCD patients (10%), as compared to the general population. When combined with subclinical obsessions and compulsions, symptom prevalence rates approach 20% in first-degree relatives. Interestingly, familial rates of OCD are significantly higher in patients with childhood OCD than in patients with adult OCD. This may be related to a heritable tic-related form of OCD with onset in childhood. Although there have been no systematic twin studies of sufficient size to draw conclusions, 65–85% of monozygotic twin pairs with one twin having OCD are concordant for OCD symptoms, whereas only 15–45% of dizygotic twin pairs are so concordant.

OCD has been linked to the proposed autosomal dominant Tourette syndrome *(TS)* gene. This gene is associated with chronic motor tics, vocal tics, and OCD. Under this genetic model, males carrying the *TS* gene have a 90–95% probability of developing at least one of these behaviors. Females carrying the *TS* gene have a lower expression rate (approximately 60%), but a higher proportion will develop OCD. The exact locus of the *TS* gene has not been identified. Some familial forms of OCD with partial penetrance do not appear to be related to the *TS* gene. The genetic determinant of this form has not been identified.

Geller DA, Biederman J, Jones J, Shapiro S, Schwartz S, Park KS: Obsessive–compulsive disorder in children and adolescents: A review. *Harv Rev Psychiatry* 1998;5:260.

Jenike MA, Golding JM, Sorenson SB, Burnam MA: *Obsessive Compulsive Disorders: Theory and Management,* 2nd edn. Mosby Year-Book, 1990.

Karno M, et al.: The epidemiology of obsessive–compulsive disorder in five US communities. *Arch Gen Psychiatry* 1988;45:1094.

Pauls DL: The genetics of obsessive compulsive disorder and Gilles de la Tourette's syndrome. *Psychiatr Clin North Am* 1992;15:759.

Rasmussen SA, Eisen JL: The epidemiology and differential diagnosis of obsessive compulsive disorder. *J Clin Psychiatry* 1994;55(10 Suppl):5.

Swedo SE, Leonard HL, Rapoport JL: Childhood-onset obsessive compulsive disorder. *Psychiatr Clin North Am* 1992;15:767.

Swedo SE, Leonard HL, Garvey M, et al.: Pediatric autoimmune neuropsychiatric disorders associated with streptococcal infections: Clinical description of the first 50 cases. *Am J Psychiatry* 1998;155:264.

Clinical Findings

A. Signs & Symptoms

The clinical hallmarks of obsessions are aversive experiences of dread and uncertainty, or the disturbing sense that something is not right or is incomplete. Obsessive thoughts are the particular ideas associated with obsessive experiences. They are often bizarre or inadequate as explanations for these experiences. Obsessions can take the form of aversive mental images, dread and disgust related to perceived defilement, feelings that something very bad has either happened or is about to happen, or an urgent sense that something that needs to be done has not yet been completed. A sense of immediacy and urgency is almost always associated with the aversive experiences. Obsessions can be present without compulsions, most frequently when the individual recognizes that no action can alleviate the aversive experience. Under such circumstances the individual may only seek reassurance that his or her fears are unfounded or unrealistic.

Compulsions take the form of willed responses directed at reducing the aversive circumstances associated with the obsessive thoughts. They are generally carried out in concordance with the ideation surrounding the obsessions. They can take the form of overt behaviors or silent mental acts such as checking, praying, counting, or some other mental ritual. Mental compulsions differ from obsessive experiences in that they are willed mental acts performed for a purpose, rather than sensory or ideational experiences. Compulsions are usually carried out in a repetitive or stereotyped fashion, although they can be situation specific, dependent on the content of the obsessive thought. Compulsions can also be carried out in the absence of specific obsessive thoughts. In such cases they are usually responses to an urgent sense that something is not right or is incomplete.

Most adults with OCD recognize that their fears and behaviors are unrealistic or excessive. Insight in OCD can vary, however, from states of full awareness that the symptoms are absurd, with a few lingering doubts, through equivocal acknowledgment, to a delusional state in which the individual is convinced of the validity of his or her fear and the necessity of the consequent behavior. Some adults lose insight only during exacerbations of their illness. Others, often with schizotypal personalities, may have true insight only early in the illness, or transiently when their illness is quiescent. The term "overvalued idea" was used in the past to denote an obsessive thought firmly held to be valid. This term is no longer accepted as a construct, because it cannot be practically differentiated from delusional ideation. Patients who have lost insight in regard to their symptoms are considered to belong to a diagnostic subclass of OCD.

Avoidance may be a prominent secondary symptom in OCD. The OCD patient will avoid circumstances that trigger particularly aversive obsessions or lead to time-consuming compulsions. Avoidance, itself, is not a compulsion; but when the illness is severe it can be a prominent clinical feature. In the course of treatment, as avoidance is reduced, a temporary, paradoxical increase in compulsions can occur because of increased exposure to circumstances that trigger them.

B. Associated Experiences

OCD stands out among psychiatric disorders in the degree to which the patient's thoughts and concerns diverge from their awareness of reality. Most OCD patients recognize the absurd nature of their behavior and are acutely aware of demeaning perceptions that others might have if they knew the degree to which they were affected by their illness. They have a strong fear that they will be considered crazy. Ashamed and embarrassed, they are reluctant to disclose their symptoms to anyone who might not understand their illness. As a result, individuals with OCD tend to be highly secretive.

Early in the illness, they will try to hide their symptoms from those who know them. They may delay seeking treatment until their symptoms are noticed by those around them. Many patients will not reveal their illness to their primary physicians. Therapists sometimes will care for a patient for several years before discovering that the patient has OCD. This is particularly true for patients who experience horrific sexual, blasphemous, or violent thoughts and images. These individuals fear that the therapist will believe that they want these scenarios to occur and that they might act inappropriately in concordance with their obsessive thoughts. In short, they fear that the physician will confirm their own fears and self-condemnation. They may leave a therapeutic relationship if they sense that the therapist does not understand the illness.

The combination of secrecy, avoidance of contact with others, and the time-consuming nature of the compulsions may lead to social isolation and secondary depression. Most patients with OCD also experience a heightened sense of internal tension and distress. When their OCD is worse they will describe feelings of desperation and despair, as they are unable to relieve their feelings of dread and uncertainty. It is these feelings that may lead the patient to seek initial treatment.

Patients with OCD may also have an unreasonable fear of losing control. These feelings can be exacerbated by a perceived inability to control their compulsive behavior. The individual with OCD fears that he or she will lose control of natural inhibitions and act in a socially or personally maladaptive manner. Patients with obsessive–compulsive personality disorder (OCPD) have different issues with control; they want control for the positive sense of mastery that it engenders. Patients with OCD often shun true control and responsibility because of their unrealistic fears that they might misuse or abuse it.

C. Pathologic Relationships

Patients with OCD frequently have a parent or life partner who is involved in the illness. There are two pathologic forms of such involvement. The first involves facilitation. By pleading, nagging, demanding, or threatening, the patient will induce others to accommodate to his or her fears and concerns. The facilitator may perform rituals for the patient or permit the patient to control the environment or common time. Facilitation allows the illness to flourish without normal constraints.

The second pathologic interaction is the antagonistic–defensive dyad. Such relationships are adversarial. The antagonistic partner acts in a caustic, demeaning manner and does not understand or accept the nature of the illness. The OCD symptoms are viewed as willful antagonism. The patient reacts in a hostile, defensive manner that aggravates the partner. The hostility, instability, loss of self-esteem, and stress in these interactions exacerbate the symptoms of OCD and lead to further antagonism.

In both forms of pathologic relationship, the patient may use his or her symptoms to control the other person. This can be an unconscious or pseudoconscious process. Facilitating interactions can lead to circumstances in which the patient uses his or her illness to obtain material and emotional benefits. In antagonistic–defensive interactions, symptoms may serve to irritate and frustrate the hostile partner—one of the few mechanisms available to the patient to "get back at" that partner. In both pathologic interactive modes, the secondary gains associated with the symptoms can further ingrain the disorder.

D. Psychological Testing & Instruments for Diagnosis & Measurement

There is no good diagnostic instrument for OCD. The Structured Interview for DSM-IV-TR Diagnosis has only rudimentary questions regarding OCD symptoms, and good clinical judgment is required if the proper diagnosis is to be made. Psychological testing has little value in the diagnosis of OCD or in predicting treatment outcome or course of the illness.

Valid, reliable, and sensitive scales for the measurement of OCD symptom severity have been available only since the late 1980s. The best is the Yale–Brown Obsessive Compulsive Scale (YBOCS). This semistructured interview consists of three parts: a symptom checklist, a symptom hierarchy list, and the YBOCS. The rating scale evaluates severity of obsessions and compulsions on an ordinal scale from 0 to 4 (on the basis of time spent, interference, distress, resistance, and degree of control). The maximum score for this scale is 40. Patients with scores above 31 are considered to have extreme symptoms. Scores of 24–31 indicate severe symptoms, and scores of 16–23 indicate moderate symptoms. Patients with scores below 16 are considered to have mild to subclinical symptoms that often do not require treatment. The average YBOCS score for individuals with untreated OCD who are entering an OCD clinic is typically 23–25. The YBOCS also rates certain ancillary symptoms for informational purposes and provides for global assessments of severity and improvement.

Other scales that rate severity of symptoms include the Comprehensive Psychopathological Rating Scale and the obsessive–compulsive subsection of the Hopkins Symptoms Checklist-90 (SCL-90). Neither of these is sensitive to changes in symptom intensity. Both scales include measures that are highly influenced by other factors such as mood. The Clinical Global Scale and the National Institute of Mental Health global rating scale belong to another class of scales that involve clinical judgments of either global or OCD-specific illness severity or changes in severity. They are based on categories such as mild, moderate, much improved, and so on. An older group of scales (e.g., Leyton Obsessional Inventory or the Maudsley Obsessive and Compulsive Inventory) consist of lists of obsessions and compulsions, without true measures of severity.

E. Laboratory Findings & Imaging

Studies using MRI or computerized tomography (CT) have reported decreased gray matter volume either unilaterally or bilaterally in the head of the caudate nucleus. Positron emission tomography (PET) studies have found increased resting metabolic activity in the orbitomedial prefrontal cortex, especially in the right hemisphere. Increased metabolic activity has also been found in the basal ganglia, particularly in the anterior caudate nucleus. Effective treatment of OCD by either pharmacologic or behavioral means can be associated with regionally specific decreases in resting metabolic activity. This has led to the suggestion that neural circuits between the orbitomedial prefrontal cortex and the basal ganglia are hyperactive in OCD, and that treatments that modulate this activ-

ity may be effective in OCD. Imaging procedures are primarily of research interest, however, and have little diagnostic or therapeutic value at this time.

Other studies have found biochemical, neuroendocrine, and physiologic alterations associated with the neurotransmitter serotonin. Again, no clinically useful tests have resulted from this work. Finally, neurologic soft signs, eye-tracking results, and electroencephalogram (EEG) measurements have sometimes been found to be abnormal in patients with OCD. These observations have little clinical value, although the severity of soft signs may correlate with the severity of OCD.

Goodman WK, et al.: The Yale-Brown Obsessive Compulsive Scale. I. Development, use, and reliability. *Arch Gen Psychiatry* 1989;46:1006.

Hollander E, et al. (eds): *Current Insights in Obsessive Compulsive Disorder.* John Wiley & Sons, 1994.

Pato MT, Eisen JL, Pato CN:Rating scales for obsessive compulsive disorder, pp. 77–92. In

Schwartz JM, Stoessel PW, Baxter LR, Martin KM, Phelps DE: Systematic changes in cerebral glucose metabolic rate after successful behavior modification treatment of obsessive–compulsive disorder. *Arch Gen Psychiatry* 1996;53:109.

Stein DJ, et al.: The neuropsychiatry of OCD. In: Hollander EH, Stein D (eds). *Obsessive Compulsive Disorders.* Marcel Dekker, 1996.

Differential Diagnosis of Obsessions & Compulsions

The differential diagnosis of OCD is one of the most complex in psychiatry because of confusion over the meanings of the terms "obsessions" and "compulsions," a confusion made worse by the fact that OCPD is associated with a cognitive style and behavior unrelated to OCD. It is important to recognize cognitive and behavioral phenomena that are often confused with true obsessions and compulsions. Table 21–1 summarizes these phenomena, and they are described in more detail in the next several sections.

A. Cognitive Differentiations

Numerous intrusive or persistent mental experiences have no relation to OCD. The experiences listed in this section are often confused with obsessions but can be distinguished on the basis of careful examination.

1. Anxious ruminations & excessive worries—Anxious ruminations and excessive worries are persistent intrusive concerns about adverse circumstances in the future. They are characterized by preparative cognitive processing designed to deal with those circumstances. They differ from obsessions in that they are realistic in their nature, although they may be excessive. Worries can be fleeting or semiconscious mental experiences associated with feelings of anxiety, whereas anxious

Table 21–1. Differential Symptomatology

Cognitive Differentiations	Behavioral Differentiations
Anxious ruminations and excessive worries	Impulsions
Pathologic guilt	Meticulousness or perfectionism
Depressive ruminations	Pathologic atonement
Aggressive ruminations	Repetitive displacement behavior
Fantasies	Perseverative behavior
Paranoid fears	Stereotypic behavior
Flashbacks	Self-injurious behavior
Pathologic attraction	Pathologic overinvolvement
Rigid thinking	Pathologic persistence
Pathologic indecision	Hoarding
Realistic fears or concerns	Complex tics

ruminations are drawn out in time as the mind reviews potential adverse scenarios. They are not associated with rituals. In contrast to anxious ruminations, obsessions are immediate, aversive sensory experiences, often accompanied by incongruous dreadful mental images and specific unrealistic fears that those circumstances might occur or might have already occurred. While an individual may take preparatory actions in association with anxious ruminations, the experience lacks the dreadful immediacy of obsessive fears and the sense of urgency that drives the compulsive behaviors. Obsessions and worries can coexist when an obsession triggers not only an immediate sense of dread but also cognitive mental processing related to future untoward consequences of the dreaded event. Excessive worries and anxious ruminations also occur in generalized anxiety disorder and in OCPD. They are generally responsive to benzodiazepines. Obsessions, as a rule, are not.

2. Pathologic guilt—Pathologic guilt involves a heightened experience of responsibility for misfortune or harm. The perceived responsibility is usually excessive for the circumstance and can be delusional in nature. It is almost always associated with depressed mood. It differs from an obsession in that the individual truly believes that he or she bears responsibility for an adverse circumstance and experiences excessive remorse. Patients with OCD may have fears that they are responsible for horrific circumstances but usually recognize that their fears are un-

realistic. Their experience is one of dread or horror at the notion that they might have done something harmful, often accompanied by significant anxiety relating to future ramifications of such events. Except in cases of delusional OCD, patients with OCD rarely experience remorse or regret in association with their obsessions, because they recognize at some level the absurdity of their concern. Many patients with OCD do become depressed and may have both obsessive concerns and pathologic guilt. Pathologic guilt can occur in patients with low self-esteem and almost always occurs in patients with significant depression.

3. Depressive ruminations—Depressive ruminations involve the persistent cognitive reprocessing of past memories and experiences, associated with sadness, a sense of loss, or regret. These ruminations are active, continuous mental processes, drawn out in time. The individual ponders past events and often experiences significant guilt or remorse, without dread or uncertainty. If a sense of incompletion is present, it is associated with regret that things were not done satisfactorily in the past. There is no sense of urgency that the situation must be remedied.

4. Aggressive ruminations—Aggressive ruminations are anger-related mental processes involving either past or future ego injuries. Individuals perceive rightly or wrongly that they either were or will be offended in some way, and they replay the events surrounding these circumstances over and over in their minds. Aggressive ruminations may be associated with vengeful fantasies and paranoid ideation. Ruminations may involve envisioning past events as the individual would have preferred them to have occurred. In ruminating about the future, the individual may envision an anticipated scenario in which he or she will be slighted or wronged and may envision various responses to such indignities. In some cases the individual may have difficulty escaping from the ruminative process, leading to interference in the individual's ability to function effectively. Aggressive ruminations differ from aggressive obsessions in that the former are ego-syntonic processes, associated with anger, in which the individual is cognitively involved as an active participant. By contrast, aggressive obsessions involve horrific sensory images or unrealistic fears of acting on destructive impulses, unaccompanied by feelings of anger. The individual tries to avoid these horrific images or fears by putting the thoughts out of mind or by taking steps to make sure that they do not occur. Aggressive ruminations typically occur in individuals with personality disorders (e.g., paranoid, obsessive–compulsive, or narcissistic personality disorders) and in individuals with passive–aggressive personality traits. They may also occur in certain patients with psychotic disorders.

5. Fantasies—Fantasies are mental stories that the individual entertains, extending over a period of time. Fantasies almost always have an attractive component; however, the individual usually realizes that imagined events are unlikely to occur. In pathologic cases, the individual feels locked into the fantasies, envisioning complicated sequences of events, and is unable to withdraw from the mental experience. This may result in mental absences, delays, or impaired performance. Erotic, angry, persecutory, or paranoid fantasies should not be confused with sexual, violent, or aggressive obsessions. Erotic fantasies are associated with a sense of pleasure or captivation and are not experienced as horrific and aversive. Paranoid and anger-related fantasies involve escalating vengeful interactions with an imagined adversary and are not accompanied by doubt, dread, or uncertainty that the acts have occurred in reality. Unlike obsessions, fantasies do not drive the individual to carry out compulsions in the real world. Excessive fantasies can occur in patients with cluster A personality disorders or with OCPD.

6. Paranoid fears—Paranoid fears are concerns that somebody else harbors malevolent intent toward the affected individual. They may be associated with anger and may lead to avoidant, preparatory, or violent preemptive measures, designed to protect the individual from attack. Preventive measures are taken in order to prepare for or protect against attack, not to alleviate the circumstances causing the fear. Patients with OCD sometimes have fears of being harmed by others, as in fears of being poisoned; however, these patients fear that they may be random victims and not specific targets of someone harboring malevolence against them in particular. Violent acts do not occur as a primary consequence of the obsessions of uncomplicated OCD.

7. Flashbacks—Flashbacks are intense, intrusive experiences associated with memories of past traumatic events. The individual usually reexperiences these events in association with a related trigger. Flashbacks often occupy the individual's entire awareness, as though the individual were reliving these events in the here and now. They differ from obsessions in that they spring from memories of past experiences and not from inexplicable horrific images unrelated to previous experience. During the flashback, the individual behaves appropriately within the context of the flashback. The individual may not be aware that the behavior is inappropriate in the present time. In some circumstances traumatic events can lead to time-consuming rituals that are excessive or unrealistic in relation to the degree of psychological trauma. Such rituals should be considered compulsions.

8. Pathologic attraction—Pathologic attraction occurs as cognitive and visceral experiences draw an individual toward a maladaptive behavior. It can be associated with feelings of desire, longing, yearning, or a need for the release of tension. It is usually accompanied by an urge to satisfy or gratify that desire. Pathologic attraction differs from an obsession in that the latter is by nature an intensely aversive experience and triggers behavior based on escape rather than gratification. Pathologic attraction is often associated with impulsions (see "Behavioral Differentiations" section later in this chapter) and is generally present in patients with impulse-control disorders.

9. Rigid thinking—Rigid thinking occurs when an individual is unable to switch sets and adopt a new perspective. It is usually ego-syntonic and may be delusional in nature. People with rigid thinking may be argumentative, repeat themselves, or return to the same point again and again. They are generally unable to adopt the perspective of another individual and cannot be dissuaded from their point of view. Rigid thinking differs from obsessional concerns in that in the former there is no uncertainty or dread and little or no awareness of defect. Rigid thinking can occur in OCPD, in individuals with reduced intelligence, in geriatric populations, and in patients with organic and psychotic illness.

10. Pathologic indecision—Pathologic indecision occurs when an individual is unable to make choices with potential outcomes of unknown or mixed valence. In some cases individuals become paralyzed because they cannot make any decisions. Although there can be a sense of dreadful uncertainty associated with not knowing the outcome, in OCD the sense of dread tends to motivate decisions (including the decision not to act). Pathologic indecision can be seen in the setting of depression and is common in some forms of OCPD in which the individual wants to optimize an outcome without sufficient information. Such a condition can lead to significant procrastination and delayed commitments.

11. Realistic fears or concerns—Individuals with realistic fears or concerns may simulate a picture of OCD. Individuals with a history of violence or pathologic absent-mindedness or inattention may have realistic concerns that these problems will recur and may take special steps appropriate for their own circumstances (e.g., removing dangerous weapons, checking the stove to be sure it is off) to reduce such recurrences. The clinician must establish that such fears or concerns have no realistic basis, or are clearly excessive, before diagnosing such concerns as obsessions.

B. BEHAVIORAL DIFFERENTIATIONS

1. Impulsions—Impulsions are maladaptive behaviors that an individual is attracted to or feels impelled to perform. They are associated with an urge for gratification, satisfaction, or release of tension. The individual may derive a sense of pleasure from the completion of the act. Impulsions can take the form of violent or destructive behaviors that release the tension associated with poorly controlled anger. Impulsions differ from compulsions in that in the former the individual is drawn to the act and derives inherent (not secondary) pleasure, satisfaction, gratification, or release of tension from its completion. By contrast, compulsions are performed to escape aversive circumstances or to prevent something terrible from happening. Compulsions in uncomplicated OCD never involve the willful performance of violent or harmful acts. Impulsions cross diagnostic lines in that maladaptive acts such as drug abuse, binge eating, serial homicide, sexual paraphilias, and impulse-control disorders all fall into this category on the basis of their underlying motivation. Some behaviors can have both gratifying and compulsive components, such as hot showers extended for both pleasure and a sense of incompletion. The clinician must separate impulsions from OCD symptoms.

2. Meticulousness or perfectionism—Meticulousness, or perfectionism, is motivated by a positive sense of accomplishment in completing activities in the proper or optimal manner. The individual achieves a sense of satisfaction and believes that the act is beneficial or rewarding in some way. The individual often believes that others should behave in a similar manner regardless of whether their behavior affects the perfectionist. Perfectionism differs from obsessions with symmetry, exactness, or order in that the former is reinforced by favorable consequences. The ordering, arranging, and "just-right" compulsions of OCD are carried out because of a sense that something is, or will be, very wrong if they are not done. These patients with OCD are intensely disturbed by a sense of misalignment, and experience an aversive sense of incompletion while the behavior is in progress. They generally recognize the absurd and uniquely personal nature of the behavior and do not believe that others need to carry out the same behavior, unless it directly affects their own circumstances. Perfectionism is often associated with OCPD.

3. Pathologic atonement—Pathologic atonement is motivated by guilt or fear of punishment. Individuals may regret past actions and seek to reduce their discomfort in the performance of penitent behavior. Pathologic atonement can take the form of religious rituals, self-punitive tasks, or in severe cases, self-injurious acts, such as flagellation or self-mutilation. This behavior differs from a compulsion of OCD in that the behavior is not motivated by doubt or incompletion but is willfully carried out to reduce the experience of guilt or to avoid an anticipated punishment of greater significance.

Under certain circumstances, an individual may have pathologic uncertainty as to whether the atonement was sufficiently or properly completed and will carry out the behavior repeatedly or excessively for that reason. In such cases the behavior is not driven so much by guilt as it is by the unreasonable sense that the action has not been carried out properly or completely. In such cases a diagnosis of OCD may be considered. Pathologic atonement can be observed in patients with severe depression, hyperreligiosity, severe personality disorders, or psychosis.

4. Repetitive displacement behavior—Repetitive displacement behavior is performed to escape or numb an aversive experience associated with an affective state such as depression or extreme anxiety. The process of carrying out and focusing attention on the act reduces the individual's awareness of the primary aversive condition. Repetitive displacement behavior can mimic OCD, as in cases where depressed or anxious individuals engage in repetitive cleaning or straightening to reduce their affective experience. Although repetitive and seemingly purposeless, the function of the behavior is to numb the psychic distress associated with the primary condition. In contrast to the compulsions of OCD, consequences of the behavior are relatively unimportant. Repetitive displacement behavior can be observed in avoidant, anxious, or depressed individuals and in patients with OCPD.

5. Perseverative behavior—Perseverative behavior involves the repetition of thoughts, speech, or brief behavioral sequences. Perseverative behavior can be carried out without conscious thought or may occur because it reduces an awareness of anxiety or other aversive experiences. It may occur in response to an urge without any affective component. It differs from repeating compulsions in that it is carried out without purpose. Perseverative behavior is not performed as a corrective or preventive measure nor is it driven by a sense of incompletion.

6. Stereotypic behavior—Stereotypic behavior is a form of perseverative motor behavior that is rhythmic in nature. Typically simpler than other perseverative behavior, it may be associated with primary reward or with a reduction of awareness of anxiety or another aversive experience. Stereotypic behavior is frequently seen in the mentally retarded, in patients with organic illnesses, and in very disturbed individuals, often with schizophrenia. It also may occur in normal children.

7. Self-injurious behavior—Self-injurious behavior can occur in several psychological settings. It frequently occurs as an escape behavior to reduce the intensity of a highly aversive–affective experience. It can also occur as a pathologic–manipulative process. Finally, as mentioned earlier, it may be carried out as a self-punitive process in pathologic atonement. When carried out as an escape behavior, the individual will describe a release of tension associated with the act, particularly upon visualization of the self-injurious process. The pain or shock of the injury appears to reduce or block out the awareness of the aversive affective experience that triggers the behavior. By contrast, compulsions of uncomplicated OCD never involve direct self-harm. Self-injurious behavior is observed in patients with borderline personality disorder, severe depression, or some organic or psychotic syndromes.

8. Pathologic overinvolvement—Pathologic overinvolvement occurs when an individual is preoccupied with a single process or set of processes to the exclusion of others. Overinvolvement is generally ego-syntonic as the individual carries out the process upon which attention is focused. Each step of the process leads to the desire to carry out the next step. The individual experiences gratification from the process as it is occurring or upon completion, and the behavior is carried out because the individual values the achievement. The original purpose of the behavior may be lost. Overinvolvement becomes pathologic when the individual neglects or is unable to attend to more important tasks or social responsibilities. Pathologic overinvolvement differs from OCD in that the individual is attracted to the engagement and is not motivated by aversive experience. It can be prominent in patients with stimulant intoxication and hypomania and can occur in patients with OCPD.

9. Pathologic persistence—Pathologic persistence is observed when an individual continues to pursue an endeavor or interaction despite repeated failure or rebuff. It can be associated with rigidity of thought or related to an individual's inability to accept unwanted circumstances. It is often associated with an overvaluing of a personal agenda, relative to the agendas of others. It can result in mutually irritating interactions with those around the individual. Pathologic persistence is goal-directed, and although there may be a concomitant sense of incompleteness or unfinished business, the behavior is motivated by some other purpose, such as a desire to win, have one's own way, or accomplish one's goals. Pathologic persistence differs from OCD in that the former behavior is ego-syntonic. The individual seeks a favorable resolution of his or her pursuits and is not trying to escape an experience of dread or uncertainty. Pathologic persistence occurs in patients with OCPD, narcissistic personality disorder, borderline personality disorder, and hypomania; and in some cases of stimulant intoxication.

10. Hoarding—Hoarding is observed in numerous syndromes other than OCD. These include anorexia nervosa, Tourette syndrome, autism, Prader–Willi syndrome, OCPD, stimulant abuse, schizotypal personality disorder, and schizophrenia. In Prader–Willi syndrome, anorexia nervosa, and some cases of autism, hoarding occurs in secrecy. These patients have hidden stashes of items that they have collected, often by stealing or other surreptitious means. Collected items may have little tangible importance to the individual, as in food collected by the anorexic individual that will never be eaten. Collecting in OCPD is performed because of a sense that items may have positive value at some point in the future. The accumulation of possessions itself is important. The possessions are an extension of the individual, and the individual feels a sense of loss or waste if called upon to discard them. In OCD, by contrast, collecting is motivated by one of two different processes. It may be associated with an unreasonable urge to obtain an item, without any underlying reason (e.g., picking up bird feathers or empty bottles on the street). Such collecting can be indistinguishable from that seen in Tourette syndrome, autism, schizophrenia, and schizotypal personality disorder. The diagnosis is made on the basis of other associated pathology. Alternatively, hoarding or collecting in OCD may be associated with an unreasonable concern that the item, although unimportant now, might be needed in the future. The patient with OCD has a sense that there may be a time when not having the item will result in a distressing circumstance that should be protected against.

11. Complex tics—Complex tics occur in the setting of a tic disorder and are usually motivated by unwanted urges without rational motivation. Although some complex tics are confined to localized muscle groups, others can mimic the compulsions of OCD. Most often these latter tics involve "just-right" perceptions, accompanied by urges to order, align, or arrange. In addition, patients with Tourette syndrome can have obsessions associated with their tics, such that they fear something terrible will happen if they do not give in to the urge to tic. These tics can be indistinguishable from the compulsive behavior of OCD. In such cases it is best to classify the behavior as both a tic and a compulsion (an OCD–tic). Because treatment decisions can be affected by the presence of tics, the clinician should always observe the patient for such processes and should ask the patient about distinctive habits or mannerisms they might have or might have had previously, particularly in childhood.

Baer L, Jenike MA: Personality disorders in obsessive compulsive disorder. *Psychiatr Clin North Am* 1992;15:803.

Pigott TA, L'Heureux F, Dubbert B, Bernstein S, Murphy DL: Obsessive compulsive disorder: Comorbid conditions. *J Clin Psychiatry* 1994;55(10 Suppl):15.

Swedo SE, Leonard HL, Garvey M, et al.: Pediatric autoimmune neuropsychiatric disorders associated with streptococcal infections: clinical description of the first 50 cases. *Am J Psychiatry* 1998;155:264. [Published erratum appears in *Am J Psychiatry* 1998;155:578.]

Differential Psychiatric Diagnoses

A number of psychiatric disorders have been confused with OCD on the basis of some common phenomenologic components. The differential psychiatric diagnosis for OCD is summarized in Table 21–2.

Table 21–2. Differential Psychiatric Diagnosis for Obsessive–Compulsive Disorder

Anorexia nervosa
Body dysmorphic disorder
Hypochondriasis
Obsessive–compulsive personality disorder
Pathologic skin-picking
Specific phobias
Trichotillomania

A. OBSESSIVE–COMPULSIVE PERSONALITY DISORDER

OCPD is an Axis II disorder that has a name that sounds similar to OCD but is associated with meticulousness, persistence, rigidity, and personal isolation. As noted earlier in this chapter, only a small minority of OCD patients have concurrent OCPD. This confusion may relate historically to Sigmund Freud's characterization of obsessions and compulsions in his work with the "Rat Man." Unfortunately, the Rat Man had both OCD and OCPD, leading Freud to entangle the two entities in his interpretations. The key difference between elements of OCPD and OCD is the ego-syntonic nature of the experiences and behavior in OCPD. There is no dread but rather a desire that others conform to the individual's standards or desires.

B. SPECIFIC PHOBIAS

Specific phobias involve excessive fears of specific situations or circumstances. They often involve fears of situations that others might experience as mildly aversive or anxiety provoking (e.g., contact with snakes or spiders), but the phobic individual has an excessive reaction to those circumstances. Avoidance is prominent and effective in allaying anxiety. In OCD, fears can be situation specific; however, there is usually a sense of doubt or uncertainty associated with the dread (e.g., uncertainty whether germs are present), as the individual cannot be certain he or she has successfully avoided the aversive circumstance. No rituals are involved in simple phobias.

C. HYPOCHONDRIASIS

Hypochondriasis is an unreasonable, persistent concern that something is wrong with the body. It can lead to repeated requests for medical care or reassurance. Hypochondriasis can mimic the obsessions of OCD; however, hypochondriacal concerns are limited to the body, and there are no other obsessions and compulsions. The individual is usually not delusional and may recognize that the behavior is excessive. Patients with hypochondriasis usually lack the sense of immediacy that exists in OCD. The individual experiences worries about long-term health rather than short-term immediate dread. Hypochondriasis can be associated with abnormal somatic perceptions, which are unusual in OCD.

D. BODY DYSMORPHIC DISORDER

Body dysmorphic disorder (BDD) involves the unreasonable sense that something about the body is malformed, inadequate, or offensive to others. The individual may spend excessive time looking at, or seeking medical or surgical treatment for the affected area. BDD differs from OCD in the degree of insight, as the individual with BDD truly believes that the body area is abnormal. There is no sense of incompletion or dread that something terrible will happen. The driven behaviors associated with BDD involve corrective measures to hide or alter an imagined defect and are not carried out with a sense that something has not been completed. The distinction between BDD and OCD can be difficult when the individual experiences "just-right" perceptions related to the body or when the individual has a fear of having an offensive body odor. In such cases the diagnosis of OCD may be warranted.

E. TRICHOTILLOMANIA

Trichotillomania is characterized by urges to pull hairs from the body. The hair is most frequently pulled out singly, and the act of pulling is associated with an experience of pleasure or a release of tension. Binges of hair pulling result in large bald patches. Trichotillomania differs from OCD in that the former involves no obsessions, and the behavior is rewarding.

F. PATHOLOGIC SKIN-PICKING

Pathologic skin-picking can occur as an unconscious habit or as a response to an exaggerated concern about the texture of the skin. The individual may be drawn to the behavior by an attractive process that is hard to overcome. Skin-pickers are typically aware that what they are doing is destructive; however, they are unable to overcome the desire to carry out the behavior. Such picking is similar to trichotillomania in this regard. It differs from OCD in that in pathologic skin-picking there is no sense of dread, uncertainty, or incompletion, and the behavior is not carried out to prevent something bad from happening. It also differs from OCD in that pathologic skin-picking has a self-destructive or mutilative component that is rarely seen in uncomplicated OCD.

G. ANOREXIA NERVOSA

Anorexia nervosa involves an excessive concern with body image, accompanied by a refusal to eat, with purposeful behavior directed at maintaining a low body weight. In anorexia nervosa, there is a delusional perception that the body is overweight. Unlike in OCD, the anorexic individual has no insight regarding this concern. Feelings of dread, uncertainty, or incompletion are absent or are not prominent. Driven behaviors are performed with the intention of maintaining or exacerbating a desired condition. Although hoarding may be observed, no true compulsions are associated with the primary illness. Individuals with OCD can experience significant weight loss in conjunction with fears associated with food contamination. These individuals, however, do not typically have concerns about their body image and often acknowledge the absurdity of their condition.

Complications and Secondary Diagnoses

As mentioned earlier in this chapter, OCD has been shown to be associated with diseases of the basal ganglia. A significant number of children who developed Economo disease after an influenza epidemic early in the twentieth century experienced OCD symptoms, and there was a significant increase in the prevalence of chronic OCD in survivors of the epidemic. OCD has also been described in Huntington disease, parkinsonism, and carbon monoxide poisoning associated with destruction of the globus pallidus. There is a higher incidence of rheumatic fever in family members of patients with OCD. Adults with a history of Sydenham chorea have a higher incidence of OCD than does the population at large.

There is a high prevalence of vocal and motor tics in OCD (20%) and in the families of patients with OCD (20%). The full-fledged Tourette syndrome is present in only 5–7% of adult patients with OCD. Over 60% of children with OCD will experience at least transient tics, and as many as 15% will develop the full Tourette syndrome. For children with an early onset of symptoms, OCD may be the first manifestation of Tourette syndrome. OCD symptoms occur in 40–70% of individuals with Tourette syndrome and in 12% of family members of Tourette syndrome patients who do not themselves have Tourette syndrome.

OCD patients often have comorbid Axis I disorders. Depression is the most common secondary diagnosis in OCD. Approximately 50% of individuals with OCD will develop a major depressive episode in their lifetime. The depression occurs because OCD symptoms prevent the individual from carrying out activities important for self-esteem, and because attempts to resist the symptoms, or adequately meet the demands of the illness, inevitably fail. OCD can engender continual conflict with significant others and is often associated with social isolation.

Effective treatment of the OCD in these cases often leads to resolution of the depressive episode.

Patients with OCD also have a high prevalence of panic disorder, secondary agoraphobia, social phobia, and alcohol and other substance abuse. Agoraphobia can result from a patient's attempts to avoid circumstances that trigger obsessions. In some cases the patient may be trapped at home because he or she is unable to tolerate the obsessions and compulsions that are triggered by contact with the outside world.

Anxiety can complicate OCD, as the individual worries about both the consequences of having OCD and the consequences of being unable to complete compulsions. Patients with OCD may describe panic-like attacks that are not true panic attacks. Rather, they are attacks of severe anxiety related to violation of an obsessive concern. For example, when an individual who has contamination fears discovers that he or she has been severely contaminated, the individual may experience an overwhelming sense of dread, anxiety, and despair, related to the impossible task of decontaminating everything that he or she has defiled. This patient might mislabel these experiences as panic attacks. The clinician must be aware of this process to avoid unnecessarily complicating the patient's diagnostic picture.

There is also a high prevalence of personality disorders in patients with OCD (50–70%). Avoidant, dependent, borderline, histrionic, and schizotypal personality disorders occur most frequently. OCPD occurs in only a small minority of patients, with estimates as low as 6% of OCD cases. This observation argues against an older view that OCD was an extreme variant of OCPD. Interestingly, although personality disorder symptoms are thought to be life-long fixed traits, effective treatment of OCD will eliminate personality disorder symptoms in a majority of OCD patients, suggesting that the dysfunctional Axis II symptoms may in part be secondary to stress and tension associated with the Axis I disorder.

The diagnosis of avoidant personality disorder may be secondary to the individual's primary pathology, combined with an ambiguity in the DSM-IV-TR diagnostic criteria for the personality disorder. An unreasonable concern of being the target of disapproval of others is a DSM-IV-TR criterion for avoidant personality disorder. Individuals with OCD who fear they may be responsible for something bad happening may also fear that they will be the subject of consequent disapproval or ridicule. These patients have unreasonable concerns that they might in fact be at fault. Individuals with the true personality disorder (i.e., those who do not have OCD) are unreasonably hypersensitive to the criticism itself. As individuals with OCD improve they often no longer meet criteria for this diagnosis.

Likewise, the dependent personality disorder can occur in patients with OCD who feel that they need assistance from others in carrying out their compulsions or who need reassurance that their obsessive concerns are not valid. Such assistance relieves them of the responsibility for carrying out acts that might have dreadful consequences. These individuals are dependent on their significant other, and they experience significant discomfort when that person is not available for these purposes. These patients will meet criteria for this personality disorder as a result of the nature of their OCD. As their OCD improves, many will no longer meet criteria for this diagnosis.

Treatment

Treatment ranges from simple stress reduction to neurosurgery (Tables 21–3 and 22–4). Mild forms of OCD (i.e., with YBOCS scores of less than 16) that occur in association with temporary stress may respond to stress reduction and supportive measures. Most OCD patients seen by psychiatrists, however, require more definitive treatment.

A. PSYCHOTHERAPEUTIC INTERVENTIONS

Behavioral therapy for OCD involves exposure and response prevention. According to learning theorists, patients with OCD have learned an inappropriate active avoidance response to anxiety associated with circumstances that trigger their OCD symptoms. The clinician must encourage the patient to experience the aversive condition (exposure) without performing the compulsion (response prevention). Chronic exposure alone will reduce the anxiety associated with the exposure, but the compulsions will remain if not specifically restricted. Response prevention is critical. Typically, the individual is asked to hierarchally order his or her fears. A decision is then made as to which obsessive–compulsive dyad will be addressed. The patient is exposed by increasing degrees to the feared stimulus and is prohibited from carrying out the compulsive behavior. Anxiety with initial exposure is usually intense and enduring; however, with repeated exposure, the intensity and duration decrease. When it is not possible to expose the patient in the office, the therapist may accompany the patient to a location, such as the home or the street, where the feared stimuli are more prevalent. In an outpatient session the patient is typically instructed to repeatedly expose himself or herself to a specified set of circumstances on a proscribed number of occasions as "homework" between sessions. The patient should be encouraged to assess or question the validity of his or her obsessive thoughts as an adjunct to treatment. Such a cognitive approach may increase compliance, and when no compulsions are present, or when exposure is impractical, it may be the primary adjunct to treatment. In other cases, exposure to the actual fear (e.g., killing one's child) is not practicable, and the patient must engage in imaginal exposure. Typically, the therapist and patient will work on one symptom complex until the symptom has been reduced to an agreeable level or until a joint decision is made to address another symptom.

Many physicians have neither the time nor the experience to carry out behavioral therapy themselves and should refer the patient to a specialist in this area. Symptoms most amenable to behavior therapy involve contamination concerns and fears that evoke behavior that can be elicited in the office. Behavioral therapy is most difficult to carry out with individuals who have only obsessions or whose compulsions involve only mental activities such as counting or mental checking. Individuals with poor insight, and those who cannot tolerate exposure, tend to have more difficulty with this treatment method.

Behavioral therapy is effective in roughly 70% of individuals who agree to undergo the process. However, approximately 30% of individuals with OCD will decline this form of treatment. Behavioral therapy may be better tolerated if the patient has appropriate pharmacologic treatment. In some circumstances symptoms can disappear completely; however, they often return over a 6-month period, and an additional short course of behavioral therapy may be needed to effectively treat the symptoms.

B. PSYCHOPHARMACOLOGIC INTERVENTIONS

1. Preferential serotonergic reuptake inhibitors—Preferential serotonergic reuptake inhibitors (PSRIs), the medications most effective in treating OCD, mainly inhibit there uptake of serotonin into nerve cells (see Table 21–3). These medications include clomipramine, fluoxetine, sertraline, paroxetine, citalopram, escitalopram, and fluvoxamine. Medications with noradrenergic reuptake inhibition produce no benefit and may counteract or diminish the efficacy of serotonergic reuptake inhibition. Among the PSRIs, clomipramine alone is a tricyclic antidepressant and has significant anticholinergic, antihistaminic, and anti-α-adrenergic side effects. Clomipramine is also metabolized to desmethyl clomipramine, a metabolite that will inhibit the uptake of noradrenaline. Meta-analyses of efficacy suggest that clomipramine may be more effective than other PSRIs in treating OCD; however, there is no direct evidence that any one of the PSRIs is more effective than any other. Except in the case of fluvoxamine, each of the multicenter trials for PSRIs showed nonsignificant trends for higher doses to be more effective in treating OCD, suggesting that the optimal doses for these medications may be at the higher end of the permissible prescription range.

While PSRIs exert their main effects in depression after 3–6 weeks of treatment, in OCD they must be

Table 21–3. Pharmacologic Treatments for Obsessive–Compulsive Disorder

First line—PSRIs	Dosage (mg/d)
SSRIs	
Fluvoxamine	100–300
Fluoxetine	20–80
Sertraline	75–225
Paroxetine	20–60
Citalopram	20–60
Clomipramine	150–250
Escitalopram	20–40
Adjuncts	
SSRI/clomipramine	Various
Neuroleptics* (tics, family history of tics, schizotypal personality disorder)	
Risperidone	1–3
Olanzapine	2.5–7.5
Pimozide	0.5–4
Ziprasidone	40–120
Aripiprazole	5–15
Haloperidol	0.5–4
Clonazepam* (seizures, panic, anxiety, insomnia)	1–6
For nonresponders	
MAOIs (panic, phobias, refractory depression)*	
Phenylzine	60–90
Tranylcypromine	20–60
Venlafaxine* (refractory depression)	150–300
Mirtazepine* (refractory depression, anxiety)	15–30
Trazodone* (high-dose; refractory depression)	400–600
Clonazepam* (high-dose; for seizures, panic, anxiety)	5–10
Carbamazepine* (abnormal EEG)	Blood-level dependent

* Special circumstances that might favor this treatment option.

administered for up to 12 weeks to determine their full range of benefits. Withdrawal from medication is frequently associated with relapse within 2–3 weeks; patients need, therefore, be advised to stay on their medication to prevent relapse. Tolerance to the beneficial effects of PSRIs rarely occurs.

The medications used to treat OCD rarely eliminate the OCD syndrome; symptoms typically are reduced by 35% in aggregate and by 50–70% in most responders. Clinical practice suggests that these figures underestimate the full benefits received by patients taking the medications. Although symptom levels may fall by less than

Table 21–4. Other Treatments for Obsessive–Compulsive Disorder

Interactive treatments
Behavioral therapy (exposure and response prevention)*
Family therapy (e.g., contracts, positive reinforcement, defacilitation)
Neurosurgical treatments (extreme, refractory cases only)*
Anterior cingulotomy
Limbic leukotomy
Anterior capsulotomy
Subcaudate tractotomy
Experimental treatments
Intravenous clomipramine
Plasmapheresis (autoimmune-related OCD)*
Immunoglobulin (autoimmune-related OCD)*
Chronic penicillin (streptococcal autoimmune-related OCD)*

* Special circumstances that might favor this treatment option.

half of their baseline levels, such patients can experience a significant improvement in the quality of their lives and can function more effectively in society. Approximately 50–60% of those initially undertaking a trial of a PSRI will achieve a clinically significant response. These medications give patients the chance to tolerate their obsessions, and their urges to carry out the compulsions, without acting on them. The combination of behavioral therapy with medication appears to be optimal for most OCD patients, as up to 25% of patients who fail one modality will respond to joint treatment.

If a patient has no response to medication after 8 weeks, or has an inadequate response after 12 weeks, the clinician should consider trying a different PSRI. Approximately 20% of patients who do not respond to one PSRI will respond to another. If the patient has not responded to a second PSRI, a third PSRI trial should be attempted. One of the three PSRI trials should involve clomipramine.

2. Adjunctive medications—If a patient does not achieve an adequate response with proper trials of PSRIs, a second medication should be added. The combination of an SSRI and clomipramine should be considered first in this context. The combination of clomipramine and fluvoxamine may significantly augment serotonin uptake inhibition because fluvoxamine can inhibit the conversion of clomipramine to its noradrenergic desmethyl

metabolite. Alternatively, low-dose, high-potency neuroleptics (e.g., risperidone, olanzapine, ziprasidone, aripiprazole, pimozide, haloperidol) may be used to augment PSRI treatment, particularly if the patient has comorbid tics, a family history of tics, or features of a schizotypal personality disorder. OCD symptoms in the latter group of patients can be refractory to conventional treatments, but show a response to augmentation with a neuroleptic. For patients whose OCD has a significant anxiety component, patients with a history of seizures, and patients with additional symptoms consistent with partial complex seizures, the addition of clonazepam (0.5–6 mg) should be considered. Clonazepam can also be considered as an adjunct to high-dose clomipramine treatment (greater than 250 mg daily) as a means of reducing the potential for seizures. Both low-dose neuroleptics and clonazepam should be added after the patient has been taking the optimal PSRI for at least 6–8 weeks and is on the maximal dose tolerated. These adjuncts may have beneficial effects within 1 week; however, an adequate adjunctive trial should be 4–6 weeks. Other medications that have been used as adjunctive treatments include tryptophan, pindolol plus tryptophan, mirtazapine, gabapentin, and fenfluramine. Lithium, buspirone, and pindolol appear to have little benefit as augmenting agents in the treatment of OCD.

3. Alternative pharmacologic monotherapies—Alternative medication trials must be considered for those patients who fail to respond to adequate trials of PSRIs and adjunctive medications in conjunction with behavioral therapy. A trial of a monoamine oxidase inhibitor (MAOI) should be considered for patients with panic or phobic symptoms. Patients with a seizure history, an abnormal EEG, or suspected partial complex seizures might be considered for a trial of clonazepam or carbamazepine as a monotherapy. High-dose clonazepam (5–10 mg daily) as a monotherapy has a success rate of 20–30% in the treatment of OCD. Low-dose clonazepam does not appear to be effective as a monotherapy. Clonazepam treatment can trigger or exacerbate a depressive episode. If this occurs, the trial should be discontinued because it will not alleviate OCD symptoms. Clonazepam treatment may also interfere with the efficiency of a behavioral therapy. Other medications known to affect serotonergic neurotransmission may also be efficacious as monotherapies in isolated cases. These medications include mirtazapine, venlafaxine, high-dose trazodone, and buspirone. Clonidine has no benefit for adults with OCD; however, it has been used effectively to reduce OCD symptoms in children who have combined Tourette syndrome and OCD. Lithium, methylphenidate, neuroleptics, other heterocyclic antidepressants, and other benzodiazepines including alprazolam, have little benefit as monotherapies in OCD.

C. FAMILY THERAPY

Family members can unwittingly interfere with the success of traditional treatments. As mentioned earlier in this chapter, families can facilitate the OCD symptoms or antagonize the patient. In such cases, family therapy can be helpful. At the very least, education regarding the patient's condition and the appropriate responses to that condition should be attempted. In general, family members should not assist the patient in the OCD rituals, nor should they significantly alter or compromise the quality of their lives to accommodate the symptoms of the illness. The family should be supportive of reductions in symptoms but not critical of exacerbations. Family members should avoid disparaging remarks related to the OCD. More extensive family therapy involves mutually acceptable contracts between the patient and affected family members regarding behaviors targeted for suppression. OCD behaviors outside the contract that do not compromise the lives of family members should be dealt with only in a positive and constructive manner. Family members should be aware that behavior therapy is a stepwise process and that behavior that is currently not a part of the contract can be addressed in the future. In addition to interventions directed at the OCD, internal family conflicts may need to be addressed in therapy because they can exacerbate the OCD symptoms and impair the quality of life of all concerned.

D. NEUROSURGERY

Neurosurgery is the treatment of last resort. Neurosurgical procedures include bilateral cingulotomy, limbic leukotomy, anterior capsulotomy, and subcaudate tractotomy. Estimates of clinically significant improvement range from 25% to 90%, although controlled studies have not been undertaken. There is some disagreement regarding the optimal site of the lesion. In intractable cases, however, neurosurgery is a treatment that may offer relief from disabling symptoms and from extreme psychic pain. Improvement after surgery is not immediate but may occur over a period of up to 1 year. Adverse effects include seizures, disinhibition syndromes, and the attendant risks of general anesthesia.

Patients should not be referred for surgery unless they have had full trials of at least three PSRIs at appropriate dosages, including one trial of clomipramine, as well as trials of both a neuroleptic and clonazepam as adjunctive medications. A trial of an MAOI should have been attempted. The patient should have had a course of behavioral therapy with a qualified therapist, preferably occurring while the patient was receiving optimal pharmacologic treatment. Additionally, the OCD or its complications should have life-threatening consequences for the patient or cause extreme dysfunction or severe psychic pain. Patients should be referred to centers that have stringent presurgical entrance criteria and extensive experience with this treatment modality.

E. EXPERIMENTAL TREATMENTS

1. Intravenous clomipramine—It is ironic that intravenous clomipramine treatment is considered an experimental treatment when most of the early work in Europe demonstrating the efficacy of clomipramine was completed using this parenteral preparation. Intravenous clomipramine treatment is currently receiving attention in the United States and may have significant promise in the treatment of OCD that does not respond to PSRIs. Specific clinical recommendations for this treatment modality are not yet available.

2. Immunosuppressant & antistreptococcal treatment—Recurrent, episodic, postinfectious OCD in children has been treated with immunosuppressive measures including steroids, plasmaphoresis, and immunoglobulin treatment. In addition, children with repeated poststreptococcal episodes have been placed experimentally on prophylactic penicillin treatment. Although initial trials of immunosuppressants seem positive, specific clinical recommendations regarding these treatments are not available. As a rule, these treatments are not effective in treating OCD in adults.

Allen AJ, Leonard HL, Swedo SE: Case study: A new infection-triggered, autoimmune subtype of pediatric OCD and Tourette's syndrome. *J Am Acad Child Adolesc Psychiatry* 1995;34:307.

Baer L: *Getting Control: Overcoming Your Obsessions and Compulsions.* New York: Penguin, 1991.

Foa EB: *Stop Obsessing: How to Overcome Your Obsessions and Compulsions,* New York: Bantam Books, 1991.

Hewlett WA: Novel pharmacologic treatments of obsessive compulsive disorder. In: Hollander EH, Stein D (eds). *Obsessive Compulsive Disorders.* Marcel Dekker, 1996.

Koran LM, Sallee FR, Pallanti S: Rapid benefit of intravenous pulse loading of clomipramine in obsessive–compulsive disorder. *Am J Psychiatry* 1997;154:396.

March JS, et al.: The Expert Consensus Guideline Series: Treatment of obsessive compulsive disorder. *J Clin Psychiatry* 1997;(suppl 4):3.

Marks I: Behavior therapy for obsessive–compulsive disorder: A decade of progress. *Can J Psychiatry* 1997;42:1021.

McDougle CJ: Update on pharmacologic management of OCD: Agents and augmentation. *J Clin Psychiatry* 1997;12:11.

Mindus P, Rasmussen SA, Lindquist C: Neurosurgical treatment for refractory obsessive–compulsive disorder: Implications for understanding frontal lobe function. *J Neuropsychiatry Clin Neurosci* 1994;6:467.

Ravizza L, Barzega G, Bellino S, Bogetto F, Maina G: Predictors of drug treatment response in obsessive–compulsive disorder. *J Clin Psychiatry* 1995;56:368.

Prognosis

There is no cure for OCD. The best that can be expected is a temporary remission of certain symptom complexes with appropriate behavioral therapy, and partial remission of symptoms with pharmacotherapy or neurosurgery. Even such partial remission is a welcome relief for patients plagued by this illness and often allows them to function with some effort at a full capacity. Overall, 75–85% of patients seeking treatment will achieve a significant clinical response with optimal combination treatments. Individuals with schizotypal features or neurologic soft signs have a poorer response prognosis, and the former group may not respond to either pharmacotherapy or behavioral interventions. Individuals who will not or cannot tolerate medications and behavioral measures likewise have a poor prognosis. Most biological research on OCD has been carried out only in the past decade, and new treatments such as immunosuppressive therapy, prophylactic penicillin, and intravenous clomipramine show promise for the future. The clinician should be optimistic that although at present there is no cure, the future may provide far more effective treatments.

Somatoform Disorders

22

Charles V. Ford, MD

Patients who somatize psychosocial distress commonly present in medical clinical settings. Approximately 25% of patients in primary care demonstrate some degree of somatization, and at least 10% of medical or surgical patients have no evidence of a disease process. Somatizing patients use a disproportionately large amount of medical services and frustrate their physicians, who often do not recognize the true nature of these patients' underlying problems. Somatizing patients rarely seek help from psychiatrists at their own initiative, and they may resent any implication that their physical distress is related to psychological problems. Despite the psychogenic etiology of their illnesses, these patients continue to seek medical care in nonpsychiatric settings where their somatization is often unrecognized.

Somatization is not an either-or proposition. Rather, many patients have some evidence of biological disease but overrespond to their symptoms or believe themselves to be more disabled than objective evidence would indicate. Medical or surgical patients who have concurrent anxiety or depressive disorders use medical services at a rate two to three times greater than that of persons with the same diseases who do not have a comorbid psychiatric disorder.

Despite the illusion that somatoform disorders are specific entities, as is implied by the use of specific diagnostic criteria from the *Diagnostic and Statistical Manual of Mental Disorders*, 4th edition (DSM-IV), the symptoms most of these patients experience fail to meet the diagnostic criteria of the formal somatoform disorders. Further, over time, patients' symptoms tend to be fluid, and patients may be best described as having one disorder at one time and another disorder at some other time. Somatization is caused or facilitated by numerous interrelated factors (Table 22–1), and for an individual patient a particular symptom may have multiple etiologies. In other words, these disorders are heterogeneous both in clinical presentation and in etiology.

Somatoform disorders are generally multidetermined, and because they represent final common symptomatic pathways of many etiologic factors, each patient must be evaluated carefully so that an individualized treatment plan can be developed.

Barsky AJ, Ettner SL, Horsky J, et al.: Resource utilization of patients with hypochondriacal health anxiety and somatization. *Med Care* 2001;39:705–715.

Ford C: Somatization and fashionable diagnoses: Illness as a way of life. *Scand J Work Environ Health* 1997;3(23 suppl):7–16.

CONVERSION DISORDER

 ## ESSENTIALS OF DIAGNOSIS

DSM-IV-TR Diagnostic Criteria

A. One or more symptoms or deficits affecting voluntary motor or sensory function that suggest a neurological or other general medical condition.

B. Psychological factors are judged to be associated with the symptom or deficit because the initiation or exacerbation of the symptom or deficit is preceded by conflicts or other stressors.

C. The symptom or deficit is not intentionally produced or feigned (as in factitious disorder or malingering).

D. The symptoms or deficit cannot, after appropriate investigation, be fully explained by a general medical condition, or by the direct effects of a substance, or as a culturally sanctioned behavior or experience.

E. The symptom or deficit causes clinically significant distress or impairment in social, occupational, or other important areas of functioning or warrants medical evaluation.

F. The symptom or deficit is not limited to pain or sexual dysfunction, does not occur exclusively during the course of somatization disorder, and is not better accounted for by another mental disorder.

Table 22–1. Causes of Somatization

Illness allows a socially isolated person access to an auxiliary social support system.
The sick role can be used as a rationalization of failures in occupation, social, or sexual roles.
Illness can be a means of obtaining nurturance.
Illness can be used as a source of power to manipulate other people or social situations.
Somatic symptoms may be used as a communication or as a cry for help.
The somatic symptoms of certain psychological disorders (e. g., major depression and panic disorder) may be incorrectly attributed to physical disease.
Because physical illness is less stigmatizing than psychiatric illness, many patients prefer to attribute psychological symptoms to physical causes.
Some individuals may be hypersensitive to somatic symptoms and amplify them. Such hypersensitivity is often related to concurrent emotions such as depression and anxiety.
Somatic symptoms can represent behavior learned in childhood, in that some parenting styles may emphasize attention to illness.
The sick role can provide incentives such as disability payments, the avoidance of social responsibilities, and solutions to intrapsychic conflicts.
Trauma, particularly childhood physical or sexual abuse, appears to predispose individuals to the use of somatic symptoms as a communication of psychosocial distress.
Physicians can inadvertently reinforce the concept of physical disease by symptomatic treatment or through so-called fashionable diagnoses, such as multiple chemical sensitivities or reactive hypoglycemia.

Specify type of symptom or deficit:

With motor symptom or deficit. This subtype includes such symptoms as (impaired coordination or balance, paralysis, or localized weakness, difficulty swallowing or "lump in throat," aphonia, and urinary retention).

With sensory symptom or deficit. This subtype includes such symptoms as (loss of touch or pain sensation, double vision, blindness, deafness, and hallucinations).

With seizures or convulsions. This subtype includes such symptoms as seizures or convulsions with voluntary motor or sensory components.

With mixed presentation. This subtype is used if symptoms of more than one category are evident.

(Reprinted, with permission, from *Diagnostic and Statistical Manual of Mental Disorders*, 4th edn. Text Revision. Washington DC: American Psychiatric Association, 2000.)

General Considerations

Conversion disorder previously known as hysteria or hysterical conversion reaction is an ancient medical diagnosis: described in both the Egyptian and Greek medical literature. Although often thought to have disappeared with the Victorian age, these disorders continue to the present but often with more subtlety and sophisticated mimicry than characterized by the dramatic symptoms of the past.

A. Epidemiology

The reported incidence of conversion symptoms varies widely depending on the populations studied. The lifetime incidence of conversion disorder in women is approximately 33%; however, most of these symptoms remit spontaneously, and the incidence in tertiary-care settings is considerably lower. The incidence in men is unknown. Patients with conversion symptoms comprise 1–3% of patients seen by neurologists. Conversion is diagnosed in 5–10% of hospitalized medical or surgical patients who are referred for psychiatric consultation. Conversion symptoms occur in all age ranges from early childhood to advanced age. The disorder occurs with an approximately equal frequency in prepubertal boys and girls, but it is diagnosed much more frequently in adult women than in men.

Conversion symptoms appear to occur more frequently in people of lower intelligence, in those with less education or less social sophistication, and in those with any condition or situation in which verbal communication may be impeded.

B. ETIOLOGY

Some authors have viewed conversion as more of a symptom than a diagnosis, with the implication that another underlying psychiatric disorder is usually present. It is likely that conversion is heterogeneous and that for some patients there is more than one cause. Among proposed etiologies are suggestions that the symptoms resolve an intrapsychic conflict expressed symbolically through a somatic symptom. For example, a person with a conflict over anger may experience paralysis of a right arm. Interpersonal issues have also been implicated. That is, the symptom may manipulate the behavior of other persons and elicit attention, sympathy, and nurturance.

Conversion often follows a traumatic event and may be a psychological mechanism evoked to cope with acute stress. Conversion symptoms are frequently found in patients receiving treatment on neurologic services and in patients with cerebral dysfunction. It seems likely that underlying neurologic dysfunction facilitates the emergence of conversion symptoms, perhaps as a result of impairment in the patient's ability to articulate distress. Conversion may also be viewed as a learned behavior. For example, a person who has genuine epileptic convulsions may learn that seizures have a profound effect on others and may develop pseudoseizures. In this case, the individual may have both genuine epileptic seizures and pseudoseizures, and distinguishing between the two may be difficult.

Current theories about the etiology of conversion emphasize the role of communication. People who have difficulty in verbally articulating psychosocial distress, for any reason, may use conversion symptoms as a way of communicating their distress.

C. GENETICS

According to one nonreplicated Scandinavian study, relatives of patients with conversion disorder were at much higher risk for conversion symptoms. Polygenic transmission was proposed.

Clinical Findings

A. SIGNS & SYMPTOMS

A conversion symptom, by definition, mimics dysfunction in the voluntary motor or sensory system. Common symptoms include pseudoseizures, vocal cord dysfunction (e. g., aphonia), blindness, tunnel vision, deafness, and a variety of anesthesias and paralyses. On careful clinical examination and with the aid of laboratory investigations, these symptoms prove to be nonphysiologic. A clinical example is the presence of normal deep tendon reflexes in a person with a "paralyzed" arm.

Contrary to popular belief, patients with conversion disorder may be depressed or anxious about the symptom. Some phenomena that have traditionally been associated with conversion, such as symbolism, *la belle indifference* (an inappropriate lack of concern for the disability), and histrionic personality, do not reliably differentiate conversion from physical disease.

B. PSYCHOLOGICAL TESTING

Psychological tests often demonstrate comorbid psychiatric illness associated with tendencies to deny or repress psychological distress. A characteristic finding on the Minnesota Multiphasic Personality Inventory-2 (MMPI-2) is the presence of the "conversion V," in which the hypochondriasis and hysteria scales are elevated above the depression scale, forming a "V" in the profile. However, such a finding is not pathognomonic for conversion.

C. LABORATORY FINDINGS

Most conversion symptoms are, by definition, pseudoneurologic. Laboratory examinations, such as nerve conduction speed, electromyograms, and visual and auditory evoked potentials, demonstrate that the sensory and nervous system is intact despite the clinical symptoms. Simultaneous electromyographic and video recording of a patient with pseudoseizures can be diagnostic when the patient has epileptic-like movements while the simultaneous electroencephalogram (EEG) tracing demonstrates normal electrical activity in the brain.

D. NEUROIMAGING

Consistent with observations that conversion symptoms are more likely to involve the non-dominant side of the body is the finding that the majority of conversion disorder patients have unilateral right hemisphere structural or physiological abnormalities demonstrated by neuroimaging. Functional neuroimaging has demonstrated decreased activity in cortex and subcortical circuits reflecting cerebral representation of peripheral symptoms (e. g., decreased activation of visual cortex during "hysterical" blindness). These decreases have been frequently shown to be associated with concurrent activation in limbic regions such as the cingulate or orbitofrontal cortex. In general, there appears to be similarity of functional neuroimaging findings of conversion disorder and hypnosis.

E. COURSE OF ILLNESS

Most conversion symptoms remit quickly, often spontaneously. They are frequently transient reactions to acute psychosocial stressors. Prolonged symptoms are generally associated with environmental reinforcers (e. g., the symptom provides a solution to a chronic family conflict and/or disability payments). Conversion symptoms, either similar to the original symptoms or a new symptom,

Table 22–2. General Guidelines for the Treatment of Somatizing Disorders

1. The clinician must remain vigilant to the possibility that the patient has covert physical disease and may develop physical disease during the course of treatment for his or her somatization.
2. A patient with somatization should not be conceptualized from an either-or perspective. Most somatizing patients have some degree of concurrent physical disease.
3. To the greatest extent possible, medical or surgical care should be coordinated by one primary care physician. Psychiatric consultation, however, is often valuable in helping the primary care physician formulate a treatment plan for the patient.
4. The somatizing patient frequently has a comorbid psychiatric disorder. When identified, such disorders should be treated because the somatization may represent the symptomatic expression of one of these disorders.
5. The somatizing patient should not be told that his or her symptoms are psychogenic or "all in your head." Such comments are almost inevitably rejected and destroy therapeutic rapport, and they may be inaccurate.
6. Invasive diagnostic or therapeutic procedures for the somatizing patient should be initiated only for objective signs and symptoms, not for subjective complaints.
7. The acute onset of a somatoform disorder may be associated with an acute stressor in the patient's life (e. g., physical or sexual abuse).
8. Chronic somatization is rarely responsive to traditional insight-oriented psychotherapy, but behavioral modification techniques are often useful in modifying the patients' illness behavior.
9. The treatment of somatization disorders generally requires multiple treatment techniques provided by a multidisciplinary treatment team.
10. Somatization is often a chronic condition (i.e., "illness as a way of life"), and cure is improbable. Somatizing patients require ongoing management using techniques that reduce the risk of iatrogenic complications.

may occur with recurrence of stressors. This is particularly true with pseudoseizures.

Differential Diagnosis (Including Comorbidity)

The differential diagnosis of conversion disorder always involves the possibility of physical disease. Even when conversion is obvious, the patient may have underlying neurologic or other disease that he or she has unconsciously amplified or elaborated. Table 22–2 lists conditions that often cause errors in diagnosis.

Malingering must also be considered. The primary difference between malingering and conversion is that the degree of conscious motivation is higher in malingering. Systematic studies of conversion disorder suggest that it is often accompanied by other psychiatric disorders. Depression is common; and schizophrenia has also been reported, though rarely. Patients with conversion disorder may be responding to overwhelming environmental stressors that they cannot articulate, such as concurrent sexual or physical abuse or the feeling of being overwhelmed with responsibilities. Dissociative syndromes are also often associated with conversion, particularly pseudoseizures (which are regarded by some clinicians to be dissociative episodes). Some clinicians have proposed that dissociative disorders and conversion disorders involve the same mechanisms: dissociation reflects mental symptoms and conversion represents somatic symptoms. Conversion is grouped with the dissociative disorders

in *International Classification of Disease*, tenth edition (ICD-10).

Treatment

The treatment of conversion disorder is often multimodal and varies according to the acuteness of the symptom. If the symptom is acute, symptom relief often occurs spontaneously or with suggestive techniques. If the symptom is chronic, it is often being reinforced by factors in the patient's environment; therefore, behavioral modification techniques are necessary.

A. Psychopharmacologic Interventions

There are no specific psychopharmacologic interventions for conversion disorder. However, when comorbid conditions are identified (e. g., depression), these conditions must be treated with the appropriate medications (see Chapter 18 and 19).

B. Psychotherapeutic Interventions

Acute conversion symptoms may, on occasion, respond to insight-oriented psychotherapy techniques. On the whole, insight-oriented therapies have not been effective for chronic conversion symptoms, which generally require behavioral modification for symptom relief. Behavioral therapy can be offered in the context of physical or speech therapy and this offers the patient a face-saving mechanism by which the patient can gradually discard their symptoms. Patients also receive positive reinforcement for symptomatic improvement and are ignored, to avoid reinforcement, at times of symptom expression.

C. OTHER INTERVENTIONS

Hypnosis and Amobarbital Interviews: An acute conversion symptom may remit with suggestions through hypnosis or by the use of an Amytal (or lorazepam) interview that creates an altered state of consciousness. Such techniques may be useful in determining underlying psychological stressors, but caution must be exercised so that patients do not incorporate the interviewer's suggestions as a part of their own history.

D. ENVIRONMENTAL MANIPULATION

When the conversion symptom represents "a cry for help" because of environmental pressures, it may be necessary to manipulate these stressors in order to produce symptomatic relief. For example, the pseudoseizures of a teenage girl might be a cry for help because she is involved in an incestuous relationship with her stepfather. Obviously, symptom relief will require attention to the sexual abuse.

E. TREATMENT OF COMORBID DISORDERS

When identified, comorbid disorders must be treated concurrently. Conversion symptoms may respond, for example, to treatment for an underlying depression.

Complications/Adverse Outcomes of Treatment

Remission, with treatment of a conversion symptom, does not rule out the possibility that the patient has an underlying physical disease to which he or she was reacting with exaggeration or elaboration. Thus each patient must receive a careful medical evaluation. Conversely, a failure to consider conversion disorder and to continue to provide treatment as though the patient has a physical disease reinforces the symptom and can lead to permanent invalidism.

Prognosis

Most conversion symptoms remit quickly, those which persist are often associated with environmental reinforcers and are more resistant to treatment. Factors associated with a good prognosis are symptoms precipitated by stressful events, preceded by good premorbid psychological health, the absence of comorbid neurologic or psychiatric disorders.

In the past, an underlying neurologic disease would later emerge in about 25% of patients. However, at the present, with more sophisticated neurologic diagnostic tests, the subsequent emergence of previously undetected neurologic disease is uncommon.

Ford CV: Conversion disorder and somatoform disorder not otherwise specified In: Gabbard GO (ed). *Treatment of Psychiatric Disorders*, 3rd edn. Washington, DC: American Psychiatric Press Inc., 2001, pp. 1755–1776.

Varilleunier P: Hysterical conversion and brain function. In: Laureys S (ed). *Progress in Brain Research*, Vol. 150. Amsterdam Elsevier, 2005;309–329.

■ SOMATIZATION DISORDER & UNDIFFERENTIATED SOMATOFORM DISORDER

 ESSENTIALS OF DIAGNOSIS

DSM-IV-TR Diagnostic Criteria
Somatization Disorder

A. *A history of many physical complaints beginning before age 30 years that occur over a period of several years and result in treatment being sought or significant impairment in social, occupational, or other important areas of functioning.*

B. *Each of the following criteria must have been met, with individual symptoms occurring at any time during the course of the disturbance:*

(1) *four pain symptoms: a history of pain related to at least four different sites or functions (e. g., head, abdomen, back, joints, extremities, chest, rectum, during menstruation, during sexual intercourse, or during urination)*

(2) *two gastrointestinal symptoms: a history of at least two gastrointestinal symptoms other than pain (e. g., nausea, bloating, vomiting, other than during pregnancy, diarrhea, or intolerance of several different foods)*

(3) *one sexual symptom: a history of at least one sexual or reproductive symptom other than pain (e. g., sexual indifference, erectile or ejaculatory dysfunction, irregular menses, excessive menstrual bleeding, vomiting throughout pregnancy)*

(4) *one pseudoneurological symptom: a history of at least one symptom or deficit suggesting a neurological condition not limited to pain (conversion symptoms such as impaired coordination or balance, paralysis or localized weakness, difficulty swallowing or lump in throat, aphonia, urinary retention,*

hallucinations, loss of touch or pain sensation, double vision, blindness, deafness, seizures; dissociative symptoms such as amnesia; or loss of consciousness other than fainting)

C. Either (1) or (2):

(1) after appropriate investigation, each of the symptoms in Criterion B cannot be fully explained by a known general medical condition or the direct effects of a substance (e. g., a drug of abuse, a medication)

(2) when there is a related general medical condition, the physical complaints or resulting social or occupational impairment are in excess of what would be expected from the history, physical examination, or laboratory findings

D. The symptoms are not intentionally produced or feigned (as in factitious disorder or malingering).

DSM-IV-TR Diagnostic Criteria
Undifferentiated Somatoform Disorder

A. One or more physical complaints (e. g., fatigue, loss of appetite, gastrointestinal complaints).

B. Either (1) or (2):

(1) after appropriate investigation, each of the symptoms in Criterion B cannot be fully explained by a known general medical condition or the direct effects of a substance (e. g., a drug of abuse, a medication)

(2) when there is a related general medical condition, the physical complaints or resulting social or occupational impairment are in excess of what would be expected from the history, physical examination, or laboratory findings

C. The symptoms cause clinically significant distress or impairment in social, occupational, or other important areas of functioning.

D. The duration of the disturbance is at least 6 months.

E. The disturbance is not better accounted for by another mental disorder (e. g., another somatoform disorder, sexual dysfunction, mood disorder, anxiety disorder, sleep disorder, or psychotic disorder).

F. The symptom or deficit is not intentionally produced or feigned (as in factitious disorder or malingering).

(Reprinted, with permission, from *Diagnostic and Statistical Manual of Mental Disorders*, 4th edn. Text Revision. Washington DC: American Psychiatric Association, 2000.)

General Considerations

The syndrome of multiple unexplained physical symptoms was traditionally known as "hysteria" or "grand hysteria." It also received the eponym "Briquet's syndrome" for a brief time prior to being defined and renamed Somatization Disorder by the *Diagnostic and Statistical Manual of Mental Disorders*, third edition (DSM-III) in 1980. There have been repeated efforts to refine diagnostic criteria but recent phenomenological studies indicate that there is considerable overlap with hypochondriasis.

A. EPIDEMIOLOGY

Reports of the incidence of somatization disorder in the general population vary widely, depending on the populations studied and the techniques used. According to the Epidemiologic Catchment Area (ECA) studies, the incidence of somatization disorder is 0.1–0.4%. However, in one investigation of an academic family practice, 5% of patients met criteria for somatization disorder. A similarly high incidence has been demonstrated for hospitalized medical or surgical patients. Of note, most patients with somatization disorder are not diagnosed as such, and because of their "doctor-shopping" behavior they see multiple physicians, often simultaneously. The prevalence of undifferentiated somatoform disorder (the subsyndromal form of the disorder) is much higher than that of somatization disorder and may affect as much as 4–11% of the general population. Individuals who meet the full criteria for somatization disorder tend to be female, unmarried, nonwhite, poorly educated, and from rural areas.

B. ETIOLOGY

There are no well-accepted theories as to the etiology of somatization disorder. Patients with this disorder often come from chaotic, unstable, and dysfunctional families in which alcohol was abused. These patients often use physical symptoms as a coping mechanism. The high rate of psychiatric comorbidity associated with somatization disorder suggests that the disorder may represent a common final symptomatic pathway for different psychiatric problems, particularly major depression and personality disorder.

C. GENETICS

The evidence for a genetic influence in the development of somatization disorder is limited but suggestive of a common genetic tendency associated with criminality. Women are more likely to express this genetic tendency as somatization disorder, and men more likely to express it as antisocial personality disorder. It is difficult to delineate precise genetic mechanisms in the face of massive environmental influences.

Clinical Findings

A. SIGNS & SYMPTOMS

Patients with somatization disorder, by definition, present to physicians with multiple unexplained physical symptoms. These presentations are often accompanied by a sense of urgency. Thus, these patients are subjected to numerous invasive diagnostic or treatment procedures. Symptoms are multisystemic in nature and frequently involve chronic pelvic pain, atypical facial pain, and nonspecific subjective complaints such as dizziness. Medical care costs for these patients may run as high as two to eight times that of age-matched control subjects. Patients with somatization disorder also have a number of psychological symptoms, including depression, anxiety, suicidal gestures, and substance abuse. They may be addicted to prescribed medications, and at times they may exhibit drug-seeking behaviors.

B. PSYCHOLOGICAL TESTING

There are no specific psychological tests for somatization disorder, but patients with this disorder usually score high on MMPI-2 scales 1 (hypochondriasis) and 3 (hysteria) and on the somatization scale of the Symptom Check List-90, revised version. Because of high co-morbidity (see below), psychological testing is not consistent for the group as a whole.

C. LABORATORY FINDINGS

There are no specific laboratory findings for somatization disorder. The diagnosis is based on a lack of objective evidence to substantiate physical disease.

D. NEUROIMAGING

Studies reporting neuroimaging results in patients with Somatization Disorder have been inconsistent, suggesting that Somatization Disorder is a poorly defined disorder which may be the final common symptomatic pathway of several different underlying psychiatric disorders.

E. COURSE OF ILLNESS

These patients, by definition, develop multiple unexplained physical symptoms beginning in adolescence or early adulthood. Symptomatic presentation, which can be quite dramatic, is frequently associated with concurrent psychosocial stressors. The number, and intensity, of symptoms may wax and wane over time but rarely does a year or two pass without some symptomatic complaints. These patients characteristically undergo numerous invasive diagnostic and therapeutic procedures which, in retrospect, had vague indications. Somatization Disorder frequently persists into late life.

Differential Diagnosis (Including Comorbidity)

Organic physical disease is always part of the differential diagnosis for these multisymptomatic patients who often carry poorly documented diagnoses of systemic diseases (e. g., systemic lupus erythematosus). Many of these patients have received one or more "fashionable diagnosis" such as fibromyalgia, dysautonomia, chronic fatigue syndrome, or total allergy syndrome. Few physicians have the means or the energy to make complete reviews of these patients' medical records, but such reviews generally fail to demonstrate objective evidence for any of these diagnoses.

Patients with somatization disorder almost always have one or more comorbid Axis I psychiatric diagnosis and almost always meet criteria for at least one personality disorder. Despite the multiplicity of psychiatric signs and symptoms, and a medical history of multiple unexplained physical complaints, patients with somatization disorder are often unrecognized.

Treatment

Patients with somatization disorder perceive themselves as being medically ill and are unlikely to seek psychiatric care for their distress. They may resent any implication that their problems are psychogenic and may reject referrals for psychiatric treatment. Thus the primary management of these patients falls on the primary care physician and his or her capability to coordinate care with multiple medical specialists.

A. PSYCHOPHARMACOLOGIC INTERVENTIONS

There is no specific psychopharmacologic treatment for Somatization Disorder. These patients do, however, frequently suffer from comorbid psychiatric disorders such as panic disorder or depression, which should be appropriately treated (see Chapters 9, 18 and 19).

B. PSYCHOTHERAPEUTIC INTERVENTIONS

The provision of group experiences, particularly those that are supportive rather than insight-oriented, may significantly reduce medical care utilization. Group support allows these patients to feel socially connected and reduces their need to reach out to the medical system for assistance.

C. MANAGEMENT PRINCIPLES

Primary care physicians can use several simple management techniques to significantly lower medical care utilization by patients with somatization disorder. These principles include the following: (1) schedule frequent appointments without requiring development of a new symptom, (2) avoid statements that the symptoms are "all in your head," (3) undertake invasive diagnostic or therapeutic procedures only if objective signs or symptoms are present, and (4) prescribe all medications and coordinate medical care.

Complications/Adverse Outcomes of Treatment

Patients with somatization disorder are at risk for iatrogenic complications of invasive or therapeutic procedures (e. g., peritoneal adhesions resulting from multiple abdominal operations). Habituation to prescribed analgesics or anxiolytics also occurs frequently. Clinicians must exercise caution when prescribing any potentially lethal medication for these patients because they are prone to impulsive acting-out behaviors including suicide attempts. Conversely, an approach that is too confrontational about the basic psychological issues underlying the medical care–seeking behaviors may motivate these patients to find a physician who is less psychologically minded and more accommodating to requests for medications and operations.

Prognosis

Somatization disorder is a chronic problem that continues throughout the patient's life. Management principles are aimed at reducing symptoms and containing medical care costs, not at cure. These patients frequently experience iatrogenic complications from medications and surgical procedures. However, one long-term study found no evidence of reduced longevity, which suggests that these patients do not have any underlying biological disease.

Mai F: Somatization disorder: A practical review. *Can J Psychiatry* 2004;49:652–662.

Fink P, Rosendal M, Toft T: Assessment and treatment of functional disorders in general practice: The extended reattribution and management model-an advanced educational program for non-psychiatric doctors. *Psychosomatics* 2002;43:93–131.

■ HYPOCHONDRIASIS

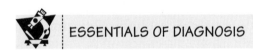 ESSENTIALS OF DIAGNOSIS

DSM-IV-TR Diagnostic Criteria

A. *Preoccupation with fears of having, or the idea that one has, a serious disease based on the person's misinterpretation of bodily symptoms.*

B. *The preoccupation persists despite appropriate medical evaluation and reassurance.*

C. *The belief in Criterion A is not of delusional intensity (as in delusional disorder, somatic type) and is not restricted to a circumscribed concern about appearance (as in body dysmorphic disorder).*

D. *The preoccupation causes clinically significant distress or impairment in social, occupational, or other important areas of functioning.*

E. *The duration of the disturbance is at least 6 months.*

F. *The preoccupation is not better accounted for by generalized anxiety disorder, obsessive–compulsive disorder, panic disorder, a major depressive episode, separation anxiety, or another somatoform disorder.*

Specify if:

With poor insight: if, for most of the time during the current episode, the person does not recognize that the concern about having a serious illness is excessive or unreasonable.

(Reprinted, with permission, from *Diagnostic and Statistical Manual of Mental Disorders*, 4th edn. Text Revision. Washington DC: American Psychiatric Association, 2000.)

General Considerations

Hypochondriasis which literally means "below the cartilage" reflects the abdominal symptoms and concerns of these patients. Hypochondriasis was once considered to be the male equivalent of "hysteria" but it is now recognized as having equal gender distribution. Recent phenomenological research suggests that there is considerable overlap between Somatization Disorder and Hypochondriasis.

A. EPIDEMIOLOGY

The incidence of hypochondriasis in the general population is not known. Between 4–6% of the patients in one internal medicine clinic met DSM-IV criteria for hypochondriasis. The typical age at onset is young adulthood, and the disorder occurs with an approximately equal frequency in men and women. Contrary to popular belief, it is not more prevalent among the elderly. Transient hypochondriasis frequently follows acute illness or injury and may be viewed as a normal hypervigilant scanning of bodily functions for detection of further injury.

B. Etiology

Hypochondriasis has been interpreted from a psychodynamic perspective as the turning inward of unacceptable feelings of anger. An alternative explanation is that hypochondriasis is learned behavior resulting from a childhood in which family members were excessively preoccupied with illness and bodily functions. Other proposed etiologies include the view that hypochondriasis is a form of depression or obsessive–compulsive disorder (OCD), with a symptomatic focus on bodily function. Hypochondriasis is likely a multidetermined disorder.

C. Genetics

Hypochondriasis is a familial disorder, but there is no direct evidence of genetic input. The increased incidence in family members can be explained on the basis of learned behavior or the indirect influence of psychiatric disorders that do have genetic input (e.g., major depression) and that occur in both the patient and family members.

Clinical Findings

A. Signs & Symptoms

The hypochondriacal patient typically presents with fear and concern about disease rather than with dramatic symptoms. The fears may emanate from the misinterpretation of normal bodily sensations. Sensations regarded as normal aches and pains by most people are interpreted by the hypochondriacal patient as evidence of serious disease. The hypochondriacal patient characteristically relates his or her history in an obsessively detailed manner, often with relatively little affect. These patients tend to be emotionally constricted and are limited in their social, occupational, and sexual functions. Many hypochondriacal patients keep their own personal medical records. They often own the Physicians' Desk Reference or the Merck Manual. They feel transient relief when reassured that they do not have serious disease but, within hours or days, begin to obsessively doubt that assurance and may return for another visit.

B. Psychological Testing

Psychological testing (e.g., The MMPI-2) generally demonstrates a preoccupation with somatic symptoms in association with underlying depression and anxiety.

C. Laboratory Findings

No laboratory findings are diagnostic of hypochondriasis. The diagnosis is often made by exclusion when all tests for physical diseases are normal.

D. Neuroimaging

There are no reported studies of neuroimaging of patients with Hypochondriasis.

E. Course of Illness

Hypochondriasis is a condition that characteristically begins in early adulthood and continues to late life. Symptoms wax and wane and symptomatic exacerbation may occur at times of occupational or interpersonal stress, with learning about an acquaintance's illness, or reading about a disease in a magazine. Worry or concern about relatively minor symptoms such as those associated with irritable bowel syndrome may escalate into an obsessional conviction of having a malignancy. At times, the patient may become so preoccupied with disease fears/conviction that interpersonal relationships are adversely impacted. Interestingly, these patients often handle genuine physical disease in an appropriate and realistic manner.

Differential Diagnosis (Including Comorbidity)

The hypochondriacal patient must be reevaluated continually for the possibility that physical disease may underlie each new symptomatic complaint. Hypochondriacal patients may have concurrent relatively benign polysymptomatic illnesses that they interpret as evidence of more severe disease. They also have a higher prevalence of major depression, panic disorder, and OCD than is expected for the general population. These patients may interpret the physiologic symptoms of major depression or panic disorder as evidence of disease.

Treatment

Treatment of hypochondriasis falls predominantly to the primary care physician to whom these patients repeatedly return; hypochondriacal patients see their problems as medical, not psychiatric. Although some patients ultimately accept referral to a psychiatrist, premature referral may destroy rapport and make management more difficult.

A. Psychopharmacologic Interventions

Symptomatic improvements of hypochondriacal symptoms have been demonstrated after administration of selective serotonin reuptake inhibitors (SSRI). This is independent of the effects of treating comorbid psychiatric illness and suggests the possibility that, at least for some patients, Hypochondriasis may be a subtype of OCD.

B. Psychotherapeutic Interventions

Hypochondriacal patients are usually not good candidates for traditional insight-oriented psychotherapy because they tend to be alexithymic (unable to express feelings in words). However, a recently developed psychotherapeutic intervention based on the principles of cognitive–behavioral therapy (CBT) appears to hold promise. The approach is based on the provision of new information, discussion, and exercises intended to modulate the sensations of benign bodily discomfort that are due to normal physiology and to help patients reattribute these sensations to their appropriate cause rather than to fears of serious illness. This combined behavioral intervention can be used by the primary care physician or by staff working within the medical setting.

Group therapy techniques can also meet these patients' needs for relationships and can be a vehicle by which cognitive–behavioral approaches are used to modify these patients' illness behavior.

C. TREATMENT OF COMORBID DISORDERS

Hypochondriasis is often accompanied by depression, anxiety, or OCD. When one or more of these disorders are present, appropriate treatment should be initiated. Hypochondriacal patients tend to be inordinately sensitive to medication side effects. They continually scan their bodies in a hypervigilant fashion for bodily sensations. It is often necessary to initiate pharmacologic treatment with very low dosages—while encouraging the patient to tolerate side effects—and then to gradually increase the dosage into the therapeutic range as tolerated.

D. MANAGEMENT PRINCIPLES

Within the primary care setting, patients should be seen at regularly scheduled intervals. Each new complaint or worry should be accompanied by a limited evaluation to ensure that it does not represent the development of organic disease. Invasive procedures should not be undertaken without clear indication. The doctor–patient relationship should be warm, trusting, and empathetic and should gradually enable these patients to express their emotional feelings more openly.

Complications/Adverse Outcomes of Treatment

Failure to recognize hypochondriasis may result in needless expense due to exhaustive medical evaluation. Purely medical management may reinforce the symptoms, and iatrogenic complications may result from unneeded invasive procedures.

Prognosis

Hypochondriasis is characterized by a chronic fluctuating course. With few exceptions, cure is not to be anticipated for these long-term patients. Patients whose hypochondriasis is related to a defined depressive episode or to panic disorder often experience a significant relief of hypochondriacal symptoms when the comorbid condition is treated effectively. A few patients with more severe chronic comorbid depression or OCD will deteriorate; some become invalids for life. Patients with good pre-

morbid psychological health who demonstrate transient hypochondriasis in response to acute illness or life stress have a good prognosis and may show complete remission of symptoms.

Margariños M, Zafar U, Nessenson K, Blanco C: Epidemiology and treatment of hypochondriasis. *CNS Drugs* 2002;16:9–22.

Creed F, Barsky F: A systematic review of the epidemiology of somatization disorder and hypochondriasis. *J Psychosom Res* 2004;56:391–408.

Barsky AJ, Ahern DK: Cognitive behavioral therapy for hypochondriasis: A randomized controlled trial. *JAMA* 2004;291:1464–1470.

■ BODY DYSMORPHIC DISORDER

 ESSENTIALS OF DIAGNOSIS

DSM-IV-TR Diagnostic Criteria

- **A.** Preoccupation with an imagined defect in appearance. If a slight physical anomaly is present, the person's concern is markedly excessive.
- **B.** The preoccupation causes clinically significant distress or impairment in social, occupational, or other important areas of functioning.
- **C.** The preoccupation is not better accounted for by another mental disorder (e. g., dissatisfaction with body shape and size in anorexia nervosa).

(Reprinted, with permission, from *Diagnostic and Statistical Manual of Mental Disorders*, 4th edn. Text Revision. Washington DC: American Psychiatric Association, 2000.)

General Considerations

Dysmorphophobia was originally described in the 19th century and has been regarded as closely related to other monosymptomatic hypochondriacal disorders (e.g., delusions of bromosis). It was first included in the *Diagnostic and Statistical Manual of Mental Disorders*, third edition, revised (DSM-III-R) in 1987. Patients with body dysmorphic disorders (BDD) are characterized by their preoccupations with perceived defects in appearance—"imagined ugliness" (a term coined by K. A. Phillips in 1991).

A. EPIDEMIOLOGY

Studies in the general population have found an incidence of BDD in the range of 1–5%. However, there are higher rates among dermatology and cosmetic surgery patients. There is probably a dimensional rather than a categorical quality to BDD that ranges from relatively normal concern with one's body (in a society preoccupied with appearance) to a delusional intensity to the preoccupation that becomes totally incapacitating.

Of those individuals who present for clinical attention, there is a roughly equal distribution between men and women. Most patients are 20–40 years old. A high percentage of these patients have never married or are unemployed.

B. ETIOLOGY

Theories of the etiology of body BDD are closely tied to issues of comorbidity (see later section). Many clinicians believe that BDD is a part of obsessive–compulsive spectrum of disorders but it is also closely related to social anxiety disorder and major depression. Cultural values that emphasize personal appearance may also contribute to the development of BDD.

C. GENETICS

No studies have reported evidence for a genetic influence in the development of BDD.

Clinical Findings

A. SIGNS & SYMPTOMS

Patients with BDD are most commonly preoccupied with hair or facial features such as the shape of the nose. Other parts of the body such as breasts or genitalia can also be the source of preoccupation. For example, a man may become preoccupied with the size of his penis. Patients may spend hours each day gazing in a mirror or other reflective surfaces. Fears of humiliation, because of the imagined defect, may cause these patients to become housebound, unable to use public transportation or attend social functions or work. These patients may visit physicians multiple times seeking treatment, particularly surgical intervention to correct defects that are imperceptible to the normal observer. Most patients with BDD spend considerable time, hours per day, in repetitive behaviors attempting to improve or hid the perceived defect. There behaviors may include attempts to camouflage the defect such as engaging in excessive grooming or behaviors such as picking at the skin. Patients with BDD, on the whole, have little insight into their condition and a considerable proportion can be described as delusional.

B. PSYCHOLOGICAL TESTING

One simple screening question, "Are you concerned about your appearance?" may lead to other questions that confirm the diagnosis. Psychological testing such as the MMPI-2, or projective testing can help determine the presence of comorbid disorders. Tests may indicate depression, OCD, social phobia, or an underlying psychotic process.

C. LABORATORY FINDINGS

No specific laboratory findings establish a diagnosis of BDD.

D. NEUROIMAGING

One study utilizing single photon emission computerized tomography (SPECT) demonstrated a broad range of findings that did not support the view of BDD as being in either the OCD or MDD spectrum of disorders. It did, however, suggest some involvement of parietal regions, consistent with cerebral areas involved in facial recognition.

E. COURSE OF ILLNESS

Patients generally have the onset of BDD in adolescence. In the more extreme forms it is associated with complete social withdrawal and a high incidence of suicide. Because of the pain from their imagined ugliness, persons with BDD are highly impaired in interpersonal relationships and their occupations; often unable to work because they are housebound. They frequently seek multiple consultations from dermatologists or plastic surgeons. The course of BDD is chronic with low rates of remission even with treatment.

Differential Diagnosis (Including Comorbidity)

The differential diagnosis of BDD includes delusional disorder, somatic type, in which the patient has a clear-cut noninsightful distortion of reality; anorexia nervosa, in which the patient has a distorted body image and refuses to maintain body weight at or above a minimally normal weight for age and height; and gender identity disorder, in the which the patient is preoccupied with his or her body, thinking that it reflects the wrong gender (i.e., transsexualism).

The large majority of patients with BDD have a comorbid psychiatric disorder, most commonly major depression, social phobia, psychotic disorders, OCD, substance abuse disorders, and personality disorders (most commonly cluster C). Persons with BDD have high rates of suicidal ideation and attempts.

Treatment

BDD can best be conceptualized as a syndrome of heterogeneous etiology rather than as a specific entity. As such, one must keep in mind the high incidence of psychiatric comorbidity and the various underlying psychiatric disorders that are manifested as a preoccupation with appearance. Many of these patients seek surgery, and the psychiatrist may be asked to render an opinion as to whether surgery is contraindicated (see below). Physicians must remain alert to the increased risk of suicide in patients with BDD.

A. Psychopharmacologic Interventions

A SSRI should be the first choice as an antidepressant medication. The SSRIs are of proven efficacy in treating BDD but are, as of yet, an "off-label" prescription; there are no FDA approved medications for BDD. Positive responses to SSRIs have been reported in patients whose symptoms have a delusional intensity, lending further credence to the opinion that BDD is in the OCD spectrum of disorders. Similar to the treatment of OCD patients being treated with SSRIs treatment response for BDD may require 10–12 weeks, at relatively high dosages.

B. Psychotherapeutic Interventions

CBT provided in either individual or group format has been demonstrated to be an effective treatment for BDD. Techniques emphasize cognitive restructuring, exposure with response prevention (e.g., exposing the perceived defect in social situations and preventing avoidance behaviors) and behavioral experiments such as empirically testing hypotheses involving dysfunctional thoughts and beliefs.

There are no reports concerning psychodynamic psychotherapy but it is unlikely that this modality would be helpful in patients with so little insight about these disorders.

C. Non-Psychiatric Medical Interventions

Although the majority of BDD patients seek non-psychiatric treatment from dermatologists and cosmetic surgeons these treatments are rarely effective and at times may worsen the disorder.

D. Treatment of Comorbid Conditions

Comorbid psychiatric conditions such as major depression and social phobia should be treated.

Complications/Adverse Outcomes of Treatment

It is important to recognize the intensity of the BDD patient's distress. These patients are at risk for suicide or the development of psychosis. Patients who receive surgical interventions are frequently displeased with the result and continue to seek further operations.

Prognosis

The long-term outcome of BDD is unknown. Diagnostic criteria for the disorder have been formulated relatively recently, and data are preliminary. Earlier reports on dysmorphophobia (an earlier described syndrome similar to BDD) suggest that a significant proportion of these patients develop psychotic processes and that most are severely disabled from their disorder. Suicide rates are markedly elevated. Recent reports of success in treating BDD with SSRIs may portend a more favorable long-term prognosis.

Looper KJ, Kirmayer LJ: Behavioral medicine approaches to somatoform disorders. *J Consult Clin Psychol* 2002;70:810–827.

Phillips KA, Pagano ME, Menaid W, Stout RL: A 12-month follow-up study on the course of body dysmorphic disorder. *Am J Psychiatry* 2006;163:907–912.

Grant JE, Phillips KA: Recognizing and treating body dysmorphic disorder. *Ann Clin Psychiatry* 2005;17:205–210.

■ PAIN DISORDER

 ESSENTIALS OF DIAGNOSIS

DSM-IV-TR Diagnostic Criteria

  A. *Pain in one or more anatomical sites is the predominant focus of the clinical presentation and is of sufficient severity to warrant clinical attention.*

  B. *The pain causes clinically significant distress or impairment in social, occupational, or other important areas of functioning.*

  C. *Psychological factors are judged to have an important role in the onset, severity, exacerbation, or maintenance of the pain.*

  D. *The symptom or deficit is not intentionally produced or feigned (as in factitious disorder or malingering).*

  E. *The pain is not better accounted for by a mood, anxiety, or psychotic disorder and does not meet criteria for dyspareunia.*

   Pain disorder associated with psychological factors

   Pain disorder associated with both psychological factors and a general medical condition

Specify if:

  Acute: duration of less than 6 months.

  Chronic: duration of 6 months or longer.

(Reprinted, with permission, from *Diagnostic and Statistical Manual of Mental Disorders*, 4th edn. Text Revision. Washington DC: American Psychiatric Association, 2000.)

General Considerations

Pain syndromes are categorized based on whether they are associated primarily with (1) psychological factors, (2) a general medical condition, or (3) psychological factors and a general medical condition. The second categorization is not considered to be a mental disorder but is related to the differential diagnosis. This classification of pain appears to be superior to previous systems because it takes into account underlying physical disease to which the patient may be reacting in an exaggerated form. Thus the clinician can avoid the either-or dualism that prevailed earlier. Most patients probably have some degree of physical disease that initiates painful sensations, and it is the response to these sensations that constitutes abnormal illness behavior.

A. Epidemiology

Pain is the most common complaint with which patients present to physicians. It is estimated that the cost to the United States economy (direct and indirect costs) for pain related disability is in the range of 100 billion dollars. A well-constructed European epidemiologic study found that pain disorder is the most common of the somatoform disorders; The incidence over one year was 8.1% and life-time incident was 12.7%. According to one U.S. study, 14% of internal medicine private patients had chronic pain. Those who seek medical care for chronic pain may be a subgroup of those who experience it.

B. Etiology

Pain is a heterogeneous disorder. No single etiologic factor is likely to apply to all patients. Among the proposed etiologies are psychodynamic formulations that pain represents an unconsciously determined punishment to expiate guilt or for aggressive feelings or an effort to maintain a relationship with a lost object. Consistent with psychodynamic theories, some patients with pain syndromes demonstrate masochistic, self-defeating personality characteristics.

Another etiologic theory proposes that pain represents learned behavior. It is hypothesized that the patient's previous experiences of personal pain have led to changes in other persons' behavior, thereby reinforcing the experience of pain and pain behaviors. Consistent with

this theory are observations that some pain patients have experienced medical illnesses or injuries associated with pain or lived in childhood homes where disease, illness, and pain were present. It has also been proposed that pain represents a somatic expression of depression. There is a high incidence of depression in pain patients and among their family members and depression often precedes pain symptoms. Another important dysphoric affect is anger which often precedes the onset of chronic pain symptoms and/or be an important factor in maintaining the pain complaints.

Because pain is a subjective symptom, it is easy to simulate. A substantial percentage of litigants who claim pain have been shown to exaggerate or outright malinger the symptom.

C. Genetics

No studies have related genetic factors to pain disorder.

Clinical Findings

A. Signs & Symptoms

Patients who repetitively seek treatment for pain may represent a subset of individuals with pain who have certain patterns of illness behavior, rather than reflecting psychological characteristics of all persons who have pain per se. Pain syndromes include fibromyalgia, atypical facial pain, chronic pelvic pain, chronic low back pain, recurrent or persistent headaches, and so on. These patients' descriptions of pain are often dramatic and include vivid descriptions such as "stabbing back pain" or "a fire in my belly."

B. Psychological Testing

Psychological tests such as the MMPI are often used to evaluate pain patients. Common findings include somatic preoccupation, underlying depression or anxiety, and a tendency to deny psychological symptoms. The McGill Pain Questionnaire, a patient self-report test, frequently discloses that the patient uses idiosyncratic and colorful words to describe his or her pain experience.

C. Laboratory Findings

In experimental settings, pain disorder patients often have a lower threshold for pain than do normal subjects. It is difficult to determine if this greater sensitivity is the result of physiologic or psychological differences.

D. Neuroimaging

Elucidation of brain mechanisms involved in pain is evolving rapidly through techniques of functional neuroimaging. Interpretations of findings remain at the investigational stage but there is promise for future clinical applications. Available information, to date, implies that the anterior cingulate cortex plays a critical role in the emotional component of pain. Chronic pain syndromes have been associated with increased activity in the somatosensory cortices, anterior cingulate cortex and the prefrontal cortex and decreased activity in the thalamus.

E. Course of Illness

No common symptoms or psychological features describe all pain patients. Despite this heterogeneity, pain patients share some features. Pain patients tend to focus on their pain as an explanation for all their problems; they deny psychological problems and interpersonal problems, except as they relate to pain. These patients frequently describe themselves as independent, yet observations of them suggest that they are dependent on others. They frequently demand that the doctor remove the pain, and they are willing to accept surgical procedures in their search for pain relief. "Doctor shopping" is common. Family dynamics are altered in a manner that makes the pain patient the focus of the family's life.

Pain patients often see themselves as disabled and unable to work or perform usual self-care activities. They demand, and often receive, a large number of medications, particularly habituating sedatives and analgesics. The pain persists despite chronic and often excessive use of these medications, on which these patients may become both psychologically and physiologically dependent.

Differential Diagnosis (Including Comorbidity)

The differential diagnosis of pain disorder inevitably involves underlying disease processes that may cause the pain. The coexistence, however, of such disease does not rule out the diagnosis of pain disorder if psychological factors are believed to exacerbate or intensify the pain experience. Patients with chronic pain have a high frequency of comorbid psychiatric disorders, including depressive spectrum disorders, anxiety disorders, conversion disorder, and substance abuse disorders. Many of these patients meet diagnostic criteria for a personality disorder, most commonly dependent, passive-aggressive, or histrionic personality disorders.

Treatment

The treatment of acute pain disorder is generally aimed at reducing the patient's underlying anxiety and the acute environmental stressors that exacerbate the patient's personal distress. Psychiatrists are much more likely to be involved in the evaluation than in the treatment of chronic

pain syndromes. Psychiatrists may see patients with these syndromes on referral or as a part of a multidisciplinary pain treatment team. Because patients with chronic pain often resent implications that their pain has psychological causes, psychiatrists are usually most effective when serving as consultants to other health care providers. Chronic pain characteristically leads to changes in behavior that are reinforced by environmental factors. These patients have often assumed an identity as a chronically disabled person and have taken a passive stance toward life. The major objectives for treatment must be to make the patient an active participant in the rehabilitation process, to reduce the patient's doctor shopping, and to identify and reduce reinforcers of the patient's pain behaviors.

A. Psychopharmacologic Interventions

Patients with chronic pain have generally received prescriptions for multiple analgesics, often including opiate medications. These patients may demand increasingly larger dosages of medication if they have become dependent, and they may exhibit considerable resistance to discontinuing or decreasing medications. Clinicians must explain to these patients that medications have not been successful in relieving pain and that other techniques are indicated. Medications may play a limited role as part of the overall treatment. As a general rule, nonsteroidal anti-inflammatory agents rather than opiates should be the first choice in medication. When more potent analgesics are indicated, they should be prescribed on a fixed-dosage schedule rather than on a variable-dosage schedule. Patients who are prescribed medication on an as-needed basis are much more likely to engage in pain behaviors to indicate the need for medication. The use of a fixed-dosage schedule enables the extinction of pain behaviors as a means of communicating the need for more medication. Patients who have been prescribed opiates either over a long period of time or in high dosages may require a detoxification program rather than abrupt discontinuation.

Antidepressant medications are often helpful to pain patients, particularly when symptoms of major depression are present. Clinical experience suggests that dual-reuptake inhibitors (serotonin and norepinephrine) such as duloxetine or venlafaxine are more effective than the specific serotonin reuptake inhibitors. Tricyclic antidepressants such as nortriptyline continue to have a role in the treatment of chronic pain patients and patients may have a beneficial response to dosages lower than those used to treat depression. Caution must be utilized in prescribing potentially habituating medications (e. g., benzodiazepines) for sleep or anxiety because these patients are at high risk for prescription drug abuse/dependency. Anecdotal reports suggest that "off label" use of the atypical antipsychotic medications (e. g., olanzapine) or antiepileptic medications (e. g., gabapentin) may be useful in some patients.

B. Psychotherapeutic Interventions

Insight-oriented psychotherapy may be helpful for the few patients who have identified unconscious conflictual issues. However, the vast majority of patients with chronic pain are not psychologically oriented, and insight psychotherapy is not efficacious. Supportive psychotherapy may be helpful in reassuring and encouraging these patients and in improving their compliance with other aspects of the treatment program. As a general rule, behavioral therapy is the most effective type of psychotherapy in the treatment of pain disorders. Both operant conditioning and CBT are widely used (see Chapter 10).

Operant conditioning is based on the concept that certain learned behaviors develop in response to environmental cues. Thus the patient has learned a variety of pain behaviors that are elicited in certain situations. Patients often communicate their pain to others (e. g., by grimacing) to elicit responses. Behavioral analysis identifies both the stimuli and the response-altering reinforcements to these behaviors. The behavioral therapist works to substitute new behaviors for previously learned pain behaviors. Patients are praised for increasing their activity and are not rewarded for pain. Behavioral techniques are most useful when the patient's family is included in the overall treatment program, so that pain behavior is not reinforced when the patient returns home.

CBT techniques focus on identifying and correcting the patient's distorted attitudes, beliefs, and expectations. One variety of this treatment involves teaching the patient how to relax or refocus thinking and behavior away from the preoccupation of pain.

C. Pain Clinics & Centers

Chronic pain patients are often disabled and receive fragmented medical care from multiple specialists. A pain clinic provides comprehensive integrated medical care. These clinics seem to work best when a strong behavioral therapy component is associated with a comprehensive evaluation and when treatment interventions include the patient's spouse, family, and when applicable, employer. The therapeutic focus of pain clinics is to transfer the patient's sense of responsibility for treatment from physicians and medications to the patient himself or herself and to work actively within a rehabilitation program to restore self-care and social and occupational functioning. The focus is on rehabilitation more than it is on pain relief. The message provided is that the patient must learn how to "play hurt." These techniques are often useful for short-term improvement in

function. Limited data are available regarding long-term outcome.

D. Treatment of Comorbid Disorders

Treatment of the symptom of pain often involves attention to coexisting or secondary psychiatric disorders. Major depression should be treated pharmacologically, and anxiety disorders should be treated as indicated with relaxation techniques, behavioral therapy, or pharmacotherapy. Substance abuse problems frequently require detoxification and appropriate rehabilitation techniques to maintain abstinence. Patients whose pain appears to be related to symptoms of posttraumatic stress disorder may require treatment for that disorder; specialized treatment programs for the survivors of violent crimes or sexual abuse may be indicated.

Complications/Adverse Outcomes of Treatment

Pain disorder patients are at risk for iatrogenic addiction to opiate compounds or benzodiazepines. These patients often sabotage their treatment programs, proclaim that psychiatric treatment was not successful, and then use this as proof that their pain has a physical cause.

Prognosis

Surprisingly little information is available concerning prognosis for chronic pain patients. Clinicians may see patients who have complained of chronic pain for many years, even decades, and who, in the interim, have been subjected to multiple surgical procedures and have experienced iatrogenic complications. Factors known to be of poor prognostic significance include ongoing litigation related to the pain (e.g., when the illness or accident that caused the pain was associated with a potentially compensable injury), unemployment, loss of sexual interest, or a history of somatization prior to the onset of chronic pain.

Eisendrath SJ: Psychiatric aspects of chronic pain. Neurology 1995;45(Suppl A):S26.

Fishbain DA et al.: Chronic pain-associated depression: Antecedent or consequences of chronic pain? A review. *Clin J Pain*, 1997;13:116.

deLeeuw R, Albuquerque R. Okeson J, Carlson C: The contribution of neuroimaging techniques to the understanding of supraspinal pain circuits: Implications for orofacial pain. *Oral Surg Oral Med Oral Pathol Oral Radiol Endod* 2005;100:308–314.

Fallon BA. Pharmacotherapy of somatoform disorders. *J Psychosomatic Res* 2004;56:455–460.

Dersh J, Polatin PB, Gatchel RJ. Chronic pain and psychopathology: research findings and theoretical considerations. *Psychosom Med* 2002;64:773–786.

■ SOMATOFORM DISORDER NOT OTHERWISE SPECIFIED

The diagnostic category of somatoform disorder not otherwise specified consists of a widely varied group of disorders that mimic physical disease or have an uncertain psychological relationship to physical disease. Included among these disorders are false pregnancy, psychogenic urinary retention, and mass psychogenic illness (so-called mass hysteria).

General Principles for the Treatment of Somatizing Patients

As noted earlier in this chapter, the somatizing disorders display considerable phenomenological overlap and fluidity of symptomatic expression over time. Relatively few somatizing patients fit clearly into one of the somatoform disorder categories described in this chapter. Table 22–2 provides general guidelines for the management of somatizing disorders.

Factitious Disorders and Malingering 23

Charles V. Ford, MD

▉ FACTITIOUS DISORDERS

 ESSENTIALS OF DIAGNOSIS

DSM-IV-TR Diagnostic Criteria

A. *Intentional production or feigning of physical or psychological signs or symptoms.*

B. *The motivation for the behavior is to assume the sick role.*

C. *External incentives for the behavior (such as economic gain, avoiding legal responsibility, or improving physical well-being, as in malingering) are absent.*

(Reprinted, with permission, from *Diagnostic and Statistical Manual of Mental Disorders,* 4th edn. Text Revision. Washington DC: American Psychiatric Association, 2000.)

Factitious disorders are consciously determined surreptitious simulations or productions of diseases. Factitious illness behavior is relatively uncommon, but when present it consumes large amounts of professional time and medical costs. The Munchausen syndrome by proxy is a particularly malignant form of child abuse that physicians must identify and manage in order to save the health or lives of children.

DSM-IV-TR lists the following four diagnostic subtypes of factitious disorder:

1. Factitious Disorder with Predominantly Psychological Signs & Symptoms

Patients with factitious disorders may simulate psychological conditions and psychiatric disorders. For example, a patient may feign bereavement by reporting that someone to whom he or she was close has died or been killed in an accident. Patients may simulate symptoms of posttraumatic stress disorder or provide false reports of previous trauma (e.g., a civilian accident or combat experience). Closely related to factitious posttraumatic stress disorder is the false victimization syndrome, in which the patient falsely claims some type of abuse. For example, a woman may falsely report that she had been raped. Other simulated psychological disorders include various forms of dementia, amnesia, or fugue; multiple personality disorder; and more rarely, schizophrenia.

2. Factitious Disorder with Predominantly Physical Signs & Symptoms

The production of physical symptoms or disease is probably the most common form of factitious disorder. Essentially all medical diseases and symptoms have been either simulated or artificially produced at one time or another. Among the most common of these disorders are factitious hypoglycemia, factitious anemia, factitious gastrointestinal bleeding, pseudoseizures, simulation of brain tumors, simulation of renal colic, and more recently, simulation of AIDS.

3. Factitious Disorder with Combined Psychological & Physical Signs & Symptoms

A patient may be admitted to the hospital with factitious physical symptoms and, in the course of hospitalization, perhaps in an attempt to obtain more sympathy or interest, may report or simulate a variety of psychological symptoms such as having experienced the recent loss of a close relative or friend or having been raped in the past.

4. Factitious Disorder Not Otherwise Specified

This category is reserved for forms of factitious disorder that do not fit one of the other categories. It includes the Munchausen syndrome by proxy, in which one person surreptitiously induces disease or reports disease in another person. Most commonly, this is the behavior of a mother in reference to a young child.

General Considerations

Factitious illnesses have been known since the Roman era and were described in Galen's textbook of medicine. Modern interest in this surreptitious production of symptoms presented to physicians was spurred by Ashers 1951 description and naming of "The Munchausen Syndrome;" subsequently over 2000 articles in professional journals have described, and tried to explain, this perverse form of illness behavior.

A. EPIDEMIOLOGY

The true incidence of factitious illness behavior is unknown but is probably more common than is recognized. One Canadian study estimated that approximately 1 in 1000 hospital admissions is for factitious disease. However, another investigation of an entirely different type determined that approximately 3.5% of renal stones submitted for chemical analysis were bogus and represented apparent attempts to deceive the physician. A study of patients referred with fever of unknown origin to the National Institutes of Health found that almost 10% had a factitious fever. One can conclude that the incidence of factitious disorder, except in certain specialized clinical settings, is relatively uncommon but may be more frequent than is recognized.

Age and gender distribution varies according to the clinical syndromes described in the next section. Patients with the full-blown Munchausen syndrome are most frequently unmarried middle-aged men who are estranged from their families. Patients with common factitious disorder are most likely to be unmarried women in their 20 s or 30 s who work in health-service jobs such as nursing. Perpetrators of the Munchausen syndrome by proxy are most often mothers of small children who themselves may have previously engaged in factitious disease behavior or meet the criteria for somatization disorder.

B. ETIOLOGY

Explanations for the apparently nonsensical and bizarre behavior of factitious disorder are largely speculative. Underlying motivations for this behavior are probably heterogeneous and multidetermined. The following explanations have been suggested:

1. The search for nurturance—Individuals in the sick role are characteristically excused from societal obligations and cared for by others. When alternative sources of care, support, and nurturance are lacking, a person may deliberately induce illness as a way of seeking such support. Many patients with factitious disorder are themselves caretakers. Factitious illness behavior allows for a reversal of roles: instead of caring for others, the patient assumes the dependent cared-for role.

2. Secondary gains—Patients with factitious disorders sometimes use illness to obtain disability benefits or release from usual obligations such as working. Their illnesses may elicit from family members attention that might not otherwise be forthcoming. When litigation is involved, the boundary between factitious disorder and malingering becomes blurred or disappears.

3. The need for power & superiority—A person who successfully perpetuates a ruse may have a feeling of superiority in his or her capacity to fool others. This has been described as "putting one over" or "duping delight." Thus, the individual can experience a transformation from feeling weak and impotent to feeling clever and powerful over others. Simultaneously the individual may devalue others whom he or she regards as stupid or foolish because they have been deceived.

4. To obtain drugs—Some patients have used factitious illness to obtain drugs. Even those patients who have sought controlled substances appear to have done so more for the thrill of fooling the physician than because of addiction.

5. To create a sense of identity—A patient with severe characterological defects may have a poor sense of self. The creation of the sick role and the associated pseudologia fantastica (pathologic lying) may provide the patient with a role by which his or her personal identity is established. Such a person is no longer faceless but rather the star player in high drama.

6. To defend against severe anxiety or psychosis—A patient with overwhelming anxiety due to fears of abandonment or powerlessness may use a factitious illness to defend against psychological decompensation. Through the perpetuation of a successful fraud and the simultaneous gratification of dependency needs, the patient feels powerful, in control, and cared for.

C. GENETICS

No information is available regarding a relationship between factitious disorders and heredity.

Clinical Findings

A. SIGNS & SYMPTOMS

DSM-IV-TR diagnostic criteria do not adequately describe the different clinical syndromes of persons who present with factitious disorder. Three major syndromes have been identified, although some overlap may exist.

1. Munchausen syndrome (peregrinating factitious disorder)—The original Munchausen syndrome, as first described by Asher in 1951, consists of the simulation of disease, pseudologia fantastica, and peregrination (wandering). Some patients with this disorder have achieved great notoriety. These patients typically present to emergency rooms at night or on the weekends when they are more likely to encounter inexperienced clinicians and when insurance offices are more likely to be closed. Their symptoms are often dramatic and indicate the need for immediate hospitalization. Once hospitalized, they become "star patients" because of their dramatic symptoms, the rarity of their apparent diagnosis (e.g., intermittent Mediterranean fever), or because of the stories that they tell about themselves (e.g., tales of being a foreign university president or a former major league baseball player). These patients confuse physicians because of inconsistencies in their physical and laboratory findings and because of their failure to respond to standard therapeutic measures. They rarely receive visitors, and it is difficult to obtain information concerning prior hospitalizations; their frequent use of aliases makes it difficult to track them. When confronted with their factitious illness behavior, they often become angry, threaten to sue, and sign out of the hospital against medical advice. They then travel to another hospital, where they once again perpetuate their ruses.

Personal historical information about Munchausen syndrome patients is limited because they are unreliable historians and are reluctant to divulge accurate personal information. What is known may be somewhat selective in that it is derived from a subgroup of patients who have allowed themselves to be studied. These individuals often come from chaotic, stressful childhood homes. They sometimes report that they were institutionalized or hospitalized during childhood, experiences that were not regarded as frightening but rather were considered a reprieve from stress at home. Childhood neuropathic traits (e.g., lying or fire setting) are often reported. Many of these patients have worked in health-related fields (e.g., as a hospital corpsman in the military). Many have a history of psychiatric hospitalization and legal difficulties.

2. Common factitious disorder (non-peregrinating) —The most common form of factitious disorder is common factitious disorder. Disease presentations may involve dermatologic conditions from self-inflicted injuries or infections, blood dyscrasia from the surreptitious use of dicumarol or self-phlebotomy, hypoglycemia from the surreptitious use of insulin, and other diseases. The patient generally has one primary symptom or finding (e.g., anemia) and is characteristically hospitalized on multiple occasions, but the physician or hospital staff never learns the true nature of the underlying "disease." In the process of their hospitalizations, these patients become the object of considerable concern from physicians, colleagues, and family members, with whom they typically have conflicted relationships.

Patients with common factitious disorder often lie, exaggerate, and distort the truth but not to the same extent, or with the degree of fantasy, as those with the Munchausen syndrome. Patients with common factitious disorder may perpetuate the ruse for years before being discovered. Unmasked, these patients typically react with hostility, eliciting angry disbelief from treating physicians, nurses, and other staff. Even in the face of incontrovertible evidence, these patients often continue to deny the true nature of their problems.

Patients with common factitious disorder typically come from dysfunctional families and exhibit histrionic or borderline personality characteristics.

3. Munchausen syndrome by proxy —This invidious disorder, in which a mother produces disease in her child, was first described in 1978. Subsequently, hundreds of case reports from all over the world have confirmed this form of child abuse. Every major children's hospital will see several cases per year.

In the Munchausen syndrome by proxy, the perpetrator (usually the mother) presents a child (usually an infant) for medical treatment of either simulated or factitiously produced disease. For example, the child may have collapsed after the mother surreptitiously administered laxatives or other medications, or the child may have experienced repeated attacks of apnea secondary to suffocation (e.g., by pinching the nostrils). After the child has been hospitalized, the mother is intensely involved in her child's care and with the ward staff. Interestingly, the mother is surprisingly willing to sign consent forms for invasive diagnostic procedures or treatment. The child may inexplicably improve when the mother is out of the hospital for a period of time. The child's father is usually uninvolved or absent.

When the mother is confronted with suspicions (or proof) that she has caused the child's illness, she often reacts with angry denial and hospital staff may also express disbelief. Reasonable suspicion of Munchausen syndrome by proxy mandates reporting, as a form of child abuse, to the appropriate child protective services. Children who have been victims of Munchausen syndrome by proxy have a high mortality rate (almost 10% die before reaching adulthood). Studies of their siblings show a similarly high mortality rate because this disease-producing behavior may be perpetrated on subsequent children. These children may need to be placed outside the home (e.g., with other relatives or in a foster-care setting).

B. PSYCHOLOGICAL TESTING

Psychological test results of Munchausen syndrome patients reflect severe characterological problems often of the sociopathic, narcissistic, or histrionic type. Approximately 30% of Munchausen syndrome patients have some form of cerebral dysfunction. This dysfunction is most commonly demonstrated by the patient's verbal IQ score being significantly greater than his or her performance IQ score, a finding possibly related to pseudologia fantastica.

Test results of patients with common factitious disorder are consistent with histrionic or borderline personality traits, somatic preoccupation, and conflicts about sexuality.

Test results of the perpetrators of Munchausen syndrome by proxy may reflect personality disorders (e.g., narcissistic) and concurrent Axis I disorders (e.g., major depression). Frequently they demonstrate no clear-cut abnormality.

C. LABORATORY FINDINGS

Laboratory testing may disclose inconsistent findings, not typical of known physical diseases (e.g., the pattern of hypokalemia that occurs with surreptitious ingestion of diuretics). The presence of toxins or medications, the use of which the patient denies, may establish the diagnosis of factitious disease behavior. For example, phenolphthalein may be present in the stool of a baby who is experiencing diarrhea as a result of Munchausen syndrome by proxy.

D. NEUROIMAGING

No neuroimaging studies have been reported specifically for factitious disorder. However, in view of the extensive lying in which these persons engage and some similarities to malingering, it would be reasonable to expect similarities to findings with lying/malingering (see below).

E. COURSE OF ILLNESS

The deceptive nature of persons with factitious illness behavior precludes good data concerning either the course of the disease or the prognosis. We do know that some patients with common factitious disorder may persist in their symptom production for years. They may give it up spontaneously or perhaps after being "caught" and confronted. Persons with Munchausen syndrome may perpetrate their simulation of disease for decades, often traveling widely and using aliases to make tracking more difficult. Some patients die as a result of miscalculations in their illness productions. Other patients trade the drama of the hospital for the drama of the courtroom and sue physicians for causing the very disease that the patient him/herself created (e.g., suing a surgeon for postoperative infections that were self-induced).

Differential Diagnosis (Including Comorbidity)

As with all somatizing disorders, the diagnosis of factitious disorders involves ruling out the presence of a genuine disease process. Patients with factitious disorder often have physical disease, but the disease is the result of deliberate and surreptitious behavior such as self-phlebotomy. Occasionally, a patient with a genuine physical disease (e.g., diabetes mellitus) will learn how to manipulate symptoms and findings in such a way as to create a combination of physical disease and factitious disorder. In such cases, both the disease process and the behavior will require therapeutic attention.

Factitious disorder must also be distinguished from malingering; the difference here is one of motivation. The person with malingering has a definable external goal that motivates the behavior, such as disability payments from an insurance company, whereas with factitious disorders, the patient's goal is to seek the sick role for the psychological needs it fulfills. Malingering and factitious disorders often overlap.

Patients with factitious disorders may also meet the criteria for other somatoform disorders, particularly somatization disorder or other Axis I disorders such as major depression or, more rarely, schizophrenia. Most patients with factitious disorders are comorbid for one of the cluster B personality disorders (i.e., antisocial, borderline, histrionic, narcissistic).

Treatment

Therapeutic approaches to factitious disorder must be different from those used to treat specific disease states. A factitious disorder represents disordered behavior that is determined by widely varied and often multiple motivations. The clinician must evaluate and develop a separate treatment plan for each patient. Further, because factitious behavior is often associated with severe personality disorders the clinician must avoid splitting and other manipulative behaviors by the patient. Thus, a multidisciplinary management strategy involving attorneys, nurses, social workers, and other professionals is essential. Unfortunately, for many patients with factitious disorder, the goal must be to contain symptoms and avoid unnecessary and expensive medical care rather than to effect a cure.

A. PSYCHOPHARMACOLOGIC INTERVENTIONS

There are no pharmacologic treatments that are specific for factitious diseases.

B. PSYCHOTHERAPEUTIC INTERVENTIONS

The overwhelming majority of patients with factitious illness have severe underlying personality disorders. Despite their superficial confidence and, at times, braggadocio, these patients are fragile. They are not candidates for confrontative insight-oriented psychotherapy and may decompensate in such treatment. The techniques described in this section are suggested for use by either psychiatrists or other members of the medical treatment team as indicated. Many patients completely reject any psychiatric treatment, and therapeutic efforts must be made by nonpsychiatric personnel.

1. Individual psychotherapy—Psychotherapy needs to be supportive, empathic, and nonconfrontative. At times just "being there" and allowing the patient to talk, even if much of the talk consists of pseudologia fantastica, provides sufficient support for the patient to no longer have the immediate need to engage in factitious illness behavior. Such treatment is not curative but helps prevent further iatrogenic complications and high medical utilization.

2. Face-saving opportunities—At times the patient will discard the symptom if he or she does not need to admit the behavior. For example, the patient may be told that the problem will resolve with physical therapy, medications, or other treatment techniques. The patient may use such an opportunity to discard symptoms in a face-saving manner and behavior without ever overtly acknowledging culpability for factitious illness behavior.

3. Inexact interpretations—Insight-oriented psychotherapy is almost always contraindicated. However, it may be useful to make interpretations without direct confrontation. For example, a patient whose factitious illness behavior is tied to losses or separation might be told in a very general way that it seems that he or she has difficulty in dealing with disappointments in life.

4. Therapeutic double-binds—The patient who is suspected of factitious illness behavior might be told that such suspicions exist—and that if symptoms fail to respond to a proposed treatment then such a failure would be confirmation of factitious illness. Although this technique may be symptomatically effective, there are obvious questions as to its ethical appropriateness. For example, is it ethical to lie to a lying patient in order to effect change?

5. Family therapy—Patients with simple factitious disorder often come from dysfunctional families and are experiencing current conflicted interpersonal relationships. The patient's factitious illness behavior may be a way of controlling or manipulating the family in order to obtain a sense of power or gratification of dependency needs. Family therapy may be one way to address distorted communications in the family and provide for the more appropriate expression of needs.

C. OTHER INTERVENTIONS

1. Staff meetings—When factitious disorder is suspected, the treating physician must recruit a multidisciplinary task force to assist with ethics and management. Such a task force, and associated staff meetings, educate all health care personnel as to the nature of the disorder, facilitate communication in such a manner as to defuse attempts by the patient to split staff, and ensure a united front for treatment. The multidisciplinary task force might include hospital administrators, the hospital attorney, a chaplain or ethicist, the patient's primary physician, a psychiatrist, and representatives from the nursing staff. Although this degree of involvement may seem like overkill, it is necessary in order to anticipate medicolegal complications.

2. Confrontation—When factitious disorder is suspected or has been confirmed, the medical staff must confront the patient. Such confrontation is generally best accomplished with several of the multidisciplinary staff members present. The staff should communicate to the patient that they know he or she has been surreptitiously producing or simulating the disease and that such behavior is indicative of internal distress. The staff should suggest to the patient that it is time to reformulate the illness from a physical disease to a psychological disorder. The patient should be told that the treatment team is concerned and that appropriate help and treatment can be made available. Despite such a supportive approach, many patients will continue to deny that they have contributed to their illness and will angrily reject any referral for psychological help.

3. Treatment of comorbid disorders—Patients must be evaluated carefully for comorbid psychiatric disorders such as major depression or schizophrenia. The presence of another Axis I disorder is relatively uncommon but when present must be treated before proceeding with psychotherapy and other management.

D. TREATMENT ISSUES IN MUNCHAUSEN SYNDROME BY PROXY

When the victim of Munchausen syndrome by proxy is a child, it may be necessary to place the child in foster care in order to protect his or her health and life. The child will require supportive psychological assistance to deal with separation from the parent and changes in his or her environment.

Perpetrators of Munchausen syndrome by proxy, usually mothers, generally have severe personality disorders, which are very difficult to treat. This is especially true when the perpetrator continues to deny her behavior. Many psychiatrists believe that return of the child to the mother must depend on the mother's acknowledgment of her behavior, the requirement that she stop it, and her recognition of the needs and rights of the child. These mothers may have severe narcissistic personality disorder. They may view others merely as objects to be manipulated rather than as separate persons with feelings, needs, and rights. When there is a history of an unexplained death of a sibling, extra care must be taken to ensure the safety of the child.

E. ETHICAL & MEDICOLEGAL ISSUES

Many ethical and medicolegal issues are raised in treating factitious disorders. Some physicians may believe that because patients with these disorders are liars, they can treat them in a cavalier manner. The following discussion demonstrates that this is not the case.

1. Confidentiality—Because a patient with factitious disorder has presented himself or herself to the physician fraudulently, violating the traditional doctor-patient relationship, a legitimate question can be raised as to whether this invalidates the physician's obligation of confidentiality. To what extent should such an individual be allowed to perpetuate fraud, as it may affect family members, friends, and other physicians? This question is not easily answered, but from a medicolegal standpoint any violation of confidentiality must be in the interest of protecting the patient's health or significantly reducing the damage to others. Such violations should not occur capriciously but only after careful consideration and consultation with the multidisciplinary task force.

2. Surreptitious room searches—The medical literature on factitious disorders contains multiple descriptions of searches of patients' rooms after they have been sent off for testing or for other reasons. Syringes and other paraphernalia may have been found, thereby confirming the diagnosis. Such searches, however, violate patients' civil rights and should be undertaken only after careful consideration and consultation with the multidisciplinary task force.

3. Withdrawal of medical care—The physician who finds that he or she has been the object of the fraudulent seeking of medical care is likely to react with anger and possibly rejection. The expenditure of professional time and the use of scarce medical supplies for patients with factitious disorders may be questioned. However, an analogy can be drawn to the question of whether medical care should be withdrawn from a patient with liver cirrhosis who continues to drink alcohol or from a patient with emphysema who continues to smoke cigarettes. The point at which one starts to enter the "slippery slope" is always an issue for debate. Medical care should be withdrawn only after careful consideration of the medicolegal ramifications.

4. Involuntary psychiatric treatment—Many patients with factitious disorder engage in self-injurious behavior that could permanently affect body function or cause death. Involuntary psychiatric treatment has been suggested but is generally rejected by the courts. In one case, a judge provided an "outpatient commitment" for a patient and ordered that all of her (publicly funded) medical care be coordinated by a guardian. Such an approach seems eminently reasonable, but it may be difficult to effect in many states, especially if the patient is covered by private insurance.

5. Malpractice Lawsuits—On the surface, one might ask how or why a patient might ever initiate a malpractice lawsuit against a physician when the patient is responsi-

ble for the medical illness. Such lawsuits, however, have occurred and can emerge in one of two different forms. One form of lawsuit can occur because many of these patients have severe borderline personality disorder. Such individuals are likely to idealize a physician initially and then later devalue him or her. With such devaluation comes rage and a resort to malpractice suits as a way of inflicting injury. The lay people who comprise juries are not knowledgeable about factitious disorders and may side with the patient.

Another form of lawsuit can occur when the patient admits factitious disorder and sues the physician for failure to recognize it. In other words, "I was lying to you, but this is a recognized medical illness, and you were incompetent not to have recognized my fraudulent behavior." One such lawsuit was settled out of court with a payment to the patient.

6. Reporting Requirements—If the health of another individual is involved (particularly that of a child), the clinician is legally required to report his or her suspicions to the appropriate authorities. In the case of children, this is a legal requirement equivalent to that of reporting any suspected child abuse. Insofar as the report is made in good faith, the physician is exempt from prosecution for the violation of confidentiality.

Complications/Adverse Outcomes of Treatment

Patients with factitious disorder have a remarkable ability to obtain hospitalization and to be treated with invasive procedures. As a result, these patients often experience unnecessary operations such as nephrectomies and even pancreatectomies. They are at risk for a number of iatrogenic complications, and physicians may contribute to drug dependence. Hundreds of thousands of dollars, millions in some cases, may be spent in the diagnosis and treatment of surreptitious and self-induced illness. The physician is also at risk. When angered, patients with these disorders may initiate lawsuits and, at the very least, will generally create disarray and dissension among their medical caretakers.

For the victim of the Munchausen syndrome by proxy, the clinician's failure to recognize the disorder or to take decisive action may result in continued medical treatment, medical complications, or even death.

Prognosis

Relatively little is known about the long-term outcome of factitious disorder. Some patients die as a result of their factitious illness behavior, and others experience severe medical complications including the loss of organs (e.g., pancreas or kidney) or limbs. If the factitious disorder is the outgrowth of, for example, a psychotic depression, the prognosis is better than if the factitious illness results from severe personality disorder, as is usually the case. Although there are reports of successful psychotherapeutic intervention with some patients, there is no evidence of continued remission on follow-up. Munchausen syndrome appears to be relatively refractory to treatment, although the ultimate outcome for most of these patients is unknown. When confronted, some patients with common factitious disorder enter psychotherapy and appear to improve and demonstrate fewer symptoms. Some patients deny their illness and merely change physicians, continuing their factitious illness behavior elsewhere; other patients deny their illness but apparently cease their behavior after being confronted with it.

The long-term prognosis of Munchausen syndrome by proxy is not encouraging. Victims have a high mortality rate during childhood, and those who survive childhood may develop somatoform disorders or factitious disorders upon reaching adulthood. Because this is a recently recognized disorder, long-term follow-up information is not yet available.

Asher R: Munchausen syndrome. *Lancet* 1951;1:339.

Krahn LE, Li H, O'Connor MK: Patients who strive to be ill: Factitious disorder with physical symptoms. *Am J Psychiatry* 2003;160:1163–1168.

Ford CV: Deception Syndromes: Factitious disorders and malingering. In: Levensen JL (eds). *Textbook of psychosomatic Medicine.* Washington, DC: American Psychiatric Publishing, 2005, pp. 297–309.

Sheridan MS: The deceit continues: An updated literature review of Munchausen Syndrome by proxy. *Child Abuse Negl* 2003;27:431–451.

Eisendrath SJ, McNeil DE: Factitious physical disorders, litigation and mortality. *Psychosomatics* 2004;45:350–352.

■ MALINGERING

General Considerations

Malingering differs from factitious disorder in that it is a deliberate disease simulation with a specific goal (e.g., to obtain opiates). Malingering is underdiagnosed, often because of the physician's fear of making false accusations. However, covert surveillance has indicated that as many as 20% of pain clinic patients misrepresent the extent of their disability.

Malingering may include the deliberate production of disease or the exaggeration, elaboration, or false report of symptoms. The essential diagnostic issue for malingering is the determination that the person is willfully simulating disease for a defined purpose. But no physician is a mind reader. Thus conscious intent must be inferred from other behaviors and psychological testing.

Malingering is not a medical/psychiatric diagnosis but rather a situation in which someone is deliberately using a bogus illness to obtain a recognizable goal. The goal may be deferment from military service, escape from incarceration (e.g., not guilty by reason of insanity), procurement of controlled substances, or monetary compensation in a personal injury lawsuit.

The judgment of the morality of malingering is largely a matter of the observer and circumstances. Most people would regard the defraudment of an insurance company, through a false injury, as an antisocial act. In contrast, the malingering of a prisoner of war, who is attempting to manipulate his or her captors, would be seen by most compatriots as a skillful coping mechanism.

A. EPIDEMIOLOGY

Malingering is most frequently seen in settings in which there may be an advantage to being sick (e.g., in the military or in front of worker's compensation review boards). The prevalence of malingering is not known, but it is most likely underdiagnosed.

B. ETIOLOGY

Malingering, by definition, is determined by a person's willful behavior to use illness for an external goal. It has been proposed, however, that malingering is one extreme of a continuum of conscious–unconscious motivation that is anchored at the other extreme by conversion symptoms. Many simulated symptoms lie somewhere between these extremes and have both conscious and unconscious components.

Patients with antisocial personality disorder are believed to be more inclined to malinger, using physical symptoms as one of their means to manipulate or defraud others. All personality types, however, have been described in association with malingering, and it can be viewed as a coping mechanism when other coping strategies are ineffective. For example, a malingered symptom may be one mechanism for an exploited laborer to get out of an intolerable work situation.

C. GENETICS

There are no reported studies that have linked malingering with heredity.

Clinical Findings

A. SIGNS & SYMPTOMS

Malingering may involve either exaggeration or elaboration of genuine illness for secondary gain (e.g., continued disability after a mild industrial injury) or the simulation of disease (e.g., faked injuries after a contrived automobile accident). Malingering may be inferred in persons who behave differently and demonstrate different function when they think they are not being observed. For example, insurance companies may covertly videotape "disabled workers" who water ski on weekends. Psychiatric disorders may also be malingered. Perhaps the most common of these are posttraumatic stress disorder and postconcussive syndrome. These disorders are characterized by subjective, often difficult to quantify, symptoms and a higher probability of being associated with potential compensable injuries.

B. Psychological Testing

Malingered psychological symptoms can often be detected from psychological testing. The validity scales of the Minnesota Multiphasic Personality Inventory-2 (MMPI-2) may demonstrate changes indicative of false reporting. Mental status examinations and psychological testing may reveal findings that are inconsistent with, or clearly not typical of, the simulated disorder. Forced choice tests may indicate that the suspected malingerer has in a statistically significant manner answered questions in an incorrect way thereby demonstrating he/she actually knew the correct answer.

C. Laboratory Findings

There are no specific laboratory tests for malingering. Some diagnostic tests may be abnormal if the person is deliberately exacerbating an existing disease or creating a new disease (e.g., surreptitious use of a diuretic).

D. Neuroimaging

Although no specific test utilizing neuroimaging to detect malingering has yet been standardized, there is considerable evidence that deception does induce brain activation. In one recently reported study of feigned memory impairment findings included bilateral activation of prefrontal cerebral regions with both genders, and different mother tongues, suggesting the importance of these regions during malingering and deception in general. This finding is consistent with a number of other studies that suggest attempted deception is associated with greater activation of executive brain functions (anterior cingulate and prefrontal cortices) as compared to truthfulness.

E. Course of Illness

A malingering symptom is generally discarded when the desired goal (e.g., financial compensation) is achieved or if the malingerer suspects that the deception has been detected. On occasion, with long standing simulated symptoms, the symptom may persist; perhaps to save face or because it has been incorporated into the person's identity.

Differential Diagnosis

The differential diagnosis of malingering includes physical disease; factitious disorder (i.e., with no discernible motive); somatoform disorders, particularly conversion disorder (in which the motive is unconscious); and pseudo-malingering. In the latter situation the patient believes that he or she is in conscious control of a symptom but actually has a disease (e.g., a person who is psychotic pretends to be psychotic in order to hide from himself the fact that he is not in control of his mental processes).

Treatment

"Treatment" of malingering is, in a sense, a contradiction in terms because the "patient" does not want to be well until the desired goal (e.g., financial compensation) is achieved. The physician must be alert in order to avoid becoming an accomplice in the malingerer's manipulations.

A. Psychopharmacologic Interventions

There are no known psychopharmacologic interventions for malingering.

B. Psychotherapeutic Interventions

There are no known psychotherapeutic interventions for malingering.

C. Subtle Confrontation

At times, subtle hints to the malingerer that the ruse has been detected will motivate the malingerer to drop the malingered symptom in a face-saving manner.

Complications/Adverse Outcomes of Treatment

It is commonly believed that malingered symptoms disappear when the malingering has achieved the patient's goal. In the process of the illness, the malingerer may experience iatrogenic complications of diagnostic or therapeutic procedures. A psychological complication occurs when, after years of litigation, the malingerer has come to believe in the illness (i.e., through learned behavior) and does not relinquish the symptom after successful resolution of the lawsuit.

Prognosis

Little is known about the prognosis of malingering. Persons who are successful at perpetuating disease simulations do not come to medical attention.

Kay NR, Morris-Jones H: Pain clinic management of medico-legal litigants. *Injury* 1998;29:305.

Pankratz L: *Patients Who Deceive: Assessment and Management of Risk in Providing Health Care and Financial Benefits.* Springfield, IL: Charles C Thomas, 1998.

Lee TMC, Liu HL, Chan CCH, et al.: Neural correlates of feigned memory impairment. *Neuroimage* 2005;28:305–313.

Miller LS, Donders J: Subjective symptomatology after traumatic head injury. *Brain Inj* 2001;15:297–304.

Dissociative Disorders

Barry Nurcombe, MD

ESSENTIALS OF DIAGNOSIS

Types of dissociative disorders according to DSM-IV-TR

Dissociative amnesia

Dissociative fugue

Dissociative identity disorder

Depersonalization disorder

Dissociative disorder not otherwise specified

(Reprinted, with permission, from *Diagnostic and Statistical Manual of Mental Disorders*, 4th edn., Text Revision. Washington DC: American Psychiatric Association, 2000.)

General Considerations

The cardinal feature of the dissociative disorders is an acute or gradual, transient or persistent, disruption of consciousness, perception, memory or awareness, not associated with physical disease or organic brain dysfunction, and severe enough to cause distress or impairment. Four types are described in DSM-IV-TR, and there is a miscellaneous fifth group. The distinction between these types may be blurred, particularly when patients exhibit symptoms from more than one type.

A. Epidemiology

Epidemiologic data on dissociative disorders are patchy. Studies of combat soldiers have found a prevalence of dissociative amnesia of 5–8%. There are no reliable data on dissociative fugue. The prevalence of dissociative identity disorder is disputed but probably low. Case reports suggest a female-to-male ratio of at least 5:1. This ratio might be exaggerated, because males with dissociative disorder, who are likely to be episodically violent, are likely to be directed to the correctional system. Dissociative identity disorder is found in all ethnic groups, though mainly in whites, and in all socioeconomic groups. Depersonalization is a frequent concomitant of anxiety disorders,

posttraumatic stress disorder, and severe depression. Up to one half of college students claim to have experienced depersonalization at some time in their lives. It has been reported that 80% of psychiatric inpatients suffer from depersonalization, but in only 12% is the symptom long lasting, and in no case is it the only symptom. The sex ratio is equal.

B. Etiology

Normal dissociation is an adaptive defense used to cope with overwhelming psychic trauma. It is commonly encountered during and after civilian disasters, criminal assault, sudden loss, and war. In normal dissociation, the individual's perception of the traumatic experience is temporarily dulled or dispelled from consciousness. Normal dissociation prevents other vital psychological functions from being overwhelmed by the traumatic experience. The capacity to dissociate, as evidenced by susceptibility to hypnosis, is widely distributed among normal people. However, it is unclear whether pathologic dissociation is an extreme or more enduring form of normal dissociation (i.e., whether there is a continuum of dissociation between normal and abnormal) or whether the pathologic form is distinctive. Recent studies of trauma subjects have found only a low correlation between hypnotizability and measures of dissociation.

Theories concerning the basis of pathologic dissociation can be classified as psychological, neurocognitive, traumagenic, and psychosocial.

1. Psychological theories—Janet postulated that some people have a constitutional "psychological insufficiency" that renders them prone to dissociate in the face of frightening experiences. At that time, memories associated with "vehement emotions" become separated or dissociated from awareness in the form of subconscious fixed ideas, which are not integrated into memory. Rather, they remain latent and are prone to return to consciousness as **psychological automatisms** such as hysterical paralyses, anesthesias, and somnambulisms (trance states).

Breuer and Freud suggested that hysterical patients harbor inadmissible ideational "complexes" resulting in a splitting of the mind and the emergence of abnormal (hypnoid) states of consciousness. Pathologic associations formed during hypnoid states fail to decay like ordinary memories but reemerge to disrupt somatic processes in the form of hysterical sensorimotor symptoms or disturbances of consciousness. Breuer and Freud disputed Janet's concept that dissociation is a passive process reflecting a hereditary degeneracy. They introduced the concept of an active defensive process that energetically deflects the conscious mind from disruptive ideas. Out of this theory emerged the later psychoanalytic concepts of repression and ego defense.

Dissociative amnesia and dissociative fugue characteristically arise in a setting of overwhelming stress, particularly in time of war or civilian catastrophe. Murderers, for example, often claim amnesia for the crime long after it would be legally advantageous to do so. Money problems, the impending disclosure of a sexual misdemeanor, marital conflict, or the death of a loved one are the usual precipitants of amnesia and fugue. Sometimes, the dissociative state is precipitated by an intolerable mood, such as severe depression with intense guilt. Dissociation blots out the unendurable memory; and a fugue represents an attempt to get away and start a new life.

It is unclear whether depersonalization represents a minor variant of global dissociation or a different process. In depersonalization, affect and the sense of being connected is split off from the individual's sense of self and perception of the outside world, giving rise to the feeling of being detached, like a robot or in a dream. Depersonalization may be the subjective component of a biological mechanism that allows an animal to function in a terrifying situation, whereas dissociation is represented by the freezing behavior that enables hunted animals to escape detection. These extreme survival maneuvers are subject to overload. Learned helplessness in animals, for example, may represent a breakdown of those neural circuits that modulate the sensitivity of the brain to incoming stimuli.

2. Neurocognitive theories—**Episodic memory** is a form of explicit memory involving the storage of events, which then have access to conscious awareness. Episodic memory is usually recounted in words, as a narrative. If significant enough, episodic memories become part of **autobiographical memory**, the history of the self. The medial temporal lobe, particularly the hippocampus, is essential to the encoding, storage, and retrieval of episodic memory. Dissociation may represent an interference with the encoding, storage, or retrieval in narrative form of traumatic episodic memories.

The locus coeruleus is an important source of noradrenergic fibers that project to the cerebral cortex, hypothalamus, hippocampus, and amygdala. The amygdala and orbitofrontal cortex select out those stimuli that have been primary reinforcers in the past. The amygdala projects to the hippocampus (via the entorhinal cortex), to the sensory association cortex, and to the hypothalamus and brain stem, coordinating a central alarm apparatus that scans sensory input for stimuli the animal has learned to fear, and sounds an alert when such stimuli are encountered. Evidence indicates that serotonin acts postsynaptically in the amygdala to provoke the synthesis of enkephalins, which modulate or dampen the affect associated with fearful experience and may interfere with the consolidation of traumatic memories. If the amygdaloid alarm system becomes overloaded and breaks down, the animal will be at the mercy of raw fear. Thus, whenever reminders of trauma are perceived in the environment, or whenever fragments of traumatic episodic memory threaten to emerge into awareness, an alarm is sounded and the fail-safe, last-resort defense of dissociation must be invoked.

Traumatic memories are stored in two systems: (1) the hippocampal explicit episodic memory system and (2) the amygdaloid implicit alarm system. The amygdaloid system can disrupt storage and retrieval via the hippocampal system. Research suggests that immature animals exposed to early inescapable stress or gross deprivation of cospecies contact are particularly vulnerable to subsequent trauma. In primates, morphine decreases (and naloxone increases) the amount of affiliative calling of an animal separated from its mother, whereas diazepam reduces freezing and hostile gestures in reaction to direct threat, probably through the prefrontal cortex. Animal research has suggested that high circulating corticosteroid levels in stressed juveniles are associated with a reduction in the population of glucocorticoid receptors in the hippocampus. Furthermore, neuroimaging studies of veterans with chronic posttraumatic stress disorder have demonstrated an apparent shrinkage in hippocampal volume.

3. Traumagenic theories—Clinical evidence for the linkage between emotional trauma and dissociation is derived from the following observations: (1) the high prevalence of histories of childhood trauma reported by patients with dissociative disorder; (2) elevated levels of dissociation in people who report child abuse; (3) elevated levels of dissociation in combat veterans with posttraumatic stress disorder; (4) the prevalence of acute dissociative reactions in war or disaster; and (5) the observation that marked dissociation during a traumatic experience predicts subsequent posttraumatic stress disorder. Almost all adults with dissociative identity disorder report significant trauma in childhood, particularly incest, physical abuse, and emotional abuse. These patients commonly report repeated abuse, sometimes of an extremely sadistic, bizarre nature.

4. Psychosocial theories—The difficulty of corroborating retrospective accounts of abuse has provoked much controversy. Are these reports false, unwittingly created by clinical interest and the recent explosion of coverage in the media? The possibility of iatrogenic facilitation cannot be excluded. The more dramatic forms of dissociative disorder—particularly fugue and multiple identity—may represent, at least in part, forms of abnormal illness behavior, distorted attempts by emotionally needy patients to elicit care and protection from therapist-parent surrogates, or bids to retain the interest of therapists in the context of an intense transference relationship. Traumagenic and psychosocial theories are not necessarily mutually exclusive.

DISSOCIATIVE AMNESIA & DISSOCIATIVE FUGUE

 ESSENTIALS OF DIAGNOSIS

DSM-IV-TR Diagnostic Criteria

Dissociative Amnesia

A. *The predominant disturbance is one or more episodes of inability to recall important personal information, usually of a traumatic or stressful nature, that is too extensive to be explained by ordinary forgetfulness.*

B. *The disturbance does not occur exclusively during the course of dissociative identity disorder, dissociative fugue, posttraumatic stress disorder, acute stress disorder, or somatization disorder and is not due to the direct physiological effects of a substance (e.g., a drug of abuse, a medication) or a neurological or other general medical condition (e.g., amnestic disorder due to head trauma).*

C. *The symptoms cause clinically significant distress or impairment in social, occupational, or other important areas of functioning.*

DSM-IV-TR Diagnostic Criteria Dissociative Fugue

A. *The predominant disturbance is sudden, unexpected travel away from home or one's customary place of work, with inability to recall one's past.*

B. *Confusion about personal identity or assumption of a new identity (partial or complete).*

C. *The disturbance does not occur exclusively during the course of dissociative identity disorder and is not due to the direct physiological effects of a substance (e.g., a drug of abuse, a medication) or a general medical condition (e.g., temporal lobe epilepsy).*

D. *The symptoms cause clinically significant distress or impairment in social, occupational, or other important areas of functioning.*

(Reprinted, with permission, from *Diagnostic and Statistical Manual of Mental Disorders*, 4th edn., Text Revision. Washington DC: American Psychiatric Association, 2000.)

Clinical Findings

A. SIGNS & SYMPTOMS

The amnesia for distressing events can be localized (i.e., complete amnesia for events during a circumscribed period of time), selective (i.e., failure to remember some but not all events during a circumscribed period of time), generalized (i.e., affecting an entire period of life), or continuous (i.e., failure to remember anything after a particular date). Patchy amnesia is prevalent among people exposed to military or civilian trauma. A common sequence is for the patient to progress from a first stage, characterized by an acute altered state of consciousness (mental confusion, headache, and preoccupation with a single idea or emotion), to a second stage in which he or she loses the sense of personal identity. At this point the patient may be found wandering in a fugue state, unable to give an account of himself or herself. Rarely, the patient enters a third stage in which he or she assumes a new identity, usually one more gregarious and uninhibited than previously. The diagnostic separation of amnesia from fugue may be illusory, because the two conditions are probably on a continuum. During the first stage of confusion and altered consciousness, some patients report audiovisual hallucinations and a preoccupation with quasidelusional ideas. This condition, originally known as hysterical twilight state, lacks the disorganization of thought processes and affective incongruity found in schizophrenia. The patient operates at a higher level of consciousness than is associated with epilepsy or other organic brain dysfunctions.

B. PSYCHOLOGICAL TESTING

Table 24–1 lists tests that are useful screens in the diagnosis of dissociative disorders.

Table 24–1. Screening Tests for Dissociative Disorders

Test	Description
Dissociative Disorders Interview Schedule (DDIS)	A structured interview that examines for dissociative disorder, somatoform disorder, depression, borderline personality disorder, substance abuse, and physical and sexual abuse
Structured Clinical Interview for the DSM-IV Dissociative Disorders (SCID-D)	A semistructured interview derived from the SCID
Dissociative Experiences Scale (DES)	A 28-item self-report questionnaire that screens for dissociative symptoms in adults (age 18 years and older)
Adolescent Dissociative Experiences Scale (A-DES)	A 30-item self-report screening questionnaire for adolescents (age 12–20 years)
Child Dissociative Checklist (CDC)	A 20-item screening checklist to be completed on children (age 5–12 years) by a parent or adult observer
Structured Interview for Reported Symptoms (SIRS)	A structured interview designed to detect the malingering of psychosis

Differential Diagnosis (including comorbid conditions)

Dissociative amnesia and dissociative fugue must be differentiated from delirium or dementia. The clinician must exclude amnestic disorders due to such medical conditions as vitamin deficiency, head trauma, carbon monoxide poisoning, and herpes encephalitis as well as amnestic disorders secondary to alcoholism (Korsakoff syndrome); to anxiolytic, anticonvulsant, sedative, and hypnotic drugs; and to steroids, lithium, or β-blockers. The clinician must also distinguish other organic disorders such as the retrograde amnesia of head injury, seizure disorder (particularly the dreamy state of temporal lobe epilepsy), and transient global amnesia due to cerebral vascular insufficiency.

Differential diagnosis is based on a full history, a detailed mental status examination, physical and neurologic examination, and when appropriate, special investigations such as a toxicology screen, laboratory testing, electroencephalography, brain imaging, and neuropsychological testing. The most difficult diagnostic problems arise when dissociation is superimposed on organic disease (e.g., pseudoseizures coexisting with epilepsy). The differentiation of dissociative disorders from malingering is discussed later in this chapter.

Treatment

Patience and the expectation that memory loss will soon clear are usually enough to help the amnestic patient recover. The key to treatment is a safe environment (e. g., hospitalization) removed from the source of stress and a trusting therapeutic relationship. Hypnotherapy or narcoanalysis (e. g., using amobarbital, benzodiazepines, or methylamphetamine) are sometimes required to facilitate recall.

Prognosis

Dissociative amnesia and dissociative fugue are usually short lived; however, after restoration of memory and identity, the patient must deal with the source of the problem.

■ DISSOCIATIVE IDENTITY DISORDER

DSM-IV-TR Diagnostic Criteria

A. *The presence of two or more distinct identities or personality states (each with its own relatively enduring pattern of perceiving, relating to, and thinking about the environment and self).*

B. *At least two of these identities or personality states recurrently take control of the person's behavior.*

C. *Inability to recall important personal information that is too extensive to be explained by ordinary forgetfulness.*

D. *The disturbance is not due to the direct physiological effects of a substance (e.g., blackouts or chaotic behavior during alcohol intoxication) or*

a general medical condition (e.g., complex partial seizures).

Note: In children: the symptoms are not attributable to imaginary playmates or other fantasy play.

(Reprinted, with permission, from the *Diagnostic and Statistical Manual of Mental Disorders*, 4th edn., Text Revision. Washington DC: American Psychiatric Association, 2000.)

Clinical Findings

A. Signs & Symptoms

Dissociative identity disorder (DID) is usually not diagnosed until patients are in their late twenties, but retrospective evidence indicates that it begins much earlier, usually in childhood. Some patients with DID have had years of treatment before the correct diagnosis is made. These patients commonly exhibit transient depression, mood swings, sleep disturbance, nightmares, and suicidal behavior. They are often self-injurious and exhibit a host of dissociative symptoms including amnesia, episodes of "lost time" (i.e., amnesia varying from several minutes to several days), depersonalization, fugue, and hallucinations. Anxiety and its somatic concomitants (e.g., dyspnea, palpitations, chest pain, choking sensations, faintness, tremors) commonly herald a switch of alter personalities. Quasineurologic symptoms such as headache, syncope, pseudoseizures, numbness, paresthesia, diplopia, tunnel vision, and motor weakness are sometimes encountered. Symptoms referable to the cardiorespiratory, gastrointestinal, or reproductive systems may dominate the clinical presentation.

Questioning will reveal that most patients have audiovisual hallucinations and quasidelusions. The auditory hallucinations may be fragments of conversations heard during traumatic experiences or metaphoric expressions of self-disgust in the form of hostile voices that revile and derogate the patient or command her to harm herself, commit suicide, or attack others. Other voices may be conversations between people about the patient, people offering solace, and the weeping and crying of distressed children. Some patients report a sense of being controlled, alterations in their body image, or the conviction that they are being followed or that their lives are threatened by shadowy enemies (e.g., the former perpetrators of alleged "ritual abuse"). Occasional discontinuities of thought and thought "slippages" may be the result of alter switching or the intrusion of traumatic themes into the stream of consciousness, causing microdissociations.

As mentioned earlier in this chapter, these patients may have had many medical and neurologic investigations. Many have been treated for mood disorder, anxiety disorder, or schizophrenia. Some wander from job to job, place to place, and doctor to doctor. Many are prone to repeated victimization by virtue of their poor choice of occupation or consorts.

The cardinal feature of DID is multiple personalities, two or more entities, each of which has a characteristic and separate personality, history, affect, values, and function. The number of alters is usually about 10, though it may be many more. Typically, the alters are somewhat two-dimensional in quality and include such entities as the host personality; a variety of child personalities (e.g., innocent child, traumatized child, "Pollyanna"); a persecutor; a cross-sex alter; an internal helper; a brazen, promiscuous "hussy;" a variety of demons; and "no one." The entities usually first emerge during childhood, in the form of imaginary protectors or companions that help the child cope with recurrent experiences of abuse and fear. The alter personalities often switch abruptly, producing a bewildering change in demeanor, sometimes with anxiety and apparent disorganization of thought. Sometimes one alter or several alters will be unaware of the other alters. Often alters will communicate with each other. The complete dramatis personae usually emerge only after therapy.

It can be difficult to elicit alter personalities. The clinician must have a reasonable suspicion that DID is present (e.g., in a patient who exhibits abrupt changes in demeanor, "lost time," total amnesia for childhood, and many physical symptoms). The exploration of puzzling events or lost time will often elicit an alter. Sometimes the clinician must ask directly to speak to "that part of you" that did something or experienced something.

B. Psychological Testing

See discussion of dissociative amnesia and dissociative fugue.

Differential Diagnosis (including comorbid conditions)

DID is most likely to be confused with the following conditions: partial complex seizures, schizophrenia, bipolar disorder, major depression with psychotic features, Munchausen syndrome, Munchausen syndrome by proxy, and malingering. Partial complex seizures, which usually last no more than a few seconds, may be confused with alter switching; however, other cardinal signs of DID are not seen in epilepsy. Occasionally, telemetry is required.

Patients with DID frequently report the following phenomena: quasidelusions; ideas of being externally controlled; auditory hallucinations involving conversations; comments about the patient cast in the third person; commands; and ideas of thought loss. When these phenomena are associated with the disruption of thinking coincident with alter switching or microdissociation, it is not surprising that patients with DID have often been mistakenly diagnosed as having schizophrenia. DID should be differentiated from schizophrenia by the lack of emotional incongruity; the dramatic, care-eliciting presentation; the history of severe trauma; the alter personalities; and high scores on dissociation scales. Hypnosis is sometimes helpful in distinguishing DID from schizophrenia.

Rapid-cycling bipolar disorder is sometimes confused with the apparent mood swings caused by alter switching in DID. However, the term "rapid-cycling" refers to brief intervals between episodes of mania or depression, not to the brevity of the episodes themselves.

Major depression with psychotic features can be confused with DID if only a superficial diagnostic evaluation has been completed, particularly because many patients with DID have an associated depressive mood. In major depression with psychotic features, the auditory hallucinations and delusions are consistent with the prevailing depressive mood. For example, the patient hears voices derogating him or her for being a bad person, and is convinced that he or she has committed an unpardonable sin, is impoverished, is being hounded by tax officials, or is rotting inside. In DID, the hallucinations are often derogatory, but they convey the theme of helpless victimization and command patients to hurt others or themselves.

In some cases of Munchausen syndrome, the pseudopatient has presented himself or herself for medical attention with the symptoms of DID. In some cases of Munchausen syndrome by proxy, a mother presents her child with the symptoms of DID. The imposture is deliberate, but the gain obscure. Satisfaction is apparently obtained from being the center of medical investigations and therapeutic attention, or from being the brave parent of a child with dramatic psychopathology. In malingering, the gain is less enigmatic: The pseudopatient is usually a criminal defendant seeking exculpation on the grounds of insanity.

Treatment

The treatment of DID is the subject of much controversy. A powerful body of opinion questions the validity of this diagnosis and questions therapeutic approaches that seek to integrate alters. Kluft describes four approaches to treatment: (1) integrate the alters; (2) seek harmony between the alters; (3) leave the alters alone and focus on improving adaptation to the here-and-now; and (4) regard the alters as artifacts, ignoring them and treating other symptoms (e.g., depression).

The last of these approaches is adopted by those who believe that DID is a fictive condition generated or reinforced by the clinicians who treat it. The first three approaches are not mutually exclusive and are adopted in accordance with the patient's capacity to tolerate the stress of integrating the alter personalities.

Excessively rapid movement in the assessment or treatment of DID will generate resistance. Once DID is identified and the diagnosis communicated, the patient will experience anxiety. Patients with DID tend to be profoundly distrustful of others and may themselves be deceptive. Patients are likely to be hypersensitive to deceit, impatience, or authoritarianism. Clinicians must be able to tolerate uncertainty, normalize any anomalous experiences that patients divulge, and eschew premature reassurance.

Many patients report complete amnesia for early and middle childhood. Most are also confused about current experience and are able to report the past in only a piecemeal fashion. Clinicians should inquire about instances of lost time, depersonalization, out-of-body experiences, flashbacks, and hallucinations. Most patients with DID are able to suppress alter switching during brief contact, but they are likely to manifest the phenomenon if the interview session extends over an hour.

Hypnosis can be useful when rapid diagnosis is required, although it may be preferable to allow the alters to emerge spontaneously. The clinician should explore each alter with regard to the following information: name, age, and sex; developmental origin; dominant affect and perceptual style; survival functions; and unique symptoms and dysfunctions. The clinician should ask to speak to a particular alter identified by name or behavior and should ask for a signal (e.g., a lifted finger) as a signal of the alter's willingness to appear. Rapport must be developed with each alter. After conducting the appropriate interview, the clinician should ask the alter to resubmerge. Although initially the clinician must treat each alter as if he or she is a separate person, it is important to convey the understanding that each alter is but a dissociated element of the client as a whole.

It can be useful to draw maps, diagrams, or family trees of the internal system of alters, identifying the components by name, age, and sex. These maps must be revised regularly throughout treatment. When a particular alter acknowledges lost time, another alter may have been internally active during that period. The internal helper alter may be the most reliable informant in the clinician's attempt to conceptualize the structure of personality fragments.

Treatment is either supportive or integrative. Integrative therapy is likely to be more complex and concomitantly more risky. A number of issues should be considered before embarking on integrative therapy. Table 24–2 lists situations in which integrative therapy is contraindicated.

If supportive therapy is pursued because the patient has a limited potential for integration, the clinician

Table 24–2. Contraindications for integrative therapy

Severe ego defect related to early neglect and trauma, and a lifelong reliance upon dissociative defenses.

Severe, pervasive comorbid pathology, particularly borderline personality disorder, histrionic personality disorder, depression, substance abuse, and eating disorder.

Poor environmental support. If the patient is involved in dysfunctional and nonsupportive relationships, retraumatization is likely to occur. There must be at least a moderate level of environmental stability and support.

The incapacity of the clinician to tolerate devaluation, acting-out behavior, suicidality, self-injury, and deceptiveness.

The inability of patient and clinician to establish and maintain a therapeutic alliance. The therapist must provide a flexible balance between support and interpretation, and maintain stable boundaries in interaction with the patient. The patient is likely to test the limits by acting out, seduction, failing to appear for appointments, or devaluing the clinician.

---

attempts to rehabilitate the patient by strengthening the ego of the host personality and by helping the patient to cope with reality. The emphasis is on stabilization, control of affect and impulse, increased responsibility in everyday behavior, and palliation of distress.

If prognostic factors are favorable, integrative therapy can be attempted. Integrative therapy aims to uncover dissociated and repressed traumatic experiences, integrate personality functioning, and replace dissociation with other defenses. Whenever the patient is overwhelmed in the course of therapy, the clinician must revert to supportive therapy. Whether the treatment is supportive or integrative, attention must be given to the shame and low self-esteem associated with sexual victimization.

Alters should be directed toward verbal and creative affective expression instead of impulsive, destructive, self-defeating acting out. Each alter represents the expression of a fixed idea: images, thoughts, or associations related to a particular traumatic experience that retains a pristine emotional charge because it has been sequestered from the normal processes of memory decay. The therapist must relate effectively to each of these internal fragments, seeking to improve the contribution of each fragment to overall functioning. The superordinate aim of integrative therapy is to promote the confluence of the entire system, not to strengthen dissociation between alters. The amount of time devoted to the development of greater general ego strength should

exceed the amount of time spent in strengthening separate alters.

Persecutory and malevolent alters are best dealt with by patient rechanneling of hostile impulses in more appropriate directions, particularly by expressing rage in words or artistic productions rather than in deeds. Malevolent alters should be confronted gently with the identity confusion that leads them to consider themselves as part of the abuser rather than as part of the patient.

The internal helper alter is a useful ally in treatment and can serve as a consultant to the therapist, providing information about the total system. The ultimate aim of integrative therapy is to reverse the pervasive attachment disruption and splitting that have accompanied abuse. As the patient improves, he or she may begin to grieve for a lost childhood and for normal attachment experiences that were lost or never provided.

The therapist should help the patient develop effective coping skills, using a gentle, educative approach, modeling accurate perception, management of affect, containment of impulse, and the consideration of alternative responses to stress. Inhibited, withdrawn alters will benefit from the encouragement of self-expression and self-assertion. Shame-based alters require the supportive resolution of shame. As the patient becomes more aware of different traumata, a dialogue may occur between the different alters. The therapist should emphasize the need for cooperation. The aim is toward increased dialogue and mutual cooperation.

The **abreaction of emotion** is an essential component of therapy and is aimed at resolving dissociation and restoring integration. The therapeutic component of abreaction may not be catharsis of feeling but rather the consequent reformulation of traumatic memories. Some patients revert to dissociative trances when they are about to remember and disclose particular traumatic experiences, and spontaneous abreaction may be triggered by reminders of trauma such as anniversaries. However, abreaction without reformulation is unproductive. During abreaction, the therapist's task is to keep the patient safe, nudge him or her toward reality, and keep him or her in the abreaction until it is concluded. Abreaction is followed by debriefing and exploration of the meaning of the experience. Successful abreaction requires full experience of the affect associated with the event, not just a disembodied memory. Premature initiation of abreaction, or the induction of abreaction in patients who cannot tolerate it, is counterproductive. Table 24–3 summarizes the sequential stages in psychotherapy with these patients.

Late in the therapy, the spontaneous fusing of alters signals readiness for personality unification. Usually this proceeds as two or more alters combine at a time. The therapist must be patient and not press for premature fusion. Full integration involves (1) reduced reliance on the dissociative segregation of experience, (2) the blending

Table 24–3. Stages in the integrative psychotherapy of dissociative identity disorder

1. Establish a working alliance.
2. Make the diagnosis, inform the patient, and maintain the therapeutic alliance.
3. Make contact with the different alters.
4. Explore the structure of the system of alters.
5. Understand the particular "fixed idea" behind each alter.
6. Work with the problems of particular alter states.
7. Help the patient develop increasing cooperation between alter states.
8. Help the patient develop nondissociative coping skills.
9. Confront dissociation and support the patient's integration of memory, affect, and identity via the abreaction of traumatic experience.
10. Help the patient develop and consolidate a new identity.

B. *During the depersonalization experience, reality testing remains intact.*

C. *The depersonalization causes clinically significant distress or impairment in social, occupational, or other important areas of functioning.*

D. *The depersonalization experience does not occur exclusively during the course of another mental disorder, such as schizophrenia, panic disorder, acute stress disorder, or another dissociative disorder, and is not due to the direct physiological effects of a substance (e.g., a drug of abuse, a medication) or a general medical condition (e.g., temporal lobe epilepsy).*

(Reprinted, with permission, from the *Diagnostic and Statistical Manual of Mental Disorders*, 4th edn., Text Revision. Washington DC: American Psychiatric Association, 2000.)

Prognosis

DID is a chronic condition that does not remit. It usually begins in childhood as a form of dissociative hallucinosis (see "Miscellaneous Types of Dissociation" section later in this chapter), but the full syndrome does not coalesce until adolescence. Some patients develop histrionic or borderline personalities, with a stormy adulthood. Others are introverted, depressed, and socially avoidant. Males are more likely than females to have a history of episodic violence in the correctional system. Many patients with DID manage to conceal their symptoms for years.

of alters into a single nondissociative personality, and (3) the harmonious coexistence of different aspects of the patient's personality. Integration is relative. Some patients are able to tolerate complete fusion and unification. Others are not capable of full unification but benefit from improved functional integration.

◼ DEPERSONALIZATION DISORDER

DSM-IV-TR Diagnostic Criteria

A. *Persistent or recurrent experiences of feeling detached from, and as if one is an outside observer of, one's mental processes or body (e.g., feeling like one is in a dream).*

Clinical Findings

A. SIGNS & SYMPTOMS

The onset of depersonalization disorder is usually sudden and typically occurs in a setting of anxiety. Derealization is commonly associated with depersonalization. Patients feel numb and out of touch with their feelings, bodies, and surroundings. Sometimes they feel as if they are observing themselves or as though they are automatons in a dream. Depersonalization is difficult to describe, and patients may express concern about "going crazy," particularly if the condition is accompanied by déjà vu experiences and distortions in the sense of time. Depression and anxiety are commonly associated with depersonalization.

B. PSYCHOLOGICAL TESTING

See discussion of dissociative amnesia and dissociative fugue.

Differential Diagnosis (including comorbid conditions)

Dissociative disorders in which depersonalization is the cardinal symptom probably merge imperceptibly with other disorders in which depersonalization is a subsidiary symptom. For example, depersonalization is likely to be elicited from patients with anxiety disorders (particularly panic disorder), other dissociative disorders, depressive disorder, and borderline personality disorder. Depersonalization has been reported in 11–42% of schizophrenic patients. In schizophrenia, depersonalization tends to become incorporated into the prevailing delusional system. Depersonalization may also be encountered in substance abuse, particularly with alcohol, marijuana, hallucinogens, cocaine, phenylcyclidine, methylamphetamine, narcotics, and sedatives. Depersonalization has also been reported after medication with indomethacin, fenfluramine, and haloperidol.

In epilepsy, particularly temporal lobe epilepsy, depersonalization may be encountered as an aura, as part of the seizure itself, or between seizures. Depersonalization in epilepsy is more likely to be associated with stereotypic movements (e.g., lip smacking), senseless words or phrases, and loss of consciousness than in dissociative disorders, in which it is likely to be more highly elaborated. Depersonalization may also be evident in postconcussive disorder, Meniere disease, cerebral atherosclerosis, and Korsakoff syndrome.

Treatment

If depersonalization is a subsidiary symptom, the primary disorder should be treated. There have been no controlled studies of treatment for depersonalization disorder proper. The relative effectiveness of supportive psychotherapy, hypnosis, exploratory psychotherapy, family therapy, and cognitive–behavioral therapy is not known. Psychotherapy focuses on the recovery of the traumatic experience from which the pathologic dissociation is thought to have arisen. Hypnosis may help in this regard. Cognitive–behavioral desensitization, flooding, and exposure have also been used.

Prognosis

Some depersonalization syndromes, particularly after acute stress, are transient. However, depersonalization can evolve into a chronic, intractable, disabling disorder.

■ DISSOCIATIVE DISORDER NOT OTHERWISE SPECIFIED

ESSENTIALS OF DIAGNOSIS

DSM-IV Diagnostic Criteria

A. *Includes dissociative symptomatology that does not fit all the criteria for the other four types of dissociative disorder.*

B. *Includes dissociative hallucinosis, dissociative states following torture or political*

indoctrination, somnambulism, "out-of-body" experiences, dissociative trances that are part of culturally sanctioned rituals, culture-bound "possession" states (e.g., amok), and the Ganser syndrome (hysterical pseudodementia).

Clinical Findings

A. SIGNS & SYMPTOMS

Dissociative hallucinosis is a form of posttraumatic stress disorder commonly encountered in sexually or physically abused adolescents, particularly in inpatient settings. Patients, usually female, experience recurrent, dramatic episodes of audiovisual hallucinosis, dissociative trances, autohypnoid states, suicidal behavior, and self-injury (e.g., wrist cutting). Male patients with this condition are often subject to intermittent explosive outbursts during which they are assaultive or self-injurious (e.g., by punching their fists against a wall) and are apparently out of touch with their surroundings. The dissociative episodes are usually precipitated by experiences that reactivate traumatic memories of sexual coercion, helplessness, humiliation, or rejection.

Dissociative trances may be part of the rituals of some religions. Culture-bound syndromes such as amok, latah, malgri, and koro are usually preceded by intense emotion (e.g., fear, humiliation), associated with the conviction of being possessed by a demon or spirit, and accompanied by dissociated, out-of-control behavior.

The **Ganser syndrome** (hysterical pseudodementia) is a condition in which the patient exhibits symptoms of an apparent dementia or psychosis that are too exaggerated or inconsistent to fit such a diagnosis. For example, the patient may exhibit **vorbeireden**, a phenomenon in which the patient's incorrect answers imply knowledge of the correct answer (e.g., Question: "How many legs has a cow?" Answer: "Five."). Several of Ganser's original cases probably had delirium. Vorbeireden can also occur in organic brain disease such as stroke or cerebral tumor. The psychogenic variety is most often encountered in a legal setting and must be differentiated from malingering. It is usually associated with global amnesia for a crime and a dissociative shut-down of intellectual processes, producing apparent dementia.

B. PSYCHOLOGICAL TESTING

See discussion of dissociative amnesia and dissociative fugue.

Differential Diagnosis (including comorbid conditions)

Dissociative hallucinosis, with its dramatic, recurrent audiovisual hallucinosis, fear of attack, explosive violence, suicidality, and self-injurious behavior must be differentiated from schizophrenia, substance-induced psychosis, major depression with psychotic features, and epilepsy.

Treatment

In many adolescents with dissociative hallucinosis, rudimentary or nascent forms of DID may be noted. In such cases, clinicians should avoid reinforcing the development of alters and relate to the patient as a whole. Hospitalization may be necessary in order to provide safety, prevent suicide and self-injury, and contain episodic dyscontrol. Individual, group, and family therapy are helpful. Pharmacotherapy, judiciously prescribed, can be a useful adjunct to treatment.

Prognosis

The prognosis for acute episodes of dissociative hallucinosis is good. However, the long-term outlook depends on the quality of family support and the patient's personality.

PHARMACOTHERAPY IN DISSOCIATIVE DISORDERS

Pharmacotherapy is adjunctive in the treatment of dissociative disorders. Neuroleptic medication is contraindicated: Not only is it ineffective, but it aggravates dissociation. Antidepressant medication, particularly serotonin reuptake inhibitors, can be helpful in counteracting insomnia, impulsiveness, depersonalization, and comorbid depression. Benzodiazepines can be helpful in acute dissociation and panic but should be avoided in the long term because of the danger of addiction.

DISSOCIATION FOLLOWING ACUTE TRAUMA

Following acute trauma, such as that associated with a civilian catastrophe or criminal assault, dissociation is commonly encountered as a part of acute stress disorder and emerging posttraumatic stress disorder (see Chapter 20). Treatment involves the provision of a safe environment, individual psychotherapy, and when required, group therapy. When children are involved, following a civilian catastrophe, preventive intervention can be provided in schools.

Briere J: Dissociative symptoms and trauma exposure: Specificity, affect dysregulation, and posttraumatic stress. *J Nerv Ment Dis* 2006;194:78–82.

Hornstein NL, Putnam FW: Clinical phenomenology of child and adolescent dissociative disorders. *J Am Acad Child Adolesc Psychiatry* 1992;31:1077.

Isaac M, Chand PK: Dissociative and conversion disorders: Defining boundaries. *Curr Opin Psychiatry* 2006;19:61–66.

Lowenstein RJ, Putnam FW: Dissociative disorders. In: Sadock BJ, Sadock VA (eds). *Comprehensive Textbook of Psychiatry*, 8th edn. Philadelphia: Lippincott, Williams & Wilkins, 2005, pp. 1844–1901.

McHugh PR, Putnam FW: Resolved: Multiple personality is an individually and socially created artifact. *J Am Acad Child Adolesc Psychiatry* 1995;34:957.

Michelson LK, Ray WJ: *Handbook of Dissociation: Theoretical, Empirical and Clinical Perspectives*. New York: Plenum Publishing Corp, 1996.

Nurcombe B: Dissociative hallucinosis and allied conditions. In: Volkmar F (ed). *Psychoses of Childhood and Adolescence*. Washington DC: American Psychiatric Press, 1996, pp. 107–128.

Putnam FW: *Dissociation in Children and Adolescents*. New York: Guilford Press, 1997.

Sexual Dysfunction and Paraphilias 25

Richard Balon, MD & R. Taylor Segraves, MD, PhD

INTRODUCTION

Sexual dysfunctions and paraphilias are disorders of either disturbance of processes in sexual functioning (sexual dysfunctions) or sexual behavior(s) (paraphilias). Human sexuality presents a very complex interaction of biology and psychology, which is reflected in complex physiological responses. A seemingly very simple event, such as erection, is regulated on the central nervous system and peripheral nervous system level, modified by various hormones, impacted by vascular changes, and influenced by various expectations, interpersonal issues, intrapsychic processes, not to mention the influences of medications and substances of abuse, the aging processes, diseases and personal habits. While there is a substantial body of literature on human sexuality in general and sexual dysfunctions and paraphilias in particular, there is mostly a lack of good evidence-based literature on most aspects of these disorders. The focus has definitely moved from psychology to biology and medicalization of human sexuality. The biological sciences, such as pharmacology, have contributed enormously to the developments in this area. However, an exclusive focus on biology and medical aspects of human sexuality is unwarranted and may trivialize a very complex area of human behavior. Even the clearly "biological" treatment approaches to sexual dysfunction may fail in certain situations due to various psychological factors. Thus, we caution the reader to always consider all factors, biological and psychological, in making the diagnosis and in planning treatment. In most cases, the judicious combination of biological and psychological treatment approaches will yield the most satisfactory results.

The diagnoses of sexual dysfunctions and paraphilias are mostly descriptive, no diagnosis specific tests or examinations are usually available. The classification of sexual dysfunctions is based on the notion of connected yet separate and clearly defined phases of the sexual response cycle—desire, arousal/excitement, orgasm, and resolution. Thus, sexual dysfunctions are classified according to impairments of one of the first three "phases" (no impairment of the resolution phase has been identified). However, clinically these disturbances are not so clearly separated and frequently overlap or coexist (e.g., lack of libido with impaired orgasm). Interestingly, the present classification defines and uses only one end of the sexual functioning spectrum, the "lack" of functioning (e.g., lack of libido), though imprecisely and vaguely. Hypersexuality is not well-defined and not conceptualized as a dysfunction, but rather at times (if at all) as related to addiction, compulsivity, or impulsivity. Another important point in classifying and diagnosing sexual dysfunctions and paraphilias is the use of clinically significant distress or impairment as one of the defining criteria of these disorders. Thus, if the lack of sexual desire does not cause any distress or impairment, one should not qualify it as a dysfunction. There seem to be some individuals who have no interest in sex and are not distressed by it, thus they do not suffer from any sexual disorder according to the currently used diagnostic systems (they may present just one end of the spectrum of certain behavior, similar to rapid vs. absent ejaculation, discussed later).

The current diagnostic system employs similar specifiers through the entire system, and thus sexual dysfunctions (not paraphilias, though) may be further subclassified as lifelong or acquired, generalized or situational, and due to psychological factors or due to combined factors. The diagnostic system also uses categories of sexual dysfunctions due to general medical condition (e.g., diabetes mellitus) or substance-induced sexual dysfunction, which may be useful to consider in formulating the diagnosis and treatment plan.

◼ SEXUAL DYSFUNCTIONS

HYPOACTIVE SEXUAL DESIRE DISORDER

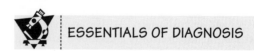 ESSENTIALS OF DIAGNOSIS

The DSM-IV-TR criteria for the diagnosis of hypoactive sexual desire disorder (HSDD) are:

A. *Persistently or recurrently deficient (or absent) sexual fantasies or desire for sexual activity. The judgment of deficiency or absence is made by the clinician, taking into account factors that affect sexual functioning, such as age and the context of the person's life.*

B. *The disturbance causes marked distress or interpersonal difficulty.*

C. *The sexual dysfunction is not better accounted for by another Axis I disorder (except another sexual dysfunction) and is not due exclusively to the direct physiological effect of a substance (e.g., a drug of abuse, a medication) or a general medical condition.*

HSDD should also be diagnosed according to subtypes: Generalized vs. situational; lifelong vs. acquired; due to psychological factors vs. due to combined factors.

(Reprinted, with permission, from the *Diagnostic and Statistical Manual of Mental Disorders*, 4th edn. Text Revision. Washington, DC: American Psychiatric Association, 2000, p. 541.)

General Considerations

There are no specific duration or severity criteria for the diagnosis of HSDD. The clinician should take into consideration such factors as the patient's age and life circumstance and use clinical judgment whether a problem should be diagnosed as a psychiatric disorder. If the individual is not stressed by the absence of libido and it does not cause interpersonal distress, a disorder cannot be diagnosed. The report of a high frequency of coital activity does not rule out the presence of HSDD in one member of a couple. The patient may agree to sexual activity in the absence of desire in order to stabilize a relationship. In the past HSDD has been labeled inhibited sexual desire, generalized sexual dysfunction, and frigidity. Lifelong HSDD is usually due to psychological factors. Situational HSDD is suggestive of interpersonal discord.

A. EPIDEMIOLOGY

Epidemiological studies in Europe, the United States, South America and Asia have found that the prevalence of complaints of low sexual desire is approximately 25–30% in females and approximately 12–25% in males. The number meeting the diagnostic criteria of this causing marked distress is probably less.

B. ETIOLOGY

HSDD may due to a general medical condition such as hypothyroidism, hyperprolactinemia, or hypogonadism.

In males, hypogonadism may be responsible for decreased libido. It is suspected, but unproven, that decreased androgenic activity in females is responsible for decreased libido in women who are post oophorectomy. Substance-induced HSDD may be related to the use of serotonin reuptake inhibitors (SSRIs) and antipsychotic drugs. HSDD may be due to other psychiatric disorders such as depressive and anxiety disorders as well as schizophrenia. Oral contraceptives have been reported to be associated with decreased libido although evidence from controlled studies is inconclusive.

Psychological factors such as social anxiety, interpersonal conflict, negative attitudes toward sexuality, and problems with sexual intimacy may be etiological factors.

C. GENETICS

There is no information concerning the genetics of this disorder.

Clinical Findings

A. SIGNS & SYMPTOMS

The major symptom is the absence of desire for sexual activity.

B. PSYCHOLOGICAL TESTING

Psychological testing is not required to make this diagnosis. A structured diagnostic method has been shown to have good reliability between expert diagnosticians in sexual medicine and novices in this area and well-validated psychometric instruments may help to validate the diagnosis and monitor progress in treatment.

C. LABORATORY FINDINGS

In male hypogonadism, serum free testosterone will be low. In both sexes, HSDD may be a sign of hypothyroidism or hyperprolactinemia. There is no definitive laboratory testing for endocrinological causes of female HSDD.

D. NEUROIMAGING

Neuroimaging does not contribute to the diagnosis of this disorder.

Course of Illness

Lack of desire related to environmental factors such as transient stress or transient interpersonal conflict may resolve as the conflict resolves. Lack of desire, which is lifelong or chronic, has a poor prognosis for recovery.

Differential Diagnosis

In general, if the disorder is situational as opposed to global, HSDD due to psychological factors is suspected.

Most lifelong cases of HSDD will be due to earlier experiences, and thus psychogenic in etiology.

Low sexual desire may be part of the symptomatic presentation of mood disorder, various anxiety disorders, and schizophrenia. In these cases, the appropriate Axis I disorder would be diagnosed. Substance induced sexual disorder should be ruled out. Many pharmacological agents such as anticonvulsants, narcotics, antipsychotics, tricyclic antidepressants (TCAs), monoamine oxidase inhibitors (MAOIs), and SSRIs may be associated with low sexual desire. Bupropion, duloxetine, and nefazodone have lower incidence of sexual dysfunction than the SSRIs. Among antipsychotics, olanzapine and aripiprazole appear to have lower rates of sexual dysfunction. Low desire for sexual activity with the designated partner disorder may also reflect the presence of a paraphilias. In such cases, a careful history would reveal normal libido for paraphilic behavior but decreased desire for nonparaphilic behavior. In such cases, the specific paraphilia would be the diagnosis. If an organic etiology is found, the diagnosis would be hypoactive sexual desire disorder due to a specified medical condition (e.g., hypogonadism). There is some evidence that thyroid disorders and temporal lobe lesions may be associated with disorders of desire. A chronic debilitating or painful medical condition may be associated with low sexual desire. Desire discrepancies, in which both members of a relationship have normal libido but one member wishes that the other had higher libido, obviously would not meet diagnostic criteria. Relationship discord must always be considered in the differential diagnosis.

Treatment

A. PSYCHOPHARMACOLOGICAL INTERVENTIONS

Bupropion has been reported to increase various indices of sexual responsiveness in women with HSDD. There have been no controlled trials of bupropion in males with this disorder.

B. HORMONAL INTERVENTIONS

If hypogonadism is detected in male patients, hormone replacement therapy is indicated (goal is the physiological level of testosterone). High-dose testosterone therapy in females has been shown to increase libido in postmenopausal women. There is no evidence supporting the efficacy of dehydroepiandrosterone (DHEA) in this disorder.

C. PSYCHOTHERAPEUTIC INTERVENTIONS

Psychological treatment usually involves cognitive behavior therapy (CBT) combined with behavioral sex therapy. Negative cognitions are challenged. The patient may be taught how to not distract himself or herself form erotic stimuli. The patient may be taught how to develop sexual fantasies. A major goal will be to educate the patient how to communicate his or her sexual preferences to the partner. Sensate focus is usually employed to decrease sexual anxiety. There is evidence for the efficacy of CBT in HSDD.

Complications

Bupropion lowers the seizure threshold. Rarely, changing libido in one member of a relationship may destabilize the relationship. The risks of androgen therapy include polycythemia, exacerbation of sleep apnea and altered serum lipids. The presence of breast or prostate carcinoma is a contraindication to androgen therapy.

Methylated-testosterone may cause liver toxicity. This is rarely an issue with transdermal testosterone preparations. Androgen therapy in females may be associated with hirsutism. The long-term safety of testosterone therapy in women is unknown.

Prognosis

The prognosis for idiopathic HSDD is poor.

American Psychiatric Association: *Diagnostic and Statistical Manual of Mental Disorders*. 4th edn. Text Revision. Washington, DC: American Psychiatric Association, 2000.

Basson R: Female hypoactive sexual desire disorder. In: Balon R, Segraves RT (eds). *Handbook of Sexual Dysfunction*. Boca Raton, FL: Taylor & Francis, 2005, p. 43.

Davis A, Castano P: Oral contraceptives and sexuality. In: Goldstein I, Meston C, Davis S, et al. (eds). *Women's Sexual Function and Dysfunction*. New York, NY: Taylor & Francis, 2006, p. 290.

Davis S, Guay A, Shifren J, et al.: Endocrine aspects of female sexual dysfunction. *J Sex Med* 2004;1:82.

Laumann EO, Nicolosi A, Glasser D: Sexual problems among women and men aged 40–80 years: Prevalence and correlates identified in the global study of sexual attitudes and behaviors. *Int J Impot Res* 2005;17:39.

McCabe MP: Evaluation of a cognitive behaviour therapy program for people with sexual difficulties. *J Sex Marital Ther* 2001;27:259.

Morales A, Buvat J, Gooren I, et al.: Endocrine aspects of sexual dysfunction in men. *J Sex Med* 2004;1:69.

Rosen R, Barsky J: Psychological assessment and self-report questionnaires in women: Subjective measures of female sexual dysfunction. In: Goldstein I, Meston C, Davis S, Traish A (eds). *Women's Sexual Function and Dysfunction*. New York, NY: Taylor & Francis, 2006, p. 434.

Schifren J, Braunstein G, Simon J, et al.: Transdermal testosterone treatment in women with impaired sexual function after oophorectomy. *N Engl J Med* 2000;343:682.

Segraves RT, Clayton A, Croft H, et al.: Bupropion sustained release for the treatment of hypoactive sexual desire disorder in premenopausal women. *J Clin Psychopharmacol* 2004;24:339.

Segraves RT: Female sexual disorders: Psychiatric aspects. *Can J Psychiatry* 2002;4:419.

SEXUAL AVERSION DISORDER

 ESSENTIALS OF DIAGNOSIS

The DSM-IV-TR criteria for the diagnosis of sexual aversion disorder (SAD) are:

A. *Persistent or recurrent extreme aversion to, and avoidance of, all (or almost all) genital sexual contact with a sexual partner.*

B. *The disturbance causes marked distress or interpersonal difficulty.*

C. *The disorder is not better accounted for by another Axis I disorder (except another sexual dysfunction).*

The SAD could also be diagnosed according to subtypes: Generalized vs. situational; lifelong vs. acquired; due to psychological factors vs. due to combined factors.

There is some controversy among clinicians as to whether sexual aversion disorder should be classified as a disorder separate from HSDD and/or panic disorder. There is minimal literature concerning the presentation and treatment of this disorder.

(Reprinted, with permission, from the *Diagnostic and Statistical Manual of Mental Disorders*. 4th edn. Text Revision. Washington, DC: American Psychiatric Association, 2000, p. 542.)

General Considerations

A. EPIDEMIOLOGY

There is no epidemiological data concerning this diagnosis.

B. ETIOLOGY

It is hypothesized but unproven that prior sexual abuse may be of etiological significance.

C. GENETICS

There is no evidence concerning the genetics of this disorder.

Clinical Findings

A. SIGNS & SYMPTOMS

The major sign of this disorder is severe anxiety and/or disgust associated with any attempt to have genital contact with a sexual partner.

B. PSYCHOLOGICAL TESTING

No psychological tests are available for this disorder.

C. LABORATORY TESTING

No laboratory tests are available for this disorder.

D. NEUROIMAGING

Neuroimaging is not used to make this diagnosis.

Course of Illness

Course is usually chronic. Some patients will respond to a combination of pharmacotherapy and psychotherapy.

Differential Diagnosis

One must first exclude panic disorder. In some patients, sexual aversion may be related to panic attacks occurring during sexual activity. One must exclude aversion secondary to dyspareunia. If dyspareunia is present, that would be the primary diagnosis. The essential difference between HSDD and aversion disorder is the presence of active avoidance rather than disinterest.

Treatment

A. PSYCHOPHARMACOLOGICAL TREATMENT

Case reports suggest that both monoamine oxidase inhibitors and SSRIs may be effective in this disorder.

B. PSYCHOTHERAPEUTIC TREATMENT

The goal of psychotherapy is to extinguish the pairing of anxiety with sexual activity. This is usually attempted by in vivo desensitization. This may be combined with attempts to augment sexual desire and assessment of psychodynamic issues. The therapist needs to enlist the sexual partner's cooperation with treatment.

Complications /Adverse Outcomes of Treatment

Rarely, successful treatment of a sexual disorder in one member of a couple may destabilize a relationship.

Prognosis

In general, prognosis is poor. Clinicians report a better prognosis for motivated patients in stable relationships.

Janata J, Kingberg S: Sexual aversion disorder. In: Balon R, Segraves RT (eds). *Handbook of Sexual Dysfunctions*. New York, NY: Taylor & Francis, 2005, p. 111.

Kingsberg S, Janata J: The sexual aversions. In: Levine S, Risen C, Althof S (eds). *Handbook of Clinical Sexuality for Mental Health Clinicians*. New York, NY: Brunner/Routledge, 2003, p. 153.

Noll J, Trickett P, Putnam F: A prospective investigation of the impact of childhood sexual abuse on the development of sexuality. *J Consult Clin Psychol* 2003;71:575.

FEMALE SEXUAL AROUSAL DISORDER

 ESSENTIALS OF DIAGNOSIS

The DSM-IV-TR criteria for the diagnosis of female sexual arousal disorder (FSAD) are:

A. *Persistent or recurrent inability to attain, or to maintain until completion of the sexual activity, an adequate lubrication–swelling response of sexual excitement.*

B. *The disturbance causes marked distress or interpersonal difficulty.*

C. *The sexual disorder is not better accounted for by another Axis I disorder (except another sexual dysfunction) and is not due exclusively to the direct physiological effect of a substance (e.g., a drug of abuse, a medication) or a general medical condition.*

Again, FSAD should also be diagnosed according to subtypes: Generalized vs. situational; lifelong vs. acquired; due to psychological factors vs. due to combined factors.

(Reprinted, with permission, from the *Diagnostic and Statistical Manual of Mental Disorders*. 4th edn. Text Revision. Washington, DC: American Psychiatric Association, 2000, p. 544.)

General Considerations

A. EPIDEMIOLOGY

The 1-year prevalence of problems with lubrication in the U.S. females aged 18–59 years is approximately 20%. Epidemiological studies in European populations have reported a 10–15% prevalence increasing to 25–35% after age 50 years, suggesting a positive relationship between problems of lubrication and aging.

B. ETIOLOGY

Problems with lubrication in the perimenopause and menopause are due to a hypoestrogenized vaginal vault. Various psychological factors also interfere with sexual arousal. Radiation therapy and cancer chemotherapy often result in diminished lubrication. Any lesion to the nervous innervation of the genitalia (e.g., spinal cord lesion, multiple sclerosis, alcoholic neuropathy) may result in decreased vaginal lubrication. Pelvic vascular disease can also result in diminished vaginal lubrication. Isolated complaints of difficulties with arousal in premenopausal women who have normal libido are rare).

C. GENETICS

There are no studies of the genetics of FSAD.

Clinical Findings

A. SIGNS & SYMPTOMS

Although the criteria for this disorder specify lack of genital responsiveness to sexual stimuli, most women with this disorder complain of decreased or absent subjective sexual arousal and many are not aware of the degree of their genital response.

B. PSYCHOLOGICAL TESTING

A structured diagnostic method has been shown to have good reliability. The Female Sexual Function Index was specifically developed to assess female arousal disorder.

C. LABORATORY TESTING

No useful, reliable laboratory tests are available for this disorder.

D. NEUROIMAGING

Neuroimaging studies of women experiencing sexual arousal have identified various subcortical and paralimbic areas which are activated during sexual arousal.

Course of Illness

Little is known about the natural history of this disorder if untreated. However, most sexual problems present in women who are relatively inexperienced sexually will improve over time in a stable, committed relationship.

Differential Diagnosis

In postmenopausal women not on estrogen replacement, one needs to consider FSAD due to hypogonadism as the primary diagnosis. Other medical disorders and the possibility of drug-induced sexual dysfunction must also be considered. The specific effects of drugs on female lubrication have been minimally studied. One always suspects a substance induced disorder if the difficulty began after starting a new agent or after dose increases of the agent. A trial off the agent may establish the diagnosis. Lack of adequate foreplay and relationship issues are part of the differential diagnosis.

Treatment

A. Psychopharmacological Treatment

Dopamine receptor agonists (e.g., apomorphine) have been minimally studied in women to date. Topical lubricants may also facilitate coital activities.

B. Psychotherapeutic Treatment

Psychotherapeutic treatment usually consists of sensate focus exercises combined with masturbation exercises. The patient is taught to be more self-focused and assertive about what she finds pleasurable sexually. Uncontrolled clinical reports suggest that this disorder may be responsive to CBT. Some clinicians augment CBT with mechanical devices and/or botanical oils. Most of these treatments are not evidence-based.

C. Other Treatment

Estrogen treatment can reverse sexual symptoms related to the menopause. Estrogen can be applied locally in the form of vaginal creams or by the use of vaginal rings containing estrogen. Estrogen can also be administered systemically either orally or by transdermal patches.

There is some evidence that a small battery operated device that is applied to the clitoris causing increased blood flow into the clitoris and labia is effective in the treatment of female arousal disorder. One double-blind, controlled study found that a botanical massage oil applied to the genitals improved sexual arousal.

Complications of Treatment

Systemic estrogen therapy is associated with an increased risk of breast cancer and cardiovascular disease. Local irritation can be produced by the use of the mechanical vacuum device, or botanical oils.

Prognosis

Psychiatric comorbidity and marital conflict are predictors of a poor outcome.

Altman C, Deldon-Saltin D: Available therapies and outcome results in transition and postmenopausal women. In: Goldstein I, Meston C, Davis S, et al. (eds). *Women's Sexual Function and Dysfunction*. New York, NY: Taylor & Francis, 2006. p. 539.

Billups KL, Berman L, Berman J, et al.: The role of mechanical devices in treating female sexual dysfunction and enhancing the female sexual response. *World J Urol* 2002;20:137.

Dennerstein L: The sexual impact of menopause. In: Levine S, Risen C, Althof S (eds). *Handbook of Clinical Sexuality for Mental Health Professionals*. New York: Brunner/Routledge, 2003, p. 187.

Ferguson D, Steidle C, Singh C, et al.: Randomized, placebo-controlled, double-blind, crossover design trial of the efficacy and safety of Zestra for women in women with and without female sexual arousal disorder. *J Sex Marital Ther* 2003;29(suppl 1):33.

Fourcroy J: Female sexual dysfunction: Potential for pharmacotherapy. *Drugs* 2003;63:1.

Fugl-Meyer A, Fugl-Meyer K: Prevalence data in Europe. In: Goldstein I, Meston C, Davis S, et al. (eds). *Women's Sexual Function and Dysfunction*. New York, NY: Taylor & Francis, 2006, p. 34.

Kang J, Laumann E, Glasser D, et al.: Worldwide prevalence and correlates In: Goldstein I, Meston C, Davis S, et al. (eds). *Women's Sexual Function and Dysfunction*. New York, NY: Taylor & Francis, 2006, p. 42.

Laan E, Everaerd W, Both S: Female sexual arousal disorder. In: Balon R, Segraves RT (eds). *Handbook of Sexual Dysfunction*. New York, NY: Taylor & Francis, 2005, p. 123.

Maravilla K: Blood flow magnetic resonance imaging and brain imaging for evaluating sexual arousal in women. In: Goldstein I, Meston C, Davis S, et al. (eds). *Women's Sexual Function and Dysfunction*. New York, NY: Taylor & Francis, 2006, p. 368.

Paik A, Laumann E: Prevalence of women's sexual problems in the USA. In: Goldstein I, Meston C, Davis S et al. (eds). *Women's Sexual Function and Dysfunction*. A. New York, NY: Taylor & Francis, 2006, p. 23.

Rosen R, Brown C, Heiman J, et al.: The female sexual function index: A multidimensional self-report instrument for the assessment of female sexual function. *J Sex Marital Ther* 2000;26:191.

Rossouw J, Anderson G, Prentice R, et al.: Risks and benefits of estrogen plus progestin in healthy postmenopausal women: Principal results from the Woman's health Initiative randomized controlled study. *JAMA* 2004;291:1701.

Utian W, MacLean D, Symonds T, et al.: A methodological study to validate a structured diagnostic method used to diagnose female sexual dysfunction and its subtypes in postmenopausal women. *J Sex Marital Ther* 2003;31:271.

MALE ERECTILE DISORDER

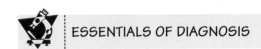 ESSENTIALS OF DIAGNOSIS

The DSM-IV-TR criteria for the diagnosis of male erectile disorder (MED) are:

A. *Persistent or recurrent inability to attain, or to maintain until completion of sexual activity, an adequate erection.*

B. *The disturbance causes marked distress or interpersonal difficulty.*

C. *The erectile dysfunction is not better accounted for by another Axis I disorder (except another sexual dysfunction) and is not due exclusively to the direct physiological effect of a substance (e.g., a* *drug of abuse, a medication) or a general medical condition.*

Again, MED should also be diagnosed according to subtypes: Generalized vs. situational; lifelong vs. acquired; due to psychological factors vs. due to combined factors.

(Reprinted, with permission, from the *Diagnostic and Statistical Manual of Mental Disorders.* 4th edn. Text Revision. Washington, DC: American Psychiatric Association, 2000, p. 547.)

General Considerations

A. Epidemiology

The prevalence of problems with erections is 1–9% below the age of 40 years, increasing to as high as 20–40% after the age of 60 years. Major correlates of erectile problems include age, depression, smoking, diabetes, and hypertension.

B. Etiology

Major depressive disorder, social anxiety, and posttraumatic stress disorder may be associated with MED. Embarrassment and apprehension about possible erectile failure in the future after an initial episode of erectile failure are felt to be involved in the genesis of psychogenic erectile disorder. After an episode of failure, a negative cognitive set and unwitting self-distraction from erotic cues may perpetuate the problem.

A variety of disease including diabetes mellitus, multiple sclerosis, and hypogonadism may be associated with organic erectile problems. Various medications, (namely, antihypertensives and psychiatric) may be associated with erectile problems.

C. Genetics

There is no evidence concerning the genetics of erectile dysfunction.

Clinical Findings

A. Signs & Symptoms

The major symptom of MED is the failure to obtain erections in a situation in which they were anticipated. This is usually accompanied by embarrassment, self-doubt, and loss of self-confidence.

B. Psychological Testing

The most commonly employed questionnaire used to measure improvement over time is the International Inventory of Erectile Function.

C. Laboratory Testing

Standard laboratory testing includes serum free testosterone and serum prolactin, especially if complaints of libido are also present. Other commonly ordered screening laboratory examinations include fasting glucose and lipids. Nocturnal penile tumescence (NPT) testing is sometimes used to differentiate psychogenic from organic impotence. Some clinicians have employed waking erections to erotic audiovisual material to try to distinguish between MED due to psychological factors and MED due to a general medical disorder. However, both of these procedures are used infrequently because of the lack of specificity. Evaluation of erection after intracavernosal injection of erectogenic drugs is sometimes used as a general screening procedure. However, the specificity of this procedure is also unclear. Specialized assessment of vascular function involves dynamic infusion cavernosography, duplex Doppler penile ultrasound, and arteriography. Specialized neurological testing might include dorsal nerve conduction latency and bulbocavernous reflex latency testing.

D. Neuroimaging

Neuroimaging studies are not useful in diagnosis at this time. Several studies of brain processing during penile erections in response to visual sexual stimuli have found that the claustrum had one of the highest activations. Other activations occurred in the paralimbic areas, striatum and hypothalamus. Studies using direct stimulation of the penis found that activation of the insula is prominent. A complex neural circuit associated with sexual arousal involving the anterior cingulate, insula, amygdale hypothalamus and secondary somatosensory cortices has been proposed.

Course of Illness

Brief episodes of erectile failure in sexually inexperienced males frequently remit without intervention. A small number of cases of chronic psychogenic erectile dysfunction will remit without intervention.

Differential Diagnosis

The major issue in differential diagnosis is to establish whether the disorder is due to another Axis I disorder or is exclusively a substance induced disorder or exclusively due to a general medical condition. Although a variety of laboratory assessments are available, the most important element in the differential diagnosis is a careful psychiatric evaluation including a sexual history. If the erectile problem is part of the symptomatic presentation of a major depressive disorder, one would diagnose it as an Axis I disorder. The next major element in the differential diagnosis is to rule out a substance-induced disorder. Many drugs such as antidepressants and antipsychotics have been reported to be associated with erectile dysfunction. If the history establishes that the disorder began after a drug was administered or after a dose adjustment, a trial off the suspected drug is in order. Erectile dysfunction may be associated with hyperprolactinemia or hypogonadism, both of which can be detected by laboratory assays. In general, these causes of erectile dysfunction are also associated with a complaint of decreased libido. By history one would establish the presence or absence of diseases likely to cause erectile problems. For example, erectile dysfunction is common in diabetes mellitus and multiple sclerosis. It also can be a result of pelvic surgery or radiation therapy.

Cases with a situational or lifelong pattern are suggestive of a psychogenic etiology. Most organic etiologies are global and acquired. The presence of erections under any circumstances, especially erections upon awakening, is suggestive of a psychogenic etiology. Since the advent of safe oral therapies, extensive laboratory examinations to determine the etiology of erectile complaints are uncommon.

Treatment

A. Psychopharmacological Treatment

First line pharmacological interventions include sildenafil, tadalafil, and vardenafil, all phosphodiesterase type 5 inhibitors. These agents have been used both in psychogenic and organic impotence with success. In psychogenic impotence, indications for the use of oral vasoactive drugs include (1) failure of psychotherapy, (2) low self-confidence, (3) chronicity, (4) alexithymia, and (5) a coexisting contributing biological factor.

B. Psychotherapeutic Treatment

Psychological treatment is usually behavioral and involves graduated sexual homework assignments, a temporary cessation of attempts at coitus, modification of unrealistic expectations and cognitions, and supportive psychotherapy. The preferred technique is conjoint couple behavioral psychotherapy.

C. Other Treatment

Vacuum erection devices, intracavernosal and intraurethral prostaglandins E1 have been used in men with both psychogenic and organic impotence. As a last resort, vascular surgery or microsurgery, or penile prosthesis implantation can be employed.

Complications/Adverse Outcomes of Treatment

Phosphodiesterase type 5 inhibitors may have the following side effects: Priapism, facial flushing, nasal stuffiness, visual disturbances, dyspepsia, and syncope. These drugs are contraindicated with the use of nitrates and should be used in caution in individuals with unstable angina or who are on multiple antihypertensive drugs.

Both intraurethral and intracavernosal prostaglandins E1 can be associated with pain at the site of injection as well as the risk of priapism. There are operative risks with penile prosthesis implantation including hemorrhage and infection.

Prognosis

The prognosis in acquired psychogenic erectile dysfunction is excellent. The prognosis in lifelong global erectile dysfunction is poor. In organic problems of mild to moderate severity, the prognosis is good with the use of oral agents. In MED with combined psychological and organic features, the prognosis for return of sexual activity is less promising unless psychotherapy is combined with pharmacotherapy.

Althof S: Erectile dysfunction: Psychotherapy in men and couples. In: Leiblum SR, Rosen R (eds). *Principles and Practice of Sex Therapy.* New York, NY: Guilford, 2000, p. 133.

Althof S: Therapeutic weaving: The integration of treatment techniques. In: Levine S, Risen C, Althof S (eds). *Handbook of Clinical Sexuality for Mental Health Professionals.* New York, NY: Brunner-Mazel, 2003, p. 359.

Fagan P: Psychogenic impotence in relatively young men. In: Levine S, Risen C, Althof S (eds). *Handbook of Clinical Sexuality for Mental Health Professionals.* New York, NY: Brunner-Routledge, 2003, p. 217.

Ferretti A, Caulo M, DelGratta C, et al.: Dynamics of male sexual arousal: Distinct components of brain activation revealed by fMRI. *Neuroimage* 2005;26:1086.

Georgiadis J, Holstege G: Human brain activation during stimulation of the penis. *J Comp Neurol* 2005;493:33.

Lewis R, Fugl-Meyer K, Bosch R, et al.: Epidemiology of sexual dysfunction. In: Lue T, Basson R, Rosen R, et al. (eds). *Sexual Medicine. Sexual Dysfunctions in Men and Women.* Plymouth, UK: Health Publications, 2004, p. 37.

Redoute J, Stoleru S, Greguire M, et al.: Brain processing of visual sexual stimuli in human males. *Hum Brain Mapp* 2000;11:162.

Rosen R, Cappelleri J, Gendrano N: Erectile function (IIEF): A state of the science review. *Int J Imp Res* 2002;14:226.

Rosen R, Hatzichristou D, Broderick G, et al.: Clinical evaluation and symptom scales: Sexual dysfunction assessment in men. In: Lue T, Basson R, Rosen R, et al. (eds). *Sexual Medicine. Sexual Dysfunctions in Men and Women.* Plymouth, UK: Health Publications, 2004, p. 173.

Segraves RT: Recognizing and reversing sexual side effects of medication. In: Levine S, Risen C, Althof S (eds). *Handbook of Clinical Sexuality for Mental Health Professionals.* New York, NY: Brunner-Routledge, 2003, p. 377.

Stoleru S: Neuroanatomical correlates of visually evoked sexual arousal in human males. *Arch Sex Behav* 1999;28:1.

Wylie K, MacInnes I: Erectile dysfunction. In: Balon R, Segraves RT (eds). *Handbook of Erectile Dysfunction.* New York, NY: Taylor & Francis, 2005, p. 155.

FEMALE ORGASMIC DISORDER

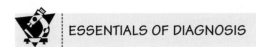 ESSENTIALS OF DIAGNOSIS

The DSM-IV-TR criteria for the diagnosis of female orgasmic disorder (FOD) are:

A. *Persistent or recurrent delay in, or absence of, orgasm following a normal sexual excitement phase. Women exhibit wide variability in the type or the intensity of stimulation that triggers orgasm. The diagnosis of FOD should be based on clinician's judgment that the woman's orgasmic capacity is less than what would be reasonable for her age, sexual experience, and adequacy of sexual stimulation she receives.*

B. *The disturbance causes marked distress or interpersonal difficulty.*

C. *The orgasmic dysfunction is not better accounted for by another Axis I disorder (except another sexual dysfunction) and is not due exclusively to the direct physiological effect of a substance (e.g., a drug of abuse, a medication) or a general medical condition.*

The FOD should also be diagnosed according to subtypes: Generalized vs. situational; lifelong vs. acquired; due to psychological factors vs. due to combined factors.

(Reprinted, with permission, from the *Diagnostic and Statistical Manual of Mental Disorders*. 4th edn. Text Revision. Washington, DC: American Psychiatric Association, 2000, p. 549.)

General Considerations

In the past, FOD has been referred to as inhibited sexual orgasm or anorgasmia.

A. EPIDEMIOLOGY

In a national epidemiology study of U.S. females aged 18–59 years, approximately 24% of U.S. females complained of difficulty reaching orgasm.

B. ETIOLOGY

The etiology may be psychogenic, drug-induced (e.g., antidepressants), or due to a general medical condition. Orgasmic capacity appears to be an earned response, with a lower rate in younger women. Lack of an advanced degree and report of religious affiliation is related to a lower frequency of orgasm attainment during masturbation. There is some evidence that early separation from the father may be related to problems achieving orgasm in heterosexual activities. Substance induced orgasmic disorder may be caused by TCAs, SSRIs, alpha-blockers, D-2 blockers and benzodiazepines. Diseases, accidents, or surgical events, which affect the nervous innervation of the genitalia, such as spinal cord lesions, multiple sclerosis, diabetes mellitus, surgical lesions, and alcoholic peripheral neuropathies, may cause FOD. Anorgasmia may be part of the symptomatic presentation of severe depression or social anxiety.

C. GENETICS

Twin studies in Australia indicate that genetics probably account for 31% of the variance in the frequency of orgasm during coitus and 51% of the variance in the frequency of orgasm during masturbation. The higher percentage of the variance in the frequency of orgasm explained by genetic factors during masturbation than coitus may be due to the absence of relationship variables during masturbation.

Clinical Findings

A. SIGNS & SYMPTOMS

The typical patient will complain of normal libido and sexual excitement without the capacity to reach orgasm.

B. PSYCHOLOGICAL TESTING

Psychological testing is rarely required to make this diagnosis. Psychometric instruments that can be used to measure progress in treatment include the Changes in Sexual Functioning Questionnaire and the Female Sexual Function Index.

C. LABORATORY TESTING

Laboratory testing is rarely indicated in the investigation of FOD. Nerve conduction studies can be obtained if one has reason to suspect neurogenic anorgasmia.

D. NEUROIMAGING

One study in women with spinal cord injury found that orgasm elicited by self-stimulation of the vaginal-cervical region included the hypothalamic paraventricular nucleus, medial amygdala, anterior cingulate, frontal, parietal, and insula cortices as well as the cerebellum. Female orgasm differed from male ejaculation in that the amygdala was not deactivated and the periaqueductal gray area was activated.

Course of Illness

Most women who have difficulty reaching orgasm in early sexual experiences gain better orgasmic capacity after sexual experience in a long-term committed relationship.

Differential Diagnosis

A careful sexual history will usually establish the presence or absence of disease capable of causing FOD. A careful pharmacological history may reveal a probable substance induced female orgasmic disorder. Serotonergic antidepressants such as paroxetine, sertraline, fluoxetine, citalopram, and es-citalopram may be associated with FOD. It is less common with bupropion, nefazodone and duloxetine. Both traditional and atypical antipsychotics may be associated with anorgasmia either because of alpha-adrenergic blockade or dopamine D-2 blockade. Benzodiazepines may also cause orgasmic delay. FOD may also be associated with relationship discord.

If FOD is global and lifelong, a psychological etiology is probable. If the problem is acquired and situational, relationship discord is a probable etiology. If the problem is acquired and global, one should carefully rule out FOD due to a general medical condition and substance-induced FOD.

Treatment

A. PSYCHOPHARMACOLOGICAL TREATMENT

There are no known therapies for FOD due to a general medical condition. In substance induced FOD, change of medication or the use of antidotes may reverse the disorder. If the patient is on an SSRI, one can substitute bupropion, nefazodone or duloxetine or use high-dose buspirone (60 mg/d) as an antidote. It is unclear whether sildenafil can reverse SSRI-induced orgasmic delay. If the patient is on a typical antipsychotic or risperidone, one can try substituting aripiprazole, quetiapine, or olanzapine. One unreplicated, controlled study found that sildenafil had a significant positive effect in orgasm attainment in young women with high libido who were in committed long-term relationships. Another unreplicated, controlled study found that bupropion improved orgasmic capacity in women with HSDD. It is unclear whether bupropion is effective in women with a primary diagnosis of FOD.

B. PSYCHOTHERAPEUTIC TREATMENT

CBT appears to be effective in the treatment of lifelong FOD due to psychological factors, but not in acquired FOD. CBT involves changing of negative sexual thoughts and attitudes. Directed masturbation homework assignments are commonly employed. Most women can learn to achieve orgasm by self-stimulation. A smaller number learn to transfer this to partner-related activities.

C. OTHER TREATMENT

There is some anecdotal evidence that the use of mechanical clitoral vacuum devices may augment orgasmic capacity in women with FOD.

Complications/Adverse Outcomes of Treatment

The use of buspirone with serotonergic antidepressants may increase the risk of a serotonin syndrome. Bupropion lowers the seizure threshold. Drug substitution always carries the risk of relapse or emergence of comorbid psychiatric illness.

Prognosis

The prognosis for FOD due to psychological factors is good. CBT combined with masturbation homework assignments is usually successful in teaching women how to achieve orgasm through masturbation. A smaller number of women are able to transfer this skip to partner related activities.

Caruso S, Intelsano G, Lupo L, et al.: Premenopausal women affected by sexual arousal disorder treated with sildenafil: A double-blind, cross-over, placebo-controlled study. *BJOG* 2001;108:623.

Dawood K, Kirk KM, Bailey JM, et al.: Genetic and environmental influences on the frequency of orgasm in women. *Twin Res Hum Genet* 2005;8:27–33.

Ellison C: Facilitating orgasmic responsiveness. In: Levine S, Risen C, Althof S (eds). *Handbook of Clinical Sexuality for Mental Health Clinicians.* New York, NY: Brunner-Routledge, 2003, p. 167.

Keller A, McGarvey E, Clayton A: Reliability and construct validity of the changes in sexual functioning questionnaire short form. *J Sex Marital Ther* 2006;32:43.

Komisaruk BR, Whipple B, Crawford A, et al.: Brain activation during vaginocervical self-stimulation and orgasm in women with complete spinal cord injury: FMRI evidence of mediation by the vagus nerves. *Brain Res* 2004;1024:77.

Laumann E, Gagnon J, Michael R, et al.: *The Social Organization of Sexuality.* Chicago, IL: University of Chicago Press, 1994.

Meston CN, Levine R: Female orgasm dysfunction. In: Balon R, Segraves RT (eds). *Handbook of Sexual Dysfunction.* New York, NY: Taylor & Francis, 2005, p. 193.

Salonia A, Briganti A, Rigatti P, et al.: Medical conditions associated with female sexual dysfunction. In: Goldstein I, Meston C, Davis S, et al. (eds). *Women's Sexual Function and Dysfunction.* New York, NY: Taylor & Francis, 2006, p. 263.

Segraves R: Role of the psychiatrist. In: Goldstein I, Meston C, Davis S (eds). *Women's Sexual Function and Dysfunction.* New York, NY: Taylor & Francis, 2006, p. 696.

MALE ORGASMIC DISORDER

 ESSENTIALS OF DIAGNOSIS

The DSM-IV-TR criteria for the diagnosis of male orgasmic disorder (MOD) are:

A. *Persistent or recurrent delay in, or absence of, orgasm following a normal sexual excitement phase during sexual activity that the clinician, taking into account the person's age, judges to be adequate in focus, intensity, and duration.*

B. *The disturbance causes marked distress or interpersonal difficulty.*

C. *The orgasmic dysfunction is not better accounted for by another Axis I disorder (except another sexual dysfunction) and is not due exclusively to the direct physiological effect of a substance (e.g., a drug of abuse, a medication) or a general medical condition.*

Again, the MOD should also be diagnosed according to subtypes: Generalized vs. situational; lifelong vs. acquired; due to psychological factors vs. due to combined factors.

(Reprinted, with permission, from the *Diagnostic and Statistical Manual of Mental Disorders*. 4th edn. Text Revision. Washington, DC: American Psychiatric Association, 2000, p. 552.)

General Considerations

MOD refers both to delayed orgasm and absence of orgasm. The diagnosis depends on clinician judgment as there are no guidelines concerning severity or duration of the problem before it reaches the threshold for diagnosis. A variety of terms have been used in the literature to refer to this disorder. They include retarded ejaculation, inhibited ejaculation, *ejaculatio retarda, impotencia ejaculandi*, and anejaculation among others.

A. EPIDEMIOLOGY

In a national epidemiological study, approximately 8% of U.S. males aged 18–59 years complained of an inability to reach orgasm.

B. ETIOLOGY

Similar to FOD, the etiology of MOD may be due to psychological factors, drug-induced or due to a general medical condition. Substance-induced MOD may be caused by TCAs, MAOIs, SSRIs, drugs causing alpha-adrenergic blockade, dopamine D-2 blockers, and benzodiazepines. Diseases, accidents or surgical procedures, which interrupt the nerve supply of the ejaculatory apparatus, can interfere with the ability to reach orgasm. Spinal cord lesions, pelvic surgery as well as peripheral neuropathies can cause anorgasmia. Difficulty reaching orgasm can be part of the presentation of severe depression. Anger at women in general or to the sexual partner in specific has been hypothesized to be responsible for male anorgasmia due to psychological factors. This hypothesis is unproven. There is minimal evidence concerning the etiology and treatment of this disorder when it is due to psychological factors.

C. GENETICS

There are no studies of the genetics of this disorder.

Clinical Findings

A. SIGNS & SYMPTOMS

The typical patient reports either that he is unable to ejaculate or that it takes an inordinately long amount of sexual stimulation in order to ejaculate. Some men may struggle to ejaculate such that they deny sexual pleasure both to themselves and their partners.

B. PSYCHOLOGICAL TESTING

Psychological testing is not available for this disorder.

C. LABORATORY TESTING

If a neurological etiology is suspected, pudendal nerve conduction studies and evoked potential studies can be ordered.

D. NEUROIMAGING

Research has been conducted concerning the cortical areas activated during ejaculation. This research does not have a clinical application. Areas activated include the ventral tegmental area, central tegmental field, zona incerta, subparafascicular nucleus and thalamic nuclei as well as the lateral putamen and claustrum.

Course of Illness

MOD due to psychological factors is rarely encountered in clinical practice and there is minimal evidence regarding its clinical course. Most clinicians regard this as chronic condition.

Differential Diagnosis

A careful medical history is taken to rule out MOD due to a general medical condition such as multiple sclerosis, diabetes mellitus, or surgical lesion affecting the nerve supply to the genitalia. A careful pharmacological history should focus on the use of opioid drugs, benzodiazepines, serotonergic drugs or drugs with significant alpha or dopamine D-2 blockade.

A careful review of the presenting symptoms may indicate probable etiologies. For example, if the difficulty is situational (i.e., partner or sex specific), one should suspect psychological factors. If the problem is acquired and global, one should carefully rule out MOD due to a general medical condition and substance-induced MOD.

Treatment

A. PSYCHOPHARMACOLOGICAL TREATMENT

There is no pharmacological treatment for MOD due to a general medical condition. Substance-induced MOD can be reversed depending on the offending agent. Serotonergic antidepressants can be replaced with antidepressants with a decreased likelihood of causing orgasm delay. Buspirone at a dose of 60 mg/d can be used as an antidote. If MOD is due to antipsychotic agents, one can substitute aripiprazole, quetiapine or olanzapine.

B. PSYCHOTHERAPEUTIC TREATMENT

There is no evidence-based therapy for MOD due to psychological factors. Most clinicians would attempt behavioral therapy using a vibrator for intense stimulation. Once ejaculation can be reliably achieved in solitary masturbation homework assignments, the clinician might try to gradually phase this new skill into partner related activities.

C. OTHER TREATMENT

If infertility is a primary concern in MOD due to a general medical condition, sperm can be obtained by the stimulation of the internal ejaculatory organs by a transrectal electrical probe.

Complications/Adverse Outcomes of Treatment

In cases of substance-induced MOD, drug substitution carries the risk of recurrence of the psychiatric disorder being treated.

Prognosis

The prognosis is substance-induced MOD is good. The prognosis of MOD due to psychological or medical conditions is poor.

Holstege G, Georgiadis J, Paans A, et al.: Brain activation during human male ejaculation. *J Neurosci* 2003;23:9185.

McMahon C, Abdo C, Incrocci L, et al.: Disorders of orgasm and ejaculation in men. In: Lue T, Basson R, Rosen R, et al. (eds). *Sexual Medicine. Sexual Dysfunctions in Men and Women.* Plymouth UK: Health Publications, 2004, p. 409.

Waldinger M: Male ejaculation and orgasmic disorders. In: Balon R, Segraves RT (eds). *Handbook of Sexual Dysfunction.* New York, NY: Taylor & Francis, 2005, p. 215.

PREMATURE EJACULATION

 ESSENTIALS OF DIAGNOSIS

The DSM-IV-TR criteria for the diagnosis of premature ejaculation (PE) are:

A. *Persistent or recurrent ejaculation with minimal sexual stimulation before, on, or shortly after penetration and before the person wishes it. The clinician must take into account factors that affect duration of excitement phase, such as age, novelty of the sexual partner or situation, and recent frequency of sexual activity.*

B. *The disturbance causes marked distress or interpersonal difficulty.*

C. *The PE is not due exclusively to the direct effect of a substance (e.g., withdrawal from opioids).*

PE could also be diagnosed according to subtypes: Generalized vs. situational; lifelong vs. acquired; due to psychological factors vs. due to combined factors.

(Reprinted, with permission, from the *Diagnostic and Statistical Manual of Mental Disorders.* 4th edn. Text Revision. Washington, DC: American Psychiatric Association, 2000, p. 554.)

General Considerations

Diagnostic criteria do not specify the exact ejaculatory latency necessary for this diagnosis. In the absence of normative data on ejaculatory latency in the general population, most clinicians would not diagnose premature ejaculation unless the intravaginal ejaculatory latency (IVEL) is less than 1 or 2 minutes. One Dutch study found that most men complaining of PE had an IVEL of less than 1 minute. A study of U.S. men diagnosed as having PE found that the median IVEL was less than 2 minutes.

A. EPIDEMIOLOGY

Approximately 28% of U.S. males aged 18–59 years complained of problems with rapid ejaculation in the preceding year. In epidemiological studies, significant correlations have been found between measures of anxiety and PE. In one Scandinavian study, only 2–3% of men reported that they had a problem with rapid ejaculation. In contrast, 18–22% of the women reported that their male partners had problems with rapid ejaculation. Interestingly, two thirds of the men surveyed stated that their partners took too long to reach orgasm. Later cohorts of women reported rapid ejaculation in their partners more often that earlier cohorts, suggesting that changing societal expectations may play a role in defining when rapid ejaculation is considered to be a problem.

B. ETIOLOGY

There are several major hypotheses concerning the etiology of patterns of lifelong PE. Psychoanalytically oriented clinicians hypothesized that unconscious anger toward women was an etiological factor. Cognitive–behavioral clinicians posited that rapid ejaculation is a pattern learned in adolescence and then maintained by performance anxiety. In spite of the wide acceptance of the cognitive–behavioral hypothesis, there is minimal evidence to support this hypothesis. Other clinicians have hypothesized that PE is the result of abnormalities in either spinal or central nervous system mechanisms controlling ejaculatory thresholds. Waldinger hypothesized that ejaculatory speed is hereditarily determined, normally distributed in the general population, and represents a normal variation and thus is not a psychiatric disorder. He further hypothesized that the set point of the ejaculatory threshold is related to hyposensitivity of the serotonin 5HT2c receptor and hypersensitivity of the 5HT1 a receptor. This hypothesis is consistent with the effects of various pharmacological influences on ejaculatory latency. There is evidence that rapid ejaculation is more common in men with panic disorder and social anxiety.

There is minimal evidence concerning the etiology of acquired PE. There appears to be a higher incidence of acquired PE in men with chronic prostatitis and after certain brain and spinal cord injuries. Premature ejaculation has been report to occur upon heroin and methadone withdrawal.

C. GENETICS

There is some evidence of a familial pattern.

Clinical Findings

A. SIGNS & SYMPTOMS

Men with lifelong PE will report ejaculating rapidly since their first experience with a sexual partner. They may be able to delay ejaculation during masturbation but not with a sexual partner. Often, they seek treatment at the insistence of their sexual partner.

B. PSYCHOLOGICAL TESTING

Psychological testing is not required to establish this diagnosis.

C. LABORATORY TESTING

The most frequent diagnostic procedure utilized in clinical trials is IVEL measured by stopwatch during sexual activities at home. The partner is the one who uses the stopwatch. How much this procedure influences ejaculatory latency is unknown.

If a neurological lesion is suspected, specialized procedures such as measurement of pudendal nerve latency and the characteristics of cortical evoked potentials from pudendal nerve stimulation or urethral stimulation are possible, These procedures are rarely used in the evaluation of men with complaints of rapid ejaculation.

D. NEUROIMAGING

Neuroimaging is not useful in diagnosis of PE.

Course of Illness

The pattern of rapid ejaculation in the absence of treatment is considered to be lifelong. There is no evidence of improvement with aging.

Differential Diagnosis

Cases of lifelong global rapid ejaculation are predominantly devoid of organic pathology. One should establish if the problem is secondary to a panic disorder or social anxiety disorder. If the man reports rapid ejaculation with one partner and not another, one obviously would investigate the differences in sexual patterns with the two partners.

If the problem is acquired, the possibility of a relationship issue or an organic pathology should be considered.

Treatment

A. PSYCHOPHARMACOLOGICAL TREATMENT

Many clinicians employ serotonergic drugs in the treatment of rapid ejaculation. The two agents used most frequently are paroxetine and clomipramine. Paroxetine usually requires chronic dosing at 20 mg. An occasional patient will respond to as-needed dosing after 2 weeks of daily dosing. Clomipramine can be used on an as-needed basis ingesting the drug 4–6 hours prior to sexual activity. Other serotonergic drugs such as fluoxetine and sertraline are used less frequently. Some investigators have reported success with benzodiazepines.

B. PSYCHOTHERAPEUTIC TREATMENT

Behavioral approaches are usually employed. These include the "start–stop" and squeeze technique. Both techniques involve repeated episodes of manual penile stimulation stopped prior to ejaculatory inevitability. The "squeeze technique" involves a firm squeeze of the frenulum before the next episode of stimulation. Clinical experience suggests that the technique requires the participation of the sexual partner to be successful. The mechanism by which these techniques work is unclear. It is assumed that in the absence of performance pressure that the man learns to monitor his level of sexual stimulation, and thus modulate his level of excitement. Behavioral treatment of PE has been shown to be more effective than a waiting-list control and equally as effective as sertraline therapy.

C. Other Treatment

Psychodynamic psychotherapy is rarely utilized in the treatment of this condition. Topical anesthetics, such as a prilocaine–lidocaine mixture, can be used to delay ejaculation.

Complications/Adverse Outcomes of Treatment

Use of serotonergic drugs with short half-life can result in a withdrawal syndrome. This has been most often reported with the immediate release form of paroxetine. Topical anesthetics can result in penile anesthesia and there is a risk of vaginal absorption.

Prognosis

The short-term prognosis with behavioral therapy and pharmacotherapy is excellent. However, the problem recurs if the drug is stopped and there is a high-relapse rate after successful behavioral therapy.

Abdel-Hamid IA, El Naggar E, Gilani A-HEL: Assessment of an as needed use of pharmacotherapy and the pause-squeeze technique in premature ejaculation. *Int J Impot Res* 2001;13:41.

Atikeler M, Gecit I, Senol F: Optimum use of prilocaine-lidocaine cream in premature ejaculation. *Andrologia* 2002;34:356.

Dunn KM, Croft P, Hacket G: Association of sexual problems with social, psychological and physical problems in men and women in a cross sectional population survey. *J Epidemiol Comm Health* 1999;53:144.

Figeira I, Possidente E, Arques C, et al.: Sexual dysfunction: A neglected complication of panic disorder and social phobia. *Arch Sex Behav* 2001;30:369.

Haavio-Mannila E, Kontula O: *Sexual Trends in the Baltic Sea Area.* Helsinki: Family Federation of Finland, 2003.

Nkangineme I, Segraves RT: Neuropsychiatric aspects of sexual dysfunction. In: Schiffer R, Rao S, Fogel B (eds). *Neuropsychiatry*, 2nd edn. Philadelphia, PA: Lippincott Williams & Wilkins, 2003, p. 338.

Patrick D, Althof S, Pryor J, et al.: Premature ejaculation: An observational study of men and their partners. *J Sex Med* 2005;2:358.

Screponi E, Carosa E, Di Stasi M, et al.: Prevalence of chronic prostatitis in men with premature ejaculation. *Urol* 2001;58:198.

Simpson G, McCann B, Lowy M: Treatment of premature ejaculation after traumatic brain injury. *Brain Inj* 2003;17:723.

Waldinger M: Rapid ejaculation. In: Levine S, Risen C, Althof S (eds). *Handbook of Clinical Sexuality for Mental Health Professionals.* New York, NY: Bruner-Routledge, 2003, p. 257.

DYSPAREUNIA (NOT DUE TO A GENERAL MEDICAL CONDITION)

 ESSENTIALS OF DIAGNOSIS

The DSM-IV-TR criteria for the diagnosis of dyspareunia (DYS) are:

A. *Recurrent or persistent genital pain associated with sexual intercourse in either a male or a female.*

B. *The disturbance causes marked distress or interpersonal difficulty.*

C. *The disturbance is not caused exclusively by Vaginismus or lack of lubrication, is not better accounted for by another Axis I disorder (except another sexual dysfunction) and is not due exclusively to the direct physiological effect of a substance (e.g., a drug of abuse, a medication) or a general medical condition.*

The DYS should also be diagnosed according to subtypes: Generalized vs. situational; lifelong vs. acquired; due to psychological factors vs. due to combined factors.

(Reprinted, with permission, from the *Diagnostic and Statistical Manual of Mental Disorders.* 4th edn. Text Revision. Washington, DC: American Psychiatric Association, 2000, p. 556.)

General Considerations

A number of terms are used to describe dyspareunia in females including chronic pelvic pain, vulvodynia, vulvovestibulitis, and vestibulodynia. These terms do not have precise definitions. Vulvar vestibulitis refers to pain experienced in the vulvar vestibule upon contact whereas vulvodynia usually refers to chronic vulvar pain that may occur with or without sexual contact. However, many patients cannot describe the location of their pain with precision. Some men will complain of painful ejaculation, testicular pain after ejaculation, penile sensitivity or muscle cramps after sexual activity.

In most cases of dyspareunia, psychological and relationship factors will be evident. It is often impossible to determine if theses issues preceded or were the result of dyspareunia.

A. Epidemiology

Approximately 14% of U.S. females and 8% of U.S. males aged 18–59 years complained of painful coitus in the preceding year.

B. Etiology

There is little definitive information concerning the etiology of dyspareunia in women. Even less is known about dyspareunia in males.

C. Genetics

There have been no genetic studies of dyspareunia.

Clinical Findings

A. Signs & Symptoms

The typical female patient with dyspareunia first consults her primary care physician or gynecologist. The diagnosis is made by history. The patient may describe superficial or deep pain upon penetration, which may persist only during sexual activity or she may describe a chronic throbbing pain, which lasts hours after sexual contact. After several invasive and painful evaluations, they may be told that a physical etiology cannot be found and then are referred to mental health professionals. Most complaints of sexual pain cannot be adequately diagnosed. Male patients often present initially to urologists. We have little information concerning the typical presentation of male patients with dyspareunia.

B. Psychological Testing

Psychological testing is of little use in the diagnosis of dyspareunia.

C. Laboratory Testing

Yeast cultures, testing for venereal disease, and evaluation for endometriosis may be performed by gynecologists prior to referral to mental health professional. Hormonal assays and cytological examination may also be performed. Most gynecologists will use a cotton swab during the pelvis examination to locate areas where touch elicits pain.

D. Neuroimaging

There have been no neuroimaging studies of patients with dyspareunia.

Course of Illness

There is little evidence concerning the course of this illness. Idiopathic dyspareunia is described by most clinicians as having a chronic and unremitting course.

Differential Diagnosis

The major differential is between dyspareunia due to psychological factors and dyspareunia due to combined factors or due to a general medical condition. This differential diagnosis is often impossible to make with precision. Dyspareunia due to psychological factors is a diagnosis of exclusion. As knowledge regarding physical causes of sexual pain is limited, one assumes that many cases of dyspareunia due to medical causes are erroneously designated as psychogenic. Most women with severe dyspareunia will also have personal psychological distress as well as relationship discord.

The first issue in differential diagnosis is to identify treatable organic etiologies. A gynecologist experienced in the diagnosis of dyspareunia will try to replicate the pain upon physical examination.

Treatment

A. Psychopharmacological Treatment

There are no specific pharmacotherapies for this disorder. Antidepressants (e.g., duloxetine) may help if depression accompanies dyspareunia.

B. Psychotherapeutic Treatment

One of the most helpful psychotherapeutic interventions in female dysparunia is to acknowledge the reality of the pain. Typical psychotherapy consists of cognitive behavioral pain management. Pelvic floor biofeedback may be employed.

C. Other Treatment

Dyspareunia due to atrophic vaginitis can be alleviated by vaginal creams and nonhormonal vaginal lubricants may be helpful. Treatment of yeast infections may be necessary. Acupuncture and hypnotherapy have been advocated. For idiopathic dyspareunia, gynecologists may suggest sitz baths, topical lidocaine, corticosteroid creams, or physical therapy. Rarely, vestibulectomy may be performed.

Complications/Adverse Outcomes of Treatment

There are no known complications to the psychological treatment of this condition.

Prognosis

The prognosis is variable and most often poor.

Bergeron S, Meana M, Binik Y, et al.: Painful genital sexual activity. In: Levine S, Risen C, Althof S (eds). *Handbook of Clinical Sexuality for Mental Health Professional.* New York, NY: Brunner-Routledge, 2003, p. 131.

Goldstein I: Medical management: Perspective of the sexual medicine physician. In: Goldstein I, Meston C, Davis S, et al. (eds). *Women's Sexual Function and Dysfunction.* New York, NY: Taylor & Francis, 2006, p. 508.

Herman H: Physical therapy for female sexual dysfunction. In: Goldstein I, Meston C, Davis S, et al. (eds). *Women's Sexual Function and Dysfunction.* New York, NY: Taylor & Francis, 2006, p. 496.

Payne K, Bergeron S, Khalife J, et al.: Assessment, treatment strategies and outcome results: Perspective of pain specialists. In: Goldstein I, Meston C, Davis S, et al. (eds). *Women's Sexual Function and Dysfucntion.* New York, NY: Taylor & Francis, 2006, p. 471.

Pukall C, Payne K, Kao A, et al. Dyspareunia. In: Balon R, Segraves RT (eds). *Handbook of Sexual Dysfunction.* New York, NY: Taylor & Francis, 2005, p. 249.

VAGINISMUS (NOT DUE TO A GENERAL MEDICAL CONDITION)

 ESSENTIALS OF DIAGNOSIS

The DSM-IV-TR criteria for the diagnosis of vaginismus (VAG) are:

A. *Recurrent or persistent involuntary spasm of the musculature of the outer third of the vagina that interferes with sexual intercourse.*

B. *The disturbance causes marked distress or interpersonal difficulty.*

C. *The disturbance is not better accounted for by another Axis I disorder (e.g., somatization disorder) and is not due exclusively to the direct physiological effect of a general medical condition.*

The VAG should also be diagnosed according to subtypes: Generalized vs. situational; lifelong vs. acquired; due to psychological factors vs. due to combined factors.

(Reprinted, with permission, from the *Diagnostic and Statistical Manual of Mental Disorders.* 4th edn. Text Revision. Washington, DC: American Psychiatric Association, 2000, p. 558.)

General Considerations

Clinically, one may encounter this syndrome in women attempting coitus for the first time. It may also be a cause for "unconsummated marriage". In the later case, patients may present for treatment when pregnancy is desired. Many women with vaginismus are able to experience sexual pleasure as long as vaginal penetration is not attempted.

A. EPIDEMIOLOGY

There is minimal evidence concerning the epidemiology of this condition.

B. ETIOLOGY

It is hypothesized to be a conditioned anxiety reaction, which results in spasm of the entrance to the vagina. This may be the result of previous painful sexual encounters including sexual abuse or excessive fear about penetration. Studies concerning history of child sexual abuse, personality traits, marital conflict, and presence of sexual dysfunction in the partner have been inconsistent. Studies about abnormalities in pelvic floor physiology have been inconsistent. There is comorbidity with anxiety disorders.

C. GENETICS

There is no information concerning the genetics of this disorder.

Clinical Findings

A. SIGNS & SYMPTOMS

The patient usually reports inability to achieve vaginal penetration. The gynecologist may have observed that the patient was unable to assume or maintain the dorsal lithotomy position for a pelvic examination.

B. PSYCHOLOGICAL TESTING

Psychological testing is not helpful in establishing this diagnosis.

C. LABORATORY TESTING

Many but not all women with vaginismus will have spasm of the vaginal musculature during a gynecological examination. Physical therapists have been reported to be able to differentiate women with vaginismus from normal controls on the basis of muscle tone of the pelvic floor.

D. NEUROIMAGING

There are no neuroimaging studies of women with vaginismus.

Course of Illness

There is minimal evidence concerning the natural history of untreated vaginismus.

Clinicians believe that some cases spontaneously remit in long-term committed relationships.

Differential Diagnosis

The major differential is a physical cause for pain during coitus. This requires careful gynecological examination.

Treatment

A. PSYCHOPHARMACOLOGICAL TREATMENT

Individual case reports suggest that benzodiazepine-assisted systematic desensitization may be successful in reversing this condition.

B. PSYCHOTHERAPEUTIC TREATMENT

Behavioral approaches are the preferred treatment. The patient is taught to relax. Then over weeks, she gradually introduces objects of increasing diameter into her vagina. These objects can be her fingers or vaginal dilators. The size of the object she introduces into her vagina is increased until the vagina can comfortably accommodate a size approximately the diameter of her partner's erect penis. Once she can comfortably introduce a large object into her vagina without painful spasm, she then asks her partner to do the same. Gradually, this progresses to vaginal penetration. Although this approach is common clinical practice, there are no controlled trials demonstrating its efficacy.

C. OTHER TREATMENT

In the past, perineal plasty or levatorplasty was performed. A surgical approach is rarely utilized today. There are also case reports of successful use of botulinum toxins. Some cases are treated by physical therapists who teach the patient to control the muscle tone of the pelvic floor.

Complications/Adverse Outcomes of Treatment

There are no reported complications of the behavioral treatment of vaginismus.

Prognosis

With appropriate treatment, the prognosis is good. However, it should be emphasized that successful treatment requires empathy and patience. The simple application of vaginal dilators is seldom successful in reversing this condition.

Basson R, Schultz W, Binik Y, et al.: Women's sexual desire and arousal disorders and sexual pain. In: Lue T, Meston C, Davis S, et al. (eds). *Sexual Medicine. Sexual Dysfunction in Men and Women.* Plymouth, UK: Health Publications, 2005, p. 851.

Schultz WCM, Van de Wiel HBM: Vaginismus. In: Balon R, Segraves RT (eds). *Handbook of Sexual Dysfunction.* New York, NY: Taylor & Francis, 2005, p. 273.

Stewart E: Physical examination in female sexual dysfunction. In: Goldstein I, Meston C, Davis S, et al. (eds). *Women's Sexual Function and Dysfunction.* New York, NY: Taylor & Francis, 2006, p. 347.

■ PARAPHILIAS

Paraphilias are deviations from what are conventionally considered normal human sexual interests and behaviors. The term paraphilia literally means love (philia) beyond the usual (para). The essential features of paraphilias are recurrent, intense, sexually arousing fantasies, sexual urges, or behaviors involving either nonhuman objects; or the suffering or humiliation of oneself or one's partner, or children or other nonconsenting persons, or also any combination of urges or behaviors over the period of at least 6 months and causing significant distress or impairment in social and other functioning. The wide category of paraphilias not otherwise specified includes, among others, rare entities such as telephone scatophilia (obscene phone calls), necrophilia (sexual acts with corpses), partialism (exclusive focus on one body part), zoophilia (sexual activity involving animals), coprophilia (including feces), urophilia (urine, urination), klismaphilia (enemas) and others.

Studies of paraphilias, especially treatment studies, are difficult to conduct, as (1) paraphilias are rare and are not socially acceptable (and thus, treatment is usually not sought by individuals with paraphilias), (2) comorbidity with other disorders is high, and (3) ethical considerations frequently do not allow for rigorous studies. There is no FDA approved treatment for paraphilias.

Men with paraphilias seem, in general, to have difficulties with attachment and intimacy and are self-centered, antagonistic, have higher levels of neuroticism, lower agreeableness and lower conscientiousness.

Treatment of paraphilias is challenging, as no good data exist and patients usually avoid treatment unless forced by law. Treatment should always include both pharmacotherapy (when evidence available) and psychotherapy. There is no evidence that either of these two modalities is better than the other one. Treatment should progress from modalities associated with fewer side effects and complications, such as cognitive–behavioral therapy and relapse prevention and later antidepressants, to treatments with a higher risk of severe complications such as antiandrogens and other hormones.

EXHIBITIONISM

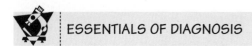

ESSENTIALS OF DIAGNOSIS

The DSM-IV-TR criteria for the diagnosis of exhibitionism are:

A. *Over a period of at least 6 months, recurrent, intense sexually arousing fantasies, sexual urges, or behavior involving the exposure of one's genitals to an unsuspecting stranger.*

B. *The person has acted on these sexual urges, or the sexual urges or fantasies cause marked distress or interpersonal difficulty.*

(Reprinted, with permission, from the *Diagnostic and Statistical Manual of Mental Disorders.* 4th edn. Text Revision. Washington, DC: American Psychiatric Association, 2000, p. 569.)

General Considerations

The onset is usually before the age of 18 years, but it can begin at an older age. Most persons suffering from exhibitionism are heterosexual.

A. Epidemiology

The incidence and prevalence of exhibitionism is unknown. Exhibitionism, like other paraphilias, is more frequent among males.

B. Etiology

The etiology of this disorder is unknown. Some have speculated that males suffering from exhibitionism are shy and unable to establish a normal sexual relationship. In the psychoanalytic view, male exhibitionism is associated with a dominant, seductive mother and a distant father. The assault on masculinity and adequacy is resolved in feelings of power and gratification when female reacts to his genital displays. Deviant arousal may also play a role in the etiology of exhibitionism.

C. Genetics

There is no information about the genetics of exhibitionism.

Clinical Findings

A. Signs & Symptoms

Persons suffering from exhibitionism usually display their genitals hoping to shock or excite the victim. They are usually unable to control the urge to expose themselves. They expose themselves in various places, for example, while driving. The exposure is usually accompanied or followed by masturbation. Various triggers (stress, interpersonal conflict, boredom) may elicit the urge to expose oneself. The exposure may make the subjects excited, turned on, wanted, desired, and calm.

B. Psychological Testing

Psychological testing is not helpful in establishing the diagnosis of exhibitionism.

C. Laboratory Findings

There are no specific laboratory tests for exhibitionism.

D. Neuroimaging

Neuroimaging is not useful in the diagnosis of exhibitionism.

Course of Illness

The duration of exhibitionism is long, usually with no asymptomatic periods, and the course is chronic if untreated. The disorder possibly becomes less severe after the age of 40.

Differential Diagnosis (Including Comorbid Conditions)

The differential diagnosis includes other paraphilias. Exhibitionism should be distinguished from nudism—persons with exhibitionism do not usually have interest in exposure at nudist places.

Comorbidity of exhibitionism with other disorders is high (up to 92%), especially with current and lifetime sexual disorders, other paraphilias, impulse control disorders, and substance abuse disorders. Major depression and substance abuse appear largely secondary to exhibitionism.

Treatment

A. Psychopharmacological Interventions

Serotonergic antidepressants (e.g., fluvoxamine, paroxetine, clomipramine) have been found helpful in some cases. More severe cases (e.g., repeat offenders, failure with other treatments) may be helped with hormonal preparations, such as long-acting agonists of luteinizing hormone-releasing hormone (LHRH) and antiandrogens in special settings. Treatment with LHRH agonists and other antiandrogens requires appropriate initial and follow-up laboratory testing as serious side effects are not uncommon (discussed later). Buspirone hydrochloride has also been successfully used in a case of exhibitionism.

B. PSYCHOTHERAPEUTIC INTERVENTIONS

Psychotherapy is important in fostering compliance and ameliorating attitudinal problems. Cognitive–behavioral therapy, private exposure and covert sensitization have been described as useful in this condition.

Complications/Adverse Outcomes of Treatment

Side effects of treatment using (antidepressants, e.g., include headaches, gastrointestinal disturbances, and prolonged ejaculation. Antiandrogens can produce more serious side effects, including feminization, fatigue, liver damage, and decreased bone density, among others. Comorbid or secondary depression and substance abuse need to be treated vigorously.

Prognosis

Prognosis of treated exhibitionism is probably fair to good. Untreated exhibitionism is usually chronic.

Grant JE: Clinical characteristics and psychiatric comorbidity in males with exhibitionism. *J Clin Psychiatry* 2005;66:1367–1371.

Osborne CS, Wise TN: Paraphilias. In: Balon R, Segraves RT (eds). *Handbook of Sexual Dysfunction.* New York: Taylor & Francis, 2005, p. 293.

Segraves RT, Balon R: *Sexual Pharmacology. Fast Facts.* New York, NY: WW Norton & Company, Inc., 2003.

FETISHISM

 ESSENTIALS OF DIAGNOSIS

The DSM-IV-TR criteria for the diagnosis of fetishism are:

A. *Over a period of at least 6 months, recurrent, intense sexually arousing fantasies, sexual urges, or behavior involving the use of nonliving objects (e.g., female undergarments).*

B. *The fantasies, sexual urges, or behaviors cause clinically significant distress or impairment in social, occupational, or other important areas of functioning.*

C. *The fetish objects are not limited to articles of female clothing used in cross-dressing (as in transvestic fetishism) or devices designed for the purpose of tactile genital stimulation (e.g., a vibrator).*

(Reprinted, with permission, from the *Diagnostic and Statistical Manual of Mental Disorders.* 4th edn. Text Revision. Washington, DC: American Psychiatric Association, 2000, p. 570.)

General Considerations

Fetishism is usually considered relatively harmless. It frequently occurs in the frame of other paraphilias (e.g., sadomasochism).

A. EPIDEMIOLOGY

The incidence and prevalence of fetishism is unknown.

B. ETIOLOGY

The etiology of fetishism is unknown. According to psychoanalytical theories, male child experiences anxiety about mother's missing penis, for which he finds a symbolic object, and thus resolves this fear. The fetish may be linked to someone else whom the person was close to during childhood.

C. GENETICS

There are no genetics findings regarding fetishism available.

Clinical Findings

A. SIGNS & SYMPTOMS

Fetishism is usually egosyntonic and rarely causes distress. There are numerous objects that could serve as fetish. Frequent fetishes include women's underpants, bras, shoes and other apparel. The person usually either masturbates while holding, rubbing or smelling the fetish, or asks the sexual partner to wear it.

B. PSYCHOLOGICAL TESTING

Psychological testing is not helpful in establishing the diagnosis of fetishism.

C. LABORATORY FINDINGS

There are no laboratory findings specific to fetishism.

D. NEUROIMAGING

There are no known imaging studies of fetishism.

Course of Illness

The course of fetishism tends to be chronic.

Differential Diagnosis (Including Comorbid Conditions)

Differential diagnosis includes transvestic fetishism and other paraphilias. Fetishism is frequently comorbid with other paraphilias.

Treatment

A. Psychopharmacological Interventions

Very little is known about psychopharmacological treatment of fetishism, as many people with fetishism live healthy, happy lives and consider their sexual interest or preoccupation to be a "gift." Several case reports describe treatment of fetishism with either antidepressants (fluoxetine), or antiandrogens and anxiolytics.

B. Psychotherapeutic Interventions

Again, very little is known about psychotherapy of fetishism. Possibly useful modalities include psychoeducation, cognitive–behavioral therapy and individual psychodynamic psychotherapy, if distress present.

C. Other Interventions

Classical conditioning paradigm with erections elicited by vibrator was used in one case.

Complications/Adverse Outcomes of Treatment

If antidepressants or antiandrogens are used, their various side effects mentioned previously may occur.

Prognosis

Prognosis is unknown as most patients do not seek treatment and there are no outcome studies.

Fedoroff JP: The paraphilic world. In: Levine S, Risen C, Althof S (eds). *Handbook of Clinical Sexuality for Mental Health Professionals.* New York, NY: Bruner-Routledge, 2003, p. 333.

FROTTEURISM

 ESSENTIALS OF DIAGNOSIS

The DSM-IV-TR criteria for the diagnosis of frotteurism are:

A. *Over a period of at least 6 months, recurrent, intense sexually arousing fantasies, sexual urges, or behaviors involving touching and rubbing against a nonconsenting person.*

B. *The person has acted on these sexual urges, or the sexual urges or fantasies cause marked distress or interpersonal difficulty.*

(Reprinted, with permission, from the *Diagnostic and Statistical Manual of Mental Disorders.* 4th edn. Text Revision. Washington, DC: American Psychiatric Association, 2000, p. 570.)

General Considerations

The behavior usually occurs in crowded places (e.g. public transportation), which are conducive to this behavior and from which escape of arrest is easier. Frotteurism tends to be a crime of opportunity or an example of social incompetency, and is rarely preferred over other sexual activities.

A. Epidemiology

There are no data on the epidemiology of frotteurism. Again, frotteurism occurs more frequently in males.

B. Etiology

The etiology of frotteurism is unknown. Frotteurism is viewed by some as a disturbance of one of the phases of courtship.

C. Genetics

There are no data available on genetics of frotteurism.

Clinical Findings

A. Signs & Symptoms

The person suffering from frotteurism usually rubs his or her genitalia against the victim's thighs or buttocks, or fondles the victim's genitalia or breasts with hands ("toucherism"). The person usually fantasizes about an exclusive relationship with the victim.

B. Psychological Testing

Psychological testing is not useful in diagnosing frotteurism.

C. Laboratory Findings

No specific laboratory findings have been reported in frotteurism.

D. Neuroimaging

There are no reports of neuroimaging in individuals with frotteurism.

Course of Illness

Frotteurism peaks between 15–25 years of age and then gradually declines in frequency.

Differential Diagnosis (Including Comorbid Conditions)

Differential diagnosis includes other paraphilias, social phobia, brain damage, and mental retardation.

Frotteurism is frequently associated with Asperger syndrome.

Treatment

A. Psychopharmacological Interventions

Little is known about the pharmacological treatment of frotteurism. SSRIs (fluoxetine) may be helpful in frotteurism. One study of a case refractory to other treatments used leuprolide acetate, a gonadotropin-releasing hormone agonist.

B. Psychotherapeutic Interventions

No good data on the use of psychotherapeutic interventions exist. Cognitive–behavioral therapy may be useful, as persons with frotteurism frequently use cognitive distortions in justification of their behavior.

Complications/Adverse Outcomes of Treatment

If hormones are used, their side effects (in case of leuprolide acetate erectile dysfunction, decreased bone mineral density) may occur.

Prognosis

The prognosis, especially in cases of comorbidity with conditions such as Asperger syndrome, is poor.

PEDOPHILIA

 ESSENTIALS OF DIAGNOSIS

The DSM-IV-TR criteria for the diagnosis of pedophilia are:

A. *Over a period of at least 6 months, recurrent, intense sexually arousing fantasies, sexual urges or behaviors involving sexual activity with a prepubescent child or children (generally age 13 or younger).*

B. *The person has acted on these sexual urges, or the sexual urges or fantasies cause marked distress or interpersonal difficulty.*

C. *The person is at least age 16 years and at least 5 years older than the child or children in Criterion A.*

Note: Do not include an individual in late adolescence involved in an ongoing sexual relationship with a 12- or 13-year old.

(Reprinted, with permission, from the *Diagnostic and Statistical Manual of Mental Disorders*. 4th edn. Text Revision. Washington, DC: American Psychiatric Association, 2000, p. 570.)

General Considerations

The diagnosis of pedophilia should specify whether the patient is attracted to males, female or both, and whether it is limited to incest. Other subtyping includes exclusive type (attracted only to children) and nonexclusive type. Pedophilia usually develops during adolescence, though it could start at any age. The frequency of pedophilic behavior fluctuates and worsens with stress. It is important to note that the diagnosis of pedophilia cannot be assigned to a child. Not all child sexual offenses are necessarily pedophilic, some of them could be indiscriminate in partner choice due to excessive drive, poor impulse control, intoxication, dementia, mental retardation and others.

A. Epidemiology

The prevalence of pedophilia in the general population is unknown. Pedophilia has also been reported in women, but is rare.

B. Etiology

The etiology of pedophilia is unknown. Numerous factors such as brain abnormalities (e.g., attention-deficit hyperactivity disorder, dementia, mental retardation, seizure disorder), biological abnormalities (hormonal levels, or neurotransmitter changes), comorbidity and clinical similarities (e.g., with OCD), developmental (sexual abuse during childhood etc.), environmental, psychological (psychodynamic theories), and other factors have been considered in the etiology of pedophilia. However, none of these factors can fully explain pedophilia or any other paraphilia, and neither can the response to treatment modality (e.g., SSRIs, hormones).

C. Genetics

Though the possibility of familial transmission of pedophilia has been suggested, there are no solid data on the genetics of pedophilia available. There are reports of association between pedophilia and Klinefelter syndrome.

Clinical Findings

A. SIGNS & SYMPTOMS

Sexual arousal by children—either in sexual fantasies, by watching child pornography, by contacting children via the internet, or by sexually abusing children—is the central behavioral manifestation of pedophilia.

B. PSYCHOLOGICAL TESTING

Differences between pedophiles and other subjects on various psychological tests (e.g., Millon, neuropsychological batteries, Rorschach) have been reported. However, no psychological test is useful in diagnosing pedophilia.

C. LABORATORY FINDINGS

Phalloplethysmography has been used in diagnosing pedophilia. It is a psychophysiological technique in which the person's penile blood volume is monitored during exposure to a standardized set of sexual stimuli involving, among others, male and female children and adolescents. The sensitivity of this test in detecting pedophilia in nonadmitters is ≥55%, and the specificity is around 95%. Nevertheless, its usefulness is still considered questionable, and is limited to research or comprehensive assessment of pedophiles, which includes other testing. It is probably more reliable and useful than psychological testing.

Other laboratory testing (though occasional abnormalities may occur) has not been found useful in diagnosing pedophilia.

D. NEUROIMAGING

There are no solid neuroimaging data of pedophilia.

Course of Illness

The course of pedophilia is usually chronic, especially in those attracted to males.

Differential Diagnosis (Including Comorbid Conditions)

Other paraphilias, personality disorders, psychosis, dementia, mental retardation, brain injury, and seizure disorder should be considered in the differential diagnosis of pedophilia. Pedophiles frequently meet the criteria for personality disorder(s), namely, antisocial personality disorder. Nevertheless, the diagnosis of personality disorder does not explain or supplant the diagnosis of pedophilia.

Treatment

Treatment of pedophilia is usually done in a specialized setting. It is recommended that the treatment is comprehensive and designed to

1. reduce pedophilic interests,
2. establish adult sexual interests, and
3. decrease attitudes and beliefs supportive of pedophilic behaviors.

These goals could be achieved by psychopharmacological, psychological, or, in extreme cases, partially by surgical approaches.

A. PSYCHOPHARMACOLOGICAL INTERVENTIONS

Various serotonergic antidepressants (e.g., fluoxetine, sertraline), antipsychotics (e.g., chlorpromazine, risperidone) and mood stabilizers (e.g., carbamazepine, lithium) have been reported as useful in the treatment of pedophilia, mostly in case-reports or small series of patients. Antidepressants are especially useful in reducing compulsive urges.

Interestingly, naltrexone, a long-acting opioid, was reportedly useful in the treatment of adolescent pedophiles and other sexual offenders.

Hormones such as cyproterone acetate (CPA, not available in the United States), methylprogesterone acetate (MPA) and leuprolide acetate (LPA) (Schober et al., 2005) have been successfully used in the treatment of pedophilia. CPA and MPA are available in IM and oral forms, LPA only in an IM form. These hormones are useful in reducing sexual drive, erotic fantasies, sexual activity, possibly aggressiveness, and NPT.

B. PSYCHOTHERAPEUTIC INTERVENTIONS

Numerous psychological interventions have been used in pedophilia with more or less success. Covert sensitization, olfactory aversion, satiation strategies (e.g., masturbation till orgasm to nondeviant fantasies with continuing masturbation focusing on pedophilic fantasies), and imaginal desensitization have been used to reduce pedophilic interests. Fading (gradual replacement of pedophilic visual stimulus with adult sexual stimulus), exposure and masturbatory conditioning have been used to establish adult sexual interests. Finally, cognitive restructuring, externalization of cognitive distortions, victim empathy training, and developing a prosocial behavior have been used to decrease attitudes and beliefs supportive of pedophilic behavior.

Individual psychodynamic psychotherapy was used in pedophilia in the past. CBT may be useful in cognitive restructuring, but also in ameliorating or management of comorbid conditions, resolution of other life issues and relapse prevention.

C. OTHER INTERVENTIONS

Surgical castration and/or stereotactic neurosurgery are quite successful in the treatment of pedophilia, with recidivism rates below 5%. However, these interventions are not usually used in the United States for ethical reasons.

Complications/Adverse Outcomes of Treatment

Antidepressant treatment could be complicated by the usual side effects of antidepressants (nausea, headaches, and others), including prolonged ejaculation or anorgasmia. Hormonal treatment could be complicated by numerous side effects such as weight gain, thrombophlebitis, pulmonary embolism, changes of sperm count and motility, hypertension, nausea, liver damage, erectile failure, elevated risk for depression, diabetes, insomnia, and others. Thus, various tests (blood pressure, blood glucose, weight, complete blood count (CBC), liver function tests, hormonal levels, bone density) should be done before treatment and monitored through the treatment.

[margin note: uthor: Please fine CBC.]

Prognosis

The prognosis of untreated pedophilia is poor.

Abel GG, Osborn C, Phipps AM: Pedophilia. In: Gabbard GO (ed). *Treatment of Psychiatric Disorders,* 3rd edn. Washington DC: American Psychiatric Press, Inc., 2001, p. 1981.

Bebbington PE: Treatment of male sexual deviation by use of vibrator: Case report. *Arch Sex Behav* 1977;6:21–24.

Bradford JM: Organic treatment for the male sexual offender. *Ann N Y Acad Sci* 1988;528:193–202.

Freund K, Blanchard R: Phallometric diagnosis of pedophilia. *J Consult Clin Psychol* 1989;57:100–105.

Gaffney GR, Lurie SF, Berlin FS: Is there familial transmission of pedophilia? *J Nerv Ment Dis* 1984;172:546–548.

Perilstein RD, Lipper S, Friedman LJ: Three cases of paraphilia responsive to fluoxetine treatment. *J Clin Psychiatry* 1991;52:169–170.

Ryback RS: Naltrexone in the treatment of adolescent sexual offenders. *J Clin Psychiatry* 2004;65:982–986.

Schober JM, Kuhn PJ, Kovacs PG, Earle JH, Byrne PM, Fries RA: Leuprolide acetate suppresses pedophilic urges and arousability. *Arch Sex Behav* 2005;34:691–705.

SEXUAL MASOCHISM

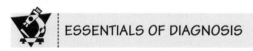 ESSENTIALS OF DIAGNOSIS

The DSM-IV-TR criteria for the diagnosis of sexual masochism are:

A. *Over a period of at least 6 months, recurrent, intense sexually arousing fantasies, sexual urges or behaviors involving the act (real, not simulated) of being humiliated, beaten, bound, or otherwise made to suffer.*

B. *The fantasies, sexual urges or behaviors cause clinically significant distress or impairment in social, occupational, or other important areas of functioning.*

(Reprinted, with permission, from the *Diagnostic and Statistical Manual of Mental Disorders.* 4th edn. Text Revision. Washington, DC: American Psychiatric Association, 2000, p. 573.)

General Considerations

Sexual masochism is frequently linked to sexual sadism. Sigmund Freud was the first one to combine these two terms into sadomasochism. Individuals with masochism do not seek help frequently, unless they have marital problems or concerns about being harmed.

A. EPIDEMIOLOGY

The prevalence of sexual masochism in the general population is unknown. Some suggest that sexual masochism occurs more often among middle and upper socioeconomic class individuals.

B. ETIOLOGY

The etiology of masochism is unknown. Various psychoanalytical explanation exist, nevertheless, none provides a satisfactory explanation.

C. GENETICS

There are no data regarding the genetics of sexual masochism.

Clinical Findings

A. SIGNS & SYMPTOMS

The behavior of sexual masochist's behavior may range from mild forms (such as being spanked) to more severe ones (such as being bound and beaten, whipped, receiving electrical shocks, being cut and having objects inserted in the orifices). Other forms of humiliation, such as being urinated or defecated on, being forced to crawl and bark like a dog may also be involved. Some individuals may just invoke masochistic fantasies during masturbation or intercourse. Hypoxyphilia or asphyxiophilia (sexual arousal by oxygen deprivation by strangling, mask etc.) is considered the most extreme and the most dangerous variation of masochism.

B. PSYCHOLOGICAL TESTING

Psychological testing is not helpful in establishing the diagnosis of sexual masochism.

C. LABORATORY FINDINGS

There are no laboratory findings specific to masochism.

D. NEUROIMAGING

There are no specific neuroimaging studies of sexual masochism.

Course of Illness

Masochistic fantasies are likely present during childhood. Sexual masochism's behavior usually starts during early adulthood. The course is usually chronic, with repetition of the same sexual behaviors.

Differential Diagnosis (Including Comorbid Conditions)

The differential diagnosis of sexual masochism includes other paraphilias. Sexual masochism frequently coexists with sexual sadism, fetishism, and transvestic fetishism.

Treatment

A. PSYCHOPHARMACOLOGICAL INTERVENTIONS

There is not much information on psychopharmacology of sexual masochism available. There have been cases of sexual masochism treated with lithium and with leuprolide acetate.

B. PSYCHOTHERAPEUTIC INTERVENTIONS

Individual psychotherapy and cognitive–behavioral therapy could be used in treatment of sexual masochism, but no specific data is available.

C. OTHER INTERVENTIONS

No other treatments are available.

Complications of Treatment

Hormonal treatment of paraphilia could be associated with side effects specific to a selected hormone mentioned before (see "Pedophilia" section).

Prognosis

Prognosis is unknown and is probably poor.

SEXUAL SADISM

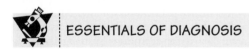

ESSENTIALS OF DIAGNOSIS

The DSM-IV-TR criteria for the diagnosis of sexual sadism are:

A. *Over a period of at least 6 months, recurrent, intense sexually arousing fantasies, sexual urges or behaviors involving the act (real, not simulated) in which the psychological or physical suffering (including humiliation) of the victim is sexually exciting to the person.*

B. *The person has acted on these sexual urges with a nonconsenting person, or the sexual urges or fantasies cause marked distress or interpersonal difficulty.*

(Reprinted, with permission, from the *Diagnostic and Statistical Manual of Mental Disorders.* 4th edn. Text Revision. Washington, DC: American Psychiatric Association, 2000, p. 574.)

General Considerations

The central feature sexual sadism is sexual arousal due to suffering of the victim. Some individuals may fantasize sadistic facts during sexual activity and do not act on them. Sexual sadism may occur with a consenting (e.g., in sadomasochism) or with a nonconsenting partner. Sexual sadism may vary from mild forms, such as spanking, to much more severe acts, such as beating and humiliation of the victim, and may involve rape or killing of the victim.

A. EPIDEMIOLOGY

There is no reliable data on the prevalence of sexual sadism available. Serious forms of sexual sadism attract a lot of media and general public attention, but are relatively rare.

B. ETIOLOGY

As with other paraphilias, the etiology of sexual sadisms is unknown. There are various psychoanalytic theories of sadism. Sexual sadists frequently meet the criteria for personality disorder(s). None of the theories or associations explains the etiology of sexual sadism.

C. GENETICS

There are no genetic studies of sexual sadism.

Clinical Findings

A. SIGNS & SYMPTOMS

Sexual sadist's behavior, parallel to sexual masochism, may vary from mild forms, such as spanking the partner, to more severe, such as tying and beating, whipping, cutting, stabbing the partner and inserting objects into partner's orifices. Other forms of humiliation, such as forcing the victim to crawl and bark like a dog, or keeping the victim in a cage may also be involved. Some individuals may just invoke sadistic fantasies during masturbation or intercourse.

B. Psychological Testing

Psychological testing is not helpful in diagnosing sexual sadism. Homicidal sexual offenders scored higher on Psychopathy Checklist-Revised, and portrayed themselves better in the areas of sexual functioning (Derogatis Sexual Functioning Inventory) and aggression/hostility (Buss–Durkee Hostility Inventory).

C. Laboratory Findings

No specific laboratory tests for sexual sadism are available. It is unclear whether phallometric testing can help in diagnosing sexual sadism.

D. Neuroimaging

There are no neuroimaging findings specific to sexual sadism and no known neuroimaging studies of sexual sadism.

Course of Illness

The age of onset of sexual sadism varies, but it usually starts during early adulthood. Sadistic fantasies are likely to occur in childhood. The course of sexual sadism, especially untreated, is usually chronic.

Differential Diagnosis (Including Comorbid Conditions)

The differential diagnosis of sexual sadism includes other paraphilias, personality disorders (especially cluster B), psychosis, mental retardation and organic brain syndrome.

Persons with sexual sadism frequently meet the criteria for antisocial personality disorder.

Treatment

A. Psychopharmacological Interventions

Treatment of sexual sadism should be executed in specialized settings involving a team of specialists familiar with the treatment of this paraphilia (especially in cases involving legal issues). Serotonergic antidepressants (e.g., fluoxetine) have been occasionally used in the treatment of sexual sadism. Hormonal preparations such as cyproterone acetate (not available in the United States), leuprolide acetate and medroxyprogesterone acetate have been used in the treatment of sexual offenders. These hormones are useful in reducing sexual drive, erotic fantasies, sexual activity, possibly aggressiveness, and NPT. In the past, some of the antipsychotics were also used in the treatment of sexual sadism.

B. Psychotherapeutic Interventions

Individual psychotherapy has been used in many cases of sexual sadism. Cognitive–behavioral approach with a focus on control and management of problematic thoughts, urges and behaviors, modification of paraphilic arousal, amelioration or management of comorbid conditions, resolution of other life issues and relapse prevention may also be useful. Various techniques described for the treatment of pedophilia (discussed earlier) could also be useful. Evidence for psychotherapy of this condition in an organized fashion is lacking.

C. Other Interventions

Surgical castrations of sexual sadists have been performed in other countries, but are not condoned in the United States.

Complications/Adverse Outcomes of Treatment

Hormonal treatment of paraphilias could be associated with side effects specific to the selected hormone mentioned before (see section on "Pedophilia").

Prognosis

The prognosis of sexual sadism is unknown, but is probably poor, especially in untreated cases.

Firestone O, Bradford JM, Greenberg DM, Larose MR: Homicidal sex offenders: Psychological, phallometric and diagnostic features. *J Am Acad Psychiatry Law* 1998;26:537–552.

TRANSVESTIC FETISHISM

 ESSENTIALS OF DIAGNOSIS

The DSM-IV-TR criteria for the diagnosis of transvestic fetishism are:

A. *Over a period of at least 6 months, in a heterosexual male, recurrent, intense sexually arousing fantasies, sexual urges, or behaviors involving cross-dressing.*

B. *The fantasies, sexual urges, or behaviors cause clinically significant distress or impairment in social, occupational, or other important areas of functioning.*

(Reprinted, with permission, from the *Diagnostic and Statistical Manual of Mental Disorders*. 4th edn. Text Revision. Washington, DC: American Psychiatric Association, 2000, p. 575.)

General Considerations

The diagnostic consideration should consider whether transvestic fetishism is associated with gender dysphoria, that is, discomfort with one's gender role or identity. Transvestic fetishism is not necessarily heterosexual. The majority of transvestites who have been treated or volunteered for research are Caucasian, well-educated, currently or previously married, in their forties, and began cross-dressing before the age of 12.

A. Epidemiology

In a random sample general population study from Sweden, 2.8% males and 0.4% of females reported at least one episode of transvestic fetishism. No similar data from the United States are available.

B. Etiology

The etiology of transvestic fetishism is unknown. The psychoanalytic explanation of this paraphilia frequently entertains the idea of unconscious fantasy of merging or identification with the mother.

C. Genetics

No genetic studies of transvestic fetishism are available. There is some evidence for familial occurrence of transvestic fetishism.

Clinical Findings

A. Signs & Symptoms

Cross-dressing leads not only to sexual arousal, but also decreases anxiety and elevates the mood of the person with transvestic fetishism. Transvestites may pass as a woman for a short period of time. Cross-dressing is a complex psychosexual phenomenon, and orgasm does not necessarily occur during all cross-dressing activities. The initial cross-dressing may be total or partial, with partial cross-dressing later progressing into full cross-dressing.

B. Psychological Testing

Psychological testing does not contribute to the diagnosis of this paraphilia.

C. Laboratory Findings

There are no laboratory tests useful for the diagnosis of transvestic fetishism.

D. Neuroimaging

There are no neuroimaging findings specific to transvestic fetishism available.

Course of Illness

Transvestic fetishism usually begins during the first decade of life. The course is chronic.

Differential Diagnosis (Including Comorbid Conditions)

The differential diagnosis includes other paraphilias, gender identity disorder and personality disorders. Transvestic fetishism frequently occurs together with fetishism and sexual masochism. Other comorbid conditions include erectile dysfunction, alcohol abuse or dependence, marital discord, dysthymia, major depression, and psychosis infrequently.

Treatment

A. Psychopharmacological Interventions

Various psychotropic medications (e.g., buspirone, serotonergic antidepressants such as sertraline, lithium) have been successfully used in cases of transvestic fetishism. Hormones, such as estrogens and antiandrogens (diethylstilbestrol, medroxyprogesterone acetate) have also been successfully used in some cases of this paraphilia. However, no studies of any treatment modality are available.

B. Psychotherapeutic Interventions

Psychodynamic psychotherapy has been the treatment of choice for transvestic fetishism for a long time. It still remains an important part of a comprehensive treatment plan. Cognitive–behavioral therapy could probably be useful in transvestic fetishism, too, but reports on its usefulness in this paraphilia are not available. Marital therapy may be useful in cases of marital discord. Attendance of self-help groups and treatment of spouse should also be included in the treatment of transvestic fetishism.

C. Other Interventions

Electrical aversion techniques to apply operant conditioning was used in the past, but are not considered ethical at present. Posthypnotic suggestion has also been used in transvestic fetishism.

Complications/Adverse Outcomes of Treatment

Complications of treatment include the various side effects of antidepressants and hormones (see "Pedophilia" section).

Prognosis

The prognosis of transvestic fetishism, especially untreated one, is rather poor.

Brown GR: Transvestism and gender identity disorder in adults. In: Gabbard GO (ed). *Treatment of Psychiatric Disorders*, 3rd edn. Washington DC: American Psychiatric Press, Inc., 2001, p. 2007.

Langstrom N, Zucker KJ: Transvestic fetishism in the general population: Prevalence and correlates. *J Sex Marital Ther* 2005;31: 87–95.

VOYEURISM

 ESSENTIALS OF DIAGNOSIS

The DSM-IV-TR criteria for the diagnosis of voyeurism are:

A. *Over a period of at least 6 months, recurrent, intense sexually arousing fantasies, sexual urges, or behaviors involving the act of observing an unsuspecting person who is naked, in the process of disrobing, or engaging in sexual activity.*

B. *The person has acted on these sexual urges, or the sexual urges or fantasies cause marked distress or interpersonal difficulty.*

(Reprinted, with permission, from the *Diagnostic and Statistical Manual of Mental Disorders*. 4th edn. Text Revision. Washington, DC: American Psychiatric Association, 2000, p. 575.)

General Considerations

The act of looking is for the purpose of achieving sexual excitement, and sexual activity with the observed person is usually not sought. Sexual satisfaction is achieved via masturbation, either during looking or later in response to the memory of whatever was witnessed.

A. Epidemiology

There is no data on the epidemiology of voyeurism.

B. Etiology

The etiology of voyeurism is unknown. Some experts view voyeurism as a disorder of courtship (finding a partner phase).

C. Genetics

There is no evidence regarding heritability of this condition.

Clinical Findings

A. Signs & Symptoms

Sexual satisfaction is achieved via masturbation either during observation of the unsuspecting individual, or

later in response to the memory of the observation. The victim's lack of suspicion and the risk of being caught are central to the person's arousal.

B. Psychological Testing

There is no psychological testing available for diagnosing voyeurism.

C. Laboratory Findings

There are no voyeurism-specific laboratory findings.

D. Neuroimaging

There are not known neuroimaging studies of voyeurism.

Course of Illness

The onset of voyeurism is usually before age 15. The course tends to be chronic.

Differential Diagnosis (Including Comorbid Conditions)

The differential diagnosis of voyeurism includes other paraphilias, personality disorders and psychosis.

Treatment

A. Psychopharmacological Interventions

Successful treatment of voyeurism with antidepressants such as paroxetine and fluoxetine (for example, 75) has been reported.

B. Psychotherapeutic Interventions

Cognitive–behavioral therapy, individual psychotherapy and behavioral modification may be useful in the treatment of voyeurism. No solid data is available on their usefulness in this condition.

C. Other Interventions

There have not been other interventions reported in this condition.

Complications/Adverse Outcomes of Treatment

Antidepressant side effects such as diarrhea, headaches, prolonged ejaculation may occur when these medications are used in voyeurism.

Prognosis

Prognosis of untreated voyeurism is probably poor.

Eating Disorders

26

Harry E. Gwirtsman, MD, James E. Mitchell, MD, & Michael H. Ebert, MD

The eating disorders, anorexia nervosa and bulimia nervosa, may be classified as true psychosomatic illnesses, inasmuch as an underlying biological vulnerability interacts with a particular cultural stress in order to produce behavioral and psychological symptoms. For example, anorexia and bulimia nervosa are more prevalent in industrialized societies, where there is an overabundance of food and where attractiveness in women is linked with being thin, than in agriculturally-based societies. Immigrants from cultures in which anorexia nervosa is rare are more likely to develop the illness as they assimilate the ideals of a thin body appearance.

■ ANOREXIA NERVOSA

 ### ESSENTIALS OF DIAGNOSIS

DSM-IV-TR Diagnostic Criteria

A. *Refusal to maintain body weight at or above a minimally normal weight for age and height (e.g., weight loss leading to maintenance of body weight less than 85% of that expected; or failure to make expected weight gain during a period of growth, leading to body weight less than 85% of that expected).*

B. *Intense fear of gaining weight or becoming fat, even though underweight.*

C. *Disturbance in the way in which one's body weight or shape is experienced, undue influence of body weight or shape on self-evaluation, or denial of the seriousness of the current low body weight.*

D. *In postmenarcheal females, amenorrhea, i.e., the absence of at least three consecutive menstrual cycles. (A woman is considered to have amenor-*

rhea if her periods occur only following hormone, e.g., estrogen, administration.)

Specify type:

Restricting type: during the current episode of anorexia nervosa, the person has not regularly engaged in binge-eating or purging behavior (i.e., self-induced vomiting or the misuse of laxatives, diuretics, or enemas).

Binge-eating/purging type: during the current episode of anorexia nervosa, the person has regularly engaged in binge-eating or purging behavior (i.e., self-induced vomiting or the misuse of laxatives, diuretics, or enemas).

(Reprinted, with permission, from *Diagnostic and Statistical Manual of Mental Disorders,* 4th edn, Text Revision. Copyright 2000 American Psychiatric Association.)

General Considerations

In some ways, the term anorexia nervosa is a misnomer, because the affected individual's appetite and craving for food are usually preserved. Nevertheless, the individual will actively counter the feelings of hunger with disordered thinking, leading to self-imposed starvation. The threshold for defining the amount of weight loss considered to be serious enough to qualify for the diagnosis of anorexia nervosa is computed on the basis of the Metropolitan Life Insurance tables or pediatric growth charts. A body mass index less than or equal to 17.5 kg/m^2 (calculated as weight in kilograms/height in meters^2) represents an alternative guideline accepted by many researchers. Nevertheless, these standards are only suggested guidelines, and clinicians should also consider the individual's body build and weight history.

A. EPIDEMIOLOGY

Lifetime prevalence rates for anorexia nervosa in females are approximately 0.5–1.0, or 1 in 100–200 individuals.

Many more individuals exhibit symptoms that do not meet the criteria for the disorder (i.e., eating disorder not otherwise specified; see later in this chapter), but this is an area for continued research. More than 90% of affected individuals are female, and data concerning the prevalence of the illness in males are scant. Worldwide, the disorder appears to be most common in the United States, Canada, Europe, Australia, Japan, New Zealand, and South Africa; but few systematic studies of the illness have been conducted in other countries.

The onset of illness is bimodal: One peak occurs in early adolescence (age 12–15 years) and another in late adolescence and early adulthood (age 17–21 years); the mean age at onset is approximately 17 years. The illness rarely appears de novo before puberty or after age 40 years. Often an associated life event, such as moving away from home, precedes the first episode of anorexia nervosa. Although the prevalence of this disorder showed marked increases in the latter half of the twentieth century, more recently this rate of increase has slowed.

B. ETIOLOGY

The incidence and prevalence of eating disorders have increased greatly in the latter half of the 20th century. This increase is due in part to cultural pressures in industrialized societies (placed largely on women), including an overemphasis on a slim female figure with an almost prepubescent shape. This emphasis is depicted in magazines, the entertainment industry, and beauty contests. Nevertheless, anorexia nervosa cannot be completely culturally based, because it appears to have been described almost 300 years ago, when cultural pressures were different. Consequently, part of the etiology of eating disorders must be biological, with the degree of phenotypic expression determined by cultural factors. Disturbances in central nervous system monoamines, particularly norepinephrine and serotonin, and in certain neuropeptides have been reported in the acute phase of anorexia nervosa. Few of these abnormalities persist into the weight-restored phase of the illness, and those that do may be at least partially related to the state of malnutrition.

C. GENETICS

Concordance rates for monozygotic twins with anorexia nervosa are higher than those for dizygotic twins. Among first-degree biological relatives, there is an increased risk for anorexia nervosa and for mood disorder, the latter found particularly among the relatives of individuals with the binge-eating/purging type. More recent studies have identified a susceptibility locus on chromosome 1. There is at least preliminary evidence for certain candidate genes which confer susceptibility, including the norepinephrine transporter (NET) gene, the monoamine oxidase A (MAO-A) gene, and the serotonin transporter (SERT) gene.

Clinical Findings

A. SIGNS & SYMPTOMS

Weight loss is frequently accomplished by reduction in total food intake and also involves the exclusion of highly caloric foods, leading to an extremely restricted diet. Patients may lose weight by purging (via either self-induced vomiting or misuse of laxatives and diuretics) or by exercising excessively. As weight continues to decline, the patient's fear of becoming fat may increase, as do feelings of being overweight. The body image distortion that these individuals experience has a wide range, from the fervently held belief that one is globally overweight, to a realization that one is thin but that certain body parts such as the abdomen, buttocks, or thighs are too big. Such disturbed self-perceptions may be modified by cultural factors and may not present prominently. Instead, the patient may complain of a distaste for food or epigastric discomfort as the expressed motivation for food restriction.

Self-esteem in patients with anorexia nervosa is overly dependent on body shape and weight, and these patients seem obsessed with employing a wide variety of techniques to estimate body size, including frequent weighing, measuring of body parts, and looking in the mirror for perceived fat. Losing weight is judged to be an admirable achievement of unusual self-discipline, whereas weight gain is regarded as an unacceptable failure of self-control. Meanwhile, patients typically deny the serious medical implications of malnutrition.

Most patients with anorexia nervosa have food-related obsessions. They frequently hoard food or collect recipes and may be involved in food preparation for the family or in food-related professions (e.g., waitress, cook, dietitian, nutritionist). They may also have fears of eating in public. Such obsessions have also been observed in other forms of starvation, including experimental starvation.

Signs of starvation account for most of the physical findings in anorexia nervosa. These signs include emaciation; significant hypotension, especially orthostatic; bradycardia; hypothermia; skin dryness and flakiness; Lanugo, or the presence of downy body hair on trunks or extremities; peripheral edema, especially ankle edema; petechiae on extremities; sallow complexion; salivary gland hypertrophy, particularly of the parotid gland; dental enamel erosion; osteoporosis (which results from reduced estrogen secretion, increased cortisol secretion, and inadequate calcium intake); and Russell's sign, or scars and calluses on the back of the hand. Amenorrhea may precede the onset of appreciable diminished weight, because it may be related to the loss of body fat stores

Table 26–1. Laboratory Abnormalities in Anorexia Nervosa

Category	Common	Uncommon/Rare
Hematology	Leukopenia	Thrombocytopenia
Chemistry	Abnormal luteinizing hormone (LH) release Elevated cortisol Elevated liver functions Elevated serum bicarbonate Hypercarotenemia Hypercholesterolemia Hypochloremia Hypokalemia Hypozincemia Low estrogen (females) Low normal thyroxine (T_4) Low triiodothyronine (T_3)	Hyperamylasemia Hypomagnesemia Hypophosphatemia Metabolic acidosis
Miscellaneous	Positive stool for occult blood	
Electrocardiogram	Sinus bradycardia	Arrhythmias
Electroencephalogram	Diffuse abnormalities	
Resting energy expenditure	Significantly reduced	
Brain imaging	Increased ventricular/brain ratio	
	Widened cortical sulci	

rather than decrease of body mass. Menarche may be delayed in prepubertal females.

Among patients who frequently engage in purging behaviors, many do not binge eat. Instead, they regularly vomit after consuming small meals.

It is not clear which of the many psychological manifestations seen in anorexia nervosa are a cause or consequence of malnutrition, as studies of forced starvation in volunteers have reported symptoms of food preoccupations, food hoarding, binge eating, unusual taste preferences, as well as other personality changes, such as depression, obsessionality, apathy, and irritability. Such symptoms remit with nutritional rehabilitation.

B. PSYCHOLOGICAL TESTING

Although extensive psychological testing is not used in the diagnosis of anorexia nervosa, screening tests can be extremely valuable in identifying eating psychopathology in community samples. Two such tests are the Eating Disorders Inventory and the Eating Attitudes Test. These tests are also useful in documenting improvement during treatment. It is also important to assess coexisting Axis I and Axis II psychiatric illness with relevant instruments such as the Structured Clinical Interview for the *Diagnostic and Statistical Manual of Mental Disorders*, fourth edition (DSM-IV) or the Beck Depression Inventory. It

is felt that deficits on neuropsychological tests that persist after refeeding are associated with poorer outcomes.

C. LABORATORY FINDINGS & IMAGING

Most organ systems are affected by malnutrition, and a variety of physical disturbances can be noted (Table 26–1). Coexisting dehydration may be indicated by an elevated blood urea nitrogen. If induced vomiting is part of the clinical picture, then metabolic alkalosis may ensue, with elevated serum bicarbonate, hypochloremia, and hypokalemia. Laxative abuse may cause metabolic acidosis and a positive stool for occult blood. Neuroendocrine abnormalities are also common.

Amenorrhea is the result of abnormally low levels of estrogen secretion, which is due to a diminution of pituitary release of follicle-stimulating hormone and luteinizing hormone. For patients who have been amenorrheic for 6 months or more, a bone density examination is recommended.

Differential Diagnosis

General medical conditions such as chronic inflammatory bowel disease, hyperthyroidism, malignancies, and AIDS can cause serious weight loss; however, it is rare for patients with these disorders to have a distorted body image, a fear of becoming obese, or a desire for further weight loss. Such medical conditions are also usually not associated with increased exercise and activity, except for hyperthyroidism. Superior mesenteric artery syndrome, a disorder characterized by postprandial vomiting secondary to intermittent gastric outlet obstruction, may precede or occur concurrently with anorexia nervosa when significant emaciation is present.

Coexisting major depressive disorder may present a difficult differential diagnosis. Most individuals with uncomplicated major depression do not have an excessive fear of gaining weight; however, even after weight restoration, anorexic patients may experience episodes of depression that require intervention. Individuals with schizophrenia may present with fluctuating weight patterns and bizarre beliefs related to food, but rarely demonstrate the body image disturbance and fear of fat associated with anorexia nervosa.

Because the diagnostic criteria for social phobia, obsessive–compulsive disorder, and body dysmorphic disorder overlap with those of anorexia nervosa, additional diagnoses of these disorders should be made only if individuals with anorexia nervosa have fears, obsessions, or body distortions unrelated to eating, food, or body shape and size.

Treatment

Anorexic individuals seldom seek professional assistance on their own, but instead are persuaded or coerced by family members to be evaluated for treatment. These individuals rarely complain about the weight loss per se but rather will describe the somatic or psychological distress related to the consequences of starvation, such as cold intolerance, muscle weakness or loss of stamina, constipation, abdominal pain, and mental depression. Frequently patients deny the core problem, and the history obtained from such patients is unreliable. Consequently it is advisable for the clinician to obtain information from family members or other outside sources to accurately evaluate features of the illness, such as the degree of weight loss.

A multidisciplinary approach utilizing multiple modalities is essential in treating anorexia nervosa. This is because no controlled treatment studies exist to determine the comparative efficacy of any particular management model for any eating disorder, nor have any potential adverse effects of psychosocial stratagems been systematically assessed. The Psychiatrist may coordinate a treatment team that includes other disciplines, such as psychologists, social workers, registered dietitians, and other physicians and dentists. Educational materials, including self-help workbooks; information on community-based and Internet resources; and direct advice should be provided to patients and their families by trained professionals. Such materials also help to counter other misinformation disseminated over the Internet by

'pro-ana' websites that promulgate a permissive attitude towards eating disorder lifestyles.

Patients may require acute intensive medical intervention to correct fluid and electrolyte imbalances, cardiac problems, and organ failure. It may be beneficial to the patient to institute such intensive treatment earlier rather than later in the course of the illness, when the consequences of malnutrition, such as cortical gray matter loss, osteoporosis, or delayed physical growth and development, have become evident. Hospitalization should most certainly occur prior to the development of medical instability, such as orthostatic hypotension, heart rhythm abnormalities, or hypothermia.

The advent of behavior therapies has reduced markedly the morbidity and mortality of the illness; these therapies are now the centerpiece of most inpatient therapeutic programs. There is general agreement that weight restoration should be a central goal for seriously underweight adult patients, and for children and adolescents who are well below their expected height and weight, and most of these patients will require inpatient management, during which controlled conditions can be achieved. In such an environment, patients are encouraged to consume increased numbers of calories in order to earn specific privileges, such as increased activity, decreased need for staff supervision, visits from relatives, and therapeutic sessions. During this phase, it is felt by clinicians that patients must be engaged in individual and family therapy in order to secure their cooperation and alliance with the treatment program. In some cases, forced nasogastric or parenteral feeding is necessary, but such invasive medical procedures have considerable risk of inducing refeeding syndrome, or infection. Although family therapy is felt to be essential in children and adolescents, adults who have had the illness for more than 5 years rarely demonstrate much response to this modality, or any other form of psychotherapeutic intervention. Group psychotherapy is frequently utilized as a therapeutic modality, but its efficacy has not been adequately assessed in any scientific study to date.

Careful attention must be paid to caloric intake, so that these patients are not fed too quickly, but they must receive enough food to overcome their metabolic resistance (occasionally reaching 70–100 kcal/kg per day, especially in male patients), both during and immediately after the weight-gaining phase. This curious phenomenon of resistance to weight gain has been linked to energy wasting and relatively higher resting energy expenditure (REE) in malnourished patients. Most clinicians attempt to achieve weight goals of 2–3 lbs/week for hospitalized patients, and 0.5–1 lb/week in partial or outpatient programs. For seriously underweight patients, exercise should be be carefully monitored and supervised, and in some cases restricted, as there is considerable risk of pathological fracture with high-impact activities, such as running or jumping. Care should be taken to avoid refeeding syndrome, consisting of hypophosphatemia, hypomagnesemia, hypocalcemia, and fluid retention. This is especially true in patients who have abruptly been withdrawn from diuretics or laxatives, as they have elevated aldosterone levels due to chronic dehydration, a consequence of abusing such substances. Hypothyroidism in underweight patients is a physiological reaction to malnutrition, and should not be treated with exogenous hormone replacement, as it will reverse with weight restoration. Nutritional status may be monitored with serum complement 3 and 4, and serum transferrin levels.

Healthy target weights for female patients should be determined by the weight at which normal menstrual function returns, which may be higher than the weight at which such patients first experienced amenorrhea. Usually, this weight is at least 90% of average body mass index (i.e., 20–25). For male patients, a target weight should be determined by the restoration of normal testicular function. In prepubertal children and adolescents, growth curves should be followed. It has been reported that anorexic patients who achieve their target weights prior to discharge from the hospital have lower rehospitalization rates than those patients who are discharged before achieving their target weight.

Pharmacologic agents, such as antidepressants, second generation antipsychotics, cyproheptadine, and lithium, may be helpful adjuncts, especially for patients who have coexisting depressive or psychotic features. Some patients may show some response to pro-motility agents, such as metoclopramide, during the refeeding phase of their treatment. Antianxiety agents have also been given before mealtimes by clinicians to mitigate anticipatory anxiety. No specific psychopharmacologic agent has been discovered that can induce an anorexic patient to eat and gain weight outside of a structured behaviorally oriented program. Medications should be utilized with caution in malnourished patients, as they are much more susceptible to their potential side effects.

However, there is some evidence that certain medications, such as olanzapine may aid in weight gain in adult and adolescent underweight anorexics, and that fluoxetine in dosages of up to 60 mg/day, may have some utility in preventing relapse in patients whose weight has been restored. Some patients have also benefited from zinc-containing supplements. Although hormone replacement therapy is frequently prescribed, there is no evidence that estrogen replacement, biphosphonates (e.g. alendronate), or calcium or vitamin D supplementation can reverse the reduced bone mineral density caused by malnutrition in anorexic patients.

Controlled trials and clinical consensus suggest that cognitive–behavioral therapies (CBT) and interpersonal psychotherapies (IPT) may be helpful to patients with anorexia nervosa in maintaining weight and healthy eating behaviors. It is felt that ongoing psychotherapeutic treatment is indicated for one or more years following weight restoration.

Complications/Adverse Outcomes of Treatment

Medical complications of anorexia nervosa are common, especially if the disease has been present for 5 years or more. Complications include anemia, which is usually normochromic and normocytic (i.e., with normal erythrocyte indices); impaired renal function, which is associated with chronic dehydration and hypokalemia, or the direct toxicity of laxatives; cardiovascular complications such as arrhythmias and hypotension; osteoporosis, resulting from diminished dietary calcium, increased cortisol, and decreased estrogen secretion; and dental decay.

Many patients with anorexia nervosa exhibit symptoms of depressed mood, social withdrawal, obsessional symptoms, irritability, insomnia, and diminished interest in sex. Almost 50% meet criteria for major depressive disorder, but these features may be complications of starvation rather than a truly comorbid condition. Such depressive symptoms should be reassessed after weight restoration, because they persist in a subset of patients. Patients with the bulimic type of anorexia nervosa are more likely to abuse alcohol or other drugs, exhibit labile mood, be sexually active, and have other impulse-control problems. If anorexia nervosa develops prior to puberty, it may be associated with more severe comorbid mental disturbances.

Obsessive–compulsive symptoms unrelated to food, body shape, or weight may be present and may warrant a diagnosis of obsessive–compulsive disorder in up to one-quarter of anorexic patients. Other psychological symptoms, such as feelings of ineffectiveness, a need to control one's environment, inflexible thinking, limited social spontaneity, and overly restrained initiative and emotional expression, may also be observed during the course of the illness (Table 26–2).

Table 26–2. Comorbidity of Anorexia Nervosa

Disorder	Percentage
Anxiety disorders	60–65
Phobia	40–61
Obsessive–compulsive disorder	26–48
Mood disorders	36–68
Substance abuse	23–35
Personality disorders	23–35
Cluster A	<5
Cluster B	15–55
Cluster C	15–60

Prognosis

Reviews of follow-up studies show that about 45% of patients have an overall good outcome, about 30% have an intermediate outcome (i.e., still having considerable difficulty with the symptoms of the illness), and about 25% have poor outcome and rarely achieve a normal weight. Between 5% and 10% of patients with anorexia nervosa die as a result of complications. Patients who have had the illness chronically or intermittently for 12 years or more have death rates as high as 20%. Most commonly death results from the consequences of starvation, suicide, or electrolyte imbalance. Risk factors for mortality include lower weight during the acute phase of the illness, longer duration of illness, and alcohol dependence. Approximately 40% of patients are able to give up the peculiarities related to food consumption acquired during the anorexic episode, such as binge eating, laxative abuse, or other obsessive food rituals. More than one-half of patients with the restricting type of anorexia nervosa alter their eating patterns, change to the binge eating/purging category, and may eventually meet the criteria for bulimia nervosa. Compulsive excessive exercise may be the most persistent behavior pattern associated with all eating disorders. Only about 25% of anorexia nervosa patients will be able to give up the weight phobias and distorted body image associated with the disorder. These observations indicate that the psychological sequelae of anorexia nervosa are perhaps the most enduring and resistant to treatment. Some research suggests that an onset during early adolescence (i.e., age 13–15 years) may be associated with a better prognosis. Despite advances in treatment, the prognosis for this illness has not improved over the past half century. Although the evidence is not completely convincing, it is thought that early intervention may prevent a chronic course in anorexia nervosa, as adolescents with this disorder have a better outcome following intensive structured programs than adults.

■ BULIMIA NERVOSA

ESSENTIALS OF DIAGNOSIS

DSM-IV-TR Diagnostic Criteria

A. *Recurrent episodes of binge eating. An episode of binge eating is characterized by both of the following:*

(1) eating, in a discrete period of time (e.g., within any 2-hour period), an amount of food that is definitely larger than most people would eat during a similar period of time and under similar circumstances

(2) a sense of lack of control over eating during the episode (e.g., a feeling that one cannot stop eating or control what or how much one is eating)

B. *Recurrent inappropriate compensatory behavior in order to prevent weight gain, such as self-induced vomiting; misuse of laxatives, diuretics, enemas, or other medications; fasting; or excessive exercise.*

C. *The binge eating and inappropriate compensatory behaviors both occur, on average, at least twice a week for 3 months.*

D. *Self-evaluation is unduly influenced by body shape and weight.*

E. *The disturbance does not occur exclusively during episodes of anorexia nervosa.*

Specify type:

Purging type: during the current episode of bulimia nervosa, the person has regularly engaged in self-induced vomiting or the misuse of laxatives, diuretics, or enemas.

Nonpurging type: during the current episode of bulimia nervosa, the person has used other inappropriate compensatory behaviors, such as fasting or excessive exercise, but has not regularly engaged in self-induced vomiting or the misuse of laxatives, diuretics, or enemas.

(Reprinted, with permission, from *Diagnostic and Statistical Manual of Mental Disorders*, 4th edn. Copyright 2000 American Psychiatric Association.)

General Considerations

The term bulimia has a Greek derivation meaning "ox hunger" and connotes a state in which an individual repetitively consumes a feast-like quantity of food. For this condition to be classified as a psychiatric disorder, some emotional distress must be associated with the habit of binge eating. More recently, the subjective quality of a feeling of loss of control over the eating has become integrally associated with the illness.

The modern definition of bulimia first appeared in the *Diagnostic and Statistical Manual of Mental Disorders*, third edition (DSM-III), which relied on a series of descriptive criteria to characterize the disorder. Many of the descriptors were mostly accurate, such as "inconspicuous

Table 26–3. DSM-IV-TR Research Diagnostic Criteria for Binge-Eating Disorder

---

A. Recurrent episodes of binge eating. An episode of binge eating is characterized by both of the following:
   (1) eating, in a discrete period of time (eg, within any 2-hour period), an amount of food that is definitely larger than most people would eat in a similar period of time under similar circumstances
   (2) a sense of lack of control over eating during the episode (eg, a feeling that one cannot stop eating or control what or how much one is eating)
B. The binge-eating episodes are associated with three (or more) of the following:
   (1) eating much more rapidly than normal
   (2) eating until feeling uncomfortably full
   (3) eating large amounts of food when not feeling physically hungry
   (4) eating alone because of being embarrassed by how much one is eating
   (5) feeling disgusted with oneself, depressed, or very guilty after overeating
C. Marked distress regarding binge eating is present.
D. The binge eating occurs, on average, at least 2 days a week for 6 months.
E. The binge eating is not associated with the regular use of inappropriate compensatory behaviors (eg, purging, fasting, excessive exercise) and does not occur during the course of anorexia nervosa or bulimia nervosa.

(Reprinted, with permission, from *Diagnostic and Statistical Manual of Mental Disorders*, 4th edn. Copyright 1994 American Psychiatric Association, pp. 729–731.)

eating" and "frequent weight fluctuations." However, the criteria lacked specificity because no measure of the severity or frequency of binge eating had been set. Additionally, a poorly formulated conceptualization of comorbidity mandated the presence of depressed mood and excluded the possibility of an association with anorexia nervosa. Many binge eaters do not necessarily have concomitant depression, and a number of patients with food-restrictive anorexia nervosa eventually develop bulimic behaviors. Consequently, an enormous overlap exists between anorexia and bulimia nervosa, approaching 50% of patients with anorexia.

The revised diagnostic criteria (DSM-IV-TR) have provided solutions to many of these problems. First, the disorder was renamed bulimia nervosa, distinguishing it from the activity of binge eating. The severity criterion now requires at least two binge-eating episodes for a period of 2 months or more. Additionally, a previous history or concurrent diagnosis of anorexia nervosa does not exclude the diagnosis of bulimia nervosa. Finally, the symptom of purging one's food has been incorporated as a required criterion.

This classification method set up an interesting dilemma: How does one diagnose repetitive binge eating that is out of control in patients who do not purge their food? DSM-IV has proposed research diagnostic criteria for binge-eating disorder (Table 26–3). The new definition has incorporated a severity criterion (Criterion C) of two binge-eating episodes per week for a 6-month period of time. The characteristics of binge-eating disorder bear a striking resemblance to those of bulimia in DSM-III. To add more specificity to the diagnosis, the concurrent appearance of frequent purging behavior, as seen in bulimia nervosa, and diet pill abuse are exclusionary criteria.

A. EPIDEMIOLOGY

Prevalence rate estimates for bulimia are based predominantly on surveys carried out in high school and college populations. Table 26–4 summarizes the results of 22 studies of approximately 18,000 high school and college individuals. The behavior of binge eating was found to be extremely common, appearing in 36% of respondents across studies. This prevalence rate declines as progressively restrictive definitions are applied. Only 1–3% of respondents engaged in binge-purge behavior so severe that it met the criteria for a psychiatric illness as defined in DSM-IV. Nevertheless, as Table 26–4 illustrates clearly, the reservoir of individuals who engage in binge-eating behavior is quite large. This provides a population

Table 26–4. Prevalence Rate Estimates for Bulimia

	Mean	Range
Binge eating	36%	7–75%
Weekly binge eating	16%	5–39%
DSM-III bulimia	9%	3–19%
DSM-III-R bulimia nervosa	2%	1–3%

(Modified and reproduced, with permission, from Devlin MJ et al: Is there another binge eating disorder? A review of the literature on overeating in the absence of bulimia nervosa. *Int J Eating Dis* 1992;11:333; Fairburn CG, Beglin SJ: Studies of the epidemiology of bulimia nervosa. *Am J Psychiatry* 1990;147:401; and from Mitchell JE: *Bulirnia Nervosa*. Minneapolis, MN: University of Minnesota Press, 1990.)

of susceptible candidates whose behaviors may intensify, provided that current cultural stressors, such as the overvaluation of an excessively thin appearance, continue unabated.

The Epidemiologic Catchment Area study, the largest survey of psychiatric disorders in the United States to date, was carried out before the criteria for bulimia or bulimia nervosa were available and, therefore, was unable to assess the prevalence of this disorder. However, at a prevalence rate of 1–3%, bulimia nervosa is at least as common in the female population as other major psychiatric disorders such as schizophrenia (1.5%) and major depressive disorder (1.3%). Furthermore, available evidence indicates that the prevalence of bulimia nervosa, which showed dramatic increases in the latter half of the twentieth century, has more recently had a slight decrease in the United States.

Reported frequencies of Bulimia Nervosa have been similar in the industrialized world, such as the United States, Canada, Europe, Australia, Japan, New Zealand, and South Africa. Caucasians and Asians are racially preponderant in most studies.

Most surveys that have examined the sex ratio of patients with bulimia or bulimia nervosa have found the overwhelming preponderance (98–100%) to be female. The average age at onset of the disorder is 18–20 years, and most patients are seen for psychiatric consultation after 3–5 years. Thus epidemiologic research demonstrates complete unanimity in reporting that bulimia, like anorexia nervosa, is almost exclusively a disorder of young women. In general, individuals with bulimia nervosa are of normal weight, but occasionally they can be significantly overweight. Some research suggests that patients with bulimia nervosa are frequently overweight prior to the onset of the illness.

B. Etiology

The cultural pressures described previously for anorexia nervosa also operate in the etiology of bulimia nervosa, namely the excessive idealization of thinness and the prejudice against obesity. These pressures are particularly evident when career choices involve public display of the body, such as in dancing, fashion modeling, acting, and so on. Bulimic symptomatology is especially prevalent in women who have chosen such careers.

Preexistent trauma such as sexual or physical abuse may be a risk factor for eating disorders, as it occurs in approximately one-third of the patients; however, a recent review of the literature was unable to find a specific causal relationship between early abuse experiences and bulimia nervosa.

As with anorexia nervosa, some research has linked aberrant central nervous system monoamine metabolism with bulimia nervosa, particularly serotonin deficiency. Whether these biological abnormalities are the cause or consequence of the binge-purge behaviors has yet to be determined. However, it is of interest that fluoxetine, a pharmacologic agent that presumably makes more serotonin available at the synapse, has demonstrated efficacy in this disorder.

C. Genetics

Studies have reported an increased risk of substance abuse, alcoholism, and mood disorders in the first-degree relatives of patients with bulimia nervosa. A large study has found a higher concordance rate for bulimia nervosa in monozygotic than dizygotic female twin pairs. It is less well established that there is an increased frequency of obesity in first-degree relatives of bulimic individuals. The D_2 dopamine receptor has emerged as a possible candidate gene meriting further study, but the field currently lacks animal models that might illuminate further genetic and biological research.

Clinical Findings

A. Signs & Symptoms

It is very important to be able to differentiate a clinically defined binge from what would normally be considered a feast during holidays such as Thanksgiving. In one study, bulimic patients were asked to engage in binge-eating and purging behavior while in a controlled hospital environment. Bulimic subjects consumed over 3000 calories during each binge, and this food was ingested in less than 40 minutes, followed by a purge. Frequently, individuals with bulimia nervosa will engage in repetitive binge-purge activity. Typically bulimic individuals will consume high-caloric, easily ingested foods such as ice cream or cake, but this is not always the case. Individuals who snack throughout the day on small amounts of food are not considered to be binge eaters.

Vomiting is by far the most widely used compensatory behavior to control weight, probably because it is also the most efficient means of preventing weight gain. Vomiting is used by 80–90% of bulimic individuals. Frequently, fingers, hands, or instruments are inserted into the oropharynx to induce vomiting by stimulation of the gag reflex, but individuals who have become experienced at purging may be able to vomit spontaneously. Rarely, emetics are abused in order to induce vomiting, with the possibility of resultant cardiotoxicity. Approximately one-third of patients with bulimia nervosa abuse laxatives; enemas and diuretics are used much less frequently.

Self-esteem in patients with bulimia nervosa is inordinately dependent on body shape and weight but not to the degree observed in patients with anorexia nervosa. Although bulimic patients generally feel that they cannot control the binge-purge behavior, they are frequently able to engage in the behavior only surreptitiously, and plan binges around important daily activities such as work and school.

The stimuli or triggers for binge eating may include: dysphoric mood states, interpersonal stress, dietary restraint with ensuing hunger pangs, or dissatisfaction with body shape or size. Although the binge-purge activity may be anxiolytic and may temporarily reduce depressed feelings, self-critical feelings and intense bouts of depression may occur following binge-purge episodes.

So-called 'nonpurging' bulimics may employ fasting, excessive exercise, or overuse of thyroid hormones, prescription and over the counter diet preparations, and substances of abuse (e.g. amphetamines, cocaine) to inhibit appetite or increase metabolism. When patients with bulimia nervosa have coexisting diabetes mellitus, they may skip doses of oral hypoglycemic medication or injectable insulin in order to promote the inefficient metabolism of glucose.

B. PSYCHOLOGICAL TESTING

As with anorexia nervosa, the diagnosis of bulimia nervosa does not depend on the results of psychological tests, although the tests mentioned in the discussion of anorexia nervosa are useful for screening purposes and for monitoring treatment response. The Eating Disorders Examination is perhaps the most extensively used comprehensive interview-based assessment instrument for the clinical characterization of an eating disorder. As with anorexia nervosa, it is helpful to use the appropriate psychological tests to characterize and quantify comorbid depression, anxiety, or Axis II disorders.

C. LABORATORY FINDINGS & IMAGING

Vomiting leads to a loss of gastric hydrochloric acid, which results in hypochloremia and, via renal compensatory mechanisms, hypokalemia. Serum electrolytes frequently demonstrate metabolic alkalosis, with elevations in serum bicarbonate. Serum amylase has also been mildly elevated, predominantly the S amylase fraction, derived from the salivary glands. Hypomagnesemia is another common finding in the purging type of bulimia. In bulimic individuals who abuse laxatives, chronic diarrhea may lead to metabolic acidosis, hypophosphatemia, and hyponatremia.

Differential Diagnosis

Few medical syndromes mimic the major features of bulimia nervosa. Most of these syndromes are rare neurologic illnesses such as the Kluver-Bucy syndrome, the Kleine-Levin syndrome, or brain tumors originating near or invading the hypothalamic area. Occasionally patients develop bulimic symptoms in the context of certain types of epilepsy or in the course of progressive dementias. None of these syndromes is associated with the overconcern with body shape and weight characteristic of bulimia.

DSM-IV rules out the diagnosis of bulimia nervosa if patients meet the weight criterion for anorexia nervosa; however, the course of an eating disorder may exhibit sequential episodes of both disorders. Patients with major depression often exhibit atypical features, including overeating during the winter time; however, such patients rarely engage in compensatory behaviors in order to control weight. Patients with borderline personality disorder may exhibit impulsive binge eating and purging, and can fulfill the criteria for both illnesses simultaneously. The eating disorder most commonly seen in an office-based practice is eating disorder not otherwise specified (see later in this chapter). This disorder presents a challenge to clinicians who are unfamiliar with the specific criteria for bulimia nervosa. These criteria must all be met before the patient can be diagnosed with a particular form of bulimia nervosa.

Most patients with bulimia nervosa are normal weight, but a certain percentage may be overweight. The interface between eating disorder and obesity is discussed in the section on binge-eating disorder (BED).

Treatment

Treatment of bulimia nervosa is currently accomplished by a variety of approaches. Patients who demonstrate major electrolyte disturbance, who have depression with suicidal ideation, or who have not responded to outpatient management are candidates for inpatient treatment. Hospitalization is rarely required for uncomplicated bulimia nervosa. Partial hospitalization and residential programs are also options for patients with bulimia nervosa, and the best results have been reported by high intensity programs that engage patients in treatment at least 40 hours/week (5 days/week for 8 hours/day). Many outpatient psychosocial approaches also have value in the treatment of this disorder, and current research strongly emphasizes the short-term effectiveness of individual CBT and interpersonal psychotherapy (IPT). However, psychodynamic psychotherapeutic approaches may also be associated with reasonable outcomes. Group psychotherapy has also been found to be a superior form of treatment. Although patients with bulimia nervosa have normal weight, and do not require nutritional rehabilitation, nutritional counseling has been found to be useful in helping patients develop nutritionally balanced meal plans that minimize the cycle of binge-purge activity and food restriction. Support groups such as overeaters anonymous (OA) may be helpful as adjunctive modalities, but should not be substituted for professional medical and nutritional therapies.

Antidepressants of every class, including tricyclics, monoamine oxidase inhibitors, trazodone, and selective serotonin reuptake inhibitors, have demonstrated efficacy in reducing bulimic symptoms, even in the absence of coexisting depression. Fluoxetine at 60 mg/day is the only FDA approved treatment for this disorder, and sertraline has also been shown to be effective in one controlled trial. Bupropion has been associated with an increased incidence of seizures in bulimia nervosa patients, and an FDA warning in the package insert limits the use of this agent. Several medication trials are sometimes required to establish the proper medication for a given patient. Approximately 15–20% of patients may require only a pharmacologic agent to achieve a response. It is recommended that pharmacotherapy with an SSRI be added to the therapeutic regimen if the results of psychotherapy are suboptimal after a 3–4 month period, since the best outcomes have been achieved when antidepressant medications are combined with CBT. Nevertheless, relapse may occur not infrequently both during treatment with fluoxetine, and when this agent is discontinued. The anti-convulsant topiramate may have some usefulness in helping to diminish binge-purge episodes in bulimic patients. Ondansetron, an anti-emetic which acts by inhibiting peripheral 5-hydroxytrypamine type-3 (5-HT$_3$) receptor activity, has also been effective in diminishing bulimic behaviors. Additionally, bright light therapy in certain controlled trials has reduced binge-purge frequency in bulimia nervosa patients.

Complications/Adverse Outcomes of Treatment

Binge eating is a dangerous behavior pattern, and it becomes even more hazardous when coupled with purging. Complications may affect almost every bodily system ranging from the integument to glandular regulation by the neuroendocrine system (Table 26–5). Even so, many bulimic individuals are able to continue their aberrant eating behaviors for many years before seeking treatment. Frequently the appearance of a medical complication, such as gastrointestinal bleeding, dental caries, or loss of dental enamel from the lingual surfaces of the incisors, initiates the process of psychiatric referral and treatment. By the time bulimic individuals become patients, however, their metabolic disturbances are quite advanced. Investigations have revealed that more than 50% of patients with diagnosed bulimia nervosa exhibited signs of dehydration and an electrolyte abnormality, 25% had metabolic alkalosis and diminished serum chloride, and 14% had demonstrable hypokalemia. Associated laxative abuse may result in severe diarrhea, leading to a metabolic acidosis. Such metabolic abnormalities are usually associated with muscle fatigue and general malaise and can also be responsible for the pathogenesis of dangerous cardiac tachyarrhythmias. Though not common, patients with bulimia nervosa may develop potentially serious or even fatal complications such as cardiac arrhythmias, orthostatic hypotension, seizures, esophageal tears, or gastric rupture.

A frequently noted physical sign is the chipmunk appearance of the face, caused by marked hypertrophy of the salivary glands, and elevations of the salivary amylase isoenzyme. Another hallmark of the illness is Russell's sign, consisting of abrasions, calluses, or scars on the back of the hand used to manually induce vomiting. In general, medical complications are more common in patients with the purging type of bulimia than in those with the nonpurging type.

Patients with bulimia nervosa have high rates of coexisting psychopathology (Table 26–6). Rates of mood disorder range from 24% to 88%, although the symptoms of major depression with melancholic features are observed less frequently. Concomitant personality disorder may also complicate bulimia nervosa, with rather

Table 26–5. Medical Complications of Bulimia Nervosa

Cardiovascular
Cardiomyopathy (with ipecac abuse)
Electrocardiogram changes and arrhythmias
Orthostatic hypotension

Dehydration and electrolyte abnormalities
Hypokalemia
Metabolic acidosis
Metabolic alkalosis

Dental
Increased caries
Upper incisor erosions

Dermatologic
Hand abrasions (Russell's sign)
Petechial hemorrhages

Endocrine
Irregular menses and amenorrhea

Gastrointestinal
Cathartic colon (with laxative abuse)
Constipation
Esophageal/gastric perforations
Esophagitis/gastritis
Gastrointestinal bleeding
Salivary gland hypertrophy

Neurologic
Increased seizure frequency

Table 26–6. Comorbidity of Bulimia Nervosa

Disorder	Percentage
Mood disorders	24–88
Anxiety	2–3
Obsessive-compulsive disorder	3–80
Substance abuse	9–55
Personality disorders	
Cluster A	<10
Cluster B	2–75
Cluster C	16–80

low rates of the cluster A (schizoid, schizotypal, paranoid) subtypes but significantly higher rates of comorbid cluster B (histrionic, borderline, narcissistic, antisocial) and cluster C (avoidant, obsessive–compulsive, dependent, passive–aggressive) forms. Obsessive–compulsive disorder is also noted, but studies show considerable variation in reports of coprevalence rates, ranging from 3% to 80%. Rates of other anxiety disorders (e.g., generalized anxiety, phobias, panic disorder) are lower, ranging from 2% to 31%. Significant degrees of impulsivity are associated with the illness, and substance abuse with either stimulants, cocaine, or alcohol occurs in more than 30% of patients with Bulimia Nervosa.

Prognosis

Much less is known about the natural history or long-term outcome of bulimia nervosa than for anorexia nervosa. Community surveys indicate that only modest degrees of spontaneous improvement in binge eating, purging, and laxative abuse. Approximately 50–70% of those who complete short-term psychosocial treatment programs and/or medications report substantial reduction of bulimic symptoms. However, longer-term follow-up studies indicate a 60% ate of recovery, the term "recovery" has not yet been fully defined for bulimic disorders, and it varies from study to study. Nevertheless, the data thus far argue strongly that treatment for bulimia nervosa is only partially effective and that relapse is quite common (30–85%). Patients with bulimia nervosa may require more prolonged therapy in order to experience a sustained remission. Bulimia nervosa patients rarely go on to develop anorexia nervosa. The death rate for bulimia nervosa is much lower than that for anorexia nervosa. Patients who remain in remission for more than one year have a better long-term outcome, but

there is no evidence that early enrollment in a treatment program results in a more sustained remission.

EATING DISORDER NOT OTHERWISE SPECIFIED (NOS)

DSM-IV-TR Diagnostic Criteria

The eating disorder not otherwise specified category is for disorders of eating that do not meet the criteria for a specific eating disorder. A sizeable percentage (>50%) of patients who receive treatment for eating disorder from clinicians are relegated to this category. For example, up to 28% patients in one diagnostic study of anorexia nervosa denied that they feared weight gain, and accurately appraised their bodies as emaciated.

Other examples include:

1. *For females, all of the criteria for anorexia nervosa are met except that the individual has regular menses.*

2. *All of the criteria for anorexia nervosa are met except that, despite significant weight loss, the individual's current weight is in the normal range.*

3. *All of the criteria for bulimia nervosa are met except that the binge eating and inappropriate compensatory mechanisms occur at a frequency of less than twice a week or for a duration of less than 3 months.*

4. *The regular use of inappropriate compensatory behavior by an individual of normal body weight after eating small amounts of food (e.g., self-induced vomiting after the consumption of two cookies).*

5. *Repeatedly chewing and spitting out, but not swallowing, large amounts of food.*

6. *Binge-eating disorder: recurrent episodes of binge eating in the absence of the regular use of compensatory behaviors characteristic of bulimia nervosa (see Table 26–3).*

(Reprinted, with permission, from *Diagnostic and Statistical Manual of Mental Disorders*, 4th edn. Text Revision. Copyright 2000 American Psychiatric Association.)

Patients with Eating Disorder NOS (ED-NOS) in general do not differ in their clinical course, level of impairment, nor treatment response from those who fulfill DSM-IV criteria for anorexia nervosa or bulimia nervosa. For example, patients who fulfill criteria for anorexia nervosa but who have not lost enough weight to meet the weight criterion, or who do not have amenorrhea, should have a similar plan of care as those with DSM-IV-TR diagnosable anorexia nervosa.

Recently, an area of intensive research has begun to delineate a group of circadian eating disorders known collectively as the 'night eating syndrome (NES)'. The symptoms of this condition include: morning anorexia, evening hyperphagia, and insomnia. A variant of this disorder involves a somnambulistic sleep disorder characterized by recurrent awakenings, often accompanied by eating or drinking, sometimes with a reduced awareness or ability to recall the events of the nocturnal eating episodes. Further studies of the phenomenology, potential causalities, and treatment of these disorders are underway.

BINGE-EATING DISORDER (BED)

 ESSENTIALS OF DIAGNOSIS

DSM-IV Diagnostic Criteria (Research)
  See Table 26–3

General Considerations

Although, as mentioned earlier in this chapter, the female population in the industrialized world yearns to emulate the slimmest appearing models, in reality an extremely high proportion of women are overweight. BED was incorporated in the DSM-IV as an example of eating disorders not otherwise specified and provisional criteria were offered to guide research on this condition. Since that time a sizeable literature has accumulated on BED suggesting that this may be a valid diagnostic entity, although to some extent the criteria remain controversial.

A. EPIDEMIOLOGY

Over 18 million women (27.1%) in the United States are overweight, and over 7 million (10.8%) are severely overweight. Furthermore, obesity appears to be most prevalent in minorities, especially in African Americans and Hispanics. A field study of binge-eating disorder has found that this is an extremely prevalent problem. Two

percent of individuals in a community sample identified themselves as having had the disorder. In treatment seeking obese individuals the rate of BED appears to be between 10% and 20%, and in the severely obese such as those who are seeking surgery for obesity BED is as high as 30–50%. The prevalence rate of binge-eating disorder may be as high as 70% in self-help groups such as OA. According to available studies, 60–75% of patients with binge-eating disorder are female, and the disorder typically begins during adolescence.

B. ETIOLOGY

No major etiologic theories have been promulgated that are specific to the construct of binge-eating disorder. Studies indicate that factors that increase the risk of both psychiatric disorders in general and obesity help to predict the development of binge-eating disorder. Family studies of probands with binge-eating disorder are inconsistent.

C. GENETICS

Although little work has been done in this area, the available research suggests that BED is a familial disorder, and there is a strong suggestion of a probable genetic component.

Clinical Findings

A. SIGNS & SYMPTOMS

Although in the DSM-IV the binge-eating episodes in patients with BED are described exactly as they are in bulimia nervosa, research has shown that the binge-eating episodes tend to be somewhat different. Usually they are lower in calorie content and the criterion that individuals eat more rapidly than usual has not always been demonstrated in research studies. Fairly consistently BED has been shown to be associated with more severe obesity, with earlier onset of obesity, and with greater levels of psychopathology than is seen in other obese individuals.

Relative to the assessment of obese individuals, the initial evaluation should include a complete history and physical examination with a careful ascertainment of BMI and waist circumference. Generally a BMI ≥ 25 is considered overweight and a BMI > 30 obese. Waist circumference for overweight is greater than 35 in females and greater than 40 in males.

Differential Diagnosis

Two subtypes of disordered eating appear to primarily affect overweight and obese individuals. These include BED and NES. NES is characterized by a phase delay in the circadian pattern of eating manifested by (1) awakenings during the night, often accompanied by ingestion of food, (2) evening hyperphagia, or (3) both of the above. Although this disorder was originally described in 1955 it has only received research attention in recent years. Although NES is uncommon in the general population (perhaps 1–2%) the prevalence increases in those being seen for the treatment of obesity (approximately 10–15%) and is highest for those undergoing assessment for obesity surgery procedures (approximately 40%). NES has been associated with increased rates of affective disorders compared to non-NES obese subjects, and NES appears to be familial with a high rate of NES symptoms in first-degree relatives of affected individuals.

Treatment

There have been three major treatment approaches to BED: psychotherapy generally using cognitive behavioral techniques, medication management, and behavioral weight loss programs. There is now a sizeable literature suggesting that cognitive behavioral therapy is an effective treatment for many patients with BED. IPT and dialectical behavioral therapies have been shown effective as alternative treatments. However, despite dramatic improvements in binge-eating symptoms, most patients lose little weight, which is of concern to patients and their physicians. Very-low-calorie diets have resulted in significant weight loss in BED, but only 1-year follow-up studies are available, and it is well known that the 5-year outcomes for obesity following very-low-calorie diets are extremely poor.

The SSRIs and venlafaxine (a serotonin/norepinephrine reuptake inhibitor) at high dosages appear to be effective in reducing the frequency of or eliminating binge eating, and there is also literature suggesting that the weight loss agent sibutramine and the anticonvulsants topiramate and zonisamide result in decreases in binge eating, and, of equal importance, in more robust weight loss. Unfortunately, the combination of antidepressants with either behavioral weight control measures and/or CBT does not significantly improve reductions in binge eating, although additional weight reduction may be achieved, especially with the fat blocker orlistat. Nutritional counseling and dietary management are other empirically supported behavioral stratagems which focus upon weight loss. Of note, traditional behavioral weight loss treatments also appear to be effective in reducing binge eating and inducing weight loss, a finding that was in some ways surprising, since some investigators had speculated that weight reduction techniques might actually worsen binge eating. This has not been found to be the case.

Since there is no evidence to suggest that BED patients should receive treatment different from obese individuals who do not binge eat, we review below the general treatment of obesity. In individuals who are modestly overweight (BMI 25–26.9) who have evidence of obesity related comorbidities, a dietary intervention combined with increased physical activity and the use of behavioral techniques can be helpful. For those with a BMI of 27–27.9 who have comorbidities or in those with a BMI > 30, the diet, physical activity and behavior therapy may be supplemented by the use of medications such as sibutramine and orlistat. In those with a BMI greater than 35 who have comorbidities, or in all subjects with a BMI > 40, bariatric surgery procedures should be strongly considered. The most common procedure performed in the United States is currently the Roux-n-Y gastric bypass, although gastric banding procedures, which are technically much easier to accomplish and usually completely reversible, are gaining in popularity. However, the amount of weight loss with the latter type of procedure is more modest than is seen with gastric bypass.

Complications/Adverse Outcomes of Treatment

Accumulating evidence indicates that patients with binge-eating disorder have increased psychopathology compared to obese control subjects who do not engage in binge eating. The disorders most frequently associated with binge-eating disorder appear to be major depression, panic disorder, borderline personality disorder, and avoidant personality disorder. It is also important to focus on certain possible medical comorbidities, such as hypertension, Type II diabetes and dyslipidemias, as most individuals with binge-eating disorder who have the illness for more than 5 years develop at least moderate obesity.

Prognosis

Little information is available on the outcome of binge-eating disorder, but the available evidence indicates that the course of this disorder is variable over time, and the outcome of treatment appears to be similar to that of bulimia nervosa. However, it is well known that obesity in general has an extremely poor long-term outcome.

American Psychiatric Association: Practice guidelines for eating disorders. *Am J Psychiatry* 1993;150:212.

American Psychiatric Association: *Diagnostic and Statistical Manual of Mental Disorders*. 4th edn, Text Revision. Washington, DC: American Psychiatric Association, 2000.

Anderson AE: *Practical Comprehensive Treatment of Anorexia Nervosa and Bulimia*. Baltimore: Johns Hopkins University Press, 1985.

Brownell KD, Fairburn CG (eds): *Eating Disorders and Obesity: A Comprehensive Textbook*. New York: Guilford Press, 1995.

Fairburn CG, Wilson GT (eds): *Binge Eating: Nature, Assessment, and Treatment*. New York: Guilford Press, 1993.

Garner DM, Garfinkel PE (eds): *Handbook of Treatment for Eating Disorders,* 2nd edn. New York: Guilford Press, 1997.

Halmi K (editor): *Psychobiology and Treatment of Anorexia Nervosa and Bulimia.* Washington, DC: American Psychiatric Press, 1992.

Kaye WH, Gwirtsman HE (eds): *A Comprehensive Approach to the Treatment of Normal Weight Bulimia.* Washington, DC: American Psychiatric Press, 1985.

Mitchell JE: *Bulimia Nervosa.* Minneapolis, MN: University of Minnesota Press, 1990.

Munsch S, Beglinger C: Obesity and binge eating disorder. In: Riecher-Rössler A. Steiner M. (eds). *Bibliotheca Psychiatrica.* New York: Karger, 2005.

Pope HG, Hudson JI: Is childhood sexual abuse a risk factor for bulimia nervosa? *Am J Psychiatry* 1992;149:455.

Yager J, Gwirtsman HE, Edelstein CK (eds): *Special Problems in Managing Eating Disorders,* Washington, DC: American Psychiatric Press, 1992.

Yager J, Devlin MJ, Halmi KA, et al.: *Practice Guideline for the Treatment of Patients with Eating Disorders,* 3rd edn. American Psychiatric Association, 2006. Available online at http://www.psych.org/psych_pract/treatg/pg/prac_guide.cfm

Wadden TA, Stunkard AJ, Berkowitz RI (eds).: *Obesity: A Guide for Mental Health Professionals, Psychiatric Clinics of North America.* Philadelphia, PA: WB, Saunders Company, 2005.

Sleep Disorders

27

Camellia P. Clark, MD, Polly J. Moore, PhD, & J. Christian Gillin, MD

This chapter primarily focuses on sleep and sleep disorders in adults. While many basic and clinical aspects are similar in children, developmental issues and some disorders not present in adults, for example, sudden infant death syndrome, are beyond the scope of this chapter. For further information the reader is referred to *Principles and Practice of Sleep Medicine in the Child* (Ferber and Kryger, 1995).

GENERAL APPROACH TO THE PATIENT

Office Evaluation

Clinicians should ask routinely about sleep and wakefulness. A thorough sleep history lays the foundation for accurate diagnosis and effective treatment of sleep disorders (Table 27–1). Patients' sleep complaints will usually fall into four general categories: Complaints of difficulty initiating sleep or staying asleep (insomnia), difficulty staying awake during the day (hypersomnia); abnormal movements or behavior during sleep (parasomnia), timing of the sleep–wake cycle at undesired or inappropriate times over a 24-hour day (circadian rhythm disorder), or a combination of the above (see Figure 27–1).

During the evaluation, the patient's bed partner or other informants should be included whenever possible. Since the patient may be unaware of sleep and wakefulness difficulties, bed partners often initiate the sleep evaluation for sleep apnea, periodic limb movements (PLMs) during sleep, or excessive daytime sleepiness (EDS). Sleep disorders can be disruptive to a household, not just the patient (e.g., sleepwalking, loud snoring).

The clinician should take a thorough history of all pertinent medical and psychiatric problems and family history, review medications, personal relationships, environmental stressors, and review of systems and complete a physical examination including a thorough neurologic examination.

Sleep Laboratory Evaluation

Most sleep complaints can be managed by the nonspecialist, with the motivation and cooperation of the patient, through behavioral modification, treatment of underlying and comorbid diagnoses, and appropriate use of medication for symptomatic relief of sleep-related symptoms.

For sleep apnea, PLMs during sleep, narcolepsy, parasomnias with potential for serious injury, or intractable insomnia, referral to a sleep disorder center should be considered.

Nocturnal polysomnography (PSG) records the patient's sleep overnight in a sleep laboratory. Polygraphic sleep recordings are obtained in a quiet, dark, comfortable laboratory environment. Surface electrodes are affixed to the skin to monitor the electroencephalogram (EEG), bilateral eye movement activity or electrooculogram (EOG), and chin muscle tonus or electromyogram (EMG). Sleep staging is determined by a scanning of these tracings visually. The anterior tibial EMG reflects PLMS when present. Additional physiologic monitoring includes respiratory effort monitoring of the chest and abdomen, airflow such as end tidal CO_2 or nasal-oral thermistor, blood O_2 saturation, and electrocardiogram.

Changes in EEG frequencies discriminate waking and nonrapid eye movement (non-REM) sleep stages; the concurrent presence of eye movements in the EOG. A dramatic decrease in muscle tone in the EMG and a desynchronized EEG distinguish rapid eye movement (REM) sleep. Table 27–2 defines terms commonly used in sleep studies.

OVERVIEW OF SLEEP

Sleep Stages & Architecture

Normal sleep involves two states: REM sleep and non-REM sleep. REM sleep is often associated with dreaming. Non-REM sleep is a period of decreased physiologic and psychological activity and is further divided into stages 1, 2, 3, and 4 on the basis of visually scored EEG patterns.

Sleep normally begins with non-REM stage 1, before progressing successively into non-REM stages 2 through 4, during which the EEG generally declines in frequency and increases in amplitude. Stages 3 and 4 sleep, also called slow-wave sleep (SWS), are typically most intense early in the sleep period. The amount of SWS declines across the night. REM sleep is characterized by high-frequency; low-amplitude EEG, loss of muscle tone in the major antigravity muscles, and REMs (see Figure 27–2).

Table 27–1. Office Evaluation of Chronic Sleep Complaints

1. Detailed history and review of the sleep complaint, as well as predisposing, precipitating, and perpetuating factors
2. Review of the difficulties falling asleep, maintaining sleep, and awakening early
3. Timing of sleep and wakefulness over the 24-h day
4. Evidence of EDS and fatigue
5. Bedtime routines, sleep setting, preoccupations, anxiety, beliefs about sleep and sleep loss, fears about consequences of sleep loss, nightmares, enuresis, and sleepwalking
6. Medical and neurologic history and examination and routine laboratory examinations
7. Review of use of prescription and nonprescription medications, hypnotics, alcohol, and stimulants
8. Evidence of sleep-related breathing disorders: Snoring; orthopnea, dyspnea; headaches; falling out of bed; nocturia; obesity; short, fat neck; enlarged tonsils; narrow upper oral airway; and foreshortened jaw (retrognathia)
9. Abnormal movements during sleep; "jerky legs," leg movements, myoclonus, "restless legs," leg cramps, and cold feet
10. Psychiatric history and examination
11. Social and occupational history, marital status, living conditions, financial and security concerns, and physical activity
12. Sleep environment—ambient noise, light, and temperature
13. Sleep–wake diary for 2 weeks
14. Typical exposure to light (sunlight and artificial) and darkness across a 24-h day
15. Interview with bed partners or persons who observe the patient during sleep
16. Tape recording of respiratory sounds during sleep to screen for sleep apnea

(Adapted from Gillin JC, Ancoli-Israel S: The impact of age on sleep and sleep disorders. In: Salzman C (ed). *Clinical Geriatric Psychopharmacology*, 4th edn. Baltimore: Lippincott Williams & Wilkins, 2005, p. 492.)

The Neurobiology of Sleep

The neurophysiologic underpinnings of sleep and wakefulness are incompletely understood. Aspects of REM sleep such as periodic REMs and atonia are generated within the brain stem. Non-REM sleep is partially controlled by rostral brain regions such as the hypothalamus, basal forebrain, and thalamus.

A variety of neurotransmitter systems and brain regions appear to regulate sleep and wakefulness. The arousal network involves the activity of neurons containing acetylcholine, norepinephrine, serotonin, orexin (hypocretin), and dopamine (DA), whereas Gamma aminobutyric acid (GABA)-ergic mechanisms figure prominently in initiating non-REM sleep (Table 27–3).

Sleep & Circadian Rhythms

The rhythm of sleep and wakefulness is governed by one or more internal biological "clocks," by environmental stimuli, and by a host of processes that promote or inhibit arousal (see Table 27–4.) In the absence of *zeitgebers* (time cues such as social activities, meals, and bright lights), humans tend to self-select a sleep–wake cycle of about 25 hours from wake time to wake time. In other words, if a person lives in an experimental environment free of time cues and is allowed to go to bed and arise at will, that person will tend to go to sleep about an hour later each "night" and wake up about an hour later each "morning." For this reason, shifts in the sleep–wake

cycle activity are usually easier when the cycle is lengthened rather than shortened—in traveling west rather than east, for example—or when rotating from an afternoon to an evening work shift, rather than from an afternoon to a morning work shift.

Normally, the circadian oscillator is entrained to the 24-hour environment by zeitgebers such as social activities and meals, and especially by environmental light. Information about light reaching the retina is conveyed to the suprachiasmatic nuclei (SCN) in the anterior hypothalamus. The SCN are important oscillators that maintain the circadian rhythm of sleep–wakefulness.

In addition to synchronizing the circadian oscillator with the environment, the timing of light exposure can also shift the phase position of the oscillator (i.e., the temporal relationship between rhythms or between one rhythm and the environment). Bright light (1500 lux) in the evening hours (6–9 pm) coupled with darkness from 9 pm to 9 am tends to cause a phase delay in sleep–wake and other biological oscillators (i.e., one would go to bed later and wake up later). In contrast, exposure to bright light in the early morning hours (5–7 am) coupled with darkness in the evening tends to advance the phase position of the oscillator (i.e., one would go to bed earlier and wake up earlier). Furthermore, bright light during daylight hours can enhance the amplitude of the circadian rhythm, thereby demarcating the periods of both nocturnal sleep and daytime wakefulness. Bright light has been reported to have antidepressant effects in seasonal depressions occurring in the winter and in some

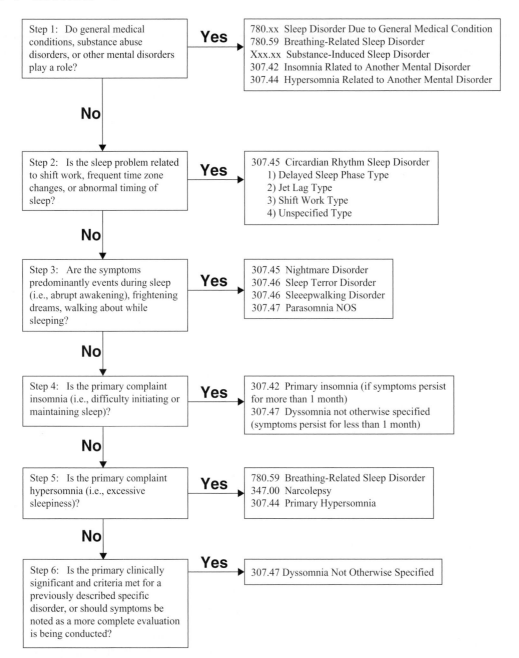

Figure 27–1. Steps for a sleep disturbance algorithm. (Adapted from Gillin JC, Ancoli-Israel S, Erman M: Sleep and sleep–wake disorders. In: Tasman A, Kay J, Lieberman JA (eds). *Psychiatry.* 2nd edn. Philadelphia: Saunders, 1996, pp. 1217–1248.)

Table 27–2. Glossary of Terms Used in Sleep Studies

Term	Definition
Polysomnography (PSG)	Multi channel physiologic recording of sleep
REM sleep	Rapid eye movement sleep, characterized by bursts of rapid eye movements, low-voltage fast EEG, and atonia; associated with dreaming
NREM sleep	Non-Rapid eye movement sleep; consists of four stages
Stage 1	A transitional state of lighter sleep between wakefulness and full sleep; characterized by low voltage, mixed frequency EEG and slow rolling eye movements
Stage 2	Sleep characterized by EEG waveforms called K-complexes and spindles, usually around 50–75% of TST
Stage 3	Sleep characterized by 20–50% high amplitude slow EEG waves (25–50%)
Stage 4	Sleep characterized by > 50% high amplitude slow EEG waves
Total sleep time (TST)	Total minutes of NREM sleep + total minutes REM sleep
Sleep latency	Elapsed time from "lights out" to onset of sleep
REM latency	Elapsed time from sleep onset to REM onset; normally varies from 70–100 min (in young adults) to 55–70 min (in elderly); may be abnormally short in narcolepsy, depression and other conditions
Sleep efficiency (SE)	Time asleep divided by total time in bed; usually expressed as a percentage, normally $\geq$ 90% in young adults; decreases somewhat with age
Wakefulness after sleep onset (WASO)	Time spent awake after sleep onset
Respiratory disturbance index (RDI)	Respiratory events (apneas + hypopneas) per hour of sleep; sometimes referred to as apnea-hypopnea index (AHI)
Apnea	A cessation of airflow of 10 s or longer
Hypopnea	A reduction by 50% in airflow of 10 s or longer
Multiple Sleep Latency Test (MSLT)	An objective measure of EDS in which sleep latency and REM latency are measured during four to five 20-min nap opportunities spaced 2 h apart across the day
Periodic Limb Movements (PLMs)	Intermittent (every 20 –40 s) leg jerks or leg kicks during sleep

(Adapted from Gillin JC, Ancoli-Israel S: The impact of age on sleep and sleep disorders.In: Salzman C (ed). *Clinical Geriatric Psychopharmacology,* 4th edn. Baltimore: Lippincott Williams & Wilkins, 2005, p. 484.)

patients with major depressive disorder or premenstrual depression.

Sleep Changes with Development & Aging

Sleep–wake states change dramatically across the life span, not only with regard to the amount of sleep, but also to circadian timing. With advancing age, REM latency tends to decrease and the length of the first REM period tends to increase.

The amount of time spent each night in SWS is high in childhood, peaks in early adolescence, and gradually declines with age until it nearly disappears around the sixth decade of life. Young adults typically spend about 15–20% of total sleep time (TST) in SWS. Sleep tends to be shallower, more fragmented, and shorter in duration in middle-aged and elderly adults compared to young adults. In addition, daytime sleepiness increases. The relative amount of "shallower" stages 1 and 2 sleep tends to increase as the "deeper" stages 3 and 4 sleep tend

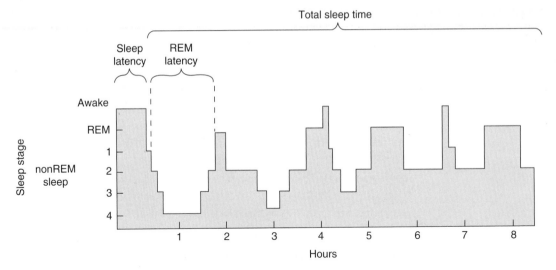

Figure 27–2. Hypnogram of sleep stages in young versus old. (Adapted from Gillin JC, Ancoli-Israel S: The impact of age on sleep and sleep disorders. In: Salzman C (ed). *Clinical Geriatric Psychopharmacology*, 4th edn. Baltimore: Lippincott Williams & Wilkins, 2005.)

to decrease. Men tend to lose SWS at an earlier age than women do.

After the age of 65, about one in three women and one in five men report that they take over 30 minutes to fall asleep. Wakefulness after sleep onset (WASO) and number of arousals increase with age, an increase that may be due at least in part to the greater incidence of sleep-related breathing disorders, PLMS, and other physical conditions in these age groups. WASO may also increase with age because older people are more easily roused by internal and external stimuli.

Changes in the circadian rhythm may lead to daytime fatigue, napping, and poor nocturnal sleep. Related to a phase-advanced temperature rhythm, elders tend to retire and arise earlier than younger adults. Psychosocial alterations can disrupt zeitgebers and light exposure. Napping also increases with age, but the TST per 24 hours does not change with age.

Clinical Syndromes

This section follows the system in the *International Classification of Sleep Disorders*, Revised (ICSD-2). which groups sleep complaints by primary symptomatology: Insomnia, or disorders of initiating and maintaining sleep; hypersomnia, or disorders of EDS; parasomnias; and circadian rhythm disorders. The section also comprises of a brief discussion of sleep alterations associated with psychiatric disorders, substance use, medical conditions, and the reproductive cycle.

■ INSOMNIA

 ESSENTIALS OF DIAGNOSIS

DSM-IV-TR Diagnostic Criteria 307.42
Primary Insomnia

A. The predominant complaint is difficulty initiating or maintaining sleep, or nonrestorative sleep, for at least 1 month.

B. The sleep disturbance (or associated daytime fatigue) causes clinically significant distress or impairment in social, occupational, or other important areas of functioning.

C. The sleep disturbance does not occur exclusively during the course of Narcolepsy, Breathing-Related Sleep Disorder, Circadian Rhythm Sleep Disorder, or a Parasomnia.

D. The disturbance does not occur exclusively during the course of another mental disorder (e.g., Major Depressive Disorder, Generalized Anxiety Disorder, a delirium).

E. The disturbance is not due to the direct physiological effects of a substance (e.g., a drug of abuse, a medication) or a general medical condition.

Table 27–3. Neurotransmitters and Neuromodulators that may Regulate Sleep–wake States

Substance	Involved in Control of Wakefulness
Acetylcholine	Cholinergic neurons of the dorsal midbrain and pons densely innervate the thalamus and thus regulate alertness and cortical activation.
Serotonin	Dorsal raphe neurons (DRN) are active during waking, less active during NREM sleep, and virtually inactive during REM sleep.
Norepinephrine	Noradrenergic neurons in locus coeruleus (LC) are very active during waking, and are thought to promote wakefulness. These neurons cease firing in REM sleep.
Dopamine	Extracellular levels of DA are elevated during waking. D_1 and D_2 antagonists (typical antipsychotics) tend to promote sleep.
Histamine	Histaminergic neuronal activity is high during wakefulness, and H_1 antagonists produce drowsiness and sleep.
Hypocretin/orexin	Orexin neurons are most active during waking and locomotor activity. Deficiencies in this system are presumed to cause narcolepsy.
	Involved in control of NREM or REM sleep.
GABAergic	Preoptic anterior hypothalamic neurons appear to promote sleep by inhibiting wakefulness via GABAergic projections. Hypnotic effects of BZDs may be mediated by enhancement of GABA.
Melatonin	Melatonin is secreted by the pineal gland and is best established as a marker of circadian rhythm. MEL may hasten sleep or ease jet lag.
Interleukins and other immune modulators	Interleukins promote SWS in animals, and immune modulators may be increased in plasma at sleep onset in normal control subjects. NREM sleep measures may correlate with natural killer cell activity in humans.
Adenosine	Adenosine appears to promote sleep. Alerting effects of caffeine may be mediated by blockade of adenosine receptors.
Serotonin	l-tryptophan has hypnotic effects, increases delta sleep. Serotonergic neurons in DRN cease firing in REM sleep and may inhibit cholinergic neurons in laterodorsal tegmentum-pedunculopontine tegmentum (LDT-PPT), ponto-geniculo-occipital (PGO) waves, and REM sleep.
Prostaglandins	Prostaglandins D_2 and E_2 increase sleep and wakefulness, respectively, in animals.
Endogenous sleep factors	Putative hypnotoxins include delta sleep inducing peptide (DSIP), uridine, arginine vasotocin, and muramyl peptides.

(Reprinted, with permission, from *Diagnostic and Statistical Manual of Mental Disorders*, 4th edn. Text Revision. Copyright 2000 American Psychiatric Association.)

General Considerations

Insomnia is the complaint of difficulty initiating or maintaining sleep or of nonrestorative sleep (not feeling well-rested after sleep that is adequate in amount). Insomnia is more common in women than in men; more common with age; and often associated with medical and psychiatric disorders or use of alcohol, drugs, and medication.

Clinical Findings

Transient insomnia is much more common than chronic (> 1 month) insomnia. It generally results from acute stress. Many such cases resolve without intervention. PSG abnormalities have been documented in acute bereavement. However, persistent insomnia should raise the consideration of depression, adjustment disorder, or other psychiatric disorders. Psychophysiologic insomnia is a "disorder of somatized tension and learned sleep-preventing associations that result in a complaint of

Table 27–4. Glossary: Terms Commonly used in the Study of Circadian Rhythms

Term	Definition
Chronobiology	**The Study of Circadian Rhythms**
Circadian rhythms	Refers to biological rhythms having a cycle length of about 24 h. Derived from Latin: *circa dies*, "about 1 day." Examples include the sleep–wake cycle in humans and temperature, cortisol, and psychological variation over the 24-h day. Characterized by exact cycle length, amplitude, and phase position.
Phase position	Temporal relationship between rhythms or between one rhythm and the environment. For example, the maximum daily temperature peak usually occurs in the late afternoon.
Phase-advanced rhythm	Patient retires and arises early.
Phase-delayed rhythm	Patient retires and arises late.
Zeitgebers	Time cues such as social activities, meals, and bright lights.

(Adapted from Gillin JC, Ancoli-Israel S: The impact of age on sleep and sleep disorders. In: Salzman C (ed). *Clinical Geriatric Psychopharmacology,* 4th edn. Baltimore: Lippincott Williams & Wilkins, 2005, p. 485.)

insomnia" (ICSD-2 1997). All patients with chronic insomnia probably develop learned sleep-preventing associations, such as marked overconcern with the inability to sleep. The frustration, anger, and anxiety associated with trying to sleep or maintain sleep serve only to arouse them further as they struggle to sleep. These patients can acquire aversive associations with their bedrooms, often sleeping better in other places such as in front of the television set, in a hotel, or in the sleep laboratory. Psychophysiologic insomnia can become chronic.

Differential Diagnosis

Because chronic insomnia is so commonly caused by medical, psychiatric, or substance use comorbidity or in association with medication, the clinician should always look carefully for other conditions and treat the primary disorder. Although 780.59 Breathing-Related Sleep Disorder is classified as a hypersomnia, apneic episodes can cause insomnia. Insomnia can also be associated with sleep-related movement disorders, for example, restless legs syndrome (RLS) and PLMS (discussed separately).

Treatment

Nonpharmacologic treatment includes education about sleep hygiene (see Table 27–5, Stimulus-Control Treatment) as well as identifying and correcting faulty beliefs, for example, the fear of not being able to function at all without 8 hours uninterrupted sleep.

Sleep restriction therapy involves gradually improving sleep consolidation (minimizing interruptions of the nocturnal sleep period) by limiting the time patients spend in bed. Many insomniac patients underestimate

Table 27–5. Stimulus Control Treatment

Keep bedtimes and awakening constant, even on the weekends.
Do not use the bed for watching television, reading a book, or working. If sleep does not begin within a period of time, say, 30 min, leave the bed and do not return until drowsy.
Avoid napping.
Exercise regularly (3–4 times per week), but try to avoid exercising in the early evening if this tends to interfere with sleep.
Discontinue or reduce alcohol, caffeine, cigarettes, and other substances that may interfere with sleep.
"Wind down" before bed with quiet or relaxing activities.
Maintain a cool, comfortable, and quiet sleeping environment.

Table 27–6. Non-BZD Hypnotics

Generic	Trade	Half-life (h)	Onset	Dose, Adult (mg)	Mechanism
Zolpidem	Ambien	1.5–2.4	Fast	5–10	$GABA_A$ Agonist
Zaleplon	Sonata	1	Fast	5–10	$GABA_A$ Agonist
Eszopiclone	Lunesta	5–7	Medium	2–3	$GABA_A$ Agonist
Ramelteon	Rozerem	1–2.6	Fast	8	Melatonin Agonist

actual sleep time ("sleep state misperception") and have poor sleep efficiency (SE). If the patient reports sleeping 6 hours per night, he or she is required to limit time in bed to 6 hours or slightly more. This simple maneuver usually produces mild sleep deprivation, shortens sleep latency, and increases SE. As sleep becomes more consolidated, the patient is allowed gradually to increase time in bed. It may be helpful to counsel for acute stressors and break the "vicious cycle" of psychophysiological insomnia.

A. Psychopharmacologic Interventions

Benzodiazepines (BZDs) have been the most widely prescribed true sedative-hypnotics, being safer than barbiturates. They generally reduce sleep latency, minutes awake after sleep onset, SWS, and REM while increasing Stage 2. The choice of BZD depends on onset and duration of action (in relation to the timing of sleep complaints) and anxiolytic properties if needed. In the absence of substance abuse history or concomitant abuse of other substances, short-term use of BZDs to treat insomnia is usually safe and effective. The long-term efficacy is not clear; physiologic tolerance can occur.

Non-BZD hypnotics include zolpidem, zaleplon, eszopiclone (the S-isomer of zopiclone), and ramelteon (see Table 27–6.) Compared to BZDs, these drugs tend to have less risk of misuse, rebound insomnia, and withdrawal symptoms and can generally be given to recovering addicts. Zolpidem can be taken in doses larger than described. Aside from ramelteon, these are $GABA_A$ receptor agonists, which probably explains their less marked motor and cognitive side effects. Onset and duration of action should be considered. Some nonBZDs can cause morning "hangovers" if taken too late in the night. Controlled-release zolpidem, is now The U.S. Food and Drug Administration (FDA) approved and has shown efficacy in long-term use as well.

Ramelteon, a selective melatonin (MEL) agonist (active at MT1 and MT2 sites), does not bind to GABA receptors, nor does it possess activity within the brain reward system. It is being marketed as "addiction proof"; if this claim stands the test of time, it will provide an impor-

tant option for many patients in recovery. Its rapid onset of action and melatonergic mechanisms appear promising for initial insomnia, especially in the context of a delayed circadian phase.

Other medications prescribed for insomnia in the absence of psychiatric comorbidity include trazodone, other sedating antidepressants, and the more sedating atypical antipsychotics.

Over-the-counter (OTC) sleeping pills usually consist of or contain histamine 1 antagonists (e.g., diphenhydramine). Their efficacy is dubious. "Natural" remedies include valerian and MEL, the latter which has been used for many years and probably does have some efficacy.

Complications/Adverse Outcomes of Treatment

The liability for tolerance, withdrawal, and abuse must be considered in regard to all the BZDs, although many patients with anxiety disorder and insomnia take them long-term without misuse, particularly after proper patient education and supervision. However, withdrawal from prolonged high-dose BZDs can cause seizures, psychosis, delirium or even death. Rebound insomnia can also occur even with well-planned tapering.

The "war on drugs" increasingly leads many clinicians to prescribe medication with less favorable safety profiles than BZDs, (e.g., risk of priapism with trazodone and metabolic complications with atypical antipsychotics). Elderly patients are particularly vulnerable to the anticholinergic side effects of antihistamines.

Many people think "natural" products are safer, not knowing that the FDA classifies them as dietary supplements and does not regulate them as closely as "manufactured" pharmaceuticals. Serious problems have resulted from unsafe processing (e.g., L-tryptophan byproducts causing an eosinophilia-myalgia syndrome). Recently, an analysis of MEL tablets bought at "reputable" pharmacies, supermarkets, and health food stores found widely varying actual doses of MEL as well as adulterants such as BZDs. Potential drug interactions are less well-known for complementary medicine products, particularly in regard to botanicals which contain multiple chemical compounds.

Prognosis

Depends on the underlying cause of insomnia as well as the prevention of secondary complications such as substance misuse in the context of self-medication.

■ RESTLESS LEGS SYNDROME/PLMS IN SLEEP

Insomnia associated with RLS, PLMS, or other sleep-related movement disorders is coded as 307.47 Dyssomnia Not Otherwise Specified.

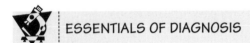 ESSENTIALS OF DIAGNOSIS

DSM-IV-TR Criteria 307.47
Dyssomnia Not Otherwise Specified
The Dyssomnia Not Otherwise Specified category is for
  insomnias, hypersomnias, or circadian rhythm dis-
  turbances that do not meet criteria for any specific
  Dyssomnia.

(Reprinted, with permission, from *Diagnostic and Statistical Manual of Mental Disorders*, 4th edn. Text Revision. Copyright 2000 American Psychiatric Association.)

General Considerations/Clinical Findings

Restless leg syndrome (RLS) and PLMS are often discussed together because they overlap in presentation and symptoms. RLS is an uncomfortable "creeping, crawling" sensation or "pins and needles feeling" (described as similar to akathisia by patients who have had both) in the limbs, especially in the legs. RLS tends to occur during waking and at sleep onset, whereas PLMS occurs during sleep. Patients with RLS sometimes also have PLMS, but patients with PLMS often do not have RLS. For most patients with RLS, being recumbent increases leg discomfort and leads to difficulty sleeping. Further sleep disruption may occur if movement of the affected limb becomes the only way to relieve the dysesthesia.

PLMS are involuntary, rhythmic (roughly every 20–40 seconds over periods up to hours) twitches, typically ankle dorsiflexion. Each movement may lead to a brief arousal; PLMS can provoke tremendous sleep fragmentation, yet patients commonly are not consciously aware of the movements and may present with hypersomnia alone. They may present after accidentally kicking their bedmates or drastically disarranging the bed linens. PLMS increases with age, the prevalence being about 30% over 50 years and 50% over 65.

Differential Diagnosis

The differential diagnosis of RLS and PLMS includes akathisia, neurologic diseases (e.g., neuropathies, myelopathies, spinal cord problems) as well as systemic illness (e.g., anemia, nutritional/metabolic disturbances, cancer, and particularly chronic renal disease with dialysis). Similar symptoms can result from the discontinuation of illicit substances or medications, particularly antidepressants.

Treatment

Treatment should include correcting underlying disorders (e.g., iron deficiency anemia) and (if possible) discontinuing the medications which cause RLS and PLMS. Most treatments reduce either the muscle activity or the sleep disruption. Treatment generally involves one of three drug categories: Dopaminergic agents (ropinirole, pramipexole); GABAergic agents (e.g., baclofen, gabapentin and other anticonvulsants, and BZDs, especially clonazepam); and opioids such as propoxyphene or codeine preparations (e.g., Tylenol 3). It is not uncommon to have to switch from one drug class to another after a previously effective medication loses efficacy; conversely, it can be helpful to switch to a previously effective medication in a different drug class.

Some sleep experts consider dopaminergic agents the treatment of choice for RLS, although their long-term effects have not been well studied, even in nonpsychiatric populations. Ropinirole (the only FDA-approved RLS treatment) and pramipexole (previously used in Parkinson's disease [PD]) have more benign side effects than older agents (e.g., levodopa/carbidopa), and fewer peripheral side effects. Patients should be encouraged to use BZDs or opioids on alternate nights if possible. Anticonvulsants may be an option for recovering substance abusers, particularly if psychiatric comorbidity (e.g., psychosis) is a relative contraindication to dopaminergic agents.

Prognosis

Prognosis depends on the underlying cause, the degree of sleep disruption, and the extent to which treatment complications can be prevented.

■ HYPERSOMNIAS

 ESSENTIALS OF DIAGNOSIS

DSM-IV-TR Diagnostic Criteria 780.59
Breathing-Related Sleep Disorder

A. Sleep disruption, leading to excessive sleepiness or insomnia, that is judged to be due to a sleep-related breathing condition (e.g., obstructive or central sleep apnea syndrome or central alveolar hypoventilation syndrome).

B. The disturbance is not better accounted for by another mental disorder and is not due to the direct physiological effects of a substance (e.g., a drug of abuse, a medication) or another general medical condition (other than a breathing-related disorder).

Coding note: *Also code sleep-related breathing disorder on Axis III.*

(Reprinted, with permission, from *Diagnostic and Statistical Manual of Mental Disorders*, 4th edn. Text Revision. Copyright 2000 American Psychiatric Association.)

DSM-IV-TR Diagnostic Criteria 347.00
Narcolepsy

A. Irresistible attacks of refreshing sleep that occur daily over at least 3 months.

B. The presence of one or both of the following:

    (1) cataplexy (i.e., brief episodes of sudden bilateral loss of muscle tone, most often in association with intense emotion)

    (2) recurrent intrusions of elements of rapid eye movement (REM) sleep into the transition between sleep and wakefulness, as manifested by either hypnopompic or hypnagogic hallucinations or sleep paralysis at the beginning or end of sleep episodes

C. The disturbance is not due to the direct physiological effects of a substance (e.g., a drug of abuse, a medication) or another general medical condition.

(Reprinted, with permission, from *Diagnostic and Statistical Manual of Mental Disorders*, 4th edn. Text Revision. Copyright 2000 American Psychiatric Association.)

DSM-IV-TR Diagnostic Criteria 307.44
Primary Hypersomnia

A. The predominant complaint is excessive sleepiness for at least 1 month (or less if recurrent) as evidenced by either prolonged sleep episodes or daytime sleep episodes that occur almost daily.

B. The excessive sleepiness causes clinically significant distress or impairment in social, occupational, or other important areas of functioning.

C. The excessive sleepiness is not better accounted for by insomnia and does not occur exclusively during the course of another Sleep Disorder (e.g., Narcolepsy, Breathing-Related Sleep Disorder, Circadian Rhythm Sleep Disorder, or a Parasomnia) and cannot be accounted for by an inadequate amount of sleep.

D. The disturbance does not occur exclusively during the course of another mental disorder.

E. The disturbance is not due to the direct physiological effects of a substance (e.g., a drug of abuse, a medication) or a general medical condition.

Specify if:
Recurrent: *If there are periods of excessive sleepiness that last at least 3 days occurring several times a year for at least 2 years.*

(Reprinted, with permission, from *Diagnostic and Statistical Manual of Mental Disorders*, 4th edn. Text Revision. Copyright 2000 American Psychiatric Association.)

General Considerations/Clinical Findings

The term hypersomnia encompasses pathologically increased sleep duration (e.g., the patient with atypical depression who sleeps 14 hours a day), "sleep attacks" (abrupt involuntary onset of sleep), EDS, or a combination of these). It is important to note that hypersomnia or EDS can also be associated with poor nocturnal sleep (such as sleep disrupted by PLMs in sleep or other parasomnias) and with circadian rhythm disorders. The most common cause of EDS in the general population is chronic lack of sleep. It is important to differentiate between fatigue and EDS.

Treatment

The treatment of hypersomnia depends on diagnosis. When possible, treatment should attempt to correct an aspect of the pathophysiology itself. Supportive therapy may help patients adjust to the illness and its social sequelae (e.g., being fired for falling asleep on the job).

Prognosis

Prognosis depends on the nature of the underlying disorder, neurological causes of hypersomnia other than narcolepsy being generally more difficult to treat. Early diagnosis and treatment is vital for all hypersomnias to minimize psychosocial sequelae and potentially fatal results (e.g., falling asleep at the wheel of a vehicle).

BREATHING-RELATED SLEEP DISORDER

General Considerations

This disorder is defined as sleep disruption due to abnormal ventilation during sleep, usually presenting as EDS but sometimes as insomnia. This category includes sleep apnea and central alveolar hypoventilation. Obstructive sleep apnea, the most common pathological cause of EDS, is present in 1–2% of the general population.

Because snoring is a common symptom and can cause significant sleep disturbance (with arousals on PSG) even if criteria for sleep apnea are not met, it is described in this section.

Clinical Findings

Sleep apnea is manifested as abnormal breathing during sleep, commonly associated with snoring (often loud enough to disturb bed partners or people in other rooms) and gasping or other evidence of increased respiratory effort. PSG involves apneas (actual cessations of breathing) and hypopneas (shallow, ineffective breaths). The apnea-hypopnea or respiratory disturbance index (RDI) consists of the total of these events per hour: 10 is abnormal, and 15 almost invariably requires treatment. Based on thoracic and abdominal strain gauges, each period of apnea or hypopnea can be classified as central, obstructive, or mixed, sleep apnea being diagnosed according to the preponderance and pattern of events. PSG often also reveals dysrhythmia and decreased oxygen saturation. Untreated patients are at increased risk of pulmonary hypertension, right-sided heart failure, stroke, myocardial infarction, sudden death, impotence, cognitive problems, and a depressive syndrome that generally remits with treatment.

In central sleep apnea, respiratory drive governed by the brain stem "shuts off" during sleep. This condition may occur in a variety of neurologic and cardiovascular disorders.

Central alveolar hypoventilation, which occurs with "mechanically normal" lungs, produces hypoxia and often hypercarbia even if apneas or hypopneas are not present. It is often encountered in the morbidly obese.

Snoring may be associated with conditions causing airway turbulence (e.g., deviated septum). The upper airway resistance syndrome (UARS) entails nonocclusive airway collapse associated with negative intrathoracic pressure; PSG confirmation requires the use of an esophageal pressure transducer. Sleep apnea should be ruled out.

Differential Diagnosis (Including Comorbid Conditions)

The differential diagnosis includes other respiratory disorders which can worsen with the physiologic changes of sleep (e.g., asthma), comorbid neurological disorders, and some anxiety disorders. Comorbid PLMS is also common and requires disorder-specific treatment if it does not resolve with treatment of apnea.

Treatment

Treatment focuses on achieving and maintaining airway patency. The treatment of choice for Obstructive Sleep Apnea (OSA) is continuous positive airway pressure (CPAP) delivered through a mask. This treatment "props" open the airway with room air delivered at low pressures (typically 5–15 cm H_2O). Numerous variations help make this as comfortable as possible for the patient, including a variety of nasal and oral masks, humidifiers, variations on pressure control and timing (e.g., bilevel positive airway pressure (BiPAP), which provides different pressures for inhalation and exhalation).

A number of dental devices have been developed to hold the tongue forward and the airway open. Surgical procedures have been developed, including the uvulo-palatopharyngoplasty (UPPP), which enlarges the upper airway by removing soft tissue. Bony dysmorphology can be corrected surgically. Obese patients should be encouraged to lose weight; weight loss, even if much less than that required to reach ideal weight, can be very helpful.

If snoring is positional, devices such as pillows to discourage the patient from sleeping in a supine position may be helpful. Laser-assisted uvulo-palatoplasty (LAUP), which can be performed under local anesthesia as an outpatient and can be repeated as necessary, may control snoring.

Theophylline, medroxyprogesterone, and some antidepressants have been recommended as respiratory stimulants for central apnea with mixed results.

Complications/Adverse Outcomes of Treatment

The risks of cardiovascular and respiratory sequelae (as well as EDS-related accidents) are obvious. While CPAP is very effective, noncompliance is common. Many patients, especially those with concomitant anxiety, feel "claustrophobic." They may benefit from a supportive, behavioral desensitization as well as the correction of faulty beliefs.

When a LAUP is performed without prior PSG, OSA may go undiagnosed when snoring resolves. However, unresolved silent apnea will continue to disrupt sleep and lead to persistent EDS as well as cardiovascular comorbidity.

Prognosis

Early treatment can prevent cardiovascular comorbidity.

NARCOLEPSY
Clinical Findings

Narcolepsy is associated with uncontrollable sleep attacks in inappropriate, embarrassing, and even dangerous situations (e.g., while driving). Although sleep attacks have been described as brief (e.g., lasting 15–20 minutes) and refreshing, this is not always true. Most narcoleptics experience related symptoms, particularly *cataplexy* (a sudden loss of muscle tone), *hypnagogic hallucinations* (dreamlike experiences while falling asleep), and sleep paralysis (brief paralysis associated with the onset of sleep or wakefulness). However, only 10–15% of narcoleptic patients have all four major symptoms. Many narcoleptic patients report having performed complex behavior (such as walking from one place to another or writing) without recalling it.

Even in the absence of serious consequences, these symptoms can be frightening and frustrating for patients and vexing for family members, coworkers, and others. Cataplexy (which can involve the whole body but at times is confined to one area, (such as the hand) is often associated with emotions such as surprise or anger. The symptoms can be misinterpreted or misidentified by lay people and unwary clinicians. For example, mild episodes of cataplexy (dropping a cup upon hearing a joke) may be attributed to carelessness or clumsiness. A patient may be misdiagnosed as psychotic if the doctor mistakenly assumes the hypnagogic hallucinations have occurred during full wakefulness or have the same significance as waking hallucinations.

Narcolepsy is associated with defective REM sleep regulation. Cataplexy and sleep paralysis can be thought of as atonia without REM, whereas hypnagogic hallucinations and sleep attacks have been likened to REM intrusion. Though the absolute risk of developing narcolepsy is only 1–2% in first-degree relatives of accurately diagnosed probands, an increased prevalence of certain histocompatibility locus antigen (HLA) subtypes has been reported. Recently, animal models of narcolepsy have shown hypocretin neuron deficiencies. Decreased cerebrospinal fluid (CSF) hypocretin levels have been reported in human narcolepsy.

The diagnosis of narcolepsy is confirmed by a positive Multiple Sleep Latency Test (MSLT) (with the finding of REM onset during two daytime nap opportunities) following a night of PSG ruling out other causes for abnormal MSLT. Sleep-onset REM periods are often present on nocturnal PSG.

Differential Diagnosis (Including Comorbid Conditions)

Sleep attacks and cataplexy-like episodes have been reported in neurological disorders such as traumatic brain injury (e.g., Harriet Tubman). These are coded as DSM-IV 780.54 Sleep Disorder due to a General Medical Condition, Hypersomnia Type. Some experts believe that narcolepsy-like syndromes without cataplexy are almost always produced by comorbid neurologic disorder. When no such neurologic disorder is found, such a syndrome would be coded as DSM-IV 307.44 Primary Hypersomnia.

Narcolepsy patients are not exempt from other causes of hypersomnia. If narcolepsy worsens in a patient with previously well-controlled symptoms careful questioning should be conducted about other possible causes of hypersomnia (medications, sleep apnea, and PLMS). Some patients fabricate a history of narcolepsy to obtain stimulants. Obtaining PSG confirmation or previous medical records will protect against this.

Treatment

Although some patients with narcolepsy achieve reasonable control of sleep attacks with scheduled naps, many require medication. Modafinil is the treatment of choice for EDS and may be helpful for EDS related to neurologic comorbidity, medications (e.g., sedating antipsychotics such as clozapine), and obstructive sleep apnea in which EDS persists despite optimization of all disorder-specific treatments. The exact mechanisms by which modafinil is effective are unknown. It is not related to the amphetamines and appears to have less risk of side effects (e.g., insomnia, psychosis) and misuse than "scheduled" stimulants, (e.g., methylphenidate, amphetamines) which are still used. Pemoline, a longer acting, non-scheduled stimulant, is also effective but is no longer recommended given its "black box" warning for hepatotoxicity. Sodium oxybate (gamma hydroxybutyrate

[GHB]), an endogenous GABA metabolite, is the only medication for cataplexy approved by the FDA. Its exact anticataplectic mechanisms are unknown, although other anticataplectic medications (tricyclic antidepressants [TCAs], monoamine oxidase inhibitors [MAOIs], selective serotonin reuptake inhibitors [SSRIs]) may act via serotonergic mechanisms or by increasing norepinephrine through decreased reuptake or increased release. GHB also alleviates sleep attacks somewhat, perhaps indirectly by alleviating disturbed nocturnal sleep by inducing SWS and consolidating sleep. Because of frequent use as a "club drug" with catastrophic consequences (neurological sequelae and death from intoxication and life-threatening withdrawal not treatable with BZDs), GHB is scheduled and available only through a tightly regulated distribution program.

The treatment of cataplexy and the other cardinal symptoms of narcolepsy was previously based on REM sleep inhibition, which is still useful.

Complications/Adverse Outcomes of Treatment

Although the misuse of stimulants is rare in the absence of a comorbid substance abuse history, withdrawal symptoms, physiological tolerance, and, occasionally, psychosis can develop, particularly with amphetamines and sometimes with methylphenidate. Dramatic cataplexy rebound is to be expected if any anticataplectic agent is stopped, with TCAs being generally more dangerous than SSRIs in this regard.

■ PARASOMNIAS

(See Table 27–7.)

Table 27–7. A Comparison of Parasomnias by Symptoms and Findings

Characteristic	Nightmare Disorder	Sleep Terror Disorder	REM Behavior Disorder	Sleepwalking Disorder
Sleep stage	REM	NREM	REM	NREM
Dream recall	Yes	No	Yes	No
Motor activity	No	Screaming, motoric agitation	Yes	Yes
On awakening	Alert	Confused, disoriented	Alert	Confused, disoriented
Time of night	Last third	First third	Second half	First half
Prevalence	Children 20%, adults 5–10%	Children, 5%, adults < 1%	Unknown	Children 1–20%, adults < 1%
Autonomic activation	Slight, secondary to fear	Extreme, with sweating and vocalizations	Associated with REM and motor activity	Not present
Danger to self	No	No	Patient acts out dream, may accidentally injure bed partner	Patient walks anywhere
Treatment	Monitor; symptoms usually decrease with age; if severe consider psychotherapy and/or suppress REM (MAOIs or other antidepressants)	Monitor; symptoms usually decrease with age; if severe consider low dose tricyclic or BZD	Safe environment for all; clonazepam; consider if triggered by antidepressants; treat neurological comorbidity (common) or watch for future development; not uncommon in narcolepsy	Maintain a safe environment and monitor symptoms; if severe consider suppress SWS (BZDs, TCAs)

(Adapted from Gillin JC, Ancoli-Israel S: The impact of age on sleep and sleep disorders. In: Salzman C (ed). *Clinical Geriatric Psychopharmacology,* 2nd edn. Baltimore: Williams & Wilkins, 1992.)

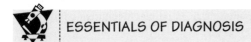
ESSENTIALS OF DIAGNOSIS

DSM-IV-TR Diagnostic Criteria 307.47

Nightmare Disorder

A. Repeated awakenings from the major sleep period or naps with detailed recall of extended and extremely frightening dreams, usually involving threats to survival, security, or self-esteem. The awakenings generally occur during the second half of the sleep period.

B. On awakening from the frightening dreams, the person rapidly becomes oriented and alert (in contrast to the confusion and disorientation seen in Sleep Terror Disorder and some forms of epilepsy).

C. The dream experience, or the sleep disturbance resulting from the awakening, causes clinically significant distress or impairment in social, occupational, or other important areas of functioning.

D. The nightmares do not occur exclusively during the course of another mental disorder (e.g., a delirium, Posttraumatic Stress Disorder) and are not due to the direct physiological effects of a substance (e.g., a drug of abuse, a medication) or a general medical condition.

(Reprinted, with permission, from *Diagnostic and Statistical Manual of Mental Disorders*, 4th edn. Text Revision. Copyright 2000 American Psychiatric Association.)

DSM-IV-TR Diagnostic Criteria 307.46

Sleep Terror Disorder

A. Recurrent episodes of abrupt awakening from sleep, usually occurring during the first third of the major sleep episode and beginning with a panicky scream.

B. Intense fear and signs of autonomic arousal, such as tachycardia, rapid breathing, and sweating, during each episode.

C. Relative unresponsiveness to efforts of others to comfort the person during the episode.

D. No detailed dream is recalled and there is amnesia for the episode.

E. The episodes cause clinically significant distress or impairment in social, occupational, or other important areas of functioning.

F. The disturbance is not due to the direct physiological effects of a substance (e.g., a drug of abuse, a medication) or a general medical condition.

(Reprinted, with permission, from *Diagnostic and Statistical Manual of Mental Disorders*, 4th edn. Text Revision. Copyright 2000 American Psychiatric Association.)

DSM-IV-TR Diagnostic Criteria 307.46

Sleepwalking Disorder

A. Repeated episodes of rising from bed during sleep and walking about, usually occurring during the first third of the major sleep episode.

B. While sleepwalking, the person has a blank, staring face, is relatively unresponsive to the efforts of others to communicate with him or her, and can be awakened only with great difficulty.

C. On awakening (either from the sleepwalking episode or the next morning), the person has amnesia for the episode.

D. Within several minutes after awakening from the sleepwalking episode, there is no impairment of mental activity or behavior (although there may initially be a short period of confusion or disorientation).

E. The sleepwalking causes clinically significant distress or impairment in social, occupational, or other important areas of functioning.

F. The disturbance is not due to the direct physiological effects of a substance (e.g., a drug of abuse, a medication) or a general medical condition.

(Reprinted, with permission, from *Diagnostic and Statistical Manual of Mental Disorders*, 4th edn. Text Revision. Copyright 2000 American Psychiatric Association.)

DSM-IV-TR Diagnostic Criteria 307.47

Parasomnia Not Otherwise Specified

The Parasomnia Not Otherwise Specified category is for disturbances that are characterized by abnormal behavioral or physiological events during sleep or sleep–wake transitions, but that do not meet criteria for a more specific Parasomnia. Examples include

1. *REM sleep behavior disorder:* Motor activity, often of a violent nature, that arises during rapid eye movement (REM) sleep. Unlike sleepwalking, these episodes tend to occur later in the night and are associated with vivid dream recall.

2. *Sleep paralysis:* An inability to perform voluntary movement during the transition between wakefulness and sleep. The episodes may occur at sleep onset (hypnagogic) or with awakening (hypnopompic). The episodes are usually associated with extreme anxiety and, in some cases, fear *of impending death. Sleep paralysis occurs commonly as an ancillary symptom of Narcolepsy and, in such cases, should not be coded separately.*

3. *Situations in which the clinician has concluded that a Parasomnia is present but is unable to determine whether it is primary, due to a general medical condition, or substance induced.*

(Reprinted, with permission, from *Diagnostic and Statistical Manual of Mental Disorders*, 4th edn. Text Revision. Copyright 2000 American Psychiatric Association.)

General Considerations/Clinical Findings

Parasomnias are sleep-related disorders characterized by unusual events or behavior occurring either during sleep or during sleep–wake transitions. Parasomnias occurring during non-REM sleep are more often associated with being difficult to arouse, confusion upon awakening, and a lack of memory for the event. REM parasomnias generally involve waking clearly and rapidly, with recall for the event. These features are important in obtaining a proper diagnosis.

Differential Diagnosis (Including Comorbid Conditions)

Frequent nightmares should always raise the possibility of psychiatric comorbidity (particularly mood or anxiety disorder). REM sleep behavior disorder can present as a reversible complication of several antidepressants; otherwise, it is generally associated with current or future neurologic comorbidity, such as narcolepsy and PD. Criminal defendants may allege REM behavior disorder as a defense, particularly for violent or egregious actions; however, it is believed that REM behavior disorder cannot be simulated on PSG.

Treatment

Treatment depends on the particular disorder. The reassurance that children do not suffer during sleep terrors or recall them afterward can be very helpful for families. It is especially important in sleepwalking and REM behavior disorder to maintain a safe environment for the patient and others. Lock balcony doors. Use special precautions when sleeping in unfamiliar surroundings such as hotels. Move the bedmate into a separate room if needed. Careful instruction in sleep hygiene is important in all parasomnias. Bruxism (tooth grinding) can be treated with dental devices. Behavioral measures without sham-

ing or punishing are important for enuretic children (see Chapter 10).

Some authorities believe that sudden infant death syndrome is a parasomnia. Parents should be aware that the risks of sudden infant deaths are reduced when infants are put to bed supine (e.g., the "Back to Sleep" campaign).

Complications/Adverse Outcomes of Treatment

Are often the result of inadequate treatment but may result from medication side effects, ill-fitting dental devices producing pain, etc.

Prognosis

Depends on the underlying disorder and the prevention of accidents.

■ CIRCADIAN RHYTHM DISORDERS

See Table 27–4.

 ESSENTIALS OF DIAGNOSIS

DSM-IV-TR Diagnostic Criteria 307.45
Circadian Rhythm Sleep Disorder

A. *A persistent or recurrent pattern of sleep disruption leading to excessive sleepiness or insomnia that is due to a mismatch between the sleep–wake schedule required by a person's environment and his or her circadian sleep–wake pattern.*

B. *The sleep disturbance causes clinically significant distress or impairment in social, occupational, or other important areas of functioning.*

C. *The disturbance does not occur exclusively during the course of another Sleep Disorder or other mental disorder.*

D. *The disturbance is not due to the direct physiological effects of a substance (e.g., a drug of abuse, a medication) or a general medical condition.*

Specify type:

Delayed Sleep Phase Type: *A persistent pattern of late sleep onset and late awakening times, with an inability to fall asleep and awaken at a desired earlier time*

Jet Lag Type: *Sleepiness and alertness that occur at an inappropriate time of day relative to local time, occurring after repeated travel across more than one time zone*

Shift Work Type: *Insomnia during the major sleep period or excessive sleepiness during the major awake period associated with night shift work or frequently changing shift work*

(Reprinted, with permission, from *Diagnostic and Statistical Manual of Mental Disorders*, 4th edn. Text Revision. Copyright 2000 American Psychiatric Association.)

General Considerations/Clinical Findings

In disturbances of circadian rhythm, there is a misalignment between the timing of sleep–wake patterns and the desired or normal pattern. These patients may complain of either insomnia or hypersomnia (or both at different times of the 24-hour day). Two processes appear to mediate the propensity to sleep: a homeostatic process by which the propensity to sleep is related directly to the duration of prior wakefulness, and a circadian process that regulates the propensity across a 24-hour day. In persons living on a normal sleep schedule, the circadian sleep propensity is greatest at night and mid-afternoon.

DELAYED SLEEP PHASE TYPE

The major symptoms are prolonged sleep latency and difficulty waking up at the desired time. Most common in adolescence, it can also be encountered with "jet lag" and shift work.

THE JET LAG TYPE

Is characterized by sleepiness and alertness out of synchrony with the "new" time zone. It may be encountered with delayed or advanced sleep phase. Eastward travel (entailing a phase advance of the biological clock) usually takes longer to adjust to than does westward travel (which entails a phase delay).

THE SHIFT WORK TYPE

Involves insomnia, hypersomnia, or both, at inappropriate times, in relationship to work schedules (e.g., rotating or permanent shift work, or irregular work hours). Complications include gastrointestinal or cardiovascular symptoms, increased use of alcohol, disruption of family and social life, low morale and productivity, and high absenteeism. Many individuals never adjust completely to the work schedule because they try to revert back to a normal sleep–wake schedule on weekends and holidays in order to participate in family and social activities.

UNSPECIFIED TYPE

(DSM-IV) includes *advanced sleep phase syndrome* and *non-24-hour sleep–wake syndrome*. Common in older persons, advanced sleep phase syndrome is characterized by early evening sleepiness, early sleep onset, and early morning awakening. In non-24-hour sleep–wake syndrome, patients live on a free-running rest-activity cycle continuously shifting in and out of phase with real-world time. This disorder can complicate chronic poor sleep–wake hygiene. It is usually found in the blind, probably because light does not properly synchronize the SCN with the environment.

Differential Diagnosis

Includes other disorders involving circadian disruption (e.g., depression) but is usually not difficult given the history.

Treatment

Involves patient education, the promotion of sleep hygiene, and an attempt to synchronize sleep and wakefulness with the underlying phase position of the circadian clock. Because the natural cycle length of the circadian clock is longer than 24 hours, it is usually easier to phase-delay the clock than to phase-advance it. Shift workers, for example, tend to do better when shifting in a "clockwise direction" (i.e., from day to evening to night work schedules) than when shifting in a counterclockwise direction. This kind of schedule shift should be implemented in personnel planning for shift workers as much as possible. Many schools are starting later in the morning to minimize tardiness, accidents driving to school, and suboptimal performance related to the near-ubiquitous delayed sleep phase in teenagers.

Appropriate time cues (zeitgebers and timed exposure to bright light) can be very helpful in readjusting and synchronizing the sleep–wake rhythm and the internal clock.

Bright light in the evening produces a phase delay (e.g., retiring later and arising later) and can be very helpful for advanced sleep phase syndrome. In contrast, early-morning bright light phase advances the sleep–wake cycle and is helpful in delayed sleep phase syndrome. It is important to maintain darkness during the desired sleep period: Blackout curtains and sunglasses may be helpful. Light administration using sunlight and additional indoor lighting is very useful even if a proper light box is not available. In addition, it is important to maintain the desired sleep–wake schedule and prevent a rapid "relapse" to the previous pattern.

MEL is more effective as a "resynchronizing" agent than as a soporific per se. It can be administered in carefully timed doses to ameliorate jet lag, but unforeseen changes in travel plans can bring severe discomfort. Treatment with both bright light and MEL must be carefully timed, because the sensitivity of the biological clock undergoes a circadian variation.

Treatment of Shift Work Sleep Disorder depends on the individual's symptoms and timing. It may involve judicious use of bright light, MEL, hypnotics, caffeine, and modafinil in any combination. In general, bright light promotes alertness and should be utilized in shift work environments where possible.

Complications/Adverse Outcomes of Treatment

Include the potential "overcorrection" of the circadian phase, "overtreatment" of a given symptom (e.g., if the patient drinks coffee at the end of the shift in order to stay awake long enough to drive home, sleep latency is prolonged), and maladaptive behaviors (e.g., using alcohol as a hypnotic) arising from attempts to self treat. Excessive doses of MEL have been reported to trigger free running, which is very difficult to treat.

Prognosis

Depends on the underlying disorder and the minimization of safety risks (e.g., preventing drowsy driving during jet lag).

■ SLEEP & OTHER DISORDERS

SLEEP & PSYCHIATRIC DISORDERS (SLEEP DISORDERS RELATED TO ANOTHER MENTAL DISORDER)

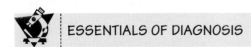

ESSENTIALS OF DIAGNOSIS

DSM-IV-TR Diagnostic Criteria 307.42
Insomnia Related to Another Mental Disorder [Indicate the Axis I or Axis II disorder]

A. *The predominant complaint is difficulty initiating or maintaining sleep, or nonrestorative sleep, for at least 1 month that is associated with daytime fatigue or impaired daytime functioning.*

B. *The sleep disturbance (or daytime sequelae) causes clinically significant distress or impairment in social, occupational, or other important areas of functioning.*

C. *The insomnia is judged to be related to another Axis I or Axis II disorder (e.g., Major Depressive Disorder, Generalized Anxiety Disorder, Adjustment Disorder With Anxiety) but is sufficiently severe to warrant independent clinical attention.*

D. *The disturbance is not better accounted for by another Sleep Disorder (e.g., Narcolepsy, Breathing-Related Sleep Disorder, a Parasomnia).*

E. *The disturbance is not due to the direct physiological effects of a substance (e.g., a drug of abuse, a medication) or a general medical condition.*

(Reprinted, with permission, from *Diagnostic and Statistical Manual of Mental Disorders*, 4th edn. Text Revision. Copyright 2000 American Psychiatric Association.)

DSM-IV-TR Diagnostic Criteria 307.44
Hypersomnia Related to Another Mental Disorder [Indicate the Axis I or Axis II disorder]

A. *The predominant complaint is excessive sleepiness for at least 1 month as evidenced by either prolonged sleep episodes or daytime sleep episodes that occur almost daily.*

B. *The excessive sleepiness causes clinically significant distress or impairment in social, occupational, or other important areas of functioning.*

C. *The hypersomnia is judged to be related to another Axis I or Axis II disorder (e.g., Major Depressive Disorder, Dysthymic Disorder) but is sufficiently severe to warrant independent clinical attention.*

D. *The disturbance is not better accounted for by another Sleep Disorder (e.g., Narcolepsy, Breathing-Related Sleep Disorder, a Parasomnia) or by an inadequate amount of sleep.*

E. *The disturbance is not due to the direct physiological effects of a substance (e.g., a drug of abuse, a medication) or a general medical condition.*

(Reprinted, with permission, from *Diagnostic and Statistical Manual of Mental Disorders*, 4th edn. Text Revision. Copyright 2000 American Psychiatric Association.)

Many psychiatric disorders and substance use disorders are associated with subjective and objective sleep abnormalities. Psychotropic medications frequently have effects on sleep and sleepiness. The high prevalence of comorbid psychiatric and substance use disorders mandates careful attention to diagnosis in every case. (Sleep and Substance Use will be discussed in the next section.)

It is important to remember that psychiatric patients can also have "nonpsychiatric" sleep disorders. For example, the disorganized psychotic patient may practice such poor sleep hygiene that his sleep–wake cycle becomes completely irregular. A depressed patient may develop comorbid RLS or PLMS related to antidepressant medication. A patient with bipolar disorder who gains weight on medications may present with new or aggravated symptoms of snoring or obstructive sleep apnea.

Even when sleep/wake difficulties are related to the psychiatric disorder itself or cannot be adequately controlled by optimizing medication, most psychiatric patients can benefit from education and periodic reminders about general sleep hygiene. Simple cognitive and behavioral techniques related to insomnia can be applied at "medication visits" very easily. Judicious timing of light exposure (not necessarily requiring a light box or light visor) can also assist in optimizing sleep wake schedules. For example, the patient who has difficulty awakening may benefit from allowing more natural light to come in the windows; the patient with early retiring and terminal insomnia may benefit from exposure to evening light during walks before dusk.

■ MOOD DISORDERS

General Considerations

It is important to note that sleep disturbances (particularly insomnia) are often the earliest symptoms of depressive, hypomanic, or manic episodes and are also common in cyclothymia, dysthymia, and episodes of minor depression. Approximately 70% of depressed patients complain of insomnia, which involves initial, middle, or terminal insomnia and subjectively nonrestorative sleep in any combination. Mania can be precipitated by seemingly minor amounts of sleep deprivation or by jet lag. Thus, insomnia and jet lag must be treated aggressively or avoided in bipolar patients.

In unipolar patients, sleep disturbance is often the earliest sign of an impending recurrence or relapse as well as one of the most persistent and distressing residual symptoms during periods of remission. There is evidence that insomnia may be a risk factor for subsequent depressive episodes even in those with no previous history of depression.

Clinical Findings

Most patients are able to report symptoms of sleep disturbance. One possible exception is subjective hypersomnia, common in atypical and bipolar depression. The few polysomnographic studies depression with hypersomnia have not shown decreased sleep latency on the MSLT or a longer TST, although time in bed is increased.

Mania is characterized by diminished TST and other abnormalities on PSG. In major depression, PSG abnormalities reported include shortened REM latency and increased amounts of REM as well as prolonged sleep latency, reduced TST and SE, and decreased SWS.

Differential Diagnosis

Comorbid anxiety and substance use are common in unipolar and especially bipolar patients; together with medication side effects, these are the most common other causes of insomnia and hypersomnia.

Treatment

Psychopharmacologic Interventions

Antidepressants are the pharmacological mainstay of treatment for unipolar depression. They are used in bipolar depression together with mood stabilizers or atypical antipsychotics. Most antidepressants suppress REM sleep; many affect SWS and sleep continuity measures. Virtually all antidepressants have been reported to exacerbate RLS and PLMS.

Sedating antidepressants can be helpful in treating depression associated with severe insomnia. "Activating" antidepressants are used for hypersomnic or anergic depressions. "Activating" antidepressants can exacerbate insomnia and are generally given early in the day; they include bupropion, most SSRIs, MAOIs, and venlafaxine. Sedating antidepressants are taken at bedtime and include trazodone, mirtazepine, maprotiline, and TCAs, particularly the tertiary amines.

All mood stabilizers except lithium are anticonvulsants and can cause EDS, especially in combination with other medication; however, they generally have few effects on PSG. Lithium, like many antidepressants, may increase REM latency and decrease REM; it also may increase SWS in mania. Atypical antipsychotics (see below) are increasingly used as mood stabilizers to augment antidepressants.

Psychotherapeutic Interventions

Careful attention to regular scheduling and optimization of zeitgebers (social rhythm therapy) is very helpful, especially in bipolar disorders.

Complications/Adverse Outcomes of Treatment

It is important to remember that any psychotropic agent can cause unwanted sedation in a given patient. Many effective antidepressants worsen insomnia and are frequently given in conjunction with anti-insomnia drugs, sedating antidepressants (particularly trazodone), and the more sedating atypical antipsychotics. Given the risks of priapism and other cardiovascular complications with trazodone, and the risks of diabetes and weight gain with atypical antipsychotics, these decisions must be made carefully.

Prognosis

It is well known that manic episodes are best treated early with aggressive prescription of sedating medications, especially atypical antipsychotics and BZDs. For mood disorders in general, prognosis is a function of treatment compliance, the presence or absence of comorbidities, and the aggressive treatment of prodromal or residual symptoms (e.g., insomnia).

ANXIETY DISORDERS

General Considerations

Patients with anxiety disorders commonly complain of insomnia. Nightmares are common in posttraumatic stress disorder (PTSD) (civilian or military); some PTSD patients develop a phobic avoidance of sleeping which further aggravates the disorder. In panic disorder, panic attacks are not uncommon during SWS. If sleep panic attacks are mistaken for dangerous cardiac events, the patient may become very afraid of sleep.

Clinical Findings

Most patients with anxiety disorder report symptoms of insomnia and panic attacks directly. However, many patients have faulty beliefs which may be elicited only by direct questioning or after psychoeducation. They may fear that they will die or "go crazy" if they do not get enough sleep. Polysomnographic abnormalities have been found in generalized anxiety disorder, panic disorder, PTSD, and obsessive–compulsive disorder (OCD).

Differential Diagnosis

Mood disorders and substance use disorders are commonly comorbid. PLMS and sleep-disordered breathing are common in PTSD. Obstructive sleep apnea and other respiratory disorders should be considered in cases involving sleep panic attacks.

Treatment

Appropriately tailored psychotherapy can be extremely helpful and may be absolutely necessary in anxiety disorders. Patient education and brief cognitive/ behavioral interventions around sleep are used.

Among the most common medications prescribed for anxiety disorders are the SSRIs and venlafaxine. BZDs are also helpful in many cases, although the best choice for anxiety symptoms may not resolve insomnia. Buspirone is a nonsedating anxiolytic that is not associated with dependence. Atypical antipsychotics are increasingly used in treatment-resistant anxiety disorders.

Complications/Adverse Outcomes of Treatment

Liability for tolerance, withdrawal, and abuse must be considered for all the BZDs, although many anxiety disorder patients take them long term without misuse, particularly with proper education and supervision. Unfortunately, the "war on drugs" has led to a reluctance to prescribe and take BZDs. Many patients, particularly those with anxiety disorders, are terrified of "getting hooked"; the author of this chapter (C. P. Clark) has seen severe consequences of anxiety disorders patients taking less than the prescribed dose, stopping "cold turkey," etc.

Prognosis

As with most psychiatric disorders, prognosis is best with early diagnosis and treatment. Disorders such as OCD, PTSD, and panic disorder (especially with agoraphobia) can cause major suffering and disability. Untreated anxiety (whether as part of an anxiety disorder or not) is increasingly recognized as a risk factor for suicide.

PSYCHOTIC DISORDERS

General Considerations

Sleep disturbance is common in schizophrenia and schizoaffective disorder, often becoming increasingly severe as an acute episode develops. The effective treatment of insomnia can help agitation and positive symptoms to some extent.

CLINICAL FINDINGS

Disorganized patients may have difficulty reporting their symptoms; in this case information from caregivers can be helpful. The most common PSG findings in schizophrenia are decreased SWS measures and evidence of sleep disruption.

Differential Diagnosis (Including Comorbid Conditions)

Comorbid substance misuse is common and can frequently exacerbate or mimic psychotic disorders. The author (C. P. Clark) has seen one patient on depot medications who remained abstinent from illegal drugs but repeatedly induced psychotic mania with very large amounts of caffeine and "energy drinks" (e.g., 7–8 cans Red Bull/ day).

Comorbid anxiety disorders are common in psychotic patients. Anxiety symptoms in this population are often underdiagnosed and improperly treated; many clinicians assume anxiety reflects paranoia or worsening psychotic symptoms. Increasing the dose of antipsychotic medication is not particularly helpful for panic attacks. In fact, severe anxiety can be related to akathisia, which can be worsened by increasing the dose of an antipsychotic drug. Careful questioning is required to determine the exact nature of symptoms; patients may not recognize akathisia as a side effect or realize its characteristic "physical restlessness" is different from "pure" anxiety or agitation. Patients may complain of "paranoia" when they have fear or GAD-like pathological worry (e.g., that their car will break down and require expensive repairs) rather than believing that someone is persecuting them.

Finally, bizarre complaints of "dying several times every night" may reflect apneic episodes. OSA is common in psychotic patients, who may have special difficulties tolerating and complying with CPAP.

Treatment

Antipsychotic medications are the cornerstone of treatment, although psychotherapy and psychosocial rehabilitation are often necessary as well. Other classes of medication are utilized for augmentation or treatment of specific symptoms (e.g., lithium for chronic suicidality).

Complications/Adverse Outcomes of Treatment

The risks of extrapyramidal side effects (EPSE) and tardive dyskinesia (TD) in with conventional antipsychotics

has led to more frequent use of atypical antipsychotics which are associated with weight gain, onset or worsening of diabetes mellitus, and other metabolic sequelae. Patients have suffered severe exacerbations after unilaterally discontinuing medication such as olanzapine based on TV ads for malpractice suits.

For conventional antipsychotics, sedation generally increases with decreasing potency. Atypical antipsychotics, particularly olanzapine, quetiapine, and clozapine, can be sedating; clozapine is also associated with enuresis and drooling during sleep.

Prognosis

Is generally guarded but can be improved by treatment compliance, sobriety, quality of treatment, and the availability of social supports and services.

◼ DEMENTIA

General Considerations

Dementia is one of the most common health problems in older people, and Alzheimer's disease (AD) is the most common type of dementia. Given the neural pathophysiology of dementing disorders (e.g., cholinergic degeneration and dysfunction in AD), it is not surprising that sleep disturbance is a common feature. Related problems such as disruptive nocturnal behavior are a common precipitant of institutionalization.

Clinical Findings

Recognizing the presence of dementia is generally not difficult; however, all demented patients should be regularly screened for sleep/wake symptoms. Profound sleep fragmentation and disruption of the sleep–wake cycle have been documented by activity. PSG may show prolonged sleep latency; lowered SE; and decreased TST, SWS, and non-REM sleep. In severe dementia (e.g., AD), the EEG may be so abnormal (e.g., slow waves during waking) that it is difficult to score PSG.

Differential Diagnosis (Including Comorbid Conditions)

Efforts should be made to rule out treatable causes of dementia (e.g., some cases of normal pressure hydrocephalus) and to look for related neurological disorders (e.g., PD). Many demented patients will have comorbid symptoms of anxiety, depression, and/or psychosis. Sudden onset of symptoms and a fluctuating sensorium are cues to rule out delirium.

Sleep-disordered breathing and PLMS are common in dementia. Untreated sleep apnea can worsen symptoms and accelerate neuronal degeneration; CPAP can improve functioning particularly if applied with special measures to improve tolerability by patients who have early AD.

Treatment

A. PSYCHOPHARMACOLOGIC INTERVENTIONS

Cholinesterase inhibitors mitigate deficient cholinergic activity in AD; they are being used increasingly in other dementias as well. Other agents are used to target specific symptoms (e.g., antipsychotics for hallucinations, SSRIs for comorbid depression or anxiety, sedative medications for insomnia).

B. PSYCHOTHERAPEUTIC INTERVENTIONS

It is crucial to intervene to preserve remaining cognition and help maintain socialization and independence (e.g., with adult day programs). Behavioral measures can be very helpful even in advanced disease and decrease the risks of "overmedication". Support and counseling are crucial for caregivers, who are at increased risk for medical and psychiatric disorder.

C. CHRONOTHERAPEUTIC INTERVENTIONS

Regular routines and schedules are important, with the provision of a sleep-conducive environment at night and appropriate activities and stimulation to enhance daytime wakefulness. Evening bright light and MEL can partially restore a normal circadian rhythm and improve sleep consolidation and behavior.

Complications/Adverse Outcomes of Treatment

Medication side effects are of particular concern. In some studies, BZDs and other sedating medications have been associated with increased falling. On the other hand, such agents may help keep the patient sleeping through the night, indirectly decreasing the risk of falling by preventing night wandering. Cholinergic agents commonly carry sleep–wake and other side effects. Tacrine and donepezil can worsen insomnia; rivastigmine can produce somnolence.

Demented patients are especially prone to EPSE and TD, yet atypical antipsychotics have been linked to cardiovascular sequelae. The latter risk is especially difficult to determine given the high prevalence of cardiovascular disease in dementia, especially mixed and vascular types. No medication is FDA-approved for treatment of psychosis or agitation in dementia.

Prognosis

The overall poor prognosis may improve gradually with improved treatment.

Terminal dementia patients need to be palliated no less than patients dying from cancer, heart failure, or other "medical" disorders.

■ SOMATOFORM & RELATED DISORDERS

Chronic fatigue syndrome (CFS) and fibromyalgia involve disturbed or nonrestorative sleep, loss of energy, severe fatigue, tiredness, and easy fatigability. In PFS, pain may be the predominant symptom; in CFS, fatigue and cognitive impairment are predominant. Both disorders have a high comorbidity with depression, yet these PSG patterns are distinct from those observed in major depression.

■ SLEEP & SUBSTANCE USE

Because of their common features, Substance Induced Sleep Disorders are discussed in general, with further information pertinent to specific substances described below.

 ESSENTIALS OF DIAGNOSIS

DSM-IV Diagnostic Criteria 292.89
  Substance-Induced Sleep Disorder

  A. *A prominent disturbance in sleep that is sufficiently severe to warrant independent clinical attention.*

  B. *There is evidence from the history, physical examination, or laboratory findings of either (1) or (2):*

   (1) the symptoms in Criterion A developed during, or within a month of, Substance Intoxication or Withdrawal

   (2) medication use is etiologically related to the sleep disturbance

  C. *The disturbance is not better accounted for by a Sleep Disorder that is not substance induced. Evidence that the symptoms are better accounted for by a Sleep Disorder that is not substance* *induced might include the following: The symptoms precede the onset of the substance use (or medication use); the symptoms persist for a substantial period of time (e.g., about a month) after the cessation of acute withdrawal or severe intoxication or are substantially in excess of what would be expected given the type or amount of the substance used or the duration of use; or there is other evidence that suggests the existence of an independent non-substance-induced Sleep Disorder (e.g., a history of recurrent non-substance-related episodes).*

D. *The disturbance does not occur exclusively during the course of a delirium.*

E. *The sleep disturbance causes clinically significant distress or impairment in social, occupational, or other important areas of functioning.*

Note: *This diagnosis should be made instead of a diagnosis of Substance Intoxication or Substance Withdrawal only when the sleep symptoms are in excess of those usually associated with the intoxication or withdrawal syndrome and when the symptoms are sufficiently severe to warrant independent clinical attention.*

Code [Specific Substance]-Induced Sleep Disorder:

(291.89 Alcohol; 292.89 Amphetamine; 292.89 Caffeine; 292.89 Cocaine; 292.89 Opioid; 292.89 Sedative, Hypnotic, or Anxiolytic; 292.89 Other [or Unknown] Substance)

Specify type:

Insomnia Type: *If the predominant sleep disturbance is insomnia*

Hypersomnia Type: *If the predominant sleep disturbance is hypersomnia*

Parasomnia Type: *If the predominant sleep disturbance is a Parasomnia*

Mixed Type: *If more than one sleep disturbance is present and none predominates*

Specify if:

With Onset During Intoxication: *If the criteria are met for Intoxication with the substance and the symptoms develop during the intoxication syndrome*

With Onset During Withdrawal: *If criteria are met for Withdrawal from the substance and the symptoms develop during, or shortly after, a withdrawal syndrome*

(Reprinted, with permission, from *Diagnostic and Statistical Manual of Mental Disorders*, 4th edn. Text Revision. Copyright 2000 American Psychiatric Association.)

General Considerations

Any psychoactive compound will generally affect sleep, particularly in pathologic use, abuse, or dependence. The effects of a drug on sleep are multifaceted and determined by drug type, frequency, dosage and duration of (chronic or acute) use, degree of intoxication, and comorbidity with medical or psychiatric disorders, as well as by possible gradual changes in the brain in response to the drug(s). A systematic description of sleep disturbances associated with substance abuse is complicated because polysubstance abuse is common and can involve drugs with different or opposite effects on sleep. An example is acute intoxication with alcohol while withdrawing from cocaine. In general, the effects of withdrawal are roughly opposite those for intoxication or current use (e.g., hypersomnia in caffeine withdrawal). Within a particular class of drugs, substances with a faster onset of action generally convey greater risk of misuse and withdrawal symptoms than those with a slower onset.

Many people without a substance use disorder use substances (particularly alcohol, nicotine, and caffeine) in ways that affect the sleep wake cycle. They are often unaware of the effects these substances can have. For example, many people may use alcohol as a hypnotic without realizing it can disrupt sleep later in the night. Sleep disturbances can also occur following appropriately prescribed medication taken as directed.

In general, the sleep–wake effects of withdrawal are roughly opposite those for intoxication or current use of the particular substance (e.g., hypersomnia in caffeine discontinuation).

Clinical Findings

Depend on the substance(s) used and its amount, timing, and chronicity.

Differential Diagnosis (Including Comorbid Conditions)

The drinking of alcohol with recreational (or misused/ diverted prescription) drugs or the simultaneous use of multiple illicit drugs very common. Even during prolonged abstinence, many patients with substance abuse or dependence have psychiatric comorbidity such as mood, anxiety, or psychotic disorder. Caffeine commonly produces or exacerbates anxiety. Nicotine use is more common in mood, anxiety, and psychotic disorders than in the general population and is common in patients who use drugs or alcohol.

Treatment

Continued abstinence is the ultimate goal. A variety of psychotherapeutic interventions are aimed at relapse prevention or preventing a "slip" from developing into prolonged use. Twelve Step groups (e.g., Alcoholics Anonymous, Narcotics Anonymous) can be extremely helpful. The treatment of true comorbid disorders (and in some cases other substance-induced disorders such as psychosis) is important to improve the chances of abstinence.

Complications/Adverse Outcomes of Treatment

Risks of treatment are small compared to the risks of untreated substance use or dependence.

Prognosis

Depending on the type of symptoms and the substance that caused them, substance-induced sleep disorders can persist long into abstinence and be associated with considerable morbidity. For example, chronic insomnia is a risk factor for relapse into alcohol abuse.

ALCOHOL

Is probably the most frequently used sleeping aid in the general population. In normal controls, alcohol at bedtime shortens sleep latency, increases non-REM sleep, and reduces REM sleep. However, when alcohol is metabolized in the middle of the night, a "mini-withdrawal" ensues, with shallow, disrupted sleep and REM rebound, often with indigestion and nocturia. Nightly alcohol use produces some tolerance to REM suppression and initial sedation. Sleepiness potentiates the sedative effects of alcohol, increasing risks of motor vehicle accidents.

At different stages of the illness, alcoholics may experience insomnia, hypersomnia, parasomnias, and even circadian rhythm disturbances. Sleep disordered breathing and PLMS are especially common long into abstinence.

BZDs are used to treat withdrawal and patients in detoxification programs, but are rarely used otherwise because of the increased risk of abuse and dependence in patients with a history of substance use disorder. Disulfiram, naltrexone, and acamprosate have been used to treat alcoholism.

AMPHETAMINE, OTHER STIMULANTS, AND COCAINE

Cocaine and stimulants such as the amphetamines activate the dopaminergic arousal system. Withdrawal is usually characterized by hypersomnia and depression. PSG shows increased TST as well as depression-like findings (increased REM and shortened REM latency). Insomnia as a side effect, tolerance, and physiological withdrawal can occur with the appropriate use of amphetamine and methylphenidate (e.g., for narcolepsy and Attention-deficit hyperactivity disorder [ADHD]). Even modified-release amphetamine and methylphenidate can be abused (e.g., by snorting the crushed capsule content). Despite frequent concerns by parents, ample evidence shows that appropriately treating ADHD in children and adolescents, even with amphetamine or methylphenidate, decreases rather than increases the risk of abusing substances (perhaps by enhancing impulse control and reducing the risk of school dropout).

CAFFEINE

There are large interindividual differences regarding the effects of caffeine. The extent of caffeine's effects may last 8–14 hours; thus, afternoon intake can disturb sleep. Many OTC analgesics and cold remedies contain caffeine.

NICOTINE

Chronic nicotine use is associated with increased SL and arousals in smokers. Withdrawal may be associated with initial insomnia or hypersomnia, although these are generally minor compared to other symptoms. An exception is heavy dependence, in which withdrawal symptoms awaken the smoker until more nicotine is smoked. Nicotine patches have been associated with increased dreaming and insomnia. Smoking accelerates the metabolism of many drugs. Evidence suggests that smoking increases the risk of sleep-disordered breathing.

OPIOIDS

Though the acute administration of morphine, heroin, and other opioids to normal subjects or abstinent addicts reduces TST, SE, SWS, and REM sleep, opioids can indirectly improve sleep by their analgesic effect in patients with painful conditions. Methadone can be used in detoxification programs, although chronic use of methadone disrupts sleep and can increase the frequency of central apneas. Methadone, buprenorphine, and naltrexone are also used in the long-term treatment of opioid dependence.

SEDATIVES, HYPNOTICS, & ANXIOLYTICS

BZD abuse and dependence generally occurs with simultaneous misuse of alcohol or other drugs, particularly stimulants. Patients with history of abuse or dependence are at increased risk for addiction to BZDs. Barbiturate misuse and withdrawal are sometimes seen in migraine patients taking combination products; withdrawal is generally more severe than BZDs.

BZDs shorten sleep latency, improve sleep continuity, elevate stage 2 sleep, and decrease SWS, and REM sleep. True withdrawal may produce long-lasting effects on anxiety and sleep. Withdrawal must be differentiated from rebound or the reemergence of anxiety or insomnia symptoms. Patients should be cautioned not to stop BZDs abruptly or without medical guidance, although this still occurs iatrogenically in general hospitals with surprising frequency.

For short-term use (e.g., acute treatment of insomnia) and when used for PLM/RLS, patients should avoid taking BZDs for several consecutive nights. Even the tapering of chronic BZDs often produces insomnia and should be undertaken gradually whenever possible, with individualized dose adjustment. Switching to longer acting BZDs may facilitate taper in some settings and is best when it becomes necessary to detoxify a patient from barbiturates and BZDs. While anticonvulsants generally prevent seizures during BZD withdrawal, they are not helpful for the associated autonomic dysregulation.

SLEEP & MEDICAL CONDITIONS

 ESSENTIALS OF DIAGNOSIS

DSM-IV-TR Diagnostic Criteria 780.xx

Sleep Disorder Due to . . . [Indicate the General Medical Condition]

A. *A prominent disturbance in sleep that is sufficiently severe to warrant independent clinical attention.*

B. *There is evidence from the history, physical examination, or laboratory findings that the sleep disturbance is the direct physiological consequence of a general medical condition.*

C. *The disturbance is not better accounted for by another mental disorder (e.g., an Adjustment Disorder in which the stressor is a serious medical illness).*

D. *The disturbance does not occur exclusively during the course of a delirium.*

E. *The disturbance does not meet the criteria for Breathing-Related Sleep Disorder or Narcolepsy.*

F. *The sleep disturbance causes clinically significant distress or impairment in social, occupational, or other important areas of functioning.*

Specify type:

.52 Insomnia Type: *if the predominant sleep disturbance is insomnia*

.54 Hypersomnia Type: *if the predominant sleep disturbance is hypersomnia*

.59 Parasomnia Type: *if the predominant sleep disturbance is a Parasomnia*

.59 Mixed Type: *if more than one sleep disturbance is present and none predominates*

Coding note: *Include the name of the general medical condition on Axis I, e.g., 780.52 Sleep Disorder Due to Chronic Obstructive Pulmonary Disease, Insomnia Type; also code the general medical condition on Axis III (see Appendix G for codes).*

(Reprinted, with permission, from *Diagnostic and Statistical Manual of Mental Disorders*, 4th edn. Text Revision. Copyright 2000 American Psychiatric Association.)

General Considerations

Sleep complaints are often encountered in a variety of medical-surgical conditions, especially in the hospital. Virtually any type of pain, anxiety, or discomfort can cause insomnia, as can the restriction of normal movement (e.g., in traction), lack of normal circadian zeitgebers in an intensive care unit, noisy monitors, round-the-clock neurologic checks, and so on (Tables 27–8 and 27–9).

Clinical Findings

These disorders can present with insomnia, hypersomnia, parasomnias, or a mixture of these and are coded accordingly in the DSM-IV.

Table 27–8. Symptoms and Disorders that May Cause Sleep Disturbance

Seizures
Involuntary movements
Dyspnea/respiratory symptoms
Palpitations
Nocturia
gastroesophageal reflux
Chronic hemodialysis (severe PLMs in sleep)
Trauma (even concussion) or neurological disorders disrupting circuits regulating sleep and wakefulness

Differential Diagnosis (Including Comorbid Conditions)

Patients with medical disorders may have comorbid depression, anxiety, or substance use disorder. Adjustment disorders can also cause insomnia. Furthermore, almost any class of medication can be associated with insomnia, hypersomnia, or sedation; small case series may not be reflected in the *Physicians' Desk Reference.* Medications exert their effects through direct effects on sleep stages (e.g., pindolol-associated nightmares), through effects on sleep disorder (e.g., aggravation of PLMS caused by the dopamine antagonist metoclopramide), and through seemingly unrelated physiologic effects (e.g., diuretic medication leading to nocturia).

Treatment

Behavioral measures for insomnia and in some cases supportive psychotherapy can be helpful. Diagnosing the underlying disorder and optimizing its treatment is crucial. For remaining symptoms, medications otherwise useful for insomnia, hypersomnia, and some parasomnias may be helpful.

Complications/Adverse Outcomes of Treatment

As in patients without comorbid disorders, drugs used to treat insomnia, hypersomnia, and parasomnias can have side effects. Patients with sleep apnea or heavy snoring must not be given drugs that depress respiration.

Prognosis

Depends primarily on that of the underlying medical disorder.

Table 27–9. Effects of Sleep and Wakefulness on Medical Disorders

Respiratory	Position
	Decreased Respiratory drive
	Decreased airway tone
Cardiovascular	Position
	Sleep related autonomic changes in blood pressure, heart rate
	Dysrhythmias in susceptible patients
	Myocardial infarction (MI), sudden death more common in morning (high REM propensity)
Epilepsy	Sleep deprivation may trigger seizures
	REM may be somewhat protective
Headache	Sleep deprivation may trigger migraines, cluster headaches

■ SLEEP & THE REPRODUCTIVE CYCLE

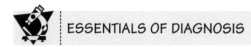

ESSENTIALS OF DIAGNOSIS

DSM-IV-TR Diagnostic Criteria 307.47
Dyssomnia Not Otherwise Specified
The Dyssomnia Not Otherwise Specified category is for insomnias, hypersomnias, or circadian rhythm disturbances that do not meet criteria for any specific Dyssomnia.
(Sleep disorders due to pregnancy, menopause, perimenopause, or other aspects of the reproductive cycle are coded 307.47 Dyssomnia Not Otherwise Specified.)

(Reprinted, with permission, from *Diagnostic and Statistical Manual of Mental Disorders*, 4th edn. Text Revision. Copyright 2000 American Psychiatric Association.)

General Considerations

Because stages of the reproductive cycle and normal pregnancy are not medical disorders, related sleep disturbances would be coded as 307.47 Dyssomnia Not Otherwise Specified. Exceptions might include sleep disorders due to premenstrual dysphoric disorder or a variety of psychiatric disorders that worsen premenstrually.

Physical discomfort disrupts sleep at any stage of pregnancy. The first trimester (with its increased progesterone) is generally associated with daytime sleepiness. The mechanical, physiologic, and hormonal effects of pregnancy are also associated with an increased incidence and severity of snoring. Obstructive sleep apnea develops in some cases. Many gravid women develop PLMS or experience an aggravation of it.

Babies disrupt parental sleep. The postpartum period is a time of potential risk for more serious conditions (e.g., affective disorder and psychosis) that can be triggered by sleep loss. Little research has attempted to separate the physical and hormonal effects of lactation on sleep or to examine the implications of sleeping arrangements (e.g., infant cosleeping) on the mother's sleep.

During menopause, hot flashes can disrupt sleep. The PSG may show decreased REM and TST and increased sleep latency.

American Psychiatric Association: *Diagnostic and Statistical Manual of Mental Disorders*, 4th edn. Text Revision. 2000.

Arendt J, Deacon S: Treatment of circadian rhythm disorders—melatonin. *Chronobiol Int* 1997;14:185.

Ballenger JC, et al.: Consensus statement on panic disorder from the International consensus group on depression and anxiety. *J Clin Psychiatry* 1998;59(Suppl 8):47.

Benca RM: Sleep in psychiatric disorders. *Neurol Clin* 1996;14:739.

Casey DE: Side effect profiles of new antipsychotic agents. *J Clin Psychiatry* 1996;57(Suppl 11):40.

Diagnostic Classification Steering Committee, Thorpy MJ (Chairman): *The International Classification of Sleep Disorders: Diagnostic and Coding Manual.* American Sleep Disorders Association, 1990.

Ferber R, Kryger MH (eds). *Principles and Practice of Sleep Medicine in the Child.* Philadelphia: W. B. Saunders, 1995.

Gillin JC, Ancoli-Israel S: The impact of age on sleep and sleep disorders In: Salzman C (ed). *Clinical Geriatric Psychopharmacology,* 4th edn. Baltimore: Lippincott Williams & Wilkins, 2005, pp. 483–511.

Harding SM: Sleep in fibromyalgia patients: Subjective and objective findings. *Am J Med Sci* 1998;315:367.

Kryger MH, Roth T, Dement WC (eds).: *Principles and Practice of Sleep Medicine,* 4th edn. Philadelphia: Elsevier Saunders, 2005.

Obermeyer WH, Benca RM: Effects of drugs on sleep. *Neurol Clin* 1996;14:827.

Rechtschaffen A, Kales A (eds): *A Manual of Standardized Terminology, Techniques, and Scoring System for Stages of Human Subjects.* Washington, DC: US Government Printing Office, 1968.

Sharpley AL, Cowen PJ: Effect of pharmacologic treatments on the sleep of depressed patients. *Biol Psychiatry* 1995;37:85.

US Modafinil in Narcolepsy Multicenter Study Group: Randomized trial of modafinil for the treatment of pathological somnolence in narcolepsy. *Ann Neurol* 1998;43:88.

Impulse-Control Disorders

28

John W. Thompson, Jr., MD, & Daniel K. Winstead, MD

Although impulse-control disorders are often thought to be rare conditions, a recent replication of the National Comorbidity Study demonstrated a 12-month prevalence rate of 8.9%. This percentage however also included disorders such as oppositional defiant disorder (1%), conduct disorder (1%), and attention-deficit/hyperactivity disorder (ADHD) (4.1%). Intermittent explosive disorder was reported at 2.6% of the surveyed population. Intermittent explosive disorder and pathological gambling (0.2–3.3% of populations surveyed) are much more common than the other disorders in this group.

Kessler RC, Chiu WT, Demler O: Walters EE: Prevalence, Severity, and Comorbidity of 12-month DSM-IV Disorders in the National comorbidity survey replication. *Arch Gen Psych* 2005;62:617–627.

■ INTERMITTENT EXPLOSIVE DISORDER

ESSENTIALS OF DIAGNOSIS

DSM-IV-TR Diagnostic Criteria

A. Several discrete episodes of failure to resist aggressive impulses that result in serious assaultive acts or destruction of property.

B. The degree of aggressiveness expressed during the episodes is grossly out of proportion to any precipitating psychosocial stressors.

C. The aggressive episodes are not better accounted for by another mental disorder (e.g., antisocial personality disorder, borderline personality disorder, a psychotic disorder, a manic episode, conduct disorder, or ADHD) and are not due to the direct physiological effects of a substance (e.g., a drug of abuse, a medication) or a general medical condition (e.g., head trauma, Alzheimer's disease).

(Reprinted, with permission, from *Diagnostic and Statistical Manual of Mental Disorders,* 4th edn. Text Revision. Washington DC: American Psychiatric Association, 2000.)

General Considerations

A. EPIDEMIOLOGY

The National Comorbidity Study replication reported a 12-month prevalence rate of 2.6%. This is more common than previously realized.

B. ETIOLOGY

The outbursts associated with intermittent explosive disorder (sometimes referred to as episodic dyscontrol) were initially viewed as the result of limbic system discharge or dysfunction or even as interictal phenomena. The *Diagnostic and Statistical Manual of Mental Disorders,* 4th edition (DSM-IV) does now exclude those patients in whom an aggressive episode was thought to be related to a general medical condition (e.g., temporal lobe seizures, delirium) or to the direct psychological effects of a substance, whether a drug of abuse or a prescribed medication. Disorders that can be identified as resulting from neurological insult or a seizure disorder are now classified elsewhere. Nevertheless, neurological soft signs, nonspecific electroencephalogram anomalies, or mild abnormalities on neuropsychological testing have been noted in patients given this diagnosis.

Psychodynamic explanations have also been proposed. Childhood abuse is thought to be a risk factor for the development of this disorder. Others postulate narcissistic vulnerability as a possible mechanism that triggers these attacks. Thus, one can conceptualize the "explosive" episodes as resulting from a real or perceived insult to one's self-esteem or as a reaction to a perceived threat of rejection, abandonment, or attack.

C. GENETICS

Little is known about the genetics of intermittent explosive disorder. Family studies of individuals with this disorder have shown high rates of mood and substance-use disorders in first-degree relatives.

Clinical Findings

A. SIGNS & SYMPTOMS

Aggressive outbursts occur in discrete episodes and are grossly out of proportion to any precipitating event. Furthermore, there is often a lack of rational motivation or clear-cut gain to be realized from the aggressive act itself. The patient expresses embarrassment, guilt, and remorse after the act and is often genuinely perplexed as to why he or she behaved in such a manner. Some patients have described periods of exhaustion and sleepiness immediately after these acts of violence.

B. PSYCHOLOGICAL TESTING

Neuropsychological testing may reveal minor cognitive difficulties such as letter reversals. A careful history may reveal developmental difficulties such as delayed speech or poor coordination. A history of febrile seizures in childhood, episodes of unconsciousness, or head injury may be reported.

C. LABORATORY FINDINGS

Laboratory findings are nonspecific. Nonspecific EEG findings may be noted. Several research projects have found signs of altered serotonin metabolism in cerebrospinal fluid or platelet models.

Differential Diagnosis

If the behavior can be better explained by an underlying neurological insult, then the correct diagnosis would be personality change due to general medical condition, aggressive type. The clinician must decide whether the aggressive or erratic behavior would be better explained as a result of a personality conduct disorder. Purposeful behavior with subsequent attempts to malinger must be distinguished from intermittent explosive disorder. Recent studies suggest a high rate of combined lifetime mood and substance-use disorders in patients with this disorder.

Treatment

Both psychotherapy and pharmacotherapy have been described as treatments for intermittent explosive disorder; however, no double-blind, randomized, controlled trials have been conducted. There are case reports or open trials of the use of anticonvulsants, antipsychotics, antidepressants, benzodiazepines, β-blockers, lithium carbonate, stimulants, and opioid antagonists. Novel anxiolytics such as buspirone have been efficacious in individual cases. Current scientific data are insufficient and inconclusive regarding treatment of the disorder; therefore, clinicians must proceed with individualized treatment plans based on their best clinical judgment.

Complications/Adverse Outcomes of Treatment

Intermittent explosive disorder can be complicated by legal difficulties, job loss, difficulties with interpersonal relationships, and divorce. Although patients may have been prone to lose their temper repeatedly over a long period of time, they may not seek medical attention until a major life disruption has resulted from one of these outbursts.

Adverse outcomes of treatment are related to the side effects of particular medications used to treat this disorder.

Prognosis

Intermittent explosive disorder is thought to have its onset in adolescence or young adulthood and to run its course by the end of the third decade of life. Here again, the data for such conclusions are quite limited.

Kim SW: Opioid antagonists in the treatment of impulse-control disorders. *J Clin Psychol* 1998;59:159.

McElroy SL, Soutullo CA, Beckman DA, et al.: DSM-IV intermittent explosive disorder: A report of 27 cases. *J Clin Psychol* 1998;59:203.

■ KLEPTOMANIA

 ESSENTIALS OF DIAGNOSIS

DSM-IV-TR Diagnostic Criteria

A. Recurrent failure to resist impulses to steal objects that are not needed for personal use or for their monetary value.

B. Increasing sense of tension immediately before committing the theft.

C. Pleasure, gratification, or relief at the time of committing the theft.

D. The stealing is not committed to express anger or vengeance and is not in response to a delusion or a hallucination.

E. The stealing is not better accounted for by conduct disorder, a manic episode, or antisocial personality disorder.

(Reprinted, with permission, from *Diagnostic and Statistical Manual of Mental Disorders,* 4th edn. Text

Revision. Washington DC: American Psychiatric Association, 2000.)

General Considerations

Although kleptomania has been recognized since the early nineteenth century as an egodystonic impulse to steal, little systematic study has been undertaken to understand this disorder. The individual with kleptomania often feels guilty and fears apprehension and prosecution. Several psychiatric disorders have been linked to kleptomania; the most recent studies point to eating disorders and compulsive spending.

A. EPIDEMIOLOGY

Because most shoplifters steal for profit, fewer than 5% of shoplifters meet criteria for kleptomania. It is a rare disorder of unknown prevalence, although the disorder may be more common than thought. Kleptomania is more common in women than in men.

B. ETIOLOGY

The etiology of kleptomania is unknown. It may be a symptom rather than a disorder.

C. GENETICS

Little is known about the genetics of kleptomania. Family studies have demonstrated high rates of mood, substance-use, and anxiety disorders in first-degree relatives.

Clinical Findings

A. SIGNS & SYMPTOMS

The hallmark of kleptomania is the failure to resist the impulse to steal useless objects that have little monetary value. This behavior is not usually purposeful but is performed to relieve a sense of inner tension. There is often a sense of relief upon completion of the theft. The theft usually occurs in retail stores or work locations or from family members. Some patients report feeling high or euphoric while stealing. Most feel guilty after the act and may donate stolen items to charity, return items to the location from which they were stolen, or pay for the stolen items.

A comprehensive history may reveal other compulsive behavior that does not meet full criteria for obsessive–compulsive disorder (OCD). Symptoms of mood disorders, substance-use disorders, anxiety disorders, and eating disorders may also be common in this population.

B. PSYCHOLOGICAL TESTING & LABORATORY FINDINGS

Neuropsychological testing and laboratory data are nonspecific.

Differential Diagnosis

The diagnosis of kleptomania should not be given if the patient's behavior is better accounted for by antisocial personality disorder, bipolar disorder, or conduct disorder or if stealing occurs as a result of anger or vengeance or as the result of a hallucination or delusional belief. Other important diagnoses to consider include major depression, anxiety disorder, and substance-use disorders.

Treatment

Psychotherapy and pharmacotherapy have been found useful in single reports. Selective serotonin reuptake inhibitors (SSRIs) and lithium are the agents used most frequently to treat kleptomania. Response rates are confounded by the high rates of comorbid mood and eating disorders.

Complications/Adverse Outcomes of Treatment

The majority of patients with kleptomania have a lifetime diagnosis of major mood disorder. Anxiety disorder is also common, as are substance-use and eating disorders. Complications include apprehension, arrest, and conviction for stealing with shame and embarrassment to the patient, friends, and family members. Other risks might include self-destructive behavior associated with major mood disorders and substance use. Adverse outcomes of treatment are related to the side effects of medication and failure to recognize comorbid conditions that may be treated easily.

Prognosis

Kleptomania is thought to begin in adolescence and can continue into the third or fourth decades of life. The course is not well studied and includes a spectrum from brief and episodic to chronic.

Black DW: Compulsive buying: A review. *J Clin Psychol* 1996;57(Suppl 8):50.

McElroy SL, Keck PE, Jr., Phillips KA: Kleptomania, compulsive buying, and binge-eating disorder. *J Clin Psychol* 1995;56(Suppl 4):14.

Goldner EM, Geller J, Birmingham CL, Remick RA: Comparison of shoplifting behavior in patients with eating disorders, psychiatric control subjects, and undergraduate controls. *Can J Psychiatry* 2000;45(5):471–475.

■ PYROMANIA

 ESSENTIALS OF DIAGNOSIS

DSM-IV-TR Diagnostic Criteria

A. Deliberate and purposeful fire setting on more than one occasion.

B. Tension or affective arousal before the act.

C. Fascination with, interest in, curiosity about, or attraction to fire and its situational contexts (e.g., paraphernalia, uses, consequences).

D. Pleasure, gratification, or relief when setting fires, or when witnessing or participating in their aftermath.

E. The fire setting is not done for monetary gain, as an expression of sociopolitical ideology, to conceal criminal activity, to express anger or vengeance, to improve one's living circumstances, in response to a delusion or hallucination, or as a result of impaired judgment (e.g., in dementia, mental retardation, substance intoxication).

F. The fire setting is not better accounted for by conduct disorder, a manic episode, or antisocial personality disorder.

(Reprinted, with permission, from *Diagnostic and Statistical Manual of Mental Disorders*, 4th edn. Text Revision. Washington DC: American Psychiatric Association, 2000.)

General Considerations

Pyromania strikes fear in the hearts of mental health professionals, because there is a serious potential for harm to the patient and to society. The therapist must balance carefully the issues surrounding confidentiality and the duty to protect third parties from the danger presented by these patients.

A. Epidemiology

The epidemiology of pyromania is unclear. After other causes of fire setting are ruled out, only a small population of pyromaniac individuals remains. Pyromania is thought to be rare. In clinical populations, however, fire-setters are not uncommon. Between 2% and 15% of psychiatric inpatients are fire-setters. The peak age of fire-setters is 13 years, and 90% of fire-setters are male. Many are from emotionally and economically deprived families.

B. Etiology

The etiology of pyromania is not well understood. There is little research to support any hypotheses.

C. Genetics

Little is known about the genetics of pyromania.

Clinical Findings

A. Signs & Symptoms

The signs and symptoms of true pyromania may be indistinguishable from other forms of fire setting. Diagnosis is by exclusion. Most fire setting cannot be classified as an impulse-control disorder, but impairment in the ability to control impulses is recognized in most cases of arson. Patients are usually identified after legal charges have been filed.

B. Psychological Testing

Psychological testing of fire-setters reveals a significant amount of psychiatric comorbidity; however, studies on pure populations of pyromaniacs are not available. Among fire-setters, suicidal behavior has been reported. Screening for suicide is warranted for this population.

C. Laboratory Findings

Lower cerebrospinal fluid concentrations of 3-methoxy-4-hydroxyphenylglycol and 5-hydroxyindoleacetic acid have been reported in fire-setters as compared to control subjects.

Differential Diagnosis

The diagnosis of pyromania should not be given if fire setting can be accounted for more appropriately by motives of profit, crime concealment, revenge, or as a symptom of another psychiatric disorder. Fire setting has been found in over half of children with conduct disorder. It may be a harbinger of adult antisocial personality disorder.

Treatment

Early intervention programs with adolescent fire-setters have reported success in deterring fire setting. Other comorbid psychiatric disorders such as schizophrenia and bipolar disorder should be treated aggressively.

Complications/Adverse Outcomes of Treatment

A significant number of fire-setters will repeat this behavior. While they are working with such patients, therapists must be constantly aware of the potential for harm to third parties. Little is known about the comorbidity of pyromania with other psychiatric disorders Fire setting is quite common among psychiatric inpatients: The most common associations are psychotic disorders, mood disorders, and severe personality disorder. Two thirds of fire-setters are intoxicated at the time of the index offense. Female fire-setters have a high degree of psychiatric comorbidity, as high as 92% in one study.

Prognosis

The prognosis and course of illness are unclear. Early detection and the treatment of comorbid psychiatric disorders are recommended.

Barnett W, Richter P, Sigmund D, et al.: Recidivism and concomitant criminality in pathological firesetters. *J Forensic Sci* 1997;42:879.

Geller JL: Arson in review. From profit to pathology. *Psychiatr Clin N Am* 1992;15:623.

Puri BK, Baxter R, Cordess CC: Characteristics of fire-setters. A study and proposed multiaxial psychiatric classification. *Br J Psychiatry* 1995;166:393.

Lindberg N, Holi MM, Tanip, Virkkunen M: Looking for Pyromania: Characteristics of a conservative sample of Finish male criminals with histories of fire-setting between 1973 and 1993. *BMC Psychiatry* 2005;5:47.

■ PATHOLOGIC GAMBLING

 ESSENTIALS OF DIAGNOSIS

DSM-IV-TR Diagnostic Criteria

A. *Persistent and recurrent maladaptive gambling behavior as indicated by five (or more) of the following:*

   (1) is preoccupied with gambling (e.g., preoccupied with reliving past gambling experiences, handicapping or planning the next venture, or thinking of ways to get money with which to gamble)

   (2) needs to gamble with increasing amounts of money in order to achieve the desired excitement

   (3) has repeated unsuccessful efforts to control, cut back, or stop gambling

   (4) is restless or irritable when attempting to cut down or stop gambling

   (5) gambles as a way of escaping from problems or of relieving a dysphoric mood (e.g., feelings of helplessness, guilt, anxiety, depression)

   (6) after losing money gambling, often returns another day to get even ("chasing" one's losses)

   (7) lies to family members, therapist, or others to conceal the extent of involvement with gambling

   (8) has committed illegal acts such as forgery, fraud, theft, or embezzlement to finance gambling

   (9) has jeopardized or lost a significant relationship, job, or educational or career opportunity because of gambling

   (10) relies on others to provide money to relieve a desperate financial situation caused by gambling

B. *The gambling behavior is not better accounted for by a manic episode.*

(Reprinted, with permission, from *Diagnostic and Statistical Manual of Mental Disorders*, 4th edn. Text Revision. Washington DC: American Psychiatric Association, 2000.)

General Considerations

A. Epidemiology

The prevalence of pathological gambling has been estimated at 0.2–3.3%, increasing with the number of gaming venues available. Roughly two thirds of gamblers are male. Pathologic gambling is a growing problem in adolescent and elderly populations.

B. Etiology

The etiology of pathologic gambling is unknown. Biochemical, behavioral, psychodynamic, and addiction-based theories have been proposed.

C. Genetics

Family studies of pathologic gamblers reveal higher rates of pathologic gambling in first-degree relatives than in the general population. The rates of mood disorder and substance-use disorder in first-degree relatives are many times that of the general population.

Clinical Findings

A. SIGNS & SYMPTOMS

Pathologic gamblers spend excessive amounts of time at gaming establishments or obtaining money to gamble. They deplete family bank accounts, borrow money from family members, lie about their gambling, and attempt to recoup their losses with large bets. They repeatedly promise to cut back on their gambling and make unsuccessful attempts to do so. Pathologic gamblers usually present to mental health professionals after they have been forced into treatment because of illegal activity to obtain funds. For example, they write bad checks, embezzle money, or engage in insurance fraud. Up to 75% of the members of Gamblers Anonymous admit to engaging in illegal activity.

The gambler's spouse is likely to be depressed. Some studies have reported higher rates of child abuse by the gambler and particularly by the spouse. This is more likely to occur when the spouse confronts the gambler about depletion of family resources. The clinician should interview the extended family to understand the full extent of the patient's borrowing. The clinician also should take a careful history of mood symptoms and suicidal ideation, because 20% of individuals in treatment for pathologic gambling have reported attempting suicide.

Differential Diagnosis

Pathologic gambling must be separated from social gambling. Social gambling usually occurs with friends, and the amount of money to be spent is determined before gambling starts. Social gambling is time-limited and does not cause significant financial constraints on the family. Professional gambling, in contrast to pathologic gambling, involves calculated bets without significant attempts to recoup losses (called "chasing losses"). Other differential diagnoses include manic episodes and antisocial personality disorder. Many gamblers appear to be hypomanic while gambling and depressed when on a losing streak, thus making bipolar II disorder particularly difficult to differentiate.

Prognosis

The typical pathologic gambler goes through several phases before coming to the attention of mental health professionals. Onset is usually in adolescence or early adulthood. The winning phase begins after the patient has a large windfall that equals half of a normal year's salary. The gambler then starts betting regularly, feeling euphoric as he or she does so, seeking more and more "action." At first, many gamblers are adept at winning money.

The losing phase usually begins as a streak of bad luck (referred to by Gamblers Anonymous populations as the "bad beat"). Losing begins a cycle of chasing losses with foolish bets that plunge the gambler further and further into debt. As the bets become more and more risky, the gambler enters a phase of desperation when illegal sources of money are considered. Desperation usually occurs after the family bank account and retirement savings are depleted. The gambler may contemplate or attempt suicide at this point.

Another clinical presentation of gambling has been described as "the escape artist" who gambles to pass time and avoid boredom. Women and the elderly are overrepresented in this group.

Treatment

Several treatment approaches are available, from Gamblers Anonymous to inpatient psychiatric treatment. Some programs involve a multidisciplinary 12-step addiction-based model designed specifically for the pathologic gambler. The gambler must take responsibility for his or her debt, cut up credit cards, and allow someone else to handle his or her money. Medication management can be helpful if comorbid psychiatric disorders are present. SSRIs and opiate antagonists have been studied in controlled trials with some efficacy.

Complications/Adverse Outcomes of Treatment

Complications of treatment include continued gambling, side effects of medication, and suicide. Comorbid conditions include substance-use disorder, depression, bipolar disorder, and attention-deficit/hyperactivity disorder. Antisocial and narcissistic personality disorders may be present. Outcomes vary depending on the population studied and the method used. Some surveys report a 55%-response rate 1 year after inpatient treatment. Surveys of Gamblers Anonymous groups show lower and possibly more accurate response rates, in the 10% range at 1-year follow-up.

DeCaria CM, Hollander E, Grossman R, et al.: Diagnosis, neurobiology, and treatment of pathological gambling. *J Clin Psychol* 1996;57(Suppl 8):80.

Lesieur HR, Rosenthal RJ: Pathological gambling: A review of the literature. *J Gambl Stud* 1991;7:5.

Grant JE, Potenza MN, Hollander E, et al.: Multicenter investigation of the opioid antagonist nalmefene in the treatment of pathological gambling. *Am J Psychiatry* 2006;163(2):297–302.

TRICHOTILLOMANIA

ESSENTIALS OF DIAGNOSIS

DSM-IV-TR Diagnostic Criteria

A. Recurrent pulling out of one's hair resulting in noticeable hair loss.

B. An increasing sense of tension immediately before pulling out the hair or when attempting to resist the behavior.

C. Pleasure, gratification, or relief when puling out the hair.

D. The disturbance is not better accounted for by another mental disorder and is not due to a general medical condition (e.g., a dermatological condition).

E. The disturbance causes clinically significant distress or impairment in social, occupational, or other important areas of functioning.

(Reprinted, with permission, from *Diagnostic and Statistical Manual of Mental Disorders*, 4th edn. Text Revision. Washington DC: American Psychiatric Association, 2000.)

General Considerations

A. EPIDEMIOLOGY

The incidence of trichotillomania in the general population is unknown, but estimates have placed its prevalence in the United States as high as 8 million people. A recent survey of 2579 college freshmen indicated that 0.6% would have met criteria for trichotillomania at some point in their lifetimes. Trichotillomania appears to be more prevalent in females (although males may predominate in patients under age 6 years).

B. ETIOLOGY

The etiology of trichotillomania is unknown; however, different theories have been proposed about the pathogenesis of this complex disorder. Psychoanalytic theory views pathologic hair pulling as a manifestation of disrupted psychosexual development, often due to pathologic family constellations. In contrast, behavioral theory conceptualizes hair pulling as a learned habit similar to nail biting or thumb sucking. Recently, a biological theory has been postulated as several researchers have

proposed a serotonergic abnormality in trichotillomania and have suggested that the disorder may be a pathologic variant of species-typical grooming behaviors. Neuropsychological abnormalities, treatment response to some antidepressants, and frequent comorbidity with OCD have led to speculation regarding a neurobiological etiology, perhaps involving frontal lobe or basal ganglia dysfunction.

C. GENETICS

Family studies are suggestive of a genetic predisposition for trichotillomania but may reflect environmental learning and are inconclusive.

Clinical Findings

A. SIGNS & SYMPTOMS

Patients, particularly young ones, frequently deny that they pull their hair intentionally. Others typically describe pulling their hair when alone, but they may pull it openly in front of immediate family members. These episodes tend to occur during sedentary activities such as watching television, reading, studying, lying in bed, or talking on the telephone, and they may be more frequent during periods of stress. Patients may be unaware that they are pulling their hair until they are in the middle of an episode. Some patients report being in a trance-like state when they pull their hair. These episodes may last a few minutes or a few hours. Patients may pull a few hairs or many hairs per episode. Many patients do not feel pain when the hair is pulled; some patients report that it feels good.

Patients frequently engage in oral manipulation of the hair once it is pulled including nibbling on the roots or swallowing the hair. The later behavior can lead to a rare but serious complication, a trichobezoar (hair ball) in the gastrointestinal tract. The consequences of a trichobezoar can be life-threatening: obstruction, bleeding, perforation, pancreatitis, and obstructive jaundice.

Patients typically pull hair from their scalp, causing diffuse hair thinning or virtual baldness. The typical patient demonstrates patchy areas of alopecia without inflammation that spare the periphery. Many patients are adapt at hiding areas of hair loss by judicious hair styling, but may ultimately resort to hairpieces and wigs when the areas become too large or too numerous to hide. Patients may also pull hair from other parts of their body, including eyelashes, eyebrows, pubic region, or from face, trunk, extremities, or underarms.

B. PSYCHOLOGICAL TESTING & LABORATORY FINDINGS

Although psychological testing may not be useful in confirming a diagnosis of trichotillomania, a punch biopsy may be of some help in this regard. The biopsy results typically reveal increased catagen hairs along with melanin pigment casts and granules in the upper follicles and infundibulum.

Differential Diagnosis

According to DSM-IV-TR diagnostic criteria, a diagnosis of trichotillomania is not warranted if the condition can be better accounted for by another mental disorder or is due to a general medical condition. For example, if a patient has another significant Axis I psychiatric disorder (e.g., a condition with delusions or hallucinations) that might account for the hair pulling, then the diagnosis of trichotillomania would not be warranted. When patients deny that they pull their hair intentionally, dermatologic consultation may be required to rule out other causes of hair loss. Most notable among these conditions is alopecia areata, but tinea capitis, traction alopecia, androgenic alopecia, monilethrix, and other dermatologic conditions should also be considered. A punch biopsy may be indicated particularly when one of these disorders is suspected.

Treatment

An initial double-blind cross-over trial compared clomipramine to desipramine in 13 patients with trichotillomania screened to rule out neurologic disorder, mental retardation, primary affective disorder, psychosis, and OCD. Clomipramine produced improvement in clinical symptoms (33–53% reduction in severity scores) on each of three rating scales designed to assess trichotillomania symptomatology and clinical improvement; scores on two of the three scales were statistically significant. Two subsequent placebo-controlled, double-blind cross-over studies failed to show efficacy for fluoxetine.

Little rigorous research has been conducted concerning the differential effectiveness of treatments for trichotillomania. Clomipramine and behavior therapy probably constitute the current treatments of choice, but this conclusion is tempered by the paucity of treatment outcome studies. Habit renewal training is the most effective form of behavioral therapy. Trichotillomania occurs with variable levels of severity in terms of hair pulling and comorbid psychopathology. As a result, response to treatment is highly variable and rather unpredictable.

Complications/Adverse Outcomes of Treatment

Although hair loss is self-induced, patients are often particularly sensitive to comments about their appearance and go to great lengths to hide their disfigurement. These patients are often fearful that their shameful "secret" will be discovered and that they will be ridiculed in public. If the disorder is protracted, the patient's self-esteem can suffer drastically. Some individuals develop avoidant behavior and become socially withdrawn in order to avoid exposure. Trichobezoar is a rare complication. Little is known about the comorbidity of trichotillomania. Aside from the possibility that the disorder may be related to anxiety or mood disorder, there has been much speculation that it is a variant of OCD. Some research lends support to this hypothesis; however, the studies that failed to show efficacy for fluoxetine would argue against such a relationship.

Trichotillomania in preadolescents (particularly in those younger than 6 years of age) is thought to be associated with little psychopathology. In adolescent and adult patients, however, an association with other mental disorders has been demonstrated. In a study of 60 adult chronic hair-pullers (50 of whom met strict criteria for trichotillomania), only 18% did not demonstrate a current or past diagnosis of an Axis I psychiatric disorder other than trichotillomania. The lifetime prevalence of mood disorders was 65%, and 23% met criteria for current major depressive episode. Lifetime prevalence of anxiety disorders was 57%, and 10% demonstrated a current diagnosis of OCD and 5% a history of OCD. Another 18% endorsed present or past obsessions and compulsions not meeting the full criteria for OCD. Lifetime prevalence of panic disorder with or without agoraphobia was 18%, generalized anxiety disorder 27%, simple phobia 32%, eating disorder 20%, and substance abuse disorder 22%.

A smaller study that used standardized assessment techniques found that 45% of the trichotillomania patients studied met criteria for current or past major depression, 45% had generalized anxiety disorder, 10% had panic disorder, and 35% had alcohol or substance abuse. Unfortunately, patients with OCD were excluded from the study.

Adverse outcomes of treatment are limited to the usual side effects experienced with clomipramine or other antidepressants.

Although there might be adverse consequences of psychodynamic psychotherapy or a behavioral treatment approach, such adverse outcomes are generally thought to be rare and unpredictable.

Prognosis

The prognosis and course of illness generally can be predicted from the age at onset. Trichotillomania begins most often in childhood or young adolescence. Hair pulling in very young children is frequently mild and remits spontaneously. Patients with a later age at onset tend to have more severe symptoms that run a chronic course. These patients are thought to have a higher incidence of comorbid anxiety and depressive disorders.

Keuthen NJ, O'Sullivan RL, Goodchild P, et al.: Retrospective review of treatment outcome for 63 patients with trichotillomania. *Am J Psychiatry* 1998;155:560.

Minichiello WE, O'Sullivan RL, Osgood-Hynes D, et al.: Trichotillomania: Clinical aspects and treatment strategies. *Harv Rev Psychiatry* 1994;1:336.

■ IMPULSE-CONTROL DISORDERS NOT OTHERWISE SPECIFIED

This category is for disorders of impulse control (e.g., skin picking) that do not meet the criteria for any specific impulse control disorder or for another mental disorder having features involving impulse control described elsewhere in the DSM-IV-TR (e.g., substance dependence, a paraphilia).

McElroy SL, Hudson JI, Pope, HG Jr., et al.: The DSM-III-R impulse control disorders not elsewhere classified: Clinical characteristics and relationship to other psychiatric disorders. *Am J Psychiatry* 1992;149:318.

Grant TE, Levin L, Kim D, Polenta MN: Impulse control disorders in adult psychiatric inpatients. *Am J Psychiatry* 2000;162(11):2184–2188.

Adjustment Disorders

Ronald M. Salomon, MD, & Lucy Salomon, MD

The diagnosis of adjustment disorder would seem relatively straightforward, provided the clinician considers a wide range of stressors and other Axis I diagnoses, but it can present a number of pitfalls. Challenging diagnostic situations can arise when the stressor is subtle, for example, in a change of a previously stable life situation without any obvious stressor. The clinician should exclude any specified symptom complex that meets diagnostic criteria for another Axis I disorder even if it may be related to a specific stressor. Only the other Axis I diagnoses should be recorded if its criteria are met. However, if a discrete recent stressor has been identified, an adjustment disorder diagnosis may be more appropriate than, for example, anxiety disorder not otherwise specified or depressive disorder not otherwise specified.

The normal challenges of a life cycle are usually taken in stride with socially and culturally prescribed ranges of expected responses. However, commonly encountered events can disrupt an unusually crucial part of an individual's self-view (Table 29–1), and provoke symptoms outside of expected norms. Stressors leading to adjustment disorders are often termed "problems in coping." Among adolescents, adjustment disorders frequently emerge following disappointment(s) in relationships with family members or friends. Especially complex difficulties may be encountered among homosexual teens. In adult crime victims, early detection of adverse responses was shown to improve outcome.

Individuals of all ages may encounter adjustment disorders following psychiatric hospitalization, or after treatment for another, otherwise unrelated, psychiatric disorder. For example, after being hospitalized for severe obsessive–compulsive disorder (OCD), a patient may express a conduct disturbance that is otherwise atypical for OCD. It may then be appropriate to add the diagnosis of adjustment disorder. Exceptionally severe or extreme stressors may precipitate maladaptive responses. Retirement and aging can bring feelings of loss, depleted health and vigor, and fear of the future. If the symptoms and gravity of the stressor are less than those required for acute stress disorder, the diagnosis of adjustment disorder may be appropriate.

Diagnostic Validity

Lacking clear behavioral or emotional symptom criteria, the validity of the diagnostic label of adjustment disorder is sometimes questioned. Diagnostic recording allows communication with patients, insurers, and other clinicians. It assists in disease control by focusing research and guiding therapeutic selection. Contemporary knowledge of differential diagnosis, prognosis, course, and future risks may be illuminated by naming a disorder. Even though more studies are needed, the adjustment disorder diagnosis fulfills these expectations. The therapist will find criteria easily met, defensible, and practical. However, the adjustment disorder diagnosis must not become a conciliatory label aimed to avoid controversies. A diagnostic label cannot reconcile societal and individual standards of response to a stressor. Examples include the societal acceptance of requests for death, euthanasia, or "rational suicide;" the differentiation between biological and functional (purely psychological) disorders; or other similar contemporary issues. They must remain foci of controversy rather than indications of underlying psychopathology. When used with poor specificity or to evade controversy, the application of a diagnosis of adjustment disorder effectively undermines psychological and organic pathological correlates and diminishes the credibility of psychiatric nosology.

Clinical use of the diagnosis of adjustment disorder diagnosis may be less prevalent in other countries, even though the true prevalence is similar. The description of these symptoms in *International Classification of Diseases*, 10th edition, (ICD-10) largely overlaps with *Diagnostic and Statistical Manual of Mental Disorders*, fourth edition, Text Revision (DSM-IV-TR). In ICD-9, the term "adjustment reaction" was used for disturbances lasting weeks to months, and symptoms lasting hours to days were labeled "acute reaction to stress." This system required a retrospective view because duration cannot be established at the onset of symptoms. There are other possible reasons for intercultural differences in the use of the diagnosis of adjustment disorder. In some European countries, reimbursement for treatment does not cover extensive care for minor conditions. Culture-specific syndromes, such as the Latino *ataque de nervios*, apply to a variety of symptom presentations, many of which

Table 29–1. Commonly Observed Precipitants for Adjustment Disorders

College or university adjustments
Conscription into military service
Death of parent or companion
Natural disaster
New marriage or cohabitation
Pregnancy
Recent or anticipated combat
Recent or anticipated loss
Retirement
Terminal illness in self, parent, or companion

do not come to psychiatric attention. Appendix I of DSM-IV-TR is devoted to cultural syndromes. In addition, substance abuse and alcoholism are often comorbid in patients with adjustment disorders. Because thresholds for the diagnosis of substance abuse are interpreted differently from one country to the next, an international standardization of the diagnosis may be difficult to achieve.

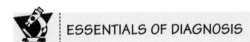 ESSENTIALS OF DIAGNOSIS

DSM-IV-TR Diagnostic Criteria

A. *The development of emotional or behavioral symptoms in response to an identifiable stressor(s) occurring within 3 months of the onset of the stressor(s).*

B. *These symptoms or behaviors are clinically significant as evidenced by either of the following:*

(1) marked distress that is in excess of what would be expected from exposure to the stressor

(2) significant impairment in social or occupational (academic) functioning

C. *The stress-related disturbance does not meet the criteria for another specific Axis I disorder and is not merely an exacerbation of a preexisting Axis I or Axis II disorder.*

D. *The symptoms do not represent bereavement.*

E. *Once the stressor (or its consequences) has terminated, the symptoms do not persist for more than an additional 6 months.*

(Reprinted, with permission, from *Diagnostic and Statistical Manual of Mental Disorders*, 4th edn. Text Revision. Washington DC: American Psychiatric Association, 2000.)

General Considerations

A. Epidemiology

In the United States, adjustment disorder diagnoses are quite common. Among psychiatric admissions, one estimate suggests that 7.1% of adults and 34.4% of adolescents had adjustment disorders. Among adults in France seen in general practice settings, a similar rate of 13.7% of those with psychological problems was observed. This was 1% of all patients consecutively seen with or without psychological problems. Many of these individuals merit substance abuse and conduct disorder diagnoses. Among university students receiving psychiatric assessments, a very high proportion was diagnosed as having adjustment disorders. Large population studies such as the Epidemiologic Catchment Area study have not assessed adjustment disorders because of a lack of sensitivity in the instrument used, that is, the Diagnostic Interview Schedule. Further studies are needed to better understand cultural, reimbursement, and records-confidentiality influences on true population rates and clinician utilization rates for the adjustment disorder diagnosis.

B. Etiology

Adjustment disorders appear to occur more often in individuals who are at risk for other psychiatric disorders, implying that etiologic factors may be shared. As in posttraumatic stress disorder (PTSD), neurobiological characteristics (e.g., elevated corticosteroid blood levels in response to stress) have been associated with the development of adjustment disorders.

A commonplace stressor may not be immediately clear, or it may be paradoxical. Adaptation difficulties in marriage, pregnancy, or childbirth can provoke feelings of guilt because the experience "should" be welcomed, not shunned. Natural preferences for lifestyle stability may be difficult to reconcile with goals requiring change. For example, a stably married individual unexpectedly confronted by parenthood faces role change, increased responsibility, and loss of freedom. Improved coping may result if the individual develops insight into a long-standing fear of being thrust into the role of single parent, as may have happened in his or her own family.

C. RISK FACTORS FOR THE GENERAL POPULATION

Major early risk factors include prior stress exposure, stressful early childhood experiences, and a history of mood or eating disorder. Family unity disruptions or frequent family relocations predispose children to adjustment disorders. The incidence of adjustment disorders is greater in children of divorced families following a subsequent, independent stressor. The death of a parent predisposes children to adjustment disorders. A high-suicide risk has been reported, especially after the loss of the father. Adjustments to living with the extended family (e.g., in-laws, step-parents) are additional predisposing factors. The outlet of symptom expression—be it depressed mood, conduct disturbance, or anxiety—may be determined by prior experience or biological constitution. Prior exposure to war, without meeting criteria for PTSD; (see Chapter 20), is a risk factor.

Factors that increase susceptibility in one situation can decrease it in another. For example, a high educational level can protect an individual who faces one stressor, but it can pose a risk factor for adjustment disorders in another context. Small-town life can predispose by providing too much shelter from stress yet limited support networks.

D. RISK FACTORS IN SPECIAL POPULATIONS

Immigrant populations are at risk for adjustment disorder. It is simplistic to regard the entire immigration process as a precipitant; rather, precipitant stressors should be identified separately. For example, among new immigrants to Israel, stress responses to missile attacks during the Gulf War could be predicted by the immigrants' adaptation prior to the attacks. Laotian Hmong immigrants in Minnesota were the focus of highly informative investigations that showed the need for studies of preventive intervention. Acculturation may be similar to other novel situations in many ways, but it also presents a large number of unique difficulties, all at the same time (Table 29–2). Any or all of these factors may require attention in treatment.

Among prison populations, adjustment disorder contributes heavily to suicide, which is frequently preceded by inmate-to-inmate conflict, disciplinary action, fear, physical illness, and the receipt of bad news. For a substantial number, the provision of mental health services within 3 days of the event was not sufficient to prevent suicide.

Chronic illness increases the need for medical contact and may constitute a major challenge to usual coping.

Table 29–2. Stressors Among Immigrant Populations[1]

Isolation from family and ethnic supports
Longing for familiar environments, all the while teaching hosts about the culture
Novel cognitive styles, task expectations
Reordering of developmental sequences, social expectations, and milestone assessments
Social and language challenges
Trauma of the journey for self and immigrant cohort
Unfamiliar time concepts and spatial orientation

[1] Reprinted, with permission, from Zipstein D, Hanegbi R, Taus R: An Israeli experience with Falasha refugees. In: Williams CL, Westermeyer J (editors): *Refugee Mental Health in Resettlement Countries.* Hemisphere, 1986.

Illness appears to be a precipitant rather than a predisposing factor. Adjustment disorders are not more prevalent among those with medical illnesses. On the other hand, should an adjustment disorder occur, it will often affect the clinical course of a somatic illness. The detection of adjustment disorder is remarkably poor, even on oncology services. It might improve with universal screening on admission. Early psychiatric consultation is associated with shorter length of stay. The course of asthma, chronic obstructive pulmonary disease, diabetes mellitus, end-stage renal disease, systemic lupus erythematosus, stroke, coronary artery disease, HIV/AIDS, chronic pain or headache, or cancer can be affected by the individual adjustment. Illness behavior, the give and take between patient and caregiver, and secondary gain all affect assessments of adjustment. The distinction between lifestyle versus coping style and then the setting of expectations for treatment compliance require skilled clinical judgment. For example, the asthmatic adolescent who rebels by skipping a scheduled inhaler dose does not need as rigid a guideline as one with "brittle" diabetes who skips insulin shots.

Also observed in the medical setting, complaints or lawsuits against physicians frequently result in adjustment disorder.

E. GENETICS

Other than a global suggestion that a family history of psychiatric disorder is a risk factor for adjustment disorder, little is known about genetic inheritance or determinants of this condition, not surprising given the potential heterogeneity of a disorder defined by stressor rather than symptom.

Clinical Findings

A. SIGNS & SYMPTOMS

In the primary care setting, distress reported by individuals, friends, or family members must be carefully assessed. Individual distress is variably reported and interpreted. Adjustment disorder diagnoses derive solely from expressed emotional and behavioral symptoms that may not be expressed clearly or may be minimized, masking distress. Symptoms themselves may contribute further to the individual's loss of confidence and disrupted sense of safety and well-being. Maladaptive behavior, fear, and uncertainty arise from losing control as customary defenses fail. The gravity of the stressor is interpreted in a context of past encounters with similar events and cannot be evaluated solely by the therapist's or society's standards. Stress must be evaluated in terms of the individual's subjective perception, giving perceptions a degree of validity. Adjustment will be facilitated when the therapist shows flexibility and accepts the individual's needs and distress. Careful listening and sensitivity are required because, with its paucity of somatic symptoms, individuals with adjustment disorder can masquerade as fairly stable, hiding high fragility and even suicidal risk. Clinicians may not appreciate the importance of a seemingly minor stressor, but they must give utmost respect to the individual, scheduling an interview that is long enough to understand the patient's subjective perceptions.

The distress experienced with adjustment disorder may include dissimilar emotions and behaviors. Such distress is beyond the expected response to the identified stressor (as can be identified on Axis IV). Suspicion of heightened severity, intensity (e.g., suicidal risk), or duration beyond that manageable by the primary care clinician indicates a need for professional psychiatric assessment and treatment, as does the failure of supportive intervention. Symptoms can be delayed, especially in women, and may change over time. Chronic stress can elicit chronic adjustment disorders. Clinical observation of the course of adjustment disorder reveals a strong association with suicidality, personality disorder, and drug use. A lack of suicide attempt in a first episode does not protect from future attempts. Completed suicide appears to be more frequent after an earlier attempt, or in the presence of personality disorder. The severity and lethality of suicide attempts often increase over time. Individuals with adjustment disorder are no less a suicide risk than those with major depressive disorder.

B. PSYCHOLOGICAL TESTING

Psychological testing (e.g., using the Minnesota Multiphasic Personality Inventory) has documented adjustment disorder risk factors (see "General Considerations" section earlier in this chapter) and comorbidity with type A personality style and other personality disorders (especially cluster B). Psychological testing can help the clinician to identify suicidal individuals, the degree of depression, and the level of hopelessness. Testing suggests that adjustment disorders are more likely in individuals with socially prescribed perfectionism—a tendency toward the exaggerated perception that others have inordinately high expectations of them. On neuropsychological testing, no impairment is observed in patients with adjustment disorders; impairments are found in patients with depression and other disorders.

C. LABORATORY FINDINGS

Pathophysiologic studies of adjustment disorders show little evidence of somatic involvement, although different mechanisms may be involved among different symptom groups. Patients with adjustment disorders resemble normal control subjects in most physiologic studies, with the nonspecific exception of elevated cortisol response to stress, decreased sensitivity to pain and decrease in delta sleep (e.g., following marital separation or soon after divorce). In comparison to patients with adjustment disorder and controls, individuals with major depressive episodes exhibit more physiologic markers of change (e.g., event-related potentials, decreased heart rate, and cortisol and ACTH suppression following dexamethasone).

D. NEUROIMAGING

Treatment-refractory adjustment disorder may be an indication for imaging with a goal of differential diagnosis. One study, for example, revealed temporal lobe epilepsy after the patient had had 2 years of failed psychotherapy for misdiagnosed adjustment disorder. In another case, Hallervorden–Spatz disease was revealed by MRI in a presentation initially presumed to be a severe adjustment disorder.

Course of Illness

The symptoms of adjustment disorder usually resolve quickly, with or without resolution of the stressors. Generally, inpatient stays are shorter for adjustment disorders than for depression, and improvement takes place during the first 3 weeks of admission. Long-term outcome surveys suggest cautious optimism in the prognosis for treated children and adults. Adjustment disorders may reoccur in children and adolescents with greater frequency than in adults. Clearly adolescence is fraught with many somatic changes and social adjustment requirements. For a first-time diagnosis, the majority of adults will fare very well after suicide risks abate. Adjustment disorders in children and adolescents predict future episodes of adjustment disorder but do not predict future affective episodes. Recovery is not greatly affected by comorbidity; the prognosis of an adjustment disorder alone is the same as for an adjustment disorder with co-morbid diagnoses.

Differential Diagnosis (Including Comorbid Conditions)

A. Relationship to Other Entities

When symptoms do not resolve quickly and therapy reveals other psychopathology or personality disorder, the initial diagnosis of adjustment disorder is often revised. When the diagnosis is uncertain, a provisional diagnosis accommodates individuals who may otherwise resist treatment because of preconceived expectations or fears of psychiatric labeling. Patients may accept more readily a temporary and minimal diagnosis, one that permits further assessment. It is often appealing to view a new patient as healthy, with a milder diagnosis. The temporary and relatively vague nature of "adjustment disorder" allows for changes in the primary admission diagnosis. Emergency room diagnoses of adjustment disorder are often changed to conduct disorder or substance abuse. This broadly inclusive diagnosis allows symptoms to be addressed while relatively mild, before a major syndrome develops, such as a major depressive episode. Given these properties, some vagueness and ambiguity are unavoidable.

B. Reactions to Stress

Normal grief reactions or bereavement may show cultural variability and be difficult to differentiate from adjustment disorders. Suicide risks may be present following bereavement, no matter which diagnosis is ultimately given. If the reaction to the stressor is within expectable and culturally acceptable norms, a nonpathologic reaction to stress should be recorded.

The diagnoses of Acute Stress Disorder and PTSD differ from adjustment disorder in accordance with the extreme severity of the stressor. Acute stress disorder follows an extreme stressor, more severe than stressors in adjustment disorder, and is associated with severe, specific symptoms (see Chapter 20). Acute stress disorder differs from PTSD in that the former remits after 1 month. The adjustment disorder diagnosis differs from both stress disorder diagnosis in that it is applicable to a wider range of presentations than these very specific and severe disorders. Furthermore, the emotional and behavioral responses in adjustment disorder are out of proportion to the stressor. In PTSD, the stressor leads to symptoms that are specific, severe, enduring, and handicapping (see Chapter 20).

In the impulse-control disorders, particularly intermittent explosive disorder, the precipitant stressor is minute in significance.

C. In Medical Settings

Adjustment disorder diagnoses may be applicable when the psychological stress of a physical illness causes psychiatric symptoms. For example, recently introduced implantable cardioverter defibrillators, have been associated with considerable psychological stress. In a way, adjustment disorder is the converse of the diagnosis of psychological factors affecting physical illness, in which a defensive coping style (e.g., repression) might worsen a systemic problem (e.g., peptic ulcer). It may be appropriate to give both diagnoses.

General medical conditions can cause psychiatric symptoms physiologically (and not psychologically as in adjustment disorder) and should be reported as such (e.g., mood disorder due to general medical condition). Individuals with chronic medical conditions may merit a second diagnosis of psychological factors affecting physical condition, reflecting both directions of the mind–body interaction.

D. Comorbidity

The symptoms of cluster B personality disorders often overlap with those of adjustment disorder, so that an adjustment disorder diagnosis is redundant in most cases. By definition, behavioral and emotional disturbances are excessive in personality disorders; these individuals would almost all be diagnosed as having adjustment disorder. However, according to DSM-IV-TR, adjustment disorder should be specified under circumstances in which the observed adjustment disorder is atypical for that personality disorder type.

Other, often comorbid, diagnoses that need to be assessed include substance or alcohol abuse or dependence, somatoform and factitious disorders, and psychosexual disorder.

Treatment

Individuals who have adjustment disorder will often appear relatively healthy compared to others with psychiatric disorders, sometimes deceptively so. Although successful treatment rates are greater than 70% in adjustment disorders, about one third of patients do not fare well. Timely intervention can prevent later, more serious problems and point to an underlying weaknesses that can be a focus of treatment. As with patients with almost any psychiatric diagnosis, and possibly especially so for adjustment disorders, effective referral for follow-up care has a greater impact on frequency of ER visits than the diagnosis itself.

According to the patient's capacities, different therapeutic techniques can be chosen that may challenge erroneous beliefs and help the patient develop a psychological understanding of the problem. Adjustment difficulties worsen in the face of novel stressors when strong

Table 29–3. Treatment of Adjustment Disorders

Treatment Approach	Primary Method	Secondary Methods
Behavioral	Psychodynamac psychotherapy	Cognitive-behavioral, interpersonal, or supportive psychotherapy
Pharmacologic	Antidepressant (e. g., sertraline, 25–75 mg daily)	*Only if patient has no history of alcohol abuse:* hypnotics (e. g., zolpidem, 5–10 mg at bedtime for 10 days) or anxiolytics (e. g., clonazepam, 0.5 mg at bedtime for 10 days)

emotions are harbored but are poorly recognized or awkwardly expressed. Early intervention is probably more important than a particular therapeutic approach. As in other disorders, the building of an alliance in the course of diagnostic interviewing is critical to the success of future therapy. The prudent interviewer will patiently avoid judgmental inflection and allow the individual wide latitude for emotional expression. An expeditious identification of the stressor in a permissive environment, allowing open expression of the fears and perceived helplessness, helps build an alliance focused on management of emotions resulting from the stressor. Table 29–3 summarizes psychotherapeutic and pharmacologic approaches to the treatment of adjustment disorders.

A. PSYCHOTHERAPEUTIC INTERVENTIONS

1. Psychoanalytic & psychodynamic approaches— There are numerous viewpoints from which psychological disturbances can be modeled in the effort to create treatment approaches. Historically, psychoanalytic and psychodynamic approaches have taken a leading role in the interpretation of behavior and emotion. In this view, individuals with adjustment disorder struggle unsuccessfully with effects of a stressor that most would manage more adaptively. Different forms of stress, difficult as they are to quantify, affect individuals in markedly different ways. Each individual has coping skills and mechanisms, some of which are used out of habit. Patients accommodate more easily to currently unmanageable stress when a history of similar difficulties is brought to light. Such a history can be examined in the transference, where perceptions of the relationship between the patient and the therapist are contaminated by attributes from prior relationships despite therapeutic neutrality. As therapy unfolds, the therapist becomes a target for misdirected anger and resentment, which is pointed out and examined as a

means of exploring the problem. The work of therapy is to help the patient recognize and understand the unconscious struggle that arises when the pursuit of pleasure and relief from irritants (the pleasure principle) stands in the way of grasping reality (the reality principle), as pursued within the transference relationship.

Trauma or loss may be perceived as an assault on a strongly developed self-perception, too noxious to be accessible to grief-coping mechanisms. Inflated perceptions of the self and unreasonable expectations of others are usually strongly guarded secrets. In analytic treatment, transference may contain the perception that the therapist is a harbinger of these demands. The overburdening super-ego (internal conscience) can then be revealed as the true aggressor, alleviating the exaggerated sense of the loss. Although the loss remains a reality, its importance then diminishes to a more acceptable level. Being able to project the cause of discomfort away from inappropriate self-blame onto a realistic outside agent will relieve the patient's sense of responsibility for the loss. For example, irrational guilt can arise over having been away on a trivial errand when a parent dies of cancer. The patient, after expressing a feeling that even the therapist blames him or her, is able to examine the need to accept cancer as the cause of loss.

Other, briefer types of therapies are encouraged in the current managed care environment. Although good comparison studies are lacking, certain individuals will probably do as well with briefer approaches. Psychodynamic, crisis-focused, time-limited psychotherapies require careful patient selection based on strong past interpersonal relationships, good premorbid functioning, and the absence of personality disorder. Some authors limit the use of these more confrontational techniques to situations in which there is a circumscribed focus, high motivation and capacity for insight, and a powerful degree of involvement in the interview. The time-structure of this technique is set out clearly at the beginning, with planned termination emphasized and treated as a new stressor to be managed throughout. Goals must be defined clearly. For example, self-deprecating patients may perceive parents as simultaneously irreproachable yet harsh and over-demanding. Such patients may have recurrent, severe (but brief) emotional disturbances after any confrontation with their bosses. They may benefit from a better understanding of emotional similarities to maladaptive but customary rules of relationships from childhood. Such therapy allows recognition of relationship patterns without focusing primarily on the transference. Brief dynamic therapy has been shown to be effective compared to other therapies.

2. Cognitive–behavioral approaches—Cognitive–behavioral therapy provides the patient with tools for the recognition and modification of maladaptive beliefs regarding the stressor and the patient's ability to cope with it. Adjustment disorders can be addressed in this way because the importance of the stressor is often unrealistically overestimated in the patient's perception. In a cognitive–behavioral therapy the patient learns to recognize connections between emotions and maladaptive perceptions or beliefs, and then learns to challenge those beliefs. Cognitive–behavioral therapy has demonstrated utility in occupational health. It has been successfully used in telepsychiatry for adjustment disorders in patients with cancer.

3. Interpersonal psychotherapy—Some clinicians prefer interpersonal therapy, especially for patients who have chronic medical illness or HIV infection. Many patients with severe medical illness shun intrapsychic introspection and benefit more from a psychoeducational approach. This is true for many adolescents. Discussion remains in a here-and-now about the sick role, which is a complicated balance of needs, independence, and becoming a more or less willing target for the caring of other individuals. Open discussions ensue about who does what for whom in which way, and about how the illness and its consequences will affect the self and others. The modeling of coping mechanisms can be helpful. Humor can be effective, if introduced carefully. Death and dying become more approachable. These individuals often benefit from a reframing of problems from an interpersonal perspective and welcome discussions of ways to change dysfunctional behavior. The therapist may be able to address issues inaccessible to a medical–surgical team. The patient may be reluctant to seem ungrateful to, and fearful of losing a relationship with, the primary care physician. Such a patient may regard the medical caregiver's purpose as one that provides medical treatment alone.

4. Supportive therapy—Supportive therapy is sometimes erroneously written off as hand-holding and comforting, whereas "real therapy" involves confrontation, analysis, and intellectualization. Supportive therapy should involve specific strategies and careful planning. Interventions have the goal of shoring up inadequate defense mechanisms. Intervention gently guides the individual to a verbalization of emotions regarding the stress. Communication, relaxation, and anger control (e.g., "counting to 10") are emphasized. In an acute crisis involving loss, or in medical settings where new information brings acute distress, a skilled supportive intervention can be eminently appropriate and effective.

5. Family therapy—Family therapy is often recommended. It can be among the most effective approaches to alleviating adjustment disorder by identifying the role the family plays in promoting a maladaptive coping response. However, some families are ill-prepared to participate in treatment for the "identified" patient. In family sessions, lines of support can be examined and reestablished by skillful work to minimize distortions, blame, and isolation.

B. Psychopharmacologic Interventions

Pharmacotherapy is often used to treat adjustment disorders. It may be useful when specific symptoms merit a medication trial. Drug selection is based on symptoms; for example, a short course of a benzodiazepine for adjustment disorder with anxious mood. The treatment goal is rapid symptom relief and prevention of a chronic problem, such as generalized anxiety disorder. Antidepressants are used frequently, even more frequently now with the advent of direct-to-consumer marketing (Samuelian, 1994). Selective serotonin reuptake inhibitors are generally well-tolerated and appear to be beneficial for some patients, but double-blind, placebo-controlled studies are lacking. They are probably under-prescribed for adolescents, males, those on welfare, and those in rural areas. Short-term trials of benzodiazepines and alprazolam are often prescribed, for example, for adjustment disorder involving anticipatory anxiety prior to chemotherapy. Hypnotics, such as zolpidem, should be considered for short-term use. The use of herbal preparations, such as St. John's Wort, merits further study.

C. Nontraditional Approaches

In association with other treatments, nontraditional approaches can provide added benefit. Relaxation techniques, yoga, massage, and progressive muscle relaxation have been reported as helpful. Guided exposure or guided imagery can help with anticipatory stressors. Acupuncture has been used to treat adjustment disorders; but the results are unclear. Sleep deprivation, effective in treating endogenous and reactive depressions, may be useful in treating adjustment disorders.

The financing of treatment for adjustment disorders will depend increasingly on the recognition that treatment improves outcome and quality of life, prevents more serious reactions from developing, and reduces the risk of recurrences. There is little to be gained by waiting for the advent of disorders that are difficult to treat. Adjustment disorder should be treated actively, assuring restored premorbid functioning. Even so, brief therapies will need to be used. To justify treatment, third-party payers typically require information about symptoms that indicate risk, treatment goals, therapeutic methods, and outcome monitoring.

Complications/Adverse Outcomes of Treatment

Recovery from adjustment disorders can be complicated by a variety of poor outcomes. It is all too easy to overlook risk factors in the clinical setting. For example, persistent denial of the importance of a stressor may result in masked or displaced anger with a strong risk of suicidality. In the patient's distorted view, denial will sometimes justify deceit in order to conceal issues such as physical safety and suicidality. Highly ambivalent, mixed emotional struggles (e.g., terminal illness in an unfaithful spouse, relationship problems among adolescents) require the clinician to be extra attentive and cautious. Among adolescents with adjustment disorder, suicidal ideation, threat, or attempt are associated with previous psychiatric treatment, poor psychosocial functioning, suicide as a stressor, dysphoric mood, and psychomotor restlessness. Notably, the suicidal process—evolution of ideation to completion—is short and rapid in adjustment disorder, and often comes with little warning in the form of prior emotional or behavioral problems. Adolescents in urban areas who were diagnosed as having adjustment disorder made more serious suicidal attempts than those with other disorders. Assessing suicide risk in the presence of adjustment disorder is extremely important.

In the presence of a comorbid personality disorder, adjustment disorder episodes frequently reoccur, to the point where diagnosing them separately is not necessary. However, it is still necessary to treat adjustment disorder in this common context. According to one study, 15% of individuals with adjustment disorder also meet criteria for one of the cluster B personality disorders (antisocial, histrionic, borderline, or narcissistic personality disorders). A personality disorder diagnosis predicts poor acute outcome and the likelihood of chronic impairment in social support among individuals with an adjustment disorder.

Comorbid substance abuse is common in individuals with a primary diagnosis of adjustment disorder. Although, alcoholism may "protect" people from stress (see discussion on cultural norms, earlier in this chapter), it clearly diminishes coping skills, promotes social isolation, and adds a suicide risk factor.

Some adverse outcomes are iatrogenic. Although helpful for some patients, the risks of somatic treatment must be explained carefully. Medications carry side effects and other risks (e.g., suicide by overdose of tricyclic antidepressants), and for these disorders the potential for benefit has not been demonstrated against placebo. Hypomanic or manic switches occur occasionally even with modern antidepressants, and individual risk for this response cannot be predicted reliably. Movement disorder has been reported after single doses of neuroleptics. Benzodiazepines may impair judgment and pose risks of abuse and dependence.

Prognosis

Although short-term prognosis is quite good in adjustment disorder, there may be an increased frequency of Axis I or Axis II diagnoses in the longer term. Further research is needed to identify individual prognostic factors and appropriate treatments.

Al-Ansari A, Matar AM: Recent stressful life events among Bahraini adolescents with adjustment disorder. *Adolescence* 1993;28:339.

Chess S, Thomas A: *Origins and Evolution of Behavior Disorders.* New York: Brunner/Mazel, 1984.

Greenberg WM, Rosenfeld DN, Ortega EA: Adjustment disorder as an admission diagnosis. *Am J Psychiatry* 1995;152:459.

Kovacs M, Gatsonis C, Pollock M, Parrone PL: A controlled prospective study of DSM-III adjustment disorder in childhood. Short-term prognosis and long-term predictive validity. *Arch Gen Psychiatry* 1994;51:535.

Greenberg WM, Rosenfeld DN, Ortega EA: Adjustment disorder as an admission diagnosis. *Am J Psychiatry* 1995;152:459.

Gur S, Hermesh H, Laufer N, Gogol M, Gross-Isseroff R: Adjustment disorder: A review of diagnostic pitfalls. *Isr Med Assoc J* 2005;7(11):726–731.

Leigh H: Physical factors affecting psychiatric condition. *Gen Hosp Psychiatry* 1993;15:155.

Newcorn JH, Strain J: Adjustment disorder in children and adolescents. *J Am Acad Child Adolesc Psychiatry* 1992;31:318.

Rickel AU, Allen L: *Preventing Maladjustment from Infancy Through Adolescence.* Thousand Oaks, CA: Sage, 1987.

Schatzberg AF: Anxiety and adjustment disorder: A treatment approach. *J Clin Psychiatry* 1990;51(Suppl 11):20.

Semaan W, Hergueta T, Bloch J, Charpak Y, Duburcq A, Le Guern ME, Alquier C, Rouillon F: Cross-sectional study of the prevalence of adjustment disorder with anxiety in general practice. (French) *Encephale* 2001;27:238.

Speer DC: Can treatment research inform decision makers? Nonexperimental method issues and examples among older outpatients. *J Consult Clin Psychol* 1994;62:560.

Strain J, Hammer JS, Huertas D, Lam HT, Fulop G: The problem of coping as a reason for psychiatric consultation. *Gen Hosp Psychiatry* 1993;15:1.

Oquendo MA: Differential diagnosis of *ataque de nervios. Am J Orthopsychiatry* 1995;65:60.

World Health Organization: *International Statistical Classification of Diseases and Related Health Problems,* 10th rev. World Health Organization, 1992.

Personality Disorders

30

David Janowsky, MD

■ PERSONALITY DISORDERS IN GENERAL

 ESSENTIALS OF DIAGNOSIS

DSM-IV-TR Diagnostic Criteria

A. An enduring pattern of inner experience and behavior that deviates markedly from the expectations of the individual's culture. This pattern is manifested in two (or more) of the following areas:

    (1) cognition (i.e., ways of perceiving and interpreting self, other people, and events)

    (2) affectivity (i.e., the range, intensity, lability, and appropriateness of emotional response)

    (3) interpersonal functioning

    (4) impulse control

B. The enduring pattern is inflexible and pervasive across a broad range of personal and social situations.

C. The enduring pattern leads to clinically significant distress or impairment in social, occupational, or other important areas of functioning.

D. The pattern is stable and of long duration and its onset can be traced back at least to adolescence or early adulthood.

E. The enduring pattern is not better accounted for as a manifestation of another mental disorder.

F. The enduring pattern is not due to the direct physiological effects of a substance (e.g., a drug of abuse, a medication) or a general medical condition (e.g., head trauma).

(Reprinted, with permission, from the *Diagnostic and Statistical Manual of Mental Disorders*. 4th edn. Text Revision. Washington, DC: American Psychiatric Association, 2000.)

General Considerations

A. EPIDEMIOLOGY

The prevalence of diagnosable personality disorders in the general population has been estimated at 10–20%. This rate is much higher in mental health treatment settings, with as many as 50% of psychiatric patients meeting criteria for one or more personality disorders.

Some personality disorders are diagnosed more frequently in men, and some are more prevalent in women. Thus, for example, borderline personality disorder appears to be more common in women. Antisocial personality disorder predominates in men.

B. ETIOLOGY

The causes of personality disorders are not well understood. As with essentially every other type of psychiatric disorder, they probably involve various combinations of biologic, temperamental, and social etiologies. Historically, classic psychoanalytic theory suggests that personality disorders occur when a person fails to progress through the usual stages of psychosexual development. Fixation at the oral stage (i.e., the infantile stage) is considered to cause a personality characterized by demanding and dependent behavior, the current parallel being the dependent personality disorder. Fixation at the anal stage (i.e., the stage of toilet training) is thought to lead to obsessionality, rigidity, and emotional aloofness. The current diagnostic parallel is obsessive–compulsive personality disorder. Fixation at the phallic stage (early childhood) is thought to lead to shallowness and difficulty sustaining intimate relationships, the diagnostic parallel being histrionic personality disorder.

Related to the above, developmental and environmental problems have been a major focus of interest to scholars of personality. This is in part because onset occurs early in life and is frequently associated with real and perceived disruptive childhood experiences. Of particular interest has been the extremely high rate of reported neglect and childhood sexual, physical, or emotional abuse in patients with certain personality disorders, especially borderline personality disorder and histrionic personality disorder.

C. GENETICS

Genetic factors are often influential in the etiology of personality disorders. For example, family, twin, and adoption studies suggest that schizotypal personality disorder is linked to a family history of schizophrenia. Similar studies have delineated genetic factors related to antisocial and borderline disorders.

Clinical Findings

A. SIGNS & SYMPTOMS

In the United States of America, Personality disorders are coded on Axis II of the American Psychiatric Association's *Diagnostic and Statistical Manual of Mental Disorders,* Fourth Edition, Text Revision (DSM-IV-TR), so as to separate them from the major mental disorders (i.e., bipolar disorder, schizophrenia, panic disorder), which are coded on Axis I. Both Axis I and Axis II disorders can and frequently do coexist.

Personality disorders as currently described in DSM-IV-TR are described as "an enduring manifestation of inner experience and behavior that deviates markedly from the expectations of the individual's culture, is pervasive and inflexible, has an onset in adulthood, is stable over time, and leads to distress or impairment." DSM-IV-TR Personality disorders are representative of long-term functioning and are not limited to episodes of illness.

For purposes of DSM-IV-TR classification, there are 10 personality disorders and these are grouped into three major categories or clusters. Cluster A (paranoid, schizoid and schizotypal) is composed of individuals who are generally odd or eccentric. They may have abnormal cognitions, such as being overly suspicious or exhibiting peculiar expressions or odd speech. Cluster B personality disorders (antisocial, borderline, histrionic, and narcissistic) consist of individuals with dramatic, acting-out behaviors. Cluster C disorders (avoidant, dependent, obsessive–compulsive) include those personality disorders generally marked by prominent anxiety and avoidance of novelty.

Co-occurrence of several personality disorders in a given individual within a given cluster is common, as is co-occurrence across clusters. Furthermore, a patient meeting criteria for a particular personality disorder will also often exhibit some features of other disorders within the same cluster, as well as across clusters. In addition to the 10 personality disorders, DSM-IV-TR includes criteria for two additional disorders, these being the passive–aggressive and the depressive personality disorder. There is also a category entitled personality disorders, not otherwise specified.

As a group, the personality disorders are one of the most difficult and complicated emotional disorders to diagnose and to treat. Diagnosis is difficult in part because the disorders are often difficult to differentiate from each other, due to overlapping symptoms, and because the boundary between normality and psychopathology for each diagnosis is not distinct. Treatment of personality disorders is also difficult. Almost by definition, they are well-established behaviors and/or ways of thinking that are not perceived by the afflicted individual as abnormal or aberrant.

Manifestations of personality disorders are frequently evident early in life. Some behaviors in children such as aggressiveness and stealing predict later personality problems, such as antisocial personality disorder. However, other behaviors, such as childhood social isolation and shyness seem to be of little value in predicting later cluster C disorders.

B. PSYCHOLOGICAL TESTING

A number of psychological tests have been developed to assess personality traits and disorders. Of particular prominence are the Millon Clinical Multiaxial Inventory (MCMI), and the Minnesota Multiphasic Personality Inventory (MMPI).

The MCMI is a self-administered, true-false inventory that provides information on personality style, significant personality patterns and associated clinical disorders. The inventory includes 344 items, grouped into 22 overlapping scales. These consist of 4 validity scales, 11 clinical scales, 5 treatment issue scales, and 2 interpersonal scales. Unlike the MCMI, the Minnesota Multiphasic Personality Inventory was developed to aid in the diagnosis of mental disorders. However, it is often used to describe individuals more globally. It consists of over 500 items and includes nine basic clinical scales (i.e., hypochondrias, depression, hysteria, psychopathic deviance, masculinity/femininity, paranoia, anxiety, schizophrenia, and mania). Validity scales are also included. Other assessment instruments have been developed, as have various semistructured interview protocols such as the Structured Clinical Interview for DSM-IV-TR, which can be used to diagnose personality disorders.

C. LABORATORY FINDINGS

There are no proven biological markers that are highly specific for the personality disorders. However, certain associations have been reported. For example, low platelet monoamine oxidase activity has been found in patients who have schizotypal personality disorder. Also, low 5-hydroxyindoleacetic acid is found in the cerebrospinal fluid of patients who have borderline personality disorder associated with suicide attempts and aggressive behavior.

Hypersensitivity to an acetylcholine-enhancing drug is characteristic of borderline personality disorder patients who have mood lability. In addition, abnormal dexamethasone suppression tests are less likely to be found in personality disorder patients with depression than in patients with pure major depressive disorder. More recently, certain genetic profiles are being defined for specific personality disorders.

Differential & Coexisting Diagnoses

Personality disorders frequently are associated with Axis I disorders of nearly all types. Mood, anxiety, and substance-abuse disorders are the most common correlates. Conversely, it has been reported that over 50% of patients hospitalized with major depressive disorder also have a diagnosable personality disorder. In many cases a personality disorder is thought to predispose the individual to the recurrence and greater intensity of an Axis I disorder, thus indicating a poorer prognosis. Also, the presence of an Axis I diagnosis can complicate the process of establishing a personality disorder diagnosis, since common symptoms of personality disorders (e.g., interpersonal withdrawal or dependency) can be influenced by mood state. Furthermore, the personality disorders are not mutually exclusive. The majority of patients meeting criteria for one personality disorder will also meet criteria for other personality disorders.

Dimensional Considerations

Although useful for purposes of communication between professionals, the categorical classification of personality disorders presented in the DSM-IV-TR is considered by many professionals to be deeply flawed, and possibly irrelevant.

Thus, although DSM-IV-TR offers clinical criteria-based personality disorder subtypes, many professionals believe that these are artificial constructs.

The idea that mental illness generally and personality disorder specifically can be accurately defined categorically is currently in dispute. The arbitrariness of having a specific set and number of characteristics necessary to make a diagnosis may be too exclusive, or not exclusive enough. Similarly, the question of whether certain personality disorders such as schizotypal, avoidant, and borderline personality disorders are actually a part of a continuum of Axis I disorders remains very much an open and controversial question. How one draws the line between being normal and having a pathologic condition is also a question not erased by arbitrarily classifying disorders, based on reaching a threshold number of symptoms.

Considering personality and personality disorders to be a grouping of symptoms of core traits or temperaments, measured on a continuum, represents a viable or at least an additional alternative to the current categorical diagnostic standards of DSM-IV-TR. Indeed, such a strategy is the norm in normal personality research, where dimensional evaluations show greater reliability and correlations than do categoric ones.

There are several ways to consider a dimensional approach to diagnoses. One is to measure the actual characteristics of a given personality diagnosis (i.e., rating each component as not present to highly present) and then deriving a total score. Another approach has been to show the relative presence of each symptom, as related to the others, or to present a relative profile on each personality disorder (i.e., high schizoid, low paranoid, low borderline, high avoidant, etc.). Alternatively, core personality traits or temperament variables can be measured, and the various characteristics related to specific personality disorders.

Many different scales have been developed to classify trait/temperament variables. One popular scale is the NEO-PI or five-factor model of personality. Here, personality is divided into five major components, each with a set of subordinate facets. The five major components are: neuroticism (the predisposition to experience anxiety, depression, and hostility), extroversion (the tendency to be outgoing or gregarious as opposed to shy), openness to experience, agreeableness, and conscientiousness.

Another frequently utilized scale is the Cloninger Tridimensional Personality Questionnaire. This Questionnaire divides into four major components: novelty seeking, harm avoidance, reward dependence, and persistence. Other scales are designed to measure impulsiveness and the tendency to engage in dangerous activities.

There is evidence that certain personality patterns and traits, especially in the extreme, are associated with specific categorically defined personality disorders and psychopathology.

However, some personality traits change over time. Thus, with aging, individuals become less extroverted, more agreeable and show less neuroticism and are more conscientious. Over time, individuals become less emotional and better socialized. Although there are differences in the expression of traits between different personality diagnoses, the trait differences between diagnoses are considerably less than those between individuals who have and do not have a personality disorder.

Treatment

Personality disorders are difficult to treat, in part because they often do not cause personal distress. Because the personality disorders are experienced as a fundamental part of the individual, rather than as a distressing symptom, the affected individual often has limited insight into the nature of his or her problems. Therefore, people with personality disorders are likely to present for treatment only during times of crisis or with the resurgence of major psychiatric symptoms such as depression or anxiety, or when others such as family or coworkers are disturbed by their behavior.

Patients with personality disorders tend to be challenging to their therapists. They are often angry, manipulative, demanding, or defensive. However, improvement in personality disorders often occurs over time.

Specific psychotherapy techniques, either in individual or group settings, including behavioral, cognitive, or interpersonal therapies may be effective. Here, the alliance and collaboration between therapist and patient or patient and group appears to be a critical component of successful treatment.

Prognosis

Personality disorders in general are highly associated with disability in the general population, and generally, when coexistent, worsen the prognosis and relapse rates of Axis I disorders.

Although limited evidence confirms that certain personality disorder diagnoses are stable over time, it is not clear that this is a valid assumption overall. Indeed, several personality disorders (i.e., borderline personality disorder, antisocial personality disorder) are likely to improve over time, or change from one disorder to another, with some features of a disorder replaced by others as the patient ages. Thus, personality disorders characterized by impulsivity and anger, such as borderline and antisocial personality disorders tend to show some reduction in these features as the individual reaches middle age.

■ INDIVIDUAL PERSONALITY DISORDERS

CLUSTER A PERSONALITY DISORDERS

PARANOID PERSONALITY DISORDER

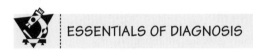

ESSENTIALS OF DIAGNOSIS

DSM-IV-TR Diagnostic Criteria

A. *A pervasive distrust and suspiciousness of others such that their motives are interpreted as malevolent, beginning by early adulthood and present*

in a variety of contexts, as indicated by four (or more) of the following:

(1) *suspects, without sufficient basis, that others are exploiting, harming, or deceiving him or her*

(2) *is preoccupied with unjustified doubts about the loyalty or trustworthiness of friends or associates*

(3) *is reluctant to confide in others because of unwarranted fear that the information will be used maliciously against him or her*

(4) *reads hidden demeaning or threatening meanings into benign remarks or events*

(5) *persistently bears grudges, i.e., is unforgiving of insults, injuries, or slights*

(6) *perceives attacks on his or her character or reputation that are not apparent to others and is quick to react angrily or to counterattack*

(7) *has recurrent suspicions, without justification, regarding fidelity of spouse or sexual partner*

B. *Does not occur exclusively during the course of schizophrenia, a mood disorder with psychotic features, or another psychotic disorder and is not due to the direct physiological effects of a general medical condition.*

(Reprinted, with permission, from the *Diagnostic and Statistical Manual of Mental Disorders.* 4th edn. Text Revision. Washington, DC: American Psychiatric Association, 2000.)

General Considerations

A. EPIDEMIOLOGY

The prevalence of paranoid personality disorder has been estimated at 0.5–4.5% of the general population. It is relatively common in clinical settings, particularly among psychiatric inpatients. Individuals with a paranoid personality disorder typically rarely seek treatment on their own. They are usually referred by family members, coworkers or employers. The disorder appears to be slightly more common in women than in men.

B. ETIOLOGY

Although the etiology of paranoid personality disorder is uncertain, both genetic and environmental aspects are thought to play an etiologic role. For example, the risk of developing the disorder is somewhat enhanced in families with a history of schizophrenia and delusional disorders.

Environmentally, the risk for this disorder appears to be increased if the individual's parents exhibited irrational outbursts of anger, and where the frequent fear the individual experienced as a child is projected onto others later in life.

C. GENETICS

Although the finding is not a strong one, paranoid personality disorder patients do have more biological relatives with schizophrenia than with controls. The link between paranoid personality disorder and schizoid personality disorder is quite weak, although measurable.

There is some evidence that paranoid personality disorder is more common among individuals with a family history of schizophrenia or delusional disorder, persecutory type, compared to controls. However, this is not a particularly strong finding.

Clinical Findings

A. SIGNS & SYMPTOMS

The cardinal feature of paranoid personality disorder is the presence of generalized distrust or suspiciousness. Individuals feel that they have been treated unfairly, are resentful of this mistreatment, and bear long-lasting grudges against those who have slighted them. They place a high premium on autonomy and react in a hostile manner to others who seek to control them and they can be violent. These patients are often unsuccessful in intimate relationships because of their suspiciousness and aloofness.

When interviewed, patients with a paranoid personality disorder are formal, businesslike, skeptical, and mistrustful, and exhibit poor or fixated eye contact. They consistently project blame for their difficulties onto others, externalizing their own emotions while paying keen attention to the emotions and attitudes of others. Underlying their formal and at times moralistic presentation is considerable hostility and resentment.

Differential Diagnosis

There is considerable overlap between patients with paranoid personality disorder, patients with schizoid personality disorder, and those with schizotypal personality disorder. Of those patients with schizoid personality disorder, 47% were also diagnosed as also having a paranoid personality disorder. In addition, the disorder often appears in combination with schizotypal personality disorder, although this in part is because of the shared feature of paranoid ideation. Other common personality disorder comorbidities include the borderline and narcissistic personality disorders. When paranoid personality disorder is comorbid with narcissistic personality disorder, the paranoid features serve to justify the patient's delusions of persecution, with the obstructions of others seen as evidence of the merit of the patient's overvalued ideas. Paranoid personality disorder is similar to several Axis I disorders. These include delusional disorder—persecutory type, schizophrenia, and paranoid type. Paranoid personality disorder is distinguished from the above Axis I disorders by the absence of delusions, hallucinations, and defective reality testing, although differentiation is not always easy.

Treatment

A. PSYCHOPHARMACOLOGIC INTERVENTIONS

There is little available data to suggest that pharmacologic interventions are of significant benefit in paranoid personality afflicted individuals. Although not demonstrated by controlled clinical trials, low-dose antipsychotic medications may decrease the patient's paranoia and anxiety. Under situations of stress, some patients decompensate, and the paranoid ideation reaches delusional proportions. In such cases antipsychotic medication can be of obvious benefit.

B. PSYCHOTHERAPEUTIC INTERVENTIONS

1. **Group/marital interventions**—Group therapy can be quite difficult for patients with paranoid personality disorder. Their lack of basic trust and their suspiciousness often prevent them from being integrated fully into groups. Their wariness and suspiciousness may become self-fulfilling, as their hostility makes other members uncomfortable and rejecting. Paranoid personality disorder patients sometimes present for treatment as couples or as a family. Working with them in this context is also difficult, since such patients often feel that the therapist and family members are working against them.

2. **Individual psychotherapies**—Patients with paranoid personality disorder represent a unique challenge to the psychotherapist. They lack trust, and thus, rarely enter treatment unless there is another coexisting emotional disorder, such as a mood or anxiety disorder, or coercion from a family member or employee. They have difficulty relinquishing control, and may not tolerate the ambiguity associated with the less directive interventions. Among behavioral techniques used, social skills role playing, particularly involving appropriate expression of assertiveness has been reported. No therapeutic techniques have actually been proven efficacious in treating paranoid personality disorder patients. However, clinical wisdom suggests that cognitive techniques that focus on the patient's overgeneralizations (e.g., "That person didn't talk to me; therefore, he hates me.") and their propensity to dichotomize the social world into trustworthy and hostile are useful. With psychodynamic and interpersonal approaches, interpretations are used sparingly, and

treatment focuses on the gradual recognition of the origins and negative consequences of the patient's mistrust.

Prognosis

Little is known about the long-term outcome of paranoid personality disorder. Although the disorder is difficult to treat, patients generally appear to have a greater adaptive capacity than do those who have personality disorders associated with severe social detachment. However, under stress, patients with paranoid personality disorder usually withdraw and avoid interpersonal attachments, thus perpetuating their mistrust, and they may become overtly psychotic.

SCHIZOID PERSONALITY DISORDER

 ESSENTIALS OF DIAGNOSIS

DSM-IV-TR Diagnostic Criteria

A. *A pervasive pattern of detachment from social relationships and a restricted range of expression of emotions in interpersonal settings, beginning by early adulthood and present in a variety of contexts, as indicated by four (or more) of the following:*

(1) neither desires nor enjoys close relationships, including being part of a family

(2) almost always chooses solitary activities

(3) has little, if any, interest in having sexual experiences with another person

(4) takes pleasure in few, if any, activities

(5) lacks close friends or confidants other than first-degree relatives

(6) appears indifferent to the praise or criticism of others

(7) shows emotional coldness, detachment, or flattened affectivity

B. *Does not occur exclusively during the course of schizophrenia, a mood disorder with psychotic features, another psychotic disorder, or a pervasive developmental disorder and is not due to the direct physiological effects of a general medical condition.*

(Reprinted, with permission, from the *Diagnostic and Statistical Manual of Mental Disorders.* 4th edn. Text Revision. Washington, DC: American Psychiatric Association, 2000.)

General Considerations

A. EPIDEMIOLOGY

Estimates of the prevalence of schizoid personality disorder in the general population vary with the criteria used, ranging from 0.5–7% and individuals with this disorder are relatively uncommon in clinical settings. The disorder occurs more often in men than in women and may be more severe in men. The general withdrawal of patients with schizoid personality disorder means that they rarely disturb others, and in part this accounts for their rare appearance in treatment settings.

B. ETIOLOGY

The diagnosis of schizoid personality disorder has become restricted to people with a profound defect in the ability to form personal relationships and to respond to others in a meaningful way.

The causes of schizoid personality disorder are not well understood. Genetic factors are suspected, and some reports suggest that patients with this disorder often come from environments that are deficient in emotional nurturing. There is also evidence that famine may be associated with schizoid personality disorder, as it appears to be with schizophrenia.

C. GENETICS

The symptoms of schizoid personality disorder resemble the negative symptoms of schizophrenia. Thus, an increased prevalence of schizoid personality disorder among individuals with a family history of schizophrenia might be expected.

However, schizoid personality disorder does not appear to have a strong genetic relationship to schizophrenia. Finally, many of the features of Asperger syndrome also resemble schizoid personality disorder, and the possibility of a relationship to autism exists.

Clinical Findings

A. SIGNS & SYMPTOMS

In the case of the schizoid personality, the individual is not necessarily distressed or disturbing of others. Thus, the life history of patients with schizoid personality disorder is typically characterized by a preference for solitary pursuits. These individuals may have none or only a few intimate relationships, and show little apparent interest in people, outside of internal fantasy. Social detachment and restricted emotional expressivity, i.e., affective constriction, make these patients appear aloof, distant, and difficult to engage. Schizoid personality patients are more likely to demonstrate interest when describing abstract pursuits that require no emotional involvement. Although reality testing is generally intact, schizoid personality disorder patients' lack of social contact precludes the correction of their somewhat idiosyncratic interpretations of social transactions.

Differential Diagnosis

Patients with schizoid personality disorder resemble individuals with avoidant personality disorder (to be described later). They can be distinguished from those with avoidant personality disorder by their indifference to others. They also may be confused with patients with schizotypal personality disorder. In contrast to schizotypal personality disorder, the schizoid personality disorder patient is affectively flat and unresponsive, rather than behaviorally eccentric, with odd thoughts, although both disorders often co-occur. Finally, the schizoid personality disorder patient may share a number of symptoms in common with patients with Asperger syndrome.

Treatment

A. Psychopharmacologic Interventions

Little is known about the effective pharmacologic treatment of schizoid personality disorder. Thus far, effective pharmacotherapy has not been demonstrated for the disorder as such, although associated anxiety and depression when it occurs may be treated with antidepressant and other medications.

B. Psychotherapeutic Interventions

1. Group/family techniques—Often individuals with schizoid personality disorder come to treatment at the request of family members. In some cases, family-based interventions may be helpful in clarifying for the patient the family's expectations, and perhaps in addressing any intolerance and invasiveness on the part of the family that could be worsening the patient's withdrawal.

Group therapy can also be helpful as a source of directed feedback from others that would otherwise be missed or ignored. Such a setting can also allow for the modeling and acquisition of needed social skills. However, the initial participation of the schizoid personality disorder patient will invariably be minimal, and the therapist may sometimes need to act to prevent the patient from being the hostile target of other group members. However, as with so many therapies, the above assertions are based on clinical wisdom, and have not been proven experimentally.

2. Individual psychotherapies—Psychotherapeutic interventions tend to be difficult to accomplish in the patient with schizoid personality disorder. Such patients are often not psychologically minded and typically experience little perceived distress. The tendency of these patients to intellectualize and distance themselves from emotional experience can also restrict the impact of treatment.

The therapeutic alliance is often impeded by the low value that these individuals place on relationships. However, clinical wisdom suggests that more cognitively based treatment approaches may receive greater initial acceptance. Distorted expectancies and perceptions about the importance and usefulness of relationships with others can be explored.

Prognosis

Patients with schizoid personality disorder display problems at an earlier age, i.e., in early childhood, than do patients with other personality disorders. Social disinterest tends to self-perpetuate isolation, as does flattened affect. However, relative to patients with other personality disorders, those with schizoid personality disorder are less likely to experience anxiety or depression, particularly if they are not in social, educational, or occupational situations that tax their limited social skills. Also, the number of individuals with schizoid personality disorder who are not in mental health care may be large, and such individuals may be relatively well-adjusted to their lives.

SCHIZOTYPAL PERSONALITY DISORDER

 ESSENTIALS OF DIAGNOSIS

DSM-IV-TR Diagnostic Criteria

A. A pervasive pattern of social and interpersonal deficits marked by acute discomfort with, and reduced capacity for, close relationships, as well as by cognitive or perceptual distortions and eccentricities of behavior, beginning by early adulthood and present in a variety of contexts, as indicated by five (or more) of the following:

  (1) ideas of reference (excluding delusions of reference)

  (2) odd beliefs or magical thinking that influence behavior or is inconsistent with cultural norms (e.g., superstitious, belief in clairvoyance, telepathy, or "sixth sense"; in children and adolescents, bizarre fantasies or preoccupations)

  (3) unusual perceptual experiences (including bodily illusions)

  (4) odd thinking and speech (e.g., vague, circumstantial, metaphorical, overelaborative, or stereotyped)

  (5) suspiciousness or paranoid ideation

  (6) inappropriate or constricted affect

    (7) behavior or appearance that is odd, eccentric, or peculiar

    (8) lack of close friends or confidants other than first-degree relatives

B. *Does not occur exclusively during the course of schizophrenia, a mood disorder with psychotic features, another psychotic disorder, or a pervasive developmental disorder.*

(Reprinted, with permission, from the *Diagnostic and Statistical Manual of Mental Disorders.* 4th edn. Text Revision. Washington, DC: American Psychiatric Association, 2000.)

General Considerations

A. EPIDEMIOLOGY

The prevalence rate of schizotypal personality disorder has been estimated at approximately 3–5% of the general population. Furthermore, up to 30% of general psychiatric outpatients have one or more schizotypal traits, with comorbidity existing with mood, substance-use, and anxiety disorders. Men are slightly more likely to have the disorder.

B. ETIOLOGY

Schizotypal personality disorder occurs significantly more frequently among the biological relatives of schizophrenic individuals than in the general population. This finding, together with the results of twin studies, suggests a genetic relationship to schizophrenia. Of all of the personality disorders, schizotypal personality disorder most strongly shows a continuum with schizophrenia. Thus, it is likely that those etiologic factors which induce schizophrenia are similar to those which induce schizotypal personality disorder.

C. GENETICS

The concept of schizotypal personality disorder originally developed because of the fact that relatives of schizophrenic patients often had symptoms similar to schizophrenia. There is also evidence that biologic and neuro-cognitive markers of schizophrenia are shared with patients with schizotypal personality disorder. Schizotypal personality disorder is currently thought to be a component of schizophrenia spectrum disorders (which also includes schizoaffective disorder, schizophreniform disorder, and psychotic mood disorders). As such it may not clearly be an actual personality disorder.

Clinical Findings

A. SIGNS & SYMPTOMS

Schizotypal personality disorder is characterized by peculiar behavior, odd thoughts, odd speech, unusual perceptive experiences, and magical beliefs. These patients usually have negative or poor rapport and show social dysfunction, social anxiety, and a lack of motivation. They are frequently underachievers with regard to occupational status.

    The disorder may be manifested during childhood or adolescence as social isolation and peculiar behavior or language. Although the features of the disorder resemble schizophrenia, rates of depression and anxiety are also quite high among such patients. The latter features often constitute the presenting complaint, rather than the ongoing cognitive anomalies.

Dimensional Considerations

A dimensional system can be applied to the characterization of schizotypal personality disorder patients precisively and cluster A disorders patient's in general. The components of the cluster A diagnoses, such as aloofness, mistrust, suspiciousness, eccentricity, vulnerability, anxiousness, interpersonal sensitivity, introspection and introversion, negative temperament, perceptual cognitive distortions, restricted expression, and evidence of intimacy avoidance can be considered on a continuum, allowing placement in a given individual between normalcy and psychopathology.

    Alternatively, cluster A disorders can be considered from the perspective of personality traits and temperamental characteristics. Thus, for example, schizotypal personality disorder patients are associated with high levels of neuroticism and low levels of conscientiousness, agreeableness, and extroversion. Furthermore, Cluster A personality disorder patients in general show high levels of introversion, most dramatically in individuals with schizoid personality disorder.

Differential Diagnosis

Schizotypal personality disorder is considered by some investigators to be a schizophrenia spectrum disorder. However, the relatives of schizophrenic patients who display schizotypal personality disorder more often tend to exhibit social isolation and poor rapport, rather than psychotic-like symptoms and ideas of reference. Thus, although the schizotypal personality disorder appears with relatively greater than expected frequency in the relatives of schizophrenic patients (i.e., 10%), it is not necessarily merely a milder form of schizophrenia. With respect to other Cluster A disorders, 70% of patients with schizotypal personality disorders have been found to have one or more additional Cluster A personality disorders. Furthermore, comorbidity with Axis I mood, anxiety, and substance-use disorders is also common.

Treatment

A. Psychopharmacologic Interventions

Low-dose antipsychotic medications are sometimes prescribed to treat the cognitive peculiarities, depression, odd thoughts and speech, anxiety, and impulsivity of patients with schizotypal personality disorder. First and second generation antipsychotics have been demonstrated to have clinical efficacy in placebo-controlled clinical trials. Antipsychotic medications are particularly useful in patients with moderately severe schizotypal symptoms and mild transient psychotic episodes. It is unknown whether antipsychotic medications have a prophylactic benefit for this disorder. In addition, some anecdotal evidence suggests that lithium and mood stabilizers may be helpful in treating selected schizotypal patients.

B. Psychotherapeutic Interventions

1. Group/marital interventions—Group therapy, especially social skills training, is believed to be helpful to patients with schizotypal personality disorder. This form of therapy addresses the associated social anxiety and awkwardness. However, patients with more severe symptoms may prove disruptive in group therapy, particularly if prominent paranoid ideation is present, and patients with overtly eccentric behavior may inadvertently make other group members uncomfortable.

2. Individual psychotherapies—Patients with schizotypal personality disorder are generally thought to be poorly suited for nondirective psychotherapies because of a propensity to decompensate under unstructured conditions. Often recommended is a supportive approach, with an emphasis on reality testing and attention to interpersonal boundaries, combined with directive approaches focused on problematic behavior. A cognitive focus also appears useful, with attempts made to help the patient recognize cognitive distortions, such as referential, paranoid, or magical thinking. This can be accomplished through educative interventions that teach patients to corroborate their odd ideas and thoughts with environmental evidence rather than with personal impressions.

Prognosis

Estimates of the proportion of patients with schizotypal personality disorder who go on to develop overt schizophrenia are variable. The proportion is generally thought to be relatively low, possibly around 10% or less, with some estimates as high as 20–25%. Paranoid ideation, social isolation, magical thinking, and functional decline are the most stable symptoms, and appear to be the most predictive of the eventual development of schizophrenia. These symptoms are also most associated with a poor prognosis and a more chronic outcome.

CLUSTER B PERSONALITY DISORDERS

ANTISOCIAL PERSONALITY DISORDER

 ESSENTIALS OF DIAGNOSIS

DSM-IV-TR Criteria

A. *There is a pervasive pattern of disregard for and violation of the rights of others occurring since age 15 years, as indicated by three (or more) of the following:*

   (1) failure to conform to social norms with respect to lawful behaviors as indicated by repeatedly performing acts that are grounds for arrest

   (2) deceitfulness, as indicated by repeated lying, use of aliases, or conning others for personal profit or pleasure

   (3) impulsivity or failure to plan ahead

   (4) irritability and aggressiveness, as indicated by repeated physical fights or assaults

   (5) reckless disregard for the safety of self or others

   (6) consistent irresponsibility, as indicated by repeated failure to sustain consistent work behavior or honor financial obligations

   (7) lack of remorse, as indicated by being indifferent to or rationalizing having hurt, mistreated, or stolen from another

B. *The individual is at least age 18 years.*

C. *There is evidence of conduct disorder with onset before age 15 years.*

D. *The occurrence of antisocial behavior is not exclusively during the course of schizophrenia or a manic episode.*

(Reprinted, with permission, from the *Diagnostic and Statistical Manual of Mental Disorders.* 4th edn. Text Revision. Washington, DC: American Psychiatric Association, 2000.)

General Considerations

A. Epidemiology

Antisocial personality disorder appears to be reasonably common in the general population, with its rate estimated at 2–4% in males and 0.5–1.0% in women. However, since such patients rarely seek treatment voluntarily, and generally come to treatment only when interventions are mandated, these numbers may be underestimated. Finally, there is a strong correlation between having conduct disorder as a child and developing antisocial personality disorder as an adult.

B. Etiology

It appears that both biological and environmental factors are involved as causes of antisocial personality disorder. Individuals are at increased risk for this disorder if they had an antisocial or alcoholic father (even if they were not raised by that person). Other associated variables occurring in childhood include living in a nonintact family, low parental education, hyperkinetic problems, conduct problems, and bullying and adult criminal offenses in the family.

C. Genetics

Family studies of antisocial personality disorder reveal an increased incidence of this disorder in family members. Individuals are at increased risk for this disorder if they had an antisocial or alcoholic father (even if they were not raised by that person). Twin studies also support a genetic component to the etiology of antisocial personality disorder. The primary environmental deficient appears to be the lack of a consistent person to give emotional and loving support as a young child. Surprisingly, merely living in a high crime area does not in and of itself increase the risk of antisocial personality disorder.

Clinical Findings

A. Signs & Symptoms

As described in the DSM-IV-TR, antisocial personality disorder consists of a pattern of recurrent antisocial, delinquent, and criminal behavior that begins in childhood or early adolescence and basically pervades all aspects of an individual's life. Negative job performance and marital instability are also hallmarks of the antisocial personality disorder patient.

A major feature of antisocial personality disorder is a disregard for the rights and feelings of others. This is a characteristic that leads to a variety of unacceptable behaviors, often noted during adolescence or childhood as a conduct disorder. Thus, beginning earlier than 15 years of age, patients have histories of impulsive behavior, aggression toward others, school discipline problems,

and breaking the law. Patients with antisocial personality disorders are deficient in meeting social roles and occupational obligations. Relationships are generally superficial and short-lived. Use of illegal substances is common. These individuals tend to be easily bored and impulsive. They seek novelty in their lives and seem unable to avoid behavior that has a high probability of leading to punishment. They may exploit others for personal benefit or at times for no good reason. They often rationalize their antisocial behavior as necessarily defensive, believing others are trying to exploit them.

Differential Diagnosis

Substance abuse is comorbid in two thirds of patients with antisocial personality disorder. Other comorbid conditions include the following: other personality disorders, sexual dysfunction, paraphilias, mood disorders, and anxiety disorders. Patients with antisocial personality disorder have high rates of death from natural causes and suicide.

With respect to personality traits and temperament, antisocial personality disorder patients often score low in harm avoidance, low in reward dependence and high in novelty seeking. These characteristics are associated with risk taking without fear, lack of concern for others, and impulsivity.

Treatment

A. Psychopharmacologic Interventions

Overall, there is little evidence that the pharmacologic treatment of antisocial personality disorder is effective. However, treatment of associated symptoms may be useful. Psychostimulants may be used to treat associated symptoms of attention deficit disorder. Although efficacy has not been demonstrated by controlled clinical trials, selective serotonin reuptake inhibitors (SSRIs), bupropion, and antipsychotic agents have been used to reduce impulsive aggression.

B. Psychotherapeutic Interventions

1. Group, marital, and community programs— There are no specific psychological tests that are used routinely to diagnose antisocial personality disorder. Because of the patients' lack of insight, treatments have generally been directed to affected individuals with criminal backgrounds.

Nevertheless, socially based interventions, particularly with others of similar temperaments and problems, are often considered by clinical practitioners to be the treatment of choice for patients with antisocial personality disorder. It is thought that in group contexts, rationalization and evasion can be confronted by others who recognize these patterns. Group membership and associated caring for and from others presumably allows patients with antisocial personality disorder to experience feelings of belonging that many never received from their families. Similarly, family therapy may be useful when the family system is contributing to or perpetuating the antisocial behavior. Also addressed can be issues of maintaining attachment with a spouse, parenting issues, and the impulsive aggressiveness that can lead to abuse.

Intensive community-based treatment programs may be helpful. A decrease of 20–40% in criminal behavior and recidivism, a probable marker of antisocial personality disorder, occurs with such treatment. Usually such treatments focus on improving social skills, treating substance abuse, managing impulse control, and diminishing antisocial attitudes.

2. Individual psychotherapeutic interventions— The literature generally considers the individual psychotherapy of antisocial personality disorder to be ineffective. Also, individual psychotherapists often find patients with antisocial personality disorder to be difficult, untrustworthy, manipulative, and with low frustration tolerance. Dropout rates can be as high as 70%. Traditional psychotherapy is impeded by the antisocial patient's interpersonal indifference, which hinders the formation of a true therapeutic alliance. Also, punishment based techniques have proven typical ineffective as have contingency-based behavioral techniques.

Cognitive–behavioral psychotherapy has been used with reported success in treating antisocial personality disorder. The patient's distorted cognitive constructs and attitudes toward social groups are analyzed. Specifically, cognitive approaches involve addressing distortions that are typically self-serving or that minimize the future consequences of the individual's behavior.

Prognosis

Antisocial personality disorder, as it appears in young adults, is thought to be among the most treatment refractory of the Axis II disorders. However, the behavioral problems associated with antisocial personality disorder tend to peak in late adolescence and early adulthood, and 30–40% of these individuals show significant improvement in their antisocial behaviors by the time they reach their mid-thirties and forties.

During their later years antisocial personality disorder patients are at risk for developing chronic alcoholism and late-onset depression. They often continue to be irresponsible, but without the dramatic aggressiveness of their earlier years. Possibly of significance, the core personality traits of conscientiousness and agreeableness

naturally increase with age, and this change has been suggested to be responsible for the "improvement" in antisocial personality disorder patients over time.

BORDERLINE PERSONALITY DISORDER

 ESSENTIALS OF DIAGNOSIS

DSM-IV-TR Diagnostic Criteria

A. *A pervasive pattern of instability of interpersonal relationships, self-image, and affects, and marked impulsivity beginning by early adulthood and present in a variety of contexts, as indicated by five (or more) of the following:*

(1) *frantic efforts to avoid real or imagined abandonment.*
   (Do not include suicidal or self-mutilating behavior covered in criterion 5).

(2) *a pattern of unstable and intense interpersonal relationships characterized by alternating between extremes of idealization and devaluation*

(3) *identity disturbance: Markedly and persistently unstable self-image or sense of self*

(4) *impulsivity in at least two areas that are potentially self-damaging (e.g., spending, sex, substance abuse, reckless driving, binge eating)*
   Note: Do not include suicidal or self-mutilating behavior covered in criterion 5.

(5) *recurrent suicidal behavior, gestures, or threats, or self-mutilating behavior*

(6) *affective instability due to a marked reactivity of mood (e.g., intense episodic dysphoria, irritability, or anxiety usually lasting a few hours and only rarely more than a few days)*

(7) *chronic feelings of emptiness*

(8) *inappropriate and intense anger or difficulty controlling anger (e.g., frequent displays of temper, constant anger, recurrent physical fights)*

(9) *transient, stress-related paranoid ideation or severe dissociative symptom*

(Reprinted, with permission, from the *Diagnostic and Statistical Manual of Mental Disorders*. 4th edn. Text Revision. Washington, DC: American Psychiatric Association, 2000.)

General Considerations

A. EPIDEMIOLOGY

The prevalence of borderline personality disorder in the general population is about 1–2%. However, the disorder is particularly common among psychiatric inpatients and on related medical units, such as emergency rooms, where as many as 20–30% of patients meet criteria for the disorder. Borderline personality disorder is identified more commonly in women than in men, although evidence suggests that it may be under-identified in men. The features of the disorder are more common among young adults.

B. ETIOLOGY

Borderline personality disorder patients are quite common in psychiatric settings, typically accounting for one third or more of clinical personality disorder diagnoses, and this diagnosis has been receiving considerable attention in the psychiatric and psychological literature. The causes of the disorder are uncertain. Psychoanalytic thinking commonly focuses on disturbances in the normal separation–individuation phase of development between the child and the mother, as well as other aberrant parenting patterns. Such developmental problems are thought to leave the child with problems of separation and self-identity.

Many patients with borderline personality disorder report childhood sexual, physical, and/or emotional abuse, and it is likely that such abuse or its perception has etiologic significance. This purported abuse is thought to lead to dissociation, splitting, repression, mood lability, and identity problems. Other forms of parental failure such as neglect or poor expression of affection, overcriticism, or invalidating communication have been proposed to be of etiologic importance, as has developmental trauma. Alternatively, overindulgence has been thought to lead to immature coping styles, leading to the disorder.

C. GENETICS

The possible genetic influences leading to borderline personality disorder are not well understood. However, some investigators have speculated that a genetic factor leads to the enhanced anxiety, emotional lability, and instability that characteristic of borderline personality disorder, and that it is the tendency toward emotional lability that is inherited.

Borderline personality disorder occurs relatively more often in the families of patients with the disorder and there is also some evidence from family studies that bipolar disorder and/or major depression occurs more often in families with borderline personality disorder. It may be that certain personality traits (i.e., aggression, impulsivity, affective instability) are what are genetically

determined in the borderline personality disorder patients and their families, rather than the actual syndrome. Possibly related, new evidence suggests that abnormal frontolimbic circuiting underlies borderline personality disorder.

Clinical Findings

A. SIGNS & SYMPTOMS

Borderline personality disorder as now defined in DSM-IV-TR represents a pervasive pattern of mood instability associated with unstable but intense interpersonal relationships. Commonly impulsivity, inappropriate or intense anger, recurrent suicidal threats and gestures, and self-mutilating behavior occur. There is a persistent identity disturbance, chronic feelings of emptiness or boredom, and an exaggerated attempt to avoid real or perceived abandonment. Transient paranoid ideation or dissociative symptoms may also occur. In addition, primitive defense mechanisms, such as splitting (exaggerated dichotomies of good and evil, worthy and unworthy, etc.) are often present. A general overall deficit in the ability to test reality is also characteristic of the diagnosis

Borderline personality disorder patients are also characterized by a poorly established self-image that is heavily dependent for validation on relationships, in combination with an expectation of mistreatment or exploitation. This combination of features makes those with the disorder extremely concerned about close relationships and highly sensitive to changes in these relationships. Reaction to interpersonal conflicts is characterized by dramatic emotional changes, often associated with impulsive self-destructiveness.

The borderline personality disorder patient's mood often switches between rage, despair, and anxiety over the course of a single day. Multiple suicidal gestures and self-mutilation and self-injurious behaviors are among the most striking actions of these patients. As described above, such behavior is noted primarily after interpersonal turmoil, often after rejection by an intimate. Suicidal gestures often tend to increase in lethality as they recur, and completed suicide occurs in up to 10% of borderline personality disorder patients.

Adding to the complexity of borderline personality disorder, self-injurious behavior, often beginning in childhood or adolescence, may not be a sign of suicidal intent as such. Such cutting, burning, and associated attempts to cause pain are often due to attempts to regulate dysphoric affect, guilt, tension, dissociative symptoms, and/or to communicate emotions. These self-injurious behaviors are especially associated with a history of childhood sexual abuse.

The assessment of borderline personality disorder patients is complicated by the cognitive style that these patients manifest. Although positive comments can be found, patients' evaluations of themselves and their surroundings often are negative in the extreme. Alternatively, situations and people can be overidealized. The borderline personality patient's tendency to evaluate his or her mental status negatively (i.e., more depressed or anxious) leads to self-reported clinical pictures that are more pathologic than outwardly appear.

Associated with the borderline personality symptoms as such, the patient may admit to and appear to exaggerate a wide variety of behavioral syndromes, including severe depression and anxiety, psychotic features, paranoid ideation, and somatic concerns.

Dimensional Perspectives

Borderline personality disorder can be considered from a dimensional perspective. From this perspective, characteristics of the borderline personality disorder patient are considered on a spectrum between the normal and severely symptomatic. From that perspective, therapy can be directed toward symptom complexes. Borderline personality disorder patients can also be classified with respect to their temperaments and core personality traits. On the five-factor model of personality scale, they often show high neuroticism, low agreeableness, and low conscientiousness, with no special relationship to extraversion reported. Similarly, for the Tridimensional Personality Questionnaire and its derivative, the cluster for borderline personality disorder consists of high novelty seeking (seen primarily in males), fairly high harm avoidance (primarily in females), low reward dependence, and low self-directedness.

Differential Diagnosis

Borderline personality disorder is frequently associated with a variety of Axis I disorders, and with almost all other Axis II disorders, especially those in cluster B. Major depression is commonly comorbid with borderline personality disorder. Substance-abuse disorder, alcoholism, posttraumatic stress disorder, and anxiety disorders are frequently diagnosed in patients with borderline personality disorder.

Treatment

A. PSYCHOPHARMACOLOGIC INTERVENTION

A number of psychopharmacologic strategies are useful in treating borderline personality disorder. Controlled clinical trials demonstrate the efficacy of lithium carbonate in diminishing anger, irritability, and self-mutilation. A more limited body of evidence indicates that carbamazepine increases behavioral control and diminishes anger and impulsivity. Sodium valproate has been used to treat irritability and aggressiveness in borderline patients. In open label studies, the atypical antipsychotic agent, olanzapine, improves paranoid and other psychotic ideation, impulsive aggression, and depression. Similarly, first-generation antipsychotics and some atypical antipsychotics (clozapine, risperidone, and quetiapine) have a similar therapeutic profile to olanzapine in open label studies. Several SSRI antidepressants (fluoxetine and fluvoxamine) have therapeutic efficacy with regard to mood fluctuations, aggression, and overall adaptive behavior.

Finally, any medication administered to a borderline disorder patient should be monitored carefully and prescribed cautiously because of the enhanced risks for noncompliance, development of substance abuse, and use in suicide attempts or gestures.

B. PSYCHOTHERAPEUTIC INTERVENTION

1. Group/family approaches—Group therapy has been reported to be a useful format to address the interpersonal problems of borderline personality disorder patients. In such groups patients can form attachments to the group as such or to individual group members, rather than focusing their positive and negative feelings and transferences on a single therapist. Having peers available to mediate the inevitable conflicts that develop with other group members is also helpful. Similarly, family therapy, used especially to work out dependency issues and issues of dramatic acting out, has been reported to be helpful.

2. Individual psychotherapies—Generally, psychotherapy with borderline patients is made difficult by the severity and nature of the borderline personality disorder patients' behaviors, and by the patient's ability to evoke strong negative reactions before the therapist. However, there are several structured therapies that have proven useful in the treatment of borderline personality disorder patients.

Dialectical behavior therapy is a very popular and effective form of treatment. In the initial stages of treatment, a supportive approach is used to establish a therapeutic alliance. Over time the therapist focuses on identifying and changing ineffective behaviors. The emphasis of the therapy is on stress tolerance, coping skills development, emotional regulation, self-management, and suppression of secondary gain from acting out behavior.

With treatment, patients come to recognize the pattern of self-destruction, instability, and projection that have characterized their lives and to understand its origins. Patients also explore their rigid good-versus-bad view of others, recognizing that others' motivations, like their own, are more complex than they appear, and that their sensitivity to others' untrustworthiness is often a distortion arising out of experience.

Dialectical behavioral therapy has been demonstrated to be effective in controlled trials. Treatment results in less self-injurious behavior and anger, and fewer inpatient days. Patients treated with this psychotherapy had less drug and alcohol use, and depressive symptoms were improved.

Mentalization based psychotherapy is a type of supportive interventions that uses interventions that focus on establishing an alliance. This treatment is structured, has a clear focus, and reaches agreement about the role of the therapist, phone calls, cancellations, and how emergencies are managed. Real-life issues for the patient are a major focus. In controlled clinical trials, individuals receiving mentalization-based therapy showed improvement in anxiety, social adjustment, and organizational skills.

Prognosis

Patients with borderline personality disorder repeatedly engage in self-destructive behaviors which, as mentioned above, can be lethal. Patients sometimes sabotage treatment when it seems to be going well. In part, their difficult course relates to the extreme negative reactions their demands and behaviors often elicit in their therapists and families. Undoubtedly related, the consistent stable behaviors of many symptoms are affective instability and anger. Their behavior tends to become more dramatic and dangerous as others, such as family, therapists, and significant others, reject them or habituate to their demands and crises. As a result, prognosis can be poor. Over involvement in family relations, antisocial behaviors, chronic anger, and overuse of medical facilities predict a poor outcome. Conversely, impulsive and dangerous behaviors seem to diminish as patients approach middle age. A better outcome is associated with higher intelligence, superior social supports, and increased self-discipline.

HISTRIONIC PERSONALITY DISORDER

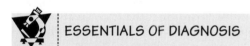 **ESSENTIALS OF DIAGNOSIS**

DSM-IV-TR Diagnostic Criteria

A. A pervasive pattern of excessive emotionality and attention seeking, beginning by early adulthood and present in a variety of contexts, as indicated by five (or more) of the following:

(1) is uncomfortable in situations in which he or she is not the center of attention

(2) interaction with others is often characterized by inappropriate sexually seductive or provocative behavior

(3) displays rapidly shifting and shallow expression of emotions

(4) consistently uses physical appearance to draw attention to self

(5) has a style of speech that is excessively impressionistic and lacking in detail

(6) shows self-dramatization, is theatric, and has exaggerated expression of emotion

(7) is suggestible, i.e., easily influenced by others or circumstances

(8) considers relationships to be more intimate than they actually are

(Reprinted, with permission, from the *Diagnostic and Statistical Manual of Mental Disorders*. 4th edn. Text Revision. Washington, DC: American Psychiatric Association, 2000.)

General Considerations

A. EPIDEMIOLOGY

The frequency of histrionic personality disorder has been estimated to be as high as 12% in females, and the overall prevalence of histrionic personality disorder has been estimated as 1–3% in the general population. Rates of the disorder are much higher in psychiatric and general medical setting, because these patients often actively pursue treatment.

Histrionic personality disorder tends to be diagnosed more frequently in women, and there is a strong possibility that the disorder may be overlooked in men. For younger adults, males and females have been reported to be equally likely to receive a diagnosis of histrionic personality disorder, whereas in middle age, women predominate. Nevertheless, epidemiologic studies indicate that overall, the gender differences in prevalence may be slight.

B. ETIOLOGY

As with most personality disorders, the etiology of histrionic personality disorder is not well understood. Some researchers speculate that problems in parent–child relationships lead to the associated low self-esteem. One possibility is that the patient uses dramatic behavior and other similar means to superficially impress others, due to their low self-concept, thinking that he or she is not worthy of attention without such special behaviors.

C. GENETICS

There is considerable evidence that there is a genetic component to histrionic personality disorder. There also appears to be a family association between histrionic and antisocial personality disorders and some have suggested that both of these disorders could be gender-related expressions of the same illness.

Clinical Findings

A. SIGNS & SYMPTOMS

The cardinal feature of histrionic personality disorder is the deliberate use of excessive, superficial emotionality and sexuality to draw attention, evade unpleasant responsibilities, and control others. Histrionic personality disorder patients feel best when they are the center of attention and they become disappointed or petulant should the attention shift. Their emotions are characteristically labile, and they may exhibit temper tantrums, tearful outbursts, or dramatic accusations when upset. These displays are often used to provoke a reaction, such as guilt, sympathy, or acquiescence from those around them.

Patients with histrionic personality disorder are often quite concerned with their physical appearance and attractiveness, and may dress and carry themselves in a seductive or provocative manner. Interactions may be dominated by flirtatious banter, interspersed with dramatic anecdotes about the patient's life and circumstances.

Unlike some other personality disorders diagnoses, patients with histrionic personality disorder place a premium on interpersonal relationships, and the quality of these relationships, at least their superficial quality, is quite important to them. However, there is often a pattern of sequential unsuccessful relationships, with a seemingly capricious flight from relationship to relationship occurring. Although descriptions of events may be passionate and colorful, they tend to be imprecise and lack detail, with the information obtained being more impressionistic than specific.

Also prominent in those with histrionic personality disorder is the repression of anger and other disturbing affects. Anger tends to be expressed either fleetingly or indirectly. More comfortable with the expression of physical rather than psychological symptoms, these patients may present with somatic entities such as somatization disorder or conversion disorder.

Dimensional Perspectives

Considered from the perspective of character traits and temperaments, histrionic personality disorder patients are found to be characterized by high levels of extraversion and marked neuroticism. High scores on novelty seeking and reward dependence and low scores on harm avoidance are also characteristic of these individuals.

Differential Diagnosis

Histrionic personality disorder especially requires differentiation from the cluster B disorders, narcissistic personality disorder, borderline personality disorder, and less so with antisocial personality disorder. The diagnosis also resembles and overlaps with bipolar spectrum disorders, eating disorders, and substance-abuse disorders

Treatment

A. PHARMACOLOGIC INTERVENTIONS

There is little or no evidence that pharmacologic treatment is effective in altering histrionic personality disorder symptoms as such. However, individuals with this disorder often have major depressive disorder and/or an anxiety disorder. For these patients, conventional antidepressants can be quite effective. Also, in some patients monoamine oxidase inhibitors have been reported to be useful. Because these patients are likely to misuse prescription medications, caution is warranted when prescribing such medications in general, and drugs of abuse specifically.

B. PSYCHOTHERAPEUTIC INTERVENTIONS

1. Group/marital interventions—It has been suggested that patients with histrionic personality disorder may derive particular benefit from group therapy, especially from groups comprised of similar patients. Such groups provide a mirror of the histrionic patient's own behavior, and can serve to confront emotional displays rather than accepting or ignoring them. Moreover, histrionic personality disorder patients have considerable need for approval from others, and thus, are more likely to accept confrontations in order to avoid being rejected.

Histrionic personality disorder patients can be challenging to work in couples or marital therapy. Their commitment to the marital relationship is often tenuous, or they may be unwilling to risk relinquishing the degree of control they maintain in the relationship.

2. Individual psychotherapies—There are no controlled clinical trials that identify the best psychotherapeutic strategies for treating histrionic personality disorder. Clinical consensus indicates that the psychotherapy should be empathic and interactive. Limit setting and identifying acting-out behavior are desirable therapeutic topics.

Histrionic personality disorder is most commonly treated with psychodynamic psychotherapy, supportive psychotherapy, and cognitive–behavioral therapy. Operationally, regardless of the therapy utilized, the tumultuous relationship history of the patient is likely to repeat itself within the psychotherapeutic relationship. Identification of the patient's true feelings, as engendered in the therapeutic relationship, and the delineation of the self-perpetuating quality of these emotions and their subsequent behaviors is an important part of the therapy. Similarly, a focus on the links between thoughts and feelings increases the patient's capacity for reflection, thereby decreasing the likelihood of impulsive acting out behaviors occurring.

Prognosis

The prognosis for histrionic personality disorder patients is relatively good. These patients tend to be reasonably effective in social settings. This allows them to be the beneficiaries of social feedback and support. In the face of abandonment, they are vulnerable to depression, but as with many of their other complaints, the dysphoria can be short-lived, and it is highly reactive to external circumstances. The prognosis is more pessimistic if the patient meets criteria for other cluster B personality disorders.

Over time, histrionic personality disorder patients tend to improve regardless of treatment. Significantly, decreases in extraversion and neuroticism often occur as one ages, and these changes have been suggested as an explanation for the above improvement over time which tends to occur.

NARCISSISTIC PERSONALITY DISORDER

 ESSENTIALS OF DIAGNOSIS

DSM-IV-TR Criteria

A. *A pervasive pattern of grandiosity (in fantasy or behavior), need for admiration, and lack of empathy, beginning by early adulthood and present in a variety of contexts, as indicated by five (or more) of the following:*

(1) *has a grandiose sense of self-importance (e.g., exaggerates achievements and talents, expects to be recognized as superior without commensurate achievements)*

(2) *is preoccupied with fantasies of unlimited success, power, brilliance, beauty, or ideal love*

(3) *believes that he or she is "special" and unique and can only be understood by, or should associate with, other special or high-status people (or institutions)*

(4) *requires excessive admiration*

(5) *has a sense of entitlement, i.e., unreasonable expectations of especially favorable treatment or automatic compliance with his or her expectations*

(6) *is interpersonally exploitative, i.e., takes advantage of others to achieve his or her own ends*

(7) *lacks empathy: Is unwilling to recognize or identify with the feelings and needs of others*

(8) *is often envious of others or believes that others are envious of him or her*

(9) *shows arrogant, haughty behaviors or attitudes*

(Reprinted, with permission, from the *Diagnostic and Statistical Manual of Mental Disorders.* 4th edn. Text Revision. Washington, DC: American Psychiatric Association, 2000.)

General Considerations

A. EPIDEMIOLOGY

Narcissistic personality disorder occurs in less than 1% in the general population. It is frequently comorbid in populations of psychiatric patients, being estimated at 2–16%. The disorder is somewhat more common in men than in women.

B. ETIOLOGY

Although the cause of narcissistic personality disorder is unknown, one hypothesis is that there has been a lack of clear parental appreciation of the child's accomplishments. This deficiency, or conversely, excessive attention and overgratification concerning accomplishments, is thought to lead the child, and later the adult to continually seek adoration, and to have difficulties in attaining self-esteem at realistic levels.

Clinical Findings

A. SIGNS & SYMPTOMS

The hallmarks of the narcissistic personality disorder are grandiosity, a notable lack of empathy and of a lack of consideration for others. There also is hypersensitivity to evaluation by others. Narcissistic individuals exaggerate their accomplishments, act egotistical and are manipulative of those around them. They have an exaggerated sense of entitlement, being convinced that they deserve special treatment and admiration. Thus, individuals with narcissistic personality disorder are frequently boastful of their accomplishments and often appear haughty and irritating, although they can be outwardly charming. Usually they have little insight into their narcissism. They are often excessively self-centered and self-absorbed and have problems with commitment. They have an exaggerated sense of uniqueness, and show devaluation, disdain, contempt, and deprecation of others.

Narcissistic personality disorder patients are prone to attribute and externalize the source of their problems to people who they think do not appreciate, support, or defer to them. Because they are highly vulnerable to criticism, any negative statements about them provokes anger, disdain, counter arguments, and devaluation of the person making the statement. Some narcissistic individuals react to criticism by becoming enraged, sometimes with acute paranoid ideation and marked deterioration in judgment.

Given the narcissistic personality disorder patient's view on life, these patients are vulnerable to depressive episodes and social withdrawal following injury to their self-image. Linked to this, envy of others is a major feature characteristic of personality disorder patients. Such envy makes it difficult for these patients to appreciate what they actually have acquired or accomplished. Individuals with narcissistic personality disorder are especially prone to dislike growing old, and thus, may become more depressed and demanding during the fourth, fifth, and later decades of life.

Dimensional Consideration

With regard to the core personality or temperamental structure of narcissistic personality disorder patients, such individuals score high on extraversion and low on cooperativeness. They also score high on novelty seeking and low on harm avoidance and reward dependence.

Differential Diagnosis

Patients with narcissistic personality disorder can be easily confused with patients with hypomania because of the grandiosity common to both disorders. Indeed, bipolar manic patients demonstrate most of the identifying criteria of narcissistic personality disorder, but generally only when manic. Although difficult to differentiate, patients with narcissistic personality disorder, rather than being overly involved in a whirl of activities, are usually more selective, participating only in those tasks that they think merit their special talents and unique abilities, and for which they can be recognized.

Narcissistic personality disorder is also often confused with and commonly associated with a diagnosis of antisocial personality disorder. Some scholars have suggested that the former is merely a less aggressive version of the latter. Both disorders are characterized by interpersonal exploitiveness and a lack of empathy. However, the patient with narcissistic personality disorder is less likely to be thrill seeking and impulsive, and more likely to exaggerate their talents and to be grandiose. It is also difficult to distinguish between patients with narcissistic personality disorder and those with borderline personality disorder. However, the obvious independence and the compulsion to exert interpersonal control in narcissistic personality disorder patients contrasts with the neediness and dependency of many patients with borderline personality disorder. Substance-abuse disorders and hypochondriasis are often comorbid with narcissistic personality disorder.

Treatment

A. PSYCHOPHARMACOLOGIC INTERVENTIONS

There is little evidence to suggest that psychopharmacotherapy is effective in the treatment of narcissistic personality disorder, except when comorbid conditions occur such as depression, anxiety, and suicidality. Under such conditions, appropriate antidepressant or other symptom specific therapies are indicated.

B. PSYCHOTHERAPEUTIC INTERVENTIONS

1. Group/marital interventions—Although controlled studies are lacking, there is a large body of clinical experience regarding the psychotherapy of narcissistic personality disorder. With respect to the group therapies, patients with narcissistic personality disorder can be disruptive if criticism by other group members precipitates rage or withdrawal. To this end, the therapist must ensure that some support for the patient is provided in order to render the inevitable confrontations more palatable. However, treatment in a homogeneous group of narcissistic personality disorder patients is thought to help these patients to increase their understanding of themselves through a mirroring of their own maladaptive patterns of behavior.

Patients with narcissistic personality disorder choose to participate in couples' therapy with some frequency. Here, the therapist must guard against unilaterally blaming the patient for the disruptions in the relationship, since the maladaptive behavior patterns of the couple are often complementary and self-sustaining. In such cases role-playing and role-reversal techniques have been considered particularly useful.

2. Individual psychotherapeutic interventions—As with group and marital treatments, psychotherapy with patients with narcissistic personality disorder is usually challenging. These patients often develop expectations of the therapist that are grandiose or expansive. They may not be able to build a trusting or working alliance. Furthermore, they usually come to treatment only following pressure from others, and thus, unless they are depressed or otherwise symptomatic, they are poorly motivated to receive psychotherapeutic help.

In treating narcissistic personality disorder patients, certain pitfalls exist. The therapist must avoid the extremes of either joining the patient in his or her self-admiration, or of strongly criticizing the patient. Although confronting the patient is often necessary, it needs to be carefully timed and presented with a tone of support and empathic acceptance.

Cognitive interventions can be directed at the cognitive distortions of self and others that are typical in these patients. Such distortions often involve a magnification of the differences between the patient and other people whereby the difference favors the patient, and others are viewed with contempt. Conversely, if the difference favors another, the patient feels worthless and humiliated. This situation can be addressed by modifying the patient's standards and goals to an internal frame of reference, rather than a comparison with others.

Prognosis

Little is known about the long-term prognosis of patients with narcissistic personality disorder. In the absence of treatment, and possibly with treatment, the features of the disorder are unlikely to diminish. Indeed, they tend to worsen during middle age and become more strongly associated with depression and despair.

The features of the disorder tend to self-perpetuate, with the patient's devaluation of others eventually driving away those who might have provided the expected admiration. The significant depression resulting from such rejections is typically resolved by an increase in defensive self-aggrandizement that repeats the cycle.

CLUSTER C PERSONALITY DISORDERS

AVOIDANT PERSONALITY DISORDER

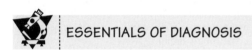

ESSENTIALS OF DIAGNOSIS

DSM-IV-TR Diagnostic Criteria

A. *A pervasive pattern of social inhibition, feelings of inadequacy, and hypersensitivity to negative evaluation, beginning by early adulthood and*

present in a variety of contexts, as indicated by four (or more) of the following:

(1) avoids occupational activities that involve significant interpersonal contact, because of fears of criticism, disapproval, or rejection

(2) is unwilling to get involved with people unless certain of being liked

(3) shows restraint within intimate relationships because of a fear of being shamed or ridiculed

(4) is preoccupied with being criticized or rejected in social situations

(5) is inhibited in new interpersonal situations because of feelings of inadequacy

(6) views self as socially inept, personally unappealing, or inferior to others

(7) is unusually reluctant to take personal risks or to engage in any new activities because they may prove embarrassing

(Reprinted, with permission, from the *Diagnostic and Statistical Manual of Mental Disorders.* 4th edn. Text Revision. Washington, DC: American Psychiatric Association, 2000.)

General Considerations

A. EPIDEMIOLOGY

The prevalence of avoidant personality disorder has been estimated at 0.5–2.4% in the general population, with larger numbers occurring in women than in men.

B. ETIOLOGY

As with all other personality disorders, the etiology of avoidant personality disorder is uncertain. Because shyness and fear of strangers is a normal component of certain developmental stages, some theorists have speculated that patients with this disorder may be stagnated in their emotional growth in this regard. Because young people may "outgrow" their social awkwardness, caution is suggested in diagnosing this disorder in children or adolescents.

Clinical Findings

A. SIGNS & SYMPTOMS

Avoidant personality disorder patients possess a persistent behavioral pattern of avoidance, created by anxiety, which leads to a restricted life-style and limited social interactions.

Individuals with avoidant personality disorder are described as introverted, inhibited, and anxious. They tend to have low self-esteem and they are sensitive to rejection. They tend to be awkward, have social discomfort, and are very afraid of being embarrassed or acting foolish.

Avoidant personality disorder patients show anxiety and discomfort when discussing their problems. Their excessive concern with evaluation by others is particularly apparent during personal questioning, during which they may interpret innocuous questions as criticism. The social anxiety associated with avoidant personality disorder leads to interpersonal withdrawal and avoidance of unfamiliar or novel social situations, primarily because of fears of rejection rather than because of disinterest in others. In those relationships that are maintained, patients tend to adopt a passive, submissive role, as they are particularly uncomfortable in situations in which there is a great deal of public scrutiny and failures are likely to be widely known.

B. DIMENSIONAL PERSPECTIVES

Temperamentally, patients with avoidant personality disorder score extremely high on neuroticism and extremely low on extraversion scales, thereby being highly introverted.

Differential Diagnosis

There has been a debate as to whether avoidant personality disorder is in the spectrum of anxiety disorders or is a separate psychopathological entity. Avoidant personality disorder has been shown in familial studies to be related to chronic anxiety.

Clearly many features of avoidant personality disorder are indistinguishable from those of the Axis I disorder, social phobia. Indeed, the latter two diagnoses may actually be alternative names for the same condition. If there is a difference, the primary distinction lies in the continuing nature of avoidant personality disorder symptoms, with characteristics such as low self-esteem and an intense desire for acceptance reflecting an enduring part of the personality rather than a transient condition. Similarly, avoidant personality disorder and generalized anxiety disorder have symptoms in common, as does avoidant personality disorder and major depression. Comorbidity, therefore, exists with major depressive disorder, dysthymia, social phobia, panic disorders, and related anxiety disorders.

Treatment

A. PSYCHOPHARMACOLOGIC INTERVENTIONS

There is some support in the literature for the use of SSRIs, monoamine oxidase inhibitors and β-blocking agents for controlling the symptoms of social phobia. This suggests that these medications may also be helpful in treating avoidant personality disorder, although controlled studies have not been performed. These medications theoretically may facilitate early efforts at increasing social risk-taking, and thus, allow the patient some successful experiences that can be built upon. Other forms of anxiolytic medication (i.e., buspirone, benzodiazepines) may also be helpful for this purpose, although the risk of addiction with benzodiazepines clearly exists.

B. PSYCHOTHERAPEUTIC INTERVENTIONS

1. Group & marital therapies—Group therapy, either supportive or cognitive in focus, may be of particular use in helping patients with avoidant personality disorder to have contact with strangers within a generally accepting and supportive environment. This helps the patient to overcome social anxiety and to develop interpersonal trust. In such group encounters, the apprehensions that invariably emerge can assist avoidant personality disorder patients in understanding the effect that their rejection sensitivity has on others. Family or couples therapy may also be of particular benefit for patients who are involved in an environment that perpetuates avoidant behavior by undermining self-esteem.

2. Individual psychotherapeutic Interventions—Patients with avoidant personality disorder often seek psychotherapy for assistance with their symptoms. However, such patients are usually reluctant to disclose personal information out of fear of rejection and humiliation. Early psychotherapeutic efforts are typically directed at establishing trust through provision of support and reassurance. Subsequent efforts may be directed at encouraging assertive behavior via assertiveness training, social skills training via cognitive therapy, and exploring distorted thoughts and attitudes and overvalued assumptions that maintain social withdrawal. Similarly, behavioral desensitization using gradual exposure to social tasks that have increasing potential for provoking anxiety can lead to positive experiences that enable patients to tolerate social risk-taking.

Prognosis

Little is known about the natural course and outcome of avoidant personality disorder. The most consistent and continuing symptoms are feelings of inadequacy and social ineptitude. The social anxiety and withdrawal associated with avoidant personality disorder is obviously long-standing and generalized. However, many patients with this disorder manage adapt to their problems and show little impairment, assuming they exist in a favorable interpersonal and occupational environment. The prognosis tends to be worse if other personality disorders are present, or if the patient is in a fixed, unsupportive environment that maintains the avoidance behaviors.

DEPENDENT PERSONALITY DISORDER

DSM-IV-TR Diagnostic Criteria

A. *A pervasive and excessive need to be taken care of that leads to submissive and clinging behavior and fears of separation, beginning by early adulthood and present in a variety of contexts, as indicated by five (or more) of the following:*

    (1) has difficulty making everyday decisions without an excessive amount of advice and reassurance from others

    (2) needs others to assume responsibility for most major areas of his or her life

    (3) has difficulty expressing disagreement with others because of fear of loss of support or approval.
    (Do not include realistic fears of retribution.)

    (4) has difficulty initiating projects or doing things on his or her own (because of a lack of self-confidence in judgment or abilities rather than a lack of motivation or energy)

    (5) goes to excessive lengths to obtain nurturance and support from others, to the point of volunteering to do things that are unpleasant

    (6) feels uncomfortable or helpless when alone because of exaggerated fears of being unable to care for himself or herself

    (7) urgently seeks another relationship as a source of care and support when a close relationship ends

    (8) is unrealistically preoccupied with fears of being left to take care of himself or herself

(Reprinted, with permission, from the *Diagnostic and Statistical Manual of Mental Disorders*. 4th edn. Text Revision. Washington, DC: American Psychiatric Association, 2000.)

General Considerations

A. Epidemiology

The prevalence of dependent personality disorder has been estimated at 0.5–3.0% in the general population. Furthermore, this disorder is heavily represented in mental health treatment settings because of the general propensity that such patients have to demonstrate help-seeking behavior. The disorder is more common in women than in men. Individuals with dependent personalities tend to be somewhat older than those with other personality disorders.

B. Etiology

Theories about the cause of dependent personality disorder often suggest a childhood environment existed in which dependent behaviors were directly or indirectly rewarded, and independent activities were discouraged. Increasing evidence from twin studies, also suggests possible, but poorly defined, genetic influences.

Clinical Findings

A. Signs & Symptoms

The hallmark of dependent personality disorder is a lifelong interpersonal submissiveness. This submissiveness can be into a particular relationship, but more commonly is a generalized style of relating to others. The dependency arises from poor self-esteem and feelings of inadequacy that drive those afflicted to rely heavily on others to get their needs met. Because abandonment is greatly feared, any expression of displeasure or anger is inhibited so as not to endanger the relationship.

B. Dimensional Perspectives

Not surprisingly, dependent personality disorder patients have been found to combine increased neuroticism with agreeableness.

Differential Diagnosis

Patients with dependent personality disorder often submerge their identity within the context of a dependency relationship, in a way that is similar to borderline personality disorder. However, the dependent personality disorder patient lacks the history of turbulent relationships that characterizes the borderline personality disorder patient. The rage and manipulativeness of the latter disorder contrast with the appeasement that is characteristic of dependent personality disorder cases. However, it is relatively common for patients to meet criteria for both disorders.

Many individuals who have Axis I disorders, particularly mood and anxiety disorders, as well as those with general medical disorders can appear quite dependent and can present with low self-esteem. For these individuals, the features may be limited to the duration of the primary disorder, and do not reflect a long-standing personality pattern. Dependent personality disorder commonly co-occurs with many Axis I and Axis II disorders, especially panic disorder and agoraphobia.

Treatment

A. Psychopharmacological Interventions

Patients who have dependent personality disorder often experience fatigue, malaise, and vague anxiety. For these symptoms, SSRI or tricyclic antidepressant therapy can be useful. Anxiolytic medication may also be useful, especially during crises that emerge after efforts at establishing autonomy, since fears of abandonment and separation may be exacerbated at these times. However, as with many other disorders, use of antianxiety medications should be time limited, and focused on specific target symptoms.

B. PSYCHOTHERAPEUTIC INTERVENTIONS

1. Group/marital interventions—Patients with dependent personality disorder have been reported to derive considerable benefit from group therapy, as it offers an opportunity for the development of supportive peer relations with a low risk for abandonment. Group members can reinforce the patient's efforts at establishing autonomy and provide a protected arena in which to try out new and more constructive interpersonal behaviors.

Family or couples therapy can also be useful. It may, however, present the challenge of working within a family system in which the patient's dependency may play an important functional role. It is therefore critical to enlist the support of other family members for the patient's efforts at autonomy, lest the patient be undermined or meet with rejection or withdrawal which perpetuates the dependency cycle.

2. Individual psychotherapeutic interventions—Patients with dependent personality disorder are generally receptive to psychological treatment as part of a more general pattern of seeking assistance and support from others. The primary goal of such interventions is to make the patient become more autonomous and self-reliant. As with the other personality disorders, a variety of individual treatments of dependent personality disorder are reported useful. Cognitive–behavioral psychotherapy is reported to be very helpful in assisting in developing assertiveness and effective decision making. Negative, cognitive constructs are challenged. Assertiveness training is a typical component of treatment. Role-playing, focusing on communication skills, particularly around negative feelings allows the patient to practice assertive behaviors. In more psychodynamically oriented treatments, exploration of past separations and their impact on current behaviors, as well as exploration of the current long-term effects of dependent behavior can help the patient arrive at a greater understanding of his or her difficulties, with self-discovery reflecting another step toward autonomy.

Prognosis

The prognosis of dependent personality disorder, in the absence of comorbid diagnoses, is generally good. Individuals with this disorder are likely to have had at least one supportive relationship in the past, and generally have a capacity for empathy and trust exceeding that observed in most of the other personality disorders. The primary obstacles to improvement involve the exacerbation of anxieties as efforts toward establishing autonomy are made, and the emergence of severe depression, should the patient's desperate clinging behaviors or attempts at autonomy ultimately lead to rejection.

OBSESSIVE–COMPULSIVE PERSONALITY DISORDER

 ESSENTIALS OF DIAGNOSIS

DSM-IV-TR Diagnostic Criteria

A. *A pervasive pattern of preoccupation with orderliness, perfectionism, and mental and interpersonal control, at the expense of flexibility, openness, and efficiency, beginning by early adulthood and present in a variety of contexts, as indicated by four (or more) of the following:*

1 *is preoccupied with details, rules, lists, order, organization, or schedules to the extent that the major point of the activity is lost*

2 *shows perfectionism that interferes with task completion (e.g., is unable to complete a project because his or her own overly strict standards are not met)*

3 *is excessively devoted to work and productivity to the exclusion of leisure activities and friendships (not accounted for by obvious economic necessity)*

4 *is overconscientious, scrupulous, and inflexible about matters of morality, ethics, or values (not accounted for by cultural or religious identification)*

5 *is unable to discard worn-out or worthless objects even when they have no sentimental value*

6 *is reluctant to delegate tasks or to work with others unless they submit to exactly his or her way of doing things*

7 *adopts a miserly spending style toward both self and others; money is viewed as something to be hoarded for future catastrophes*

8 *shows rigidity and stubbornness*

(Reprinted, with permission, from the *Diagnostic and Statistical Manual of Mental Disorders.* 4th edn.

Text Revision. Washington, DC: American Psychiatric Association, 2000.)

General Considerations

A. EPIDEMIOLOGY

The prevalence of obsessive–compulsive personality disorder has been estimated at roughly 1% in the general population. Although it is more common in clinical settings, it is seen less often there than are many other personality disorders. This is because people with this disorder often view the traits in question as desirable, rather than as a problem. The disorder appears to be more common in men than in women.

B. ETIOLOGY

Psychoanalytic theories as to the etiology of obsessive–compulsive personality disorder suggest stagnation in the "anal stages" of development of personality. It is still uncertain whether overly controlling parenting has an influence on this disorder, but this has been proposed.

C. Genetics

Genetic components underlying this disorder are uncertain, and have hardly been explored. However, there is evidence that first-degree relatives of individuals with obsessive–compulsive disorder have relatively higher rates of obsessive–compulsive disorder, which would suggest a genetic relationship.

Clinical Findings

A. SIGNS & SYMPTOMS

Obsessive–compulsive personality disorder is characterized by rigidity and affective constriction, inflexibility, obstinacy, and a penchant for orderliness. Characteristically, there is a strong pattern of perfectionism. The disorder is typically associated with overconscientiousness.

Patients with obsessive–compulsive personality disorder tend to have difficulty in personal relationships because they do not like to submit to others' ways of doing things. This can lead to occupational problems, because these individuals often will simply refuse to work with others, or will be annoying to them. In a diagnostic interview, they are usually not interested in the affective quality of relationships and have a formal and somewhat stilted style of relating. They will often describe their life in a solemn, intellectualized way, as though describing a casual acquain-

tance. Their emotional tone is likely to be muted. They often provide exceptionally detailed responses to questions.

Differential Diagnosis

Obsessive–compulsive personality disorder was long considered a prelude to obsessive–compulsive disorder, a relationship that is now considered questionable. Obsessive–compulsive personality disorder differs from Axis I obsessive–compulsive disorder in that the Axis I diagnosis of obsessive–compulsive disorder is typically associated with marked distress concerning the obsessions or compulsions. The patient with obsessive–compulsive personality disorder experiences no such distress, aside from a tendency to worry in general. Indeed, the patient with obsessive–compulsive personality disorder typically views his or her preoccupation with order and perfectionism as a positive characteristic, and one that makes him or her superior to others. As a result, the relationship between the Axis I and Axis II disorders is imperfect at best, and the available evidence suggests that fewer than half of the patients with the Axis I obsessive–compulsive disorder also have an obsessive–compulsive personality disorder. Other personality disorders, such as avoidant and dependent personality are just as common in patients with obsessive–compulsive disorder. Major depressive disorder, dysthymia, and generalized anxiety disorder are often comorbid with obsessive–compulsive personality disorder. Patients with anorexia nervosa and bulimia are sometimes diagnosed with obsessive–compulsive personality disorder.

Treatment

A. PSYCHOPHARMACOLOGIC INTERVENTIONS

Pharmacotherapy has not been demonstrated to be effective in the treatment of obsessive–compulsive personality disorder. serotonergic drugs, such as clomipramine and other SSRIs have not been shown to have the degree of usefulness seen with the treatment of Axis I obsessive–compulsive disorder. However, these drugs are thought by some to helpful in decreasing the perfectionism and the ritualizing that can occur in those with obsessive–compulsive personality disorder. Also these drugs may be useful during crises in which anxiety and depression are prominent.

B. PSYCHOTHERAPEUTIC INTERVENTIONS

1. Group/marital interventions—Group therapy is difficult to conduct in patients with obsessive–compulsive personality disorder. These patients typically attempt to ally themselves with the therapist and to treat the other group members, whom they often perceive as having the "real" problems. One advantage of treatment in using the group format is that the intellectualized explanations offered by the patient are interrupted by the other group members. This increases anxiety, but also leaves the obsessive–compulsive patient more open to new experiences.

In family or couples therapy, a major challenge involves having the patient relinquish control over other family members. This process can be assisted by prescribing homework tasks in which various roles, including decision making, are reassigned within the family. The patient's desire to conform to the authority of the therapist can be used to facilitate the loosening of control over others, as well as over himself or herself.

2. Individual psychotherapeutic interventions— Obsessive–compulsive personality disorder patients are often difficult to treat because they rarely come to psychotherapeutic treatment except when urged to do so by others. They have difficulty seeing that their personality features are maladaptive. When they do come to psychotherapy on their own, they usually do so because of their associated depression, anxiety, or somatic complaints.

The individual with obsessive–compulsive personality disorder desires to perform well as a patient, consistent with his or her general pattern of perfectionism in other life areas. However, the general constriction and distrust of affective expression creates a number of resistances for the therapist to overcome. Patients may be highly critical of themselves or of the therapy, demanding justification for every intervention offered. A central part of the treatment will involve exploring the source and the unreasonable nature of the harsh and rigid standards the patient has set for both self and others.

Given the rationalizing and intellectualizing nature of obsessive–compulsive personality disorder patient, cognitive interventions are often relatively well received. Such efforts usually focus on the inaccuracy of key assumptions held by the patient (i.e. that one must be perfectly in control of the environment, or that any failure is intolerable). Consequences of such beliefs can be explored and ways to refute the beliefs discussed. In controlled clinical trials, cognitive–behavioral psychotherapy has the most efficacy in treating obsessive–compulsive symptoms.

Prognosis

Little is known about the prognosis of obsessive–compulsive personality disorder. The most stable characteristics are rigidity and problems in delegating. In the absence of co-occurring disorders, the outlook is probably favorable for such patients. The patient's capacity for self-discipline and order precludes many of the problems typical of other personality disorders. However, not a small number of these patients go on to develop Axis I anxiety disorders, and the self-criticism and barren emotional life of these patients leave them particularly vulnerable to developing depression.

OTHER PERSONALITY DISORDERS

Two personality disorders are described in an appendix to DSM-IV-TR: They are passive–aggressive (negativistic) personality disorder and depressive personality disorder. Although officially classified as personality disorders, not otherwise specified, passive–aggressive personality disorder has been in the nomenclature for many years and depressive personality disorder has been the focus of considerable research.

Passive–aggressive personality disorder is characterized by passive resistance and negativistic attitudes toward others who place demands on the individual with the disorder. Such demands are resented and opposed indirectly, through procrastination, stubbornness, intentional inefficiency, and memory lapses. Passive–aggressive individuals tend to be sullen, irritable, and cynical, and they chronically complain of being underappreciated and cheated. Interest in interpersonal attachment is typically low, and such people tend to be unsuccessful in interpersonal relationships because of their capacity to evoke hostility and negative responses from others.

Depressive personality disorder is characterized by enduring depressive cognitions and behaviors. Some researchers have proposed that this is essentially the same concept as dysthymic disorder or possibly subsyndromal depressive disorder. Depressive personality disorder patients are gloomy, and their self-esteem is habitually low. They are harsh on themselves and tend to be judgmental of others. They are pessimistic about the future and remorseful about the past. They tend to be quiet, passive, and unassertive. The disorder can be distinguished from major depression by its long-term nature and by the absence of somatic signs of depression, such as sleep or appetite disturbance.

Andreasen NC, Black DW: *Introductory Textbook of Psychiatry,* 2nd edn. American Psychiatric Press, 1995.

Benjamin LS: *Interpersonal Diagnosis and Treatment of Personality Disorders.* Guilford Press, 1993.

Cloninger RC: *Personality and Psychopathology.* American Psychiatric Press, 1999.

Coccaro EF: Psychopharmacologic studies in patients with personality disorders: Review and perspective. *J Personal Disord* 1993;7(Suppl):181.

Hubbard JR, Saathoff GB, Barnett BL Jr.: Recognizing borderline personality disorder in the family practice setting. *Am Fam Physician* 1995;52:908.

Livesley WJ: *The DSM-IV Personality Disorders.* Guilford Press, 1995.

Maj M, Akiskal HS, Mezzich JE, Okasha, A: *Personality Disorders.* John Wiley and Sons, Ltd., 2005.

Millon T: *Disorders of Personality: DSM-IV and Beyond.* John Wiley & Sons, 1996.

Morey LC: *An Interpretative Guide to the Personality Assessment Inventory (PAI).* Psychology Resources, 1996.

Oldham JM, Skodol AK, Bender DS: *Textbook of Personality Disorders.* American Psychiatric Publishing, Inc. 2005.

Waldinger RJ: *Psychiatry for Medical Students,* 3rd edn. American Psychiatric Press, Section IV. Techniques & Settings in Child & Adolescent Psychiatry, 1997.

SECTION III

Psychiatric Disorders in Children and Adolescents

Intellectual Disability

Ludwik S. Szymanski, MD, Sandra L. Friedman, MD, MPH, & Elizabeth L. Leonard, PhD

TERMINOLOGY

The term **Intellectual Disability (ID)**, commonly used in Europe, is now becoming preferred to the previous one **Mental Retardation (MR)**, although both are still used interchangeably. **Developmental disability** is a legal term defined by the Developmental Disabilities Assistance and Bill of Rights Amendments of 1996, and is used in statutes referring to entitlements. Its requirements are: The condition is due to mental and/or physical impairment, is manifested prior to age 22, is likely to be lifelong, results in substantial functional limitations in three or more major life activities and in need for lifelong services or supports.

DEFINITION

ID does not denote an illness or a single disorder entity but a behavioral syndrome of variable etiology characterized by intellectual and adaptive functioning below level expected for the person's age, education and sociocultural context. In fact, strictly speaking, it is not a mental disorder like a mood or psychotic disorder. Formal definitions of ID have evolved over time. The modern ones are tri-factorial, requiring impairment in (1) intellectual functioning, (2) adaptive functioning, and (3) onset before age 18. In the US, the standard definition is of the *Diagnostic and Statistical Manual of Mental Disorders*, fourth edition, Text Revision (DSM-IV-TR) (American Psychiatric Association 2000).

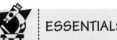 **ESSENTIALS OF DIAGNOSIS**

DSM-IV-TR Diagnostic Criteria
  Mental Retardation

A. *Significantly subaverage intellectual functioning: An IQ of approximately 70 or below on an individually administered IQ test (for infants, a clinical judgment of significantly subaverage intellectual functioning).*

B. *Concurrent deficits or impairments in present adaptive functioning (i.e., the person's effectiveness in meeting the standards expected for his or her age by his or her cultural group) in at least two of the following areas: Communication, self-care, home living, social/interpersonal skills, use of community resources, self-direction, functional academic skills, work, leisure, health, and safety.*

C. *The onset is before age 18 years*

Code based on degree of severity reflecting level of intellectual impairment:
Mental Retardation has the following levels of severity and codes:

317	Mild Mental Retardation	IQ level 50–55 to approximately 70

318.0	Moderate Mental retardation	IQ level 35–40 to 50–55
318.1	Severe Mental Retardation	IQ level 20–25 to 35–40
318.2	Profound Mental Retardation	IQ level below 20 or 25
319	Mental Retardation Severity Unspecified: When there is strong presumption of mental retardation but the person's intelligence is untestable by standard tests	

(Reprinted, with permission, from the *Diagnostic and Statistical Manual of Mental Disorders*, 4th edn. Text Revision. Copyright 2000 American Psychiatric Association.)

The second most common definition is of the American Association on MR. It also requires onset prior to age 18 and presence of significant limitations in (A) intellectual functioning (defined as an IQ score of 2 SD or more below the mean of an individually administered assessment instrument) and (B) adaptive behavior (in conceptual, social, and practical skills). For the purpose of either definition the adaptive behavior is commonly assessed clinically, but use of testing instruments such as Vineland Adaptive Behavior Scales is recommended. The American Association on Mental Retardation (AAMR) definition specifies scores on such scales of 2 SD or more below the instrument's mean.

Thus, if a person has an IQ close to the cutoff point (within the error range of the instrument, usually ±5 points), the diagnosis will depend on the level of adaptive functioning. Therefore, such person may qualify for the diagnosis of ID, for example, in school age when learning is impaired by poor academic skills but may lose this diagnosis later, with the acquisition of work skills important for an adult.

SUMMARY

1. ID is not a single disorder.
2. ID a behavioral syndrome of a triad of significant limitation in intellectual and adaptive functioning, and onset prior to age 18. It is NOT diagnosed by subaverage IQ alone.
3. The diagnosis must be made considering person's socio-cultural and linguistic diversity and associated disabilities.
4. ID does not have to be lifelong.

5. All people with ID have an ability to learn and progress and all possess strengths which must be supported in any habilitation program.

American Association on Mental Retardation: *Mental Retardation: Definition, Classification, and Systems of Supports*, 10th edn. Washington, DC: American Association on Mental Retardation, 2002.

Sparrow SS, Balla DA, Cicchetti DV: *Vineland Adaptive Behavior Scales*. Circle Pines, MN: American Guidance Series, 1984.

General Considerations

A. EPIDEMIOLOGY

Estimates of the prevalence of ID have changed over time depending on its definition. With current definition it is thought to be about 0.7–1% of the population and in about two-thirds of cases are within the mild range of severity, although there are regional differences. Persons with ID are also at increased risk for comorbid mental disorders, with the prevalence ranging between 16% and 71%, and virtually all diagnostic categories are represented.

B. ETIOLOGY

Etiologic consideration of intellectual and other developmental disabilities requires a conceptual framework that takes into account the timing of insult or risk to the developing brain and its impact on developmental functioning. There are multiple factors that may contribute to ID, with occurrence in the prenatal, perinatal, and postnatal periods. ID has many different causes, and sometimes biologic, social, behavioral, and educational factors interact to affect how a person functions (Table 31–1). There may be similarities in type of insults in all three of these time frames, such as infection, toxins, and deprivation of nutritional, environmental, and chemical substances. The timing of these insults however, often determines the degree of ID. In addition, the more significant the etiologic insult, the more likely that other types of disabilities will result, such as in motor function, communication, social, and self-help skills.

1. Perinatal insults—Perinatal insults associated with birth asphyxia has been noted to be the etiology for children with a range of intellectual disabilities and cerebral palsy. Events associated with hypoxia and ischemia can be causative, both in preterm and full term infants). Other perinatal events, such as infections and their consequences, may also contribute to developmental outcome.

2. Postnatal causes—Postnatal causes are those that are acquired. Mild MR has been associated with postnatal environmental deprivation, with lack of adequate nutritional and social support. In addition, infections, anoxia, trauma, cerebral vascular events, and malignancy and the effects of its treatment may all influence the level

Table 31–1. Intellectual Disabilities: Causes and Clinical Presentation

Etiologic Timing	Insult	Example	Clinical Presentation	Diagnostic Procedures	Complications	Prognosis
Prenatal: Genetic	Autosomal dominant	Neuro-fibromatosis	Cafe-au-lait macules, large head	Skin exam, slit lamp inspection	Seizures, bone malformations, tumors	Good, some have disabilities
	Autosomal recessive	Hurler (MPS I)	Coarse facies, hirsuitism, cloudy corneas, short stature	Skeletal X-rays, urine mucopoly- saccharides; DNA mutation analysis	Contractures, cardiac valve abnormalities, hearing impairment	ID, early death; but good with early enzyme replacement.
	X-linked	Fragile X	Large head, prominent pinnae, elongated face, prominent chin and forehead.	DNA assay for Fragile-X	Seizures; mitral valve prolapse, dilation of ascending aorta, tremors and ataxia (older)	Better with early diagnosis and education
	Chromosomal	Down syndrome: (trisomy 21, translocation)	Hypotonia, oblique palpebral fissures, simian crease	Chromosomal analysis	Congenital heart defects, hypothyroidism	Normal lifespan, possible early onset Alzheimer's dementia
	Metabolic	MSUD	Vomiting, seizures, lethargy, coma	Urine and plasma amino acids, ABG, electrolytes	Acidosis with stress or illness	Neurological damage
Prenatal: External influences	Intrauterine malnutrition	Placental insufficiency	IUGR, symmetric SGA, thin, pale, dry skin	Per standardized growth parameters	Low Apgar scores, hypoglycemia, meconium aspiration	Normal development to learning problems
	Toxins	Alcohol (fetal alcohol syndrome)	Microcephaly, smooth philtrum	History, physical examination	ADHD-like, cognitive deficiencies	Related to cognitive level
	Infections	CMV	Microcephaly, peri-ventricular calcifications, petechiae, hepatitis	Urine culture (<2 wks); maternal serology	Seizures, chorioretinitis	Hearing impairment, ID
Perinatal	Infection	Herpes virus encephalitis	Fever, vesicular rash, seizures, jaundice, respiratory distress	LP, culture of lesions	Hepatitis, pneumonia, chorioretinitis	From recovery to severe motor/cognitive impairment, death

(continued)

Table 31-1. (Continued)

Etiologic Timing	Insult	Example	Clinical Presentation	Diagnostic Procedures	Complications	Prognosis
Postnatal	Deprivation	Birth asphyxia	Respiratory distress	ABG, oxygen saturation	Seizures, CP, contractures, scoliosis	Variable, depends on level of cognition
	Infection	H. Influenzae meningitis	Hypotension, respiratory distress	LP	Seizures, HL	Good to developmental delays
	Deprivation	Nutritional	Reduced energy, attention, anemia	CBC, chem panel (including proteins)	Learning problems	Good with improved nutrition
	Trauma-emotional	PTSD	Developmental and behavioral problems	History, developmental and psychiatric evaluation	Flashbacks, nightmares	From good to long term psychiatric and learning problems
	Trauma-physical	Shaken baby syndrome	Irritability, lethargy, seizures	X-rays, MRI, fundoscopy,	Brain death	Depends on degree of trauma
	Toxins	Lead toxicity	Hyperactivity, developmental delay	CBC, blood lead level, bone X-rays	Poor compliance with treatment, continued lead exposure	From good to severe impairments: ID, ADHD, ASD
	Vascular	CVA	Reduced responsiveness, sensory, language motor, impairments	Neuroimaging, coagulation studies	Residual motor, cognitive, language impairments	Depends on timing and extent of bleeding
	Hypoxia	Near-drowning	Hypothermia, unresponsive, cardiopulmonary arrest	CXR, C-spine, mech vent, ECG, head CT, EEG, ICU support	Seizures, infection, brain death	Recovery to severe ID, CP, death

MPS: mucopolysacchridosis; MSUD: maple syrup urine disease; ABG: arterial blood gas; IUGR: intrauterine growth retardation; SGA: small for gestational age; LP: lumbar puncture; ADHD: attention deficit hyperactivity disorder; CMV: cytomegalovirus; HL: hearing loss; ID: intellectual disability; CP: cerebral palsy; CBC: complete blood count; PTSD: posttraumatic stress disorder; MRI: magnetic resonance imaging; ASD: autism spectrum disorder; CVA: cerebral vascular accident; EEG: electroencephalogram; ECG: electrocardiogram; C-spine: cervical spine imaging; CT: computed tomography; mech vent: mechanical ventilation; ICU: intensive care unit.

of cognitive function. Risk factors for mild ID have been associated with multiple births, nutritional and social deprivation, low maternal education, and teen pregnancy. While male gender has been noted to be a risk factor, this high male-to-female ratio difference is less apparent as the severity of ID increases. Other risk factors that have been associated with ID include low birth weight, and older maternal age.

C. GENETICS

Most diagnoses of ID are felt to have prenatal causes. Genetic and metabolic disorders, central nervous system malformations, congenital infections, toxic exposures, deprivation of essential elements in utero, and many idiopathic etiologies are all considered to be potential prenatal etiologic factors. Severe to profound ID is more likely associated with genetic etiologies, although genetics certainly may play a role in those with moderate and mild ID. A larger percentage of children with mild ID are also felt to have idiopathic causes.

Battaglia A, Bianchini E, Carey JC: Diagnostic yield of the comprehensive assessment of developmental delay/mental retardation in an institute of child neuropsychiatry. *Am J Med Genet* 1999;82(1):60–66.

Chapman DA, Scott KG, Mason CA: Early risk factors for mental retardation: Role of maternal age and maternal education. *Am J Ment Retard* 2002;107(1):46–59.

Crocker AC, Nelson RP: Mental retardation. In: Levine MD, Carey WB, Crocker AC (eds). *Developmental–Behavioral Pediatrics*, 2nd edn. Philadelphia: WB Saunders, 1992.

Harris JC: *Intellectual Disability*. New York: Oxford University Press, 2006.

Rubin IL: Prematurity and its consequences. In: Rubin IL, Crocker AC (eds). *Medical care for children and adults with developmental disabilities*, 2nd edn. Baltimore: Paul H. Brookes, 2006, pp. 217–232.

Szymanski L, King B: Practice parameters for the assessment and treatment of children, adolescents and adults with mental retardation and co morbid mental disorders. *J Am Acad Child Adolesc Psychiatry* 1999;38:12(Suppl):5S–31S.

Williams-Costello D, Friedman H, Minich N, Fanaroff AA, Hack M: Mproved survival rates with increased neurodevelopmental disability for extremely low birth weight infants in the 1990s. *Pediatrics* 2005;115(4):997–1003.

Winter S, Kiely M: Cerebral palsy. In: Rubin IL, Crocker AC (eds). *Medical care for children and adults with developmental disabilities*, 2nd edn. Baltimore: Paul H. Brookes, 2006, pp. 233–246.

Clinical Findings

A. SIGNS & SYMPTOMS

By definition, the onset of ID is before 18 years of age. The diagnosis, however, is usually made much earlier. Language delays often become apparent during the second year of life, with motor delay being the more common developmental concern during the first year.

Children with ID often present with delay in receptive and expressive language skills. Language and cognition are closely associated; children with severe ID are more apt to have more significant language delays. Children with more significant cognitive delay also usually present earlier than those with milder cognitive deficits. Table 31–2 provides information regarding behavioral phenotypes for specific genetic and developmental disorders.

Tests of developmental functioning in the very young child are not felt to be predictive of later cognitive skills, unless there are profound delays. The diagnosis of MR or ID is generally made after infancy, usually before the child is enrolled in school. Sometimes the diagnosis is made later, if a thorough assessment had not been performed earlier. To make the diagnosis, cognitive and adaptive abilities are assessed. Consideration also needs to be given to the environment in which a person lives, ad the manner in which he or she interacts with others on a daily basis.

There are times when the exact level of functioning cannot be determined with certainty. Sometimes a child has not yet received the needed intensive educational support and it is unclear how he or she will respond to these services. Other times, testing cannot be completed or is not felt to reflect a child's potential. In those instances, further testing is required at a future date to more accurately determine the level of functioning.

In addition to language delays, children may present with delays in play, social, and adaptive skills. Gross motor skills generally develop well, except in certain disorders associated with significant hypotonia. Fine and oral motor skills may also be affected. Developmental milestone acquisition is generally slow but steady. A child may also display developmental plateaus or regression of developmental skills. In those instances, assessment may be required to rule out the presence of metabolic, neurodegenerative, or neurophysiologic disorders.

Children with intellectual disabilities continue to learn, albeit at a rate slower than typically developing peers.

It is important to obtain a thorough medical history, which often provides etiologic information. Parental concern has been shown an important indicator of the presence of developmental problems. The history should include information about pregnancy, delivery, and the perinatal period. Information needs to be obtained regarding past and present medical issues, including illnesses and injuries. A child's response and recovery from illnesses also need to be explored. Developmental history should be obtained, including developmental milestones in the various developmental domains, as well as overall developmental trajectory. The social environment, with potential stressors, needs to be explored. Family medical history, going back three generations,

Table 31–2. Behavioral Phenotypes

Syndrome	Genetic Findings	Cognitive Features	Behavioral Features	Psychopathology
Fragile X	Full mutation: >200 CGG repeats in FMR1 on Xq27.3	IQ correlated with number of CGG repeats. Males: Mild to severe ID; females: Borderline IQ to mild ID	Gaze aversion, perseverations, repetitive speech, social withdrawal	ADHD-like, ASD-like, prone to anxiety
Smith-Magenis	Deletion on 17p11.2	Moderate ID	SIB, aggression, self-hugging, tantrums	ADHD-like, SMD
Prader-Willi	Either 15q11-q13 deletion on paternal chrom 15 or maternal uniparental disomy of chrom 15	Borderline IQ to mild ID (higher IQ with maternal disomy). Learning disability.	Compulsive hyperphagia, tantrums, aggressive behavior, skin picking	OCD, anxiety, psychotic and affective disorder, ADHD
Angelman	15q11-q13 deletion on maternal chrom 15, disomy	Severe ID	Appear happy, sociable, episodic laughter	ASD-like, ADHD-like
Williams	Deletion at 7q11.23	Borderline IQ to moderate ID	Over-friendly, social disinhibition, excessive empathy	Anxiety, ADHD, sleep disorder
Down syndrome	trisomy 21 (in 92%), translocation	Moderate-severe ID	Friendly, affectionate, some stubborn, overactive	Depression may occur; early onset Alzheimer
Rett	X-linked dominant, MECP2 mutation	Severe ID	Central "hand-wringing," poor social interaction	Early ASD features
Cornelia de Lange	No genetic marker	Severe ID	Self-injurious, compulsive, overactive, aggression	ADHD
CHARGE	Chromosome 8; CHD7 (some patients)	Mild-Moderate ID; Average IQ	Socially withdrawn, need for order	OCD, ADHD
VCFS (DiGeorge)	22q11.2 deletion	Moderate ID to average	↓ social interaction, blunt affect, poor self-esteem	ADHD, ASD, psychosis (in 25%), bipolar, schizoaffective

CGG: trinucleotides; IQ: intelligence quotient; ADHD: attention deficit hyperactivity disorder; ASD: autism spectrum disorder; ID: intellectual disability; SIB: self-injurious behavior; OCD: obsessive–compulsive behavior; FM: fine motor; exec fx: executive function.

is needed in the evaluation potential genetic factors. In addition to psychological and psychiatric assessment, the child requires a physical examination that includes a thorough neurological assessment. This examination should include assessment of growth parameters, including head circumference. Dysmorphology should be identified, as it may indicate to prenatal contributing factors. Other physical findings are important, such evaluation of integument for neurocutaneous lesions, coarse facies and/or enlarged liver and spleen for certain storage diseases, muscle distribution, bulk, or asymmetries in certain neurological disorders.

B. Psychological Testing

1. Indications for psychological assessment—Psychological assessment measures intelligence and adaptive functioning, as well as behavior and academic achievement. It aids in diagnosis, determining abilities and disabilities, treatment plan formulation, eligibility for habilitative and/or rehabilitative services and planning for other interventions. The selection of specific tests is tailored to the age and ability of the individual. Obtaining collateral information from parents, caregivers, teachers, and employers is essential for accurate assessment, since children, nonverbal individuals and persons with significant ID are unable to construct an adequate developmental and behavioral history.

The psychologist has to understand the individual's ability to sustain attention and comprehend tasks required by a particular test, in order to make an informed decision which tests yield the greatest information about cognition and behavior. Specific instruments have been developed to measure intelligence and associated cognitive abilities including attention, memory, motor function, receptive and expressive language and executive functions (planning, sequencing, organization and task management). Tests administered during childhood may be restricted to a single domain of function. With maturity it is possible to measure additional areas of cognition and behavior with greater reliability and validity. In a comprehensive assessment, a battery of tests is employed to measure multiple domains of cognition and behavior.

While personality testing is within the scope of practice for psychologists, it is less useful for individuals with significant ID who usually lack language and cognitive skills necessary for exploring intrapersonal dynamics through tests such as the Rorschach, personality inventories (Minnesota Multiphasic Personality Inventory-2 [MMPI-2]) or projective measures like picture apperception tests (Thematic Apperception Test).

2. Measurement of intelligence

The diagnosis of ID requires that intelligence, as measured on a standardized test, is two or more standard deviations below the mean, with an IQ below 70 (the other two diagnostic criteria are: Deficits in adaptive functioning and onset prior to age 18). To gain an accurate appraisal of the person's function, individual rather than group testing is required. Testing should occur in a quiet and comfortable place free from distraction. This generally precludes bedside testing except for screening tests designed for that purpose. Sufficient time should be allotted to pace the testing to the comfort level and ability of the individual. It may be necessary to provide for frequent breaks. Testing may often require several sessions over different days. The person being tested should not be fatigued. If they become hyper-aroused or extremely anxious, test data will not be valid and testing should be discontinued and administered at a later time. Tests are used for diverse populations stratified by socioeconomic status, culture, language, geographic location and gender. Individuals of low socioeconomic status may test less well than more affluent and educated persons. The low scores in such situations should not be automatically attributed to mild intellectual impairment. This is one reason why in individuals with suspected ID, measures of intelligence and adaptive behavior are critical in order not to confound lack of education, poverty or inexperience with ID. If

necessary, an interpreter should be used for persons not fluent in English. The validity of test results can be significantly affected by translation and the interpretation of results should be viewed with the caveat that tests have been normed on native English speakers. Several IQ tests have been translated into Spanish with appropriate norms for native speakers.

Psychological tests that are standardized are based on a normal distribution of scores with a mean of 100 and a standard deviation of 15 points. Normal scores range from 85–115, representing one standard deviation from the mean. Abnormal scores on standardized tests fall within 1.5–2.0 standard deviations below the mean. Subtests on intelligence tests have scores measured in scaled points ranging from 1–18 with a mean of 10 and a standard deviation of 3. Standardized tests are constructed to enable valid comparisons between scores. For example, an IQ of 85 corresponds to a scaled score of 7 on a subtest that might measure a variable like fund of knowledge (Information on the Wechsler scales) and a Z score of -1.0 standard deviations. All of these scores are at the 16th percentile and equivalently scaled for comparison.

3. Interpretation of test results

The report, prepared by the psychologist following completion of testing, lists all tests administered, raw scores and standard scores for test comparisons. It is important to stress that the summary scores, such as a Full Scale IQ, do not adequately capture individual differences enumerated by testing. The clinician needs to be aware that summary scores combine data and may lead to a false impression since they represent a mean of all tests administered. The psychologist should look at all scores, and their ranges, to gain an accurate impression of an individual's profile defining patterns of strengths and weakness across all domains evaluated. For IQ tests this means examining index or cluster scores where subtests are divided into similar constructs. Different clusters measure verbal comprehension, perceptual organization, working memory and processing speed.

Following are the other areas of importance to consider:

1. Gross and fine motor skills and coordination.
2. Language including vocabulary, syntax, pragmatics, fluency and articulation.
3. Memory including visual and verbal domains for encoding and retrieval.
4. Motor strength.
5. Visual-motor and perceptual abilities.
6. Executive skills involving planning, organization, task management, and cognitive flexibility.
7. Achievement testing including reading, arithmetic, and writing.

Commonly used psychological tests are listed in Tables 31–3 to 31–5.

4. Assessment of adaptive behavior—While adaptive behavior is often estimated clinically, preferably it should be assessed through standardized instruments, such as -II the Vineland Adaptive Behavior Scales or the American Association on Mental Retardation (AAMR) Adaptive Behavior Scales-2. These instruments are administered by interviewing parents or other caregivers, familiar with the individual. Assessment of adaptive behavior quantifies function in the major domains of development with regard to what an individual can and cannot do in comparison to age matched peers. This includes activities of daily living involving language, socialization, communication, self-care, and motor skills. Daily living activities are hierarchically evaluated to include chronological age and maturation that is the hallmark of development. For example, communication skills required for a three year-old take into account the complexity of vocabulary development for expression, comprehension and nonverbal abilities, such as gestural skills, while requisite skills for adolescents would include the ability to read, write and follow written instructions.

C. LABORATORY FINDINGS

A number of factors are considered when making the decision to perform laboratory tests. The child's presentation, medical history, developmental history, family history, physical examination, and the results of psychological testing may all influence which tests are recommended. The workup should reflect guided by the child's presentation and working hypothesis of etiologic factors, and may be done over time as certain medical disorders are ruled out. The lower the level of cognitive function, the greater is the likelihood of finding associated genetic or medical conditions.

1. Genetic testing—Genetic testing such as high resolution karyotyping and Fragile-X testing, is often performed in the assessment of children with ID, particularly when etiology is unclear. FISH studies are also frequently done to confirm or rule out a suspected genetic disorder. Newer comparative genomic hybridization (CGH), which looks at DNA at the gene level, is often being used when first line genetic testing (e.g., chromosomes and Fragile-X) are negative, yet the index of suspicion is high for a genetic disorder.

2. Metabolic screening tests—These tests are recommended by some practitioners for all children in whom etiology is unclear. Others obtain metabolic testing when the developmental trajectory is characterized by regression, particularly with common illnesses, or there is prolonged recovery from such illnesses. Children with metabolic disorders may also present with a number of signs or symptoms, including but not limited to cyclic vomiting, hearing or visual impairments, enlarged liver or spleen, coarse facies.

3. Electrophysiological testing—This testing is not a part of a routine workup for children with ID. However, these children have a higher incidence of seizures disorders compared to the general population and it increases significantly in the presence of severe ID. EEG should be obtained if there are staring episodes, paroxysmal outbursts with no identifiable precipitants, developmental regression, or behaviors consistent with seizures.

4. Evaluation of hearing acuity—This should be performed on any child with language delay, including those with ID, even in the context of a normal neonatal hearing test. If routine audiologic assessment using headphones is not feasible, visual reinforcement audiometry, in a sound field without the use of headphones, may be used to assure that hearing acuity is adequate for language development. If this test is felt to be unreliable or provides insufficient information, neurophysiologic assessment, such as auditory brainstem response (ABR) or brainstem auditory evoked response (BAER) may be performed.

5. Ophthalmologic assessment—This assessment is also important to identify specific medical conditions associated with ID, and to rule out reduced visual acuity.

D. NEUROIMAGING

Neuroimaging is not indicated for all children with the diagnosis of ID. It should be considered in the context of an abnormal neurologic exam, such as asymmetry of motor finding or abnormal reflexes. Disproportionate head growth, abnormal head size, seizures may all indicate the need for magnetic resonance imaging (MRI). The more severe the ID, the more apt positive findings will be identified on neuroimaging studies.

MRI of the brain may be obtained to identify structural abnormalities of the brain, with better resolution of brain tissue compared to the computed tomography (CT) scan. CT scan is preferred to identify osseous structures and is a quicker test, although it does provide exposure to radiation. Magnetic resonance spectroscopy (MRS) may also be used in the evaluation of metabolic disorders. PET scans and SPECT scans use radioactive tracers, based on glucose metabolism and blood flow, respectively, and may be used in the evaluation of seizure foci.

E. COURSE OF ILLNESS

The life course of ID depends on its degree, associated disabilities and etiology, as well as on psychological factors (psychopathology, behavioral traits), environmental factors (attitudes of people in immediate environment and of society at large), and services the persons receives. There are, however, common features in the life of persons who have this diagnosis. To a large extent they have

Table 31–3. Representative Tests Used to Evaluate Different Cognitive Functions at Various Ages

Name of Test	Age		
	Infant/Preschool	Child	Adult
Ability measured: Development/intelligence			
1. Bayley Scales of Infant and Toddler Development-III	●		
2. Miller Assessment of Preschoolers	●		
3. Wechsler Preschool and Primary Scale of Intelligence-III	●		
4. Wechsler Intelligence Scale for Children-IV		●	
5. Stanford-Binet 5		●	●
6. Wechsler Adult Intelligence Scale-III			●
Ability measured: Language			
1. Preschool Language Scale-4	●		
2. Peabody Picture Vocabulary Test-4		●	●
3. Expressive One-Word Picture Vocabulary Test		●	●
4. Reynell Developmental Language Scales	●	●	
5. Receptive-Expressive Emergent Language Test-3	●		
6. California Verbal Learning Test		●	●
7. Boston Diagnostic Aphasia Examination-3			●
Ability measured: Motor function			
1. Grip Strength		●	●
2. Purdue Pegboard Test		●	●
3. Grooved Pegboard Test		●	●
4. Finger Tapping Test		●	●
Ability measured: Adaptive behavior			
1. Vineland Adaptive Behavior Scales-III	●	●	●
2. AAMR Adaptive Behavior Scales-2	●	●	●
Ability measured: Executive function			
1. NEPSY-II	●	●	
2. Delis–Kaplan Executive Function System		●	●
Ability measured: Achievement			
1. Woodcock–Johnson III NU Tests of Achievement		●	●
2. Wechsler Individual Achievement Test-II			●

Table 31–4. Tests for Special Populations

Nonverbal Tests	Tests for Autism and Related Disorders
Test of Nonverbal Intelligence-3	Autism Diagnostic Interview-Revised
Leiter International Performance Scale-Revised	Autism Diagnostic Observation Scales
Raven's Progressive Matrices	Childhood Autism Rating Scale
Wechsler Nonverbal Scale of Ability	Gilliam Asperger Disorder Scale

been shaped by the *normalization* approach and currently *inclusion*. They hold that people with ID should have life opportunities as close as possible to the norms of the society at large, and that they should be included to maximally possible extent in the life of the society. They should be given supports necessary for such inclusion to occur. In most states institutionalization of a person with ID (children in particular) is not an option anymore and large state institutions are closing, their population having been reduced by about three-fourth in the past quarter century. By federal law (Individuals with Disabilities Education Act, first enacted in 1975, amended since) all children with ID are entitled to special education, mostly in regular classrooms, with all necessary ancillary services, up to age 21. Adults with ID usually receive vocational training, many have "regular" or at least sheltered jobs, and live in their communities, with their families, in small group homes or independently.

Alvarez N: Neurology. In: Rubin IL, Crocker AC (eds). *Medical Care for Children and Adults with Developmental Disabilities*, 2nd edn. Baltimore: Paul H. Brookes, 2006, pp. 249–271.

American College of Medical Genetics: Evaluation of mental retardation: Recommendations of a consensus conference. *Am J Med Genet* 1997;72(4):468–477.

Dykens E (ed): Special issue on behavioral phenotypes. *Am J Ment Retard* 2001;106(1):1–107.

Glascoe FP, Parents' concerns about children's development: Prescreening technique or screening test? *Pediatrics* 1997; 99(4):522–528.

Graham JM, Jr., Superneau D, Rogers RC, Corning K, Schwartz CE, Dykens EM: Clinical and behavioral characteristics in FG syndrome. *Am J Med Genet* 1999;85(5):470–475.

Graham JM, Jr., Rosner B, Dykens E, Visootsak J: Behavioral features of CHARGE syndrome (Hall-Hittner syndrome) comparison with down syndrome, Prader-Willi syndrome, and Williams syndrome. *Am J Med Genet* 2005;133(3):240–247.

Luckasson R, Schalock RL, Spitalnick DM, Sprent S, Tasse M, et al.: *Mental Retardation: Definition, Classification, and Systems of Support*. American Association on Mental Retardation, Washington, DC, 2002.

Summers JA, Feldman MA: Distinctive pattern of behavioral functioning in Angelman syndrome. *AJMR* 1999;104(4):376–384.

Differential Diagnosis (Including Comorbid Conditions)

In **Dementia** there is a decline in cognitive functioning from premorbid level, especially in memory. The onset may be at any age. If the onset is postnatal but prior to age 18, and premorbid development was normal, both dementia and ID might be diagnosed, but since it may be difficult to document that the premorbid development was normal, the DSM-IV-TR does not recommend diagnosing dementia in these cases before age 4–6 years, or if the condition is sufficiently described by the diagnosis of ID alone. The hallmark of **Pervasive Developmental Disorders** is a qualitative impairment in social interaction and communication: In contrast, children with ID are able to relate well to others, sometimes very affectionately, in a manner corresponding to their developmental level. However, more than half of the children with autistic disorder have a comorbid ID. By definition in **Learning Disorders** (LD) and **Communication Disorders**, there is no global intellectual impairment but skills in a specific domain are below level expected for the age, intelligence level and education. Thus, an LD may be comorbid with ID. In many **other mental disorders**,

Table 31–5. Screening Tests for Office or Bedside Evaluation

Test	Purpose	Age
Denver Developmental Screening Test-II	Overall screen for development for infants and preschool children for language, motor skills, social interaction	Birth to 6 yr
Bayley Infant Neuro-Developmental Screener	Evaluation of infant development including motor, cognitive, social/emotional skills	3 to 24 mos
Folstein Mini-Mental State Examination	Screens various mental functions involved in cognition	Adults

Table 31–6. Misconceptions about Psychopathology in People with ID

Misconception	Reality
Subaverage IQ sufficient for diagnosis	Impairments in IQ and in adaptive skills, and onset < 18 are all required
ID is lifelong	Some may lose diagnosis with improvement in adaptive skills
People with ID sooner or later stop learning	Learning is usually lifelong (like everybody's) and with appropriate services and supports their lives will improve
People with ID have unique personalities (e.g., uninhibited, aggressive)	Full range of personality types may be seen. Certain traits are more common in certain syndromes ("behavioral phenotypes"), but not unique. Low self-image and dependency are common due to environmental factors and experiences
People with ID are too retarded to have mental disorders	People with ID are at increased risk for mental disorders
People with ID have mental disorders unique to them	Full spectrum of mental disorders may be seen. Manifestations may be modified by impairments in communication skills and cognition and environmental experiences
Professionals should focus on person's deficits	Treatment and habilitation should focus on developing person's inherent strengths, compensatory strategies to overcame impairments and removing impairments if possible

such as in schizophrenia, there may be decline in both intellectual and adaptive functioning. If this occurs prior to age 18 a comorbid diagnosis of ID might be made. If the onset is at later age, the history of premorbid normal development, usually from third party informants will rule out the diagnosis of ID.

People with ID are at increased risk for developing comorbid mental disorders. There is no evidence that these disorders are different from those occurring in persons without ID, but their manifestations may differ, being modified by the level and nature of the individual's ID, as noted above. The standard DSM-IV-TR should be used, interpreted in the context of person's communication skills, intelligence, past experiences, culture and education. These will be discussed below in sections on individual disorders. In most situations DSM-IV-TR diagnosis is possible, but in some only general category of diagnosis is made and the Not Otherwise Specified (NOS) subcategory is employed. The Royal College of Psychiatrists (2001) has published a manual of psychiatric criteria for use with adults with ID complementary to International Classification of Diseases (ICD-10), quite useful, but it was not field-tested for validity. Clinicians should be aware of phenomenon of "diagnostic overshadowing": If a person has an ID, clinicians tend to ignore symptoms of a comorbid psychopathology or see it as a manifestation of ID.

The term "behavior disorder," not infrequently encountered, has not been defined and does not denote a specific diagnostic category. Persons with ID and with comorbid diverse mental disorder may have similar symptomatic behaviors. For example, aggressive behavior may be exhibited by persons who have diverse comorbid disorders such as mood, psychosis, or Posttraumatic stress disorder (PTSD). "Behavior disorder" might be used to describe nonspecific behavior that occurs in certain situations only (such as in a classroom), while a diagnosis of an underlying mental disorder has been ruled out.

A. COMORBID MENTAL DISORDER & BEHAVIORAL PROBLEMS

Professionals and general public have had many misconceptions about behavior of persons with ID. These are summarized in Table 31–6. Nevertheless, individuals with ID often have comorbid neuropsychiatric conditions that may include problems with affective regulation, anxiety and attention. They may exhibit disruptive behaviors, impulsivity, overactivity, distractibility, mood or anxiety symptoms, and more extreme and aberrant behaviors like self-injury or stereotypical motor mannerisms.

These behaviors can be evaluated during an informal observation, clinical interview, formal testing, school or work observation or home visit. There are also instruments that are used to measure behaviors associated with psychiatric and behavioral problems in individuals with ID. These usually consist of checklists identifying behaviors such as attentional problems and can be completed by parents, caregivers, or health professionals and are useful in alerting the clinician to more severe problems requiring more comprehensive evaluation.

If available, detailed behavioral data recorded at the individual's school, work or residence should be reviewed. They typically include tabulation of the frequency of behaviors in question in various settings and events that precede and follow the behaviors (antecedents and consequences). For example, temper tantrums that result in being sent out of the classroom may indicate to a person's wish to avoid a difficult classroom task. At the end of the assessment the diagnostician should be able to answer the following questions:

a. Does the person have an ID?

b. Is there a mental disorder warranting a diagnosis?

c. What is the profile of individual's strengths and impairments?

d. What are the factors causing/maintaining the problem? (biomedical, psychological, environmental)

e. Is intervention necessary?

f. What are the interventions with best benefit/risk ratio?

g. What is the predicted outcome without treatment?

In order to answer these questions, the assessment should be based on bio-psycho-social and developmental model. Even that the psychiatrists usually are not responsible for the primary diagnosis and assessment of ID,

they must do the psychiatric assessment in the context and with understanding of person's abilities, impairments and functioning in all domains. A very useful schema developed by the AAMR (2002) suggests five dimensions that should be considered:

1. Intellectual functioning and adaptive skills.
2. Adaptive behavior skills: Conceptual (language, reading and writing, money concepts, self-direction); social (such as interpersonal, responsibility, following rules and laws); practical (daily living, housekeeping, transportation, occupation, safety).
3. Participation, interaction and social roles.
4. Health (physical and mental, etiology of ID).
5. Context (environments, culture).

Thus, the first step is to review past medical, psychological, and other assessments and if these are unavailable or unreliable (e.g., only group IQ testing had been done), or outdated (e.g., old genetic testing could not diagnose Fragile-X), the patient should be referred for psychological, medical and other appropriate consultations.

The psychiatric evaluation follows usual principles, but the techniques have to be modified according to person's developmental level and communication skills, as described in Table 31–7 to 31–8.

Table 31–7. Psychiatric Assessment in ID: History

Informants	Multiple, including family, teachers, work counselors, therapists
Background history	Critically review, update if needed: Past psychological, medical, etiological, environmental assessments, school/work records
Referral history	Overt reasons for referral; why referred now (was it prompted by environmental factors); expectations of various caregivers
Presenting symptoms	Longitudinal history of symptoms, their variability with time, place, caregivers, when/where symptoms do not occur? Concrete description and examples of problem behaviors as well as strengths. Past management of problem behaviors and its effectiveness.
Past history, personality	Strengths, adaptive skills, unusual behaviors, communication patterns
Psychiatric history	Evaluations, diagnoses, hospitalizations, treatments, their results and side effects, alternative treatments
Education/work	Settings, programs, supports, results
Health	Health and developmental history, medical problems known to be associated with underlying etiology
Family history (parents, siblings, extended)	Family constellation, medical, psychiatric, and genetic history, understanding of attitudes to, and feelings about, patient's disability, appropriateness of expectations.
Environmental	Current and past services and their adequacy (medical, psychiatric, educational, work and other supports, entitlements); family's ability to advocate
Legal and cultural	Guardianship status if over 18; cultural context redisability, language environment

Table 31–8. Psychiatric Assessment in ID: Patient Interview

Setting	If possible, natural, (home, school, work, unobtrusive observation in waiting room); alone and jointly with caregivers; provide sufficient time.
Verbal techniques	Assess patient's skills: Observe communication with caregivers; use clear language, avoid leading questions or requiring yes-no answers, ascertain that questions are understood, encourage spontaneous expression
Nonverbal techniques	Observe general appearance and behavior, activity level, distractibility, eye contact, joint attention, stereotypical and other unusual behaviors, nonverbal social communication, physical clues (e.g., callus from hand-biting)
Content (if verbal)	Strengths, preferences, friendships, functioning in various settings, understanding of the evaluation and of own disability
Mental status	As much as possible avoid standard MS; preferably assess within context of general conversation

In the majority of people with ID who have a mild/moderate cognitive and communication impairment usual DSM-IV-TR diagnostic criteria can be used, although they may have to be modified to reflect the person's understanding and life context. In those whose communication skills are too low, the diagnosis is made primarily on the basis of history from caregivers and observation of patient's behavior. Modifications pertaining to more common disorders are discussed below beginning with disorders beginning in infancy and childhood.

1. Pervasive developmental disorders (PDD)—Majority of persons with a diagnosis within this category (except Asperger's and PDD NOS) have also an ID. The diagnosis is based primarily on history and clinical observations and thus standard criteria can be used. In nonverbal persons with severe/profound MR a PDD is not infrequently erroneously diagnosed on the basis of stereotypical behaviors and lack of language. However a longer observation may document that they have an ability for nonverbal social communication and relate to familiar people.

2. Learning disorders—These can be diagnosed in persons with ID, providing that the impairments in question cannot be adequately explained by the ID alone and are below level expected for person's age, education and intelligence level. Children with poor language might avoid situations demanding verbal communication through what appears as social withdrawal.

3. Feeding & eating disorders of infancy or early childhood—Pica (persistent ingestion of nonnutritive substances) is seen sometimes in children and adults with severe/profound ID and may be life threatening, as is rumination disorder. Medical assessment is essential, including testing for trace metal deficiency (which may be associated with pica), for gastro-oesophageal reflux disease (GERD) and for helicobacter pylori infection.

4. Stereotypic movement disorder (SMD)—Significant ID is often associated with variety of stereotypic movements, which appear to be self-stimulatory, and sometimes lead to self-injury (Self-Injurious Behavior [SIB]) (in which case a specifier with SIB is added) and are the reason for referral to a psychiatrist. These may also be part of behavioral phenotypes such as Lesch Nyhan syndrome, may be caused by a painful, undiagnosed medical condition or be a side effect of a medication (such as tics resulting from methylphenidate). SIB can lead to severe injury or be even life threatening. SMD is diagnosed on the basis of observable behaviors. SIB may include head banging and hitting, self-biting, eye-poking, extreme aerophagia.

5. Attention-deficit/hyperactivity disorder (ADHD)—Hyperactivity is a frequent problem with children with ID in school settings. However, a diagnosis of ADHD should not be made unless the presentation is inconsistent with the child's developmental level. Since most of DSM-IV-TR criteria for ADHD are based on observable behaviors, the standard diagnostic approaches are used. Inappropriate classroom placement and other environmental anxiety producing factors are often the cause of ADHD-like symptoms in this population. They may also be a part of a behavioral phenotype, for example, in Fragile-X and fetal alcohol syndrome (FAS) or a side effect of a medication.

6. Conduct disorder—One must ascertain that the individual is aware that the inappropriate behaviors are prohibited by societal rules (same applies to diagnosis of Antisocial Personality Disorder in adults). This may be difficult in persons with low or no language skills. Persons who are discharged from institutions without preparation might not be aware of the rules of conduct that are expected of them in the community. Children and adults with ID are also vulnerable to pressure from others and might be induced by them to break rules and laws. Sometimes they are quite willing to do it, believing that in this way they can make friends.

7. Aggression & other challenging behaviors—The term "Challenging Behavior" is often applied nonspecifically to any behavior that is inappropriate by caregiver's standards. Aggression and SIB are the most frequent referral complaints. There is no single diagnostic category, or treatment, for aggression. It may be a part of the presentation of virtually any mental disorder in this population, including psychosis, mood disorder, ADHD, conduct disorder, anxiety disorder, PTSD, personality disorder. Comprehensive diagnostic assessment is required, including information whether aggression is limited to certain persons or situations. Detailed description of actual behavior is necessary, since some caregivers tend to label any resistance they encounter as aggressive. Aggression is sometimes ascribed to seizure disorders, which many people with ID have. A more complex aggressive behavior, targeted at a specific person(s), is usually not linked to seizures.

In assessing these behaviors one should differentiate between factors that caused them and factors that maintain them. For example, a painful middle ear infection might lead to intractable head banging and self-injury. The pain may subside after a course of antibiotics but the SIB may continue if the individual has learned that it provided him with increased attention by the staff.

8. Psychotic disorders—Schizophrenia occurs in people with ID at least as often as in general population and probably more often. In persons with mild ID and good verbal skills the manifestations are similar to those in people without ID and same diagnostic criteria may be used. However, the verbal productions (e.g., description of delusions) may be simpler and concrete. The diagnosticians must be sure that their questions are understood: for example, when asked about "hearing voices' many patients will assume that they are being asked about their hearing ability. Careful interviewing and "interpreting" by a caregiver may help in differentiating poor language skills from psychotic verbalizations. In people with significant ID and poor or no language, the diagnosis will have to rely on observations of behavior and mood changes, such as behaviors becoming bizarre, and moods becoming inappropriate. In such cases diagnosing subcategories of the disorder will not be possible and the general diagnosis of Psychotic Disorder NOS might have to be used. Self-stimulatory and SIBs alone, often seen in this population should not be seen as an evidence of psychosis.

People with a velo-cardio-facial syndrome (that may be associated with mild degree of ID), are at increased risk for developing a psychotic disorder (as well as a mood disorder). Presentation corresponding to a Brief Psychotic Disorder has been seen in persons with ID who were subjected to very stressful situations beyond their control and understanding.

9. Mood disorders—People with ID may suffer of, and may be even at increased risk for, *depressive disorders*. Unfortunately they often remain undiagnosed, because depressed individuals tend to be quiet and not disruptive and may not have language abilities to verbalize depressed mood, anhedonia or thoughts of death, but may refuse to attend activities they like or even start engaging in SIB. Suicidal behavior had been described in this population. Aggressive behavior is not infrequent, especially if depressed persons are forced to attend activities required in their setting. Their complaints may be simpler, such as that they feel sick. The diagnostician will have to rely on behavioral observations, presence of vegetative signs and on mood changes as observed by caregivers. An important differential diagnosis is dementia, especially in adults with Down syndrome. These individuals are at high risk for developing Alzheimer Dementia. While neuropathological changes may occur by age 40, clinical dementia is usually not seen before 50, or even later. A person with dementia usually tries to perform a task but fails, while one with depression may not even attempt it. Persons with *bipolar disorders* comorbid with ID may exhibit irritability, aggression, and hyperactivity, masturbate excessively, may laugh and appear inappropriately happy. The changes in behavior and mood are usually observed and reported by caregivers familiar with the individual.

10. Anxiety disorders—Full spectrum of anxiety disorders has been reported in people with ID. Again here, poor communication skills may interfere with assessing subjective feelings of anxiety, obsessive thoughts, discomfort, panic, worry, etc. However, in most of these disorders the diagnosis may be made on the basis of behavioral observation. It may be difficult to decide whether perseverative and self-stimulatory behaviors often seen in people with significant ID are part of an obsessive–compulsive disorder, since in nonverbal persons it is unclear whether they are related to obsessions and whether the person recognizes that they are unreasonable. Anxiety disorders are also part of various behavioral phenotypes. *Posttraumatic stress disorder* is often missed if the individuals cannot report a traumatic event (such as an abuse) or are not believed, if they report it. On the other hand, persons with ID are at risk for abuse and victimization and PTSD should be always considered as a differential diagnosis and if otherwise unexplained behavioral changes occur. An event not considered traumatic by an average person may be traumatic for a person with ID. The modifications of DSM-IV-TR diagnostic criteria for PTSD that are aimed at children are also relevant for people with significant ID.

Harris JC: *Intellectual Disability*. New York NY: Oxford University Press, 2006.

Patja K, Iivanainen M, Raitasuo S, et al.: Suicide mortality in mental retardation: A 35-year follow-up study. *Acta Psychiatr Scand* 2001;103:307–311.

Reid AH: Schizophrenic and paranoid syndromes in persons with mental retardation: Assessment and diagnosis. In: Fletcher RJ, Dosen A (eds). *Mental Health Aspects of Mental Retardation*. New York: Lexington Books, 1993, pp. 98–110.

Szymanski LS, Kaplan LC: Mental Retardation. In: Wiener JM, Dulcan MK (eds). *Textbook of Child and Adolescent Psychiatry*, 3rd edn. Washington, DC: American Psychiatric Press, 2004, pp. 221–260.

Reiss S, Levitan GW, Szyszko J: Emotional disturbance and mental retardation: Diagnostic overshadowing. *Am J Ment Defic* 1982;86:567–574.

Treatment

A. PLANNING FOR TREATMENT & EDUCATION

Once a level of function is determined, it is important for the clinician to utilize this information to develop a plan of intervention to allow persons with ID to achieve their highest functional potential. Therefore, a psychologist will take test information and interpret it to formulate a treatment and education plan to enhance developmental strengths and determine accommodations or remedial methods to strengthen weaker skill areas. Except in cases where impairment is severe (i.e., IQ less than 55), individuals are likely to have a profile of developmental strengths and weaknesses for which an individualized treatment plan can be developed. For preschool and latency children this may include referral for early intervention or special education. For adolescents and young adults, in addition to special education, assessment aids in planning for prevocational and vocational training and preparation for independent or supported employment and living.

B. PSYCHOPHARMACOLOGIC INTERVENTIONS

Medical problems are more common in people with severe ID. Seizure disorders may present with behavioral problems or developmental regression. Their identification therefore greatly impacts on the type of treatment that is required. The aim is to treat individuals with the fewest number of anticonvulsant medications to have the best seizure control without excessive sedation. For seizures that are refractory to more conventional treatment, treatments such as the ketogenic diet, vagal nerve stimulator, and even surgery may be considered.

C. PSYCHOTHERAPEUTIC INTERVENTIONS

Behavioral management programs also may need to be developed for both the home and school settings.

D. OTHER INTERVENTIONS

Cerebral palsy is commonly associated with severe ID. Spasticity has significant impact on the spine, hips, and joints. There needs to be aggressive management to prevent or reduce contractures and to enhance mobility. These individuals generally require physical and occupational therapy. They may also require orthotic and adaptive seating devices. Muscle relaxants may be needed and sometime orthopedic surgery. Individuals with associated abnormal motor function may have problems with feeding, which may be due to difficulties with swallowing, chewing, gastric motility, and/or gastrointestinal reflux. Determination needs to be made regarding the source of the problem, which will impact on recommendations for change in consistency of foods, need for medications and/or tube feeding to avoid aspiration and promote adequate weight gain.

In terms of educational services and developmental treatments, children less than 3-years of age are eligible for Early Intervention services. With the passage of the Individuals with Disabilities Act (IDEA; PL 101–476) and its subsequent amendments, educational services in the least restrictive environment are now mandated for all children until age 21. In addition to specialized educational curricula, children often require different types of therapy. Occupational therapy addresses fine motor, sensory processing, and adaptive skills. Speech therapy works on receptive and expressive language, articulation, and oromotor problems. Both occupational therapists and speech pathologists may provide feeding therapy. Adaptive physical education may be provided for children with motor difficulties. Resource room assistance may be provided to children who are integrated into a regular classroom but require additional services for certain subject.

Alvarez N: Neurology. In: Rubin IL, Crocker AC (eds). *Medical Care for Children and Adults with Developmental Disabilities*, 2nd edn. Baltimore: Paul H. Brookes, 2006, pp. 249–271.

Friedman S: Nursing homes. In: Rubin IL, Crocker AC (eds). *Medical Care for Children and Adults with Developmental Disabilities*, 2nd edn. Baltimore: Paul H. Brookes, 2006, pp. 94–103.

Giangreco MF: Interactions among programs, placement, and services in educational planning for students with disabilities. *Ment Retard* 2001;39(5):341–350.

Treatment for Mental Disorders in People with ID

The common mistake in treatment of mental disorders in this population is to rely only on psychotropic drugs.

Yet, principles of treatment are the same as of corresponding disorders in people who do not have ID. The major modifications are based on the fact that persons with ID and comorbid mental illness are essentially multi-handicapped, have multiple needs and usually depend on others. Therefore an effective treatment program must be coordinated with treatment approaches in all domains in order to address person's comprehensive needs.

A. PRINCIPLES

Comprehensive diagnostic assessment (as delineated above) of needs, strengths, required supports, in all areas.

1. Clear goals of treatment, beyond ameliorating inappropriate behaviors that trouble the caregivers, and toward helping the patient to achieve optimal, feasible quality of life.

2. Insuring that the patient receives a comprehensive treatment, of which the psychiatric therapies are a part, and which may include medical treatment, education and habilitation, appropriate school or work, and living arrangements

3. Collaboration between professionals on treatment team.

4. Full range of psychiatric interventions, including psychotherapies, family therapy, behavior therapy, psychopharmacology, as needed.

5. Systematic, evidence-base follow-up on patient's progress and adverse effects.

6. Consideration of human rights and legal requirements.

B. PSYCHOTHERAPEUTIC TREATMENT

Persons with ID and comorbid mental disorders can be good candidates for psychotherapy, if they possess sufficient language skills to engage in interactive communication with the therapist, even on a simple level (similarly to children).

Principles of psychotherapy in this population are summarized in Table 31–9.

Group psychotherapy follows similar guidelines, but emphasis is given to helping the patients to learn from one another. In multiple-family group therapy several families, including patients and their siblings, participate and learn from one another's experience.

Table 31–9. Guidelines for Psychotherapy with Persons with ID*

Requirements of the therapist:	Motivated, experienced with people with ID, flexible, serving as role model, supportive but not paternalistic, respectful
Requirements of the patient	Willingness, basic communication skills
Verbal techniques	Adapt language level to patient's understanding; avoid too complex or too simple language; insure that the patient understands (beyond asking "do you understand?"; avoid questions requiring "yes" or "no" answers, encourage spontaneous verbalizations; explain abstract concepts using concrete examples.
Verbal content	Focus on patient's strengths first; explore understanding of own behavior and others' feelings about it; if necessary teach through concrete examples; teach understanding of own strengths and disability using examples (e.g., presence and absence of "talent"); if necessary teach concrete scripts of appropriate behavior and communication.
Nonverbal techniques	Use games, other activities, to create model situations for interpersonal interactions: for example, losing in a game; managing anger. Guide the patient to recognize appropriateness/inappropriateness of own behavior from video- or audio-tapes of self.
Family counseling	Involve family through separate, later joint, session; model how to communicate and manage patient's behavior; to create opportunities to succeed; gradually increase their active participation while decreasing therapist's; teach them to promote patient's self-image and independence; provide them with behavior management plan; help to see patient's strengths and to achieve gratification from him/her.
School/caregivers collaboration	Obtain ongoing behavioral data on follow-up: Collaborate on implementing and generalizing behavioral program; promoting patient's self-image, strengths and independence; providing opportunities to succeed (e.g., meaningful jobs, friendships and functions at school).

*Adapted from Szymanski LS, Kaplan LC: Mental retardation. In: Wiener JM, Dulcan MK (eds). *American Psychiatric Publishing Textbook of Child and Adolescent Psychiatry*, 3rd edn. Washington, DC: American Psychiatric Publishing, 2004, pp. 221–260.

Standard techniques of behavioral therapy are used (discussed in Chapter XX. The focus with people with ID should be on rewards for appropriate behaviors and minimizing what they can see as punishment (e.g., "time out"). For some individual the latter might actually be a reward if it leads to avoiding tasks they dislike. To be effective, behavioral plan has to be generalized to all situations (such as home and school) and implemented consistently by all caregivers. Baseline behavioral assessment and detailed follow up are necessary. Aversive techniques are not used, except very rarely by some, as a last resort, for a brief time, in case of intractable SIB/aggression, in well controlled situations, and only if markedly effective.

Psychopharmacological Treatment

Same principles of rational psychopharmacology as with people without ID should be followed:

a. Other treatable reasons for inappropriate behaviors should be ruled out (e.g., medical disorder, or painful condition underlying a SIB).

b. If a comorbid mental disorder has been diagnosed, it should be treated appropriately.

c. Least intrusive intervention should be tried first, for example, behavioral management, environmental changes) and medications added later as needed.

d. Behavioral data should be collected at baseline and in a regular follow-up.

e. Lowest effective dose should be employed.

f. A drug should be used only if documented effective and with good risk-to-benefit ratio. One should avoid a "Christmas tree" approach of adding new drugs to ineffective ones.

g. Polypharmacy should be avoided unless augmenting affect of a medication is clearly documented.

h. Adverse effects should be carefully monitored, bearing in mind that a person with limited language skills may not be able to report them. Drug-drug interactions should be considered as people with ID often are on multiple medications for medical reasons.

i. An overall goal must be kept in mind: Maximizing person's quality of life, rather than eliminating "challenging" behaviors solely for caregivers' convenience.

j. Legal requirements should be followed: Obtaining informed consent of the individual or the guardian or court in states that require it (e.g., Massachusetts).

Aman MG, Collier-Crespin A, Lindsay RL: Pharmacotherapy of disorders in mental retardation. *Eur Child Adolesc Psychiatry* 2000;9(Suppl 1):98–107.

Harris JC: *Intellectual Disability.* New York, NY: Oxford University Press, 2006.

Health Care Financing Administration (HCFA): General Safety Precautions for Psychopharmacological Medications in ICFs/MR, Washington, DC: HCFA, 1996, p. 3.

Reiss S, Aman MG: Psychotropic Medications and Developmental Disabilities: *The International Consensus Handbook.* Columbus OH: The Ohio State University, 1998.

Szymanski LS, Kaplan LC: Mental retardation. In: Wiener JM, Dulcan MK (eds). *American Psychiatric Publishing Textbook of Child and Adolescent Psychiatry,* 3rd edn. Washington, DC: American Psychiatric Publishing, 2004, pp. 221–260.

Szymanski LS, Kiernan WE: Multiple family group therapy with developmentally disabled adolescents and young adults. *Int J Group Psychother* 1983;33:521–534.

Complications & Adverse Outcomes of Treatment

Mortality rate for people with ID is generally considered to be comparable to the general population. Medically fragile people with severe to profound MR are also living longer but they continue to have a higher mortality rate than the general population. These individuals may be nonambulatory, dependent for all their daily needs, have seizure disorders, orthopedic problems associated with spasticity, and may require tube feeding. They may have problems handling oral secretions, increasing their risk for aspiration, or maintaining a patent airway. Chronic pulmonary problems, such as reactive airway disease or recurrent lower respiratory tract infections may occur.

Other medical problems more commonly seen in severe ID include sleep disorders, vision impairment, and hearing loss.

Botsford A: Status of end of life care in organizations providing services for older people with a developmental disability. *Am J Ment Retard* 2004;109:421–428. *Med Gen* 1999;82(1):60–66.

Strauss DJ, Shavelle RM, Anderson TW: Life expectancy of children with cerebral palsy. *Pediatr Neurol* 1998;18:143–149.

Prognosis

All children with ID need the love and support of their families, and to be included in family life. With ongoing support to meet each individual's needs, the functioning of a person with ID can be expected to improve over time.

Children do best with early identification of their developmental problems, and appropriate services and interventions. The etiology and severity of the ID also influences the level of functioning.

Approximately 80–85% of children ID fall within the mild range. They generally are able to read, write, and perform math between the 3rd and 6th grade levels. Individuals with mild ID usually live independently within the community as adults, and often the diagnosis is no longer used. Moderate ID affects about 10% of children with ID. They may learn some basic reading and writing, as well as a number of functional skills. As adults, they usually require some type of oversight or supervision. Approximately 3–5% of children with ID are in the severe range. They generally are not able to learn basic academics, although may be able to perform some self-help skills and routines. They will require supervision in their daily activities and living environment. Profound MR affects about 1–2% of children. Children with profound retardation will need intensive support for the rest of their lives. They may or may not be able to communicate by verbal or other means.

Resources

Organization of families and advocates for children and adults with intellectual and developmental disabilities, The ARC of the United States, at www.thearc.org

National Dissemination Center for Children with Disabilities, at www.nichcy.org

American Association on Intellectual and Developmental Disabilities, at www.aaidd.org

National Organization for Rare Disorders, at www.rarediseases.org

United Cerebral Palsy, at www.ucs.org

Browder DM, Xin YP: A meta-analysis and review of sight word research and its implications for teaching functional reading to individuals with moderate to severe disabilities. *J Spec Educ* 1998;32(3):130–153.

Crocker AC, Nelson RP: Mental retardation. In: Levine MD, Carey WB, Crocker AC (eds). *Developmental–Behavioral Pediatrics*, 2nd edn. Philadelphia: WB Saunders, 1992.

Meltzer LJ, Zadig JM: Educational assessment. In: Levine MD, Carey WB, Crocker AC, Gross RT (eds). *Developmental–Behavioral Pediatrics*. Philadelphia: WB Saunders, 1983.

Wolfensberger W: *Normalization: The Principle of Normalization in Human Services*. Toronto: National Institute on Mental Retardation, 1972.

American Academy of Child and Adolescent Psychiatry (AACAP): Practice parameters for the assessment and treatment of children, adolescents, and adults with mental retardation and co-morbid mental disorders. *J Am Acad Child Adolesc Psychiatry* 1999;38(suppl 12):5S–31S.

American Association on Mental Retardation: *Mental Retardation: Definition, Classification, and Systems of Supports*, 10th edn. Washington, DC: American Association on Mental Retardation, 2002

American Psychiatric Association: *Diagnostic and Statistical Manual of Mental Disorders*, 4th edn. Text Revision. Washington, DC: American Psychiatric Publishing, 2000.

Aylward G: *Bayley Infant Neurodevelopmental Screener*. San Antonio, TX: Psychological Corporation, 1955.

Bayley N: *Bayley Scales of Infant and Toddler Development*, 3rd edn. San Antonio, TX: Psychological Corporation, 2005.

Brown L, Sherbenou R, Johnson S. *Test of Nonverbal Intelligence*, 3rd edn. San Antonio, TX: Psychological Corporation, 1997.

Brownell R (ed).: *Expressive One-Word Picture Vocabulary Test*, 2000 edn. Novato, CA: Academic Therapy Publications, 2000.

Bzoch KR, League R, Brown V: *Receptive-Expressive Emergent Language Test*, 3rd edn. Austin, TX: Pro-ed, 2003.

Chaney RH Eyman RK: Patterns of mortality over 60 years among persons with mental retardation in a residential facility. *Ment Retard* 2000;38:289–293.

Cohen M: *Children's Memory Scale*. San Antonio, TX: Psychological Corporation, 1997.

Delis D, Kaplan E, Kramer J: *Delis-Kaplan Executive Function System*, San Antonio, TX: Psychological Corporation, 2001.

Crocker AC: The developmental disabilities. In: Rubin IL, Crocker AC (eds). *Medical Care for Children and Adults with Developmental Disabilities*, 2nd edn. Baltimore: Paul H. Brookes, 2006, pp. 15–22.

Delis D, Kramer J, Kaplan E, Ober B: *California Verbal Learning Test-Children's Version*. San Antonio, TX: Psychological Corporation, 1994.

Delis D, Kramer J, Kaplan E, Ober B: *California Verbal Learning Test*, 2nd edn. San Antonio, TX: Psychological Corporation, 2000.

Dunn LM, Dunn LM: *Peabody Picture Vocabulary Test*, 4th edn. Circle Pines, MN: American Guidance Service, 2006.

Folstein M, Folstein S, McHugh P, Fanjiang G: *Mini-Mental State Examination*. Lutz, FL: Psychological Assessment Resources, Inc., 2001.

Frankenburg WK, Dodds J, Archer P, Bresnick P, et al.: *Denver Developmental Screening Test*., 2nd edn. Denver, CO: Denver Developmental Materials, Inc., 1990.

Gilliam J: *Gilliam Asperger Disorder Scale*. Austin, TX: Pro-ed, 2001.

Goodglass H, Kaplan E: *Boston Diagnostic Aphasia Examination*, 3rd edn. San Antonio, TX: Psychological Corporation, 2000.

Kazuo N, Leland H, Lambert N: *AAMR Adaptive Behavior Scales*, 2nd edn. Lutz, FL: Psychological Assessment Resources, 1992.

Korkman M, Kirk U, Kemp S: for the *NEPSY*, 2nd edn. San Antonio, TX: Psychological Corporation, 2007.

Lord C, Rutter M, DiLovore P, Risi S: *Autism Diagnostic Observation Schedule*. Los Angeles, CA: Western Psychological Services, 1999.

Moldavsky M, Lev D, Lerman-Sagie T: Behavioral phenotypes of genetic syndromes: A reference guide for psychiatrists. *J Am Acad Child Adolesc Psychiatry* 2001;40(7):749–761.

Miller LJ: *Miller Assessment for Preschoolers*, San Antonio, TX: Psychological Corporation, 1982.

Raven JC: *Raven's Progressive Matrices*, San Antonio, TX: Psychological Corporation, 2003.

Reynell JK, Gruber CP: *Reynell Developmental Language Scales* (U.S. Edition), Lost Angeles, CA: Western Psychological Services, 1990.

Roid GH: *Stanford-Binet Intelligence Scales*, 5th edn. Itasca, IL: Riverside Publishing, 2003.

Roid GH, Miller L: *Leiter International Performance Scale-Revised*. Woodale, IL: Stoelting Company, 1997.

Royal College of Psychiatrists: *DC–LD, Occasional Paper OP 48*. London: Gaskell, 2001.

Rutter M, Le Couteur A, Lord C: *Autism Diagnositic Interview-Revised*. Los Angeles, CA: Western Psychological Services, 1994.

Schloper E, Reichler R, Renner B: *Childhood Autism Rating Scale*. Los Angeles, CA: Western Psychological Services, 1998.

Sparrow S, Cicchetti D, Balla D: *Vineland Adaptive Behavior Scales*, 2nd edn. New York: Pearson Assessments, 2006.

Wechsler D: *Wechsler Intelligence Scale*, 3rd edn. San Antonio, TX: Psychological Corporation, 1997.

Wechsler D: *Wechsler Memory Scale*, 3rd edn. San Antonio, TX: Psychological Corporation, 1997.

Wechsler D: *Wechsler Individual Achievement Test*, 2nd edn. San Antonio, TX: Psychological Corporation, 2001.

Wechsler D: *Wechsler Preschool and Primary Scale of Intelligence*, 3rd edn. San Antonio, TX: Psychological Corporation, 2002.

Wechsler D: *Wechsler Intelligence Scale for Children*, 4th edn. San Antonio, TX: Psychological Corporation, 2003.

Wechsler D, Naglieri J: *Wechsler Nonverbal Scale of Ability*. San Antonio, TX: Psychological Corporation, 2006.

Williams-Costello D, Friedman H, Minich N, Fanaroff AA, Hack M, Improved survival with increased neurodevelopmental disabilities for extremely low birth weigh infants in 1990s. *Pediatrics* 2005;115:997–1003.

World Health Organization: *International Classification of Diseases and Related Health Problems*, 10th Revision. Geneva: World Health Organization, 1992.

Woodcock RW, McGrew KS, Mather N: *Woodcock-Johnson III*, Normative Update. Itasca, IL: Riverside Publishing, 2006.

Zimmerman I, Steiner V, Pond R: *Preschool Language Scale*, 4th edn. San Antonio, TX: Psychological Corporation, 2002.

Learning Disorders

32

Michael G. Tramontana, PhD

DEFINITION

Terms such as learning disorder and learning disability often are used interchangeably, although the latter term is used more commonly. A major stride in the definition of learning disabilities came from the National Joint Committee for Learning Disabilities. The National Joint Committee for Learning Disabilities defined a learning disability as a generic term that refers to a heterogeneous group of disorders manifested by significant difficulties in the acquisition and use of listening, speaking, reading, writing, reasoning, or mathematical abilities. These disorders are intrinsic to the individual and presumed to be due to central nervous system dysfunction. Even though a learning disability may occur concomitantly with other handicapping conditions (e.g., sensory impairment, mental retardation, social and emotional disturbance) or environmental influences (e.g., cultural differences, insufficient/inappropriate instruction, psychogenic factors), it is not the direct result of those conditions or influences (Hammill et al. 1981, p. 336).

This definition went further than the earlier one contained in the Education for All Handicapped Children Act of 1975 (P.L. 94–142) by stipulating specifically that a learning disability must be presumed to be due to central nervous system dysfunction. Although this was implied in previous definitions, never before was it made explicit. Accordingly, the newer definition helps to resolve a good deal of confusion and ambiguity involving identification and differential diagnosis. Deficiencies in academic achievement can arise from a variety of factors, operating alone or in combination. To say that there is a learning disability, however, means that there must be a basis for inferring that some form of brain dysfunction is involved.

ESSENTIALS OF DIAGNOSIS

Diagnostic Criteria
Diagnostic and Statistical Manual of Mental Disorders, 4th edition, Text Revision (DSM-IV-TR) identifies three types of learning disorders: (1) reading disorder,

(2) mathematics disorder, and (3) disorder of written expression. In each disorder, the diagnosis depends on documentation that
- *Achievement in the area, as assessed on an individually administered standardized test, falls substantially below expectations based on the person's age, measured intelligence, and education*
- *The deficiency significantly interferes with academic achievement or daily activities requiring the particular skill*
- *The skill deficiency exceeds what usually would be associated with any sensory deficit, if present*
Inherent in these criteria are considerations pertaining to the severity, extent, and specificity of the observed deficit—whether it be in reading, mathematics, or written expression. The deficit must be nontrivial or substantial, although this is not defined further by DSM-IV-TR. It must affect relevant aspects of daily functioning. It also must be specific and not simply reflective of intellectual, sensory, or educational limitations.

The diagnostic category of learning disorder not otherwise specified refers to deficiencies in reading, mathematics, or written expression that interfere with academic achievement but do not meet criteria for a specific learning disorder. This is an ambiguous category that probably should not be viewed as representing a disorder. At best, it implies that a learning disorder is suspected but cannot be documented through ordinary means.

General Considerations

A. EPIDEMIOLOGY

Estimates have varied, but about 2–8% of all school-aged children in the United States are thought to have a learning disability. The estimates are arbitrary to some extent, as they are based on the adoption of an agreed-upon cutoff in a continuous distribution. These estimates are influenced not only by debates over what the objective criteria for identification should be (see below) but also by public policy considerations having to do with the allocation of special services.

ETIOLOGY

The issue of etiology is addressed, at least in broad terms, by the National Joint Committee for Learning Disabilities definition of learning disabilities. In one form or another, brain dysfunction is the source of a learning-disabled individual's deficit(s) in reading, mathematics, or written expression. The dysfunction may stem from genetic or congenital factors, arising especially during middle to later stages of fetal brain development. Neuropathologic studies suggest the presence of relatively subtle irregularities (e.g., focal dysplasia, abnormal cortical layering, polymicrogyria), often clustering in the left perisylvian region, although the precise pattern will vary with the type of learning disabilities involved. This observation accounts for the specific nature of learning disabilities, in that earlier or more widespread abnormalities in brain development typically would give rise to more generalized disorders such as mental retardation. Insults occurring after birth may be a factor, provided that they affect the acquisition rather than loss of a particular skill. Although similar deficits may arise, the convention is to regard a learning disability as a neurodevelopmental disorder rather than as an acquired brain injury.

There have been a number of misconceptions regarding the cause of learning disabilities. One misconception has suggested that children with disabilities are not disordered but rather delayed on certain developmental dimensions, their difficulties presumably reflecting a slower rate of maturation of an otherwise normal brain. This would explain why a fairly severe disability can exist in the absence of documented brain impairment, at least when gross indices are used. However, current research does not support such a hypothesis. There is no evidence that the brains of learning-disabled individuals are immature, or unfinished, in some way. Rather, newer and more detailed investigations have documented specific structural abnormalities. Nor is there any indication that the disabled learner's performance resembles that of a normal younger child or that the disability is eventually outgrown. The child with learning disabilities is not merely delayed but rather deviant in the performance of processes necessary for normal reading, math, or writing. The disability may be "silent" in earlier years, giving the false impression of normal brain development, only to become evident when the child enters school.

Galaburda AM, Kemper TL: Cytoarchitectonic abnormalities in developmental dyslexia: A case study. *Ann Neurol* 1979;6:94.

Hammill DD et al.: A new definition of learning disabilities. *Learn Disability Quart* 1981;4:336.

Clinical Findings

A. PSYCHOMETRIC CRITERIA

Clear operational criteria are needed in order to identify learning disabilities. For example, how does one decide whether an individual's achievement falls "substantially below expectations" (a DSM-IV-TR diagnostic criterion)? This determination is usually based on some type of discrepancy criterion that stipulates the minimum difference that must exist between scores obtained on standardized tests of the individual's intelligence quotient (IQ) and scores obtained on one or more areas of an achievement test.

In what is probably the most commonly used form of evaluation, IQ-achievement comparisons are made using standard scores. Different school systems set their own cutoffs, although the minimum discrepancy is typically one to two standard deviations (SDs), or 15–30 points for standard scores with a mean of 100 and a SD of 15. For example, for an individual with a measured IQ of 105, an achievement test score of 90 or less would be needed to meet discrepancy criteria at 1 SD, 75 or less at 2 SDs, and so forth. The problem with this method is that it does not correct for the correlation between IQ and achievement test scores. IQ and achievement test scores usually correlate moderately, so that a high score on one test will often be accompanied by a less extreme (lower) score on the other because of regression to the mean. As a result, high-IQ individuals tend to be over-identified, and low-IQ individuals under-identified, as having a learning disability.

A better approach utilizes regression-based criteria that adjust the standard test score comparisons for the correlation between IQ and achievement. A regression equation is derived for each achievement measure based on its obtained correlation with IQ (this correlation is usually available in the published test manual). This approach allows for an examination of any discrepancy between actual achievement and expected achievement predicted by the IQ measure. A cutoff between 1 and 2 standard errors of prediction (SE_{pred}) typically would be used in determining whether the discrepancy is significant.

B. SUBTYPES

Learning disabilities occur singly or in combination. Obviously, the underlying pattern of cognitive deficits will vary depending on how many types of learning disability are involved.

Each type of learning disability also can be further differentiated or subtyped based on the pattern of underlying deficits. To date, much of the research has focused mainly on reading and has identified two especially robust patterns of reading disability, or dyslexia: an auditory–linguistic subtype and a visual–spatial subtype.

For example, the problem with letter reversals and other perceptual distortions that are commonly thought to characterize dyslexia are associated with the visual–spatial subtype of reading disability. However, the auditory–linguistic subtype of reading disability is the more prevalent subtype. A common feature of most poor readers (and spellers) is a weakness in phonologic processing, which makes it difficult for the reader to phonemically segment spoken or printed words. Poor fluency in extracting words from printed material (and vice versa) is the result.

Hynd GW, Connor RT, Nieves N: Learning disabilities subtypes: Perspectives and methodological issues in clinical assessment. In: Tramontana MG, Hooper SR (eds). *Assessment Issues in Child Neuropsychology.* New York: Plenum Publishing, 1988, pp. 281–312.

Psychological Corporation: *Wechsler Individual Achievement Test.* 2nd edn. New York: Harcourt Brace Jovanovich, 2002.

Shankweiler DP, Crain S: Language mechanisms and reading disorder: A modular approach. *Cognition* 1986;24:139.

C. Assessment Procedures

The most commonly used measure of general intelligence for school-aged children is the Wechsler Intelligence Scale for Children, third edition (WISC-III). For measuring academic achievement, numerous individually administered standardized measures are available. Comprehensive or broadband batteries include the Wechsler Individual Achievement Test and the Woodcock-Johnson Psycho-Educational Battery—Revised. Both of these tests include specific subtests that assess skills in reading, mathematics, and written expression.

Wechsler D: *Wechsler Intelligence Scale for Children.* 4th edn. New York: Psychological Corporation, 2003.

Woodcock RW, Johnson MB: *Woodcock-Johnson Tests of Achievement.* 3rd edn. Itasca, IL: Riverside Publishing, 2001.

Differential Diagnosis

A key issue to consider is whether an individual's poor achievement in one or more areas is merely the result of low intelligence. That is, a child's reading skills may be poor not because of a specific processing disorder but because of generally low aptitude or learning ability. Although similar underlying deficits (e.g., poor phonology) may be involved in both mentally retarded and nonretarded disabled readers, the requirement for specificity would not be met in the case of mental retardation. By definition, discrepancy-based criteria for learning disabilities would help to make this differentiation.

Similarly, other exclusionary criteria pertaining to the diagnosis of learning disabilities (e.g., sensory impairment, cultural differences, inadequate instruction) must be considered. If such factors are present, it must be assumed that, whether operating alone or in combination, they cannot fully account for deficits exhibited by a particular child.

One of the more common differentiations to be made is between learning disabilities and attention-deficit/hyperactivity disorder (ADHD). In both disorders, poor school achievement is likely, although the underlying mechanisms differ. In ADHD, the problems have to do more with the disruptive effects of inattention and poor task persistence that result in poor learning or skill acquisition. The child's performance is generally more variable in ADHD than in learning disabilities, and close observation often will reveal that the child is capable of processing the material but becomes unfocused or distracted at times. In learning disabilities, the processing deficits persist even when attention is optimal. Of course, some children have both conditions: estimates of comorbidity are at about 25%.

Emotional factors also must be distinguished from learning disabilities. School functioning can become impaired by a significant emotional disturbance, which makes it essential for the clinician to gather a careful history of the onset of academic symptoms. Emotional factors tend to exert a generalized or nonspecific effect, usually by impeding concentration or motivation. Although not the direct cause of specific disabilities, emotional factors may often worsen or compound the disabilities. In some cases, phobic reactions may occur to certain types of material, causing significant avoidance and further decreases in achievement. Careful evaluation will almost always document an underlying pattern of relatively lower aptitude upon which specific anxiety reactions become superimposed.

Barkley RA: Attention deficit disorder with hyperactivity. In: Mash EJ, Terdal LG (eds). *Behavioral Assessment of Childhood Disorders,* 2nd edn. New York: Guilford Press, 1988, pp. 281–312.

Treatment

Generally speaking, there are three types of treatment or intervention for learning disabilities: remedial approaches, compensatory approaches, and interventions for secondary social–emotional problems.

A. Remedial Approaches

Remedial approaches are aimed directly at improving specific skills. For example, a child with poor phonologic processing may receive intensive instruction and practice with phoneme-grapheme correspondence to improve word-attack skills in reading. Although there is no age cutoff per se, remedial interventions tend to have more of an impact earlier on, usually before the child reaches about 10 years of age. Effectiveness also depends on whether the interventions appropriately target the child's particular pattern of underlying deficits. A child with dyslexia may receive intensive help with visual tracking, even though visual problems may have nothing to do with why he or she is unable to read fluently (as would be true in the vast majority of cases). There has been a proliferation of therapies for learning disabilities, many of which lack empirical validation of their effectiveness.

B. COMPENSATORY APPROACHES

Compensatory approaches help the individual to compensate, or work around, a particular deficit rather than to change it directly. These approaches are usually deferred until after an adequate course of remediation has been tried and the deficit persists. The individual should be assisted in developing strategies for containing the problem and managing to go on despite it. For example, the person with poor phonology may be taught to rely more on whole word recognition to improve reading fluency. In more severe cases, the individual may have to learn how to adapt without being a proficient reader—concentrating efforts instead on developing minimal "survival skills" (e.g., recognizing common phrases, reading a menu) while emphasizing other areas.

C. INTERVENTIONS FOR SECONDARY SOCIAL–EMOTIONAL PROBLEMS

Children with learning disabilities are at increased risk for problems with frustration, performance anxiety, negative peer interactions, school avoidance, and low self-esteem. Services may include education of parents on how to manage common emotional reactions, school-based interventions that teach positive coping skills, and individual psychotherapy for patients in whom more significant emotional problems have emerged. Pharmacotherapy should be considered when more pronounced or persistent anxiety or depressive symptoms are present and when ADHD is also present.

Prognosis

Children generally do not outgrow learning disabilities. As noted earlier in this chapter, one of the common misconceptions regarding learning disabilities was that they merely reflect a delay—the implication being that the child will catch up eventually and exhibit normal functioning. Children with learning disabilities do improve, but except in the mildest cases, a relative weakness in the affected skill will persist. Children may even improve to roughly average levels, although this achievement would still fall below the expectations for an otherwise bright individual.

Reviews of research on adult outcomes suggest that, as a group, individuals with learning disabilities attain lower educational and occupational levels. Outcomes are poorer in patients with more severe learning disabilities, lower IQ, frank neurologic impairment, and lower socioeconomic status. Evidence regarding the long-term benefits of early educational intervention is inconclusive.

Spreen O: Prognosis of learning disability. *J Consult Clin Psychol* 1988;56:836.

Motor Skills Disorder & Communication Disorders

33

Michael G. Tramontana, PhD, & Barry Nurcombe, MD

■ MOTOR SKILLS DISORDER (DEVELOPMENTAL COORDINATION DISORDER)

 ESSENTIALS OF DIAGNOSIS

DSM-IV-TR Diagnostic Criteria
- **A.** *Performance in daily activities that require motor coordination is substantially below that expected given the person's chronological age and measured intelligence. This may be manifested by marked delays in achieving motor milestones (e.g., walking, crawling, sitting), dropping things, "clumsiness," poor performance in sports, or poor handwriting.*
- **B.** *The disturbance in Criterion A significantly interferes with academic achievement or activities of daily living.*
- **C.** *The disturbance is not due to a general medical condition (e.g., cerebral palsy, hemiplegia, or muscular dystrophy) and does not meet criteria for a pervasive developmental disorder.*
- **D.** *If mental retardation is present, the motor difficulties are in excess of those usually associated with it.*

(Reprinted, with permission, from *Diagnostic and Statistical Manual of Mental Disorders*, 4th ed. Text Revision Copyright 2000 American Psychiatric Association.)

General Considerations

Recent research suggests that developmental coordination disorder can be divided into several subcategories (Table 33–1).

A. EPIDEMIOLOGY

It is estimated that 6% of schoolchildren have developmental coordination disorder. Children with perceptual motor defects have a high incidence of educational problems and psychological maladjustment.

B. ETIOLOGY

Motor development involves the gradual acquisition of central control over reflex movement. There is controversy over whether this acquisition involves the suppression of reflex and spontaneous cyclic movements of early infancy or whether infantile movements are incorporated into the elements that become voluntary motor skills.

Skilled movement requires a program of action with a specified objective or set goal. The program is composed of a sequence of hierarchically organized subroutines under executive control. Once acquired, motor skills are flexible. For example, the child who has learned to walk can do so on smooth, rugged, soft, or hard surfaces. The adaptation to different situations of the programmed subroutines requires accurate perception, central processing, executive control, and progressive feedback. Feedback monitors the approximation of the program to the set goal and modifies the timing, speed, force, and direction of movement until the desired endpoint is achieved. Initially, feedback produces jerky movements, as the child struggles to master the skill. Eventually, the skill is regulated centrally and the subroutines automated. A variety of skills can be built up from a limited number of practiced subroutines deployed in accordance with combinatorial rules. The combinatorial rules act as a kind of grammar, organizing the subroutines in hierarchical fashion. Skilled performance can be delayed or disrupted if basic reflexes are not suppressed or incorporated into the program, or if the following functions are delayed, defective, or disrupted: Perception, central processing and programming, motor function, or feedback.

The hypothesis of minimal brain damage or minimal brain dysfunction was formerly invoked to explain minor sensorimotor abnormalities or immaturities, however, there is no way to prove this hypothesis. It is unclear whether the defects or delays occur in the peripheral

Table 33–1. Subcategories of Developmental Coordination Disorder

---

Clumsiness: inefficiency in the performance of fine motor movements

Adventitious movements: synkinesis, chorea, tremor, or tics

Dyspraxia: inability to learn or perform serial voluntary movements to complete skilled acts

Material-specific dyspraxia: motor execution below expected for age with regard to writing (dysgraphia), drawing (constructional dyspraxia), or speech (verbal dyspraxia)

Neurologic soft signs: nonnormative performance on motor or sensory neurologic tests in the absence of localizable neurologic disease or defect

Pathologic handedness: left-handedness associated with left-hemispheric defect and paresis of the right hand

---

or in the central apparatus or, if so, how they relate to developmental coordination disorder.

C. GENETICS

Like many other neurodevelopmental disorders of childhood onset, it is likely that there are multiple vulnerability genes associated with this condition. None, however, have been identified as yet.

Clinical Findings

A. SIGNS & SYMPTOMS

1. Clumsiness—The clumsy child is slow, jerky, and inefficient in fine-motor performance. Agonist and antagonist muscles are poorly coordinated. Motor milestones are delayed. The child drops things, tends to lose his or her balance, and is poor at activities requiring hand-eye coordination. Clumsiness can affect a particular set of muscles (e.g., orofacial, hand and finger, shoulder girdle), several sets, or the entire body musculature. The child's social development is likely to be affected, particularly if clumsiness is associated with learning problems.

2. Adventitious movements—These movements involve one or more of the following unwilled movements during a purposeful motor activity: synkinesis, chorea, tremor, or tic.
Synkinesis refers to movement in a set of muscles other than that in which the primary motor action takes place. It may be homologous (i.e., symmetrical) or heterologous (i.e., asymmetrical). For example, while drawing with the right hand, the child with synkinesis moves his or her left hand (homologous) or tongue (heterologous). **Chorea** refers to repetitive abrupt movements of

the limbs or face. **Tremor** refers to rhythmic oscillations of a body part. A **tic** is an abrupt, involuntary, repetitive movement of a particular set of muscles, usually in the face, mouth, head, neck, or diaphragm.

3. Dyspraxia—Despite normal strength, coordination, and perception, the dyspraxic child is unable to learn or perform motor skills. Dyspraxia may involve all effector muscles or may affect mainly the orofacial musculature, hand, or trunk and lower limb. The components of the motor skill are intact, but they are combined in an incoherent manner. A clumsy child will slowly get the job done. The dyspraxic child will not get the job done at all.

4. Material-specific dyspraxia—Children with material-specific dyspraxia exhibit defective motor performance in regard to specific tasks such as handwriting (specific dysgraphia), drawing and construction (constructional dyspraxia), or the articulation of words (verbal dyspraxia).

5. Neurologic soft signs—Found normally in younger children, neurologic soft signs represent a heterogeneous group of phenomena that disappear with normal development. Soft signs are regarded as abnormal if detected beyond a normative cut-off age (8–10 years). They are usually found incidentally unless tested for specifically. Their reliability, validity, and significance are disputed. A number of studies have suggested an association with cognitive dysfunction, learning problems, and psychiatric disturbance. In some cases soft signs may be related to mild brain damage; in other cases they may be related to a genetically determined factor that also correlates with a nonspecific vulnerability to psychiatric disturbance.

6. Pathologic handedness—Pathologic left-handedness occurs following damage during early development to the left hemisphere, causing a shift from right- to left-handedness. Right-sided hypoplasia, impaired visuospatial functioning, and language impairment are often found in association with this condition.

A. ASSESSMENT PROCEDURES

After taking a developmental history, processing questions directed at elucidating motor performance, and administering a neurologic examination, the clinician can apply the specific assessment procedures described in the following sections:

1. Clumsiness—Gubbay's standardized test battery for the assessment of clumsy children, Denckla's Finger Tapping Test, and Rapin et al.'s Peg-Moving Procedures Test for Clumsiness are useful screening instruments.

2. Adventitious movements—The Fog Test and Wolff et al.'s procedure screen for synkinesis are useful. In order to elicit choreiform movements, Wolff and Hurwitz had children stand with their eyes closed; arm, wrists, and fingers extended; and wrists pronated.

3. Dyspraxia—The Lincoln-Oseretsky Test includes a subtest for dyspraxia. Dyspraxia can be tested by having the child imitate hand postures, pantomime manual activities, and use actual objects (e.g., pen, cup) in an appropriate way.

4. Material-specific dyspraxia—Dysgraphia is tested by observing handwriting. Constructional dyspraxia is tested by having the child copy drawings (e.g., the Bender-Gestalt Test) or block designs. Verbal dyspraxia is screened for using the Reynell Developmental Language Scales.

5. Neurologic soft signs—Neurologic soft signs can be screened for with the Physical and Neurological Examination for Soft Signs or the Examination for Minor Neurological Signs in Children. The Examination for Minor Neurological Signs tests the following: Digit span, visual tracking, speech, nystagmus, eye symmetry, hand dominance, crossed dominance of arm and leg, right-left self-identification, right-left identification on examiner, bilateral hand stimulation, face-hand apposition, finger localization, graphesthesia, stereognosis, synkinesis, finger-to-nose apposition, diadochokinesis, and passive head turning.

B. PSYCHOLOGICAL TESTING

Additional psychological testing should be undertaken if there is evidence of attentional difficulties or specific areas learning disability.

C. LABORATORY FINDINGS

Laboratory tests are seldom necessary in the evaluation of clumsiness unless there are abnormal findings on neurologic examination or a history of acute changes in motor skills. However, measurement of creatine kinase and lactate dehydrogenase should be performed with children who have reduced muscle mass or limited capacity for physical exertion.

D. NEUORIMAGING

Abnormal findings on neurological examination suggestive of a focal brain abnormality should have magnetic resonance imaging studies or computed tomography as part of their evaluation.

E. COURSE OF ILLNESS

Typically, mild and moderate degrees of clumsiness in early childhood improve over development. More severe clumsiness has a less favorable outcome only in regard to motor proficiencies.

Pincus JH: Neurological meaning of soft signs. In: Lewis M (ed). *Child and Adolescent Psychiatry: A Comprehensive Textbook,* 3rd edn. Philadelphia: Lippincott Williams & Wilkins, 2002, pp. 573–581.

Shafer SO, et al.: Hard thoughts on neurological "soft signs." In: Rutter M (ed). *Developmental Neuropsychiatry.* New York: Guilford Press, 1983, pp. 113–143.

Shaffer D, et al.: Neurological "soft signs": Their origins and significance for behavior. In: Rutter M (ed). *Developmental Neuropsychiatry.* New York: Guilford Press, 1983, pp. 144–163.

Wilson PH: Practitioner review: Approaches to assessment and treatment of children with DCD: An evaluative review. *J Child Psychol Psychiatry* 2005;46:806–823

Differential Diagnosis

Clumsiness is observed in chronic intoxication with neuroleptic and anticonvulsant drugs, in neuromuscular disorders (e.g., Charcot-Marie-Tooth disease, Duchenne's disease), and in upper motor neuron disorders (e.g., cerebral palsy, degenerative disorders). Children with Down syndrome, autism, Asperger's syndrome, specific dyslexia, and ADHD are sometimes more clumsy than is appropriate for their mental age.

Synkinesis is associated with agenesis of the corpus callosum, Klippel-Feil syndrome, hypogonadism, midline facial defects, and a rare familial syndrome. It may be associated with ADHD and conduct disorder. Chorea is observed in Sydenham's chorea (anti-streptolysin titer and electrocardiogram should be ordered to test for rheumatic fever), hyperthyroidism, benign familial chorea, CNS degenerations (e.g., Wilson's disease, Hallervorden-Spatz disease, homocystinuria, Huntington's disease), and tardive dyskinesia. Tremor is associated with posterior fossa tumors; neuroleptic, lithium, or phenytoin toxicity; hyperthyroidism; and benign familial tremor. Simple motor tics should be distinguished from Tourette's syndrome.

Dyspraxia is associated with subacute sclerosing panencephalitis, HIV encephalopathy, Rett's disorder, and degenerative disorders of the CNS, whether inborn or acquired. Dyspraxia can be associated with learning disorders and possibly ADHD and autism. Dysgraphia and oral-motor dyspraxia may be associated with neurofibromatosis, congenital heart disease, and homocystinuria. Constructional dyspraxia is observed in William's disease. Verbal dyspraxia has been described in galactosemia and fragile-X syndrome.

Treatment

A number of treatment methods have been proposed, but it is not clear whether any of them is effective. Ayres designed a motor training program based on the theory that motor skills disorders are caused by a failure to inhibit primitive reflexes. Kephart's motor training targets posture, balance, locomotion, manipulation, catching, and propulsion. Bobath and Connolly have designed physiotherapy and occupational therapy techniques for the remediation of motor handicaps.

Complications/Adverse Outcomes of Treatment

All children with developmental difficulties in motor coordination should receive supportive care failure to do so may lead to with increased academic, emotional, and behavioral problems.

Prognosis

Children with motor deficits that continue into adolescence and adulthood are more likely than their peers to have poor social competence, reduced academic motivation, lower self-esteem, obesity, and poorer physical fitness in part due to their reluctance to engage in physical activity and sports.

Connolly K: Motor development and motor disability. In: Rutter M (ed). *Developmental Psychiatry.* Baltimore: University Park, 1981, pp. 138–153.

Deuel RK: Motor skills disorders. In: Hooper SR, Hynd GW, Mattision RE (eds). *Developmental Disorders: Diagnostic Criteria and Clinical Assessment.* Hillsdale, NJ: Lawrence Erlbaum Associates, 1992, pp. 239–281.

Gillberg C: Deficits in attention, motor control, and perception: A brief review. *Arch Dis Child* 2003;88:904–910.

Voeller KKS: Nonverbal learning disabilities and motor skills disorders. In: Coffey CE, Brumback RA (eds). *Textbook of Pediatric Neuropsychiatry.* Washington, DC: American Psychiatric Press, 1998, pp. 719–768.

COMMUNICATION DISORDERS

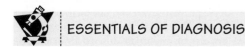 ESSENTIALS OF DIAGNOSIS

Diagnostic Criteria
DSM-IV-TR identifies the following categories of communication disorder:

- ***Expressive language disorder:*** *A disturbance manifested by symptoms such as markedly limited vocabulary, errors in grammatical relationships, or difficulties with word recall or sentence production*

- ***Mixed receptive-expressive language disorder:*** *A disturbance that includes the symptoms of an expressive language disorder together with deficits involving the processing or understanding of spoken words and sentences*

- ***Phonological disorder:*** *A disturbance, formerly known as a developmental articulation disorder, manifested by developmentally inappropriate production, use, representation, or organization of speech sounds, such as sound substitutions or sound omissions*

- ***Stuttering:*** *A disturbance in the normal fluency and temporal patterning of speech characterized by one or more of the following: Sound and syllable repetitions, whole-word repetitions, prolongations, interjections, broken words, blocking, circumlocutions, and excess tension in word production*

In each disorder, the problem must be severe enough to interfere with the patient's school or occupational achievement or with social communication. The problem also must exceed what would be expected based on the patient's age, intelligence, or dialect and on the presence of environmental deprivation or speech-motor or sensory deficits (if a sensory, speech-motor, or known neurologic deficit is present, it should be coded as an Axis III disorder). In addition, the diagnosis of either an expressive language disorder or mixed receptive-expressive language disorder requires that the criteria for a pervasive developmental disorder are not met.

The DSM-IV-TR category communication disorder not otherwise specified refers to any disturbance in communication that does not meet the criteria for a specific disorder of communication as noted in this section. Such disorders include voice disorders, cluttering (in which excessive wordiness interferes with idea expression), and so on. Although not specifically mentioned in DSM-IV-TR, deficits in pragmatic language abilities are included in this category. The term "pragmatics" refers to the use of language in a social context, with respect to either the understanding or expression of intended meanings. "Getting the message" entails more than simply a literal decoding and processing of words according to syntactic rules. It relies on the incorporation of a broader range of features, many of them nonverbal, such as prosodic and gestural cues. The interpretation of indirect meaning, humor, or sarcasm often depends heavily on these features. The same is true with respect to effective expression within a social context, which from a psychiatric standpoint is an especially important dimension of language functioning, as it often may relate to problems with interpersonal relationships and social skills development.

General Considerations

DSM-IV-TR criteria reflect a number of advancements in the conceptualization and definition of communication disorders in childhood. Many discussions on the topic make a distinction between acquired and developmental language disorders. An **acquired language disorder,** or acquired aphasia in childhood, is a syndrome involving impairment in one or more language abilities after the normal onset of speech. It usually has an identifiable neurologic basis and in general can be classified using the same terms used to classify adult aphasias. By contrast, a **developmental language disorder** (sometimes referred to as congenital aphasia) impedes the normal acquisition of language. It has no obvious point of onset, and although a neurologic basis may be suspected, it may not be verifiable. Earlier versions of DSM criteria specifically referred to developmental speech and language disorders. This distinction was dropped in DSM-IV, where the criteria were treated purely on functional grounds without implicit reference to type of onset.

Another improvement was the elimination of a category of communication disorders in childhood referring solely to receptive language impairment. The possibility of a specific disorder of receptive language, similar to Wernicke's aphasia, cannot exist in a child who has never learned to speak. Any disorder affecting receptive language, which would interfere with a child's ability to process and understand spoken input, will necessarily impede the child's ability to produce spoken language. Thus language disorders in children generally are either global or primarily expressive in nature.

A. Epidemiology

Prevalence rates for childhood speech and language deficits vary according to the classification criteria and cutoff points used in defining abnormality. Such deficits can be defined strictly on statistical grounds, as when impaired performance is defined as falling below a particular score on a standardized test. For example, if the cutoff is set at two standard deviations (SDs) below the mean, then by definition, 2% of the reference group would fall in the impaired range; this impairment rate would rise to roughly 7% if the cutoff were set at 1.5 SDs, and so forth. Shrinkage in the estimates would result if exclusionary criteria were considered.

There also appears to be an elevated rate of comorbidity with childhood psychopathology. For example, in one study 60% of children with language disorders met diagnostic criteria for ADHD.

B. Etiology

Speech and language disorder have multiple etiologies, some genetic, some congenital, and some arising from perinatal trauma such as prematurity and anoxia. Some form of underlying brain dysfunction has generally been assumed, even in disorders of the so-called developmental variety, although evidence to support this assumption may be lacking. Many studies examining children with language disorders—especially earlier studies—failed to document the presence of any CNS abnormalities.

New and important insights have begun to unfold, especially with recent technological advances in the study of brain function. For example, electrophysiologic features in the newborn—specifically involving auditory evoked responses over the left hemisphere—are predictive of language skills at 3 years of age. Such findings support a general presumption of left-hemispheric dysfunction in many speech and language disorders. Pragmatic language functions, and their dependence on various nonverbal abilities, are thought to be influenced strongly by right-hemispheric processes.

C. Genetics

Language disorders occur more frequently in families with a history of language or learning problems than in the general population and are about four times more likely in boys than girls. As genetically complex disorders it is likely that interactive relationships between multiple genetic loci will be important and lead to the degree of affectedness within specific domains of disability. However, there has been at least one autosomal dominant gene, FOXP2, on chromosome 7q31 that has been identified through the study of three generations of one family with a severe communication disorder.

Clinical Findings

A. Signs and Symptoms

Communication disorder is a broad term used to describe a variety of developmental disorders including those associated with cognitive impairment, in which speech and language also are affected. Specific disorders must be distinguished because of important differences in the approach to treatment and prognosis.

B. Psychological Testing

Several key issues must be addressed in the diagnosis and evaluation of communication disorders. First, a child's speech or language functioning must be assessed through the use of standardized, individually administered tests. Basing the diagnosis on clinical observations alone is generally insufficient, except when the nature or severity of the disorder prevents formal testing. Table 33–2 describes sample measures and instruments.

Second, cutoff points should be set in determining abnormality or impairment on specific measures. In other words, what constitutes a significant deficit? This is somewhat arbitrary, although the cutoff is typically set at about 2 SDs below the mean on any particular measure, at or below which the obtained score would be considered to reflect impairment. A slightly higher cutoff may be

Table 33–2. Assessments for Specific Speech and Language Capabilities

Capabilities measured	Tests
Word comprehension	Peabody Picture Vocabulary Test—3rd Edition
Expressive vocabulary, or naming abilities	Expressive Vocabulary Test
Listening comprehension for spoken instructions of increasing length and complexity	Token Test for Children
Multifaceted measures of language	Clinical Evaluation of Language Fundamentals—4th Edition Test of Language Development—Revised
Speech articulation	Goldman-Fristoe Test of Articulation
Pragmatic language functions	No standardized tests; Wigg has developed a series of checklists for evaluating pragmatics behaviorally in children 3 years of age and up

used (e.g., 1–1.5 SDs) if the goal pertains more to initial screening than to formal diagnosis. A more liberal cutoff may also be used when it reflects a level of performance that is clearly discrepant with the child's more general functioning. Thus a score of 85 on a standardized language measure—which technically falls in a low average range—could be viewed as reflecting a significant problem in a child with an intelligence quotient of 115 or more.

Finally, how is an unbiased estimate of a child's global abilities obtained, against which his or her language performance can be compared? DSM-IV-TR requires that this estimate be based specifically on a nonverbal measure of intellectual capacity. This is because many intelligence measures depend heavily on verbal abilities; thus their results would be unduly lowered when a specific language impairment is involved. Measures of nonverbal intelligence include the Test of Nonverbal Intelligence, the Leiter International Performance Scale, and the Performance section of the Wechsler Intelligence Scales.

C. Laboratory Findings

All children with a communication disorder should have a complete medical evaluation and formal audiologic testing to detect medical conditions or hearing loss that may contribute to their condition.

D. Neuroimaging

Abnormal findings on neurological examination suggestive of a focal brain abnormality should have magnetic resonance imaging studies or computed tomography as part of their evaluation. Functional neuroimaging in this area has also accelerated in recent years. Typically dyslexic children exhibit altered patterns of brain activation in a variety of brain regions including the left parietotemporal cortex as well as frontal regions. At present the diagnostic value of these studies has yet to be established.

E. Course of Illness

Communication disorders are usually detectable before 4 years. Severe forms may be apparent by 2 years of age. Children with communication disorders are at high risk for developing learning disabilities and experiencing academic difficulties when they enter school. Parents should develop skills to advocate for their children in order to ensure that they receive the services they need.

Differential Diagnosis

The valid diagnosis of a communication disorder requires that it be differentiated from other factors that could interfere with effective communication. Language acquisition can be impeded by environmental deprivation, although such deprivation rarely would constitute the primary cause of a language disorder. Hearing-impaired children and children with neuromotor dysfunction may exhibit slow oral language growth. However, a specific language impairment may also be inferred if the degree of impairment exceeds what would be expected due to the sensory or sensorimotor deficit(s) alone. The same is true with respect to mental retardation, if present.

It is especially difficult to distinguish language disorders from autism or other pervasive developmental disorders. A communication impairment of one kind or another is a defining characteristic in various forms of pervasive developmental disorders. Important differences that may distinguish pervasive developmental disorders include the idiosyncratic use of words, aprosodic features, deviant eye contact, and an apparent disinterest in communication as reflected in the absence of a gestural language system or other nonverbal means of communication. Also, unlike the poor auditory memory often observed in language-impaired children, many children with pervasive developmental disorders exhibit superior memory.

It is also difficult sometimes to distinguish language impairment and ADHD. In both disorders, the child may have difficulties following spoken language or in expressing ideas in a focused and goal-directed manner. In ADHD, however, the problems with efficient focusing would not be limited to verbal areas. Both disorders may coexist (indeed the comorbidity rate appears fairly high), in which case the attention deficits may be especially pronounced when verbal processing is involved.

Many forms of learning disabilities can be viewed as the extension of language processing problems into the school-age period, especially when skills such as reading, spelling, and writing are involved. These problems can be considered language-based forms of learning disorders, particularly if accompanied by broader problems with language comprehension or production. The range of learning disabilities is varied, however, in that nonverbal types of learning disabilities also exist.

Treatment

Therapeutic services in the area of communication disorders are provided by appropriately certified speech and language pathologists. Services may focus on speech impediments, including problems with voice quality, oral-motor control, and phonologic and fluency weaknesses. Receptive and expressive language processing problems may also be addressed, with exercises aimed at improving word comprehension, naming abilities, syntactic awareness, and higher-order listening comprehension and formulation skills.

Depending on the therapist's qualifications, services may be directed toward facilitating pragmatic language abilities such as interpreting indirect meanings, utilizing nonverbal cues, and applying associated skills necessary for effective social communication (e.g., taking turns, maintaining eye contact). Treating pragmatic deficits is a more specialized aspect of language intervention that is related closely to behaviorally oriented treatment approaches focusing on social skills development. Such approaches are not necessarily emphasized in the training and experience of all speech and language pathologists; thus it must be considered specifically when exploring potential referral options. The same is true with respect to identifying speech and language pathologists who are suited for remedial work in areas such as mnemonics and language-based learning disabilities.

Arthur G: *Arthur Adaptation of the Leiter International Performance Scale.* Washington, DC: Psychological Services Center, 1952.

Brown L, Sherbenou RJ, Dollar SJ: *Test of Nonverbal Intelligence.* Austin, TX: Pro-ed, 1982.

Cohen DJ, Paul R, Volkmar FR: Issues in the classification of pervasive and other developmental disorders: toward DSM-IV. *J Am Acad Child Psychiatry* 1986;25:213.

Crary MA, Voeller KKS, Haak NJ: Questions of developmental neurolinguistic assessment. In: Tramontana MG, Hooper SR (eds). *Assessment Issues in Child Neuropsychology.* New York: Plenum Publishing, 1988, pp. 249–279.

DiSimoni F: *The Token Test for Children.* Boston: Teaching Resources, 1978.

Dunn LM, Dunn LM: *Peabody Picture Vocabulary Test*—3rd edn. Circle Pines, MN: American Guidance Service, 1997.

Goldman R, Fristoe M: *Goldman-Fristoe Test of Articulation.* Circle Pines, MN: American Guidance Service, 1969.

Hammil DD, Newcomer PL: *Test of Language Development.* Austin, TX: Pro-ed, 1988.

Molfese DL: The use of auditory evoked responses recorded from newborn infants to predict language skills. In: Tramontana MG, Hooper SR (eds). *Advances in Child Neuropsychology.* Vol 1. Springer-Verlag, 1992, pp. 1–23.

Paul R, Cohen DJ, Caparulo BK: A longitudinal study of patients with severe developmental disorders of language learning. *J Am Acad Child Psychiatry* 1983;22:525.

Semel E, Wiig EH, Secord W: *Clinical Evaluations of Language Fundamentals*—4th edn. San Antonio, TX: Psychological Corporation, 2003.

Wechsler D: *Wechsler Intelligence Scale for Children,* 4th edn. New York: Psychological Corporation, 2003.

Wigg EH: *Let's Talk: Developing Prosocial Communication Skills.* Merrill, 1982.

Williams KT, *Expressive Vocabulary Test.* Circle Pines, MN: American Therapy Publication, 1997.

Autism and the Pervasive Developmental Disorders

34

Fred R. Volkmar, MD

 ## ESSENTIAL OF DIAGNOSIS

Autism and the related pervasive developmental disorders are disorders of early onset in which abnormalities in the development of social interaction and communication are associated with problems in behavior and unusual sensitivity to the inanimate environment. Autism is the best known of these conditions. DSM-IV-TR criteria for it are listed in Table 34–1. In autism a marked and sustained impairment in social interaction is associated with delayed and deviant communication and restricted, stereotyped patterns of interest and behavior. The condition was first described by Leo Kanner in 1943. Kanner emphasized two key features: autism (social disinterest) and restricted interests and trouble with change. His report underscored the importance of the lack of social interest for other aspects of development and social factors are consistently identified as central to the diagnosis of the condition. In the first decades after its description, autism was often incorrectly assumed to be a form of schizophrenia. Only in 1980 was it officially recognized as a diagnostic category (Volkmar & Klin, 2005).

DSM-IV-TR Criteria for Autistic Disorder

A. A total of at least six items from (1), (2), and (3), with at least two from (1), and one each from (2) and (3):

(1) Qualitative impairment in social interaction, as manifested by at least two of the following:

(a) Marked impairment in the use of multiple nonverbal behaviors such as eye-to-eye gaze, facial expression, body postures, and gestures to regulate social interaction

(b) Failure to develop peer relationships appropriate to developmental level

(c) A lack of spontaneous seeking to share enjoyment, interests, or achievements with other people (e.g., by a lack of show-ing, bringing, or pointing out objects of interest to other people)

(d) Lack of social or emotional reciprocity

(2) Qualitative impairments in communication as manifested by at least one of the following:

(a) Delay in, or total lack of, the development of spoken language (not accompanied by an attempt to compensate through alternative modes of communication, such as gestures or mime)

(b) In individuals with adequate speech, marked impairment in the ability to initiate or sustain a conversation with others

(c) Stereotyped and repetitive use of language or idiosyncratic language

(d) Lack of varied spontaneous make-believe play or social imitative play appropriate to developmental level

(3) Restricted repetitive and stereotyped patterns of behavior, interests, and activities, as manifested by at least one of the following:

(a) Encompassing preoccupation with one or more stereotyped and restricted patterns of interest that are abnormal either in intensity or focus

(b) Apparently compulsive adherence to specific, nonfunctional routines or rituals

(c) Stereotyped and repetitive motor mannerisms (e.g., hand or finger flapping or twisting, or complex whole body movements)

(d) Persistent preoccupation with parts of objects

B. Delays or abnormal functioning in at least one of the following areas, with onset prior to age 3: (1) social interaction, (2) language as used in social communication, or (3) symbolic or imaginative play

C. Not better accounted for by Rhett disorder or childhood disintegrative disorder

The term "pervasive developmental disorder (PDD)" was coined in 1980 as the overarching term for a class of disorders to which autism was then assigned. The term is essentially synonymous with "autism spectrum disorders." The current diagnostic system includes other conditions within this class including Asperger syndrome (social disability but with good verbal skills), childhood disintegrative disorder (a rare condition in which a condition like autism develops after a period of normal development), Rett disorder (a neurodegenerative disorder with a strong genetic basis), and pervasive developmental disorder not otherwise specified (PDD-NOS). The latter is, somewhat paradoxically, the least well defined of the PDDs and least frequent studied, yet the most common type. The clinical features of the PDDs are summarized in Table 34–1.

General Considerations

A. EPIDEMIOLOGY

The first studies of epidemiology reported a prevalence rate of 4.5 per 10,000. Subsequent studies have tended to report higher rates, on balance around 9 children per 10,000. Although there has been much interest in higher rates in recent years, that is, whether the frequency of autism is increasing, several factors make it difficult to interpret the nature of the apparent increase. For example, diagnostic criteria have changed and current approaches were designed to work well in children over the range of cognitive ability levels. Secondly, rates reported vary depending on other factors, (e.g., sample size, with highest rates in reported in the smallest samples). There is also more general awareness of the condition. Given the importance of labels for service delivery (particularly in the United States), diagnostic substitution (e.g., assignment to PDD rather than mental retardation) can be problematic particularly for studies based on reports from schools and service providers.

B. DEMOGRAPHIC, GENDER, CULTURAL, AND ETHNIC ISSUES

In Kanner's first paper, many parents of autistic children were remarkably successful, leading to the impression of an association between social class and autism. However, subsequent studies have failed to reveal such an association. It appears that Kanner's initial sample reflected referral bias. Ethnic and cultural issues have been little studied in autism. While current diagnostic criteria appear to work well, there may be major differences in

Table 34–1. Differential Diagnostic Features: Autism and Related Disorders

Feature	Autism	Asperger	Rett	CDD	PDD-NOS
Social Disturbance	Severe	Moderate–severe	Variable	Severe	Variable
Language/ Communication Impairment	Marked	Good verbal ability, poor communication	Very marked	Marked (previously normal)	Variable
Restricted interests	Marked, mannerisms, trouble with change, occasionally savant ability	Usually highly circumscribed interests (interfering with normal functioning)	Significant psychomotor retardation	Marked, as in autism	Variable—often troubled by change, Mannerisms may be less prominent
Motor issues	Often preserved early but poor later when imitation is required	Often clumsy, with fine and gross motor difficulties	Significant loss of motor abilities, hand-washing stereotypies	Often preserved but lose some self-care skills	Variable
Onset	Always before age 3 yr, often before age 1 yr. A minority regress after normal development	Problems often recognized in preschool. Motor delays may have been noted	Before age 5 yr (typically, onset with loss of skills)	By definition, child normal until age 2 yr; then major loss of skills and dramatic "autistic-like" picture	Variable

treatment. Gender differences have been consistently reported in autism, boys being 3–4 more times more likely than girls to have autism. However, this disparity is more marked at the upper end of the IQ distribution and, conversely, the ratio is less among children with more severe cognitive disability. This might either reflect a lower threshold for brain dysfunction in males or the fact that factor(s) causing autism in females must be more severe (Fombonne, 2005).

C. ETIOLOGY

In the first decades after autism was identified, there was much speculation that experiential factors might be involved in autism. However, as time went on, evidence (e.g., high rates of seizure disorder, persistence of primitive reflexes, "soft" neurological signs) suggested brain involvement. When the confusion between autism and schizophrenia was clarified, the focus began to shift toward brain and genetic mechanisms.

GENETICS

The initial impression that there was no role for genetic factors in autism was discarded when the first twin samples were collected. Twin studies have revealed high levels of concordance for monozygotic twins compared to same-sex fraternal twins (although even in the latter the rate of autism was significantly increased over the population rate). Family studies reveal prevalence rates of between 2% and 10% in siblings. Even when siblings do not have autism, they have an increased risk for language, learning, and social development problems. There are higher rates of mood and anxiety problems in family members. Although specific modes of inheritance are not yet well established, it is clear that autism is a strongly genetic disorder. Efforts are now underway to identify potential genetic mechanisms. Of the multiple genes involved, at least some of these are likely to be identified in the next few years (Rutter, 2005).

NEUROBIOLOGY

As noted, high rates of seizure disorder in autism suggest brain involvement. Although autism has been reported in association with many other conditions, these reports are based on case association rather than controlled studies with careful methodology. So, for example, what appeared to be a strong association of autism with congenital rubella became much less clear as, over time, the "autistic features" of such children markedly diminish. The strongest associations of autism with medical conditions are with two strongly genetic disorders: Fragile X syndrome and tuberous sclerosis (Minshew et al., 2005).

As the importance of genetic factors became apparent there has been less attention to studies of obstetrical risk, but some recent work has appeared. It is possible that a predisposition to autism interacts with perinatal factors in the pathogenesis of the condition. Although there has been much interest in the role of environmental factors in autism, supporting data are limited at present.

Different brain systems have been studied. Given the diversity of symptoms and clinical features it seems likely that multiple neural systems are involved. On the other hand it is clear that not all systems are involved, and sometimes autism is seen in children with good cognitive ability. Abnormalities in the limbic system, temporal and frontal lobes have been suggested. Postmortem studies have revealed abnormalities in the cortex (e.g., in the microarchitecture and cortical "minicolumns," and in neuronal packing and size). A recent finding has been the report of overall brain size increase in children with autism. It remains unclear whether the increase is generalized or local. There is much speculation that brain connectivity is adversely affected.

The possible role of immunological factors in autism has been hypothesized, for example, that maternal antibodies are directed against the fetus during the pregnancy. A recent paper reports abnormalities in the placentas of children with autism.

There has been much controversy about the role of environmental factors in autism, particularly the MMR vaccine. Persistent measles infection in combination with gastrointestinal vulnerability or the effect of thimerasol (a mercury containing compound) have been hypothesized, but larger, controlled studies have not provided consistent support. A small set of children with autism clearly do have significant developmental regression, but this may be both coincident with and unrelated to immunization. The study of "regressive" autism remains an important topic.

Clinical Findings

A. SIGNS & SYMPTOMS

Autism is characterized by a wide range of symptoms—over both age and developmental level. Less able children have significant behavioral problems and are typically mute whereas more able children are verbal and may have unusual special interests. Difficulties with social interaction are the major commonality running through this range. As first noted by Kanner, social skills are a source of major difference and impairment from early in life. Early social deficits take the form of lack of interest in joint attention, abnormalities in eye contact, and defective imitation. Social skills often do improve, but they remain a source of disability even for the most able individuals. Delays in language development are frequent concerns. When language develops it is associated with echolalia, pronoun reversal, and abnormal prosody and pragmatics. Many fail to develop symbolic–imaginative play.

In contrast to his relative lack of interest in the social environment, the nonsocial (inanimate) environment may seem highly relevant to the child with autism. Difficulties with change in routine, repetitive behavior, and unusual attachments may be observed (e.g., the child may be fascinated with spinning objects).

Autism is a disorder of early onset. Increasingly, there has been a focus early diagnosis, and autism is now often diagnosed in the first year of life. Occasionally children develop normally or near normally for a time before losing skills and developing a typical autistic profile.

Other problems are not essential diagnostic features, but are typically seen. These include problems with hyper- or hyposensitivity, problems with sleeping and eating, and difficulties with mood regulation. Self-injurious behavior is sometimes encountered.

B. Psychological Tests

Kanner's early impression of normal intellectual potential proved incorrect. It became apparent that, while children with autism often have strengths in nonverbal tasks (e.g., puzzles), they are markedly deficient in verbal cognitive abilities. Most autistic children function, overall, in the mentally retarded range, but scattered subtest scores are common. It appears that overall cognitive abilities improve with early detection and intervention. In autism areas of weakness typically include verbal concept formation, abstract thinking, and social reasoning. A different profile may be observed in individuals with Asperger disorder where verbal abilities are relatively intact.

Islets of special ability ("savant skills") are sometimes observed. Highly developed skills in special areas such as drawing, musical performance, or calendar calculation are much greater than would be expected given overall IQ. Special ability is also reflected in the relatively frequent phenomenon of hyperlexia, a precocious interest in letters and numbers (Hermelin, 2001).

C. Laboratory Findings

At this point no specific biological markers have been identified. High peripheral levels of serotonin, a central neurotransmitter, have been reported in groups of children with autism since the 1960s. The significance of this finding is unclear. Research findings on other neurotransmitter systems, such as dopaminergic, is of interest. EEG abnormalities may be seen in autism but are not diagnostic. EEG abnormalities and epilepsy are more likely in cognitive impaired autistic children. Approximately 20–25% of children with strictly diagnosed autism develop seizures; these are of diverse types. There are two peaks of seizure onset: early childhood and adolescence. Studies of evoked potentials have shown abnormalities on social tasks.

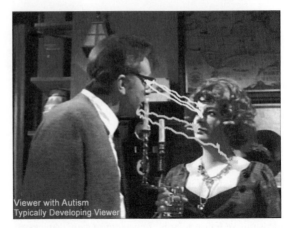

Figure 34–1. Individuals with autism look at mouths, rather than eyes in observing social interaction. (Reprinted, with permission, from Klin A, Jones W, Schultz R, Volkmar F, Cohen D: Defining and quantifying the social phenotype in autism. *Am J Psychiatry* 2002;159:895–908.)

D. Neuroimaging

MRI studies have focused both on structure and function. For example studies of the amygdala and hippocampus have not found differences in volume but fMRI studies have shown hypoactivity of the amygdala in tasks involving social and affective judgments. Probably the best replicated finding from fMRI has been the hypoactivation, relative to normal controls, of the fusiform gyrus during face perception tasks. This observation is consistent with an extensive literature on performance deficits in face processing tasks and facial expression recognition in autism, and provides an important key to understanding the core social deficits in autism. Other research has focused on the regions of the prefrontal cortex presumed to be involved in social cognitive tasks (Schultz et al., 2000). These difficulties may, in part, account for some aspects of the social difficulty in autism (see Figure 34–1).

Course of Illness

Although the outcome of autism is improving, autism is a life long disability. As many as 20% or more of autistic individuals now becoming adults may be able to function with independence and self-sufficiency. Gains can be made by individuals of all ages and levels of functioning. Positive prognostic signs for autism include some communicative speech by the age of 5 or 6 years and average nonverbal cognitive skills. As adolescents, a few individuals make gains while others lose ground. As noted previously, epilepsy sometimes has its onset in adolescence. More able individuals (e.g., those with Asperger disorder) generally have the best outcome in terms of marriage and personal self-sufficiency (Howlin, 2005).

Differential Diagnosis (Including Comorbid Conditions)

Autism must be differentiated from other developmental disorders (including related PDDs) and from sensory impairments. A detailed history and mental and physical examination are required. The early onset of problems in social interaction and communication are typical, and unusual behaviors often develop somewhat later (often around age 3 years). In mental retardation without autism, social skills are preserved and commensurate to cognitive level. In specific language disorders, language difficulties are seen in the context of good social skills. Rett disorder and childhood disintegrative disorder have highly distinctive patterns of early onset. In Asperger disorder verbal abilities are relatively preserved. It is more typical for parental concern to arise rather later in early childhood (after age 3 years); the differentiation of high-functioning autism from Asperger disorder can be problematic.

In obtaining historical information, aides to memory, such as baby books and videos, can be useful. A history of normal development followed by regression should prompt careful diagnostic investigation. Similarly, unusual features in the family history, child examination, and so forth may require specific investigation (Volkmar & Klin, 2005).

Treatment

A. EDUCATIONAL AND BEHAVIORAL INTERVENTIONS

Autism is a disorder of development. At the same time, development affects autism. The goal of treatment is to minimize the disruptive effects of autism on development and maximize normative developmental processes. Goals change with the child's age and level of functioning, but always involve an explicit focus on social, language, and adaptive (self-help) skills. A structured, comprehensive program is needed with input from various professionals. The approaches used vary on several dimensions (e.g., how much they emphasize a child-centered or a developmental approach as contrasted to an adult-centered behavioral approach); however, all approaches share many features (National Research Council, 2001).

The focus of speech and language therapy is to expand the range of the child's communication skills. This should include teaching broader communication skills and beyond more vocabulary. Children who are not yet verbal can be helped by augmentative strategies (e.g., manual signing, picture exchange, and so forth). For more advanced children, the focus is more on social language use. Behavioral interventions are used in educa-

tional program. These techniques help with management of disruptive behavior and facilitate learning. Given the tendency of children with autism to learn things in isolation, the generalization of skills is important and is an essential aim.

B. PSYCHOPHARMACOLOGICAL INTERVENTIONS

Medications do not affect the central social and communicative aspects of autism but may ameliorate the problem behavior that interfere with programming. Neuroleptic medication, particularly the atypical neuroleptics, are effective in decreasing stereotypic behavior and agitation; however, side effects may limit their usefulness. Much interest has centered on the SSRIs (selective serotonin reuptake inhibitors) given their potential for alleviating anxiety and behavioral rigidity. For adolescents with depression, antidepressants can be helpful. Mood stabilizers are sometimes useful (Scahill & Martin, 2005).

C. PSYCHOTHERAPEUTIC INTERVENTIONS

In the 1950s and 1960s, intervention often involved the psychotherapy of parents and children, with little apparent benefit. The role for dynamic psychotherapy is limited except in the case of more able individuals who can respond to supportive and directive treatment. There is a risk of depression in adolescence, which may respond to a combination of psychotherapy and pharmacology.

D. ALTERNATIVE TREATMENTS

Many different treatments have been proposed. Most lack an empirical foundation. A majority of parents engage in such treatments (although they may not always discuss them with physicians). Generally, there are no supportive data other than case report; single cures are not particularly informative. Furthermore the first follow-up studies demonstrated good outcome in a small number of cases without what, today, would be recognized as effective treatment, i.e., some children do well anyway. Furthermore there is a strong placebo (nonspecific treatment) effect. Occasionally alternative treatment is dangerous, either in terms of loss of access to effective programs or because of physical harm (Jacobson et al., 2005).

Complications/Adverse Outcomes of Treatment

Seizures are the most common medical complication. The usual risks associated with pharmacological intervention are observed. Given difficulties with judgment and cognition, there is an increased risk for injury and accidental death.

Prognosis

The earliest studies of autism suggested relatively poor prognosis, only a small number of individuals (1–2%) being able to function independently as adults. Recent research reveals major gains with early diagnosis and treatment. Outcome is significantly improved if early intervention is provided. On the other hand, some children make few gains despite appropriate programs. Some children make gains in early childhood, others in adolescence. Despite good intervention, some children do not substantively progress (Howlin, 2005).

Websites

www.aspennj.org
www.autism.fm
www.quackwatch.com

Fombonne E: Epidemiological studies of pervasive developmental disorders. In: Volkmar FR, Klin A, Paul R, Cohen DJ (eds). *Handbook of Autism and Pervasive Developmental Disorders,* 3rd edn. Vol. 1. Hoboken, NJ: Wiley, 2005, pp. 42–69.

Howlin P: Outcomes in autism spectrum disorders. In: Volkmar FR, Klin A, Paul R, Cohen DJ (eds). *Handbook of Autism and Pervasive Developmental Disorders,* 3rd edn. Vol. 1. Hoboken, NJ: Wiley, 2005, pp. 201–222.

Jacobson JW, Foxx RM, Mulick JA. (eds): *Controversial Therapies for Developmental Disabilities: Fad, Fashion and Science in Professional Practice.* Mahwah, NJ: Lawrence Erlbaum Associates, Publishers, 2005.

National Research Council: *Educating Young Children with Autism.* Washington, DC: National Academy Press, 2001.

Scahill L, Martin A: Psychopharmacology. In: Volkmar FR, Klin A, Paul R, Cohen D (eds). *Handbook of Autism and Pervasive Developmental Disorders,* 3rd edn. New York: Wiley, 2005, pp. 1102–1117.

Schultz RT, Gauthier I, Klin A, et al.: Abnormal ventral temporal cortical activity during face discrimination among individuals with autism and Asperger syndrome. [comment]. *Arch Gen Psychiatry* 2000;57(4):331–340.

Volkmar F, Cook EH, Jr., Pomeroy J, Realmuto G, Tanguay P: Practice parameters for the assessment and treatment of children, adolescents, and adults with autism and other pervasive developmental disorders. *J Am Acad Child Adolesc Psychiatry* 1999;38(12 Suppl):32S–54S.

Volkmar F, Klin A, Rutter M: Issues in classification of autism and related conditions. In: Volkmar F, Klin A Paul R, Cohen D (eds). *Handbook of Autism and Pervasive Developmental Disorders,* 3rd edn. New York: Wiley, 2005, pp. In Press.

Volkmar FR, Pauls D: Autism. *Lancet* 2003;362(9390):1133–1141.

Attention-Deficit Hyperactivity Disorder

35

Thomas Spencer, MD

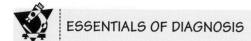

ESSENTIALS OF DIAGNOSIS

DSM-IV-TR Diagnostic Criteria
Attention-Deficit/Hyperactivity Disorder

A. Either (1) or (2):

(1) Sx (or more) of the following symptoms of **inattention** have persisted for at least 6 months to a degree that is maladaptive and inconsistent with developmental level:Inattention

  (a) Often fails to give close attention to details or makes careless mistakes in schoolwork, work, or other activities
  (b) Often has difficulty sustaining attention in tasks or play activities
  (c) Often does not seem to listen when spoken to directly
  (d) Often does not follow through on instructions and fails to finish schoolwork, chores, or duties in the workplace (not due to oppositional behavior or failure to understand instructions)
  (e) Often has difficulty organizing tasks and activities
  (f) Often avoids, dislikes, or is reluctant to engage in tasks that require sustained mental effort (such as schoolwork or homework)
  (g) Often loses things necessary for tasks or activities (e.g., toys, school assignments, pencils, books, or tools)
  (h) Is often easily distracted by extraneous stimuli
  (i) Is often forgetful in daily activities

(2) Six (or more) of the following symptoms of **hyperactivity-impulsivity** have persisted for at least 6 months to a degree that is maladaptive and inconsistent with developmental level: Hyperactivity

  (j) Often fidgets with hands or feet or squirms in seat
  (k) Often leaves seat in classroom or in other situations in which remaining seated is expected
  (l) Often runs about or climbs excessively in situations in which it is inappropriate (in adolescents or adults, may be limited to subjective feelings of restlessness)
  (m) Often has difficulty playing or engaging in leisure activities quietly
  (n) Is often "on the go" or often acts as if "driven by a motor"
  (o) Often talks excessively

Impulsivity

  (g) Often blurts out answers before questions have been completed
  (h) Often has difficulty awaiting turn
  (i) Often interrupts or intrudes on others (e.g., butts into conversations or games)

B. Some hyperactive-impulsive or inattentive symptoms that caused impairment were present before age 7 years.

C. Some impairment from the symptoms is present in two or more settings (e.g., at school [or work] and at home).

D. There must be clear evidence of clinically significant impairment in social, academic, or occupational functioning.

E. The symptoms do not occur exclusively during the course of a Pervasive Developmental Disorder, Schizophrenia, or other Psychotic Disorder and are not better accounted for by another mental disorder (e.g., Mood Disorder, Anxiety Disorder, Dissociative Disorder, or a Personality Disorder).

Code based on type:

Attention-Deficit/Hyperactivity Disorder, Combined Type: *if both Criteria A1 and A2 are met for the past 6 months*

Attention-Deficit/Hyperactivity Disorder, Predominantly Inattentive Type: *if Criterion A1 is met but Criterion A2 is not met for the past 6 months*

Attention-Deficit/Hyperactivity Disorder, Predominantly Hyperactive-Impulsive Type: *if Criterion A2 is met but Criterion A1 is not met for the past 6 months*

General Considerations

A. EPIDEMIOLOGY

Attention-deficit hyperactivity disorder (ADHD) is the most common emotional, cognitive, and behavioral disorder treated in youth. It is a major clinical and public health problem because of its associated morbidity and disability in children, adolescents, and adults. Data from cross-sectional, retrospective, and follow-up studies indicate that youth with ADHD are at risk for developing other psychiatric difficulties in childhood, adolescence, and adulthood including delinquency as well as mood, anxiety, and substance-use disorders.

Early definitions, such as the Hyperkinetic Reaction of Childhood in DSM-II, placed the greatest emphasis on motoric hyperactivity and overt impulsivity as hallmarks of the disorder. The DSM-III represented a paradigm shift as it began to emphasize inattention as a significant component of the disorder. DSM-IV now defines three subtypes of ADHD: predominantly inattentive, predominantly hyperactive–impulsive, and a combined subtype. Criteria for each DSM-IV subtype require six or greater of nine symptoms in each respective category. There are four additional criteria that include age of onset by 7 years, ADHD-specific adaptive impairments, pervasiveness, and separation from other existing conditions. The combined subtype is the most commonly represented subgroup accounting for from 50% to 75% of all ADHD individuals, followed by the inattentive subtype (20–30%), and the hyperactive–impulsive subtype (less than 15%).

Epidemiologic studies indicate that ADHD is a prevalent disorder affecting from 4% to 7% of children worldwide including the United States, New Zealand/Australia, Germany, and Brazil. Although previously thought to remit largely in adolescence, a growing literature supports the persistence of the disorder and/or associated impairment into adulthood in a majority of cases.

Prevalence estimates of childhood ADHD in the United States are estimated to be 5–8%. Estimates vary predictably depending on methodology. Definitions that require both symptom dimensions (hyperactivity/impulsivity and inattention) are more restrictive than those that require only one of these dimensions. Thus, estimates based on pre-DSM III definitions or the ICD codes of hyperkinetic disorder produce lower estimates. In addition the surveys that estimate based on symptoms alone and do not include impairment yield higher estimates. As recently by Faraone et al. (2003), other factors that affect apparent prevalence estimates include pervasiveness criteria, informants (teacher, parent, child), use of rating scales versus clinical interviews as well as ascertainment issues. Community samples have higher rates than school samples.

Gender and age of the sample also affect estimates prevalence. Girls more commonly have the inattentive type and also less commonly have accompanying ODD/CD, disruptive disorders, factors leading to lower rates of diagnosis. The original descriptions were derived from a child-focused perspective, and do not reflect what are thought to be more salient aspects of adult ADHD: the executive function disorders of poor organization, poor time management, and memory disturbance associated with academic and occupational failure. The lack of appropriate description of adult symptoms may reduce the true prevalence of ADHD in adulthood.

B. ETIOLOGY

Biological adversity—Several biologic factors have been proposed as contributors to ADHD, including food additives/diet, lead contamination, cigarette and alcohol exposure, maternal smoking during pregnancy, and low-birth weight. Although the Feingold diet for ADHD was popularized by the media and accepted by many parents, systematic studies showed that this diet was ineffective and that food additives do not cause this disorder. Several investigators have shown that lead contamination can cause symptoms of ADHD. However, lead does not account for the majority of ADHD cases, and many children with high-lead exposure do not develop ADHD. An emerging literature documents that maternal smoking and alcohol exposure during pregnancy, low-birth weight, and psychosocial adversity are additional independent risk factors for ADHD.

Pregnancy and delivery complications (i.e., toxemia, eclampsia, poor maternal health, maternal age, fetal postmaturity, duration of labor, fetal distress, low-birth weight, antepartum hemorrhage) appear to have a predisposition for ADHD. Several studies documented that maternal smoking during pregnancy is an independent risk factor for ADHD.

Psychosocial adversity—Findings of recent studies stress the importance of adverse family–environment variables as risk factors for ADHD. In particular, chronic family conflict, decreased family cohesion, and exposure to parental psychopathology (particularly maternal) are more common in ADHD families compared with control families. It is important to note that, although many studies provide powerful evidence for the importance of psychosocial adversity in ADHD, such factors tend to emerge as universal predictors of children's adaptive functioning and emotional health, rather than specific predictors of ADHD. As such, they can be conceptualized as nonspecific triggers of an underlying predisposition or as modifiers of the course of illness.

C. GENETICS

Because ADHD is believed to be highly genetic, studies of twins have been used to establish its heritability or the degree to which this disorder is influenced by genetic factors. Based on numerous studies of twins, which varied considerably in methodology and definitions of ADHD, the mean heritability for ADHD was shown to be 77%. Seven candidate genes show statistically significant evidence of association with ADHD on the basis of the pooled odds ratio (1.18–1.46) across studies: DRD4, DRD5, DAT, DBH, 5-HTT, HTR1B, and SNAP-25.

Clinical Findings

A. SIGNS & SYMPTOMS

The diagnosis of ADHD is made by careful clinical history. A child with ADHD is characterized by a considerable degree of inattentiveness, distractibility, impulsivity, and often hyperactivity that is inappropriate for the developmental stage of the child. Other common symptoms include low-frustration tolerance, shifting activities frequently, difficulty organizing, and daydreaming. These symptoms are usually pervasive; however, they may not all occur in all settings. Adults must have childhood-onset, persistent, and current symptoms of ADHD to be diagnosed with the disorder. Adults with ADHD often present with marked inattention, distractibility, organization difficulties and poor efficiency, which culminate in life histories of academic and occupational failure.

B. RATING SCALES

Rating scales are extremely helpful in documenting the individual profile of ADHD symptoms as well as assessing the response to treatments. It is important to emphasize that they should not be used for diagnosis without careful clinical confirmation and elicitation of the other criteria necessary for diagnosis. Although neuropsychological testing is not relied upon to diagnose ADHD it may serve to identify particular weaknesses within ADHD or specific learning disabilities co-occurring with ADHD.

Rating scales are available for all age groups and can be useful in assessing and monitoring home, academic and occupational performance. Increasingly, there has been a congruence of opinion in this area with a number of the most widely used scales consisting of Likert ratings of the existing DSM-IV criteria. There are two types of scales in wide use, the so-called "narrow" scales that are specific for ADHD and "broad" scales that measure additional dimensions including comorbidity. The broad scales are useful for separating straightforward and complex cases, and the narrow scales are most useful for honing in on exclusively ADHD dimensions both diagnosis and to monitor specific responses to treatment. In looking to the future, there are proposals to expand the set of diagnostic symptoms to include executive functions (such as time management and multitasking) especially in older individuals.

C. PSYCHOLOGICAL TESTING

Psychological testing is not necessary for the routine diagnosis of ADHD and does not readily distinguish children with and without ADHD. Nonetheless, psychometric testing can be valuable in narrowing the differential diagnosis and identifying comorbid learning difficulties. Many children with ADHD have difficulties with abstract reasoning, mental flexibility, planning, and working memory, a collection of skills broadly categorized as executive functioning skills. They can also present with verbal and nonverbal performance skills and/or visual–spatial processing deficits. In such circumstances, neuropsychological assessments can be valuable and may help to clarify the diagnosis. Children with learning, language, visual–motor, or auditory processing problems usually perform poorly only in their particular problem area, whereas children with ADHD may perform poorly in several areas of evaluation.

Laboratory Findings

Nonroutine laboratory studies are not indicated unless the history or physical examination is suggestive of seizures, neurodevelopmental regression, or localizing neurologic signs, or if an acute or chronic medical disorder is suspected.

NEUROIMAGING

The neurobiology of ADHD is not completely understood, although imbalances in dopaminergic and noradrenergic systems have been implicated in the core symptoms that characterize this disorder. Many brain regions are candidates for impaired functioning in ADHD. Prefrontal hypotheses in ADHD have primarily involved the dorsolateral prefrontal cortex, associated with organizational, planning, working memory, and attentional dysfunctions and Orbital lesions associated with social disinhibition and impulse control disorders.

Structural imaging studies, using computerized tomography or magnetic resonance imaging found evidence of structural brain abnormalities among ADHD patients, with the most common findings being smaller volumes in frontal cortex, cerebellum, and subcortical structures. Castellanos and colleagues found smaller total cerebral brain volumes from childhood through adolescence. This work suggested that genetic or early environmental influences on brain development in ADHD are fixed, nonprogressive, and unrelated to stimulant treatment. Numerous fMRI studies have reported Dorsal Anterior Cingulate Cortex (dACC) hypofunction in ADHD on tasks of inhibitory control

Brain imaging studies fit well with the concept that dysfunction in fronto-subcortical pathways occurs in ADHD. Three subcortical structures implicated by the imaging studies (i.e., caudate, putamen, and globus pallidus) are part of the neural circuitry underlying motor control, executive functions, inhibition of behavior, and the modulation of reward pathways. These frontal–striatal–pallidal–thalamic circuits provide feedback to the cortex for the regulation of behavior.

The fronto-subcortical systems pathways associated with ADHD are rich in catecholamines, which are involved in the mechanism of action of stimulant medications used to treat this disorder. A plausible model for the effects of medications in ADHD suggests that, through dopaminergic and/or noradrenergic pathways, these agents increase the inhibitory influences of frontal cortical activity on subcortical structures.

Imaging studies also implicate the cerebellum and corpus callosum in the pathophysiology of ADHD. The cerebellum contributes significantly to cognitive functioning, presumably through cerebellar–cortical pathways involving the pons and thalamus. The corpus callosum connects homotypic regions of the two cerebral hemispheres. Size variations in the callosum and volume differences in number of cortical neurons may degrade communication between the hemispheres, which may account for some of the cognitive and behavioral symptoms of ADHD.

Course of Illness

Samples ascertained before the publication of DSM-III relied on earlier definitions that highlighted hyperactivity as a hallmark of ADHD. Since it is hyperactivity that wanes earliest, it may be that older samples were enriched with subjects more likely to remit from ADHD than individuals identified today. There is evidence for this hypothesis in the data. In a recent analysis, the persistence rate was lowest in studies ascertained according to DSM-II ADD and highest in those studies ascertained according to DSM-III-R ADHD. The available

data also suggests a continuation of childhood behavior problems and emerging antisocial behavior among many in this group of children. For example, researchers have noted the rate of conduct disorders among children with ADHD to range between 25% and 50% at follow-up during adolescence. Reports also suggest that a majority of children with ADHD continue to exhibit deficits in attention and/or activity level in adulthood, with only about 30% of children evidencing a remission of symptoms by adolescence and early adulthood. Recent work also suggests that ADHD youth disproportionately become involved with cigarettes, alcohol, and then drugs. Individuals with ADHD, independent of comorbidity, tend to maintain their addiction longer compared to their non-ADHD peers.

Differential Diagnosis (Including Comorbid Conditions)

A. OPPOSITIONAL DEFIANT DISORDER AND CONDUCT DISORDER

There are important nosologic distinctions between attention and hyperactivity per se and that of associated symptoms common to the disruptive behavioral disorder category. Oppositional defiant disorder (ODD) is characterized by a pattern of negativistic, hostile and defiant behavior. ADHD and ODD/CD have been found to co-occur in 30–50% of cases in both epidemiologic and clinical samples. In contrast, conduct disorder (CD) is a more severe, and less common, disorder of habitual rule breaking defined by a pattern of aggression, destruction, lying, stealing, or truancy. While CD is a strong predictor of substance abuse, ODD without CD is not.

B. MOOD DISORDERS

Unipolar depression in a child may be apparent from a sad or irritable mood, a persistent loss of interest, or pleasure in the child's favorite activities. Other signs and symptoms include physiologic disturbances such as in changes in appetite and weight, abnormal sleep patterns, psychomotor abnormalities, fatigue, and diminished ability to think, as well as feelings of worthlessness or guilt and suicidal preoccupation.

Classical mania in adults is characterized by euphoria, elation, grandiosity, and increased energy. However, in many adults and most children, mania is more commonly manifested by extreme irritability or explosive mood with associated poor psychosocial functioning that is often devastating to the patient and family. In milder conditions, additional symptoms include unmodulated high energy such as a decreased sleep, over talkativeness, racing thoughts, or increased goal-directed activity (social, work, school, sexual) or an associated manifestation of markedly poor judgment such as thrill-seeking or reckless activities.

In epidemiologic studies and several controlled, prospective studies, higher rates of depression were found in ADHD. A baseline diagnosis of major depression predicted lower psychosocial functioning, a higher rate of hospitalization as well as impairments in interpersonal and family functioning. Similarly, higher rates of mania were detected in follow-up studies. ADHD children with comorbid mania at either baseline or follow-up assessment had other correlates expected in mania including additional psychopathology, psychiatric hospitalization, severely impaired psychosocial functioning as well as a greater family history of mood disorders.

C. CHILDHOOD ANXIETY DISORDERS

Childhood anxiety disorders are often not suspected in an overactive child, just as ADHD is often not assessed in inhibited children. When present, both contribute to social, behavioral, and academic dysfunction. In addition anxiety may be associated with intense intrapsychic suffering. Thus, having both ADHD and anxiety disorders may substantially worsen the outcome of children with both disorders. In the MGH follow-up study, ADHD children with comorbid anxiety disorder had increased psychiatric treatment, more impaired psychosocial functioning as well as a greater family history of anxiety disorders.

D. COGNITIVE PERFORMANCE AND LEARNING DISABILITIES

Children with ADHD perform more poorly than controls on standard measures of intelligence and achievement. In addition, children with ADHD perform more poorly in school than do controls, as evidenced by more grade repetitions, poorer grades in academic subjects, more placements in special classes, and more tutoring. The reported degree of overlap varies by definition, the more restrictive definition has a rate of 20–25%.

E. ADHD PLUS TICS

Children with ADHD have higher rates of Tic disorders that may contribute additional dysfunction due to distractions and social impairments directly attributable to the movements or vocalizations themselves. A number of studies have noted that anti-ADHD treatment is highly effective for ADHD behaviors, aggression, and social skill deficits in children with TS or chronic tics.

F. SUBSTANCE-USE DISORDERS

Combined data from retrospective accounts of adults and prospective observations of youth indicates that juveniles with ADHD are at increased risk for cigarette smoking and substance abuse during adolescence.

Treatment

The ADHD adolescent and young adult is at risk for school failure, emotional difficulties, poor peer relationships, and trouble with the law. Factors identifiable in younger youth that predict the persistence of ADHD into adulthood include familiality with ADHD and psychiatric comorbidity—particularly aggression or delinquency problems. Although the literature provides compelling evidence that the diagnosis of ADHD in childhood predicts persistent ADHD and poor outcome in adolescence, these findings also suggest that such a comprised outcome is not shared by all ADHD children. The discussion thus far has not addressed a related clinical question: Can the functioning of ADHD children normalize in the context of persistent ADHD? We analyzed data from a 4-year longitudinal study of referred children and adolescents with ADHD, to assess normalization of functioning and its predictors among boys with persistent ADHD.

Using indices of emotional, educational, and social adjustment, we found that 20% of children with persistent ADHD functioned poorly at follow-up in all three domains, 20% did well in all three domains, and 60% had intermediate outcomes. These findings suggested that the syndromatic persistence of ADHD is not associated with a uniform functional outcome but leads instead to a wide range of emotional, educational, and social adjustment outcomes that can be partially predicted by exposure to maternal psychopathology, larger family size, psychiatric comorbidity, and impulsive symptoms.

A. PSYCHOPHARMACOLOGIC INTERVENTIONS

Medications remain a mainstay of treatment for children, adolescents, and adults with ADHD. In fact, recent multisite studies support that medication management of ADHD is the most important variable in outcome in context to multimodal treatment. For example, in a large prospective and randomized long-term trial of ADHD youth, those receiving stimulants alone were observed to have similar improvement in core ADHD symptoms at 14 months follow-up compared to those randomized to receive stimulants plus psychotherapy. Of interest, both medicated groups had a better overall outcome than those receiving extensive psychotherapy without stimulants. The stimulants, specific norepinephrine reuptake inhibitors (SNRIs), certain antidepressants, and certain antihypertensives comprise the available agents for ADHD. Stimulants, SNRIs, and antidepressants have been demonstrated to have similar pharmacological responsivity across the lifespan including school-aged children, adolescents, and adult groups with ADHD.

B. STIMULANTS

The stimulants are the most commonly prescribed agents for pediatric and adult groups with ADHD.

The most commonly used compounds in this class include methylphenidate (Ritalin, Concerta, Metadate, Focalin, and others) and amphetamine (Dexedrine, Adderall). Stimulants are sympathomimetic drugs, which increase intrasynaptic catecholamines (mainly dopamine) by inhibiting the presynaptic reuptake mechanism and releasing presynaptic catecholamines. Whereas methylphenidate specifically blocks the dopamine transporter protein, amphetamines also release dopamine stores and cytoplasmic dopamine directly into the synaptic cleft. Recent data suggests that acute tolerance to stimulants may develop rapidly necessitating an ascending- or pulsing-pharmacokinetic profiles for ADHD efficacy.

Methylphenidate and d-amphetamine are both short-acting compounds, with an onset of action within 30–60 minutes and a peak clinical effect usually seen between 1 and 2 hours after administration lasting 2–5 hours. The amphetamine compounds (Adderall) and sustained release preparations of methylphenidate and dextroamphetamine are intermediate-acting compounds with an onset of action within 60 minutes and duration of 6–8 hours.

Given the need to additionally treat ADHD outside of academic settings (i.e., social, homework) and to reduce the need for in school dosing and likelihood for diversion, there has been great interest in extended release preparations of the stimulants. Extended release preparations greatly reduce untoward peak adverse effects of stimulants such as headaches and moodiness, as well as essentially eliminating afternoon wear off and rebound.

A new generation of highly sophisticated, well-developed, safe and effective long-acting preparations of stimulant drugs has reached the market and revolutionized the treatment of ADHD. These compounds employ novel delivery systems to overcome acute tolerance termed "tachyphylaxis." There are several long-acting methylphenidate formulations and a long-acting methylphenidate formulation. While Concerta is a 12-hour formulation, Metadate-CD and Ritalin LA are 8-hour methylphenidate formulations. In addition Adderall XR is a 12-hour amphetamine formulations. Methylphenidate as a secondary amine gives rise to four optical isomers: d-threo, l-threo, d-erythro, and l-erythro. Recently the active stereoisomer, d-threo-methylphenidate compound has been available in an immediate release and long-acting form as Focalin and Focalin XR.

Stimulants appear to work in all age groups of individuals with ADHD. Studies in preschoolers report improvement in ADHD symptoms, structured tasks as well as mother–child interactions; however, there may be a higher side effect burden compared to other age groups. Similarly, in adolescents response has been reported as moderate to robust, with no abuse or tolerance noted. In addition, stimulant treatment has been found to be effective in adults with ADHD.

Predictable short-term adverse effects include reduced appetite, insomnia, edginess, and GI upset. In adults, elevated vital signs may emerge necessitating baseline and on-drug monitoring. There are a number of controversial issues related to chronic stimulant use. Although stimulants may produce anorexia and weight loss, their effect on ultimate height remains less certain. While initial reports suggested that there was a persistent stimulant-associated decrease in growth in height in children, other reports have failed to substantiate this finding, and still others question the possibility that growth deficits may represent maturational delays related to ADHD itself rather than to stimulant treatment. Stimulants may precipitate or exacerbate tic symptoms in ADHD children. Recent work suggests that the majority of ADHD youth with tics can tolerate stimulant medications; however, up to one third of children with tics may have worsening of their tics with stimulant exposure. Current consensus suggests that stimulants can be used in youth with comorbid ADHD plus tics with careful monitoring for stimulant-induced tic exacerbation.

Despite case reports of stimulant misuse, there is a paucity of scientific data supporting that stimulant-treated ADHD individuals abuse their medication; however, data suggests that diversion of stimulants to non-ADHD youth continues to be a concern. Families should closely monitor stimulant medication and college students receiving stimulants should be advised to carefully store their medication. Despite the findings on efficacy of the stimulants, studies have also reported consistently that typically one third of ADHD individuals do not respond or cannot tolerate this class of agents.

1. Specific norepinephrine reuptake inhibitors (Atomoxetine)—Atomoxetine (Strattera) is one of a new class of compounds, known as SNRIs. Currently atomoxetine is the only nonstimulant that is FDA approved for ADHD. Atomoxetine may be particularly useful in stimulant failures, or when oppositionality, anxiety, or tics co-occur within ADHD. After extensive testing, atomoxetine has been found to be generally safe and well tolerated. However, there have been rare (2 out of 3 million patients) reports of liver injury.

2. Antidepressants—A subgroup of antidepressants are second-line drugs of choice for ADHD. The tricyclic antidepressants (TCAs) as well as bupropion (Wellbutrin) block the reuptake of neurotransmitters including norepinephrine. In contrast, the serotonin reuptake inhibitors are not useful for ADHD. The TCAs are effective in controlling abnormal behaviors and improving cognitive impairments associated with ADHD, but less so than the majority of stimulants. As minor increases in heart rate and the ECG intervals are predictable with TCAs, ECG monitoring at baseline and at therapeutic dose is suggested, but not mandatory.

3. Antihypertensives—The antihypertensives clonidine (Catapress) and guanfacine (Tenex) are alpha-adrenergic agonists, which have been primarily used in the treatment of hypertension. These compounds have been shown to be useful in the treatment of ADHD. Guanfacine is longer acting and less sedating than clonidine. The antihypertensives have been used for the treatment of ADHD as well as associated tics, aggression, and sleep disturbances, particularly in younger children.

4. Modafinil—Modafinil is an antinarcoleptic agent, which is structurally and pharmacologically different than other agents approved to treat ADHD. Testing in children has reported effectiveness in ADHD. While generally safe and well-tolerated there has been concerns about uncommon occurrences of a severe rash possibly related to Stevens Johnson syndrome.

C. Psychotherapeutic Interventions

The largest-scale study examining the relative and combined effectiveness of medical and nonmedical interventions for ADHD is the NIMH Multimodal Treatment Study for ADHD Study (MTA). In this 5-year, 6-site project, 579 elementary-age children with ADHD were randomly assigned to one of four 14-month treatment conditions: behavioral treatment, medication management (mostly methylphenidate), combined behavioral treatment and medication management, and a community comparison group. Children in the Behavioral Treatment arm received a very intensive combination of treatments, including school consultation, a classroom aide, an 8-week summer treatment program, and 35 sessions of parent management training. Findings from the MTA study at 14 months indicate that medical intervention was significantly more effective than behavioral and community treatments; that behavioral treatment only modestly enhanced the effect of medication alone; and that behavioral treatment alone was no more effective than the treatment received by children in the community comparison group on core symptoms of ADHD.

Complications/Adverse Outcomes of Treatment

If adult ADHD is a clinically significant disorder, then ADHD adults should show functional impairments in multiple domains. Several studies suggest this to be true.

These studies have shown that ADHD adults had lower socioeconomic status, more work difficulties, and more frequent job changes. The ADHD adults had fewer years of education and lower rates of professional employment. Similarly, others have shown that among patients with substance-use disorders, ADHD predicts social maladjustment, immaturity, fewer social assets, lower occupational achievement, and high rates of separation and divorce.

Prognosis

ADHD is a prevalent worldwide, heterogeneous disorder that frequently persists into adult years. The disorder is associated with significant impairment in occupational, academic, social, and intrapersonal domains necessitating treatment. Converging data strongly support a neurobiological and genetic basis for ADHD with catecholaminergic dysfunction as a central finding. While psychosocial interventions such as educational remediation and cognitive–behavioral approaches should be considered in the management of ADHD, an extensive literature supports the effectiveness of pharmacotherapy not only for the core behavioral symptoms of ADHD but also improvement in linked impairments including cognition, social skills, and family function.

Biederman J, Mick E, Faraone S: Normalized functioning in youths with persistent ADHD. *J Pediatr* 1998;133:544–551.

Biederman J, Faraone S, Milberger S, et al.: A prospective 4-year follow-up study of attention-deficit hyperactivity and related disorders. *Arch Gen Psychiatry* 1996;53:437–446.

Bush G, Valera EM, Seidman LJ: Functional neuroimaging of attention-deficit/hyperactivity disorder: A review and suggested future directions. *Biol Psychiatry* 2005;57:1273–1284.

Castellanos FX, Lee PP, Sharp W, et al.: Developmental trajectories of brain volume abnormalities in children and adolescents with attention-deficit/hyperactivity disorder. *JAMA* 2002;288:1740–1748.

Faraone SV, Sergeant J, Gillberg C, Biederman J: The worldwide prevalence of ADHD: Is it an American Condition? *World Psychiatry* 2003;2:104–113.

Faraone SV, Perlis RH, Doyle AE, et al.: Molecular genetics of attention deficit hyperactivity disorder. *Biol Psychiatry* 2005;57:1313–1323.

MTA Cooperative Group: A 14-month randomized clinical trial of treatment strategies for attention-deficit/hyperactivity disorder. The MTA cooperative group. Multimodal treatment study of children with ADHD. *Arch Gen Psychiatry* 1999;56:1073–1086.

Seidman LJ, Valera EM, Makris N: Structural brain imaging of attention-deficit/hyperactivity disorder. *Biol Psychiatry* 2005;57:1263–1272.

Oppositional Defiant Disorder and Conduct Disorder

36

Barry Nurcombe, MD

■ OPPOSITIONAL DEFIANT DISORDER

 ESSENTIALS OF DIAGNOSIS

DSM-IV-TR Diagnostic Criteria

A. A pattern of negative, hostile, and defiant behavior lasting at least 6 months, during which four (or more) of the following are present:

(1) often loses temper

(2) often argues with adults

(3) often actively defies or refuses to comply with adults' requests or rules

(4) often deliberately annoys people

(5) often blames others for his or her mistakes or misbehavior

(6) is often touchy or easily annoyed by others

(7) is often angry or resentful

(8) is often spiteful or vindictive

Note: Consider a criterion met only if the behavior occurs more frequently than is typically observed in individuals of comparable age and developmental level.

B. The disturbance in behavior causes clinically significant impairment in social, academic, or occupational functioning.

C. The behaviors do not occur exclusively during the course of psychotic or mood disorder.

D. Criteria are not met for conduct disorder, and, if the individual is 18 years or older, criteria are not met for antisocial personality disorder.

(Reprinted, with permission, from *Diagnostic and Statistical Manual of Mental Disorders*, 4th edn., Text Revision. Copyright 2000 American Psychiatric Association.)

General Considerations

As with conduct disorder and attention-deficit/hyperactivity disorder (ADHD) (described in previous chapter), with which it is often entangled, it is uncertain whether oppositional defiant disorder is a truly distinctive nosological category. Specifically, it is unclear whether oppositional behavior is better considered to be on a continuum between normal developmental limit-testing on the one hand and pathologically disruptive behavior on the other. The distinction between categorical disorders and dimensional psychopathology is more than a theoretical quibble. Valid categories delimit disorders that are likely to have a significantly biological (e.g., neurochemical) basis. Dimensional sets of behavior masquerading as categories may, in fact, obscure true categories that nest within their fictitious boundaries.

Oppositional defiant disorder, as defined in DSM-IV-TR, is manifest as age-inappropriate, persistent, intemperate, argumentative, defiant, deliberately annoying, irritable, resentful, vindictive behavior associated with the tendency of the subject to blame others for his or her own transgressions or omissions. The aggression of the oppositional child or adolescent is predominantly verbal rather than physical. The aggression tends to be reactive (e.g., in response to an unwelcome imposition of rules) rather than proactive (e.g., bullying), and overt (e.g., shouting) rather than covert (e.g., spreading malicious rumors).

A. Epidemiology

The prevalence of oppositional defiant disorder is uncertain, but it has been estimated at 5.7–9.9%. The average age at onset is 6 years. Oppositional defiant disorder is regarded by many researchers as a milder, precocious form of conduct disorder. The male-to-female sex ratio in childhood conduct disorder is 4:1. There is a clinical impression that childhood oppositional defiant disorder is more common among preadolescent males than females, however, the relative prevalence in females appears to rise in adolescence.

Table 36–1. The Characteristics of Coercive Parent–Child/Adolescent Interactions

Characteristic	Example
Unclear communication	Failure to address the child directly, lack of eye contact, hard-to-follow instructions
Lack of sincerity or conviction in communication	Poor eye contact; incongruity between words, gesture, and body language
Harsh, sarcastic tone of communication	"You'll do what you're told, young lady, or . . ."
Accusatory, denigrating, shaming statements	"You'll never amount to anything, you slut."
Empty threats	"If you do that once more, I'll . . ."
Bringing up the past	"I'll never forgive you for the time when you . . ."
Rigid, overgeneralized, black-and-white, "catastrophizing"	"People who smoke die young."
Preaching, moralizing, "psychologizing"	"When I was young, kids did what they were told . . ."
Failure to listen to the other person	Interrupting, changing the topic, discounting the other person's opinion ("How would you know . . . ?"), monopolizing the conversation
Capitulation, impotence, hopelessness, despair	"What's the use of talking to you? It never does any good."
Failure to praise the child's or adolescent's achievements	
Failure to follow through and monitor the child's behavior	
Inconsistent, unpredictable, excessively harsh punishment	

B. ETIOLOGY

The genesis of oppositional defiant disorder has not been studied separately from that of conduct disorder. Because conduct disorder often evolves from earlier oppositional behavior, and because the two disorders have similar risk factors, oppositional defiant disorder and conduct disorder are often discussed together.

Many young children who exhibit oppositional defiant behavior were, as infants, already temperamentally hyperreactive, irritable, difficult to soothe, and slow to adapt to new circumstances. Infants who exhibit disorganized attachment behavior are at risk of oppositional, disruptive behavior in middle childhood. Often the families of these children are highly stressed, as a result, for example, of marital discord, single parenthood, parental psychopathology, or socioeconomic disadvantage. Maternal depression may be particularly common. Preoccupied with their own problems, parents fail to provide these children with adequate praise and attention. When parents seek to set limits, they do so harshly and inconsistently. The children react defiantly, testing the limits, and the stage is set for repetitive cycles of escalating

coerciveness, with shouting and mutual accusations, often terminated by harsh physical punishment or by the capitulation of one or other of the antagonists. Children's aggressiveness is associated with how aggressive their parents were at the same age. Often parents respond to their children in the manner (and even with the same words) that their parents responded to them. In summary, a lack of positive reinforcement for acceptable behavior is associated with negative attention for oppositional behavior and with inconsistent, unpredictable, harsh punishment. Table 36–1 lists the characteristics of a coercive interaction. These factors can be targeted for therapeutic intervention (see "Treatment" section later in this chapter).

C. GENETICS

The genetics of oppositional defiant disorder has not been studied apart from that of conduct disorder. Behavioral genetic studies of aggressive behavior in children have yielded inconsistent estimates of its heritability, probably because of variations in the measurement instruments used. Most studies suggest that the trait of aggressiveness has low heritability.

Caspi A, Moffitt TE: The continuity of maladaptive behavior: From description to understanding in the study of antisocial behavior. In: Cicchetti D, Cohen DJ (eds). *Developmental Psychopathology. Risk, Disorder, and Adaptation.* Vol 2. New York: John Wiley & Sons, 1995, pp. 472–511.

Hinshaw SP, Anderson CA: Conduct and oppositional defiant disorders. In: Mash EJ, Barkley RA (eds). *Child Psychopathology.* New York: Guilford Press, 1996, pp. 113–152.

Clinical Findings

A. SIGNS AND SYMPTOMS

The persistent, recurrent aggressive and defiant behavior associated with oppositional defiant disorder may be restricted to the home or may be generalized as an antiauthoritarian attitude, for example, to teachers and other adults outside the home. It is usually evident before 8 years of age but may emerge for the first time in adolescence. Oppositional, hostile, limit-testing behavior disrupts family relationships and can interfere with learning. At school, oppositional children or adolescents may be moody, irritable, lacking in self-esteem, and often in conflict with teachers and peers. As a result, the oppositional child or adolescent often appears to have a "chip on his or her shoulder." Oppositional adolescents may be solitary or inclined to gravitate to the company of others who regard themselves as outlaws. Precocious tobacco use is likely, as is alcohol and substance abuse.

B. PSYCHOLOGICAL TESTING

Aside from questionnaires that are useful for assessing aggressive behavior (e.g., the Child Behavior Checklist and the Eyberg Child Behavior Inventory), a number of behavioral observation rating scales and questionnaires have been developed for the assessment of conflictual parent–child or family behavior (Table 36–2). These tests may be useful as monitors of the progress and effectiveness of treatment, in accordance with treatment goals and objectives.

Differential Diagnosis (Including Comorbid Conditions)

Oppositional defiant disorder should be differentiated from normal developmental limit-testing in toddlers and preschool children, and from the challenging confrontations that occur between parents and normal adolescents who are seeking to be more independent. Developmental oppositional behavior is transitory and causes no significant impairment.

Oppositional defiant disorder should be discriminated from ADHD, with which it frequently coexists, and from conduct disorder, which often succeeds it. An underlying mood disorder may be manifest, to the superficial observer, as sullen defiance. Premorbid schizophrenia or early schizophrenia is sometimes associated with

Table 36–2. Behavioral Observation Scales and Questionnaires Useful for Assessing Parent–Child or Family Interaction

Assessment Tools	Reference
The Dyadic Parent–Child Interaction Coding System	Eyberg and Robinson 1983
The Family Interaction Coding System	Reid 1978
The Marital Interaction Coding System	Robin 1988
The Interaction Behavior Code	Robin and Koepke 1985
Wahler's Standardized Observation Codes	Wahler et al. 1976
The Family Process Code	Dishion et al. 1976
The Parent Daily Report	Chamberlain and Reid 1987
The Parenting Stress Index	Loyd and Abidin 1985
The Issues Checklist	Robin and Foster 1989
The Conflict Behavior Questionnaire	Robin and Foster 1989
The Parent–Adolescent Relationship Questionnaire	Robin et al. 1986
The Family Beliefs Inventory	Vincent et al. 1986
The Family Environment Scale	Moos and Moos 1983
The Family Adaptability and Cohesion Evaluation Scales—II	Olsen and Portner 1983

negativism and marked contrasuggestibility. A comprehensive history and mental status examination will differentiate these two disorders.

Children with mental retardation, hearing loss, or impaired language comprehension are sometimes oppositional and defiant at school. Selective mutism often has oppositional features.

Oppositional defiant behavior often coexists with the following situations or conditions: Parental conflict, parental psychopathology (especially depression), physical or sexual abuse, conduct disorder, ADHD, and adolescent substance use disorder. In regard to the comorbidity of oppositional defiant disorder with ADHD and conduct disorder, it is unclear whether these disorders have mixed symptoms, whether they share risk factors, whether oppositional defiant disorder is a risk factor for other disorders, or whether it is an early manifestation of conduct disorder.

Treatment

A. CHILDREN

With children under 12 years of age, treatment is provided primarily through the parents. Whether as single parents, as parental dyads, or in parental groups, parents are educated concerning the origin and meaning of oppositional defiant behavior and are trained to replace coercive discipline with more effective child-rearing techniques. Table 36–3 describes the essentials of effective parenting.

Table 36–3. The Essentials of Effective Parenting with Oppositional Defiant Children

Provide positive attention with praise and reinforcement of desirable behavior.
Ignore inappropriate behavior unless it is serious.
Give clear, brief commands, reduce task complexity, and eliminate competing influences (e. g., television).
Establish a token economy at home with tokens or points awarded for compliance (to be "cashed in," weekly). Do not remove points for noncompliance, at first. Maintain the token economy for at least 6–8 weeks.
When the token economy is established, use response cost (removal of tokens) or time out, contingent on noncompliance, applied soon after the noncompliance (1–2 min time out per year of age). Do not release the child from time out until he or she is quiet and agrees to obey.
Extend time out to noncompliance in public places.

Adapted, with permission, from Barkley RA: *Defiant Children: A Clinician's Manual for Parent Training.* New York: Guilford Press, 1987.

Table 36–4. The Principles and Objectives of the Triple P Program

Principles

Children need a safe environment that provides opportunities for exploration and play.

Parents should respond constructively to help children solve their own problems.

Assertive discipline is more effective than coercive discipline.

Parents should take care of themselves by communicating better with each other, understanding their own emotional states, and coping with their own disruptive emotions.

Objectives

The promotion in parents of better self-regulation and problem solving.

The enhancement of child competencies that protect against adverse mental health outcomes (eg, social skills, affect regulation, problem solving).

The reduction of family conflict.

The reduction of parental distress and the promotion of parental competence.

The provision of social support.

Adapted, with permission, from Sanders MR: *Healthy Families, Healthy Nation: Strategies for Promoting Family Mental Health in Australia.* Brisbane: Australian Academic Press, 1995.

The Positive Parenting Program (Triple P) contains all these elements and has been designed as a population-based intervention strategy. Triple P is a parenting and family support program that can be delivered in five levels: level 1 targets common, everyday behavior problems; level 2 targets oppositional defiant disorder; and levels 3–5 target severe behavior problems complicated by severe family psychopathology. The program can be delivered through parent information nights; through videotapes; by information and skills training delivered through individual, self-directed, and group programs; and through three levels of intensive family therapy (requiring specific training for the clinicians who implement the therapy). Table 36–4 lists the principles and objectives of the Triple P program.

B. ADOLESCENTS

In adolescent oppositional defiant disorder, a family therapy approach has had the most success. In the Problem Solving Communication Training (PSCT) program, the family is first assessed with regard to the issues described in Table 36–5. These issues can be described as molecular (i.e., family communication problems and poor problem solving) or molar (i.e., family structural and functional problems). Molecular issues provide the specific goals

Table 36–5. Problem-Solving Communication Training: Assessment and Treatment

Assessment

What are the specific issues that provoke discord in the family?

How effective are the family's communication patterns?

Is the family involved in coercive interactions (see Table 36–1)?

Do the parents model and convey effective problem-solving techniques?

Does the family endorse negatively biased, inflexible beliefs about each other (e.g., "catastrophizing," perfectionism) (see Table 36–7)?

Are structural problems evident in the family (e.g., misalignments, coalitions, triangulation, disengagement, enmeshment, conflict, "detouring")?

What functional purpose does the adolescent's behavior serve (e.g., to distract parents who would otherwise quarrel, or to drive parents apart, or to attract attention away from a sibling regarded as more favored)?

Treatment objectives

Promote better family communication and more effective problem solving.

Help the family generalize their skills to the home.

Reverse or neutralize structural and functional problems.

Adapted, with permission, from Foster SL, Robin AL: Parent-adolescent conflict. In: Mash EJ, Barkley RA (eds): *Treatment of Childhood Disorders*, pp. 601–646. New York: Guilford Press, 1998.

and objectives of therapy, whereas molar issues inform its strategy and tactics.

The treatment objectives of PSCT are listed in Table 36–5. Family communication and problem solving are addressed by eliciting the common causes of family disagreement and then ranking them in order of seriousness or difficulty. The family is directed to address one cause of dispute per session, starting with the least acrimonious, by using a formula for problem solution (Table 36–6). As the family addresses these problems, family communication pathology can be remediated with the use of feedback, instruction, modeling, and behavioral rehearsal. Sometimes, the family's communication patterns are so adverse that they must be addressed before PSCT can begin.

Table 36–6. The Steps of Problem Solving for Families

1 Define the problem. Each family member tells the others what the problem is and why it is a problem. The other family members paraphrase the statement to check their understanding of it.

2 Generate alternative solutions, taking turns.

3 Take turns to evaluate each proposed solution. The solution with the greatest number of positive ratings wins.

4 Implement the solution and check its effectiveness.

Adapted, with permission, from Foster SL, Robin AL: Parent–adolescent conflict. In: EJ Mash, RA Barkley (editors): *Treatment of Childhood Disorders*. New York: Guilford Press, 1989, 601–646.

Table 36–7. Dysfunctional Beliefs

Parents

If my adolescent is given freedom, he or she will be ruined.

My adolescent should always obey me.

My adolescent should always make the right decision.

My adolescent is out to upset and hurt his or her parents.

If my adolescent does wrong, I must be to blame.

Adolescents

Rules are unfair.

Rules will ruin my life.

I should be allowed complete freedom.

People should always be fair to each other.

If my parents loved me, they would always trust me.

I should never upset my parents.

Adapted, with permission, from Foster SL, Robin AL: Parent–adolescent conflict. In: EJ Mash, RA Barkley (editors): *Treatment of Childhood Disorders*. New York: Guilford Press, 1989, 601–646.

In the course of treatment, the family's rigid, biased beliefs will be revealed and targeted for cognitive restructuring (Table 36–7). In cognitive restructuring, the therapist challenges each dysfunctional belief, suggests a more reasonable alternative, and helps the family to conduct an "experiment" that will disconfirm the belief.

In a severely dysfunctional family system, PSCT and cognitive restructuring are unlikely to be effective unless the family's functional and structural pathology can also be addressed. PCST can be undermined by family members who are not involved in therapy or by outside agencies that oppose it. Severe psychopathology in a family member (e.g., maternal depression, paternal alcoholism, adolescent substance abuse) may need treatment before PSCT can proceed. A minimal level of verbal ability in family members is required for PSCT to be successful. PSCT by itself is unlikely to be effective if the adolescent patient has conduct disorder.

Foster SL, Robin AL: Parent–adolescent conflict and relationship discord. In: Mash EJ, Barkley RA (eds). *Treatment of Childhood Disorders,* 2nd edn. New York: Guilford Press, 1998, pp. 601–646.

Sanders MR: The triple-P positive parenting program: Toward an empirically validated multilevel parenting and family support strategy for the prevention of behavior and emotional problems in children. *Clin Child Fam Psychol Rev* 1999;2:71–90.

Sanders MR: New directions in behavioral family intervention with children. In: Ollendick TH, Prinz RJ (eds). *Advances in Clinical Child Psychology.* Vol 18. New York: Plenum Publishing, 1996, pp. 283–330.

Prognosis

Oppositional defiant disorder is predicted by the same risk factors as is conduct disorder (e.g., marital discord, socioeconomic stress, maternal depression) but to a lesser degree. Although about 90% of children and adolescents with conduct disorder have previously met (and still meet) criteria for oppositional defiant disorder, only about 25% of children with oppositional defiant disorder go on to exhibit conduct disorder. About 50% continue to exhibit oppositional defiant disorder in late childhood and adolescence; and the remaining 25%, when assessed later, cease to meet criteria for either oppositional defiant disorder or conduct disorder.

The significance of these findings has been debated. Should oppositional defiant disorder be regarded as a precocious (albeit milder) form of conduct disorder? Or is it an extreme form of (and continuous with) normal oppositional behavior? What determines the developmental trajectory of the individual child? It has been postulated that one developmental trajectory proceeds from early oppositional-defiant behavior, along an authority conflict pathway, to serious conflict with adults during adolescence. This pathway is likely to intersect with the covert or overt antisocial trajectories described in the next section.

Oppositional behavior is common during adolescence. As described earlier in this chapter, when such behavior is severe, it is usually a manifestation of family dysfunction. The association between childhood oppositional defiant disorder and adolescent oppositional defiant disorder is unknown.

Lahey BB, Moffitt TE, Caspi A: *Causes of Conduct Disorder and Juvenile Delinquency.* New York: Guilford, 2003.

Loeber R, et al.: Developmental pathways in disruptive child behavior. *Dev Psychopathol* 1993;5:103.

CONDUCT DISORDER

 ESSENTIALS OF DIAGNOSIS

DSM-IV-TR Diagnostic Criteria

A. *A repetitive and persistent pattern of behavior in which the basic rights of others or major age-appropriate societal norms or rules are violated, as manifested by the presence of three (or more) of the following criteria in the past 12 months, with at least one criterion present in the past 6 months:*

Aggression to people and animals

(1) often bullies, threatens, or intimidates others

(2) often initiates physical fights

(3) has used a weapon that can cause serious physical harm to others

(4) has been physically cruel to people

(5) has been physically cruel to animals

(6) has stolen while confronting a victim

(7) has forced someone into sexual activity

Destruction of property

(8) has deliberately engaged in fire setting with the intention of causing serious damage

(9) has deliberately destroyed others' property (other than by fire setting)

Deceitfulness or theft

(10) has broken into someone else's house, building, or car

(11) often lies to obtain goods or favors or to avoid obligations

(12) has stolen items of nontrivial value without confronting a victim

Serious violations of rules

(13) often stays out at night despite parental prohibitions, beginning before 13 years of age

(14) has run away from home overnight at least twice while living in parental or parental surrogate home (or once without returning for a lengthy period)

(15) often truant from school, beginning before age 13 years

B. *The disturbance in behavior causes clinically significant impairment in social, academic, or occupational functioning.*

C. *If the individual is age 18 years or older, criteria are not met for antisocial personality disorder.*

Specify *type based on age at onset:* Childhood-onset type *or* adolescent-onset type.
Specify *severity:* Mild, moderate, severe.

(Reprinted, with permission, from *Diagnostic and Statistical Manual of Mental Disorders,* 4th edn., Text Revision. Copyright 2000 Washington, DC: American Psychiatric Association.)

General Considerations

As described in DSM-IV-TR, the diagnostic features of conduct disorder have evolved from earlier multivariate factor analytic studies of child and adolescent clinical populations. A former division of delinquency syndromes into undersocialized aggression and socialized aggression has been dropped in favor of the atheoretical subcategories of childhood-onset and adolescent-onset types, either of which may be mild, moderate, or severe.

It has been difficult to disentangle the taxon of conduct disorder from several other behavior disorders with which it is frequently associated (e.g., oppositional defiant disorder, ADHD, and substance use disorder). Although conduct disorder is formally described as though it were categorically distinct, it almost certainly comprises a number of associated continua.

Conduct disorder must be distinguished from transient antisocial behavior that reflects the risk-taking and group contagion that are part of normal adolescence. Antisocial behavior is common in adolescence; in most cases it requires no psychiatric attention. Conduct disorder, in contrast, represents severe, persistent, and pervasive dysfunction.

Two types of aggression have been described, variously contrasted as reactive/proactive, overt/covert, affective/predatory, defensive/offensive, socialized/undersocialized, impulsive/controlled, or hostile/instrumental. Reactive, affective, impulsive aggression is likely to be associated with child maltreatment.

A. Epidemiology

Definitive conclusions about the prevalence of conduct disorder are difficult to reach because studies have differed in the geographic areas and age ranges studied and in the methods of assessment. However, it is evident that conduct disorder is one of the most common problems in childhood and adolescence. Overall prevalence rates for conduct disorder have varied from 0.9% (Germany) to 8.7% (Missouri). Prevalence rates in adolescents have varied from 9% to 10% in boys and from 3% to 4% in girls. The prevalence of antisocial personality disorder in adults is estimated to be 2.6%. Two studies found that African-American youths were more likely to be assigned the diagnosis of conduct disorder; however, comparative studies are few.

Prospective studies have identified the following individual variables as associated with later adjudications for delinquency: drug use, stealing, aggression, general problem behavior, truancy, poor educational achievement, and lying. The following environmental variables predict delinquency: poor parental supervision, lack of parental involvement, poor discipline, parental absence, poor parental health, low socioeconomic status, and association with deviant peers. The following factors are protective: high IQ, easy temperament, good social skills, good school achievement, and a good relationship with at least one adult. Composite behavioral indices have greater predictive power than do single variables, supporting a cumulative risk model. One model of transmission postulates a genetic propensity that is triggered if the subject is exposed to parental risk factors and is subsequently expressed fully in an adverse social environment. A recent study has found that children at high genetic risk for conduct problems are more likely to develop conduct disorder following maltreatment than are those at low genetic risk. It has not been demonstrated whether genetic propensity or adverse parenting alone can generate conduct disorder. However, a Danish study found that birth complications and maternal rejection predicted antisocial violence in late adolescence.

Gender differences in prevalence and trajectory have been identified. Whereas males predominate in disruptive behavior disorders prior to adolescence, prevalence rates among the two sexes are closer by age 15 years, due to an increase in covert, nonaggressive delinquent behavior among girls. Girls are more likely to follow the nonaggressive pathway with late onset, covert offenses, and a greater likelihood of recovery. Because of the emphasis on aggressive behavior in formal diagnostic schedules for conduct disorder, it is possible that the behavioral precursors and adult outcome of female conduct disorder have been obscured. Indirect aggression (e.g., spreading malicious rumors) is more common in girls.

B. Etiology

1. Psychosis, epilepsy, & brain dysfunction—Careful history taking, mental status examination, neuropsychological testing, and electroencephalography of violent juvenile offenders often reveal hallucinatory experiences, mental absences, episodes of illogical thinking, lapses of concentration, memory gaps, suspiciousness, explosive aggression, and nonspecific electroencephalography abnormalities. These findings, along with the history of physical abuse and neglect often encountered among violent delinquents, have suggested that some antisocial youths could be experiencing covert psychosis or subclinical epilepsy caused by brain injury. An alternative explanation is that a high proportion of explosively aggressive youths harbor overt or residual posttraumatic stress disorder secondary to physical or sexual abuse and that their absences, hallucinations, lapses in concentration, and explosiveness represent dissociation stemming from unresolved trauma.

2. Psychophysiologic theories—Childhood-onset, aggressive conduct disorder (in contrast to adolescent-onset, nonaggressive conduct disorder) is associated with low tonic psychophysiologic arousal, low autonomic reactivity, and rapid habituation. These characteristics may be associated with an impairment of avoidance conditioning to social stimuli, a failure to respond to punishment, and deficient behavioral inhibition. An imbalance between central reward and inhibition systems has been postulated. It is unclear whether these psychophysiologic phenomena are inherent, whether they are secondary to disruptive experiences in early childhood, or whether they are the result of an unstable lifestyle.

3. Neuroendocrine & biochemical theories—Research into the relationship between testosterone and aggressive crime has yielded inconsistent results. Several studies have found an association between low levels of 3-methoxy-4-hydroxyphenylglycol in cerebrospinal fluid and impulsive behavior in older youths. Other abnormalities in the dopaminergic and noradrenergic systems have been described, although only in very small population samples. Low levels of cerebrospinal 5-hydroxyindoleacetic acid, a serotonin metabolite, are associated with psychopathy, aggression, and suicide; and one study correlated defiance and aggression with low levels of whole blood 5-hydroxytryptamine. Another study has suggested a relationship between disruptive behavior disorder (i.e., conduct disorder and oppositional defiant disorder) and lower concentrations of cerebrospinal fluid somatostatin. These studies must be interpreted with caution because of the following limitations: (1) They have small sample sizes, (2) they gathered data from areas (i.e., cerebrospinal fluid) that are far "downstream" from the relevant brain areas (i.e., central neurotransmitter synapses), and (3) their cross-sectional correlative nature makes it difficult to determine the direction and timing of causal sequences. Many of the children in these studies experienced severe maltreatment; moreover, conduct disorder itself may generate traumatic experiences that could affect the neurochemical systems in question.

4. Neuropsychological & neurodevelopmental theories—Associations have been found among severe and extended child maltreatment, dissociative symptoms, chronic posttraumatic stress disorder, memory defects, and reduction in hippocampal size. Low circulating cortisol has been associated with emotional numbing in chronic posttraumatic stress disorder, and high cortisol levels have been associated with flashbacks.

Delinquent populations subjected to cognitive testing have consistently exhibited IQs about eight points below those of nondelinquent populations, a difference that persists when socioeconomic status is statistically controlled. This discrepancy is primarily the result of deficits in word knowledge, verbally coded information, verbal reasoning, verbally mediated response regulation, and metalinguistic skills. The most impulsive, aggressive subjects exhibit the widest discrepancy between verbal and performance IQs. These deficits probably antedate school entry and are associated with learning problems.

Research into time-orientation, impulsivity, sensation seeking, and locus of control in youths with conduct disorder has not yielded consistent results, possibly because juvenile delinquency is not homogeneous. In terms of moral reasoning, unsocialized aggressive delinquents operate at a preconventional level and have deficient role-taking abilities. The characteristic egocentrism, hedonism, unreflectiveness, and denial of responsibility of offenders have been associated with developmental immaturity of the frontal lobe and left hemisphere.

5. Psychoanalytic & attachment theory—Early psychoanalytic theories postulated a relationship between crime and unconscious guilt. Later studies described the deficient ego and superego functioning of adult criminals, with impairment in reality testing, judgment, affect regulation, object relations, adaptive regression, and synthetic functioning. A connection has been postulated between parental psychopathology and the parent's unconscious fostering of deviant behavior in the child.

The observation that early neglect and bond disruption were prevalent in delinquents who exhibited so-called affectionless psychopathy led attachment theorists to examine the contributions of emotional neglect, attachment disruption, separation, and object loss to sociopathy. Disruptive behavior patterns are postulated to stem from three complementary processes: disorganized attachment patterns, distorted affective-cognitive structures, and the motivational consequences of insecure attachment. Disruptive behavior patterns are thought to arise ultimately from a combination of neurobiological risk factors, attachment disturbance, inappropriate parenting practices, and pathogenic family ecology.

6. Child maltreatment & adverse parenting practices—Maternal depression has been linked, via disorganized attachment, to disruptive behavior in middle childhood. Marital conflict, domestic violence, parental neglect, and child maltreatment are also associated with later antisocial behavior. The effect of divorce on child behavior is likely to be mediated mainly by exposure to marital discord before, during, and after parental separation. Physical abuse is related to later aggressive behavior and can be transferred from one generation to the next. The prevalence of sexual abuse among girls with conduct disorder is very high. According to a recent study of delinquent girls placed in therapeutic foster care, the girls first engaged in sexual activity at age 6 years, on average.

The following adverse parenting practices convey a risk for antisocial behavior: low parental involvement in child-rearing; poor supervision; and harsh, punitive discipline. Characteristic parent–child interactions involve unclear communication; lax and inconsistent monitoring; lack of follow-through; unpredictable, explosive, coercive, harsh, and overpunitive verbal or physical discipline; and a failure to provide verbal reinforcement for desirable behavior. Parents tend to back down from their child's increasingly coercive demands until, unable to tolerate them further, they lash out angrily. At such times, the parents are likely to berate the child in terms of the same undesirable characteristics that their own parents ascribed to them. Thus parents unwittingly reinforce negative behavior, fail to model and reinforce desirable behavior, and at the same time distort the child's attributional style: the child is primed to view himself or herself as bad and to expect other people, particularly authority figures, to be hostile and uncaring.

The combination of aggressive, antiauthoritarian behavior and verbal reasoning impairment causes the child to fail at school, to perceive himself or herself as rejected by teachers and peers, and to gravitate toward like-minded companions. Aggregations of high-risk youths incite and perpetuate antisocial behavior, providing a training ground for criminality and drug abuse. The parents of disruptive children are likely to have difficulty in preventing their children from mixing with rogue companions who promote delinquent behavior.

7. Attributional style—Children who are prone to conduct disorder develop a characteristic interpersonal style that reflects a complex interplay among the following factors: biological predisposition, adverse environment, distorted information processing, and the influence of peers. Aggressive children have been found to underutilize social cues, to interpret neutral or ambiguous cues as hostile, to generate few assertive solutions to social problems, and to expect that aggressive behavior will be rewarded. This is particularly likely in those children who, early in development, exhibit aggressive, hyperactive, impulsive behavior.

8. Sociologic theories—The following sociologic factors are related to antisocial behavior: severe family adversity; multiple family transitions; unemployment; socioeconomic disadvantage; disorganized, crime-ridden neighborhoods; and the prevalence of juvenile gangs. Family adversity, family transitions, and low socioeconomic status are particularly likely to be associated with childhood-onset, aggressive conduct disorder. However, the effect of low socioeconomic status is nullified when the effect of adverse parenting practices is statistically controlled. Adverse family circumstances appear to affect the child via adverse parenting.

Sociologic research has generated five main theories concerning the roots of antisocial behavior: (1) social segregation theory, (2) culture conflict theory, (3) criminogenic social organization theory, (4) blocked-opportunity theory, and (5) theories to do with differential justice and labeling.

Social segregation theory postulates that disadvantaged social or ethnic groups, particularly recent immigrants, become relegated to decaying neighborhoods ringing the inner city. Socially disorganized slums become battlegrounds for competing ethnic groups and spawn criminogenic cultural organizations such as juvenile gangs. Economically blocked from mainstream culture, many residents seek a criminal solution whereas others tolerate or adapt to the prevailing criminal tradition.

Culture conflict theory relates the antisocial behavior of the children of socially disadvantaged immigrants to the confusion and disempowerment of immigrant parents, leading to a conflict between traditional parental control and the influence of the new society. Criminogenic social organization theorists have studied the informal organization of street gangs and their focal concerns with masculinity, toughness, status, the capacity to outwit others, a hunger for excitement, and the belief that life is dictated by fate rather than planning. Blocked-opportunity theorists have emphasized the function of the gang as an illegitimate means to acquire desirable amenities in a materialistic society that accords high status to affluence.

Alternative views suggest that differential delinquency rates are related to variations in the activity of police and juvenile justice authorities: the chances for apprehension are higher in areas where there is greater police surveillance. Labeling theorists suggest that delinquency is caused by designating a juvenile as "delinquent." Evidence indicates that delinquent attitudes can be hardened by legal processing, but this is a contributory rather than a root cause of antisocial behavior.

C. Genetics

Studies have examined the concordance for adult criminality between monozygotic (MZ) and dizygotic (DZ) twins (determining heritability), the concordance for criminality between MZ twins reared apart (correcting for shared environment), and the prevalence of criminality in adopted-away offspring of adult criminals (separating environmental and genetic influences). In 10 twin comparison studies, the concordance rates for adult criminality have been up to 50% for MZ twins and 20% for DZ twins. In contrast, seven studies of adolescent antisocial behavior have demonstrated a high but equivalent concordance in MZ and DZ twins, suggesting a preponderant environmental effect. A recent metanalysis of 51 twin and adoption studies of antisocial behavior found that additive genetic and additive nonshared environmental factors were prominent. The influence of genetic and shared environmental factors may be greater during childhood, and of the non-shared environment in adolescence. Studies of the adopted-away offspring of adult criminals suggest an additive effect, for adult property crime, between biological predisposition and criminogenic environment. Interestingly, this effect does not appear to apply to aggressive crime.

Improvements in the subtyping of conduct disorder will likely lead to advances in genetic research. For example, recent studies found evidence for the heritability of an aggression trait, whereas little evidence was found for a genetic factor in adolescent-onset, nonpersisting delinquent behavior. Research into the genetics of adolescent antisocial behavior has been impeded by the tendency to regard conduct disorder as a homogeneous, categorically distinct disorder rather than as a loosely assorted conglomerate of dimensional types exhibiting multifactorial etiology (multiple causal factors), heterotypic continuity (the tendency for behavioral patterns to change over time), and equifinality (the tendency for different causal factors to result in a common phenotype).

Pedigree studies suggest an association between adult antisocial personality disorder (in men), alcoholism (in men), and hysteria (in women). Recent research suggests that antisocial personality disorder and alcoholism have separate modes of inheritance.

In summary, it appears likely that polygenic factors have a moderate influence on adult criminality, particularly in regard to recidivism for property offenses, and that adverse genetic and environmental influences interact. At this point, definitive studies have not been conducted with adolescents. Future research into the genetics of juvenile delinquency should examine subtypes of juvenile antisocial and aggressive behavior.

Three chromosomal abnormalities have been associated with antisocial behavior: 47XXY, 47XYY, and an abnormally long Y chromosome. These conditions are so uncommon as to be of little practical import. In developmentally retarded groups, the XXY anomaly may be associated with antisocial behavior. The XYY anomaly is characterized by tallness, hypotonia, hyperactivity, delayed language development, tantrums, electroencephalography abnormality, recidivism for minor property offenses, and (in one study) a sadistic sexual orientation. The long Y anomaly may also be associated with recidivism.

Bauermeister JJ, Canino G, Bird H: Epidemiology of disruptive behavior disorders. *Child Adolesc Psychiatr Clin N Am* 1994;3:177.

Jaffee SR, Caspi A, Moffitt TE, et al.: Nature X nurture: Genetic vulnerabilities interact with physical maltreatment to promote conduct problems. *Dev Psychopathol* 2005;17:67–84.

Lahey BB, Moffitt TE, Caspi A (eds). *Causes of Conduct Disorder and Juvenile Delinquency.* New York: Guilford, 2003.

Rhee SH, Waldman ID: Testing alternative hypotheses regarding the role of development on genetic and environmental influences underlying antisocial behavior. In: Lahey BB, Moffitt TE, Caspi A (eds). *Causes of Conduct Disorder and Delinquency.* New York: Guilford, 2003, pp. 305–318.

Rogeness GA: Biologic findings in conduct disorder. *Child Adolesc Psychiatr Clin N Am* 1994;3:271.

Clinical Findings

A. Signs and Symptoms

Children with conduct disorder are usually referred for evaluation during childhood or adolescence—by parents; caregivers; pediatricians; or educational, child welfare, or juvenile justice authorities—because their behavior has become intolerably disruptive or dangerous at home, in school, or in the community. Often the referral occurs in response to threatened, or actual, suspension from school.

The overlap among conduct disorder, oppositional defiant disorder, and ADHD has raised questions concerning the distinctiveness of each disorder. Furthermore, the many associated problems exhibited by these children dictate the need to gather diagnostic data from a number of informants (e.g., parents, the patient, teachers). Categorical diagnosis alone is almost useless for treatment planning. A comprehensive biopsychosocial evaluation is required with an assessment of the patient's perceptual-motor, cognitive, linguistic, academic, and social competencies; an analysis of family functioning; and an examination of the child's behavior in school, with peers, and in relation to the community. Clinical interviewing of the patient and the family allows the clinician to explore different areas in response to diagnostic hypotheses. Structured clinical interviews may be more reliable than semistructured interviews, but their rigidity and cumbersome nature virtually restrict them to research purposes.

B. Psychological Testing

Cognitive, educational achievement, and neuropsychological testing, while not helpful in categorical diagnosis, can provide important information concerning the patient's perceptual-motor, cognitive, and linguistic functioning and educational performance—data that are important in the design of a comprehensive treatment plan.

Table 36–8. Psychological Testing for Conduct Disorder

Scale	Comments
Achenbach-Conners-Quay Questionnaire (ACQ)	An expansion of the authors' respective scales, the ACQ yields two aggression factors: aggressive behavior and delinquent behavior.
Child Behavior Checklist (CBCL)	Has parent, youth, teacher, and observer versions. A multidimensional, omnibus scale analyzed separately for boys and girls age 2–3 and 4–18 years. Total behavior problem scores are broken down into externalizing and internalizing band factors and further still into aggressive and delinquent factor scores.
Conners Parent Rating Scale (CPRS) and Conners Teacher Rating Scale (CTRS)	Particularly helpful in the assessment of hyperactivity and conduct problems. All versions of the CPRS have a conduct problem or aggression factor. An abbreviated form of the scale, the Conners Abbreviated Symptom Questionnaire (CASQ), combines items relevant to conduct disorder and hyperactivity and may be useful in the monitoring of treatment in comorbid cases.
Eyberg Child Behavior Inventory (ECBI)	Designed specifically to rate aggressive behavior on a unidimensional scale. It is particularly useful as a treatment monitor.
Jessness Inventory, Carlson Psychological Survey, and Hare Psychopathy Checklist	Assess conduct-disordered behavior in adolescents.
Preschool Behavior Checklist (PBCL) and Burks Preschool and Kindergarten Behavior Rating Scale	Designed to assess behavior in younger children.
Quay's Revised Behavior Problem Checklist	Yields two factorized subscales that reflect aggressive behavior: conduct disorder and socialized aggression.

Table 36–8 lists rating scales that are useful in diagnosis and, possibly, in the monitoring of treatment.

Differential Diagnosis (Including Comorbid Conditions)

Conduct disorder is likely to coexist with oppositional defiant disorder and ADHD, and with substance use disorder, learning disorder, depression, posttraumatic stress disorder, and other anxiety disorders. In longitudinal studies, the prevalence of ADHD declines with age, whereas the prevalence of conduct disorder rises. Oppositional defiant disorder and conduct disorder are temporally continuous (see "Prognosis & Course of Illness" discussion later in this section), whereas conduct disorder and ADHD often coexist. The coexistence of conduct disorder and ADHD significantly complicates treatment and conveys a worse prognosis than the diagnosis of ADHD or conduct disorder alone.

Many youths with conduct disorder have specific developmental disorders, particularly reading disability and verbal and metalinguistic deficits. Conduct disorder is also associated with early-onset substance use and with a rapid progression to serious substance abuse. Childhood-onset conduct disorder is more likely to be associated with comorbidity than is adolescent-onset conduct disorder.

Dysthymia, major depressive disorder, and anxiety disorders have been described as comorbid with conduct disorder. Conduct problems may precede depression or become apparent after its onset. Completed or attempted suicide has often been associated with conduct problems, particularly explosive aggression. A high proportion of incarcerated delinquents have posttraumatic stress disorder, in full or subclinical form. Of patients with combined Tourette's syndrome and ADHD, 30% also have conduct disorder. Conduct disorder should be differentiated from mania, which is often associated with irritable, belligerent, and rule-breaking behavior.

Loeber R, Keenan K: Interaction between conduct disorder and its comorbid conditions. *Clin Psychol Rev* 1994;14:497.

Treatment

Conduct disorder is too complex a group of problems to be treated by a single method. Individually tailored combinations of biological, psychosocial, and ecological interventions will likely be most effective. The task is to find the most effective treatment combinations for different groups of children and adolescents with conduct problems. The following sections discuss the most common approaches to prevention and treatment.

A. EARLY INTERVENTION PROGRAMS

Early intervention programs such as Head Start may have a preventative function. Head Start programs attend to the child's physical health and provide an early education program that prepares the child for elementary school. They also educate parents about child development and offer support in times of crisis. Early mental health intervention programs, such as Triple P and Fast Track, identify aggressive children and provide intensive parent education to counteract the poor communication, inconsistency, lack of follow-through, coercive discipline, and failure to model or reward prosocial behavior that so frequently accompany nascent conduct disorder. Both Triple P and Fast Track have demonstrated promising short-term effects, however, their long-term benefits are unclear.

B. TREATMENT PROGRAMS FOR SCHOOL-AGED CHILDREN

Behavioral programs targeting parental effectiveness and the child's social problem-solving capacity, social skills, prosocial behavior, and academic functioning are more effective in the short term than are nonspecific treatment methods.

C. TREATMENT PROGRAMS FOR ADOLESCENTS

During the 1980s, a number of meta-analyses confirmed generally pessimistic impressions of the effectiveness of community and institutional interventions. During the past decade, however, several therapeutic approaches have had promising results.

The Adolescent Transition Program combines initial assessment with feedback and motivational enhancement, followed by a menu of interventions including family-focused training, family therapy, and comprehensive case management.

Evidence is accumulating that it is ineffective to treat youths who have conduct disorder in community or institutional groups. The contagious reinforcement of antisocial behavior generated by antisocial youth groups likely counteracts any benefit derived from group-oriented therapeutic programs. For that reason, therapeutic foster homes have been developed. Youths who would otherwise have been incarcerated are placed with specially trained foster parents who provide daily structure and support; institute an individualized point program; and ensure close supervision of peer associations, consistent nonphysical discipline, and social-skill-building activities supplemented by weekly individual psychotherapy. When treatment foster care was compared with group care, a significant reduction of offending was demonstrated in the 12 months following discharge. The most significant differences between treatment foster care and group care were in the capacity of treatment foster care to prevent the adolescent from associating with deviant peers and in the quality of discipline provided.

Multisystemic therapy provides home-based community treatment for violent antisocial and substance-abusing youths. Based on social ecological and family systems theory, and applying family preservation principles, multisystemic therapy aims to empower parents with parenting skills and to enable youths to cope with family, peer, school, and neighborhood problems. Multisystemic interventions target specific problems, particularly adverse sequences of behavior within and between ecological systems (e.g., between child, family, and school), and are continually evaluated from a number of perspectives. Interventions are designed to promote the generalization and long-term maintenance of therapeutic change. Strategic and structural family therapy, behavioral parent training, cognitive-behavioral therapy, and community consultation are combined in accordance with individualized treatment plans. Deviant peer contact is monitored, discouraged, and counteracted. Parent–teacher communication is promoted. Several controlled evaluation studies have demonstrated the efficacy of multisystemic therapy compared to juvenile correctional placement, conventional individual psychotherapy, and no specific treatment.

D. PSYCHOPHARMACOLOGIC INTERVENTIONS

Until recently, conduct disorder was thought to be resistant to drug treatment. Medication was thought to be useful for treating comorbid problems, for example, ADHD (using stimulants, tricyclic antidepressants, buspirone, or serotonin reuptake inhibitors), anxiety (using propranolol or bupropion), and explosive aggression (using propranolol, carbamazepine, trazodone, or neuroleptics). The rationale for medication was based primarily on hypothetical reasoning and clinical impressions. Three controlled studies have now been completed. One study has demonstrated the efficacy of methylphenidate in reducing defiance, oppositionalism, aggression, and mood changes in outpatients age 5–8 years who were diagnosed as having conduct disorder, with or without ADHD. Another controlled study has demonstrated the effectiveness of divalproex, an "antikindling" agent, in reducing hyperarousal, anger, and aggressiveness in incarcerated adolescents. Divalproex appears to be particularly effective for those adolescents whose explosive aggression is related to posttraumatic stress disorder. A third controlled study has demonstrated the effectiveness of lithium in reducing aggressiveness in inpatient adolescents with conduct disorder. In three previous controlled studies of the effectiveness of lithium in conduct disorder, two demonstrated efficacy and one did not.

Kazdin A, et al.: Cognitive-behavioral therapy and relationship therapy in the treatment of children referred for antisocial behavior. *J Consult Clin Psychol* 1989;57:522.

Steiner H: Practice parameters for the assessment and treatment of children and adolescents with conduct disorder. *J Am Acad Child Adolesc Psychiatry* 1997;36:122S.

Zavodnick JM: Pharmacotherapy. In: Sholevar GP (ed). *Conduct Disorders in Children and Adolescents*. Washington, DC: American Psychiatric Press, 1995, pp. 269–298.

Prognosis

The developmental trajectories of the disruptive behavior disorders illustrate the principle of heterotypic continuity (the tendency of behavior patterns to evolve and change with development). For example, temperamental impulsiveness and oppositional defiant behavior in infancy and the preschool period may evolve to antiauthoritarian behavior and stealing during middle childhood; to assault, breaking and entering, risky sexual behavior, and substance abuse in adolescence; and to criminality in adulthood. Such a developmental pathway is the result of a complex interplay among biological, environmental, and ecological factors.

A recent meta-analysis of factor analyses of disruptive child behavior has yielded a two-factor solution: an overt/covert factor and an orthogonal destructive/nondestructive factor, with four quadrants: property violations (e.g., fire setting, stealing, vandalism); aggression (e.g., spitefulness, bullying, assault); oppositional behavior (e.g., anger, argumentativeness, stubbornness, defiance); and status violations (e.g., truancy, rule-breaking, substance use).

Oppositional defiant disorder usually precedes conduct disorder; and conduct disorder incorporates oppositionalism, however, only about 25% of preschoolers with oppositional defiant disorder progress to conduct disorder. In view of the similar pattern of risk factors between the two disorders, it has been contended that oppositional defiant disorder and conduct disorder do not merit a separate diagnostic status. Similarly, whereas by definition all adults with antisocial personality disorder have manifested conduct disorder in adolescence, only 25–40% of adolescents with conduct disorder progress to antisocial personality disorder. Conduct disorder in adolescent girls predicts internalizing disorders (e.g., depression, somatoform disorder) and antisocial behavior.

Aside from the oppositional defiant disorder–conduct disorder–antisocial personality disorder pathway, other developmental trajectories have been identified: an exclusive substance abuse pathway; a covert, nonaggressive pathway; and an aggressive, versatile pathway. The exclusive substance abuse pathway involves progression from less serious to more dangerous illicit drugs, without aggressive or nonaggressive delinquency. The covert, nonaggressive pathway proceeds from minor theft to serious property violations. The aggressive, versatile path has an early onset, is associated with early hyperactivity and impulsivity, and involves increasingly violent behavior (e.g., from frequent fighting to assaultive behavior). A fourth pathway, authority conflict, is described as progressing from oppositionalism to serious antiauthoritarianism. Many youths with conduct disorder cross over from one trajectory to another.

Substance-Related Disorders in Adolescents

37

Yifrah Kaminer, MD, & Deborah R. Simkin, MD

 ESSENTIALS OF DIAGNOSIS

DSM-IV-TR Diagnostic Criteria
Substance Abuse

A. A maladaptive pattern of substance use leading to clinically significant impairment or distress, as manifested by one (or more) of the following, occurring within a 12-month period:

(1) recurrent substance use resulting in a failure to fulfill major role obligations at work, school, or home (e.g., repeated absences or poor work performance related to substance use; substance-related absences, suspensions, or expulsions from school; neglect of children or household)

(2) recurrent substance use in situations in which it is physically hazardous (e.g., driving an automobile or operating a machine when impaired by substance use)

(3) recurrent substance-related legal problems (e.g., arrests for substance-related disorderly conduct)

(4) continued substance use despite having persistent or recurrent social or interpersonal problems caused or exacerbated by the effects of the substance (e.g., arguments with spouse about consequences of Intoxication, physical fights)

B. The symptoms have never met the criteria for Substance Dependence for this class of substance.

(Reprinted, with permission, from *Diagnostic and Statistical Manual of Mental Disorders*, 4th edn., Text Revision. Copyright 2000 American Psychiatric Association.)

DSM-IV-TR diagnostic criteria for substance abuse and dependence are the same for adolescents and adults. Empirical data generally support the validity of the DSM-IV-TR diagnosis for substance abuse and dependence in adolescents. However, compared with adults adolescents are polysubstance users, context of use in social setting is more common than using alone, have a more rapid transition from use to dependence, are less likely to experience blackouts and have alcohol withdrawal less often. It is important to differentiate between substance abuse and dependence and not assume a natural continuity between the two. Abuse is not always a prodrome for dependence and in most instances abuse does not progress into dependence which may also develop without having gone through an abuse phase. Abuse which includes all criteria possible of abuse plus two of the dependence criteria might present a clinical situation that is more severe of dependence that is composed of merely the minimum required (i.e., 3 criteria).

Some symptoms of the dependence category may often be developmentally limited (e.g., impaired control and tolerance which is associated with the changing body mass of the individual adolescent). Another important nosological entity in youth is entitled *orphan diagnoses*, including subthreshold alcohol or other substance dependence (i.e., one or two symptoms only). A 3-year follow-up study demonstrated that this entity has a trajectory dissimilar to those of abuse and dependence. Nevertheless, adolescents who fall into this category may manifest impairment that deserves an intervention. It is expected that the development of DSM-V will take these findings into consideration and that symptom count will generate a better developmentally sound diagnostic profile for youth.

American Psychiatric Association: *Diagnostic and Statistical Manual of Mental Disorders*, 4th edn. Text Revision. Washington, DC: American Psychiatric Association, 2000.

Angold A, Costello EJ, Farmer EMZ, et al.: Impaired but undiagnosed. *JAACAP* 1999;38:129–137.

Chung T, Maisto SA: Relapse to alcohol and other drug use in treated adolescents: Review and reconsideration of relapse as a change point in clinical course. *Clin Psychol Rev* 2006;26:149–161.

Duncan BC: The natural history of adolescent alcohol use disorders. *Addiction* 2004;99(Suppl 2):5–22.

Pollock NK, Martin CS: Diagnostic orphans: Adolescent with alcohol symptoms who do not qualify for DSM-IV abuse or dependence diagnoses. *Am J Psychiatry* 1999;156:897–901.

General Considerations

The use of alcohol and other drugs are associated with the three leading causes of mortality among adolescents as a result of motor vehicle accidents, homicide and suicide. Additional morbidity under the influence of substances have contributed to violent behavior, rape, and unprotected sexual activity including unplanned pregnancy and sexually transmitted diseases.

A. EPIDEMIOLOGY

Lifetime diagnoses of alcohol and drug abuse among adolescents in different states in the US range from 3–10%. Six percent and 5.4% of youths aged between 12 and 17 were classified as needing treatment for alcohol use and illicit drug use respectively. Due to lack of motivation, limited resources, insufficient age-appropriate quality programs, and lack of a broad consensus on preferred treatment strategies, only 10–15% of adolescents in need of treatment end up receiving services.

Although any nonmedical use of drugs (including tobacco and alcohol) by adolescents is illegal and can be regarded as a form of abuse, this viewpoint ignores some key epidemiological findings. Specifically, the high prevalence of alcohol and tobacco use underscores the fact that use of alcohol and tobacco is normative, or at least not exceptionally deviant. By age 18 years, approximately 80% of youth in the United States have drunk alcohol, two thirds have smoked cigarettes, and 50% have used at least once an illicit drug. Four percent drink alcohol daily and 13% smoke half a pack of cigarettes a day. Substance use (marijuana in particular) among American youth rose alarmingly rates between 1992 and 1997. Since then, it has decreased significantly until 2002 and has since then leveled off for alcohol, tobacco, and most drug classes except for prescription opiates, the use of which continues to increase.

Most adolescents who engage in substance use do not develop substance use disorder (SUD) as defined by DSM-IV-TR criteria. It is thus imperative to understand adolescent substance use in the context of changing patterns of behavior and to distinguish normative behavior from a SUD.

Johnston LD, O'Malley IM, Bachman JG, Schulenberg JE: *Monitoring the Future. National results on adolescent drug use: Overview of key findings 2005.* Bethesda, MD: National Institute on Drug Abuse. NIH Publication No. 06–5882, 2006. http://monitoringthe/future.org/pubs/monographs/overview2005.pdf

B. ETIOLOGY

Adolescent neurodevelopment occurs in brain regions associated with motivation, impulsivity, executive functioning and addiction. Adolescent impulsivity and novelty seeking can be explained in part by maturational changes in the prefrontal cortex. These developmental processes may promote for adaptation to adulthood but also confer greater vulnerability to the drug addiction. A number of behavioral dispositions and environmental influences predict age at initiation of drug use, drug use intensity, and the experience of negative consequences during adolescence. These behavioral characteristics are impulsivity, aggression, sensation seeking, low levels of harm avoidance, inability to delay gratification, low achievement motivation, lack of a religious orientation, and psychopathology, especially conduct disorder. The most common contextual or environmental factors are stressful life events, lack of parental support, absence of prosocial peers, perception of high availability of drugs, social norms that encourage drug use, and relaxed laws and regulatory policies. Clearly, manifold risk factors, with different salience, determine overall risk. In aggregate, these risk factors determine the slope and momentum of the developmental trajectory into adulthood, culminating in substance use, abuse, or dependence. Psychiatric disorders, and temperamental precursors such as impulsivity and novelty seeking tend to peak in late adolescence or early adulthood and are predictive of SUDs.

Young adults who become problem drinkers are likely to be rebellious, nonconforming and deviant during high school. Research using difficult-temperament index to classify adolescent alcoholic patients resulted in clusters that were similar to the adult subtypes reported by Cloninger and Babor. The smaller subset of adolescents manifesting behavioral dyscontrol and hypophoria were included in Cluster 2, whereas those with primarily negative affect were included in Cluster 1. Compared with Cluster 1 subjects, Cluster 2 patients were younger at the time of first substance use, first substance abuse diagnosis, and first psychiatric diagnosis. Moreover, adolescents with difficult temperament had a high probability of having psychiatric disorders such as conduct disorder, attention-deficit/hyperactivity disorder (ADHD), anxiety and mood disorders. Cluster 1 and Cluster 2 were identified in both genders.

Babor TF, Hofman MI, Del-Boca FK, et al.: Types of alcoholics. Evidence for an empirically derived typology based on indicators of vulnerability and severity. *Arch Gen Psychiatry* 1992;49:599–608.

Cloninger CR: Neurogenetic adaptive mechanisms in alcoholism. *Science* 1987;236:410–416.

Tarter RE, Kirisci L, Mezzich A: Multivariate typology of adolescents with alcohol use disorder. *Am J Addict* 1997;6:150–158.

Zuckerman M: *Behavioral Expressions and Biosocial Bases of Sensation Seeking.* New York: Cambridge University Press, 1994

C. GENETICS

Vulnerability to engage in the use and abuse of substances involve an interaction of genetic and environmental factors (i.e., nature and nurture) over the course of development. The genetic contributions are likely to be complex traits involving multiple loci of small effect. Several individual genes that may contribute to the risk for dependence have been identified. The case of alcohol, these include genes encoding alcohol and aldehyde dehydrogenases and gamma amino butyric acid (A) receptor subunits.

Clinical Findings

A. ASSESSMENT AND SCREENING

Self-report of substance use by adolescents is generally valid and more sensitive than laboratory testing. Collateral reports of alcohol and drug abuse from parents or other adults have low to moderate sensitivity compared to self-report and urinalysis. It may be helpful, in interviewing an adolescent, to begin by asking whether illicit drugs are available at school, whether the patient has close friends who use drugs, and whether the patient has access to drugs. Examples of reliable and valid screening instruments include The Personal Experience Screening Questionnaire, the Substance Abuse Subtle Screening Inventory, the Drug Use Screening Inventory-Revised, and the Problem Oriented Screening Instrument for Teenagers and the easy to use CRAFFT. A score of 2 or higher on the CRAFFT is optimal for identifying any problem use. The **CRAFFT** questions are as follows: Have you ever ridden in a **C**ar driven by someone (including yourself) who was "high or had been using alcohol or drugs? Do you ever use alcohol or drugs to **R**elax, feel better about yourself or to fit in? Do you ever use alcohol/drugs while you are by yourself or **A**lone? Do your **F**amily/friends ever tell you that you should cut down your drinking/drug use? Do you ever **F**orget things you did while using alcohol or drugs? Have you gotten into **T**rouble while you were using alcohol or drugs?

If the self-report is positive, then it is important to assess the severity of the problem using well established semi-structured interviews such as the Teen Addiction Severity Index, the Adolescent Drug Abuse Diagnosis, or the Personal Experience Inventory. Computerized assessment is possible, for example, the Teen Addiction Severity Index was modified into a self-report administered via a telephone or a website. Modern technology also allows the telephone interactive voice response which provides a daily record of risky situations and drug use.

Brodey B, Rosen C, Winters K, et al.: Conversion & validation of the Teen-Addiction Severity Index (T-ASI) into internet and automated telephone self-report administration. *Psychol Addict Behav* 2005;19:54–61.

Knight JR, Sherritt L, Shier LA, et al.: Validity of the CRAFFT substance abuse screening test among adolescent clinic patients. *Arch Pediatr Adolesc Med* 2002;156(6):607–614.

Winters KC, Latimer WW, Stinchfield R: Assessing adolescent substance use. In: Wagner EF, Waldron HB (eds). *Innovations in adolescent Substance Abuse Interventions.* Amsterdam: Pergamon, 2001, pp. 1–29.

B. SIGNS AND SYMPTOMS

Signs and symptoms that could represent give a clue to substance include changes in social network and association with deviant peers, secretive behavior, locking of the youth room, excessive complains about violation of privacy, smell of alcohol or marijuana on clothing, the youth or in the room. Inappropriate and atypical behavior such as agitation or sedation, pupillary dilation or constriction, tachycardia, blood-shot eyes, diaphoresis, slurred speech, yawning, and unsteady gait. The presence of eye drops, prescription drugs, drug paraphernalia or drugs will make the definite confirmation.

C. LABORATORY FINDINGS

Testing for drugs of abuse can be performed on urine, blood, breath, hair, saliva, and sweat. Urine testing is most widely used because it is noninvasive, simple to obtain, and yields a detectable concentration of most drugs of abuse. The best evidence for long-term drug use is the combination of a good history and a urine toxicology screen. Screening tests for single or multiple drugs of abuse are commercially available. These tests typically screen for many possible combinations of drugs including opioids, alcohol, cocaine, marijuana, and amphetamines. Validity and reliability of urine drug test results can be compromised by tampering with the sample. Requirements for notification or permission to obtain specimens vary by jurisdiction. Patients should be asked for permission to perform testing. Self-report is highly reliable as long as it is not associated with a legal contingency. Parental report tends to be deficient or unreliable yet, should be obtained for a complete picture and to improve parental participation in the diagnostic and treatment processes.

Buchan BJ, Dennis ML, Tims FM, Diamond GS: Marijuana use: consistency and validity of self-report, on-site urine testing and laboratory testing. *Addiction* 2002;97(S1):98–108.

Burleson J, Kaminer Y: Adolescent alcohol and marijuana use: Concordance among objective-, self-, and collateral-reports. *J Child Adolesc Subst Abuse* 2006;16:53–68.

D. Neuroimaging and Neuropsychology

It is difficult to make accurate generalizations or conclusive statements about the neuropsychological and neurobiological correlates of drug use given variations in the nature or extent of deficits observed within or across different classes of agents. In any instances, however, there is evidence of impairments in prefrontally-mediated cognitive functions that underlie behavioral regulation, including decision making and inhibitory control.

Chambers RA, Taylor JR, Potenza MN: Developmental neurocircuitry of motivation in adolescence: A critical period of addiction vulnerability. *Am J Psychiatry* 2003;160:1041–1052.

Kalivas P, Volkow ND: The neural basis of addiction: A pathology of motivation and choice. *Am J Psychiatry* 2005;162(8):1403–1413.

E. Course of Illness

According to the influential "gateway" theory, there are at least four distinct developmental stages of drug use: (1) beer or wine consumption, (2) cigarette smoking or hard liquor consumption, (3) marijuana use, and (4) other illicit drug use. Approximately 25% of adolescents who use marijuana progress to the next stage, compared with only 4% who have never done so. This theory has been challenged given the increased preference for the use of marijuana with only limited or no experience with alcohol use. The best-supported hypothesis for the common comorbidity between alcohol and illicit drug dependence in adolescents is that comorbid disorders are alternative forms of a single underlying liability. The next best fitting models refer to correlated risk factors and reciprocal causation. Long-term trajectories of SUD with and without treatment are important. Youth are at increased risk for onset or worsening of SUDs until their mid 20s. Findings of long-term follow-up of adolescents with SUDs indicate that indeed adolescents have heterogeneous trajectories. A characteristic paradigm includes a small percentage of demonstrated sustained recovery, one third manifested an intermittent recovery pattern, less then 30% of low base rate of abuse at 2–8-year follow-up another one-third had sustained problems.

Abrantes AM, McCarthy DM, Aarons GA, Brown SA: Trajectories of alcohol involvement following addiction treatment through 8-year follow-up in adolescents. *Alcohol Clin Exp Res* 2003;27:258–259.

Godley SH, Dennis ML, Godley MD, Funk RR: Thirty-month relapse trajectory cluster groups among adolescents discharged from out-patient treatment. *Addiction* 2004;99(Supp 2):129–139.

Kandel DB: Epidemiological and psychosocial perspective on adolescent drug use. *J Am Acad Child Adolesc Psychiatry* 1982;20:328–347.

Differential Diagnosis (Including Comorbid Conditions)

The literature identified all psychiatric disorders, particularly disruptive behavior disorders, as an increased risk for SUD. However, the etiological mechanisms have not been systematically researched. A number of possible relationships exist between SUDs and psychopathology. Psychopathology can precede SUD, develop as a consequence of preexisting SUD, moderate the severity of substance use, or originate from a common vulnerability.

Psychiatric comorbidity is the rule rather than the exception. In 75% of cases the psychiatric comorbidity precedes the SUD. Conduct disorder is commonly associated with adolescent SUD. It usually precedes SUD. Rates of conduct disorder range from 50% to 80% in adolescent patients with SUD. ADHD is frequently observed and has been implicated as directly causing SUD as well as through the high rate of comorbid disruptive disorders which accompany ADHD. Mood disorder, especially depression, frequently precedes SUD in adolescents. The prevalence of depressive disorders ranges from 24% to more than 50%.

Several studies have found a high rate of anxiety disorder among youth with SUD. In adolescent patients with SUD, the prevalence of anxiety disorder has ranged from 7% to more than 40%. Social phobia usually precedes substance abuse, whereas panic and generalized anxiety disorder more often follow it. Adolescents with SUD often have posttraumatic stress disorder as a result of physical or sexual abuse. Bulimia nervosa and personality disorders, particularly those in Cluster B, are also commonly found. Finally, it was reported that pathological gambling in youth may be associated with substance abuse.

Grilo CM, Becker DF, Walker ML, et al.: Psychiatric comorbidity in adolescent inpatients with substance use disorders. *J Am Acad Child Adolesc Psychiatry* 1995;34:1085–1091.

Kaminer Y, Oscar OG: *Adolescent substance Abuse: Psychiatric Comorbidity & High Risk Behaviors.* New York: Taylor & Francis, 2008.

Prevention

Efforts to curtail substance abuse have historically concentrated on modifying the supply-to-demand ratio. However, reduction of supply cannot succeed as long as there is demand. Hence, reducing demand is an essential component of prevention. Laws and regulations can reduce demand. Development of effective approaches to substance abuse prevention is a national priority. The most promising prevention strategies aim to enhance social skills and drug-refusal. A school curriculum, the Life Skills Training program, was initially developed as a prevention program involving the teaching of general life skills and of skills for resisting social influences. This prevention program was led by older peers and classroom teachers. The investigators reported a lasting reduction in drug use 6 years later among the twelfth-graders in the experimental condition compared to those in the control condition. The generalizability of Life Skills Training prevention to African-American and Hispanic youth has been supported. To maximize outcome, an understanding of the heterogeneity of the adolescent population is required. Preventive efforts need to take into account the developmental staging of substance use behavior, and address the needs of adolescents in different domains of life. Prevention programs sensitive to ethnic difference must be designed. Finally, universal prevention programs may delay onset of drinking among low-risk baseline abstainers; but there is little evidence of utility for high-risk adolescents. They contend that motivational interviewing (MI) in a harm-reduction framework is well suited for secondary prevention in adolescents.

Botvin GJ, Griffin KW: Life skills training: Theory, methods, and effectiveness of a drug abuse prevention approach. In: Wagner EF, Waldron HB (eds). *Innovations in Adolescent Substance Abuse Interventions*. Amsterdam: Pergamon, 2001, pp. 31–50.

National Institute for Drug Abuse. *Preventing Substance Abuse among Children and Adolescents*—A Research-Based Guide for Parents, Educators, and Community Leaders, 2nd edn. Washington, DC: U.S. Dept. of Health and Human Services, NIH publication No. 04–4212(A), 2003.

Treatment

Significant progress has been made in conceptualizing, testing, and implementing treatment strategies and programs for adolescents with SUD. One of the challenges in the treatment of adolescent SUD has been the attempt to match the individual needs of the adolescent to appropriate treatment services and levels of care. There is a growing consensus that SUD is not an acute disorder with a potentially chronic, relapsing course. A common view of addiction treatment is that it is a linear process requiring a continuum of case management and case monitoring akin to that in chronic disease management.

A. Systems of Care for Adolescents with SUD

Eighty percent of adolescents with SUD are treated in outpatient settings. Outpatient services usually deliver episodic care utilizing group therapy without coordination or continuity of care. While many adolescents with mild to moderate severity respond to some degree to brief interventions, some do not. Moreover, the higher the severity, the less likely this is. More characteristic is a relapsing/remitting course over a prolonged period of time across several episodes of care and levels of care, with different services and interventions. Since SUD is usually a part of a dysfunction in school, family, legal, and behavioral domains, the need for service coordination and multidisciplinary teamwork is clear. There is a growing utilization of the American Society for Addiction medicine Placement Criteria for both youth and adults.

Fishman M. Treatment planning, matching, and placement for adolescent substance abuse. In: Kaminer Y, Oscar OG (eds). *Adolescent substance Abuse: Psychiatric Comorbidity & High Risk Behaviors*. New York: Haworth Press, 2007.

Libby AM, Riggs PD: Integrated services for substance abuse and mental health: Challenges and opportunities. In: Kaminer Y, Oscar OG (eds). *Adolescent Substance Abuse: Psychiatric Comorbidity & High Risk Behaviors*. New York: Haworth Press, 2007.

B. Psychosocial Treatments

Psychosocial treatments that have shown promise for adolescent SUD include the following: Multi-systemic Therapy (MST); Multi-dimensional Family Therapy (MDFT); Cognitive–Behavioral Therapy (CBT), conducted either in groups or individually; Motivational Enhancement Therapy (MET); Contingency Management Reinforcement; the Minnesota 12-Step model; and other integrative models of treatment. Twelve-step programs are often recommended. However, little is known regarding the effectiveness of this approach for adolescents.

There is little evidence to suggest that one therapy is more effective than another.

Family therapy is the most researched treatment modality for adolescent substance abuse. MST is an intensive home-based family intervention that addresses schools, peer groups, parenting skills, family communication skills, and family relations. MST combines structural and strategic family therapy with cognitive behavioral therapy. While prior reviews conclude that MST is the most promising empirically-based treatment for children with substance abuse, the conclusion was that available evidence does not support the claim that MST is more effective than usual services or other interventions for youth with social, emotional or behavioral problems. There is no evidence of harmful effects compared to alternative services. MST has several advantages in that it is comprehensive, based upon current knowledge of youth and family problems, well documented, and empirical.

MDFT is recognized as one of the most promising interventions for adolescent drug abuse. MDFT combines drug counseling with multiple systems assessment and intervention both inside and outside the family. The approach is developmentally and ecologically oriented, to the environmental and individual systems in which the adolescent resides. MDFT is manualized and delivered in 16–25 sessions over 4–6 months at home or in the office.

CBT views substance use and related problems as learned behaviors initiated and maintained by environmental factors. Most CBT approaches integrate classical conditioning, operant conditioning, and social learning theory. Recent studies involve rigorous designs, larger samples, random assignment, direct comparisons of two or more active treatments, improved measures, manualization, and longer-term outcome assessment. The focus in treatment has been on improved drug refusal skills and managing of high-risk situations. Improved self-efficacy is associated with better outcome. CBT can also be applied in group settings. Different adolescents are manageable in a group once a clearly communicated, behavioral contract for ground rules is established. Experienced therapists can address inappropriate behavior and employ "trouble shooting" techniques.

MI and MET are based on research on the process of change. MI pertains both to a style of relating and a set of techniques to facilitate that process. Five main strategies are used in applying this approach: (1) express empathy; (2) develop discrepancy; (3) avoid argumentation; (4) roll with resistance; and (5) support self-efficacy. Ever since treatment results for adolescent substance abuse have been reported, clinicians and researchers have noted the difficulty of keeping adolescents in treatment. Retention can be regarded as one successful treatment outcome. Brief motivational interventions have not been investigated until recently. A single session of MI, designed to reduce illicit drugs among young people between 16–20 years of age, produced significant decrease in cannabis use at 12-week follow-up compared with nonintervention. Several studies have successfully employed MI following a negative event (e.g., a motor vehicle accident with referral to the emergency room), an intervention exploiting a "teachable moment." MET may be suitable for adolescents because they do not have to admit to having a substance use problem in order to benefit from it. MI alone may not be sufficient for adolescents with severe AOSUD or psychiatric comorbidity. However, it may be an effective preliminary to such treatments as CBT.

The Cannabis Youth Treatment study is most probably the most important study yet conducted. This randomized prospective field experiment compared five interventions, in various combinations, across the four US implementation sites, for 600 adolescents. The study addressed the comparative efficacy of five treatments. Two group CBT interventions were offered. Both began with individual MET sessions, followed by either 3 or 10 sessions of group administered CBT. A third intervention was MET/CBT plus a 6-week family psycho-educational

intervention. A 12-session individual Adolescent Community Reinforcement Approach, and a 12-week course of MDFT were also tested. The effectiveness of five treatment models was evaluated in a community-based program and an academic medical center. Although all five models were not implemented within each treatment site, the MET plus three sessions of group CBT was replicated across all four sites, making it possible to study site differences and conduct quasi-experimental comparisons of the interventions across the study arms. All five interventions produced a significant reduction in cannabis use and negative consequences of use, from pretreatment to the 3-month follow-up. These reductions were sustained through the 12-month follow-up. Changes in marijuana use were accompanied by amelioration of behavioral problems, family problems, school problems, school absences, argumentativeness, violence, and illegal activity. Despite considerable support for family intervention in the literature, the individual Adolescent Community Reinforcement Approach and individual MET plus three sessions of group CBT produced better outcomes than the family approach in terms of days of substance use at 3 months. However, these initial differences were not sustained. The best predictor of long-term outcome was initial level of change. In terms of cost effectiveness, MDFT was better than the other interventions. One of the important contributions of the Cannabis Youth Treatment to the knowledge base is the emphasis on community effectiveness and ecological validity compared to a demonstration of efficacy in specialized research setting.

Treatment of adolescents with substance-related problems often incorporate the 12-step philosophy advocated by Alcoholics Anonymous (AA), and Narcotics Anonymous (NA). A national survey of adolescent programs found that more than two-thirds (67%) involved "12-step" concepts. Many of these programs encourage attendance at community AA and NA groups following treatment. Four studies have examined the predictors of participation in AA/NA. A retrospective study found that youth who were more hopeless, had friends who did not use drugs, and who had less parental involvement during treatment were more likely to become involved in AA. Two studies found that more severely alcohol and drug-involved youth, and those more motivated for abstinence and not by coping skills or self-efficacy, were more likely to both attend and become actively involved in AA/NA in the first 3 months posttreatment. An 8-year follow-up study found that, following inpatient treatment, more severe substance dependence, measured by the number of DSM-IV-TR dependence symptoms at the time of treatment, predicted AA/NA attendance throughout a 6-year follow-up period, but not at 8-years following treatment, after controlling for age, gender and intake substance use indices.

Developmentally-related differences between adolescents and adults suggest that 12-step programs may not be appropriate for youth. For instance, when adolescents are compared to older adult counterparts for whom AA was originally devised, adolescents on average have less addiction severity and related sequelae, and lower substance-related problem recognition and motivation for abstinence. They are significantly younger relative to the majority of other AA/NA members. Some youth are uncomfortable with the spiritual/religious emphasis of AA/NA. AA/NA may be suitable for youth whose addiction is more severe.

Treatment of substance in the context of co-occurring psychiatric disorders: the National Institute of Drug Abuse recommends integrated treatment of co-occurring psychiatric disorders as a core treatment principle. However, systemic and economic barriers impede the implementation of integrated care: Not enough treatment providers; the resistance by gatekeepers to specialty care; and financing streams. Combined treatment of psychiatric disorder and SUD may produce a better outcome than mental health or SUD treatment alone. The optimal design of integrated treatment (e.g., simultaneous or sequential), and the treatment components and dosage have yet to be determined. Psychopharmacological treatment for psychiatric comorbidity usually addresses only the psychiatric disorder.

Burleson JA, Kaminer Y, Dennis M: Absence of iatrogenic or contagion effects in adolescent group therapy: Findings from the cannabis youth treatment (CYT) study. *Am J Addict* 2006;15(Suppl 1):4–15.

Dennis ML, Godley SH, Diamond G, et al.: Main findings of the cannabis youth treatment randomized field experiment. *J Subst Abuse Treat* 2004;27:197–213.

Drug Strategies: *Treating teens: A guide to adolescent programs.* Washington, DC: Drug Strategies, 2003.

Liddle HA, Rowe CL: *Adolescent substance abuse: Research and clinical advances.* Cambridge, UK: Cambridge University Press, 2006.

Miller WR, Rollnick S: *Motivational Interviewing: Preparing people for change*, 2nd edn. New York: Guilford Press, 2002.

C. PSYCHOPHARMACOLOGICAL INTERVENTIONS

Medications are sometimes used to prevent relapse once an initial remission is secured. Pharmacotherapy is only useful when combined with counseling. Examples include naltrexone for opioid or alcohol abuse/dependence, and drugs such as disulfiram for alcohol abuse and dependence. These agents are rarely used in adolescent populations.

Waxmonsky JG, Wilens TE: Pharmacotherapy of adolescent substance use disorders: A review of the literature. *J Child Adolesc Psychopharmacol* 2005;15(5):810–825.

D. AFTERCARE

Relapse rates are over 60% 12 months after treatment. However, little has been done to link patients with aftercare. Often, there is no coordinated continuing care. The lack of posttreatment support and monitoring leaves patients vulnerable to relapse. The literature provides little guidance for aftercare programs. It is not clear who is a candidate for aftercare. Few programs describe the means of linking completers or non-completers with aftercare. Adolescents referred to residential treatment have severe SUD and are at risk both for relapse and poor linkage to aftercare. Adolescents referred from residential treatment to continuing care services are more likely to initiate and receive more continuing care services, to be abstinent from marijuana at 3 months postdischarge and to reduce 3-month postdischarge days of alcohol use provided they are assigned to an assertive continuing-care protocol providing case management, home visits, and a community reinforcement approach. Aftercare reduced the likelihood of suicidal ideations.

Many communities lack aftercare services. Even if referrals are made, many adolescents do not enter, or only participate minimally in, aftercare interventions. Godley and colleagues found that only 36% of adolescents discharged from residential treatment attended one or more aftercare sessions at community clinics. It is imperative to provide aftercare unplanned discharged adolescents because they are at the highest risk for bad outcome. At a minimum, providers should track linkage rates by type of discharge and determine whether the adolescent is referred to their own organization or another service provider to inform their linkage practice. Finally, new interventions and modalities should be tested. Telepsychiatry should be used when distance from service providers and cost effectiveness are barriers for the provision of aftercare.

Godley MD, Godley SH, Dennis ML: Preliminary outcomes from the assertive continuing care experiment for adolescents discharged from residential treatment. *J Subst Abuse Treat* 2002;23:21–32.

Kaminer Y, Burleson J, Goldston D, Haberek R: Suicidal ideation in adolescents with alcohol use disorders during treatment and aftercare. *Am J Addict* 2006;15(Suppl 1):43–49.

Complications

Substance use and abuse threatens the health and well-being of adolescents. Substance use contributes to many deaths from injuries, homicide, and suicide, the three leading causes of mortality in this age group. For example, adolescents who commit suicide are frequently under the influence of alcohol or other drugs at the time of death. Possible mechanisms underlying this relationship include the direct acute pharmacological and chronic neurological effects of psychoactive substances. Acute intoxication may be experienced as an intense dysphoric state, with behavioral disinhibition and impaired judgment. Substance use can also exacerbate preexisting psychopathology, especially impulse dyscontrol, depression, and anxiety.

Other complications include impaired school performance, school failure, unintended pregnancies, and criminal behavior. Medical complications include the toxic effects of substances on the CNS or other organ systems either as the result of chronic use, overdoses or due to the simultaneous use of multiple agents. Intravenous drug abuse can cause infections including endocarditis, hepatitis, and human immunodeficiency virus (HIV). Up to 90% of illicit injection drug users will eventually become infected with hepatitis C virus. Prostitution to support drug habits frequently leads to sexually transmitted diseases including HIV infection.

Goldston D: Conceptual issues in understanding the relationship between suicidal behavior and substance abuse during adolescence. *Drug Alch Dep* 2004;76S:S79–S91.

Prognosis

Relapse in adolescent drug abuse is commonplace. In a prospective study of adolescents, age at first use of illicit drugs did not emerge as an independent risk factor for either persistence or severity of drug use in adulthood. Alcohol and substance use increases until the early 20s, then plateaus as young adults moderate or even cease it. This decrease accompanied by a change in cognitive structure. When substance use behavior at age 18 years is controlled, there is no significant relationship between the intensity and consequences of adolescent risk and adult substance use. The effect of child and adolescent risk factors on adult substance use is likely mediated by the intensity of substance use in late adolescence.

Programs aimed at reducing risk factors during adolescence may have a more beneficial effects if they limit drug use during the peak lifetime period, at ages 18–21 years. Programs that focus on postadolescence should concentrate on concurrent risk factors that are not necessarily the same as those operating during adolescence. In early adolescence, prevention efforts should be directed at delaying onset and increase of drug use, because drug use predicts future drug use, although not in an invariant fashion. Finally, while many adolescents manifest a chronic course into adulthood some overcome their problem and transition into abstinence or normative drinking.

Bates ME, Labouvie EW: Adolescent risk factors and the prediction of persistent alcohol and drug use into adulthood. *Alcohol Clin Exp Res* 1997;21:944–950.

Depressive Disorders (in Childhood and Adolescence)

38

David A. Brent, MD, & Lisa Pan, MD

ESSENTIALS OF DIAGNOSIS

DSM-IV-TR Diagnostic Criteria
Major Depressive Episode

A. Five (or more) of the following symptoms have been present during the same 2-week period and represent a change from previous functioning; at least one of the symptoms is either (1) depressed mood or (2) loss of interest or pleasure.
Note: Do not include symptoms that are clearly due to a general medical condition, or mood-incongruent delusions and hallucinations.

  (1) depressed mood. Note: In children and adolescents, can be irritable mood
  (2) loss of interest or pleasure (anhedonia)
  (3) significant weight loss when not dieting or weight gain, or decrease or increase in appetite. Note: In children and adolescents, can be failure to make expected weight gains
  (4) insomnia or hypersomnia
  (5) psychomotor agitation or retardation
  (6) fatigue or loss of energy
  (7) feelings of worthlessness or inappropriate/excessive guilt
  (8) diminished ability to think or concentrate, or indecisiveness
  (9) recurrent thoughts of death or suicide

B. The symptoms do not meet criteria for a mixed episode.

C. The symptoms cause significant distress or impairment in social, occupational, or other important areas of functioning.

D. The symptoms are not due to the direct physiological effects of a substance (e.g., drug of abuse) or a general medical condition (e.g., hypothyroidism).

E. The symptoms are not better accounted for by bereavement (i.e., depressive/grief symptoms lasting less than 2 months).

(Reprinted, with permission, from the *Diagnostic and Statistical Manual of Mental Disorders*, 4th edn., Text Revision. Copyright 2000 American Psychiatric Association.)

In this chapter, we describe the characteristics and epidemiology of unipolar depressive disorders in children and adolescents, etiologic risk factors for depression onset and recurrence, and assessment and differential diagnosis of depressive disorders. We review recommended psychosocial and pharmacological treatments, and in conclusion, suggest areas for future investigation.

General Considerations

Child and adolescent depressive disorders are common, often recurrent, and generally continue into adulthood. These disorders are often familial, and are associated with additional morbidity and mortality from comorbid substance abuse and from suicide and suicidal behavior. Patients also suffer educational and later occupational underachievement as well as relationship difficulties. Therefore, early identification and treatment of these conditions are important public health issues.

A. Epidemiology

The estimated prevalence of MDD is 2% in children and 4–8% in adolescents. After puberty, the risk for depression increases two- to fourfold, with 20% incidence by the age of 18 years. The gender ratio in childhood is 1:1, with an increase in the risk for depression in females after puberty, when the male/female is estimated at 1:2. This may be related to higher rates of anxiety in females, changes in estradiol and testosterone at puberty, or sociocultural issues related to female adolescent development.

It is important to differentiate childhood-onset from adolescent-onset depression. Depressive disorders in adolescence are much more likely to be recurrent into adulthood. In the context of significant family adversity, prepubertal depression is most often comorbid with behavioral problems. A less common form of childhood prepubertal depression is associated with strong familial loading for depression, high rates of anxiety, high risk for bipolar outcome, and recurrent mood disorder into adolescence and adulthood.

B. Etiology

Early-onset depression is multifactorial, including, but not limited to, familial factors, early life events, neuroendocrine changes, and genetics. Twin studies show the importance of genetic and environmental factors, particularly in interaction. Familial risk factors for recurrent depressive disorders in youth include early-onset parental mood disorder. Non-familial depression has as risk factors parental substance-abuse disorder, parental criminality, family discord and low family cohesion. Abuse may also be related to an earlier onset of depressive symptoms, as well as many other comorbid conditions. The contribution of early adverse life events is much greater in the setting of familial genetic risk factors.

C. Genetics

The strongest single factor for developing MDD is familial loading for the disorder. The majority of studies including twin, adoption and high-risk studies have shown a familial pattern with interaction of environmental and genetic factors. Family studies show a two- to fourfold increased risk for depression in offspring of depressed parents. Twin studies show a heritability for depression of 40–65%. Evidence from twin studies shows greater genetic concordance in adolescent-onset depression than in childhood-onset depression, suggesting that very early onset depression is more related to environmental factors.

One model of the interaction of genes and environment indicates a strong cotransmission for depression and anxiety, with heritability of greater than 60%. Genes imparting risk for anxiety may lead to youth depression by increasing sensitivity to adverse life events, another example of gene–environment interaction. This model is further supported by the association of the genetic variant of the serotonin receptor that is less functional, contributing to early-onset depression in interaction with stressful life events.

Clinical Findings

A. Signs and Symptoms

Depressive symptoms in childhood include consistent sad or depressed mood, anhedonia, change in appetite (increase or decrease), sleep disturbance, anergia, amotivation, irritability or agitation, worthlessness or guilt, poor concentration, and morbid ideation or thoughts of suicide. Children and adolescents may present with psychomotor retardation, but more often present with disabling irritability.

Children and adolescents presenting with depressive symptoms may be classified on the basis of impairment, severity, persistence of illness, and symptom profile. In the absence of a stressor leading to time-limited adjustment disorder, depression not otherwise specified (NOS) is diagnosed when full criteria for an MDD are not met. Dysthymic disorder is pervasive and chronic, lasting at least 1 year, with fewer symptoms than MDD. Dysthymia may be complicated by major depressive episodes, and is then often referred to as "double depression." Dysthymic disorder or "minor depression," and subsyndromal depression can be disabling, and may be precursors to MDD.

Major depression involves depressed mood, irritable mood, or anhedonia, plus four other symptoms. It is the most severe of the depressive disorders, and can be associated with psychosis. Psychosis presents as auditory hallucinations of a derogatory and mood-congruent nature, but may also include morbid visual hallucinations or delusional thinking in severe cases.

B. Psychological Testing

No psychological test is diagnostic of major depressive disorder. A comprehensive psychiatric diagnostic evaluation is the most useful tool to diagnose depressive disorders in children and adolescents. The Mood and Feelings Questionnaire (short-form) can be used to screen for depression and also to monitor treatment.

C. Laboratory Findings

No laboratory studies are diagnostic of major depressive episode, however, laboratory findings are abnormal in some patients with MDD symptoms. Provocative studies of noradrenergic, hypothalamic–pituitary adrenal axis, and serotonergic systems have been found to be abnormal in depressed child and adolescent patients, but this is particularly true of patients exposed to trauma or severe life stressors.

Subclinical hypothyroidism, anemia, diabetes, and vitamin deficiencies including B_{12} and folate are associated with depressive symptoms. While these are more common in adults, screening laboratories including thyroid function testing, complete blood count, electrolytes, blood sugar, and B_{12} and folate levels may be indicated, in cases of chronic or unresponsive depression.

D. Neuroimaging

Differences in morphometric and functional magnetic resonance imaging (fMRI) have contributed to our understanding of the neural circuitry underlying the development of depressive disorders. Structural imaging studies have revealed reduced volume of the left sub-genual prefrontal cortex of both adolescents with depression and adults with family history of depression and early-onset of their own disorder. A review of imaging studies of adolescent and young adult twins suggested that this structural difference is genetically transmitted and may partially mediate the heritability of depression. Depressed adolescents also were found to have increased third and fourth ventricular volume in addition to decreased prefrontal cortical volume. In an fMRI study, depressed adolescents, like depressed adults, showed increased activity within the ventromedial prefrontal cortex and rostral anterior cingulate gyrus. Other fMRI studies have shown abnormalities in response to fearful faces, with increased amygdala activation in anxious children, and decreased amygdala activation in depressed children. In addition, MDD subjects had poorer memory for faces, and subjects who successfully encoded faces had higher activation of the left amygdala. The similarity of some of these findings to those in adults may indicate that neural circuitry contributing to depression is present in adolescence, and persist through development to adulthood.

Course of Illness

The average duration of major depressive episode in community samples is 3–6 months, with slightly longer duration in referred samples of 5–8 months. Approximately 1 in 5 adolescents will have resistant depression lasting greater than 2 years. In contrast, depressive episodes may remit spontaneously without treatment. Comorbidity, especially with dysthymic disorder, increased severity, presence of suicidal ideation, parental depression, and absence of a supportive environment contribute to longer duration and intractability of episodes.

Depression is a chronic and recurrent disorder. While childhood depression is less common, there is high likelihood of recurrence during adolescence. Adolescents remain at risk for recurrence into adulthood. Estimates of the risk for childhood recurrence from one study indicate 40% relapse by year two of remission and over 70% relapse within 5 years. Estimates of recurrence for adolescent depression are between 30–70% in 1–2 years of follow-up. Children in whom there is incomplete symptom remission, presence of dysthymia, history of abuse, continued social impairment, or parental history of early depression are more likely to experience recurrence. Children and adolescents with persistent depression are at risk for a myriad of complications including suicidal behavior, personality disorders, substance-use disorders, psychosocial dysfunction, obesity, and underachievement. Bipolar outcome occurs in 10–20% of clinical referred samples of child and adolescent depression and is most common in

psychotically depressed patients and those with a strong family history of mania.

The majority of children and adolescents presenting for treatment of depression has a co-occurring disorder. Commonly, patients suffer from comorbid anxiety disorder, which can predate the onset of depressive symptoms. This should be differentiated from dysphoria, which resolves with removal of stress. Children with a history of childhood abuse are predisposed to development of depression. In these children, posttraumatic stress disorder and other disorders of extreme stress are prevalent. Substance-use disorders can lead to depression and, conversely, self-medication of depression and anxiety can lead to substance abuse or dependence. Disruptive behavior disorders and impulse control disorders are often comorbid with depression, and can be misdiagnosed if depression is not identified. ADHD, in particular, is often diagnosed in depressed youth and may be coheritable in some families. There is evidence that depression leads to conduct disorder and the reverse.

The most serious concern in children and adolescents with depression is their increased risk for suicide and suicidal behavior. All patients should be assessed for the presence of suicidal ideation. Depressed youth with suicidal ideation require additional monitoring and treatment targeting improvement of suicidality. If suicidal ideation is present with intent, the patient requires treatment in an inpatient, restrictive setting.

Differential Diagnosis

In light of the high degree of comorbidity in child and adolescent depression, differential diagnosis is both crucial to appropriate care, and challenging. Identification and treatment of the disorder contributing to the greatest impairment is indicated. For example, treatment of a preexisting anxiety disorder may result in the resolution of depressive symptoms. Patients may not initially disclose anxiety symptoms, particularly in cases of ongoing trauma or obsessive–compulsive disorder. Such disorders require intervention beyond usual treatment for depression. Untreated ADHD may result in depressive symptoms because of its functional impairment and interpersonal difficulty. In this disorder, treatment of symptoms of inattention and impulsivity may alleviate symptoms attributed to depression. Substance-use disorders, particularly involving depressogenic substances, such as alcohol and opiates, may appear as a depressive disorder, but patients may be euthymic after detoxification and substance-abuse treatment. In the setting of psychotic disorders, affective flattening and the patient's unwillingness to share symptoms of psychosis can contribute to a misdiagnosis of depression. Finally, differential diagnosis should always include consideration of bipolar diathesis, as risk for this diagnosis in the setting of early-onset depression is as high as 10–20%. Children with a bipolar diathesis may present with decreased need for sleep, increased energy levels including marked change in behavior, flight of ideas, rapid speech, hypersexuality, grandiosity, or psychosis. In the depressed phase, some studies suggest depressive symptoms of hyperphagia, hypersomnia, and psychosis are predictive of bipolar outcome.

Treatment

Treatment approach to and response of children and adolescents with depression may vary with severity, duration, and comorbidity of the presenting illness. Treatment should always include an acute and a continuation phase, with the availability of maintenance treatment. Psycho-education, support, and involvement of family and school are fundamental to any treatment plan, and in cases of very mild depression, may be adequate. In cases of more severe depression, use of psychotherapy, pharmacotherapy, or a combination is indicated.

A. PSYCHOPHARMACOLOGIC INTERVENTIONS

In the consideration of psychopharmacologic treatment of depressed children and adolescents, it is important to note a high-placebo response rate of 30–60%. Nevertheless, there is evidence of efficacy of selective serotonin reuptake inhibitors (SSRIs) with response rates of 50–70%. Fluoxetine is the only medication approved by the FDA for the treatment of child and adolescent depression. It is the best studied and has demonstrated the greatest difference between medication and placebo. Moreover, there is evidence that fluoxetine has greater efficacy than cognitive–behavioral therapy (CBT), though combined treatment was found to have the greatest rate of response except in more severe cases, when it was equivalent to medication alone.

There are published studies demonstrating efficacy for citalopram and sertraline, though there are also unpublished negative studies. A meta-analysis of all available clinical trials, both published and unpublished, revealed that SSRIs are more efficacious than placebo, with response rates of 60% versus 49%. In some studies there are significant effects for adolescents but not for children. In addition, while tricyclic antidepressants show excellent response rates in adults, evidence does not support their use for the treatment of depression in children and adolescents.

Dosing recommendations for children and adolescents are to start at half the usual adult starting dose for 1 week (i.e., the equivalent of 10 mg of fluoxetine) and to then increase the dose to 20 mg of fluoxetine or equivalent for another 3 weeks. Dosing increases should occur

at no less than 4-week intervals to allow the medication to reach steady state. Children and adolescents may require relatively higher doses of citalopram, sertraline, or fluvoxamine, based on pharmacokinetic studies. There is evidence that, in order to prevent relapse, treatment should be continued for at least 6 months after complete symptom remission, in the case of a first episode of MDD, and for at least 12 months after a recurrent episode.

In view of its more extensive efficacy data, fluoxetine should be used as a first-line agent. In depression that has been refractory to monotherapy with adequate doses of at least two SSRIs, augmentation strategies can include buproprion, lithium, or lamotrigine. Undiagnosed comorbid conditions or misdiagnosis should first be ruled out. Psychotherapy, if not started previously, is also indicated. Other considerations in the pharmacotherapeutic treatment of depression include the management of contributing comorbidity. Milder cases may respond to psychoeducation alone or in combination with brief psychotherapy.

B. PSYCHOTHERAPEUTIC INTERVENTIONS

1. Cognitive–behavioral therapy—CBT has been shown to be one of the most efficacious psychotherapies for the management of child and adolescent depression, with or without concomitant use of pharmacotherapy. CBT is based on the premise that depressed individuals have distorted information processing, thoughts, and core beliefs. Distortion manifests itself in a negative attributional style and beliefs that lead to, exacerbate, or perpetuate depression, particularly during times of stress. CBT uses cognitive techniques and skills building to attenuate cognitive distortions and maladaptive processing. The content of various CBT treatments varies widely, ranging from the highly structured CWD-A (Coping with Depression for Adolescents), to much less structured treatments like those based on Beck's CBT, to hybrids like that used in the Treatment of Adolescent Depression Study (TADS).

Based upon TADS, CBT alone or in combination with pharmacotherapy may be best for less severe cases of depression. Predictors of poorer response to CBT, from TADS and other studies, include greater severity, history of sexual abuse, parental depression, older age of onset, and greater hopelessness.

2. Interpersonal therapy—Interpersonal Therapy (IPT) is predicated on the exploration and recognition of precipitants of depression including interpersonal loss, role disputes and transitions, social isolation, and social skills deficits. IPT for adolescents (IPT-A) is an adaptation of IPT. It begins with an "interpersonal inventory" that includes the patient's interpersonal relationships. This inventory allows therapist and patient to make collaborative decisions about goals for treatment. IPT-A may be successful because it addresses role transitions, interpersonal difficulties with peers and family, and the development of social skills—all important developmental tasks of adolescence.

In some measures of depression and functional impairment, IPT has been shown to be superior to CBT. IPT-A has been shown to be superior to "care as usual" in treatment of depression, as in regard to improvement in social adjustment, and functional status.

3. Family therapy—Family therapy is often used as an adjunct to other treatments for depression. There have been both positive and negative studies regarding the use of family therapy. Interventions such as the management of parental depression, improvement of family communication, the reduction of criticism, and the enhancement of support, are likely to be of benefit.

C. OTHER INTERVENTIONS

Light therapy has been shown to be beneficial for seasonal affective disorder and as an adjunct for MDD with a seasonal component. Light therapy involves the daily use of full spectrum light in the early morning hours to help with potential abnormality of the hypothalamic–pituitary axis. Light therapy is initiated in fall and winter months to counteract reduced daylight.

1. Electroconvulsive therapy—Although there is little controlled evidence about the use of electroconvulsive therapy (ECT) in adolescent depression, documented clinical experience supports a role for ECT in depression that is refractory to pharmacological and psychosocial management, as well as in severe psychotic depression, and life-threatening depression. There is evidence that ECT may not be effective in the case of comorbid Axis II personality disorders. It may be most efficacious in bipolar depression.

Complications/Adverse Outcomes of Treatment

One of the primary concerns in the prescription of SSRI medications in children and adolescents has been the FDA "black-box warning" concerning risk of suicidal behavior with use of these medications. FDA analysis has shown a higher rate of suicide-related events on SSRI than on placebo (at a rate of 4% compared to 2%). These adverse events occurred relatively early in treatment and did not involve any actual suicides, and few suicide attempts. In the TADS study, adverse suicidal events were almost four times more likely to occur with fluoxetine than with placebo.

In addition to concern about suicide-related behavior, antidepressants can cause side effects such as agitation, akathisia, serotonin syndrome (particularly in combination with other agents), headache, dizziness, gastrointestinal symptoms, sleep cycle disturbance, sexual dysfunction, and platelet inhibition leading to bruising. Additionally, in children at risk for bipolar disorder, it is important to consider that the risk of SSRI-induced mania has been reported as particularly high in children younger than 14 years of age. Other physicians involved in the care of child and adolescent patients should be made aware of the use of any medication. Due to platelet inhibiton, SSRIs should be stopped prior to surgery. Medications such as fluoxetine interact with many medications via the CYP-450 system, and this should be considered with each medication change or in cases of coprescription.

Prognosis

Depression is a chronic and disabling illness that often starts in childhood or adolescence. It contributes to increased risk for suicide, substance use, and other psychiatric sequelae, and interferes in the child or adolescent's personal development. While some success has been experienced in the treatment of early onset depression, up to 40% of youth with depression remain depressed at the end of clinical trials, and a higher proportion are still symptomatic. Many children and adolescents do not experience complete recovery, and all remain at risk for relapse. Further information is needed about our current methods of treatment, the management of very early onset depression, the neurobiology of depression, and the interaction of genetic and environmental contributors to depression.

Birmaher B, Brent DA: Work group on quality issues. Practice parameters for the assessment and treatment of children and adolescents with depressive disorders. *J Am Acad Child Adolesc Psychiatry* 2007;46:1503–1526.

Brent DA, Birmaher B: Adolescent depression. *N Engl J Med* 2002;347:667–671.

Bridge JA, Salary CR, Birmaher B, Asare AG, Brent DA: The risks and benefits of antidepressant treatment for youth depression. *Ann Med* 2005;37:404–412.

Caspi A, Sugden K, Moffitt TE, et al.: Influence of life stress on depression: Moderation by a polymorphism in the 5-HT gene. *Science* 2003;301:386–389.

Costello EJ, Mustillo S, Erkanli A, Keeler G, Angold A. Prevalence and development of psychiatric disorders in childhood and adolescence. *Arch Gen Psychiatry* 2003;60:837–844.

Diagnostic and Statistical Manual of Mental Disorders (DSM-IV-TR), 4th edn. Washington, DC: American Psychiatric Association, 2000.

Drevets WC, Price JL, Simpson JR Jr., et al.: Subgenual prefrontal cortex abnormalities in mood disorders. *Nature* 1997;386:824–827.

Findling RL, McNamara, NK, Stansbrey RJ, et al.: The relevance of pharmacokinetic studies in designing efficacy trials in juvenile major depression. *J Child Adolesc Psychopharmacol* 2006; (1–2):131–145.

Hammad TA, Laughren T, Racoosin J: Suicidality in pediatric patients treated with antidepressant drugs. *Arch Gen Psychiatry* 2006;63:332–339.

Pine DS: Face-memory and emotion: Associations with major depression in children and adolescents. *J Child Psychol Psychiatry* 2004;45:1199–1208.

Todd RD, Botteron KN: Family, genetic, and imaging studies of early-onset depression. *Child Adolesc Psychiatr Clin N Am* 2001; 10:375–390.

Bipolar Disorder

David A. Brent, MD, & Raymond J. Pan, MD

 ESSENTIALS OF DIAGNOSIS

DSM-IV-TR Criteria for a Manic Episode

A. A distinct period of abnormally and persistently elevated, expansive, or irritable mood for at least 1 week (or any duration if hospitalization is necessary).

B. During the period of mood disturbance, three (or more) of the following symptoms have persisted (four if the mood is only irritable) and have been present to a significant degree:

  (1) inflated self-esteem or grandiosity

  (2) decreased need for sleep (e.g., feels rested after only 3 hours of sleep)

  (3) more talkative than usual or pressure to keep talking

  (4) flight of ideas or subjective experience that thoughts are racing

  (5) distractibility (i.e., attention too easily drawn to unimportant or irrelevant external stimuli)

  (6) increase in goal-directed activity (either socially, at work or school, or sexually) or psychomotor agitation

  (7) excessive involvement in pleasurable activities that have a high potential for painful consequences (e.g., engaging in unrestrained buying sprees, sexual indiscretions, or foolish business investments)

C. The symptoms do not meet criteria for a Mixed Episode.

(Reprinted, with permission, from the *Diagnostic and Statistical Manual of Mental Disorders*. 4th edn. Text Revision. Washington, DC: American Psychiatric Association, 2000.)

DSM-IV-TR Criteria for a Hypomanic Episode

A. A distinct period of persistently elevated, expansive, or irritable mood, lasting throughout at least 4 days, that is clearly different from the usual non-depressed mood.

B. Same as B criterion for Manic Episode.

C. The episode is associated with an unequivocal change in functioning that is uncharacteristic of the person when not symptomatic.

D. The disturbance in mood and the change in functioning are observable by others.

E. The episode is not severe enough to cause marked impairment in social or occupational functioning, or to necessitate hospitalization, and there are no psychotic features.

F. The symptoms are not due to the direct physiological effects of a substance (e.g., a drug of abuse, a medication, or other treatment) or a general medical condition (e.g., hyperthyroidism).

(Reprinted, with permission, from the *Diagnostic and Statistical Manual of Mental Disorders*. 4th edn. Text Revision. Washington, DC: American Psychiatric Association, 2000.)

DSM-IV-TR Criteria for a Mixed Episode

A. The criteria are met both for a Manic Episode and for a Major Depressive Episode (except for duration) nearly every day during at least a 1-week period.

B. The mood disturbance is sufficiently severe to cause marked impairment in occupational functioning or in usual social activities or relationships with others, or to necessitate hospitalization to prevent harm to self or others, or there are psychotic features.

C. The symptoms are not due to the direct physiological effects of a substance (e.g., a drug of abuse, a medication, or other treatment) or a general medical condition (e.g., hyperthyroidism).

(Reprinted, with permission, from the *Diagnostic and Statistical Manual of Mental Disorders*. 4th edn.

Text Revision. Washington, DC: American Psychiatric Association, 2000.)

General Considerations

A. EPIDEMIOLOGY

Given the controversy in characterizing pediatric bipolar disorder (BP), there is no data on the prevalence of prepubertal BP. One published study by Lewinsohn shows a lifetime BP prevalence of approximately 1% in youths 14–18 years old (predominantly BP type II and cyclothymia). An additional 5.7% youths have subsyndromal BP symptoms. Retrospective reports of adults with BP show that 60% report the onset of BP before 20 years of age and 10–20% report BP onset before 10 years of age. BP affects both sexes equally.

B. ETIOLOGY

Contributors to the etiology and course of BP are hypothesized to include genetics, neurobiology, and family environment. Biological etiologies are suggested by correlations between genetics and neuroimaging findings and BP. A family environment including stress and abuse is associated with earlier age of onset and more difficult course.

C. GENETICS

BP is highly familial as evidenced by the increase of BP spectrum disorders in high-risk studies with offspring of BP parents. Adoption, twin, and family studies point to a familial, and most likely a genetic, etiology.

Clinical Findings

A. SIGNS & SYMPTOMS

Although the presentation of BP in mid to late adolescence is considered similar to adult BP, the presentation of pediatric BP is debated. Many children have less than the 4–7-days duration specified in the DSM-IV-TR criteria for hypomania or mania, respectively. Pediatric BP is characterized by a predominance of mixed episodes and/or rapid cycling, irritability, chronicity with long episodes, and a high rate of comorbid attention-deficit hyperactivity disorder (ADHD) and anxiety disorder. The National Institute of Mental Health Research Roundtable on pubertal BP (2001) categorized pediatric bipolar phenotypes as "narrow" (DSM-IV-TR definitions of mania and hypomania) and "broad" (including the common clinical presentation of severe irritability, mood lability, temper outbursts, depression, anxiety, hyperactivity, poor concentration, and impulsivity). The diagnosis of BP should consider the developmental context in deciding what constitutes psychopathology. For example, increased self-esteem and goal-directed activity may be consistent with normal child development. Psychosis, most commonly auditory hallucinations, has been reported in 16–60% of youth with BP. The prevalence of psychosis is lower in adolescent mania than adult mania.

In summary, it is difficult to diagnose pediatric BP because of the variability in the clinical presentation, high comorbidity, and symptom overlap with other psychiatric disorders, the role of development in symptom expression, the difficulty experienced by children in reporting their symptoms, and social context in which the BP is developing (e.g., family conflicts). However, evidence is emerging that pediatric BP is a spectrum disorder (from BP Not Otherwise Specified [NOS] through BP-I) with a consistent course and outcome.

B. Psychological Testing

Although psychological testing is not involved in the diagnosis of BP, BP often is associated with cognitive deficits in children and adolescents. A study by Dickstein and Leibenluft using the computerized Cambridge Neuropsychological Test Automated Battery (CANTAB) reported difficulties in attentional set shifting and visuospatial memory in pediatric BP. A study by McClure and Leibenluft comparing children with BP to children with anxiety disorders and healthy controls showed that children with BP misinterpreted sad, happy, and fearful child faces as angry as compared with anxious and healthy groups. Interestingly, children with BP did not misinterpret adult faces.

C. Laboratory Findings

No specific laboratory findings are diagnostic of BP in children and adolescents.

D. Neuroimaging

Although much new research exists on neuroimaging, most of the studies are preliminary. Structural magnetic resonance imaging (MRI) studies suggest that white matter hyperintensities in both cortical and subcortical brain regions and smaller amygdalar size are correlated with pediatric BP. In addition, smaller parietal and temporal lobe cortical gray matter, bilateral and left sided reductions in amygdala size, and bilateral decrease in hippocampal volume have been noted in pediatric BP. Studies have also indicated reduced gray matter volume in the dorsolateral prefrontal cortex (DLPFC). Bilateral larger basal ganglia, particularly an increase in putamen size, was identified in adolescent BP. Functional MRI studies show increased left thalamus and putamen activation and both cortical and subcortical dysfunction.

Preliminary proton magnetic resonance spectroscopy studies have suggested that substances which are markers for neuronal integrity such as N-acetyl-aspartate, choline, myoinositol, and creatine/phosphocreatine are affected in the fronto-striatal region, cingulate cortex, DLPFC, and other areas of the brain. These results are preliminary because they include small sample size and subjects in various phases of illness (e.g., depressed, hypomanic, euthymic). In addition, many subjects had comorbid disorders and were taking medication, which may have confounded the findings.

E. Course of Illness

Retrospective studies and naturalistic longitudinal studies of children and adolescents with BP report that 40–100% will recover, within 8 consecutive weeks, without meeting criteria for mania, hypomania, depression, or a mixed affective state, 1–2 years later. Of patients who recover, 60–70% show recurrence of symptoms within 10–12 months with hospitalization, psychosis, suicide attempts and completion, and poor psychosocial functioning.

As there is controversy over the presentation of pediatric BP, it is useful to study the course of the full spectrum of BP phenotypes. A recent study lead authored by Birmaher (2006) followed BP spectrum disorders (BP-I, BP-II, and BP-NOS). BP-NOS is defined as (1) elated mood plus two DSM-IV-TR BP symptoms or irritability plus three DSM-IV-TR BP symptoms; (2) at least 4 hours of symptoms in a 24 hour period; and (3) of 4 days lifetime total of symptoms. This study found that, compared with BP-I adults, BP-I youths spend significantly more time symptomatic with more mixed/cycling episodes, mood symptom changes, and polarity switches. A significant 25% of BP-NOS subjects converted to BP-I or BP-II. Furthermore, 70% of subjects with BP recovered from the index episode whereas 50% had at least one syndromal recurrence, most commonly a depressive episode. During follow-up, for 60% of the time, subjects had syndromal or subsyndromal symptoms with many changes in symptoms and shifts of polarity. Three percent of the subjects experienced psychosis. Twenty percent of BP-II subjects coverted to BP-I. Early onset, BP-NOS, long duration of mood symptoms, low-socioeconomic status, and psychosis were associated with poorer outcomes and rapid mood changes.

At this time, although suggested by familial transmission, it is not clear that pediatric BP is continuous with adult BP. In a community-based, adolescent longitudinal study, 5.7% of patients with abnormal mood, defined as persistently elevated, expansive, and irritable mood, did not go on to meet full DSM-IV-TR criteria of BP by the early twenties. In a retrospective interview of a large sample of individuals with adult BP, approximately 30% reported the onset of symptomatology before 13 years of age and approximately 40% during 13–18 years of age.

Earlier onset BP symptoms are associated with greater rates of anxiety and substance-abuse disorders, more recurrence, more rapid mood changes, shorter periods of euthymia, a higher incidence of suicide attempts, violence, and a history of abuse.

Depressed children and adolescents are at increased risk (10–20%) of developing BP, particularly if they present with psychotic symptoms, develop hypomania in response to pharmacological treatment of depression, and have a strong family loading for BP.

Differential Diagnosis (Including Comorbid Conditions)

BP shares symptoms with several other psychiatric diagnoses, which may lead to a challenging differential diagnosis. A diagnosis of BP should only be made definitively after following a patient longitudinally. ADHD is commonly associated with symptoms commonly seen in BP including irritability, talkative/pressured speech, hyperactivity, pursuit of high risk yet pleasurable activities, and distractibility. BP can be differentiated from ADHD because of grandiosity, elated mood, accelerated ideas, and hypersexuality. Thought disorder and mood-incongruent delusions and hallucinations, which are symptoms of BP, may be mistaken as schizophrenia. Irritability, mood dysregulation, and disinhibition that might be confused with symptoms of mania may be symptoms of a pervasive developmental disorder. Evaluation should exclude child abuse, non-mood-related emotional and behavioral disturbances, developmental delays, delirium, tumors, infections, and seizure disorders. Substance use should be considered, especially the use of steroids, amphetamines, and cocaine.

Most children and adolescents presenting with BP also present with other psychiatric disorders. Some of the disorders cited as comorbid with BP include ADHD, oppositional defiant disorder, conduct disorder, anxiety disorder, substance-use disorder, and pervasive developmental disorder. The risk of panic disorder may be elevated in pediatric BP. It is worth-noting that comorbidity varies with age: Pediatric BP is commonly associated with ADHD, whereas adolescent-onset BP has a greater risk of substance abuse.

Treatment

A. Psychopharmacologic Interventions

There are no controlled studies in children and adolescents of the treatment of BP-II. For acute phase medication treatment for BP-I, manic or mixed episode without psychosis, monotherapy with traditional mood stabilizers (lithium, divalproex, and carbamazepine), and atypical antipsychotics (olanzapine, quetiapine, and risperidone) is first-line treatment. The American Academy of Child and Adolescent Psychiatry (AACAP) practice parameters recommend lithium or divalproex as the first medication choice for nonpsychotic mania. Recent studies have suggested that atypical antipsychotic medication, such as olanzapine or quetiapine, are equally effective as traditional mood stabilizers and appear to yield a quicker response.

For children demonstrate only moderate to minimal improvement with monotherapy, an augmenting agent is recommended: Either another mood stabilizer or an atypical antipsychotic. The combination of two traditional mood stabilizers such as lithium and divalproex, or a traditional mood stabilizer and an atypical antipsychotic appears to be superior to mood stabilizer monotherapy for the acute treatment of manic or mixed episodes. For children having no response to initial monotherapy, or for children having intolerable side effects, monotherapy with another agent is recommended.

For children with BP-I, manic, or mixed episode without psychosis, a mood stabilizer combined with an atypical antipsychotic is recommended as the first choice, although atypical antipsychotic monotherapy may be considered as an alternative.

Children with BP experience long bouts of syndromal or subsyndromal depressive symptoms. There have been no randomized controlled treatment trials and few open-label studies of children with acute bipolar depression. In adults, monotherapy with lithium, divalproex, atypical antipsychotics, or lamotrigine and the combination of traditional mood stabilizers and atypical antipsychotics with serotonin reuptake inhibitors or bupropion is effective in the treatment of bipolar depression. Recognizing that most children and adolescents with BP have comorbid psychiatric disorders, such as ADHD, treatment should also be directed to the comorbid disorders.

Maintenance treatment consists of the same medications recommended for acute phase treatment. Medication tapering or discontinuation should be considered if the patient has been in remission for at least 12–24 consecutive months with close monitoring for symptom recurrence.

B. Psychotherapeutic Interventions

Child and family focused cognitive–behavioral therapy is effective in 8–18-year olds with BP. This therapy integrates reward-based CBT with interpersonal psychotherapy, which has a focus on empathetic validation. Psychoeducation and skills building, based in part on family systems and cognitive–behavioral intervention, has been shown to be effective in BP treatment. Psychoeducation consists of teaching parents and teachers about the symptoms, course, and treatment of BP. Skills-building focuses on communication and problem solving on symptom management, emotion regulation, and impulse control. Family-focused therapy (FFT) addresses the concerns of adolescents with BP and builds resources to manage stress and lower expressed emotion within the family.

C. Other Interventions

Case series exist on the effectiveness of electroconvulsive therapy in the treatment of acute mania and bipolar depression in adolescents. Omega-3 fatty acids (OFA) have been used in adults as well as children with BP. The U.S. Food and Drug Administration has approved the use of 3 g/day of OFA in adults. Approval for children and adolescents has not been granted.

Complications/Adverse Outcomes of Treatment

One of the concerns about pharmacologic treatment is a lack of long-term safety data available for many of the medications used for BP. Mood stabilizers and atypical antipsychotic medications are associated with weight gain and its metabolic problems (diabetes mellitus, hyperlipidemia, and elevation of liver function tests). Atypical antipsychotic medications have side effects including neuroleptic malignant syndrome, movement disorder, prolactin elevation (especially with risperidone), and cardiac conduction problems (especially with ziprasidone). Working memory deficit and cognitive dulling have been reported with mood stabilizers and atypical antipsychotics. Polycystic ovarian syndrome has been linked to the long-term use of divalproex in women. Divalproex carries a "black–box" warning about rare, but potentially life-threatening, pancreatitis. Lithium is associated with hypothyroidism, weight gain, and changes in renal function.

Selective serotonin reuptake inhibitors and other antidepressants can trigger mania, hypomania, mixed episodes, or rapid cycling, particularly when used without concomitant mood stabilizer medication. Depressed children under the age of 14 years are vulnerable. Attention should be paid for increase in agitation, suicidality, and the serotonin syndrome (see Chapter 40).

Prognosis

BP is often a chronic and disabling illness. Early childhood BP has a lower rate of recovery, with a longer duration of mixed and rapid cycling episodes, more symptoms, and more frequent polarity changes than BP of later in life. Compared with adults, adolescents with BP often have a prolonged early course and are less responsive to treatment. Youth with BP show high-lifetime rates of psychosis, which is associated with poor prognosis. Adolescents with BP are at increased risk for suicide relative to children with other psychiatric disorders. Comorbid substance abuse further increases the suicide risk. Nevertheless, open treatment studies and small randomized trials of both pharmacological and psychosocial intervention suggest reason for cautious optimism.

AACAP: AACAP official action. Practice parameters for the assessment and treatment of children and adolescents with bipolar disorder. *J Am Acad Child Adolesc Psychiatry* 1997;36:138–157.

Birmaher B, Axelson DA, Strober M, et al.: Clinical course of children and adolescents with bipolar spectrum disorders. *Arch Gen Psychiatry* 2006;63:175–183.

Caetano SC, Olvera RL, Glahn D, et al.: Fronto-limbic brain abnormalities in juvenile onset bipolar disorder. *Biol Psychiatry* 2005;58(7):525–531.

DelBello MP, Schwiers ML, Rosenberg HL: A double-blind, randomized, placebo-controlled study of quetiapine as adjunctive treatment for adolescent mania. *J Am Acad Child Adolesc Psychiatry* 2002;41(10):1216–1223.

Dickstein DP, Treland JE, Snow J, et al.: Neuropsychological performance in pediatric bipolar disorder. *Biol Psychiatry* 2004;55(1):32–39.

Geller B, Zimmerman B, Williams M, et al.: Bipolar disorder at prospective follow-up of adults who had prepubertal major depressive disorder. *Am J Psychiatry* 2001;158(1):125–127.

Kowatch RA, Fristad M, Birmaher B, et al.: Treatment guidelines for children and adolescents with bipolar disorder. *J Am Acad Child Adolesc Psychiatry* 2005;44(3):213–235.

Kowatch RA, Suppes T, Carmody TJ, et al.: Effect size of lithium, divalproex sodium, and carbamazepine in children and adolescents with bipolar disorder. *J Am Acad Child Adolesc Psychiatry* 2000;39(6):713–720.

McClure EB, Treland JE, Snow J, et al.: Deficits in social cognition and response flexibility in pediatric bipolar disorder. *Am J Psychiatry* 2005;162(9):1644–1651.

Pavuluri MN, Birmaher B, Naylor MW: Pediatric bipolar disorder: Review of the past 10 years. *J Am Acad Child Adolesc Psychiary* 2005;44:846–871.

Weller EB, Weller RA, Sanchez LE: Bipolar disorder in children and adolescents. In: Lewis M (ed). *Child and Adolescent Psychiatry: A Comprehensive Textbook*, 3rd edn. Philadelphia: Lippincott Williams and Williams, 2002.

Suicidal Behavior in Children and Adolescents

40

Robert A. King, MD

 ESSENTIALS OF DIAGNOSIS

DSM-IV-TR Diagnostic Criteria

Suicidal ideation *consists of thoughts of wishing to be dead or wishing to kill or inflict life-threatening harm on oneself.* Suicide attempt *refers to deliberate self-destructive action intended to kill oneself. Because the attempter's intention is often ambivalent, an assessment of severity of intent is a crucial part of clinical evaluation. Lethality, in contrast, refers to the actual likelihood that the attempt will cause death. The term "parasuicide" has been used to denote attempts at self-injury that are of low lethality and involve little or no wish to actually die, while deliberate self-cutting refers to non-lethal, usually repetitive self-cutting apparently motivated by feelings of tension, depersonalization, or emptiness, rather than a wish to die.*

Although mood disorders, psychosis, and substance abuse are potent risk factors for completed suicide, suicide attempts and ideation in children and adolescents can occur in a wide variety of disorders and psychopathological conditions.

Suicidal ideation—thoughts of wishing to be dead, or to kill or inflict life-threatening harm on oneself

Suicide attempt—deliberate self-destructive action intended to kill one self

Lethality—likelihood that an attempt will cause death

Parasuicide—low lethality attempts at self-injury that involve little or no wish to die

General Considerations

A. EPIDEMIOLOGY

1. Completed suicide—Completed suicide is rare in prepubertal children, with an annual rate in the US on the order of 0.6 per 100,000 for children age 5–14 in 2003. Completed suicide in adolescents, however, is the third leading causes of mortality in the U.S. in this otherwise generally healthy age group, and in 2003 accounted for the death of 7.3 teens, age 15–19, per 100,000. The most recent international data show a similar pattern of relatively low rates for youngsters age 5–14 (ranging from 0–2.4 per 100,000), with higher rates for youth age 15–24 (ranging from 2.4 to 33.1 per 100,000) (see Table 40–1). Although young male suicides substantially outnumber female suicides throughout much of the world, the pattern is reversed in rural parts of the developing world, such as India and China, perhaps due to ready access to lethal insecticides used in agriculture. Although variations in reporting practices make direct comparisons difficult, there are apparent wide international variations, with high rates of youth suicide associated with rapid political and economic changes, widespread gun availability, breakdown of traditional culture among indigenous peoples, and changes in the status of women. Reported youth suicide rates are low in many predominantly Muslim and Catholic countries.

Dramatic secular trends are also apparent internationally in the epidemiological data. According to the World Health Organization, youth suicide rates rose dramatically between the 1950s and mid-1980s in the US, much of Europe, Mexico, the Western Pacific; speculations as to the cause of this trend include rising divorce rates, increased adolescent substance use, demographic competition, erosion of religious/cultural taboos against suicide, and mass media coverage of celebrity and other suicides. The decade from 1990 to 2000 showed a decline in youth suicide rates in many, but not all countries (with Eastern Europe and Ireland being dramatic exceptions). The reasons for this decline are unclear, although greater awareness of adolescent depression and widespread availability of effective antidepressants have been speculated to play a role. In this connection, it is of note that after a decade of decline in the US, the death rate from suicide for youngsters aged 19 and under jumped 18.2% from 2003 to 2004, a period coinciding with a sharp downturn in use of antidepressants in children and adolescents due to widely publicized safety concerns.

Table 40–1. Youth suicide rates per 100,000 in selected countries[a]

Country	Year	5–14 Years All	15–24 Years All
Russia	2004	2.3	28.1
Lithuania	2004	1.6	25.5
Finland	2004	0.8	21.7
New Zealand	2000	0.7	18.2
Iceland	2004	0.0	16.2
Norway	2004	0.5	14.0
Latvia	2004	0.8	13.1
Japan	2004	0.4	12.8
Argentina	2003	0.9	12.4
Belgium	1997	0.5	12.4
China (Hong Kong SAR)	2004	0.6	12.2
Ireland	2005	0.5	11.9
Poland	2004	0.8	11.8
Austria	2005	0.4	11.8
Canada	2002	0.9	11.5
Australia	2003	0.5	10.7
Singapore	2003	0.8	10.5
United States	2002	0.6	9.9
Switzerland	2004	0.1	9.8
Sweden	2002	0.6	9.7
Hungary	2003	0.7	9.0
Czech Republic	2004	0.7	9.0
France	2003	0.4	8.1
Denmark	2001	0.3	7.5
China mainland (selected areas)	1999	0.8	6.9
Germany	2004	0.3	6.7
Mexico	2003	0.7	6.4
Israel	2003	0.2	6.0
United Kingdom	2004	0.1	5.2
Netherlands	2004	0.5	5.0
Spain	2004	0.3	4.3
Italy	2002	0.2	4.1
Portugal	2003	0.0	3.7
Greece	2004	0.2	1.7

[a] – In descending order of suicide rates, per 100,000 for 15–24 y.o. From: World Health Organization: Country Suicide Reports, (http://www.who.int/mental_health/prevention/suicide/country_reports/en/index.html) accessed 11/30/07

2. Suicidal ideation and attempts—In contrast to completed suicide, suicidal ideation and attempts are far more common. The 2005 biennial national Youth Risk Behavior Survey found that, during the preceding 12 months, 16.9% of high school students had seriously contemplated attempted suicide; 13% had made a plan to attempt suicide; 8.4% had actually attempted suicide one or more times; and 2.3% had made a suicide attempt involving an injury, poisoning, or overdose that had to be treated by a doctor or nurse. Rates of suicidal ideation and attempts among younger children, age 7–12 years, are substantially lower (on the order of 4% and 1.5%, respectively).

Suicidal ideation or behavior is a common cause for pediatric emergency room (ER) visits. During the period 1997–2002, the annual rate of ER visits in the US for deliberate self-harm was 225 per 100,000 7–24-year-olds. About 20% of such ER visits result in hospitalization. The annual hospitalization rate of youth with self-inflicted injuries is 44.9 per 100,000 5–20-year-olds. Among these hospitalized patients, the rate of cutting is 13.2%, hanging or suffocation 1.3%; and ingestion of acetaminophen 26.9%, antidepressants 14%, opiates 3.3%, salicylates 10.2%,

3. Gender—Suicidal behavior varies markedly by gender. Attempted suicide is much more common in girls aged 15–19 years than in same-aged boys. Girls in this age group attempt suicide almost twice as often as boys, while boys complete suicide about four times more often than girls. Thus, for adolescent boys, the ratio of completed to attempted suicides is about 1:517, where as it is 1:4000 for girls.

B. ETIOLOGY

1. Completed suicide

i. Major psychiatric disorder—The psychological autopsy is a procedure for reconstructing a decedent's life to understand the psychological antecedents and circumstances of the death; this process includes a review of available records and systematic interviews of knowledgeable informants regarding the decedent's lifestyle and expressed thoughts, feelings and behaviors, especially those that might provide evidence of psychopathology. Such studies find that about 90% of adolescent suicide completers have at least one diagnosable major psychiatric disorder, especially depressive, substance abuse, and conduct disorders. In about half of adolescent suicides, one or more psychiatric disorder has been present for at least three years at the time of suicide.

From a screening and prediction perspective, although these diagnostic risk factors are sensitive (i.e., which are found in most cases of adolescent suicide), they are very nonspecific, since they are found in a very large number of adolescents who do not commit suicide. The small minority of adolescent suicides without a discernable major psychiatric diagnosis still show elevated rates, compared to community controls, of family psychiatric disorder, past suicidal ideation or behavior, legal or disciplinary problems in the prior year, and firearms in the home.

ii. Psychopathological and psychosocial risk factors—Additional psychosocial risk factors for completed suicide include: Isolative or impulsive character traits; recent life stressors, such as interpersonal loss or legal or disciplinary problems (especially in youngsters with substance abuse or disruptive disorders); and family history of suicide, depression, or substance abuse. Despite variations across ethnic and racial groups, completed suicide rates do not appear to be influenced by socioeconomic status per se. Troubled parent–child relationships and nonintact family of origin appear to be associated with youth suicide, although once parental or youth psychopathology is controlled for the magnitude of this association is unclear.

iii. Media and suicide "contagion"—Clusters of apparently imitative suicide attempts and completions occur in adolescents and are estimated to account for 1–13% of youth suicides in the United States. Sensationalized media coverage of local, celebrity, or fictional suicides may provoke imitative suicidal behavior.

2. Suicidal ideation and attempts

i. Psychopathology—In community samples, adolescent suicidal ideation and attempts are associated with the presence of a psychiatric diagnosis such as substance abuse, mood, anxiety, and disruptive disorders; in adolescent girls, eating disorder also appears to be a potent risk factor for serious suicide attempts. In addition to these diagnostic risk factors, certain cognitive and personality traits, including impulsivity, aggression, hopelessness, and impaired social and problem-solving skills, are important risk factors for adolescent suicidal ideation/behavior and provide targets for therapeutic or preventive intervention.

ii. Social and problems solving skills deficits
a. Family factors— Family factors such as loss of a parent after death or divorce, residential instability, change in caretaking parent, living apart from parents (including foster care, running away from home), family conflict, and perceived low parental care and social support are all associated with adolescent suicide attempts. Sexual and physical abuse are potent risk factors for suicide attempts in youth, even after associated factors in the abusive parents such as mental disorder, impulsivity/aggression, suicidal behavior, substance abuse, parental discord, divorce and step-parenting are controlled for.

b. Problem behaviors— In light of these associations, it is not surprising that there is a high degree of overlap between adolescent suicidal ideation and attempts and the following: Impulsive, sensation-seeking, or high-risk adolescent "problem behavior," such as sub-

stance use, fighting, and antisocial behavior (even at levels below threshold for the diagnosis of a substance abuse or disruptive disorder); the early onset of sexual intercourse; and weapon carrying.

c. Gender nonconformity— Bisexual and homosexual youth, especially those who experience parental or peer rejection, stigmatization, or victimization (e.g., as part of a tumultuous "coming out" process) have an increased risk of attempted suicide, even after controlling for depression and other risk factors.

3. Precipitants
—Children and adolescents usually manifest suicidal behavior as a desperate attempt to escape from unbearable affect, such as rage, intense isolation, or self-loathing. Feelings of inner deadness, intolerable anxiety, or fear of fragmentation (in the case of psychosis) less commonly play a role. These feelings are often intensified by different forms of interpersonal discord that activate suicidal ideation or behavior. Thus, although extraordinary acute stressors, such as physical assault or sexual abuse, may precipitate suicidal feelings or behavior, the commonest immediate triggers of adolescent suicide attempts are the common-place travails of adolescence–disciplinary crises, teasing, arguments with a parent or romantic partner, or perceived failure, shame, or humiliation. Suicidal feelings and attempts can result when such upsets occur in a youngster with pessimism, hopelessness, and perceived helplessness due to depression or with poor affect regulation, impulsive decision making, impaired social and communication skills, and a propensity to aggression. In turn, the psychopathology associated with adolescent suicidality makes it more likely that the vulnerable adolescent will encounter or provoke interpersonal discord.

C. GENETIC AND BIOLOGICAL FACTORS

A family history of attempted or completed suicide is a significant risk factor for youthful suicidal behavior. Twin studies suggest that genetic factors predict 17–45% of the variance in suicidal behavior. The psychiatric disorders predisposing to suicidal behavior (especially mood disorders) have strong heritable components. Family studies suggest, however, that genetic factors contribute to the risk for suicidal behavior over and above the genetic contribution to the transmission of mood disorder. The familial transmission of suicidal behavior appears to be mediated by the transmission of a tendency to impulsive aggression; furthermore, sexual abuse in parent and child further increases the risk of suicidal behavior in the child, most likely by several mechanisms, such as shared genetic and environmental factors, and gene–environment interaction.

These associations, together with the observation that greater family loading for suicidal behavior is associated with increased risk for, and earlier onset of suicide attempts in, offspring, suggest opportunities for case finding and early intervention. Hence, prospective screening for children of parents with histories of mood disorder, suicide attempts, and childhood sexual abuse identify at-risk children who would benefit from preventive intervention.

The specific genes that contribute to suicide risk are unknown. In adults, low cerebrospinal fluid levels of the serotonin metabolite 5-hydroxyindoleacetic acid are correlated with impulsive aggression and attempted and completed suicide. Data concerning the neurobiology of adolescent suicide attempters are considerably sparser. Given the apparent centrality of impulsivity and aggression in attempted and completed adolescent suicide, genetic and neurobiological studies of adolescent suicide have focused on serotonergic regulatory genes and functioning. They have been largely inconclusive. Postmortem studies have found higher levels of 5-HT$_{2A}$ receptors and altered levels of second messenger-associated mRNA and regulatory kinases in the prefrontal cortex of adolescent suicides.

Clinical Findings

The primary goals of clinical evaluation of the suicidal child are as follows: (1) determine the degree of acute suicidal risk, (2) determine the immediate steps needed to ensure the child's safety, (3) assess the general psychiatric, psychological, family and social context of the suicidal crisis, (4) identify what internal, interpersonal, and treatment resources are available, (5) design a treatment plan to address the immediate and persistent risk factors for suicide and enhance personal resources, and (6) maximize treatment compliance and follow-up.

A. ASSESSMENT OF SUICIDE RISK

This involves systematic inquiry about the presence of suicidal ideation, whether the person had explicit plans for self-injury, and a detailed history of past incidents of actual self-harm (including their precipitants, context, and outcome). In the clinical setting, assessment is best done by means of a careful interview of the child and parents, separately and together. Careful inquiry can reveal suicidal ideation or behavior previously unsuspected by parents or other adults. A very large number of rating scales and structured instruments are available to help systematize such inquiry for research or screening purposes. Among the most commonly used are the widely translated Beck Scale for Suicidal Ideation and Suicide Intent Scale, which are useful for screening and assessing degree of intent in suicidal youngsters. The Suicidal Ideation Questionnaire and the broader and more elaborate Columbia TeenScreen have proven useful for school-based screenings. The Child Suicide Potential Index covers multiple risk domains associated with suicidal behavior and assesses risk for suicidal potential, as well as suicidality per se. The Multi-Attitude Suicide Tendency Scale Assesses conflictual attitudes towards life and death and can help discriminate suicidal youth from psychiatric and nonclinical youth.

B. ASSESSMENT OF INTENT, MOTIVATION, AND LETHALITY

Because the motivation of suicide attempts is usually ambivalent, it is important to assess the severity of intent, that is, the extent to which the youngster wished to die. Among the factors to be assessed are the following:

- *Did the patient truly wish to die?*
- *Did the patient believe the means (e.g., overdose, hanging) was lethal?*
- *How intense and persistent was the patient's suicidal ideation preceding the attempt?*
- *Did the patient plan and take premeditated steps and over how long (e.g., hoarding pills, leaving a note)?*
- *Did the patient take measures to avoid or ensure discovery and rescue (e.g., finding an isolated location; seeking help, telling immediately or not telling)?*
- *Did the suicidal ideation persist after the attempt?*

The severity of intent may range from a serious premeditated attempt of high lethality involving a clear wish to die and steps to avoid discovery, through impulsive overdoses of low lethality when someone else is either nearby or promptly sought, and the wish to die is ambivalent or passing.

To understand the motive for the suicide attempt, it is important to comprehend the interpersonal and affective context of the attempt as well as the youngster's style of interpersonal relating and emotional regulation. Although about one-half of adolescent suicide attempters endorse a wish to die (usually to obtain relief from an unbearable state of mind), one- quarter to one-half endorse interpersonal motives such as "to make people understand how desperate I was, "to show how much I loved someone," "to get help from someone," or "to find out whether someone really loved me." About a third of adolescents making serious suicide attempts are unable to describe any precipitant or motivation, stating "I don't know why I did it; I was upset." Vagueness can reflect a difficulty articulating feelings, poor emotional regulation, and impaired social problem solving skills.

The lethality of the attempt does not necessarily correspond to the intensity of a conscious intent to die. Youngsters with low suicidal intent may underestimate the toxicity of medication (e.g., a hepatotoxic acetaminophen overdose), while others with high suicidal intent can underestimate what is needed to kill themselves.

In assessing the degree of suicidal risk and the need for hospitalization, persistent suicidal ideation, high intent, high lethality of an attempt, or a history of multiple attempts are all associated with an increased risk of repetition and completion.

C. LBORATORY AND IMAGING STUDIES

Although research studies of adolescent suicide have examined neuroimaging findings and neurobiological measures (e.g., neuroendocrine provocation paradigms and platelet or cerebrospinal fluid neurotransmitter parameters), these are not useful in ordinary clinical practice. Laboratory studies such as thyroid function tests may be indicated as part of the routine pediatric evaluation of persistent adolescent depression (see Chapter 38).

Differential Diagnosis (Including Comorbid Conditions)

Having established the presence of significant suicidal ideation or behavior, the next task is to evaluate psychopathological, family, and social factors underlie the youngster's suicidality.

COMORBID PSYCHIATRIC DISORDER

Among the most potent risk factors for suicidality is the presence of mood disorder, chronic anxiety, disruptive behavior disorder (especially conduct disorder), and substance abuse. The risk of a suicide attempt increases with the number of comorbid disorders. The impact of these risk factors varies by gender, as illustrated by a landmark New York area case-control study of adolescent suicides. For boys, the risk of completed suicide was most increased by a history of a prior attempt (approximate odds ratio [OR] 22.5 compared to the general adolescent male population), followed by major depression (OR 8.6), substance abuse (OR 7.1), and previous antisocial behavior (OR 4.4). In contrast, for girls, major depression was the predominant risk factor (OR 49), followed by a history of a prior attempt (OR 8.6), and previous antisocial behavior (OR 3.2), Substance abuse did not contribute to suicidal risk in girls (OR 0.8). Although schizophrenia and bipolar disorder are major risk factors for suicide in adults, it is only in older adolescents that they play a significant role in youth suicide.

Substance abuse is an especially important risk factor, since, beyond its links to mood disorder and impaired social functioning, the depressogenic and disinhibiting effects of acute drug or alcohol intoxication facilitate the transition from suicidal ideation to impulsive action.

PSYCHOPATHOLOGICAL TRAITS

Over and above the presence of major psychiatric disorders, psychological characteristics such as hopelessness, poor impulse and affect regulation, impaired capacity to express emotion in words, and impaired problem solving and social skills are important risk factors the presence of which must be assessed and which may provide targets for clinical intervention.

Treatment

A. RISK ASSESSMENT AND DETERMINING THE LEVEL OF CARE

A crucial dispositional question in the initial evaluation of the suicidal youngster is whether immediate hospitalization is needed to insure the child's safety or whether outpatient treatment is safe and feasible. For this complex question, there are no reliable, objective algorithms. High lethality, serious intent, persistent suicidal ideation, and/or a history of multiple attempts weigh in favor of hospitalization, as do serious depression, psychosis, or persistent, current, serious life stresses. Other factors to be considered are the youngster's and parents' attitudes towards the suicidal episode. Minimization by the youngster or punitiveness by the parents regarding the episode bode ill; the quality of parental support, supervision, and commitment to treatment are important determinants of the feasibility of effective outpatient treatment. For example, can the family guarantee that firearms, dangerous medicine, and poisons in the house will be secured? Active substance abuse on a youngster's part is also problematic, since acute intoxication may cast to the winds any treatment alliance or "no harm" agreement (see below). Family turmoil, with high expressed emotion, physical or sexual abuse, active parental substance abuse, or parental psychosis make outpatient treatment risky.

When these concerns lead to hospitalization, follow-up and long-term treatment compliance must be dealt with in the transition to less restricted care. Although hospitalization is often necessary to provide a safe environment for further assessment or stabilization, there are few systematic data on the impact of hospitalization on subsequent course.

B. MEASURES TO ENSURE SAFETY AND OPTIMIZE TREATMENT COMPLIANCE AND FOLLOW-UP

If the decision is made to send the youngster home with follow-up outpatient treatment, explicit steps are needed to help ensure the child's safety and increase the likelihood of aftercare.

1. Means restriction—The presence of a firearm in the house is a potent risk factor for adolescent suicide. Parents should be educated about the importance of preventing the youngster's access to guns at home. Similarly, steps should be taken to prevent access to lethal quantities of medication or poisons.

2. Safety plans and "no harm" contracts—As part of establishing an initial treatment alliance with the youngster, the clinician should review the precipitant of the current suicidal episode and plan for the reasonable steps to be taken by the youngster and family if stresses recur. Coping measures may be devised, identifying the responsible adults who can be turned to for help, and clarifying how the clinician or other emergency mental health providers can be contacted. The culmination of the discussion should be a "no harm contract" with an explicit agreement by the youngster to try to refrain from self-harm, to employ the alternatives agreed upon, and to contact the clinician if thoughts of suicide return. It is this process that is likely to be helpful, rather than resorting to a misleading pro forma agreement to which the youngster half-heartedly agrees to in order to avoid hospitalization.

C. Steps to Maximize Compliance

About half of adolescent suicide attempters receive little or no follow-up outpatient treatment. Different interventions have been developed to improve rates of treatment adherence. If possible, definite arrangements (specifying time and therapist) should be arranged before the child leaves the ER. More patients enter and complete treatment when the referring emergency clinician personally contacts the accepting agency rather than leaving it to the patient or family to do. The building of a preliminary alliance between family and mental health care system while the family is still in the ER is useful. Innovative ER-based interventions have been developed that successfully increase adolescent attempters' adherence to outpatient treatment. These include an ER-based problem-solving intervention and a program that helps families and youngsters in the ER reframe their understanding of the child's suicidal crisis by means of a soap opera style video and participation in an initial family therapy session.

D. The Focus of Treatment

When a major psychiatric disorder is diagnosed, the primary focus is the treatment of the underlying disorder. Furthermore, the family, social, school and other stressors that precipitate, perpetuate, or exacerbate suicidal impulses must be explicitly addressed, as do hopelessness, emotional dysregulation, and impaired emotional and social problem solving. The sections that follow address treatment issues related to the presence of suicidal ideation or behavior. Since many drug and psychotherapy treatment studies of child and adolescent depression explicitly exclude suicidal subjects, the applicability of the extant treatment research is unclear. Nonetheless, despite the general correlation of depression and suicidality, the studies discussed below suggest that particular interventions can have divergent impacts on depression and suicidality.

E. Psychotherapeutic Interventions

There is a sizable research literature on psychosocial therapies for suicidal behavior in adults, including cognitive–behavioral therapy (CBT), dialectical behavior therapy, problem solving therapy, and interpersonal psychotherapy (IPT). However, despite controlled trials demonstrating the efficacy of CBT and IPT for depression in children and adolescents, the impact of these interventions on suicidal ideation and behavior (which may be independent of their impact on depression) has not been well studied. In a comparative trial of CBT, systemic-behavioral family therapy, and nondirective supportive therapy for depression, all three treatments produced comparable reductions in suicidality. However, further analysis revealed that suicidal depressed adolescents were more likely to drop out of treatment and improved less in depression than did depressed adolescents who were not suicidal. Hopelessness at intake is an important predictor of poor treatment response. Suicidal adolescents assigned to nondirective therapy did especially poorly, suggesting that specific treatment like CBT may be preferable for suicidal depressed adolescents and that treatment should specifically target hopelessness early.

Other therapeutic models, such as home-based family therapy and skills-based group treatment have yielded promising results in adolescent attempters.

F. Psychopharmacological Interventions

Although fluoxetine and other selective serotonin reuptake inhibitors (SSRIs) appear more effective than placebo for the treatment of depression in children and adolescents, the balance of risk to benefit in this age group remains controversial. Most clinical trials of these agents have not been adequately designed or sufficiently powerful to address their impact on suicidality. In the Treatment of Adolescent Depression Study, fluoxetine was markedly superior to CBT alone for the treatment of adolescent depression. However, although clinically significant suicidal ideation improved across all treatment groups (fluoxetine alone, CBT alone, CBT with fluoxetine, placebo), the groups that received CBT (either alone or with fluoxetine) showed the greatest improvement, suggesting specific beneficial effects of CBT on suicidal ideation.

Despite public and regulatory concern, the magnitude of suicidality caused by antidepressant medication appears small. Quantitative analyses suggest that the benefits of fluoxetine outweigh its risks. The Treatment of Adolescent Depression Study found a statistically significant elevated risk for harm-related adverse effects in SSRI-treated patients in contrast to non-SSRI treated patients, and evidence for the protective effect of CBT.

Epidemiological studies give an inconclusive answer as to the question of whether currently widespread SSRI treatment has had an effect on youth suicide rates. Some studies have found an inverse relationship between rates of antidepressant treatment and regional completed youth suicide rates as well as rates of adolescent suicide attempts in a large insurance database. On the other hand, an Australian population study found concurrent increases in antidepressant use and youth suicide rates, while a large UK case control study found an association between SSRI treatment and nonfatal self-harm in adolescent patients.

Prognosis

Compared to youngsters without a history of attempted suicide, youngsters with a history of attempted suicide have a markedly increased risk of completing suicide (a three-fold increase in girls and a thirty-fold increase in boys). Thus, about one-quarter to one-third of youth suicides have a prior history of a suicide attempt. Adolescent suicide attempters have high rates of subsequent repeat attempts and are also at elevated risk for motor vehicle and other accidental injuries and homicidal death. Adolescent male suicide attempters, especially those who are hospitalized, appear to have a worse prognosis than female adolescent attempters in terms of subsequent social functioning and risk of completed suicide.

Prevention

The relative rarity of completed youth suicide poses formidable statistical challenges for screening, prediction, and prevention.

Prevention efforts are best directed against risk factors that appear to play a decisive role in a significant proportion of youth suicides and that are potentially modifiable at a reasonable cost.

In the case of adolescent suicide, the most important risk factors appear to be depression, substance abuse, conduct disorder, history of prior suicide attempt, family history of suicide, and ready access to lethal means.

Universal preventive interventions for adolescent depression and/or substance abuse focused on unselected populations have produced mixed results and appear less effective than targeted programs. Such untargeted, school-based approaches include curricula teaching the warning signs of depression and suicidality, but there is not good evidence supporting their efficacy. A newer generation of universal curriculum-based programs seek to promote alternative responses to emotional distress, with a focus on improving coping and problems solving skills. Whether such programs actually produce changes in suicide-related behaviors (as opposed to attitudes) is as yet unknown.

Examples of targeted preventive interventions included those addressed to youngsters at high risk because of parental depression or identified as at-risk because of self-reported depressive symptoms. Systematic school-based screening of adolescents, using self-reports and structured interviews, such as the Columbia TeenScreen has been studied as a means of facilitating case-finding as a prologue to referral and treatment. Such screening has been shown to identify students at risk with depression and/or suicidal ideation, most of whom were not previously known to school personnel as having significant problems. Furthermore, such screening does not appear to cause an iatrogenic increase in suicidal ideation. Although promising, institutional barriers remain to implementing such programs and developing effective means of providing therapeutic intervention of teens identified as at-risk remains an unsolved problem.

Additional approaches include educating "gate keepers," such as school personnel and primary care physicians to identify at-risk youngsters.

Other community-based approaches include hotlines/crisis centers; means restriction (access to firearms or lethal quantities of medications or poisons); and minimizing contagion.

It is unclear whether hotlines reach the youngsters most in need of help as well as whether they affect outcome. There is some epidemiological evidence that stricter gun control and reduced availability of firearms decreases the youth suicide rate. On the clinical level, counseling parents of suicidal youngsters about preventing access to guns is an important intervention, although often ineffectually done. Restricting the amount of potentially lethal medications (such as acetaminophen) available per purchase or mandating the use of blister packaging (which makes it difficult to impulsively take a large number of loose pills) can successfully decrease rates of severe or fatal overdoses.

Because media publicity of suicides have been shown to increase attempted and completed suicides, school and media outlets need to implement available guidelines to avoid romanticizing or sensationalizing suicides, focusing instead on the causal connection to mental disorder.

Barbe RP, Bridge J, Birmaher B, Kolko D, Brent DA: Suicidality and its relationship to treatment outcome in depressed adolescents. *Suicide Life Threat Behav* 2004;34(1):44–55.

Brent DA: Assessment and treatment of the youthful suicidal patient. *Ann N Y Acad Sci* 2001;932:106–128; discussion 128–131.

Brent DA, Mann JJ: Family genetic studies, suicide, and suicidal behavior. *Am J Med Genet C Semin Med Genet* 2005;133(1):13–24.

Bridge JA, Goldstein TR, Brent DA: Adolescent suicide and suicidal behavior. *J Child Psychol Psychiatry.* 2006;47(3–4):372–394.

Bridge JA, Iyengar S, Salary CB, et al.: Clinical response and risk for reported suicidal ideation and suicide attempts in pediatric antidepressant treatment: A meta-analysis of randomized controlled trials. *JAMA* 2007;297:1683–1696.

Centers for Disease Control and Prevention: Youth risk behavior surveillance—United States, 2005. *Morb Mortal Wkly Rep* 2006;55(SS–5):1–108.

Comtois KA, Linehan MM: Psychosocial treatments of suicidal behaviors: A practice-friendly review. *J Clin Psychol* 2006;62(2):161–170.

Gould MS: Suicide and the Media. *Ann N Y Acad Sci* 2001;932:200–224.

Gould MS, Greenberg T, Velting DM, Shaffer D: Youth suicide risk and preventive interventions: A review of the past ten years. *J Am Acad Child Adolesc Psychiatry* 2003;42(4):386–405.

King RA, Apter A (Eds): *Suicide in Children and Adolescents.* Cambridge, UK: Cambridge University Press, 2003.

Mann JJ: Neurobiology of suicidal behavior. *Nat Rev Neurosci* 2003;4:819–828.

March J, Silva S, Petrycki S, Treatment for adolescents with depression study (TADS) team: Fluoxetine, cognitive–behavioral therapy, and their combination for adolescents with depression: Treatment for adolescents with depression study (TADS) randomized controlled trial. *JAMA* 2004;292(7):807–820.

National Center for Health Statistics: *Centers for Disease Control and Prevention.* Health, United States, 2005.

www.cdc.gov/nchs/data/hus/hus05.pdf (Last modified March 29, 2006; Accessed 8/1/8/06)

Olfson M, Gameroff MJ, Marcus SC, Greenberg T, Shaffer D: Emergency treatment of young people following deliberate self-harm. *Arch Gen Psychiatry* 2005;62:1122–1128.

Pandey GN, Dwivedi Y, Ren X, et al.: Brain region specific alterations in the protein and mRNA levels of protein kinase A subunits in the post-mortem brain of teenage suicide victims. *Neuropsychopharmacology* 2005;30(8):1548–1556.

Shaffer D, Pfeffer C, American Academy of Child and Adolescent Psychiatry Work Group on Quality Issues: Practice parameters for the assessment and treatment of children and adolescents with suicidal behavior. *J Am Acad Child Adolesc Psychiatry* (2001;40(7):24S–51S.

Shaffer D, Garland A, Gould MS, Fisher P, Trautman P: Preventing teenage suicide: A critical review. *J Am Acad Child Adolesc Psychiatry* 1988;27(6):675–687.

Winters NC, Myers K, Proud L: Ten-year review of rating scales. III: scales assessing suicidality, cognitive style, and self-esteem. *J Am Acad Child Adolesc Psychiatry* 2002;41(10):1150–1181.

World Health Organization (2007) Suicide preventioin and special programmes. Country reports and charts: http://www.who.int/mental·health/prevention/suicide/country·reports/en/ (Accessed April 29, 2007)

Anxiety Disorders in Children and Adolescents

41

Barry Nurcombe, MD

■ SEPARATION ANXIETY DISORDER

 ESSENTIALS OF DIAGNOSIS

DSM-IV-TR Diagnostic Criteria

A. Developmentally inappropriate and excessive anxiety concerning separation from home or from those to whom the individual is attached, as evidenced by three (or more) of the following:

(1) recurrent excessive distress when separation from home or major attachment figures occurs or is anticipated

(2) persistent and excessive worry about losing, or about possible harm befalling, major attachment figures

(3) persistent and excessive worry that an untoward event will lead to separation from a major attachment figure (e.g., getting lost or being kidnapped)

(4) persistent reluctance or refusal to go to school or elsewhere because of fear of separation

(5) persistently and excessively fearful or reluctant to be alone or without major attachment figures at home or without significant adults in other settings

(6) persistent reluctance or refusal to go to sleep without being near a major attachment figure or to sleep away from home

(7) repeated nightmares involving the theme of separation

(8) repeated complaints of physical symptoms (such as headaches, stomachaches, nausea, or vomiting) when separation from major attachment figures occurs or is anticipated

B. The duration of the disturbance is at least 4 weeks.

C. The onset is before age 18 years.

D. The disturbance causes clinically significant distress or impairment in social, academic (occupation), or other important areas of functioning.

E. The disturbance does not occur exclusively during the course of a pervasive developmental disorder, schizophrenia, or other psychotic disorder and, in adolescents and adults, is not better accounted for by panic disorder with agoraphobia.

Specify if:
Early onset: if onset occurs before age 6 years.

(Reprinted, with permission, from *Diagnostic and Statistical Manual of Mental Disorders*, 4th edn., Text Revision. Copyright 2000, Washington, DC: American Psychiatric Association.)

General Considerations

A. EPIDEMIOLOGY

Separation anxiety disorder (SAD) occurs in 2–4% of children and adolescents. It represents about 50% of all referrals for evaluation of anxiety disorder at this age. SAD may be slightly more prevalent in girls and in families of lower socioeconomic status. School refusal is equally common in all socioeconomic groups. Its incidence is 1–2% in school-aged children, and it may be more common in boys.

B. ETIOLOGY

SAD is linked to insecure attachment (see Chapter 45). It may be precipitated by loss, separation, or the threat of either. Parental anxiety and an enmeshed mother–child relationship is commonly associated with this condition. The combination of parental anxiety and depression is an additional risk factor. The prevalence of anxiety disorders in other family members might indicate a genetic factor.

A psychodynamic theory concerning the etiology of SAD postulates the following: (1) The mother has a hostile-dependent relationship with her own mother, (2) the mother is lonely and unsatisfied in her marriage, (3) following a threat to security, the child responds to an overly dependent relationship with the mother, (4) the mother is gratified by the child's overdependence, (5) the mother and child develop a mutually ambivalent hostile-dependent relationship, (6) the child responds to the normal stresses of school with fear and avoidance, (7) the mother is pleased by having the child at home, while at the same time annoyed by it, and (8) both mother and child focus on the somatic symptoms of anxiety and become convinced that the child has a physical disorder.

C. GENETICS

SAD, like other many other neurodevelopmental disorders of childhood onset, is likely to be associated with multiple vulnerability genes. Twin studies suggest that different genes may be playing a role in mediating this condition in males versus females. It also appears that the heritability of SAD is greater for girls than for boys.

Clinical Findings

The average age at onset is 8–9 years. Children with SAD exhibit severe distress when separated or threatened with separation from their parent, usually the mother. Fearing that harm will befall the attachment figure or themselves, they typically want to sleep in the parental bed, refuse to be alone, plead not to go to school, have nightmares about separation, and exhibit numerous somatic symptoms when threatened with separation. For example, when it is time to go to school these children complain of abdominal pain, nausea, vomiting, diarrhea, urinary frequency, and palpitations. Sometimes they have to be forced to leave the house. They may run away and hide near the home.

Differential Diagnosis (Including Comorbidity)

See end of Chapter.

Treatment

See end of Chapter.

Complications/Adverse Outcomes of Treatment

See end of Chapter.

Prognosis

See end of Chapter.

Albano AM, Chorpita BF, Barlow DH: Childhood anxiety disorders. In: Mash EJ, Barkley RA (eds). *Child Psychopathology*, 2nd edn. New York: Guilford, 2003, pp. 279–329.

■ GENERALIZED ANXIETY DISORDER

 ESSENTIALS OF DIAGNOSIS

DSM-IV-TR Diagnostic Criteria

A. *Excessive anxiety and worry (apprehensive expectation), occurring more days than not for at least 6 months, about a number of events or activities (such as work or school performance).*

B. *The person finds it difficult to control the worry.*

C. *The anxiety and worry are associated with one of the following six symptoms (with at least some symptoms present for more days than not for the past 6 months).*

   (1) restlessness or feeling keyed up or on edge

   (2) being easily fatigued

   (3) difficulty concentrating or mind going blank

   (4) irritability

   (5) muscle tension med

   (6) sleep disturbance (difficulty falling or staying asleep, or restless unsatisfying sleep)

D. *The focus of the anxiety and worry is not confined to features of an Axis I disorder, e.g., the anxiety or worry is not about having a Panic Attack (as in Panic Disorder), being embarrassed in public (as in Social Phobia), being contaminated (as in Obsessive–Compulsive Disorder), being away from home or close relatives (as in Separation Anxiety Disorder), gaining weight (as in Anorexia Nervosa), having multiple physical complaints (as in Somatization Disorder), or having a serious illness (as in Hypochondriasis), and the anxiety and worry do not occur exclusively during Posttraumatic Stress Disorder.*

E. *The anxiety, worry, or physical symptoms cause clinically significant distress or impairment in social, occupational, or other important areas of functioning.*

F. *The disturbance is not true to the direct physiological effects of a substance (e.g., a drug of abuse, a medication) or a general medical condition (e.g.,* *hyperthyroidism) and does not occur exclusively during a Mood Disorder, a Psychotic Disorder, or a Pervasive Developmental Disorder.*

(Reprinted, with permission, from *Diagnostic and Statistical Manual of Mental Disorders*, 4th edn., Text Revision. Copyright 2000, Washington, DC: American Psychiatric Association.)

General Considerations

Generalized anxiety disorder (GAD) involves excessive anxiety and worry about a number of events or activities (e.g., school performance, social relationships, clothes), causing significant impairment or distress, manifested by somatic symptoms, self-consciousness, and social inhibition.

A. EPIDEMIOLOGY

GAD occurs in about 3% of children and in 6–7% of adolescents. The sex ratio is equal. GAD is more prevalent among children of higher socioeconomic status.

B. ETIOLOGY

As with SAD, GAD is associated with a familial concentration of anxiety disorders. Parents of children with GAD have been described as anxious and hypercritical, with high expectations for their children's performance. Children with GAD are more likely to have exhibited behavioral inhibition when younger, a temperamental trait involving shyness and withdrawal from unfamiliar situations. Behavioral inhibition is probably genetically determined.

C. GENETICS

Twin studies suggest that genetic factors appear to play only a modest role in the etiology of GAD.

Clinical Findings

The average age at onset of GAD is 10 years. Children with GAD worry about their clothes, schoolwork, social relationships, and sporting performance—past, present, and future. They are exceedingly self-conscious, have low self-esteem, and complain of many somatic symptoms (particularly abdominal pain and headaches).

Differential Diagnosis (Including Comorbidity)

See end of Chapter.

Treatment

See end of Chapter.

Complications/Adverse Outcomes of Treatment

See end of Chapter.

Prognosis

See end of Chapter.

Silverman WK, Ginsberg G: Specific phobias and generalized anxiety disorder. In: March J (ed). *Anxiety Disorders in Children and Adolescents.* New York: Guilford Press, 1995, pp. 151–180.

■ AVOIDANT PERSONALITY DISORDER & SOCIAL PHOBIA

 ESSENTIALS OF DIAGNOSIS

DSM-IV-TR Diagnostic Criteria

A. Avoidant Personality Disorder: *In general, avoidant personality disorder involves pervasive social inhibition, a sense of inadequacy, and hypersensitivity to criticism, which leads to avoidance of academic and social involvement, a preoccupation with being rejected, and low self-esteem.*

B. Social Phobia: *In general, social phobia involves marked, persistent fear of social or performance situations that involve potential scrutiny by other people. The fear is sufficiently severe to interfere with normal social and academic functioning.*

(Reprinted, with permission, from *Diagnostic and Statistical Manual of Mental Disorders*, 4th edn., Text Revision. Copyright 2000, Washington, DC: American Psychiatric Association.)

General Considerations

A. EPIDEMIOLOGY

The prevalence of social phobia among children and adolescents is 0.9–1.1%. Girls predominate over boys in a ratio of about 7:3. The prevalence of social phobia has been estimated at 0.08% and 0.7% in 7-year-old and 5-year-old children, respectively. Among children in these two age groups, girls predominate over boys in a ratio of about 2:1.

B. ETIOLOGY

Adults with social phobia often report that the phobia was precipitated by a traumatic event. Compared to Attention-deficit hyperactivity disorder and to normal controls, anxiety disorders are more common among first-degree relatives of children with anxiety disorders (including avoidant personality disorder and social phobia), but there is no tendency for children with avoidant personality disorder or social phobia to have parents with the same anxiety disorder. In contrast to the development of GAD, behaviorally inhibited children show no greater tendency than do normal children to develop avoidant personality disorder or social phobia. However, the parents of behaviorally inhibited children are more likely to have, or to have had, social phobia, avoidant personality disorder, or GAD. There may be a familial predisposition to the development of fear. Social phobia has been associated with the predisposition of some children to assume a low status position in the social dominance hierarchy of their peers.

C. GENETICS

There is evidence that SAD has a strong familial basis, but there are few studies that involve cases in the pediatric age range. In addition to specific vulnerability genes contributing to this behaviorally complex phenotype, there is also the possibility that temperamental risk factors associated with the disorder may be genetically transmitted.

Clinical Findings

Children with avoidant personality disorder or social phobia experience anxiety in the company of other people or when expected to perform in some way. For example, when unfamiliar visitors arrive, they hide; they prefer single playmates to peer groups; they avoid sports events and parties; and they detest taking examinations, reading aloud in class, eating in front of others, using public toilets, answering telephones, or speaking up to people in authority. Most of these children are afraid of two or more situations. When threatened, they experience the somatic concomitants of anxiety (e.g., rapid breathing, palpitations, shakiness, chills, sweating, nausea).

Differential Diagnosis (Including Comorbidity)

See end of Chapter.

Treatment

See end of Chapter.

Beidel DC, Morris TL: Social phobia. In: March J (ed). *Anxiety Disorders in Children and Adolescents*. New York: Guilford Press, 1995, pp. 181–211.

■ PANIC DISORDER

 ESSENTIALS OF DIAGNOSIS

DSM-IV-TR Diagnostic Criteria

A. Both (1) and (2): (1) recurrent unexpected Panic Attacks; and (2) at least one of the attacks has been followed by 1 month (or more) of one (or more) of the following:
  (a) persistent concern about having additional attacks
  (b) worry about the implications of the attack or its consequences (e.g., losing control, having a heart attack, "going crazy"); or
  (c) a significant change in behavior related to the attacks

B. Absence or absence of agoraphobia (anxiety about being in specific places of situations leading to avoidance or marked distress).

C. The Panic Attacks are not due to the direct physiological effects of a substance (e.g., c. a drug of abuse, a medication) or a general medical condition (e.g., hyperthyroidism).

D. The Panic Attacks are not better accounted for by another mental disorder, such as. Social Phobia (e.g., occurring on exposure to feared social situations), Specific Phobia (e.g., on exposure to a specific phobic situation), Obsessive–Compulsive Disorder (e.g., on exposure to dirt in someone with an obsession about contamination), Posttraumatic Stress Disorder (e.g., in response to stimuli associated with a severe stressor), or Separation Anxiety Disorder (e.g., in response to being away from home or close relatives).

(Reprinted, with permission, from *Diagnostic and Statistical Manual of Mental Disorders*, 4th edn., Text Revision. Copyright 2000, Washington, DC: American Psychiatric Association.)

General Considerations

In general, panic disorder involves recurrent, unexpected panic attacks, with fear of future attacks, with or without agoraphobia (a fear of being somewhere from which escape might be difficult such as in a crowd, on a bridge, or while traveling). The disorder is manifested as acute anxiety with autonomic concomitants (e.g., racing heart; dilated pupils; rapid breathing; cold, sweaty palms), and it may present as hyperventilation, with tetany. See Chapter 19 for diagnostic criteria.

A. EPIDEMIOLOGY

Panic disorder appears to be equally prevalent in both sexes. Its base-rate prevalence is not known.

B. ETIOLOGY

In adults with panic disorder, lactate infusion provokes panic symptoms, a phenomenon not found in other anxiety disorders. Agoraphobia is probably a secondary phenomenon, produced by conditioning, when the individual is apprehensive between attacks about the next panic attack. Despite plausible hypotheses, no evidence has been found for an early history of loss or traumatic separation in adults with panic disorder, and childhood SAD is related to adult anxiety disorders generally, not to panic disorder specifically. It is not clear whether childhood SAD predisposes to adult agoraphobia; however, childhood SAD is statistically associated with the early onset of adult panic disorder. An association has been found between panic disorder and earlier traumatic suffocation experiences such as near drowning.

C. GENETICS

First-degree relatives of patients with panic disorder meet criteria for the disorder in 20–40% of cases. Twin studies also have shown a higher concordance for monozygotic than dizygotic twin pairs. No specific vulnerability genes have been identified.

Clinical Findings

Panic disorder can begin as early as the preschool years, but the peak age at onset is 15–19 years. About 25% of patients report an onset prior to 15 years of age. The condition has probably been underdiagnosed and confused with SAD. Typical symptoms are episodes of hyperventilation, trembling, palpitations, shortness of breath, sweating, numbness, depersonalization, chest pain, choking, fear of dying, dizziness, and fainting.

Treatment

See end of Chapter.

Complications/Adverse Outcomes of Treatment

See end of Chapter.

Prognosis

See end of Chapter.

Black B: Separation anxiety disorder and panic disorder. In: March J (ed). *Anxiety Disorders in Children and Adolescents.* New York: Guilford Press, 1995, pp. 212–234.

Bouwer C, Stein DJ: Association of panic disorder with a history of traumatic suffocation. *Am J Psychiatry* 1997;154:1566–1570.

■ SELECTIVE MUTISM

 ESSENTIALS OF DIAGNOSIS

DSM-IV-TR Diagnostic Criteria

A. Consistent failure to speak in specific social situations (in which there is an expectation of speaking, e.g., at school) despite speaking in other situations.

B. The disturbance interferes with educational or occupational achievement or with other social communication.

C. The duration of the disturbance is at least 1 month (not limited to the first month of school).

D. The failure to speak is not due to a lack of knowledge of, or comfort with, the spoken language required in the social situation.

E. The disturbance is not better accounted for by a communication disorder (e.g., stuttering) and does not occur exclusively during the course of a pervasive developmental disorder, schizophrenia, or other psychotic disorder.

(Reprinted, with permission, from *Diagnostic and Statistical Manual of Mental Disorders,* 4th edn., Text Revision. Copyright 2000, Washington, DC: American Psychiatric Association.)

General Considerations

A. EPIDEMIOLOGY

Selective mutism is more common in girls than boys. Prevalence estimates have varied from 0.08% to 0.7%.

B. ETIOLOGY

The cause of selective mutism is probably multifactorial. Four types of the disorder have been postulated. In symbiotic mutism, the child manipulates the environment, using shyness and clinging to avoid separation. In passive-aggressive mutism, a child scapegoated by his or her peers trenchantly refuses to speak when called on to do so. Reactive mutism is precipitated by a stressor such as illness, separation, or abuse. In speech phobic mutism, the child is afraid to hear his or her own voice.

Shyness, taciturnity and selective mutism run in families. Selective mutism may be a form of social anxiety. One study found a high prevalence of comorbid social phobia, avoidant personality disorder, and simple phobia in this condition, along with a familial aggregation of social phobia and selective mutism. Some studies suggest that selective mutism may be associated with subtle expressive language impairment.

C. Genetics

Like other many other neurodevelopmental disorders of childhood onset, it is likely that there are multiple vulnerability genes associated with this condition.

Clinical Findings

The age at onset of selective mutism is 1–5 years (average, 2.7 years). Children with selective mutism are most reluctant to speak at school, away from home, to adults, and to unfamiliar people. They are more likely to speak to peers than to teachers. One study found that 13% of children with selective mutism had a learning disorder and 10% had a history of delayed language development, but all had normal speech and language by 5 years of age. No clear association has been found between trauma and the onset of selective mutism, nor has the often-reported association with oppositional behavior been corroborated. Selective mutism may be regarded more appropriately as a symptom of social anxiety, akin to the "freezing" that some adults with social phobia experience when called on to speak in public.

Treatment

See remainder of this Chapter.

Complications/Adverse Outcomes of Treatment

See remainder of this Chapter.

Prognosis

See remainder of this Chapter.

Black B, Uhde TW: Psychiatric characteristics of children with selective mutism. *J Am Acad Child Adolesc Psychiatry* 1995;34:847.

Krysonski VL: A brief review of selective mutism literature. *J Psychol* 2003;137:29–40.
Steinhausen HC, Wachter M, Laimbock K, Metzke CW: A long-term outcome study of selective mutism in childhood. *J Child Psychol Psychiatry* 2006;47:751–756.

Differential Diagnosis (Including Comorbid Conditions)

SAD and school refusal are most likely to be confused with physical disorders when they have salient somatic anxiety equivalents. Thus gastrointestinal symptoms can be confused with peptic ulcer, esophageal reflux, abdominal emergency, or disorders associated with bowel hurry. SAD with school refusal can also masquerade as chronic fatigue syndrome, chronic muscular pain, and prolonged convalescence from infectious mononucleosis. In panic disorder, mitral valve prolapse should be investigated only if auscultation indicates the need to do so.

Selective mutism should be differentiated from deafness, mental retardation, developmental language disorder, aphonia, and the lack of understanding of a secondary language by recent immigrants. Panic disorder should be distinguished from substance-induced anxiety disorder (e.g., caffeinism), posttraumatic stress disorder, and medical disorders that cause anxiety (e.g., pheochromocytoma).

See Table 41–1 for the general and specific standard interviews and questionnaires useful in screening for and diagnosing anxiety disorders and phobias and in monitoring the treatment outcome of these disorders.

Anxiety disorders (particularly SAD) and depressive disorders frequently coincide. Anxiety disorders are also often encountered in children who have Attention-deficit hyperactivity disorder. Many children with one type of

Table 41–1. Psychological Testing for Anxiety Disorders

Standardized interviews
Schedule for Affective Disorders and Schizophrenia in School-Aged Children (K-SADS) (Puig-Antich and Chambers 1978)
Anxiety Disorders Interview for Children (ADIS-C) (Silverman and Nellis 1988)
Diagnostic Interview Schedule for Children (DISC) (Costello et al. 1985)

Questionnaires
Revised Children's Manifest Anxiety Scale (RCMAS) (Reynolds and Richman 1978)
Revised Fear Survey Schedule for Children (FSSC-R) (Ollendick 1983)
Multidimensional Anxiety Scale for Children (MASC) (March et al. 1994)

anxiety disorder have at least one other anxiety disorder (e.g., SAD with panic disorder, GAD, or avoidant personality disorder). The high degree of comorbidity may be explained on the basis of a risk hypothesis, on the basis of a hypothesis that there is a single underlying pathogenesis, or on the assumption that the symptoms of anxiety and depression overlap in a dimensional, noncategorical manner.

Curry JF, Murphy LB: Comorbidity of anxiety disorders. In: March J (ed). *Anxiety Disorders in Children and Adolescents.* New York: Guilford Press, 1995, pp. 301–320.

Treatment

A. PSYCHOTHERAPEUTIC INTERVENTIONS

Obsessive–compulsive disorder is the only anxiety disorder for which a best treatment can be recommended (see Chapter 24). With other anxiety disorders and phobias, it is reasonable to start with behavioral treatments and to try medication only if such treatments are unsuccessful. Family therapy, individual psychotherapy for unresolved conflict, and liaison with the patient's school are also commonly required.

The behavioral techniques most often used are systematic desensitization and exposure, operant conditioning, modeling, and cognitive-behavioral therapy (see Chapter 10).

B. PSYCHOPHARMACOLOGIC INTERVENTIONS

Selective serotonin reuptake inhibitors (fluoxetine, fluvoxamine, paroxetine, and sertraline), the mixed serotonin and norepinephrine reuptake inhibitor (venlafaxine), tricyclic antidepressants and high-potency benzodiazepines (e.g., alprazolam, clonazepam) hold some promise in the treatment of anxiety disorders. Fluoxetine has been recommended for the treatment of social phobia. In non-OCD anxiety disorders in the pediatric age group involving more than 1,100 patients, the overall response rate was 69% (95% CI, 65–73%) in antidepressant-treated participants versus 39% (95% CI, 35–43%) in those receiving placebo. Four placebo-controlled studies have examined the effectiveness of tricyclic antidepressants in the treatment of SAD. In only one of these studies was the experimental drug more effective than placebo. One controlled study of the effectiveness of clonazepam in treating SAD showed no superiority over placebo. Controlled trials of clonazepam in treating GAD and social phobia showed no superiority over placebo. Fluvoxamine has shown superiority to placebo in the treatment of social phobia, GAD and SAD. There are no controlled studies of the effectiveness of medication in the treatment of juvenile panic disorder. β-Blockers have shown promise in the alleviation of examination performance anxiety in undergraduate students.

Bridge JA, Iyengar S, Salary CB, et al.: Clinical response and risk for reported suicidal ideation and suicide attempts in pediatric antidepressant treatment: A meta-analysis of randomized controlled trials. *JAMA* 2007;297(15):1683–1696.

Thienemann M: Medications for pediatric anxiety. In: Steiner H (ed). *Handbook of Mental Health Interventions in Children and Adolescents.* San Francisco, CA: Jossey Bass, 2004, pp. 288–319.

Walkup JT, Labellarte MJ, Riddle MA et al.: Fluvoxamine for the treatment of anxiety disorders in children and adolescents. *N Engl J Med,* 2001;344:1279–1285.

Complications/Adverse Outcomes of Treatment

The choice of treatment should be the result of a collaborative discussion between clinician, family, and patient. Presentation of data concerning age-specific benefits should allow for an informed evaluation of the potential benefits and risks of various treatments vs. no treatment and provide a framework for the comparison of drug vs. non-drug treatments.

The predominant adverse effects of antidepressants involve either central nervous system or the gastrointestinal tract. Central nervous system side effects include headache, nervousness, insomnia, drowsiness, anxiety, dizziness, fatigue, sedation, somnolence, mania, hypomania, and irritability. Selective serotonin reuptake inhibitors-associated behavioral activation (i.e., restlessness, hyperkinesis, hyperactivity, agitation) is 2–3-fold more prevalent in children compared to adolescents; it is more prevalent in adolescents compared to adults. Other side effects include sexual dysfunction in adolescent subjects.

The U. S. Food and Drug Administration as well as British and European regulators have issued public health advisories concerning the risk of suicide and self-harm associated with the use of antidepressant medication in the pediatric population. The magnitude of this risk is small, with these medications creating a 2-fold (4% vs. 2%) increased risk for "suicidal behavior or suicidal ideation." There is a need for close monitoring. Recommended monitoring includes daily observation by caregivers, at least weekly face-to-face visits with patients or their family members or caregivers during the first 4 weeks of treatment, then every other week visits for the next 4 weeks, then at 12 weeks, and then as clinically indicated beyond 12 weeks. In addition, patients should also be monitored for associated behaviors (e.g., anxiety, agitation, panic attacks, insomnia, irritability, aggressiveness, impulsivity, akathisia, hypomania, mania). It is also clear that there is relatively little systematic data concerning the risks associated with the long-term use of these medications especially in young children.

Prognosis

The onset of SAD may be acute and precipitated by stress, or it may be gradual, without apparent precipitant. The prognosis is variable. Some children recover completely; others experience chronic or recurrent separation anxiety. These children are likely to relapse when their attachment relationships are threatened, even into maturity. Children with SAD are likely to develop panic disorder, agoraphobia, or depressive disorders in adolescence or adulthood.

The natural history of GAD is not understood. One study has shown that 65% of children diagnosed as having GAD or phobic disorder no longer carry the diagnosis after 2 years. Social phobia in childhood may become associated with alcohol abuse in adolescence. Most children with selective mutism "outgrow" it within a year of onset, although there may be residual shyness. In a minority of cases, mutism continues into late childhood or adolescence.

Child Maltreatment

William Bernet, MD

CHILD MALTREATMENT

 ESSENTIALS OF DIAGNOSIS

*The legal definitions regarding child maltreatment vary from state to state. In general, **neglect** is the failure to provide adequate care and protection for children. It may involve failure to feed the child adequately, provide medical care, provide appropriate education, or protect the child from danger. **Physical abuse** is the infliction of nonaccidental injury by a caretaker. It may take the form of beating, punching, kicking, biting, or other methods. The abuse can result in injuries such as broken bones, internal hemorrhages, bruises, burns, and poisoning. Cultural factors should be considered in assessing whether the discipline of a child is abusive or normative. **Sexual abuse** of children refers to sexual behavior between a child and an adult or between two children when one of them is significantly older or more dominant. The sexual behaviors include the following: touching breasts, buttocks, and genitals, whether the victim is dressed or undressed; exhibitionism; fellatio; cunnilingus; penetration of the vagina or anus with sexual organs or with objects; and pornographic photography. **Emotional abuse** occurs when a caretaker causes serious psychological injury by repeatedly terrorizing or berating a child. When serious, it is often accompanied by neglect, physical abuse, sexual abuse, and exposure to domestic violence.*

The psychiatric classification of abuse and neglect in the Diagnostic and Statistical Manual of Mental Disorders, Fourth Edition, Text Revision (DSM-IV-TR) appears in the chapter "Other Conditions That May Be a Focus of Clinical Attention" and in the section "Problems Related to Abuse or Neglect." The categories of abuse and neglect take a number of factors into consideration including: whether the maltreatment consisted of physical abuse, sexual abuse, or neglect; whether the victim was a child or an adult; whether the focus of clinical attention is on the victim or the perpetrator; and whether, in the case of adults, the perpetrator was the victim's partner or a person other than the victim's partner. The DSM-IV-TR categories related to child maltreatment are in given in the Box above. These conditions are coded on Axis I. DSM-IV-TR classification of child maltreatment.

995.54   Physical abuse of child if the focus of clinical attention is on the victim.

995.53   Sexual abuse of child if the focus of clinical attention is on the victim.

995.52   Neglect of child if the focus of clinical attention is on the victim.

Giardino AP, Alexander R: *Child Maltreatment: A Clinical Guide and Reference & A Comprehensive Photographic Reference Identifying Potential Child Abuse*, 3rd edn. St. Louis: GW Medical Publishing, 2005.

Hamarman S, Bernet W: Evaluating and reporting emotional abuse in children: Parent-based, action-based focus aids in clinical decision making. *J Am Acad Child Adolesc Psychiatry* 2000;39:928.

Helfer ME, Kempe RS, Krugman RD, (eds): *The Battered Child*, 5th edn. revised. Chicago: University of Chicago Press, 1999.

General Considerations

Practitioners in private practice, as well as those employed by courts or other agencies, see children who may have been emotionally, physically, or sexually abused. As a clinician, the practitioner may provide assessments and treatment for abused children and their families in both outpatient and inpatient settings. As a forensic investigator, the practitioner may work with an interdisciplinary team at a pediatric medical center and assist the court in determining what happened to the child.

A. EPIDEMIOLOGY

Each year about three million alleged incidents of child maltreatment are reported to protective services (U.S. Department of Health and Human Services, 2005). Of those reports, about one million are substantiated. Of the substantiated cases, about 60% involve neglect; about

20% involve physical abuse; about 10% involve sexual abuse; about 5% involve emotional abuse; and the rest are unspecified. About 1500 children die each year as a result of maltreatment.

B. ETIOLOGY

Child maltreatment is a tragic and complex biopsychosocial phenomenon. There are various models to explain why child abuse occurs, but generally they consider the interaction of five levels of risk factors and protective factors: (1) The individual biological and psychological makeup of the child victim is important. For example, children who are premature, developmentally disabled, and physically handicapped are more likely to be abused. (2) The individual characteristics of the adult perpetrator. For example, child abuse occurs in all strata of society, but it is associated with lower parental education, parental mental illness, and parental substance abuse, especially alcoholism. (3) The family system refers to the family environment, parenting styles, and interactions among family members. Risk factors include single parenting and domestic violence. (4) The community in which the family lives may relate to both risk and protective factors. In general, child abuse is strongly associated with poverty, financial stress, poor housing, and social isolation. However, there may be protective factors in the community related to the parent's workplace, peer groups of family members, and formal and informal social supports. (5) Finally, the values and beliefs of the culture affect the occurrence of child maltreatment. During the twentieth century, for example, there were two major societal shifts that reduced the frequency of child abuse: the concept that child behavior should be socialized primarily through love, not harsh, physical discipline; and the realization that parental authority is not absolute, that is, parents are not entitled to unrestricted authority over their children.

Myers JEB, Berliner L, Briere J, Hendrix CT, Jenny C, Reid TA, (eds): *The APSAC Handbook on Child Maltreatment*, 2nd edn. Thousand Oaks, California: Sage Publications, 2002.

U.S. Department of Health and Human Services, Administration on Children, Youth and Families: *Child Maltreatment 2005.* Washington, DC: U.S. Government Printing Office, 2007.

Clinical Findings

A. SIGNS & SYMPTOMS

Children who have been abused manifest pleomorphic symptoms in a variety of emotional, behavioral, and psychosomatic reactions. Abused children may have internalizing symptoms such as withdrawal, anxiety, depression, and sleep problems. Abused children may exhibit externalizing symptoms, such as aggression. Children who have been sexually abused are likely to display inappropriate sexual behavior. Table 42–1 lists symptoms that are associated with child abuse: they are not specific or pathognomonic; the same symptoms may occur in the absence of a history of abuse.

The parents of physically abused children have certain characteristics. Typically, they have delayed seeking help for the child's injuries. The history given by the parents is implausible or incompatible with the physical findings. There may be evidence of repeated suspicious injuries. The parents may blame a sibling or claim the child injured himself or herself.

In cases of intrafamilial sexual abuse and other sexual abuse that occurs over a period of time, there is a typical sequence of events: (1) engagement, when the perpetrator induces the child into a special relationship; (2) sexual interaction, in which the sexual behavior progresses from

Table 42–1. Symptoms Associated with Child Maltreatment

Type of Abuse	Associated Symptoms
Any abuse	Psychological symptoms related to emotional distress, such as fear, anxiety, nightmares, phobias, depression, low self-esteem, anger, and hostility More serious psychological problems such as the following: suicidal behavior; posttraumatic stress disorder; and dissociative reactions, with periods of amnesia, trance-like states, and, in some cases, dissociative identity disorder
Sexual abuse	Sexual hyperarousal (open masturbation, excessive sexual curiosity, talking excessively about sexual acts, masturbating with an object, imitating intercourse, inserting objects into the vagina or anus) Sexually aggressive behavior (frequent exposure of the genitals, trying to undress other people, rubbing against other people, and sexual perpetration) Avoidance of sexual stimuli through phobias and inhibitions In adolescents: sexual acting out may occur with promiscuity and, possibly, homosexual contact Physical symptoms (such as somatic complaints, encopresis, and eating disorders) and somatoform symptoms (such as pseudoseizures)

less intimate to more intimate forms of abuse; (3) the secrecy phase; (4) disclosure, when the abuse is discovered; and (5) suppression, when the family pressures the child to retract his or her statements (Sgroi, 1988).

The child sexual abuse accommodation syndrome is sometimes seen when children are sexually abused over a period of time. This syndrome has five characteristics: (1) secrecy; (2) helplessness; (3) entrapment and accommodation; (4) delayed, conflicted, and unconvincing disclosure; and (5) retraction (Summit, 1983). The process of accommodation occurs as the child learns that he or she must be available without complaint to the parent's demands. The child often finds ways to accommodate: by maintaining secrecy in order to keep the family together, by turning to imaginary companions, and by inducing in herself altered states of consciousness. Other children become aggressive, demanding, and hyperactive.

It is possible to distinguish the psychological sequelae of children who have experienced single-event and repeated-event trauma (Terr, 1991). The following four characteristics occur after both types of trauma: (1) visualized or repeatedly perceived intrusive memories of the event; (2) repetitive behavior; (3) fears specifically related to the trauma; and (4) changed attitudes about people, life, and the future. Children who sustain single-event traumas manifest full, detailed memories of the event; an interest in "omens," such as looking retrospectively for reasons why the event occurred; and misperceptions, including visual hallucinations and time distortion. In contrast, many children who have experienced severe, chronic trauma (e.g., repeated sexual abuse) manifest massive denial and psychic numbing, self-hypnosis, dissociation, and rage.

Sgroi SM: *Vulnerable Populations: Evaluation and Treatment of Sexually Abused Children and Adult Survivors*, Vol. 1. New York: Free Press, 1988.

Summit RC: The child sexual abuse accommodation syndrome. *Child Abuse Negl* 1983;7:177.

Terr LC: Childhood traumas: An outline and overview. *Am J Psychiatry* 1991;148:12–20.

B. Clinical Evaluation

The professional who evaluates children who may have been abused has several important tasks: finding out what happened; evaluating the child for emotional disorder; considering other possible explanations for any disorder; being aware of developmental issues, avoiding biasing the outcome with his or her preconceptions; pursuing these objectives in a sensitive manner so as not to retraumatize the child; being supportive to family members; and keeping an accurate record which may be subpoenaed for future court proceedings.

It is important to be familiar with the normative sexual behavior of children for two reasons. First, normal sexual play activities between children should not be taken to be sexual abuse. In assessing this issue, the evaluator should consider the age difference between the children; their developmental level; whether one child dominated or coerced the other child; and whether the act itself was intrusive, forceful, or dangerous. Second, sexually abused children often manifest more sexual behavior than do typical children. Sometimes they have sexual knowledge beyond what would be expected for their age and developmental level. For example, behavior such as trying to undress other people, masturbating with an object, performing fellatio, and imitating sexual intercourse are red flags that suggest a child has been sexually abused.

Patient interview—The clinical interview may need modification when assessing a child who may have been abused. The following sections describe the components of an interview that is particularly suited for forensic evaluations (Poole & Lamb, 1998; Yuille et al., 1993):

i. Build rapport and make informal observations—Build rapport with the child and make informal observations of the child's behavior, social skills, and cognitive abilities.

ii. Ask the child to describe two specific past events—In order to assess the child's memory and to model the form of the interview for the child by asking nonleading, open-ended questions, a pattern that will hold through the rest of the interview. For example, prior to interviewing the child, one can obtain specific information from the parent about a recent birthday party, trip to the zoo, etc.

iii. Establish the need to tell the truth—Reach an agreement that in this interview only the truth will be discussed, not "pretend" or imagination. For example, the interviewer can say, "If I said I'm wearing a purple hat today, would that be the truth or a lie?" Reach an agreement that it is fine to say, "I don't know." For example, the interviewer can say, "Do I have a dog named Charlie?" and the child should say, "I don't know."

iv. Introduce the topic of concern—Start with more general questions, such as, "Do you know why you are talking with me today?" Proceed, only if necessary, to more specific questions, such as, "Has anything happened to you?" or "Has anyone done something to you?" Drawings may be helpful in initiating disclosure. For example, either the child or the interviewer draws an outline of a person. Then the child is asked to add and name each body part and describe its function. If sexual abuse is suspected, the interviewer could ask, when the genitals are described, if the child has seen that part on another person and who has seen or touched that part on the child. If physical abuse is suspected, the interviewer could ask if particular parts have been hurt in some way.

v. Elicit a free narrative—Once the topic of abuse has been introduced, the interviewer encourages the child to describe each event from the beginning without leaving out any details. The child is allowed to proceed at his or her pace, without correction or interruption. If abuse has occurred over a period of time, the interviewer may ask for a description of the general pattern and then for an account of particular episodes.

vi. Pose general questions—The interviewer may ask general questions in order to elicit further details. These questions should not be leading and should be phrased in such a way that an inability to recall or lack of knowledge is acceptable.

vii. Pose specific questions, if necessary—It may be helpful to obtain clarification by asking specific questions. For example, the interviewer may follow up on inconsistencies in a gentle, nonthreatening manner. Avoid repetitive questions and the appearance of rewarding particular answers in any way.

viii. Use interview aids, if necessary—Anatomically correct dolls may be useful in developing exactly what sort of abusive activity occurred. The dolls are not used to diagnose child abuse, only to clarify what happened (Everson & Boat, 1994).

ix. Conclude the interview—Toward the end of the interview, the interviewer may ask a few leading questions about irrelevant issues (e.g., "You came here by taxi, didn't you?"). If the child demonstrates a susceptibility to suggestions, the interviewer would need to verify that the information obtained earlier did not come about through contamination. Finally, the interviewer thanks the child for participating, regardless of the outcome of the interview. The interviewer should not make promises that cannot be kept.

Parent interview—In order to evaluate a child who may have been abused, it is necessary to do more than simply interview the child and ask him or her what happened. It is also important to interview the parents and perhaps other caregivers. The parents should be able to provide information regarding the child's experiences with particular people; the duration and evolution of the child's symptoms; the child's developmental and medical history; and factors in the child's life, other than abuse, that might explain the symptoms. It may also be important to assess the parents' motivations and psychological strengths and weaknesses. For instance, some parents (who perpetrated the abuse or allowed another individual to do so) may be motivated to deny or minimize the possibility that the child was abused. Other parents (who are vengeful or overly suspicious of another person) may be motivated to exaggerate the possibility that the child was abused or may even fabricate symptoms of abuse.

C. Psychological Testing

Although psychological testing cannot diagnose child abuse, it may be a useful part of the evaluation. For example, the Child Sexual Behavior Inventory is a questionnaire to be completed by a parent, usually the child's mother. This questionnaire helps the clinician identify sexual behaviors that can be considered normative for the child's age and gender and sexual behaviors that can be viewed as relatively atypical for the child's age and gender, and which raise the suspicion of possible sexual abuse. Intellectual testing may be used to establish the child's developmental level. A general psychiatric evaluation may help with the differential diagnosis and clarify the child's treatment needs.

D. Record Review

In evaluating a child who may have been abused, it is frequently important to obtain information from outside sources such as medical, mental health, and educational records. It may be helpful to review the investigation conducted by child protective services, although those records may not be available.

Website

Johnson TC: www.TCavJohn.com has useful tools for assessment, treatment, and family education regarding child sexual abuse.

American Academy of Child and Adolescent Psychiatry: Practice parameters for the forensic evaluation of children and adolescents who may have been physically or sexually abused. *J Am Acad Child Adolesc Psychiatry* 1997;36:423–442.

Everson MD, Boat BW: Putting the anatomical doll controversy in perspective: An examination of the major uses and criticisms of the dolls in child sexual abuse evaluations. *Child Abuse Negl* 1994;18:113.

Friedrich WN, Fisher JL, Dittner CA, et al.: Child sexual behavior inventory: Normative, psychiatric, and sexual abuse comparisons. *Child Maltreat* 2001;6:37.

Poole DA, Lamb ME: *Investigative Interviews of Children: A Guide for Helping Professionals.* Washington, DC: American Psychological Association, 1998.

Yuille JC, Hunter R, Joffe R, Zaparniuk J: Interviewing children in sexual abuse cases. In: Goodman GS, Bottoms BL (eds). *Child Victims, Child Witnesses: Understanding and Improving Testimony.* New York: Guilford, 1993.

Differential Diagnosis

Children may make false statements in psychiatric evaluations. Sometimes they falsely deny abuse; sometimes they make false allegations. A number of mental processes, both conscious and unconscious, can result in false allegations. For example, a delusional mother, who believed that her ex-husband had been molesting their daughter, induces the girl to state that the father had rubbed against her in bed. By repeatedly asking leading or suggestive questions, inept interviewers have induced children to make false allegations of abuse. Some children manifest pathological lying in making false allegations. Young children may tell tall tales, making innocent statements that evolve or are molded into false allegations of abuse. Older children may lie about abuse for revenge or personal advantage. In the past, multiple allegations of abuse have been generated through group contagion or spread by parental panic and overzealous clinical investigation.

Credibility refers to the child's truthfulness and accuracy, which sometimes is an issue in assessing children who allege abuse. The following factors indicate that the child is credible: the child uses his or her own vocabulary rather than adult terms and tells the story from his or her own point of view; the child displays advanced sexual knowledge; the child reenacts the trauma in spontaneous play; sexual themes are present in play and drawings; the child's affect is consonant with the accusations; the child's behavior is seductive, precocious, or regressive; the child has good recall of details, including sensory motor and idiosyncratic details; and the child has a history of telling the truth.

The following factors indicate the child is making unreliable or fictitious allegations: the child's account is vague and lacks details, due to lack of information, not resistance or defensiveness; the child's statements are dramatic or implausible, for example, involving the presence of multiple perpetrators or situations in which the perpetrator has not taken ordinary steps against discovery; the child's statements become increasingly inconsistent over time; and the child's accounts progress over time from relatively innocuous behavior to increasingly intrusive, abusive, and aggressive activities.

Bernet W: False statements and the differential diagnosis of abuse allegations. *J Am Acad Child Adolesc Psychiatry* 1993;32:903.

Bernet W: Sexual abuse allegations in the context of child-custody disputes. In: Gardner R, Sauber S, Lorandos D (eds): *The International Handbook of Parental Alienation Syndrome: Conceptual, Clinical and Legal Considerations.* Binghamton, New York: Haworth Press. 2006.

Lamb ME, Sternberg KJ, Esplin PW, Hershkowitz I, Orbach Y: Assessing the credibility of children's allegations of sexual abuse: A survey of recent research. *Learn Individ Differ* 1997;9:175.

Ludwig S, Reece RM: *Child Abuse: Medical Diagnosis and Management,* 2nd edn. Philadelphia: Lippincott Williams & Wilkins, 2000.

Treatment

The first step in the management of child maltreatment is ensuring the child's safety and well-being. The child may need to be removed from an abusive or neglectful family. A clinician who suspects that a child has been abused should perform an assessment within the scope of the clinician's expertise—that is, the psychiatrist conducts a psychiatric evaluation, the pediatrician conducts a pediatric assessment. If the clinician continues to suspect child abuse after conducting his or her assessment, the local child protection agency must be notified (Kalichman, 1999).

Maltreated children who have significant psychological or behavioral symptoms should receive psychiatric treatment. Treatment should not be confused with forensic investigation. Although a specific treatment plan depends on the findings of a diagnostic evaluation, the psychotherapist would generally address issues such as self-esteem, worries, and fears; developing a therapeutic relationship built on trust, in which the child will not be exploited or betrayed; and gaining an understanding over time of the factors that contributed to the child's victimization.

Abused children with posttraumatic stress disorder have been successfully treated with a trauma-focused cognitive behavioral treatment (Cohen et al., 2000, 2004) that has four components: psychoeducation, anxiety management, exposure, and cognitive therapy. **Psychoeducation** includes teaching the child and the caregivers about strategies to avoid future abuse. **Anxiety management** includes teaching children how to use relaxation and other coping strategies to reduce fearful responses to memories of abuse. **Exposure** refers to mastering traumatic anxiety through talking, drawing, or writing about the abuse experiences, either in ordinary conversation or through a variety of play, artistic, or other projective techniques. **Cognitive therapy** techniques help the child replace cognitive distortions about the event or negative feelings about himself or herself.

If an abused child has no symptoms related to the maltreatment, it is appropriate to provide brief psychoeducational counseling and suggestions for recognizing any problems that arise in the future. For a child whose abuse was a transitory unpleasant experience (e.g., a single, brief episode of fondling by a stranger), it may be adaptive for the child to forget the incident and move on.

Cohen JA, Berliner L, Mannarino AP: Treating traumatized children: A research review and synthesis. *Trauma Violence Abuse* 2000;1:29.

Cohen JA, Deblinger E, Mannarino AP, Steer RA: A multi-site randomized controlled trial for children with sexual abuse-related PTSD symptoms. *J Am Acad Child Adolesc Psychiatry* 2004;43:393–402.

Kalichman SC: *Mandated Reporting of Suspected Child Abuse: Ethics, Law, and Policy,* 2nd edn. Washington, DC: American Psychological Association, 1999.

Pearce JW, Pezzot-Pearce TD: *Psychotherapy of Abused and Neglected Children.* New York: Guilford, 1997.

Runyon MK, Deblinger E, Ryan EE, Thakkar-Kolar R: An overview of child physical abuse: Developing an integrated parent-child cognitive-behavioral treatment approach. *Trauma Violence Abuse* 2004;5:65.

Complications/Adverse Outcomes of Treatment

The most serious risk in evaluating and treating victims of child maltreatment is that the child will be retraumatized. This can happen if treatment requires the child to remember and relive the traumatic experiences to an unnecessary degree or if the child and family are too emotionally fragile to cope. Although many therapists believe it can be helpful for the child to recall and share painful experiences from the past, it is not therapeutic to dwell on these events repeatedly and endlessly. Retraumatization can also occur when the child, who has already lost important people in her life, develops an attachment to a therapist and that new relationship is interrupted in a premature or painful manner. Another possible complication of therapy is the child's unwitting compulsion to reenact the aggressive or sexual aspects of the abusive relationship with new caregivers. That is, a seriously abused child may be placed with benevolent foster parents but behave in a way to provoke overly punitive behaviors by his new caregivers. Also, a seriously abused child may behave in a way to evoke rejection by an otherwise well-meaning therapist.

Treatment can have an adverse outcome if an overzealous therapist persists in looking for memories of past abuse when the abuse never happened in the first place. If a therapist repeatedly asks the patient—who can be a child or an adult—to remember abuse, the patient may "remember" it to please the therapist. To complicate the situation further, the patient may become convinced of the reality of these false memories.

Prognosis

Sometimes child maltreatment causes no long-term psychological problems at all, but sometimes it causes severe psychological problems. Child maltreatment is more likely to cause subsequent emotional and behavioral disorders if the following factors are present: greater frequency and duration of abuse; greater force; physical injury; perpetration by a family member; the child already has poor coping skills; and lack of family support. Maternal support and validation of the child's statement is correlated with better prognosis.

The long-term psychological consequences of child maltreatment have been studied prospectively by following abused children for more than 20 years (Widom, 1999; Horwitz, 2001). The long-term psychological and physical effects of childhood maltreatment were also examined retrospectively in the Adverse Childhood Experiences (ACE) Study (Dube et al., 2001). In general, individuals who experienced child maltreatment were more likely to have psychological problems—posttraumatic stress disorder, dysthymia, suicidality, alcoholism, and antisocial personality disorder—than were individuals who had not been abused.

Herman (1992) and van der Kolk (2003) have studied the long-term psychological and neurobiological effects of severe child maltreatment. Adults who were severely abused as children may develop a condition called complex posttraumatic stress disorder or a disorder of extreme stress not otherwise specified (DESNOS). The features of DESNOS are: altered regulation of affect and impulses; altered attention and consciousness; altered self-perception; altered relationships; altered systems of meaning; and somatization.

The long-term consequences of child maltreatment may be affected by the victim's genetic makeup. Caspi et al. (2002) found that children who had a variant allele of the *MAOA* gene and also had been seriously abused were much more likely to be violent and antisocial as adults. This research suggests a mechanism by which genetic makeup and life experience interact to influence psychosocial development and future attitudes and behaviors.

Caspi A, McClay J, Moffitt TE, et al.: Role of genotype in the cycle of violence in maltreated children. *Science* 2002;297:851.

Dube SR, Anda RF, Felitti VJ, Chapman DP, Williamson DF, Giles WH: Childhood abuse, household dysfunction, and the risk of attempted suicide throughout the life span: Findings from the adverse childhood experiences study. *JAMA* 2001;286:3089–3096.

Herman JL: Complex PTSD: A syndrome in survivors of prolonged and repeated trauma. *J Trauma Stress* 1992;5:377–391.

Horwitz AV, Widom CS, McLaughlin J, White HR: The impact of childhood abuse and neglect on adult mental health: A prospective study. *J Health Soc Behav* 2001;42:184–201.

Kendall-Tackett K: *Treating the Lifetime Health Effects of Childhood Victimization.* New York: Civic Research Institute, 2003.

van der Kolk BA: The neurobiology of childhood trauma and abuse. *Child Adolesc Psychiatr Clin N Am* 2003;12(2):293.

Widom CS: Posttraumatic stress disorder in abused and neglected children grown up. *Am J Psychiatry* 1999;156:1223–1229.

Posttraumatic Stress Disorder in Children and Adolescents Following a Single-Event Trauma

43

Brett McDermott, MD

 ESSENTIALS OF DIAGNOSIS

Single-event traumas experienced by children and adolescents include involvement in motor vehicle accidents, natural disasters, and other unexpected, paroxysmal events such as being assaulted or raped. In environments where the latter occur with unfortunate regularity, such as when a family experiences protracted domestic violence, ongoing sexual assault or lives in a war-zone, the individual is likely to be exposed to multiple traumatic experiences and the mental health sequelae are qualitatively different to the experience of a single-event trauma. Readers should consult the chapters on dissociative disorders, personality disorders, and references to sexual abuse to further understand the sequelae of exposure to multiple-event trauma. This chapter will focus on the mental health outcomes following exposure to a single-event trauma. Typical diagnoses include posttraumatic stress disorder (PTSD), other anxiety disorders including specific phobias, and depressive presentations. The Diagnostic and Statistical Manual, *fourth edition, Text Revision, criteria for these conditions are detailed in chapters 20, 41, and 38, respectively.*

Two diagnostic considerations influence the chapter. The overarching frame is that of developmental psychopathology. Individuals function by integration of subsystems that interact vertically (e.g., gene to cell) and horizontally (person to person). Infants, children, and adolescents also need to organize across time. Time course introduces new developmental constructs: novelty of cause and effect of inputs at different developmental stages, differential rates of development across subsystems, critical periods, and negotiating developmental challenges such as the changing relationship between parent and child. The developmental science perspective subsumes other useful heuristics such as a bio-psycho-social and a systemic perspective. Inherent is the conceptualization of an individual's trajectory over the infant–child–youth developmental span and abnormality as deviance from a normal trajectory. The concept of a normal trajectory is very useful in understanding the impact of diverse traumatic events. Repetitive traumatic events and their sequelae are discussed elsewhere in this text (see Chapter 42 on Child Maltreatment). The cumulative adversity inherent to experiencing repetitive traumatic events leads to a picture of continuity of developmental abnormality. That is, the child has been symptomatic and functionally impaired for some time. The mental health sequelae of a significant isolated, single-event trauma is seen as a developmental discontinuity—a subjective deviation from the developmental norm. For a more comprehensive account of the developmental approach see Cairns and Angold (1996). The seminal paper of Lenore Terr advocated the useful nosology of type I trauma describing the developmental discontinuity, type II the developmental continuity (Terr, 1994).

Costello EJ, Angold A: Developmental Psychopathology. In: Cairns RB, Elder GH, Costello EJ, (eds). *Developmental Science.* Cambridge UK: Cambridge University Press, 1996, pp. 168–189.

Terr L: Childhood traumas: An outline and overview. *Am J Psychiatry* 1994;148:10–20.

General Considerations

An adverse mental health outcome following a single-event trauma is not limited to PTSD. Clearly PTSD is of central importance, however, researchers have long noted other postdisaster anxiety and depressive states. Current data consistent with greater disaster-related fear of death and event exposure being more likely to have a PTSD/anxiety outcome, while greater loss and grief predisposes to a depression outcome. However, PTSD-depression symptom concordance is great and comorbid presentations are common.

The post-single-event trauma burden of mental illness is not restricted to new mental health presentations. Many individuals with preexisting mental illness will experience a postevent symptoms relapse. Reasons may be pragmatic, such as difficulty obtaining medications or access to therapy in the postdisaster environment. Systemic issues such as an increased likelihood of parent distress and/or depression may be significant. Psychopathology may be related to event phase; immediately postevent individuals and service providers are appropriately focused on physical safety, water, food, and shelter needs. Mental health presentations and service provision generally begin in the weeks following the disaster. It is often the case that mental health issues come to dominate in the months and years postdisaster. An example is major depression some months following a disaster, yet with clear temporal links to disaster-related events.

A. Epidemiology

Estimates of the prevalence of post-single-event PTSD vary greatly. Uniform PTSD rates would be unexpected given every disaster or traumatic event is unique. PTSD estimate variability is also due to disparity in research design. Published research varies in the elapsed time since the disaster, developmental stage of participants, whether the child or parent was the primary informant, and instruments used to measure psychopathology; the last mentioned range from qualitative accounts, self-report questionnaires to structured diagnostic interviews. Some early studies included data obtained from mental health professionals working for either the plaintiff or defense in lawsuits after a disaster. Design factors include bias due to selective mortality, recall and interview bias and use of convenience samples. Significant "unpackaging" of the event, both of event-related variables and the personal meaning of the event is required for a more meaningful between-event comparison.

Examples of prevalence variability include PTSD rates between 90% and 100% of children who were kidnapped and endured harrowing hours in captivity and children trapped in a school playground by sniper fire, intermediate rates of 40–60% in children who experienced major transport disasters and lower rates of 5–15% of children screened after natural disasters. Occasional studies report no children meeting diagnostic criteria for PTSD. Even in these examples limited symptom PTSD and other anxiety disorder presentations are usually reported.

Single-event trauma research is often population-based initiatives following natural disasters. Significant research initiatives have followed the devastation of Hurricanes Hugo (1989), Andrew (1992), Iniki (1992), and Katrina (2005). Research findings include female gender, younger age, high-trait anxiety, and emotional reactivity during hurricanes independently predicted PTSD symptoms more strongly than self-report hurricane exposure. Australian wildfire disasters have been subjected to similar scrutiny and surprisingly similar rates of child and adolescent PTSD have been reported, as well as high-trait anxiety as a PTSD-predictive factor and high rates of comorbid depression. Natural disasters potentially involve large numbers of individuals and/or a large proportion of a given population. An epidemiological perspective is informative and a public health approach to service provision justified. For example, a sophisticated postdisaster-intervention strategy would include screening for PTSD, the latter consistent with the National Institute for Clinical Excellence (NICE) guidelines, followed by universal and targeted responses to identified children, adolescents, and families.

B. Etiology

A potentially confusing range of causal theories have been advocated for PTSD presentations in childhood. Such theories are often extrapolated from adult research and include psychodynamic, behavioral, cognitive, and biological explanatory models. Given variations in a potential victim's integration of biological, emotional, and behavioral systems and age-appropriate differences in individual–context, individual–peer, and individual–family interactions, stressful events may affect individuals in different ways across the life span. Etiology can be divided into research findings, often from epidemiological designs, that identify risk, vulnerability, and resilience factors. PTSD is also informed at a more fundamental level by cognitive theory and neurobiological research. The area is not without complexity; seemingly simple associations such as gender, age, and PTSD have proven difficult to clarify. Published findings include no effect of age on PTSD prevalence, higher rates in older children and adolescents, and higher rates in younger children. McDermott and Palmer (2002) studied 2379 grade 4–12 students after a wildfire disaster and reported a peak prevalence of PTSD in the middle school years.

Risk factors—An overarching principle is whether the functioning of the individual with PTSD has diminished. If significant, this diminution will have rendered the individual's functioning below the normal trajectory for age. A second principle is that the impaired functioning is due to a combination of event-related, proximal factors and distal factors inherent to the individual and present before the trauma. The event-related factor with the greatest empirical evidence of association with subsequent PTSD symptoms is increased traumatic event exposure. The event-exposure–PTSD association has been demonstrated in children residing in cities subject to more earthquake damage, witnessing more hurricane damage, closer proximity to gunfire, and being closer to actual wildfire flames. Note that high exposure, while a useful summary variable, is itself a multifactorial construct that includes the perception of threat of death, concern about possible loss and bereavement, witnessing a range of disaster-related phenomena including death or serious injury, perceptual experiences such as smoke from fires, and witnessing the coping or lack of coping of parents, caregivers, and other adults. Dislocation in the immediate aftermath of a disaster has been argued as a positive factor by decreasing disaster exposure and a negative factor given the lack of continuity with family and community and removing the opportunity to constructively engage in postdisaster restorative activities. In a case-controlled study of Armenian child earthquake survivors, at 30 months postdisaster, there was no difference in PTSD and depression symptoms in a group of children removed from the disaster and those who remained, distal factors significantly associated with higher PTSD symptoms in children include high-trait anxiety, a past history of emotional problems, children with a subjective sense of low self-efficacy and low social support, children employing poor coping strategies and an internal causal attribution.

Cognitive factors—Cognitive information-processing theory postulates that there is the potential of being overwhelmed by the everyday volume of information requiring processing. To counter this, information is encoded and recalled in specific ways. Cognitive schemata are developed as a primary organizing heuristic. The schema incoming information interaction influences subsequent memory encoding and retrieval. It is postulated that trauma-related information is also encoded with relation to existing schema. Dissonance with existing schema leads to conflict and the disruption of the usual memory encoding and comprehension and memory retrieval sequence. The greater the dissonance, the greater is the likelihood of trauma symptoms and impairment.

One postulate is that there are very specific schemata, which, if violated, are more likely to precipitate trauma symptoms. Fundamental beliefs such as "good things happen to good people" may be radically undermined after a traumatic event such as the experience of being raped. Possible psychological responses to information dissonant to existing schema include assimilation, altering information to fit preconceptions and accommodation, changing existing schemata to account for, and accept the new information. The last mentioned may facilitate recovery. Unfortunately accommodation may create a secondary impairment if, for instance, new schema are punitive, self-deprecatory, undermine adaptive beliefs about safety or intimacy, and make the tasks of daily living more difficult. Child and adolescent trauma complications can be more complex given the added possibility of altered parent schema about their child's safety. An example is the double jeopardy of the child who experienced a paroxysmal, unitary (type I) sexual trauma. Such an event may lead to PTSD psychopathology. If, for a protracted period thereafter, altered parent–child safety schema leads to the child not being allowed to visit friends, go on school outings, "sleep-overs," and other events without direct parent monitoring, the normal process of child–adolescent individuation–separation may be retarded generating a secondary impairment. Further, accommodation in young children may manifest as self-blame for the event, heightened by a child's tendency to regress to a more egocentric worldview. Or by developing schema that predicts future disastrous events and ongoing extreme danger, either to themselves, friends, or family. Other changed schema may be that the event will reoccur, the event will become greater with a larger number of affected people and parents and other adults cannot protect children from traumatic events.

Biological factors—Neurobiological research including neuroimaging studies has been less active with child and adolescent participants. Studies that have been conducted are more likely to be with maltreated children than children who experienced a single-event trauma. Extrapolation from research with adults and maltreated children suggests possible decreased intracranial and cerebral volume in children who experience a single-event trauma. However, it may be that multiple insults during critical periods are needed for altered brain morphology. Neuroendocrine investigations suggest that dysregulation of the hypothalamus–pituitary stress system is likely following traumatic events. More definitive conclusions await further research.

Bremner JD: Neuroimaging of childhood trauma. *Semin Clin Neuropsychiatry* 2002;7(2):104–112.

Cohen JA, Perel JM, De Bellis MD, Friedman MJ, Putnam FW: Treating traumatized children: Clinical implications of the psychobiology of posttraumatic stress disorder. *Trauma Violence Abuse* 2002;3(2):91–108.

McDermott BM, Palmer LJ: Post-disaster emotional distress, depression and event-related variables: Findings across child and adolescent developmental stages. *Aust N Z J Psychiatry* 2002;36:754–761.

Meiser-Steadman: Towards a cognitive-behavioural model of PTSD in children and adolescents. *Clin Child Fam Psychol Rev* 2002;5(4):217–232.

Najarian LM, Goenjian AK, Pelcovitz D, Mandel FS, Najarian B: Relocation after a disaster: Posttraumatic stress disorder in Armenia after the earthquake. *J Am Acad Child Adolesc Psychiatry* 1996;35:374–383.

Genetics

Detailed understanding of the genetic aspects of an individual's response to single-event trauma is not yet available. Consistent with many psychiatric presentations, the concordance for monozygotic twins, in this case those exposed to a traumatic event and who develop PTSD, is higher than for dizygotic twins. Monozygotic twins also share their intrauterine environment and so the monozygotic twin excess may also be due to nongenetic factors. In the review of Broekman and colleagues (2007) the authors make the assumption that genetic effects are likely to be polygenetic and note a range of target endophenotypes such as alterations in the HPA axis. They also report methodological difficulties such as small sample sizes that make current findings inconclusive. Theoretical problems include differentiating potential genetic vulnerability to PTSD versus a genetic vulnerability to being exposed to a traumatic event, and so different pathways for a genetic effect to be expressed are possible. One clear advance is the gene–environment studies of early life trauma and subsequent depression or antisocial behavior at age 26 years (Caspi et al., 2003). The relationship of functional polymorphisms in the serotonin promoter region and monoamine oxidase gene modifying the long-term outcome of early traumatic experience is an exciting area of research and likely to inform our understanding of individual resilience and vulnerability to traumatic events.

Broekman BF, Olff M, Boer F: The genetic background to PTSD. *Neurosci Biobehav Rev* 2007;31(3):348–362.

Caspi A, Sugden K, Moffitt TE, et al.: Influence of life stress on depression: Moderation by a polymorphism in the 5-HTT gene. *Science* 2003;301:386–389.

Clinical Findings

A. ASSESSMENT AND HISTORY TAKING

No two single-event traumas are identical either at individual or population level. The understanding that trauma exposure can be "lumped" into a nominal variable is simplistic. It is more typical that within the event setting exposures vary widely. For the clinician it is important to "unpack" the potentially traumatic event. One useful strategy is to obtain a chronological narrative, depending on the duration of the event, at 1-, 10-, or 60-minute intervals postevent. The clinician should consider potential traumatic stimuli in all sensory modalities, for example, what did the child see, hear, smell? What were the child's thoughts at different stages of the event? What is their understanding of what occurred and the meaning they gave to the event or the roles individual's played. What were the reactions of others, especially adults in the vicinity?

The type of traumatic event, for example, experiencing a motor vehicle accident, is usually identifiable in the PTSD-symptom content including the subject matter of flashbacks, dreams, and nightmares; symbolic reminders; and, if accessible, cognitions underlying avoidance behavior. Some individuals with intellectual impairment and the very young will not have a verbal narrative of the event. In these cases, the clinicians seeks to identify behavioral discontinuities, temporally related to event exposure, in various domains such as sleep, satiety, elimination, aggression, and impulsivity. Another useful exercise is to consider the event from a non-mental-health perspective. As is often the case following natural disasters, establish, if there was environmental degradation, significant postevent economic hardship (short and long term), disruption of services (electricity, water, sewerage), and disruptions to institutions such as schools? Failure to provide services in the postevent setting emphasizes personal and collective powerlessness. Postevent concerns in these domains may have little relationship to PTSD symptoms; nevertheless, be very significant in understanding overall impairment levels.

B. SIGNS & SYMPTOMS

The clinical presentation of child and adolescent PTSD is dependant upon the child's age; given the age is a proxy for underlying developmental constructs such as cognitive, speech, and language development and sophistication of peer and societal relatedness.

Infant school children—The lack of systematic research is more pronounced in preschool and infant school children, in part because of difficulties administering questionnaires and completing semistructured interviews with young children.

Most knowledge of PTSD in this age group is from expert opinion. Young, preverbal children communicate distress by behavioral change temporally linked to a given trauma. General signs include alterations in the ease of feeding, sleeping, or generally settling the child. Parents may report regressed behavior including the child's unwillingness to explore the environment, increased stranger danger, increased aggression, or clingy behavior.

Verbal preschool children may display or voice broad emotions such as anger, sadness, and excitement. Mixed or rapidly changing emotional states are frequent. Separation anxiety is common, so too are specific trauma-related fears. Posttraumatic play, in Terr's terminology "reenactments" given the absence of the fun element of play, is typical (Terr, 1994). Reenactments are compulsive, repetitive behavioral sequences that are unconsciously linked to the traumatic event. Nontraumatized children can be involved in a traumatized child's reenactment. This involvement can place children in danger, for example, setting or playing with fire following a bushfire disaster.

Primary and high school children—With increasing age, symptomatology is more typical of adult PTSD. Age-related phenomena still exist such as aggressive or withdrawn behavior; however, behavior becomes more sophisticated. Fear of death, separation anxiety, or fear of the event recurring are common. Magical thinking and ascribing omen status to events before the trauma is common in younger children, so too are phenomena such as nightmares and sleep disturbance. Flashbacks are reported; however have a more daydream quality than the sudden, intrusive adult phenomena. A fear generalization gradient has been described such that stimuli approaching the traumatic event evoked increasing distress. For example, fear seeing any car, but greater fear seeing the same color car that was involved in a motor vehicle accident.

Denial and disavowal of the traumatic event is not often seen in childhood PTSD presentations that follow a single-event trauma. However, children do often withhold the extent of their distressing experiences from their parents, either because of perceived difficulties talking to their parents following trauma or children specifically not wanting to make their parents more anxious by the added burden of their feelings of distress. Another distinction from adult PTSD is that numbing and restriction of affect is not frequently reported by children, in part because of the difficulty in younger children understanding and discussing these concepts.

C. PSYCHOLOGICAL TESTING

Given the reticence of many children to discuss their PTSD symptoms and the low parent identification posttraumatic symptoms, rating scales can play a valuable role in postevent screening and symptom identification. Some measures such as the PTSD-reaction index can be administered by a clinician as a semistructured interview or by child self-report. Care is required to assess the developmental appropriateness of item wording; most children younger than 8 years of age will have difficulty with multiple response answer fields but can complete Yes/No formats. Questions to adolescents should include impor-

tant comorbidities such as postevent substance abuse. See chapter 41 for more details on specific measures.

D. LABORATORY FINDINGS AND IMAGING

There are currently no practice recommendations advising the routine use of specific laboratory tests or neuroimaging studies in children or adolescents who experienced single-event trauma.

Differential Diagnosis

There is a danger in equating single-event trauma with PTSD. Care should be taken to elicit or exclude PTSD diagnostic criteria as well as excluding depression and other anxiety disorders especially phobias, panic disorder with and without agoraphobia and generalized anxiety disorder. For some children the primary presenting complaint will be a sleep disorder or a restrictive eating pattern. Increased physical symptoms such as musculoskeletal complaints and alcohol and substance use have been reported in adolescents following a single-event trauma.

Treatment

Overarching treatment concerns are the need to be developmentally appropriate, especially the communication style of children at different developmental stages.

A. PSYCHOPHARMACOLOGICAL TREATMENT

The Cochrane PTSD review of Stein and colleagues (2006) identified 35 randomized controlled trials, found no trials with pediatric subjects, and concluded medication was effective in decreasing PTSD and depression symptoms and impairment in adult PTSD sufferers. Dedicated child and adolescent reviews concur with the absence of research in the pediatric domain and suggest, at the level of expert opinion, that SSRI medication may be useful for general PTSD symptoms, while alpha agonists may have a role with hyperarousal symptoms. The UK NICE guidelines advice against prescribing for children and adolescents with PTSD, with the caveat that medication may have a role in acute postevent sleep disturbance.

Donnelly CL: Pharmacologic treatment approaches for children and adolescents with post traumatic stress disorder. *Child Adolesc Psychiatr Clin N Am* 2003;12:251–269.

Stein DJ, Ipser JC, Seedat S. Pharmacotherapy for post traumatic stress disorder (PTSD). *Cochrane Database of Systematic Reviews* 2006, Issue 1. Art. no.: CD002795.DOI:10.1002/14651858. CD002795.pub2.

Taylor Tisha L, Chemtob Claude M: Efficacy of treatment for child and adolescent traumatic stress. *Arch Pediatr Adolesc Med* 2004;158(8):786–791.

B. Psychotherapeutic Interventions

Current treatment guidelines emphasize that many individuals who experience a potentially traumatic event do not become symptomatic or have mild symptoms that spontaneously remit over the first month. There is currently no evidence that a single session debriefing intervention will lead to greater or more rapid symptom reduction.

Psychological first aid—Psychological first aid (PFA) is recommended. PFA is an initiative of the National Child Traumatic Stress Network (NCTSN) and the National Centre for PTSD. The Field Operations Guide, second edition is available from the NCTSN website. This resource provides training on preparation to provide PFA and engagement issues. Core intervention areas are then covered: safety, mental status stabilization, gathering essential information, practical assistance, facilitating social connectiveness, psycho-education about emotional trauma and grief, and service linkage.

Trauma focused cognitive–behavioral therapy—If symptoms persist or cause impairment then treatment should be instigated. The current treatment of first choice is a Trauma focused cognitive–behavioral therapy (TF-CBT). While in children treatment will often include some element of play and relaxation therapy, it seems for effectiveness therapy must address the specific trauma memories and ameliorate the impact of such memories by CBT techniques such as exposure and habituation and/or cognitive restructuring. More indepth analysis is difficult given the current level of evidence, Taylor and Chemtob reported only 8 trials out of 102 identified included more than a single subject design or a control group. There is some evidence that early presentations may require brief five-session interventions. Later presentations or those that include comorbid traumatic bereavement, disability, and past history of other traumatic events may require longer intervention, that is, 8–12 sessions. TF-CBT delivery may be equally effective by group or individual therapy. Online training in TF-CBT can be obtained via the NCTSN website. One study demonstrated effectiveness of EMDR in children following a natural disaster. PTSD treatment should generally be initiated first. Comorbidities such as depressive symptoms may remit with PTSD therapy. If the severity of depressive or substance-abuse symptoms does not allow effective TF-CBT, these issues may need to be addressed first. Lastly, the usual child and adolescent strategies of parent or caregiver involvement and addressing systemic issues such as school-based initiatives to limit impairment are recommended.

National Institute for Clinical Excellence (NICE): Clinical Guideline 26. Post-traumatic stress disorder (PTSD): The management of PTSD in adults and children in primary and secondary care. The National Child Traumatic Stress Network. www.nctsnet.org/nccts/

Complications/Adverse Outcomes of Treatment

Unnecessary treatment with medication or psychotherapy can occur following the good intentions of parents and clinicians to treat children who are exposed to a traumatic event. A competent assessment should prevent undue intervention. Similarly, all screening tests have false positive and negative rates. Negative screening results should not preclude subsequent referral for diagnostic clarification. In an ideal service provision scenario, an individual with a positive screening result on a self-report measure would then be individually assessed to determine the need for an intervention.

Prognosis

Time may diminish the emotional impact and symptoms of PTSD. Possible mechanisms include habituation to the reminders of a given event and a process of more normative forgetting. However, symptom reduction may be misleading. A perception of mastery may in reality be diminished reexperiencing symptoms as a reaction to greater emotional numbing and avoidance symptoms. Over time, mastery of trauma-related fears may occur with the reestablishment of non-trauma-dependant schema. However, symptom chronicity is well described. Persistent symptoms of PTSD have been reported by children and adolescents 6 months after shipping disasters, the 2004 Indian Ocean Tsunami and wildfires, 1 year after a sniper attack on a school, 18 months after an earthquake disaster, and 2 years after bushfires. Medium-term outcome studies, defined as 1–5 years postdisaster have demonstrated symptom chronicity. Few long-term outcome studies have been undertaken. Green and colleagues conducted a 17-year follow-up of survivors of the Buffalo Creek mudslide disaster. Generalizing from the Buffalo Creek findings is difficult given the original research included data obtained retrospectively from court reports prepared for victims. Original estimates of PTSD were 32% of children experienced "probable" PTSD. At 17-year follow-up, the PTSD rate had decreased to 7%. More remaining PTSD sufferers were women. The only symptoms that increased over time were substance abuse and suicidality. Clinicians should be alert for anniversary reactions, which may increase over time and often their occurrence is not immediately attributed to the traumatic event (Terr, 1994). Anniversary symptoms may include any symptom in the PTSD spectrum as well as altered beliefs such as the view that their lives would not be full, long, and their career or marriage successful.

American Academy of Child and Adolescent Psychiatry: Practice parameters for the assessment and treatment of children and adolescents with posttraumatic stress disorder. *J Am Acad Child Adolesc Psychiatry* 1998;37(10 Suppl):4S–26S.

Green BL, Grace MC, Vary MG, et al. Children of disaster in the second decade: a 17-year follow-up of Buffalo Greek survivors. J AM Acad Child Adolesc Psychiatry 1994;33(1):71–79.

Korol MS, Kramer TL, Grace MC, Green BL: Dam break: Long-term follow-up of children exposed to the buffalo creek disaster. In: LaGreca A, Silverman WK, Vernberg EM, Roberts MC (eds). *Helping Children Cope with Disasters: Integrating Research and Practice*. Washington, DC: American Psychological Association, 2002.

Tourette Disorder and Obsessive–Compulsive Disorder in Children and Adolescents

44

Michael H. Bloch, MD, & James F. Leckman, MD

◼ TOURETTE SYNDROME AND TIC DISORDERS

 ESSENTIALS OF DIAGNOSIS

DSM-IV-TR Diagnostic Criteria

Tourette's Disorder

A. Both multiple motor and one or more vocal tics have been present at some time during the illness, although not necessarily concurrently. (A tic is a sudden, rapid, recurrent, nonrhythmic, stereotyped motor movement or vocalization.)

B. The tics occur many times a day (usually in bouts) nearly every day or intermittently throughout a period of more than 1 year, and during this period there was never a tic-free period of more than 3 consecutive months.

C. The onset is before age 18 years.

D. The disturbance is not due to the direct physiological effects of a substance (e.g., stimulants) or a general medical condition (e.g., Huntington's disease or postviral encephalitis).

Chronic Motor or Vocal Tic Disorder

A. Single or multiple motor or vocal tics (i.e., sudden, rapid, recurrent, nonrhythmic, stereotyped motor movements or vocalizations), but not both, have been present at some time during the illness.

B. The tics occur many times a day nearly every day or intermittently throughout a period of more than 1 year, and during this period there was never a tic-free period of more than 3 consecutive months.

C. The onset is before age 18 years.

D. The disturbance is not due to the direct physiological effects of a substance (e.g., stimulants) or a general medical condition (e.g., Huntington's disease or postviral encephalitis).

E. Criteria have never been met for Tourettes Disorder.

Transient Tic Disorder

A. Single or multiple motor and/or vocal tics (i.e., sudden, rapid, recurrent, nonrhythmic, stereotyped motor movements or vocalizations)

B. The tics occur many times a day, nearly every day for at least 4 weeks, but for no longer than 12 consecutive months.

C. The onset is before age 18 years.

D. The disturbance is not due to the direct physiological effects of a substance (e.g., stimulants) or a general medical condition (e.g., Huntington's disease or postviral encephalitis).

E. Criteria have never been met for Tourettes Disorder or Chronic Motor or Vocal Tic Disorder.

Tic Disorder Not Otherwise Specified

This category is for disorders characterized by tics that do not meet criteria for a specific Tic Disorder. Examples include tics lasting less than 4 weeks or tics with an onset after age 18 years.

(Adapted with permission from *Diagnostic and Statistical Manual of Mental Disorders*, 4th edn. Text Revision. Copyright 2000 American Psychiatric Association.)

General Considerations

A. EPIDEMIOLOGY

Transient tic behaviors are commonplace among school-age children. Estimates range between 4% and 24%

of school-age children experiencing tics. The number of children experiencing chronic motor tic disorders is roughly one-quarter this number. Once thought to be much rarer, the current lifetime prevalence estimates for TS ranges from 0.1% to 1%.

The prevalence of tic disorders peaks during the late first and early second decades of life due to the clinical course of the disorder. They are roughly one-third as prevalent in adulthood. Boys are about twice as likely to be affected by tic disorders as girls.

B. Etiology

The current understanding of Tourette syndrome (TS) provides a good working model for understanding the pathogenesis of other childhood neuropsychiatric disorders: a genetically determined vulnerability, age-dependent expression of symptoms reflecting maturational factors, sexual dimorphism, stress-dependent fluctuations in symptom severity, and environmental influences on the phenotypical expression of the tic.

Strong evidence implicates the basal ganglia and corticostriatal – thalamocortical (CSTC) abnormalities as central to the pathogenesis of tics. Indirect evidence for the involvement of the basal ganglia in the pathogenesis of TS comes from the association with basal ganglia pathology of other movement disorders such as Sydenham's chorea, Huntington's disease, hemiballismus and Parkinson's disease. Direct evidence supporting CSTC abnormalities in TS comes from neuroimaging, neuropathological and neurosurgical studies.

CSTC loops are multiple, parallel, but partially overlapping, neuroanatomical circuits, relaying information from most regions of the cortex to subcortical areas, particularly the striatum and thalamus, which in turn project to a subset of the original cortical areas. In CSTC loops, the basal ganglia can be viewed as a way station between intention and action (thought, affect and movement). Tics, repetitive and stereotyped movements are believed to arise from imbalances in focal populations in the basal ganglia circuits. A tic may arise through failure of inhibition of a discrete population of striatal projection neurons which become abnormally active and cause an unwanted disinhibition of a corresponding group of thalamocortical projection neurons. Thus a cortical motor pattern generator is activated so that unintended urges and motor and vocal tics are triggered.

Altered dopaminergic functioning has also been strongly implicated in the pathogenesis of TS. Evidence for abnormal dopamine neurotransmission in TS is inferred from two clinical observations. First, blockade of dopamine receptors by neuroleptic drugs suppresses tics in a majority of patients. In addition, dopamine-releasing drugs such as cocaine and amphetamines have been reported to precipitate or exacerbate tics. It has been shown that TS patients release more dopamine at dopaminer-

gic synapses in response to amphetamine. Second, the importance of dopamine in TS is supported by brain imaging using dopamine ligands in single photon emission computed tomography and positron emission tomography. In one twin study, tic severity was related to dopamine D2 receptor binding in the head of the caudate nucleus.

C. Genetics

Although the particular genetic factors responsible for TS remain largely undiscovered, there is a sizable heritable component responsible for this illness. Early twin studies have suggested that the concordance rate for TS among monozygotic twin pairs is greater than 50% while the concordance of dizygotic twin pairs is about 10%. If twins with chronic motor tic disorder are included, concordance figures increase to 77% for monozygotic and 30% for dizygotic twin pairs. Differences in the concordance of monozygotic and dizygotic twin pairs indicate that genetic factors play an important role in the etiology of TS and related conditions. These figures also suggest that nongenetic factors are critical in determining the nature and severity of the clinical syndrome.

The overall risk that an offspring of a parent with TS will develop TS is approximately 10–15%, while the risk of offspring developing a tic disorder (20–29%) or obsessive–compulsive disorder (OCD) (12–32%) is slightly higher. The risk of developing tic disorders in male offspring is higher than for females, while the risk of developing OCD is lower.

Recently, an analysis of a chromosomal anomaly in one TS patient led to the identification of two sequence variants in the *SLITRK1* gene in approximately 1% of TS cases. Specifically, among 174 unrelated probands with TS, one frameshift mutation and two identical variants in the 3' untranscribed region of this gene were identified. None of these anomalies was demonstrated in over 3,600 controls. *SLITRK1* mRNA is expressed in the human fetal brain at 20 weeks gestation in multiple neuroanatomical areas implicated in TS neuropathology including the cortical plate, striatum, globus pallidus, thalamus and subthalamic nucleus. While other genes of major effect are likely to be found, it is becoming ever clear that TS is likely to be a polygenetic disorder with complex gene–environment interactions that have yet to be fully elucidated.

D. Environmental Factors

The existence of monozygotic twins discordant for tic severity emphasizes the importance of environmental factors in the phenotypic expression of TS. In monozygotic twins discordant for tic severity, the twin with more severe tics has usually had the lower birth weight and has a greater number of dopamine receptor sites in the caudate nucleus. In observational and case control studies, low

(**A**ctivity, **P**ulse, **G**rimace, **A**ppearance, and **R**espiration); APGAR scores; stressful maternal life circumstances during pregnancy and maternal first-trimester nausea are risk factors for TS.

Tic disorders have long been identified as "stress-sensitive" conditions. Typically, symptom exacerbations follow in the wake of stressful life events. These events need not be adverse in character. Clinical experience suggests that in some unfortunate instances a vicious cycle can be initiated in which tic symptoms are misunderstood by the family and teachers, leading to active attempts to suppress the symptoms by punishment and humiliation. These efforts can lead to a further exacerbation of symptoms and an increase in stress in the child's interpersonal environment. Prospective longitudinal studies have begun to examine systematically the effect of intramorbid stress. These studies indicate that patients with TS experience more stress than matched healthy controls and that antecedent stress may play a role in subsequent tic exacerbations.

Post-infectious autoimmune mechanisms have been implicated in a small number of post-streptococcal cases of TS and OCD known as Pediatric Autoimmune Neuropsychiatric Disorder Associated with Streptococcal (PANDAS) infections. PANDAS cases are characterized by a sudden onset of symptoms, episodic course, and abrupt symptom exacerbations, sometimes accompanied by adventitious movements. The most salient differentiating factor between PANDAS and other cases of TS and OCD is an exacerbation of OCD and tic symptoms accompanied by positive streptococcal throat cultures, increased antistreptoccal and antineuronal antibodies, but no evidence of rheumatic fever. Evidence that PANDAS and post-streptococcal autoimmune factors are associated with some cases of tics and OCD comes from a variety of sources. Sydenham's chorea, a late autoimmune sequela of rheumatic fever, is often accompanied by tics, mood changes, OCD, attention-deficit hyperactivity disorder (ADHD) and anxiety. There is a large series of over 50 children in whom exacerbations of OCD or tics were accompanied by positive streptococcal throat cultures and increased antistreptoccal and antineuronal antibodies without evidence of rheumatic fever. One case-control study found an increased proportion of group A β-hemolytic streptococcal (GABHS) infections (odds ratio = 3.05) within the preceding 3 months in children *newly-diagnosed* with TS compared to well-matched controls. This suggests a role for post-streptococcal autoimmune factors in a large proportion of cases. A larger odds ratio (12.1) was demonstrated when subjects had multiple GABHS infections in the previous year, suggesting a dose-dependent effect of exposure to infection. However, prospective longitudinal studies have failed to provide evidence that newly acquired GABHS infections precede tic exacerbations. The relative prevalence of PANDAS cases and the importance of autoimmune mechanisms to TS are controversial.

Abelson JF, Kwan KY, O'Roak BJ, et al.: Sequence variants in SLITRK1 are associated with TS. *Science* 2005;310:317–320.

Findley DB, Leckman JF, Katsovich L et al.: Development of the yale children's global stress index and its application in children and adolescents with tourette's syndrome and obsessive–compulsive disorder. *J Am Acad Child Adolesc Psychiatry* 2003;42(4):450–457.

Hyde TM, Aaronson BA, Randolph C, et al.: Relationship of birth weight to the phenotypic expression of gilles de la TS in monozygotic twins. *Neurology* 1992;42:652–658.

Kalanithi PS, Zheng W, Kataoka Y et al.: Altered parvalbumin-positive neuron distribution in basal ganglia of individuals with tourette syndrome. *Proc Natl Acad Sci USA* 2005;102(37):13307–13312.

Khalifa N, von Knorring AL: Tourette syndrome and other tic disorders in a total population of children: Clinical assessment and background. *Acta Paediatr* 2005;94:1608–1614.

Leckman JF, Vaccarino FM, Kalanithi PS, Rothenberger A: Tourette syndrome: A relentless drumbeat – driven by misguided brain oscillations. *J Child Psychol Psychiatry* 2006;47(6):537–550.

Luo F, Leckman JF, Katsovich L, et al.: Prospective longitudinal study of children with tic disorders and/or obsessive–compulsive disorder: Relationship of symptom exacerbations to newly acquired streptococcal infections. *Pediatrics* 2004;113:578–585.

Mell LK, Davis RL, Owens D: Association between streptococcal infection and obsessive–compulsive disorder, TS and Tic disorder. *Pediatrics* 2005;116:56–60.

McMahon WM, Carter AS, Fredine N, Pauls DL: Children at familial risk for tourette's disorder: Child and parent diagnoses. *Am J Med Genet* 2003;121:105–111.

Peterson BS, Thomas P, Kane MJ, et al.: Ganglia volumes in patients with gilles de la tourette syndrome. *Arch Gen Psychiatry* 2003;60(4):415–424.

Scahill L, Sukhodolsky DG, Williams SK, Leckman JF: Public health significance of tic disorders in children and adolescents. *Adv Neurol* 2005;96:240–248.

Swedo SE, Leonard HL, Garvey M, et al.: Pediatric autoimmune neuropsychiatric disorders associated with streptococcal infections: Clinical description of the first 50 cases. *Am J Psychiatry* 1998;155:264–271.

Clinical Findings

A. SIGNS & SYMPTOMS

Tics are sudden, repetitive movements, gestures, or utterances that typically mimic an aspect of normal behavior. Individual tics rarely last more than a second. Many tics occur in bouts with brief inter-tic intervals of less than one second. Individual tics can occur singly or together in an orchestrated pattern. They vary in intensity or forcefulness. Motor tics, which can be viewed as disinhibited fragments of normal movement, can vary from simple, abrupt movements such as eye blinking, nose twitching, head or arm jerking, or shoulder shrugging to more complex movements that appear to have a purpose, such as facial or hand gestures or sustained looks. These two phenotypic extremes of motor tics are classified as simple and complex motor tics respectively. Similarly, phonic tics can be classified into simple and complex. Simple vocal tics are sudden, meaningless sounds such as throat clearing, coughing, sniffing, spitting, or grunting. Complex phonic tics are more protracted, meaningful utterances, which vary from prolonged throat clearing to syllables, words or phrases and to even more complex behaviors such as repeating ones own words (palalalia) or those of others (echolalia) and, in rare cases, the use of obscenities (coprolalia).

The severity of tics in TS waxes and wanes throughout the course of the disorder. The tics of TS and other tic disorders are highly variable from minute-to-minute, hour-to-hour, day-to-day, week-to-week, month-to-month, and even year-to-year. Tic episodes occur in bouts, which in turn also tend to cluster. Tic symptoms, however, can be exacerbated by stress, fatigue, extremes of temperature and external stimuli (e.g., in echolalia). Intentional movement attenuates tics in the affected area and intense involvement in activities tends to dissipate tic symptoms.

Many individuals with tics, especially those postpubertal, are aware of premonitory urges: feelings of tightness, tension, or itching that are accompanied by a mounting sense of discomfort or anxiety relieved only by the performance of a tic. Premonitory urges are similar to the sensation preceding a sneeze or an itch. Premonitory urges cause many TS patients to suffer from an endless cycle of rising tension and tic performance because the relief provided by tic performance is ephemeral. Thus, soon after tic performance the tension of the premonitory urge again rises to a crescendo. A majority of patients also report a fleeting sense of relief after a bout of tics has occurred. Most are able to suppress their tics for short intervals of time.

With increasing awareness of premonitory urges, TS patients begin to exhibit a variable degree of voluntary control over tic performance. 92% of TS subjects in one study reported that the tics they exhibited were either partially or totally voluntary. However, this voluntary control should be likened to that governing eye blinking. Eye blinking and tics can both be inhibited voluntarily, but only for a limited period of time and only with mounting discomfort. Thus, some adult TS patients are able to demonstrate nearly complete control over when their tics will occur. However, when complete or near complete control of tics is present, resistance to the mounting tension of premonitory urges can produce mental and physical exhaustion even more distracting than the tics themselves.

The tics, which are the most prominent feature of TS, may be neither the first nor the most impairing psychological disturbance TS patients endure. Children with TS have higher rates of OCD, ADHD, and disinhibited speech and behavior compared to the general population. In one study, 65% of TS patients in late adolescence regarded their behavioral problems (including ADHD and OCD) and learning difficulties to have had an equal or greater impact on their life function than the tics themselves did. In the natural course of comorbid psychiatric illness in TS, ADHD symptom, typically precede the onset of tic symptoms by a couple of years, whereas OCD symptoms typically present around the age of 12–13 after tics have reached their peak severity. Approximately 50% of children with TS experience comorbid ADHD, and an even greater proportion of children with comorbid disorders reach clinical attention. Roughly one-third to one-half of TS patients will experience clinically significant OCD symptoms during the course of their lifetime. Figure 44–1 depicts the clinical course of comorbid ADHD and OCD symptoms in children with tic disorders.

B. Instruments for Diagnosis and Measurement

Direct observational methods (e.g., videotaped tic-counting) are the most objective measures of tic severity. However, the frequency of tics varies dramatically according to setting and activity. In addition, many individuals with TS can suppress their symptoms for brief

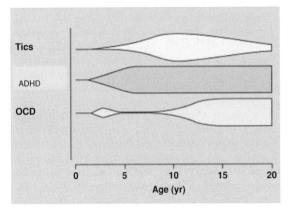

Figure 44–1. Clinical course of ADHD, OCD, and Tic Disorders. Age at which tics and coexisting disorders affect patients with TS. Width of bars shows schematically the amount the disorder affects a patient at a particular age. (Adapted from Leckman 2002.)

periods of time. Thus, clinical rating scales are the preferred method for assessing initial tic severity and measuring change in tic severity. The Yale Global Tic Severity Scale is a clinician-rated, semi-structured scale that begins with a systematic inventory of tic symptoms rated as present or absent over the past week. Current motor and phonic tics are then rated separately according to number, frequency, intensity, complexity, and interference, in accordance with 6-point ordinal scales (0 = absent; 1 through 5 for severity). Three scores are yielded: Total Motor, Total Phonic and Total Tic. Self-report inventories such as the Yale Child Study Center TS Obsessive–Compulsive Disorder Symptom Questionnaire can be completed by the family prior to their initial consultation. They are valuable ancillary tools in order to gain a long – term perspective of the child's developmental course and the natural history of the tic disorder. The Yale Global Tic Severity Scale and Yale Child Study Center TS Obsessive–Compulsive Disorder Symptom Questionnaire are freely available.

C. Laboratory Findings and Imaging

At present, no laboratory testing or neuroimaging is useful in diagnosing or treating tic disorders. However, strong evidence from neuroimaging, neuropathological and neurochemical studies implicates abnormalities in the basal ganglia and CSTC circuits in the pathogenesis of TS. On volumetric MRI, individuals with TS have smaller caudate volume than healthy controls. Reduced caudate volume in children with TS has been associated with increased tic and OCD severity in adulthood. Functional neuroimaging has revealed increased activation of the frontal cortex and caudate during willful tic suppression. This increased activation of frontal cortex and caudate is in turn correlated with decreased activity of the globus pallidus, putamen, and thalamus. Positron emission tomography studies in TS have demonstrated increased striatal dopamine receptor and transporter densities and increased amphetamine induced dopamine release in the putamen.

Bloch MH, Leckman JF, Zhu H, et al.: Caudate volumes in childhood predict symptom severity in adults with TS. *Neurology* 2005;65:1253–1258.

Bloch MH, Peterson BS, Scahill L et al.: Adulthood outcome of tic and obsessive-compulsive symptom severity in children with TS. *Arch Pediatr Adolesc Med* 2006;160:65–69.

Cheon KA, Ryu YH, Namkoong K, et al.: Dopamine transporter density of the basal ganglia assessed with [123I] IPT SPECT in drug-naive children with tourette's disorder. *Psychiatry Res* 2004;130:85–95.

Leckman JF, Riddle MA, Hardin MT, et al.: The yale global tic severity scale: Initial testing of a clinician-rated scale of tic severity. *J Am Acad Child Adolesc Psychiatry* 1989;28:566–573.

Leckman JF, Walker DE, Cohen DJ: Premonitory urges in TS. *Am J Psychiatry* 1993;150:98–102.

Leckman JF, Zhang H, Vitale A, et al.: Course of tic severity in TS: The first two decades. *Pediatrics* 1998;102:14–19.

Peterson BS, Skudlarski P, Anderson AW, et al.: A functional magnetic resonance imaging study of tic suppression in TS. *Arch Gen Psychiatry* 1998;55:326–333.

Peterson BS, Thomas P, Kane MJ, et al.: Ganglia volumes in patients with gilles de la tourette syndrome. *Arch Gen Psychiatry* 2003;60(4):415–424.

Singer HS, Szymanski S, Giuliano J, et al.: Elevated intrasynaptic dopamine release in tourette's syndrome measured by PET. *Am J Psychiatry* 2002;159:1329–1336.

Sukhodolsky DG, Scahill L, Zhang H et al.: Disruptive behavior in children with tourette's syndrome: Association with ADHD comorbidity, tic severity, and functional impairment. *J Am Acad Child Adolesc Psychiatry* 2003;42(1):98–105.

Differential Diagnosis

Tic disorders must be distinguished from movement disorders caused by general medical conditions (e.g., Huntington's disease, stroke, Lesch-Nyhan syndrome, Wilson's disease, Sydenham's chorea, multiple sclerosis, postviral encephalitis, head injury) or the direct effects of a drug (e.g. akathisia and tardive dyskinesia associated with neuroleptic medication). Table 44–1 defines the major types of movements that commonly need to be distinguished from tics. Medical and family history, movement morphology, rhythm, and modifying influences are usually sufficient for making the diagnosis. Onset of movements prior to age 18, a waxing-and-waning course of symptoms and the changing of the specific tic movements over time are characteristic of TS.

In children, tics need to be distinguished from the stereotypies of stereotyped movement disorders or pervasive developmental disorder. Stereotypies typically have an earlier age of onset than tics, are bilateral rather than unilateral, and have a soothing quality. Table 44–2 contrasts tics and stereotypies. Complex tics need to be distinguished from the compulsions of OCD. Making this particularly difficult is the high comorbidity between the two conditions. Compulsions are usually performed in response to an obsession and preceded by anxiety, worry, or concern, whereas tics are generally performed in response to a physical sensation or urges. Compulsions typically are more elaborate than tics and are more likely to resemble "normal" behavior. Often a diagnosis of both OCD and tic disorder are warranted in the same individual.

Treatment

Given the usual waxing and waning course of tic disorders, it is probable that any intervention performed in response to symptom exacerbation will lead to clinical improvement. It is usually thus most prudent to treat overall, long-term symptom severity rather than chasing individual ebbs and flows in the natural course of

Table 44–1. Differential Diagnosis of Tic Disorders

Movement	Description	Common Causes
Tics	Abrupt, stereotyped coordinated movements or vocalizations that often mimic aspects of regular behavior. Premonitory urges are common. Exacerbated by stress and relieved by distraction.	TS, Chronic Tic Disorder, Transient Tic Disorder
Stereotypies	Repetitive, purposeless, and apparently voluntary movements	Autism, Pervasive Developmental Disorder, Mental Retardation, Stereotyped Movement Disorder
Chorea	Simple, random, irregular, and nonstereotyped movements. Have no premonitory component and increase when the person is distracted. Often flows from one body part to another.	Normal in children less than 8 months of age. Cerebral Palsy, Sydenham's Chorea, Hereditary choreas, kernicteris, Lesch-Nyhan syndrome, hypoxia or stroke.
Dyskinesia	Slow, protracted twisting movements interspersed with prolonged states of muscular tension	Drug-induced, idiopathic torsion dystonia, anoxia or stroke, Wilson's disease, Huntington's Disease and Parkinson's Disease
Athetoid	Slow, irregular, writhing movements. Usually involving fingers and toes but occasionally the neck. A "slow chorea."	See chorea
Myoclonia	Brief, simple, shock-like muscle contractions that may affect individualized muscles of muscle groups.	Physiologic—hiccups, anxiety or exercise induced. Juvenile Myoclonic Epilepsy, metabolic encephalopathies, CJD, Wilson's disease and hypoxia
Synkinesis	Involuntary movement associated with a specific voluntary act, i.e., raising corner of mouth when closing one's eyes	Physiologic

the illness. Interventions should be started with the goal of reducing tics (and the side effects of treatment) to a level that minimizes social and educational impairment rather than to eliminate the tics completely (which will be unsuccessful in the majority of cases). Many cases of TS can be successfully managed without medication. When patients present with coexisting ADHD, OCD, depression, or bipolar illness it is usually better to treat these

Table 44–2. Comparison Between Tics and Stereotypies

Contrasting Features	Tics	Stereotypies
Typical age of onset	4–8 years	2–3 years
Course of symptoms	Waxing and Waning	Constant
Timing of movements	Brief and sudden	Continuous, rhythmic and prolonged
Typical movements	Eye blinking, facial grimace, throat clearing	Arm flapping, rocking
Characteristics of movements	Typically unilateral	Often bilateral
Exacerbated by	Stress, fatigue	Excitement
Premonitory urges	Present	Absent
Suppressibility	Often for short periods of time	Rare
Comorbid conditions	OCD, ADHD	PDD, Autism Spectrum Disorders
Treatment	Neuroleptic, α_2 Agonists	No response to medication

"comorbid" conditions first, as their successful treatment will often diminish tic severity.

Usual clinical practice focuses initially on educational and supportive intervention. Pharmacological treatments are typically held in reserve. The decision to employ psychoactive medication is usually made if the educational and supportive interventions have been in place for a period of months and it is clear that the tic symptoms are persistently severe and a source of impairment in terms of self-esteem, relationships with family or peers, or the child's school performance.

A. PSYCHOEDUCATIONAL INTERVENTIONS

Educating the patient, his family members, teachers, and peers is among the most important interventions available. It should be undertaken for nearly all patients with tic disorders. Family psychoeducation should focus on the following:

1. Tics are not voluntary or provocative. They typically occur in "bouts" during which tics appear in rapid succession followed by tic-free intervals.

2. Physical sensations like an itch or before a sneeze are experienced by many patients prior to tics. TS is a sensorimotor disorder. A momentary sense of relief follows the tic.

3. Many patients are able to suppress tics over the short term but often at the expense of increasing discomfort and distraction due to the premonitory urges. It is not uncommon for a child to have relatively minor tics at school and then to let loose a bout of tics after coming home.

4. Tics increase and decrease in severity over time. Due to the natural ebb and flow of symptoms, any interventions started during an exacerbation of tic severity may appear successful, because of a natural decline in symptom severity.

5. Symptoms usually improve by adulthood. This information contradicts impressions gained from the lay literature that typically focuses on the most extreme cases.

6. Tics tend to be exacerbated by fatigue, sleeplessness, stress, excitement, changes in temperature, and streptococcal infection. Tics often tend to be alleviated when a child is deeply engaged in a motor activity such as sports, playing musical instruments, or dancing. The exact exacerbating and alleviating factors are highly individualized. Good sleep and regular exercise improve tics.

7. Comorbid ADHD, OCD, learning disabilities, and disruptive or disinhibited behaviors may occur. Improving these disorders often leads to an improvement in the tics.

Resources to help educate parents about tic disorders are available at the Tourette Syndrome Association website: www.tsa-usa.org

Perhaps equally important is educating the school. By educating the educators, clinicians can promote a positive and supportive environment in the classroom. If possible, teachers should respond to outbursts of tics with grace and understanding. Repeated scolding is counterproductive. The child may develop opposition to authority figures and be reluctant to attend school. Moreover, classmates may feel free to tease the child. A useful compendium of educational accommodations is available at http://www.tourettesyndrome.net/TouretteSyndrome_Plus/

Educating peers may be equally important. Many clinicians actively encourage patients, families, and teachers to educate peers and classmates about TS. It is remarkable what can be tolerated in the classroom and on the playground when teachers and peers simply know what the problem is and learn to disregard it.

B. PSYCHOPHARMACOLOGIC INTERVENTION

Table 44–3 depicts the attributes of medications regularly used to treat tic disorder. Dopamine D_2 receptor antagonists are the most predictably effective tic-suppressing agents over the short-term. Among the typical neuroleptics, haloperidol and pimozide have the most favorable data demonstrating efficacy. Long-term experience has been less favorable, and the "reflexive" use of these agents should be avoided. Common potential side effects are tardive dyskinesia, acute dystonia, sedation, depression, school and social phobia, and/or weight gain. In many instances, by starting at low dose and adjusting the dosage upwards slowly, clinicians can avoid these side effects. The goal should be to use as little medication as possible to render the tics "tolerable." Attempts to stop the tics completely often risk over-medication.

Due to the extrapyramidal side effects associated with typical neuroleptics, atypical neuroleptics, such as risperidone, olanzapine and ziprasidone are now the most widely used medications to treat tic symptoms. These agents have potent $5\text{-}HT_2$ blocking effects as well as more modest blocking effects on dopamine D_2. Double-blind clinical trials have supported the efficacy of risperidone, olanzapine, and ziprasidone. Risperidone and olanzapine are often associated with weight gain and sedation. Ziprasidone use can be associated with QT prolongation in children, so serial monitoring with electrocardiograms may be necessary.

Clonidine and guanfacine are potent α_2-receptor agonists that are thought to reduce central noradrenergic activity. Although less effective in relieving tics compared to the neuroleptic medication, α_2-receptor agonists have the advantage of also improving comorbid

Table 44–3. Pharmacological Agents Used to Treat Tic Disorders

Medication	Starting Dose	Titration Schedule	Typical Dosage	Advantages	Side Effects
NEUROLEPTICS					
TYPICAL Haloperidol	0.25 mg/day	0.5 mg every 1–2 weeks	0.5–6.0 mg/day	Most effective medication for tics with longest record of use	Tardive dyskinesia, acute dystonic reactions, akathisia, sedation, depression, school and social phobias, and/or weight gain
Pimozide	1.0 mg/day	1.0 mg every 1–2 weeks	1–10 mg/day		
ATYPICAL Risperidone	0.25–0.5 mg/day	0.25–0.5 mg/week divided BID	1–6 mg/day	Most effective medications for tics, less side effects than typical neuroleptics, used to treat comorbid aggression and bipolar disorder	Weight gain, sedation, galactorrhea
Olanzapine	2.5–5 mg/day	2.5–5 mg every 1–2 weeks divided BID	5–20 mg/day		Weight gain, sedation, galactorrhea
Ziprasidone	5 mg/day	5mg every week with BID dosing	20–40 mg/day		Prolonged QT interval, rare heart arrhythmias
α_2-AGONISTS Guanfacine	0.5mg QHS	0.5 mg weekly to TID dosing	2–4 mg divided TID	Helps treat comorbid ADHD	Sedation
Clonidine	0.025–0.05 mcg QD or BID	0.05 mcg added on weekly to TID or QID dosing	0.05–0.25 mcg/kg TID or QID		Sedation, hypotension, rebound hypertension on withdrawal

ADHD symptoms in patients with tics. The principal side effect associated with clonidine is sedation, which occurs in 10–20% of subjects. It abates with continued use. Other side effects include dry mouth, transient hypotension, and rare episodes of worsening behavior. To reduce the likelihood of symptom or blood pressure rebound, clonidine should be tapered and not withdrawn abruptly. Guanfacine is generally preferred to clonidine because it is less sedating and not associated with rebound hypertension following withdrawal. In extreme cases, botulinum toxin injections temporarily weaken muscles associated with severe motor or vocal tics. The most common sites of injection are the neck (for motor tics) and shoulders and throat (for vocal tics).

When comorbid ADHD is the most impairing to a patient presenting with comorbid tics, the stimulants methylphenidate, d-amphetamine, and Adderall are still first line agents for the medical management of ADHD. While most patients with both ADHD and a preexisting tic disorder do well on stimulants, clinical case reports and controlled studies indicate that some children with ADHD may exhibit tics de novo or experience a worsening of tics when exposed to a stimulant. Based on a large multisite randomized, controlled clinical trial, the combination of clonidine and methylphenidate is efficacious. Nonstimulants used in ADHD include atomoxetine, tricyclic antidepressants (desipramine and nortriptyline), atypical antidepressants such as bupropion, clonidine, and guanfacine.

C. Psychotherapeutic Interventions

Habit reversal training (HRT) is the first psychotherapeutic intervention that has shown promise in reducing tic severity in patients with TS. HRT significantly reduces tic symptoms in adults with TS when compared to supportive therapy in randomized, unblinded, waitlist controlled clinical trials. HRT has shown promise in uncontrolled trials among children with TS.

HRT consists of two main components: (1) awareness training and (2) competing response practice. Awareness training consists of 4 components designed to increase an individual's awareness of his own tics. These components include (1) response description—in which the patient learns how to describe tic movements and reenacts them into a mirror; (2) response detection—in which the therapist aids the patient in tic detection by pointing out each tic immediately after it occurs in the session; (3) early warning procedure—in which an individual learns how to identify the earliest signs of tic occurrence; and (4) situational awareness training—in which an analysis is conducted to identify the high-risk situations when tics are most likely to occur. Competing response practice involves teaching individuals to produce an incompatible physical response (i.e., isometric contraction of tic-opposing muscles) upon the urge to perform a tic.

D. Neurosurgical Interventions

Neurosurgical interventions for TS are reserved for adults with intractable tics that severely affect social functioning. Originally, neurosurgical lesioning procedures were attempted to treat the most severe cases of TS. Deep brain stimulation, a relatively reversible, stereotactic technique, used to treat other movement disorders, has become the preferred method of neurosurgical treatment for medically intractable tics. Deep brain stimulation has several advantages over previous neurosurgical lesioning procedures in that it lacks many of the permanent complications typically associated with lesioning procedures (the electrodes can be removed), lends access to many surgically inaccessible sites, and allows for bilateral stimulation. It holds great promise for adult patients with intractable tics. However, in using Deep brain stimulation for tics, neither the appropriate site of electrode placement nor the electrode stimulation parameters have been established in carefully controlled clinical studies. The preferred sites of electrode placement are either the midline thalamic nuclei or the globus pallidus, pars internus (GPi). Case reports indicate a 50–80% improvement in tic frequency following the procedure. Every possible medical option to treat tics beforehand should be exhausted.

Bruggeman R, van der Linden C, Buitelaar JK, et al.: Risperidone versus pimozide in tourette's disorder: A comparative double-blind parallel-group study. *J Clin Psychiatry* 2001;62:50–56.

Mink JW: Patient selection and assessment guidelines for deep brain stimulation in tourette syndrome. *Mov Disord* in press.

Scahill L, Chappell PB, Kim YS, et al.: A placebo-controlled study of guanfacine in the treatment of children with tic disorders and attention deficit hyperactivity disorder. *Am J Psychiatry* 2001;158:1067–1074.

Shapiro ES, Shapiro AK, Fulop G, et al.: Controlled study of haloperidol, pimozide, and placebo for the treatment of gilles de la TS. *Arch Gen Psychiatry* 1989;46:722–730.

Tourette's Syndrome Study Group: Short-term versus longer-term pimozide therapy in TS: A preliminary study. *Neurology* 1999;52:874–877.

Tourette's Syndrome Study Group: Treatment of ADHD in children with tics: A randomized controlled trial. *Neurology* 2002;58(4):527–536.

Wilhelm S, Deckersbach T, Coffey BJ, et al.: Habit reversal versus supportive psychotherapy for tourette's disorder: A randomized controlled trial. *Am J Psychiatry*, 2003;160:1175–1177.

Woods DW: Habit reversal treatment manual for tic disorders. In: Woods DW, Miltenberger RG (eds). *Tic Disorders, Trichotillomania, and Other Repetitive Behavior Disorders: Behavioral Approaches to Analysis and Treatment.* Boston: Kluwer Academic Publishers, 2001, pp. 97–132.

Prognosis

The onset of TS is usually characterized by simple, transient motor tics that affect the face (typically eye blinking) around 5–7 years of age. Over time, simple motor tics generally progress in a rostrocaudal direction affecting other areas of the face, followed by the head, neck, arms, and lastly and less frequently, the lower extremities. With time, vocal tics often appear, tics become increasingly complex, and premonitory urges are experienced. TS symptoms generally peak in severity between the ages of ten and twelve. Tic severity, however, typically dissipates with the onset of adolescence. The reduction in TS severity generally ends by the early twenties. Although a small minority of TS patients experience catastrophic outcomes in adulthood, on the whole, individuals rarely experience either a sustained worsening or improvement of their symptoms after the third decade of life. One-half to two-thirds of individuals with TS experience a marked reduction of symptoms by late adolescence and early twenties, and one-third to one-half of these patients become virtually asymptomatic in adulthood. Figure 44–2 diagrams the general course of tic severity of TS patients through the first two decades of their illness.

Given that tics in children are often ephemeral, producing substantial social and educational impairment when the tics are at their worst but little afterwards, the importance of minimizing social consequences (peer teasing, poor self-esteem, and social withdrawal) and educational impairment can not be overstated in determining long-term outcome. The proper management of,

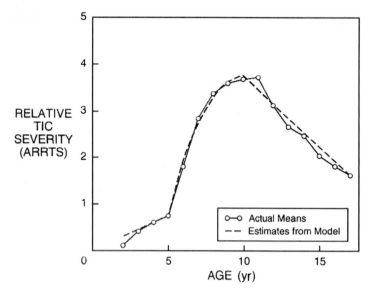

Figure 44–2. The Course of Tic Severity during the first two decades of life. The solid line connecting the small circles plots the means of the annual rating of relative tic severity scores (ARRTS) recorded by the parents. The dashed line represents a mathematical model designed to best fit the clinical data. Two inflection points are evident that correspond to the age of tic onset and the age at worst-ever tic severity, respectively. (Adapted with permission from Leckman JF, Zhang H, Vitale A, et al.: Course of tic severity in TS: The first two decades. *Pediatrics* 1998;102:14–19).

and vigilance for, psychiatric conditions highly comorbid with tic disorder, such as ADHD and OCD (that currently are more effectively treated) are also crucial. Ensuring that patients with a history of tic disorders refrain from using substances known to induce tics such as amphetamines or crack/cocaine is also likely to improve their prognosis.

■ CHILDHOOD-ONSET OCD

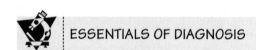 ESSENTIALS OF DIAGNOSIS

DSM-IV-TR Diagnostic Criteria
Obsessive–Compulsive Disorder

A. Either obsessions or compulsions:
Obsessions as defined by (1), (2), (3), and (4):

(1) recurrent and persistent thoughts, impulses, or images that are experienced, at some time during the disturbance, as intrusive and inappropriate and that cause marked anxiety or distress

(2) the thoughts, impulses, or images are not simply excessive worries about real-life problems

(3) the person attempts to ignore or suppress such thoughts, impulses, or images, or to neutralize them with some other thought or action

(4) the person recognizes that the obsessional thoughts, impulses, or images are a product of his or her own mind (not imposed from without as in thought insertion)

Compulsions as defined by (1) and (2):

(1) repetitive behaviors (e.g., hand washing, ordering, checking) or mental acts (e.g., praying, counting, repeating words silently) that the person feels driven to perform in response to an obsession, or according to rules that must be applied rigidly

(2) the behaviors or mental acts are aimed at preventing or reducing distress or preventing some dreaded event or situation; however, these behaviors or mental acts either are not connected in a realistic way with what they are designed to neutralize or prevent or are clearly excessive

B. At some point during the course of the disorder, the person has recognized that the obsessions or compulsions are excessive or unreasonable.

C. The obsessions or compulsions cause marked distress, are time consuming (take more than 1 hour a day), and significantly interfere with normal routine, occupational (or academic) functioning, or usual social activities or relationships.

D. If another Axis I disorder is present, the content of the obsessions or compulsions is not restricted to it (e.g., preoccupation with food in the presence of an Eating Disorder; hair pulling in the presence of Trichotillomania; concern with appearance in the *presence of Body Dysmorphic Disorder; preoccupation with drugs in the presence of a Substance Use Disorder; preoccupation with having a serious illness in the presence of Hypochondrias; preoccupation with sexual urges or fantasies in the presence of a Paraphilia; or guilty ruminations in the presence of Major Depressive Disorder).*

E. *The disturbance is not due to the direct physiological effects of a substance (e.g., a drug of abuse, a medication) or a general medical condition.*

(Reprinted, with permission, from *Diagnostic and Statistical Manual of Mental Disorders,* 4th edn., Text Revision. Copyright 2000 American Psychiatric Association.)

- *In the above-mentioned listing, item B does not apply to children.*
- *A child must have either obsessions or compulsions, but not necessarily both, to qualify for a diagnosis of OCD. Obsessions are persistent ideas, thoughts, impulses, or images, experienced as intrusive and inappropriate, that cause marked anxiety or distress. Compulsions are repetitive behaviors (e.g., hand washing, checking) or mental acts (e.g., counting, repeating words silently) the goal of which is to prevent or reduce anxiety or distress, not to provide pleasure or gratification. Obsessions or compulsions must be severe enough to cause significant distress or impairment or take up more than 1 hour a day. It is not uncommon for children, especially younger children, with OCD to have clinically significant compulsions without the insight or ability to describe obsessions. This condition is known as "OCD with poor insight."*

General Considerations

A. EPIDEMIOLOGY

Results from the Epidemiological Catchment Area study of over 18,500 adults using structured clinical interviews estimated the lifetime prevalence of OCD among adults as 1.9–3.3%. Epidemiological studies of adolescents provide similar estimates, in the range of 1.9–3.6%. The sex distribution of these epidemiologic studies suggests that OCD affects males and females equally after puberty. However, males typically have an earlier age of onset, their first presentation occurring well before puberty.

Flament MF, Whitaker A, Rapoport JL, et al.: Obsessive compulsive disorder in adolescence: An epidemiological study. *J Am Acad Child Adolesc Psychiatry* 1988;27(6):764–771.

Robins LN, Helzer JE, Croughan J, Ratcliff KS: National institute of mental health diagnostic interview schedule. Its history,

characteristics, and validity. *Arch Gen Psychiatry* 1981;38(4): 381–389.

Zohar AH, Ratzoni G, Pauls DL, et al.: An epidemiological study of obsessive–compulsive disorder and related disorders in Israeli adolescents. *J Am Acad Child Adolesc Psychiatry* 1992;31(6):1057–1061.

B. ETIOLOGY

Abnormalities in the serotonin system appear to be central to the pathogenesis of OCD. Evidence favoring the serotonin hypothesis for OCD comes from the fact that serotonin reuptake inhibitors (SSRIs) such as fluoxetine, fluvoxamine, sertraline, and paroxetine are the most effective medications for OCD. The relative effectiveness of clomipramine, a serotonin selective tricyclic antidepressant strengthens this hypothesis. Exacerbation of OCD symptoms with the administration of mCPP, a serotonin agonist lends further support. High platelet serotonin levels and high cerebrospinal fluid concentration of 5-hydroxyindoline acetic acid (a major metabolite of serotonin) are correlated with treatment response to clomipramine in children with OCD. Evidence for the presence of abnormalities in other neurotransmitter systems, specifically dopamine, is evidenced by the successful augmentation of SSRI pharmacotherapy by neuroleptic medication and the high comorbidity of childhood OCD with tic disorders.

Consistent with the serotonin hypothesis, basal ganglia–frontal lobe dysfunction has been implicated in the pathogenesis of OCD. Positron emission tomography with the glucose analog [^{18}F]fluorodeoxyglucose studies in children and adults with OCD demonstrate hypermetabolism in the caudate, orbitofrontal and anterior cingulate regions compared to normal controls during resting conditions and during periods of symptom provocation. These metabolic abnormalities were reversed with successful treatment, either behavioral or pharmacological. The high comorbidity of OCD with basal ganglia disorders such as TS and Sydenham's chorea supports this theory.

The association of obsessive-compulsive symptoms in Sydenham's chorea patients points to the importance of autoimmune processes in the pathogenesis of OCD. This observation led to the finding of a small subgroup of children with OCD or tic disorder who have pediatric autoimmune neuropsychiatric disorder associated with streptococcal infections (PANDAS). PANDAS cases have an abrupt, prepubertal onset of clinical symptoms (tic, OCD or both) after infection with GABHS. They experience symptom exacerbation with GABHS reinfection. PANDAS cases typically have a dramatic, episodic course and usually display coexisting choreiform movements if there are exacerbations. However, the prevalence of PANDAS remains controversial. PANDAS and OCD may be relatively infrequent. Nonetheless, the observation of OCD symptoms in Sydenham's chorea and the characterization of the PANDAS cohort of OCD and tic patients suggests the relevance of autoimmune and infectious factors to OCD pathogenesis.

Luo F, Leckman JF, Katsovich L, et al.: Prospective longitudinal study of children with tic disorders and/or obsessive–compulsive disorder: Relationship of symptom exacerbations to newly acquired streptococcal infections. *Pediatrics* 2004;113(6):e578–e585.

Saxena S, Rauch SL: Functional neuroimaging and the neuroanatomy of obsessive–compulsive disorder. *Psychiatr Clin North Am* 2000;23(3):563–586.

Swedo SE, Leonard HL, Mittleman BB, et al.: Identification of children with pediatric autoimmune neuropsychiatric disorders associated with streptococcal infections by a marker associated with rheumatic fever. *Am J Psychiatry* 1997;154(1):110–112.

C. GENETIC AND ENVIRONMENTAL FACTORS

OCD contains a hereditable component. The strongest evidence supporting its heritability comes from family studies and twins studies. Four family studies, each examining between 300 and 500 first-degree relatives of OCD patients, have estimated the rate of OCD to be 5–10-fold greater in first-degree relatives of OCD patients compared to the relatives of psychiatrically healthy controls. Twin studies in OCD have suggested an 87% concordance rate among monozygotic twins compared to 47% for dizygotic twins.

There is considerable evidence that TS and OCD share heritability, in other words that the same genes contribute to the phenotypic expression of both conditions. Relatives of OCD patients (without comorbid tics) have elevated rates of tic disorder compared to controls. Relatives of TS patients (irrespective of comorbid OCD diagnosis) have significantly higher rates of OCD than relatives of normal controls. An early age of onset (<18 years) is another factor associated with increased familial risk.

Studies examining potential genetic mechanisms have yet to identify unequivocally paraticular genes involved in the phenotypic expression of OCD. Among the most promising candidate genes are the serotonin transporter (*SLC6A4*) on 17q11 and the high-affinity neuronal excitatory amino acid transporter (*SLAC1A1/ECCA-1*) on 9p24.

Genetic studies of OCD have been hampered by the fact that OCD has a large degree of phenotypic heterogeneity and by a current lack of understanding into the molecular mechanisms underlying the disorder. The identification of quantitative endophenotypes with clinical, neuropsychological, imaging or electrophysiological measures, may advance the field.

With the exception of the PANDAS hypothesis, systematic efforts to identify environmental risk factors associated with OCD have lagged behind genetic studies. Current speculation focuses on perinatal adversity, parental child-rearing patterns, psychosocial stress (particularly the loss or threatened loss of close family members), traumatic brain injury, and exposure to drugs of abuse.

Hu XZ, Lipsky RH, Zhu G, et al.: Serotonin transporter promoter gain-of-function genotypes are linked to obsessive–compulsive disorder. *Am J Hum Genet* 2006;78(5):815–826.

Nestadt G, Samuels J, Riddle M, et al.: A family study of obsessive–compulsive disorder. *Arch Gen Psychiatry* 2000;57(4):358–363.

Pauls DL, Alsobrook JP, II, Goodman W, Rasmussen S, Leckman JF: A family study of obsessive–compulsive disorder. *Am J Psychiatry* 1995;152(1)76–84.

Veenstra-Vander Weele J, Kim SJ, Gonen D et al.: Genomic organization of the SLC1A1/EAAC1 gene and mutation screening in early-onset obsessive–compulsive disorder. *Mol Psychiatry* 2001;6(2):160–167

Clinical Findings

A. SIGNS AND SYMPTOMS

OCD is characterized by obsessions (unwanted and intrusive thoughts, images or impulses) and/or compulsions (repetitive behavioral or mental rituals). Since obsessions and compulsions are usually recognized by the child as nonsensical, inappropriate, or unreasonable, they are often both kept hidden from both parents and therapists. Especially in younger children, parental observation of compulsive behaviors (i.e., repeated checking of locks, washing or cleaning objects, hoarding) or physical signs of compulsive behavior (i.e., chapped hands or ulcerations from excessive washing,) can be the only definite signs of the disorder. Since the vast majority of OCD patients have insight into their condition, a detailed clinical history of obsessive and compulsive behavior from child and parents is sufficient to make a diagnosis of OCD. In order to qualify for a diagnosis of OCD, obsessions and compulsions must last more than 1 hour a day, and cause both distress and impairment.

OCD is generally considered to have a bimodal distribution in age of onset. One peak of incidence occurs in the peripubetal years and the other in early adulthood. Across the life cycle, the symptoms of OCD are similar. However, there are several important differences between pediatric and adult-onset OCD. Pediatric-onset OCD has a male predominance (unlike adult-onset OCD cases which are female-predominant), a stronger family history of OCD, and higher rates of comorbid ADHD and tic disorders. The specific content of obsessions and compulsions of OCD differ across age ranges. Children with OCD have much higher rates of aggressive obsessions (such as fear of a catastrophic event, fear of harm to self or others) and have poorer insight (i.e., being unable to recognize their obsessions and compulsions as excessive and unreasonable). Adolescents with OCD have a higher proportion of obsessions with sexual and religious themes, and cleaning and contamination-related symptoms are quite prevalent across age ranges. Patients with OCD and comorbid tics have a significantly higher rate of intrusive violent or aggressive thoughts and images, sexual and religious preoccupations, concerns with symmetry and exactness, hoarding and counting rituals, and touching and tapping compulsions compared to patients with non-tic OCD, who often suffer primarily from contamination worries and cleaning compulsions. Compulsions designed to eliminate a perceptually tinged mental feeling of unease, coined in the literature as "just right" perceptions, are particularly typical of patients with OCD and comorbid tics.

There is a very high prevalence of comorbid psychiatric illness in children with OCD. In clinical samples, around 80% of children with OCD had comorbid illness. Tic disorders, ADHD, and anxiety disorder such as separation anxiety disorder are particularly common among children receiving treatment for OCD, whereas depression and anxiety disorders are particularly common in adolescent patients. Each of these comorbidities affects one-fifth to one-third of OCD patients reaching clinical attention. Proper screening for comorbid illness of OCD patients as well as the specific content and character of each patient's individual OCD symptoms is crucial to developing a proper pharmacological and behavioral treatment strategy. Comorbid psychiatric illnesses and comorbid tic disorders are associated with poor long-term outcome in children with OCD. Furthermore, OCD patients with comorbid tics have a poorer response to SSRI pharmacotherapy but an increased likelihood of responding to antipsychotic augmentation.

Bloch MH, Landeros-Weisenberger A, Kelmendi B, Coric V, Bracken MB, Leckman JF: A systematic review: Antipsychotic augmentation with treatment refractory obsessive–compulsive disorder. *Mol Psychiatry* 2006;11(7):622–632.

Geller DA, Biederman J, Faraone S, et al.: Developmental aspects of obsessive compulsive disorder: Findings in children, adolescents, and adults. *J Nerv Ment Dis* 2001;189(7):471–477.

Leckman JF, Grice DE, Barr LC, et al.: Tic-related vs. non-tic-related obsessive compulsive disorder. *Anxiety* 1994;1(5):208–215.

Leckman JF, Walker DE, Goodman WK, Pauls DL, Cohen DJ: "Just right" perceptions associated with compulsive behavior in tourette's syndrome. *Am J Psychiatry* 1994;151(5):675–680.

B. Instruments for Diagnosis and Measurement

The Yale-Brown Obsessive Compulsive Scale (Y-BOCS) is the standard clinical rating scale for the assessment of symptom severity in adults with OCD. The Y-BOCS is a 10-item ordinal scale (0–4) that rates the severity for both obsessions and compulsions according to time occupied, degree of interference, subjective distress, internal resistance, and degree of control. The Children's Yale-Brown Obsessive Compulsive Scale (CY-BOCS) is a similar scale for use with children with OCD. CY-BOCS and Y-BOCS scales differ only according to the accompanying symptom screening checklist, the CY-BOCS being more developmentally appropriate. Both scales have been validated for use in their representative patient populations and are sensitive to changes in symptom severity following treatment. Both scales rate OCD symptoms from 0 (no symptoms) to 40 (severe OCD), a score less than 8 being considered as subclinical, over 16 as clinically significant, and over 24 as moderate to severe. Generally, a reduction in the Y-BOCS score of 25–35% with a final Y-BOCS rating of less than 16 is considered the criterion for response to treatment. The Y-BOCS rating scale takes approximately 5 minutes to complete once the patient has completed the initial symptom checklist. It serves as a good measure of symptom fluctuation in a clinical setting.

As OCD seems to be heterogeneous, with multiple genetic and environmental influences, researchers have stressed the importance of characterizing the differences between types of OCD patients so as to create more homogenous populations for genetic and neuroimaging studies. With this aim, the Dimensional Yale-Brown Obsessive Compulsive Scale (DY-BOCS) was created. The DY-BOCS uses a combination of self-report checklists and clinician ratings to assess the presence and severity of OCD symptoms in 6 thematically related symptom dimensions: aggression/harm, cleaning/contamination, symmetry/ordering, religious/sexual, hoarding, and miscellaneous. The DY-BOCS rates symptom severity according to time occupied, subjective distress, and the interference that obsessions and compulsions cause within these 6 domains.

Goodman WK, Price LH, Rasmussen SA, et al.: The yale-brown obsessive compulsive scale. II. Validity. *Arch Gen Psychiatry* 1989;46(11):1012–1016.

Goodman WK, Price LH, Rasmussen SA, et al.: The yale-brown obsessive compulsive scale. I. Development, use, and reliability. *Arch Gen Psychiatry* 1989;46(11):1006–1011.

Rosario-Campos MC, Miguel EC, Quatrano S, et al.: The dimensional yale-brown obsessive-compulsive scale (DY-BOCS): An instrument for assessing obsessive-compulsive symptom dimensions. *Mol Psychiatry* 2006;11(5):495–504.

C. Laboratory Findings and Imaging

At present, no laboratory or neuroimaging findings are useful in either making the diagnosis of OCD or in predicting its prognosis or treatment. Clinical findings are sufficient. However, neuroimaging studies of OCD patients support the hypothesis that orbitofrontal–subcortical dysfunction is central to pathogenesis. PET symptom provocation studies have demonstrated hypermetabolism in the anterior-lateral orbitofrontal cortex, caudate nucleus and paralimbic brain areas of OCD patients when they are exposed to situations that provoke OCD symptoms compared to neutral stimulus periods. PET studies have also implicated hypermetabolism in the orbitofrontal cortex and caudate nucleus in subjects with OCD compared to normal controls. Hypermetabolism in these areas reverses with successful pharmacotherapy with SSRIs or cognitive behavioral therapy. Structural volumetric MRI studies of adult subjects with OCD find increased left gray orbitofrontal volumes and reduced overall orbitofrontal volumes compared to normal controls. MRI studies examining psychotropic-naïve children with OCD find increased anterior cingulate gray matter volume, increased globus pallidus volume, and reduced striatal volume compared to normal controls.

Rosenberg DR, Keshavan MS, O'Hearn KM, et al.: Frontostriatal measurement in treatment-naive children with obsessive–compulsive disorder. *Arch Gen Psychiatry* 1997;54(9):824–830.

Saxena S, Rauch SL: Functional neuroimaging and the neuroanatomy of obsessive–compulsive disorder. *Psychiatr Clin North Am* 2000;23(3):563–586.

Szeszko PR, MacMillan S, McMeniman M, et al.: Brain structural abnormalities in psychotropic drug-naive pediatric patients with obsessive–compulsive disorder. *Am J Psychiatry* 2004;161(6):1049–1056.

Differential Diagnosis

Recurrent thoughts, images and impulses similar to the obsessions present in OCD are encountered in many other mental disorders. For instance, in Major Depressive Episodes it is not uncommon for patients to have persistent thoughts about unpleasant circumstances, personal worthlessness, or possible alternative actions. These ruminative thoughts can be distinguished from those of OCD by the fact that they are mood-congruent and ego-syntonic compared to the obsessions of OCD. There is a high comorbidity between depression and OCD; thus it is common for both ruminative depressive thoughts and obsessive thoughts to present in the same individual. The symptoms of other anxiety disorders can also mimic the symptoms of OCD. Generalized Anxiety Disorder is characterized by excessive worry, but worries can be distinguished from obsessions by the fact that the person experiences them as excessive concern about real-life circumstances, whereas obsessions are generally experienced as excessive but unreasonable. The obsessions of OCD must also be distinguished from excessive worries in mental disorders about appearance (body dysmorphic disorder, anorexia and bulimia), a specific situation or circumstance (specific phobia), or serious illness due to misinterpretation of normal bodily signals (hypochondria).

In children, OCD obsessions concerning the fear of harm to self or others must be distinguished from the fears typical of separation anxiety disorder. These two conditions can be distinguished by the observation that the obsessions of OCD are usually accompanied by stereotyped and specific compulsive rituals (i.e., checking behavior, counting), whereas in separation anxiety disorder the compulsive actions are less stereotyped. Furthermore, the occurence of other OCD symptoms besides fear of harm aids in diagnostic clarification.

The repetitive stereotypies of children with autism spectrum disorders, mental retardation and pervasive developmental disorders can resemble the compulsions of OCD. However, stereotypies can usually be easily distinguished from the obsessions of OCD because of the child's accompanying symptoms and the fact that stereotypies are usually experienced as soothing or pleasurable whereas compulsions are ego-dystonic. Stereotypies can be present in children with normal socialization skills, cognitive ability and developmental trajectory. In these cases an early onset of symptoms (less than 2 years of age) and an increase in stereotypies with excitement can be used to distinguish the two conditions. Complex tics in children with TS can mimic the compulsions of OCD. Complex tics are usually preceded by a premonitory urge, whereas compulsions are preceded by anxiety or a specific obsession. The high comorbidity between tic disorders and OCD can make this distinction difficult.

Treatment

Cognitive–Behavioral Therapy (CBT) and pharmacotherapy are effective therapies in the treatment of pediatric OCD. In one double-blind, multi-center, placebo-controlled study, the combination of CBT and Zoloft has been demonstrated to be superior to either CBT or pharmacotherapy alone. All children with OCD should be offered CBT unless there is a strong clinical reason not to do so.

A. Psychotheraputic Interventions

Cognitive behavioral therapy for children with OCD is based on exposure and response prevention. With a number needed to treat of 2.6 (95% CI: 1.7–4.2) to induce a treatment-response in children with OCD, CBT is a first-line treatment for OCD across all age ranges. In CBT for OCD, the therapist must first examine and take a detailed history of a child's specific OCD symptoms. Symptom checklists such as those that accompany the CY-BOCS and Y-BOCS rating scales are useful. The therapist, working with child and parent, designs a hierarchy of exposures, both direct and imaginary, aimed to trigger the anxiety associated with the obsessions of OCD (e.g., touching a toilet seat for a child with contamination concerns, imagining a parent in a car accident for a

Table 44–4. Pharmacotherapy for OCD

Medication	Starting Dose			Typical Dose Range	
	Child	**Adolescent**	**Adult**	**Child**	**Adult**
Clomipramine	12.5–25	25	25	50–200	100–250
Sertraline	12.5–25	25–50	50	50–200	150–250
Fluoxetine	5–10	10–20	20	10–80	40–80
Fluvoxamine	12.5–25	25–50	50	50–300	100–300
Paroxetine	5–10	10	10–20	10–60	40–60
Citalopram	5–10	10	20	10–60	40–60
Escitalopram	2.5–5	5	10	5–30	20–40

child with fears of harm coming to others). The therapist then enters into a contract with the child and parent to work on completing the exposures over a set time frame, usually a couple of months. Next, the therapist engages in the specific exposures with the child (and sometimes parent) over several treatment sessions. The child agrees not to engage in his compulsions in response to the anxiety produced. During exposures the child reports on his level of anxiety using subjective units of distress (an anxiety thermometer). Child and parent are given similar exposure assignments to complete after each session. With increased duration of exposure and with further exposures (without performing the compulsions), the child's anxiety lessens, helping him to overcome the OCD. Most CBT treatment manuals for children with OCD are freely available. They include techniques for helping children deal with stress and anxiety such as relaxation therapy. They may also include exercises to illustrate other tenets of CBT such as recognizing cognitive distortions common in OCD (e.g., overestimation of risk, all-or-nothing thinking, overcoming the need for certainty, and recognizing excessive feelings of responsibility or guilt). If a CBT therapist is not available, there are therapeutic manuals that have distilled these treatment methods in a form that can be learned by a clinician in a time-efficient manner. Moreover, self-help books are available to allow parents and children to engage in aspects of treatment themselves.

B. Psychopharmacologic Interventions

SSRIs and clomipramine are the first-line pharmacotherapy for both children and adults with OCD. Clomipramine, fluoxetine, fluvoxamine, paroxetine, sertraline and citalopram have demonstrated superior efficacy to placebo in randomized, double-blind, placebo-controlled clinical trials. Table 44–4 depicts the traditional starting and target doses for SSRIs across the age spectrum. The number of subjects needed to detect a reasonable clinical treatment response (defined by a 25–35% reduction in CY-BOCS scores) has ranged from 4 to 6 in double-blind, placebo-controlled studies. Based on cumulative studies, SSRI pharmacotherapy will lead to an average of a 6.5–9 point decline in CY-BOCS ratings and an average 30–38% reduction in symptom severity. In a meta-analysis of pharmacotherapy trials for pediatric OCD, based on meta-regression techniques, clomipramine was found superior to the SSRIs. The other SSRIs currently used to treat OCD were roughly equivalent. Clomipramine may be superior to other serotonergic agents due to its unique pharmacodynamic properties. Clomipramine is metabolized into desmethylclomipramine, a secondary amine tricyclic antidepressant identical to desipramine with a chloride atom substitution. Desipramine has been reported to be effective in treating TS and ADHD. Thus, clomipramine may be more effective in treating the disorders associated with OCD than traditional SSRIs are. These meta-regression results should be interpreted with caution. No studies have directly compared the efficacy of clomipramine to other SSRIs in children with OCD. Studies comparing these agents in adults have found no significant differences.

Despite modest evidence suggesting it might be more effective than SSRIs in children, clomipramine is rarely used as the initial pharmacological agent in OCD due to its side effect profile. In view of the potential arrythmogenic properties of clomipramine, a baseline electrocardiogram and a detailed screening for a personal and family history should be undertaken in all patients before the initiation of pharmacotherapy. The U. S. Food and Drug Administration guidelines for unacceptable EKG indices for use of clomipramine are as follows: (1) PR interval > 200 ms, (2) QRS interval > 30% increased over baseline or > 120 msec, (3) blood pressure greater than 140/90, (4) heart rate > 130 bpm, or (5) QTc > 450 msec. Moreover, clomipramine has a worse side effect profile than SSRIs, with high rates of somnolence, gastrointestinal upset, reduced seizure threshold, and anticholinergic side effects. Despite these concerns, clomipramine remains a valuable treatment for children who do not respond to one or more SSRIs.

SSRIs are the first line pharmacologic treatment for children with OCD. Based on the currently available clinical trials literature, there is no evidence that one SSRI is more effective than another. The starting and target doses for SSRIs in children are depicted in Table 44–4. Pharmacological treatment for patients with SSRIs should continue for 2–3 months at the maximal tolerated dose of medication before a child is considered a nonresponder. Many OCD patients respond only after many weeks of SSRI monotherapy.

A. AUGMENTATION STRATEGIES

Approximately half of children placed on SSRIs fail to respond despite appropriate medication. If CBT has not been conducted, it should be at this point. In adults with OCD, as many as 25% of nonresponders respond if treated with another SSRI or clomipramine. There is modest evidence that, in children with OCD, clomipramine is more effective than SSRI. Furthermore, augmentation with neuroleptic medication has been demonstrated to be an effective strategy in the treatment of adults with OCD. In adults with OCD, the number of subjects needed to detect a clinically significant treatment response (35% reduction in Y-BOCS ratings) was 4.5 (95% CI: 3.2–7.1). Neuroleptic augmentation is particularly effective in OCD patients suffering from comorbid tics (NNT = 2.3), a result that is not surprising since neuroleptic medication is the mainstay of tic treatment. The doses of neuroleptic medications used to augment SSRIs are much lower than those used to treat psychosis and aggression in children.

Bloch MH, Landeros-Weisenberger A, Kelmendi B, Coric V, Bracken MB, Leckman JF: A systematic review: Antipsychotic augmentation with treatment refractory obsessive–compulsive disorder. *Mol Psychiatry* 2006;11(7): 622–632.

Cognitive–behavior therapy, sertraline, and their combination for children and adolescents with obsessive–compulsive disorder: The Pediatric OCD Treatment Study (POTS) randomized controlled trial. *JAMA* 2004;292(16):1969–1976.

Geller DA, Biederman J, Stewart SE, et al.: Which SSRI? A meta-analysis of pharmacotherapy trials in pediatric obsessive–compulsive disorder. *Am J Psychiatry* 2003;160(11):1919–1928.

March JS, Mulle K: *OCD in Children and Adolescents: A Cognitive–Behavioral Treatment Manual.* New York: Guilford Press, 1998.

Prognosis

Results from the Pediatric OCD Treatment Study and similarly designed randomized, double-blind clinical trials of pharmacological and behavioral treatments for OCD indicate that approximately one-third to one-half of children with OCD will experience a treatment response after 12 weeks of either behavioral or pharmacological treatment for OCD. The likelihood of treatment response is significantly higher when combination therapy with both cognitive behavioral therapy and pharmacotherapy with an SSRI are initiated at the beginning of treatment. The ability of children with OCD to sustain improvement over the long-term with either of these two treatment modalities is less well studied.

A meta-analysis of long-term outcome in pediatric-onset OCD estimated that the persistence rate for full OCD was 41% and for full or subclinical OCD was 60% after 1–7 years of follow-up. Predictors of poor long-term outcome in this meta-analysis were early age of OCD onset, poor initial treatment response and comorbid psychiatric illness. The presence of a comorbid tic disorder has also been associated with poor outcome in prospective, long-term outcome studies.

Leonard HL, Swedo SE, Lenane MC, et al.: A 2- to 7-year follow-up study of 54 obsessive-compulsive children and adolescents. *Arch Gen Psychiatry* 1993;50(6):429–439.

Stewart SE, Geller DA, Jenike M, et al.: Long-term outcome of pediatric obsessive–compulsive disorder: A meta-analysis and qualitative review of the literature. *Acta Psychiatr Scand* 2004;110(1):4–13.

Developmental Disorders of Attachment, Feeding, Elimination, & Sleeping

45

Barry Nurcombe, MD

Normal infants are born with the capacity to attach to their parents and to elicit care from them. Defects in the infant's capacity to attach or elicit care, and deficiencies or disruption in the response of the caregiver, can be associated with a number of conditions such as reactive attachment disorder, rumination disorder of infancy, nonorganic failure to thrive, and psychosocial dwarfism. These conditions commence in infancy and, if not corrected, distort later social and intellectual development. Sleep problems often commence in the first 2 years of age. Pica and elimination disorders are usually first diagnosed between 2 and 5 years of age.

■ DISORDERS OF ATTACHMENT

 ESSENTIALS OF DIAGNOSIS

DSM-IV-TR Diagnostic Criteria

Reactive Attachment Disorder

A. Markedly disturbed and developmentally inappropriate social relatedness in most contexts, beginning before age 5 years, as evidenced by either (1) or (2):

　(1) persistent failure to initiate or respond in a developmentally appropriate fashion to most social interactions, as manifest by excessively inhibited, hypervigilant, or highly ambivalent and contradictory responses (e.g., the child may respond to caregivers with a mixture of approach, avoidance, and resistance to comforting, or may exhibit frozen watchfulness)

　(2) diffuse attachments as manifest by indiscriminate sociability with marked inability to exhibit appropriate selective attachments (e.g., excessive familiarity with relative strangers or lack of selectivity in choice of attachment figures)

B. The disturbance in Criterion A is not accounted for solely by developmental delay (as in mental retardation) and does not meet criteria for a pervasive developmental disorder.

C. Pathogenic care as evidenced by at least one of the following:

　(1) persistent disregard of the child's basic emotional needs for comfort, stimulation, and affection

　(2) persistent disregard of the child's basic physical needs

　(3) repeated changes of primary caregiver that prevent formation of stable attachments (e.g., frequent changes in foster care)

D. There is a presumption that the care in Criterion C is responsible for the disturbed behavior in Criterion A (e.g., the disturbances in Criterion A began following the pathogenic care in Criterion C).

(Reprinted, with permission, from *Diagnostic and Statistical Manual of Mental Disorders*, 4th edn., Text Revision. Copyright 2000, Washington, DC: American Psychiatric Association.)

General Considerations

A. Epidemiology

Although this condition is believed to be rare, it has not been included in any population-based studies and its prevalence is unknown.

B. Etiology

Bowlby conceptualized attachment as the biologically based tendency for infants to elicit care from and maintain proximity to their mothers. Babies elicit care by crying, vocalizing, reaching, sucking, making eye contact, and smiling. They maintain proximity first by clinging and following and later by using their mother as a secure base from which to explore the world. The mother, in turn, ministers to the infant's physical, emotional, and social needs and protects the infant from danger. Both mother and infant monitor proximity in the second year, so that the child's exploration is curtailed when danger is perceived by one or both attachment partners.

The infant who perceives the mother as consistently sensitive and responsive to his or her needs develops a secure relationship. In contrast, if the mother's availability is perceived as unpredictable, the child will develop a sense of insecurity. A loss or severing of the attachment relationship leads to a condition interpreted as the early equivalent of grief.

By 12 months of age, the normal infant has developed a primary attachment figure, the caregiver to whom the child preferentially seeks proximity when threatened or insecure. Infants also have one or more secondary attachment figures to whom they will go if the primary figure is unavailable. Through multiple transactions involving the dual-attachment system of mother and infant, the child constructs working models of attachment—internal representations of the self in relation to others, with perceptual, mnemonic, affective, and behavioral components. These structures have profound implications for later social relationships and for the child's capacity to trust other people. The child's working models of attachment may be associated with a sense of predictability, reliability, affection, and well-being, or with inconsistency, ambivalence, rejection, loss, rage, anxiety, or sadness.

Disordered attachment is characterized by a capacity for attachment to a primary figure, however, the attachment relationship is pervaded by excessive inhibition, heedlessness, or role reversal. In **disrupted attachment,** the mother-infant relationship has been severed, and the infant reacts with developmental arrest, disturbances of eating and sleep, loss of interest in surroundings and play, social withdrawal, and apparent depression.

Severe disturbances or disruptions of the attachment relationship are likely to disrupt or impair one or more of the following aspects of development: (1) relationships with and interest in other people, (2) the capacity to explore the world, (3) cognitive development, (4) the regulation of activity, sleep, feeding, and elimination, or (5) physical growth.

By the end of the first year of life, mother-infant attachment relationships can be characterized as secure, avoidant, resistant, or disorganized. Upon reunion with the mother after a brief separation, the infant will greet the mother and seek proximity (secure), avoid the mother (avoidant), resist the mother with irritation and ambivalence (resistant), or demonstrate freezing, confusion, stereotyped movements, and incoherent, contradictory behavior (disorganized). Disorganized attachment predicts later disruptive behavior disorder. Table 45–1 describes the factors that cause disorders of attachment.

The mother's working models of attachment, developed from her own early attachment experiences, affect her capacity to respond to the infant's attachment needs. If the mother's working models of self-other attachment are suffused with ambivalence, rage, sadness, or emptiness, and her representation of an attachment figure is characterized by rejection, sadism, explosiveness, inconsistency, or remoteness, a similar pattern of behavior is

Table 45–1. Factors That Cause Disorders of Attachment

A relative incapacity of the mother or primary caregiver to provide consistent affection, to minister to the child's physical needs, or to convey to the child that he or she will be protected from danger
A relative insensitivity or lack of attunement by the mother to the infant's affective states, with a corresponding failure to respond promptly and appropriately to the infant's needs and to provide adequate tactile stimulation
A deficiency in the infant's capacity to elicit care from the mother or to attach to her
Extremes of infant temperament—either marked sluggishness and withdrawal or excessive irritability, hypersensitivity, aversion from touch, and lack of adaptability
A combination of a lack of maternal capacity, sensitivity, or interest and a defect in the infant's capacity for attachment or self-regulation
A severance of the attachment relationship as a result of loss or separation, particularly if the infant's environment subsequently fails to provide adequate surrogate care
The exposure of the infant to multiple, changing caregivers, particularly if the care provided is perfunctory and lacking in affection

likely to be repeated with the infant. Thus when unresolved conflicts are reactivated in the parent by the demands of infant care, these "ghosts in the nursery" can disrupt or preclude good mothering.

C. GENETICS

Twin studies indicate that additive genetic effects are present in disorders of attachment, particularly among boys.

Clinical Findings

A. REACTIVE ATTACHMENT DISORDER

Reactive attachment disorder represents a failure of the infant to develop a normal attachment relationship to a primary attachment figure. The infant demonstrates one of two types of reaction: (1) socially withdrawn, emotionally constricted, anergic, and apparently unable to derive pleasure from social contact or play or (2) socially indiscriminate and emotionally shallow. Both types of reactive attachment disorder are associated with parental neglect or maltreatment or institutional child-rearing with multiple caregivers. Infants exposed to early maltreatment demonstrate disorganized attachment as toddlers and grow into socially withdrawn or aggressive, disruptive children.

B. DISORDERED ATTACHMENT

In disordered attachment, the infant has a primary attachment figure, but the attachment relationship is pathologic, with an imbalance between proximity seeking and exploration. There are three types: (1) disordered attachment with inhibition, (2) disordered attachment with self-endangerment, and (3) disordered attachment with role reversal.

In **disordered attachment with inhibition,** the infant is emotionally constricted, lacking in vitality, socially avoidant, and loath to explore the environment even when it is apparently safe to do so. The child clings persistently to the mother or avoids contact with her.

Children who demonstrate **disordered attachment with self-endangerment** are reckless, heedless, and accident-prone. Even when hurt, they rebuff their mother's attempts to comfort them. Sometimes they are self-injurious, banging their heads or biting themselves. When anxious, they are more likely to run away than to seek contact comfort from their parents.

In **disordered attachment with role reversal,** the child exhibits a precocious, overdeveloped solicitousness to the mother, alternating with punitive, bossy, controlling behavior.

C. DISRUPTED ATTACHMENT

Infants older than 6 months (the age at which the primary attachment figure is first recognized) react to separation from or loss of the attachment figure with the following sequence of behavior: (1) protest, (2) depression, and (3) detachment. Children in the stage of protest cry, demand that the parent return, and reject the attempts of others to comfort them. Depression and detachment are associated with sad face, anergia, insomnia, anorexia, loss of interest in surroundings, social withdrawal, "empty" clinging, and developmental arrest or regression. The child reacts to reminders of the primary attachment figure by ignoring or rejecting them or with a reactivation of protest.

Differential Diagnosis (Including Comorbid Conditions)

Attachment disorders should be distinguished from pervasive developmental disorder, mental retardation, and language disorder. Pervasive developmental disorder, particularly infantile autism, is characterized by delay and deviance in the development of social relationships, language, and intellect. The impairment of social relationships in autism is profound and not reversible by effective parenting. Furthermore, a history of parental failure, maltreatment, or loss is not usually encountered, and autism is associated with characteristic peculiarities of movement, language, and intellectual patterning.

Mental retardation aggravated by parental neglect or maltreatment presents a difficult differential diagnosis. Attachment relationships are intact in uncomplicated cases of mental retardation, other than in the profoundly retarded. Similarly, children with developmental language disorders do not demonstrate attachment pathology unless the language delay is associated with gross parental neglect.

COMORBIDITY

Reactive attachment disorder is a serious biopsychosocial condition. Older studies reported significant mortality and severe psychosocial morbidity associated with this disorder. However, the negative outcomes of these studies are compounded by the very poor quality of the institutions in which the studied children were housed. A number of investigations have compared the outcome of higher quality institutional rearing with that of early adoption or placement in foster care. Children raised initially in institutions tend to become more restless, distractible, disobedient, oppositional, and irritable than do control subjects. Children adopted early from institutions are better attached to their adoptive parents and siblings than are those who have been reunited with their families of origin.

For maximum benefit to intellectual development, children should probably be placed in a family well before 4 1/2 years of age. However, this question remains: Is there a watershed age beyond which the effects of early institutionalization or parental neglect are irreversible? In any case, a radical change of circumstances is required to remedy reactive attachment disorder and, despite the likelihood of individual differences in the capacity to benefit from environmental enrichment, it would be prudent to place children with adoptive families as early as possible.

Treatment

In the most egregious circumstances, parental rights must be terminated and early adoption sought. In most cases, however, remedial treatment will be appropriate.

The assessment of the family, and particularly of the parent–child interaction, has therapeutic implications, as described in Chapter 5. Parent–infant psychotherapy addresses (1) parental problems that impair caregiving, (2) the constitutional or temperamental factors in the infant that impede attachment, and (3) the match between the infant's needs and temperament and the parent's style of nurturance. Parenting problems could be related to current psychopathology (e.g., depression); unresolved conflict related to past experiences (e.g., of trauma, abuse, rejection, or neglect); or inexperience and lack of flexibility. Other, more experienced parents in mutual support groups can offer helpful advice concerning feeding, daily care, methods of consolation, and play. Nurse home visitors can work with parents to improve the quality of the match between the infant's needs and temperament and the parent's sensitivity and responsiveness, and to help parents enjoy their children.

Complications/Adverse Outcomes of Treatment

Data related to specific interventions for Reactive Attachment Disorder are limited at best. Although some treatments have advocated "holding" during periods of intense rage, coercive restraint, when applied for reasons other than imminent safety, is misdirected and may further the child's negative self-perceptions and further complicate the course of the disorder.

Prognosis

The prognosis of reactive attachment disorder and disordered and disrupted attachment has not been studied thoroughly. Insecure and, particularly, disorganized attachment during infancy have been found to predict disruptive behavior, impulse-control problems, peer relationship problems, oppositional behavior, low self-esteem, and lower social competence in preschool and school-aged children.

Lieberman AF, Zeanah CH: Disorders of attachment in infancy. *Child Adolesc Psychiatr Clin N Am* 1995;4:571.

Minnis H, Marwick H, Arthur J, McLauglin A: Reactive attachment disorder—a theoretical model beyond attachment. *Eur Child Adolesc Psychiatry* 2006; 15 (2):63–70.

Richters MM, Volkmar FR: Reactive attachment disorders of infancy and childhood. In: Lewis M (ed). *Child and Adolescent Psychiatry: A Comprehensive Textbook*, 3rd edn. Philadelphia: Lippincott Williams & Wilkins, 2002, pp. 597–602.

Zilberstein K: Clarifying core characteristics of attachment disorders: A review of current research and theory. *Am J Orthopsychiatry* 2006;17:55–64.

■ FEEDING & EATING DISORDERS OF INFANCY OR EARLY CHILDHOOD

PICA

ESSENTIALS OF DIAGNOSIS

DSM-IV-TR Diagnostic Criteria

A. *Persistent eating of nonnutritive substances for a period of at least 1 month.*

B. *The eating of nonnutritive substances is inappropriate to the developmental level.*

C. *The eating behavior is not part of a culturally sanctioned practice.*

D. *If the eating behavior occurs exclusively during the course of another mental disorder (e.g., mental retardation, pervasive developmental disorder, schizophrenia), it is sufficiently severe to warrant independent clinical attention.*

(Reprinted, with permission, from *Diagnostic and Statistical Manual of Mental Disorders*, 4th edn., Text Revision. Copyright 2000, Washington, DC: American Psychiatric Association.)

General Considerations

A. EPIDEMIOLOGY

The prevalence of pica varies widely. It is much more common among rural pregnant African-American women and among institutionalized mentally retarded patients.

B. Etiology

The cause of pica is not known. Several theories have been proposed. The nutritional theory relates pica to iron deficiency and an appetite for minerals. However, it is uncertain whether iron deficiency, which is often found in association with pica, is primary or secondary. Another theory suggests that pica, a normal phenomenon in infancy when the mouth is used as a perceptual organ, is a manifestation of delayed development; that is, it represents the retention of developmentally immature behavior, particularly in socially disadvantaged and mentally retarded children. Yet another theory, which applies to pregnant women who chew starch or clay, emphasizes the role of cultural beliefs and custom.

C. Genetics

Except as mediated by various forms of mental retardation, there are no known genetic factors specifically associated with pica.

Clinical Findings

Children with pica eat dirt, stones, ice, paint, burned match heads, starch, feces, hair, and so on.

Treatment

The proper treatment of pica is unclear. Proper supervision of young children and behavioral techniques for older children are recommended. Ferrous sulfate therapy has been recommended on the theory that the condition is caused by iron deficiency.

Complications/Adverse Outcomes of Treatment

Laboratory studies are needed to rule out lead poisoning. Aside from lead poisoning, pica can lead to excessive weight gain, malnutrition, intestinal blockage, intestinal perforation, and malabsorption.

Prognosis

Depending on the circumstances with regard to associated etiological conditions and the level of supervision the prognosis varies.

Lacey EP: Phenomenology of pica. *Child Adolesc Psychiatr Clin N Am* 1993;2:75.

McAdam DB, Sherman JA, Sheldon JB, Napolitano DA: Behavioral interventions to reduce the pica of persons with developmental disabilities. *Behav Modif* 2004;28:45–72.

RUMINATION DISORDER

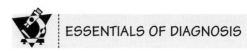 **ESSENTIALS OF DIAGNOSIS**

DSM-IV-TR Diagnostic Criteria

A. Repeated regurgitation and rechewing of food for a period of at least 1 month following a period of normal functioning.

B. The behavior is not due to an associated gastrointestinal or other general medical condition (e.g., esophageal reflux).

C. The behavior does not occur exclusively during the course of anorexia nervosa or bulimia nervosa. If the symptoms occur exclusively during the course of mental retardation or a pervasive developmental disorder, they are sufficiently severe to warrant independent clinical attention.

(Reprinted, with permission, from *Diagnostic and Statistical Manual of Mental Disorders*, 4th edn., Text Revision. Copyright 2000 Washington, DC: American Psychiatric Association.)

General Considerations

A. Epidemiology

The incidence of rumination in the general population of infants is unknown. Rumination among the mentally retarded occurs more commonly in males, particularly among the profoundly retarded. The prevalence in institutional populations is 6–10%.

B. Etiology

In infants, rumination is thought to be associated with deprivation of maternal attention or neglect. In older, mentally retarded patients, rumination has been ascribed to self-stimulation and is most often encountered in a setting of institutional neglect. Gastroesophageal reflux, hiatus hernia, or esophageal spasm may be diagnosed, but the significance of these conditions is not clear, and it should not be assumed that, even if present, they cause rumination. Rumination has been interpreted as a complex, learned behavior reinforced by maternal attention or oral sensory gratification.

C. Genetics

Except as mediated by various forms of mental retardation, there are no known genetic factors specifically associated with rumination.

Clinical Findings

Ruminators stimulate their gag reflexes manually or adopt postures that facilitate regurgitation. The frequency can vary from several times per minute to once per hour. Regurgitated food fills the cheeks and may be stirred about by the tongue before being reswallowed or spit out. Ruminators can sometimes be diverted from the practice temporarily, if they are offered interesting things to do after eating.

Differential Diagnosis

Rumination should be differentiated from other causes of vomiting and gastroesophageal reflux.

Treatment

In infants, it may be enough to provide consistent, noncontingent, contact comfort, with holding, rocking, eye contact, and soothing vocalizations. In older children (e.g., in those who are mentally retarded), or in infants for whom adequate nurturance has been insufficient to eliminate the condition, behavioral treatment will be required. The design of the specific treatment plan depends on a detailed behavioral analysis of the antecedents, the behavior, and its consequences. Usually reinforcement techniques are applied first, and aversive techniques are held in reserve in case reinforcement alone is insufficient. When the perpetuating reinforcer is intrinsic (e.g., self-stimulation in older patients) rather than extrinsic (e.g., operant vomiting reinforced by parental attention), treatment may need to be prolonged. The feeding of satiating quantities of high-caloric food is sometimes useful as a preliminary treatment in underweight patients. Habit reversal training using diaphragmatic breathing as the competing response can also lead to substantial improvement. The provision of a substitute oral stimulant such as chewing gum after meals can also be helpful.

Complications/Adverse Outcomes of Treatment

Failure to diagnose this condition and the extensive diagnostic testing in pediatric and adolescent patients prior to diagnosis can be a significant source of morbidity.

Prognosis

In general, rumination syndrome is a "benign" condition. However, there is a significant functional disability related to weight loss, school and work absenteeism, and hospitalization. In some cases rumination has a serious prognosis. Unless treated successfully, it could lead to inanition and death.

Chial HJ, Camilleri M, Williams DE, Litzinger K, Perrault J: Rumination syndrome in children and adolescents: Diagnosis, treatment, and prognosis. *Pediatrics* 2003;111:158–162.

Johnson JM: Phenomenology and treatment of rumination. *Child Adolesc Psychiatr Clin N Am* 1993;2:75.

FEEDING DISORDER OF INFANCY OR EARLY CHILDHOOD (NONORGANIC FAILURE TO THRIVE)

 ESSENTIALS OF DIAGNOSIS

DSM-IV-TR Diagnostic Criteria

A. Feeding disturbance as manifested by persistent failure to eat adequately with significant failure to gain weight or significant loss of weight over at least 1 month.

B. The disturbance is not due to an associated gastrointestinal or other general medical condition (e.g., esophageal reflux).

C. The disturbance is not better accounted for by another mental disorder (e.g., rumination disorder) or by lack of available food.

D. The onset is before age 6 years.

(Reprinted, with permission, from *Diagnostic and Statistical Manual of Mental Disorders*, 4th edn., Text Revision. Copyright 2000 Washington, DC: American Psychiatric Association.)

General Considerations

A. Epidemiology

Nonorganic failure to thrive has been found to occur in 2–5% of admissions to pediatric hospitals. It appears to be equally common in both sexes. English studies that followed birth cohorts in a socially disadvantaged London health district identified 3.5–4.6% as having nonorganic failure to thrive by 12 months of age. Most of these children had never been referred for pediatric evaluation. About 20% of families living in a socially disadvantaged inner city area will have at least one child who fails to thrive. Late birth order in a large, closely spaced family is a risk factor.

B. Etiology

Organic and nonorganic failure to thrive are not distinguished sharply. Aside from the 10% of cases of failure to thrive that are caused by clear-cut physical disease, subtle constitutional or temperamental factors in the infant often interact with a relative impairment of parenting capacity to cause this condition. However, all cases have the same final common pathway: insufficient food intake.

Among the subtle constitutional factors that interact with or trigger environmental failure are the following: hypotonic lips, poor sucking, tongue dysfunction, oral-motor impairment, poor coordination of sucking and swallowing; gastroesophageal reflux, minor forms of cerebral palsy, Sandifer's syndrome (involving tension spasm and esophageal reflux), sleep apnea, and the aftermath of nasogastric, parenteral, or gastrostomy feeding. In some cases, feeding difficulties disrupt the mother-infant interaction, engendering a vicious cycle.

Early studies implicated maltreatment and neglect as the cause of nonorganic failure to thrive. Better-controlled studies have cast doubt on the universality of this theory, however, follow-up studies of these children have demonstrated an increased risk of subsequent maltreatment and neglect.

Controlled studies of maternal characteristics have produced conflicting results. Some studies suggest an increased prevalence of depression, personality disorder, and substance abuse. Controlled observations of the mother-infant interaction have demonstrated in these mothers less reciprocity, less sensitivity to the infant's cues, greater conflict over control issues, and more negative affect; whereas infants with nonorganic failure to thrive are relatively more inhibited, less cooperative, and more likely to avert their gaze from their mothers.

C. Genetics

Organic failure to thrive occurs when there is an underlying medical cause. This may be genetically determined.

Clinical Findings

Nonorganic failure to thrive is usually noticed in the first year of life. The infant is cachectic and prone to infection. Developmental delay is the rule, but the severity of the delay is variable. These children are listless and hypotonic, exhibiting abnormal postures and intense gaze. They prefer inanimate objects to people, and they are prone to self-stimulation. They look sad and are irritable, withdrawn, or hypervigilant.

Although in clinical studies the mothers of children with nonorganic failure to thrive have seemed to demonstrate psychopathology, controlled studies have yielded inconsistent findings. One such study demonstrated increased rates of depression, substance abuse, and personality disorder. High rates of insecure and disorganized attachment were noted in the children.

Differential Diagnosis

Nonorganic failure to thrive and psychosocial dwarfism (discussed later in this chapter) must be distinguished from organic causes of failure to thrive and short stature, such as hereditary short stature, chromosomal abnormality (e.g., 46 X0, trisomy 23), dysmorphic short stature (e.g., Noonan's syndrome, Russell-Silver syndrome), skeletal dysplasia (e.g., achondroplasia, hypochondroplasia), endocrinopathy (e.g., growth hormone deficiency, growth hormone resistance, hypothyroidism, hypercortisolism, congenital adrenal hyperplasia), other causes of malnutrition, or systemic disease (e.g., chronic pulmonary disease, congenital heart disease, malabsorption syndrome, renal disease, chronic anemia). Children with nonorganic failure to thrive or psychosocial dwarfism were usually of normal size at birth.

Treatment

If the child's survival is in question, he or she must be removed from the home and hospitalized or placed into foster care. In extreme circumstances, parental rights must be terminated.

A variety of behavioral techniques have been used to counteract or remediate abnormal feeding behavior in infants. These techniques are used in tandem with individual psychotherapy aimed to enhance maternal consistency and sense of competence and to decrease maternal stress. If the mother has a diagnosable psychiatric disorder (e.g., depression or substance use disorder), it should be promptly treated. Casework can be provided in the home by a trained social worker or nurse, with attention given to financial, marital, or employment problems. Dyadic therapy involving both infant and mother is recommended when unresolved issues related to pathogenic maternal working models of attachment impede adequate childcare.

It is unclear whether or when supportive casework is preferable to dyadic therapy.

Complications/Adverse Outcomes of Treatment

Most children with nonorganic failure to thrive do not become psychosocial dwarfs. Psychosocial dwarfism is potentially reversible, if the child is removed from the noxious home environment. However, if the child is returned to an adverse situation, developmental failure will recur. The later the onset, the better the prognosis for intellectual and language functioning.

Prognosis

Children with nonorganic failure to thrive that are not treated for an extended period of time may have difficulty "catching up" developmentally and socially. About half of children who experienced failure to thrive continue to have social and emotional problems or eating problems later in life.

PSYCHOSOCIAL DWARFISM

 ESSENTIALS OF DIAGNOSIS

Diagnostic Criteria

- *Growth failure (marked linear growth retardation and delayed epiphyseal maturation)*
- *Neuroendocrine dysfunction (reversible hypopituitarism)*
- *Bizarre eating and drinking behavior (e.g., polyphagia, polydipsia, hoarding)*
- *Dramatic weight gain after hospitalization but reversion to growth failure after return to family*

General Considerations

A. Epidemiology

The incidence of psychosocial dwarfism in the general population of infants is unknown.

B. Etiology

Psychosocial dwarfism is caused by dysfunctional growth hormone secretion, which reverses when the child is hospitalized and provided with effective parental care. The condition is usually associated with severe neglect and maltreatment. It is not clear why some children respond to a noxious environment in this manner and others do not.

C. Genetics

While mutations in the growth hormone receptor gene and related genes can lead to growth failure, psychosocial dwarfism is, by definition, a condition with an environmental etiology.

Clinical Findings

Psychosocial dwarfism is usually diagnosed between 18 months and 7 years of age. Severe growth retardation with cognitive and language delays is sometimes preceded by feeding problems in infancy. The child exhibits polyphagia, food hoarding, pica, and insomnia, sometimes wandering at night apparently to look for food.

Food fads, enuresis, encopresis, and self-induced vomiting are commonly associated with psychosocial dwarfism. Mental retardation or borderline intelligence is also a concomitant. The symptoms of psychosocial dwarfism have been associated with disorders of biological rhythms, self-regulation, mood, and social relationships. Sleep, appetite, and satiety are disturbed, and these children have a deficiency in the normally pulsed release of growth hormone into the bloodstream. Sometimes these children are destructive, urinating or defecating in inappropriate places. The condition is potentially reversible, at least in part, if the child is provided with adequate, nurturant surrogate care.

Differential Diagnosis

Psychosocial dwarfism should be distinguished from short stature due to endocrine disorder, constitutional factors, or stress.

Treatment

When children with psychosocial dwarfism are provided with adequate surrogate parental care, physical and mental growth occurs within a few weeks and the eccentric behavior characteristic of the condition recedes. However, the longer that appropriate placement is delayed, the less likely it is that the child will catch up.

Complications/Adverse Outcomes of Treatment

Parental psychopathology and compliance with treatment should be monitored. There is also likely to be an increased risk of child maltreatment including overt abuse and neglect.

Prognosis

The prognosis is poor, unless adequate, surrogate parental care is provided. Short stature, delayed puberty, stunted intellectual development, and conduct problems are likely to result from untreated psychosocial dwarfism.

Benoit D: Feeding disorders, failure to thrive, and obesity. In: Zeanah CH (ed). *Handbook of Infant Mental Health,* 2nd edn. New York: Guilford Press, 2000.

Minde K, Minde R: The effect of disordered parenting on the development of children. In: Lewis M (ed). *Child and Adolescent Psychiatry: A Comprehensive Textbook,* 3rd edn. Philadelphia: Lippincott Williams & Wilkins, 2002, pp. 477–493.

Ramsey M: Feeding disorders and failure to thrive. *Child Adolesc Psychiatr Clin N Am* 1995;4:605.

Reilly SM, Skuse DH, Wolke D, Stevenson J: Oral-motor dysfunction in children who fail to thrive: Organic or non-organic? *Dev Med Child Neurol* 1999;41:115–122.

■ ELIMINATION DISORDERS

ENCOPRESIS

 ESSENTIALS OF DIAGNOSIS

DSM-IV-TR Diagnostic Criteria

A. *Repeated passage of feces into inappropriate places (e.g., clothing or floor) whether involuntary or intentional.*

B. *At least one such event a month for at least 3 months.*

C. *Chronological age is at least 4 years (or equivalent developmental level).*

D. *The behavior is not due exclusively to the direct physiological effects of a substance (e.g., laxatives) or a general medical condition except through a mechanism involving constipation.*

(Reprinted, with permission, from *Diagnostic and Statistical Manual of Mental Disorders*, 4th edn., Text Revision. Copyright 2000 Washington, DC: American Psychiatric Association.)

General Considerations

A. EPIDEMIOLOGY

A Scandinavian population study revealed a prevalence of 1.5% among children aged 7–8 years. The sex ratio was 3.4:1 in favor of boys. A British study found a prevalence of about 1.5% among children aged 10–11 years, with a sex ratio of 4.3:1 in favor of boys.

B. ETIOLOGY

The etiology of encopresis is multifactorial. Normal continence and voiding requires the following sequence of neuromuscular events: (1) sensitivity to rectal fullness, (2) constriction of the external anal sphincter, puborectalis, and internal anal sphincter, (3) rectal contraction waves, (4) increase of intra-abdominal pressure following contraction of the diaphragm and abdominal muscles, and (5) relaxation of the sphincters.

Children with encopresis exhibit abnormal anorectal dynamics, such as a weak internal sphincter, or a failure of the external sphincter to relax in concert with rectal contraction waves and abdominal straining. There are two types of encopresis: (1) with constipation and overflow incontinence and (2) without constipation and overflow incontinence.

Toilet training involves the learning of the appropriate place and time for defecation; sensitivity to rectal fullness; and the sequential coordination of withholding, finding the right place, adopting the appropriate posture, relaxing the sphincters, and increasing intra-abdominal pressure. Most children are capable of learning the sequence by 18–24 months of age, however, learning may be interrupted by several antecedent conditions or concurrent events. Particularly important are the parent's attunement to the infant's signals and the parent's capacity to introduce the child to the toilet calmly; offer praise and encouragement for a favorable result; and avoid discouragement, coercion, or punishment for failures.

A significant number of children who experience fecal retention were constipated in the first year of life. In other children, physiologic constipation has followed an attack of diarrhea. The preliminary constipation causes painful defecation, in some cases with anal fissure, which precipitates withholding. A pattern of withholding, fecal retention, and involuntary overflow may be created if withholding coincides with faulty toilet training (e.g., with coercion, harsh criticism, or physical punishment) or if the parent is emotionally unavailable or poorly attuned to the child (e.g., as a result of depression). Thus an initially physiologic condition disrupts the mother-child relationship, and psychogenic retention culminates in abnormal anorectal dynamics, megacolon, rectal insensitivity, and leakage or involuntary voiding.

A small number of children, with severe behavioral disturbance, often from neglectful or rejecting homes exhibit no retention and constipation but deliberately defecate in closets or other inappropriate places. Two other nonretentive groups of encopretics are associated with (1) an apparent insensitivity to rectal fullness and the involuntary passage of feces or (2) the passage of (often liquid) feces when emotionally aroused by anxiety, fear, or laughter.

The degree to which encopresis is associated with psychopathology in the parent or child is disputed. Enuresis, oppositional-defiant behavior, tantrums, school refusal, fire setting, and developmental immaturities have been described as concomitants, although it is uncertain to what degree these symptoms are primary or secondary to the encopresis.

C. GENETICS

Although children with some genetically determined forms of mental retardation, such as Fragile-X syndrome, are at greater risk for encopresis, this vulnerability is likely to be more related to their level of intellectual disability than a specific syndrome.

Clinical Findings

Some younger children who deliberately soil in inappropriate places do so at a time of stress or family change, for example after the birth of a sibling. Others, as described earlier in this chapter, do so in reaction to severe neglect or rejection, as in psychosocial dwarfism. A second group appears to lose sphincter control when emotionally aroused. These are often highly strung children exposed to emotional stress, for example, after a change of school.

The most serious cases are associated with constipation, retention, megarectum, megacolon, and the involuntary passage of small amounts of stool, together with liquefaction, fecal leakage, and virtually constant soiling, or the intermittent involuntary passage of large stools. Children with extreme megacolon can become disabled with abdominal distension, anorexia, and loss of weight.

Differential Diagnosis

The following causes of incontinence or constipation should be distinguished from encopresis: Hirschsprung's disease, anal stenosis, and endocrine disorder. However, the combination of soiling; constipation; a ballooned, loaded rectum; and a loaded colon occurs only in encopresis.

The clinician should evaluate the child for other developmental problems or psychiatric disorders (e.g., mental retardation, learning problems, disruptive behavior disorder, anxiety disorder).

Treatment

If the child has a loaded colon and rectum, it is likely that his or her rectum is insensitive to distension. Thus the colon should be washed out, and laxatives and stool softeners used until fecal masses can no longer be palpated and the child is passing regular stools of normal consistency. In severe cases, hospitalization is required.

Parents should be educated to administer a behavioral program. Coercion, punishment, and criticism should be avoided. It is ill-advised, for example, to punish the child by making him or her clean soiled clothes. The child should be asked to sit briefly on the toilet at the same time twice per day: after breakfast and after school. All tension should be removed from the toileting experience. The child may be read to or may read to himself or herself. The parent should make no comment if no bowel movement is passed; in contrast, the parent should praise and offer individualized reward to the child if toileting is successful. Star charts are useful both as a record and for reinforcement (see discussion on "Treatment" in Section "Enuresis").

Depressed or compulsive parents often find it difficult to institute a consistent, gentle program of this type and may need treatment in their own right. Fathers should be involved in order to provide support and to cooperate in instituting the behavioral program. Marital problems may need attention.

The child may require individual psychotherapy for associated anxiety disorder, disruptive behavior disorder, or other psychopathology. Because the possibility of relapse is high, treatment is often needed for one or more years, with a combination of laxatives, stool softeners, a high-fiber diet, parental education, parental behavior management, individual psychotherapy, and when necessary, psychiatric help for the parents. The results of this regimen are good, particularly in younger children. Success rates of 50–90% have been reported. Imipramine has been prescribed to treat encopresis, but no controlled studies of its effectiveness are available.

Complications/Adverse Outcomes of Treatment

Treatment complications are rare. Most children will improve with time and through the use of relatively innocuous interventions.

Prognosis

Most cases of encopresis resolve by adolescence. A small minority of encopretic individuals remain incontinent as adults.

Brazzelli M, Griffiths P: Behavioural and cognitive interventions with or without other treatments for the management of faecal incontinence in children. *Cochrane Database Syst Rev* 2001;(4):CD002240.

Hersov L: Encopresis. In: Rutter M, Taylor E, Hersov L (eds). *Child and Adolescent Psychiatry,* 3rd edn. Oxford, UK: Blackwell Scientific, 1994, pp. 520–528.

Mikkelson EJ: Modern approaches to enuresis and encopresis. In: Lewis M (ed). *Child and Adolescent Psychiatry: A Comprehensive Textbook,* 3rd edn. Philadelphia: Lippincott Williams & Wilkins, 2002, pp. 700–710.

ENURESIS (NOT DUE TO A GENERAL MEDICAL CONDITION)

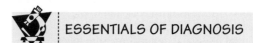 ESSENTIALS OF DIAGNOSIS

DSM-IV-TR Diagnostic Criteria

A. *Repeated voiding of urine into bed or clothes (whether involuntary or intentional).*

B. *The behavior is clinically significant as manifested by either a frequency of twice a week for at least*

3 consecutive months or the presence of clinically significant distress or impairment in social, academic (occupational), or other important areas of functioning.

C. *Chronological age is at least 5 years (or equivalent developmental level).*

D. *The behavior is not due exclusively to the direct physiological effect of a substance (e.g., a diuretic) or a general medical condition (e.g., diabetes, spina bifida, a seizure disorder).*

(Reprinted, with permission, from *Diagnostic and Statistical Manual of Mental Disorders*, 4th edn., Text Revision. Copyright 2000 Washington, DC: American Psychiatric Association.)

General Considerations

A. EPIDEMIOLOGY

The sex ratio is equal until 5 years of age, after which males predominate (2:1 at 11 years of age). Boys are more likely to develop secondary enuresis. Scandinavian and New Zealand population studies have found the prevalence of enuresis at 7 and 8 years of age to be 9.8% and 7.4%, respectively. In the United States bedwetting is more common in African-Americans and Asian immigrants than among other populations. Most enuretic children achieve continence by puberty. Approximately 3% of childhood enuretics are still incontinent at 20 years of age.

B. ETIOLOGY

The cause of enuresis is unknown. One study has found an abnormality in circadian rhythms: Enuretics did not reduce the output of urine at night, as do normal children over 12 months of age. Enuretics have low functional bladder volume, a finding that correlates with behavioral disturbance, suggesting a common etiologic factor. Indeed, enuresis correlates with other maturational delays, particularly in language, speech, motor skills, and social development. An association has been noted between the tendency to sleep for long periods each day, between 1 and 2 years of age, and later enuresis, but the significance of this finding is uncertain. Bedwetting occurs at any stage of sleep, and no abnormalities of sleep architecture have been identified.

Primary enuresis refers to enuresis without a period of continence. **Secondary enuresis** is enuresis after a period of normal bladder control. Two general population studies found that if toilet training is delayed until after 18 months, the prevalence of enuresis increases. Secondary enuresis, but not primary enuresis, is associated with psychosocial stressors. Secondary enuresis is more likely to be associated with behavioral disturbance. About 50% of enuretic children between 7 and 12 years of age have had a previous period of continence.

C. GENETICS

A genetic factor may be involved in enuresis. Bedwetting runs in families and is significantly more common in monozygotic than dizygotic twins.

Differential Diagnosis

Urinalysis, microurine, and urine culture should be ordered routinely. If daytime enuresis is present, if the patient has a history of urinary tract infections or other urinary symptoms (e.g., dysuria, urinary frequency, dribbling), or if the patient's urine grows bacteria, further urologic examinations are required in order to rule out urinary tract infection, bladder neck obstruction, urethral valves, or other structural abnormalities. Epilepsy, diabetes mellitus, diabetes insipidus, and spina bifida should be excluded by history, physical examination, and urinalysis.

Treatment

A. STAR CHARTS

The child is given a star to add to a calendar for each dry night. The star chart alone results in a cure for a minority of enuretic children. It also provides useful records of baseline and the child's progress.

B. SURGICAL TREATMENT & RETENTION CONTROL TRAINING

The efficacy of radical surgical treatments such as urethral dilatation, bladder neck repair, cystoplasty, or division of the sacral nerves has not been demonstrated. Bladder training, which involves the retention of urine for longer and longer periods of time, is no longer used.

C. PSYCHOPHARMACOLOGIC INTERVENTIONS

Heterocyclic antidepressants reduce the frequency of bedwetting in about 80% of patients and suppress it entirely in about 30%. However, most patients will relapse within about 3 months of withdrawal from the drug. The effective nighttime dosage is usually 1–2.5 mg/kg and occasionally as much as 3.5 mg/kg. This treatment essentially aims to suppress wetting while waiting for maturation in bladder control. The drug should be tapered and discontinued every 3 months and titrated back to a therapeutic level if enuresis recurs. The neuropharmacologic basis of the antienuretic effect is unknown.

The synthetic antidiuretic desmopressin acetate (desamine-D-arginine vasopressin) is an antienuretic. It may be administered intranasally or orally. Desamine-d-arginine vasopressin may operate by reducing urine volume below that which triggers bladder contraction. As with antidepressant therapy, relapse is common following withdrawal.

Sympathomimetic (e.g., ephedrine) and anticholinergic (e.g., belladonna) drugs are ineffective in treating enuresis.

D. Psychotherapeutic Interventions

The alarm-and-pad technique (in which an alarm is triggered when the first drop of urine onto a pad closes an electrical circuit) has a 75–80% rate of cure and a 30% relapse rate. It is the most effective treatment available for both primary and secondary enuresis. Children with daytime enuresis, behavioral problems, and a lack of motivation may be resistant to behavioral treatment. Optimal improvement requires at least 6–8 weeks of treatment. For maximum benefit, the alarm-and-pad technique may be combined with antidepressant or antidiuretic medication and a star chart.

If behavioral treatment is clearly the most effective method, why is it not the standard? Probably because it is cumbersome, lengthy, embarrassing, and requires good motivation. It is reasonable to begin treating enuresis with drugs and to move to behavioral treatment if medication is ineffective.

Complications/Adverse Outcomes of Treatment

Treatment complications are rare. Most children will improve with time.

Prognosis

Most cases of enuresis remit between 5 and 7 years of age or 12 and 15 years of age. A minority of cases continue into adulthood.

Glazener CM, Evans JH, Peto RE: Alarm interventions for nocturnal enuresis in children. *Cochrane Database Syst Rev* 2005;(2):CD002911.

Mikkelson EJ: Modern approaches to enuresis and encopresis. In: Lewis M (ed) *Child and Adolescent Psychiatry: A Comprehensive Textbook*, 3rd edn. Lippincott Williams & Wilkins, 2002, pp. 700–710.

■ SLEEP DISORDERS

Sleep problems often commence before 2 years of age. Sleep disorders are described more fully in Chapter 30. This section deals with the sleep disorders of infancy and early childhood. Four types of sleep problems affect this age group: (1) insomnia or dyssomnia (nightwaking), (2) hypersomnia (primary hypersomnia and breathing-related sleep disorder [sleep apnea]), (3) parasomnia (somnambulism, night terrors, nightmares, head banging, body rocking), and (4) circadian rhythm disorder (irregular sleep habits). The first three disorders are discussed in the sections that follow.

PRIMARY INSOMNIA

 ESSENTIALS OF DIAGNOSIS

DSM-IV-TR Diagnostic Criteria

Primary Insomnia

  A. *The predominant complaint is difficulty initiating or maintaining sleep, or nonrestorative sleep, for at least 1 month.*

  B. *The sleep disturbance (or associated daytime fatigue) causes clinically significant distress or impairment in social, occupational, or other important areas of functioning.*

  C. *The sleep disturbance does not occur exclusively during the course of Narcolepsy, Breathing-Related Sleep Disorder, Circadian Rhythm Sleep Disorder, or a Parasomnia.*

  D. *The disturbance does not occur exclusively during the course of another mental disorder (e.g., Major Depressive Disorder, Generalized Anxiety Disorder, a delirium).*

  E. *The disturbance is not due to the direct physiological effects of a substance (e.g., a drug of abuse, a medication) or a general medical condition.*

(Reprinted, with permission, from *Diagnostic and Statistical Manual of Mental Disorders*, 4th edn., Text Revision. Copyright 2000 Washington, DC: American Psychiatric Association.)

General Considerations

Primary insomnia is most likely to be associated with psychosocial stress, maternal depression, inconsistent limits, and anxiety. It also occurs in association with sedative medication, Tourette's syndrome, attention-deficit/hyperactivity disorder, mental retardation, autism, and Rett's syndrome.

Table 45–2. Preliminary Steps in the Treatment of Primary insomnia

1 Involve both parents in diagnosis and treatment.
2 Obtain full information about the details of the sleep disorder: its antecedents, nature, consequences, and previous treatment.
3 Inquire about other problem behaviors and about any disruptions in the child's typical day.
4 Obtain information about the parents, including their backgrounds, health, personalities, and marital relationship.
5 Have the parents keep a detailed daily record, for 2 weeks, of the child's sleep habits (e. g., bedtime, time of falling asleep, number of times awake) and daily routine (e. g., mealtimes, naptime).
6 Observe the parent-child interaction during free play: observe the parent-infant interaction during feeding.

Different parents have different tolerances for night-waking. Thus prevalence is a relative matter. Breast-fed infants wake more often than those who are bottle-fed. Waking is not associated with parity or sex, however, it is associated with perinatal adversity other than prematurity.

Clinical Findings

Nightwaking is sometimes associated with colic, a condition in which the child flexes the legs and cries paroxysmically as though in pain. The cause of colic is unknown. The condition seldom lasts beyond 4 months of age.

Treatment

Minde has proposed a treatment approach that starts with several preliminary steps (Table 45–2). Treatment should aim to help the child regulate his or her own sleep without disturbing the parents (Table 45–3). The treatment of marital problems, if any, should be reserved until a later date. Minde claims an 85% success rate with this regimen.

Table 45–3. Treatment of Nightwaking

1 Help the parents establish regular daytime and nighttime routines.
2 Ask the father to handle the nighttime routine and waking.
3 If the child is waking at night, have the father check on the child every 5–10 minutes; if the child is awake, have the father soothe the child with words but without picking up the child.
4 If the child must be weaned from the parental bed, shaping can be used. The child is moved to his or her own bed, and the mother sits on the bed soothing the child, to sleep. After 2–3 nights, she sits beside the bed. Gradually, she moves the chair further and further away, until she is outside the room.
5 Ask the parents to keep a daily journal, monitoring the progress of the sleep disturbance.
6 Schedule return visits every 2 weeks for about 8 weeks.

Complications/Adverse Outcomes of Treatment

Failures are most likely if the parents cannot establish daytime and nighttime routines, or if the father is not involved. Unfortunately, the practice of prescribing sedatives and hypnotics for pediatric insomnia is common among community-based pediatricians, especially among patients with special needs. Empirical evidence supporting this practice is limited.

Prognosis

Chronic insomnia may increase the chances of emotional and behavioral problems.

SLEEP APNEA (BREATHING-RELATED SLEEP DISORDER)

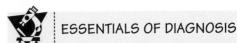 ESSENTIALS OF DIAGNOSIS

DSM-IV-TR Diagnostic Criteria

Breathing-Related Sleep Disorder (Sleep Apnea)

A. *Sleep disruption, leading to excessive sleepiness or insomnia that is judged to be due to a sleep-related breathing condition (e.g., obstructive or central sleep apnea Syndrome or central alveolar hypoventilation syndrome).*

B. *The disturbance is not better accounted for by another mental disorder and is not due to the direct physiological effects of a substance (e.g., a drug of abuse, a medication) or another general medical condition (other than a breathing-related disorder).*

(Reprinted, with permission, from *Diagnostic and Statistical Manual of Mental Disorders*, 4th edn., Text Revision. Copyright 2000 Washington, DC: American Psychiatric Association.)

General Considerations

Sleep apnea is peripheral or central in origin. Peripheral apnea is caused by oropharyngeal obstruction (e.g., by enlarged tonsilloadenoid tissue). Central apnea occurs in the sudden infant death syndrome. It may be associated with sleeping prone and excessive environmental temperature.

Clinical Findings

In obstructive sleep apnea, the sleeping child's breathing stops intermittently and is then followed by snoring respirations.

TREATMENT

Prone sleeping and excessive bedding (e.g., blankets and comforters) should be avoided. Tonsillectomy and adenoidectomy may be necessary.

Complications/Adverse Outcomes of Treatment

Children undergoing adenoidectomy (or other pharyngeal surgery) for treatment of upper airway obstruction have more frequent complications postoperatively and increased potential for serious respiratory compromise than those who undergo this procedure for other indications.

Prognosis

Chronic apnea can be associated with failure to thrive, attentional difficulties and other cognitive impairment, daytime drowsiness, and chronic headache.

PARASOMNIA

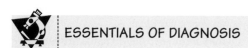 ESSENTIALS OF DIAGNOSIS

DSM-IV-TR Diagnostic Criteria

Nightmare Disorder

  A. Repeated awakenings from the major sleep period or naps with detailed recall of extended and extremely frightening dreams, usually involving threats to survival, security, or self-esteem. The awakenings generally occur during the second half of the sleep period.

  B. On awakening from the frightening dreams, the person rapidly becomes oriented and alert (in contrast to the confusion and disorientation seen in Sleep Terror Disorder and some forms of epilepsy).

  C. The dream experience, or the sleep disturbance resulting from the awakening, causes clinically significant distress or impairment in social, occupational, or other important areas of functioning.

  D. The nightmares do not occur exclusively during the course of another mental disorder (e.g., a delirium, Posttraumatic Stress Disorder) and are not due to the direct physiological effects of a substance (e.g., a drug of abuse, a medication) or a general medical condition.

Sleep Terror Disorder

  A. Recurrent episodes of abrupt awakening from sleep, usually occurring during the first third of the major sleep episode and beginning with a panicky scream.

  B. Intense fear and signs of autonomic arousal, such as tachycardia, rapid breathing, and sweating, during each episode.

  C. Relative unresponsiveness to efforts of others to comfort the person during the episode.

  D. No detailed dream is recalled and there is amnesia for the episode.

  E. The episodes cause clinically significant distress or impairment in social, occupational, or other important areas of functioning.

  F. The disturbance is not due to the direct physiological effects of a substance (e.g., a drug of abuse, a medication) or a general medical condition.

Sleepwalking Disorder

  A. Repeated episodes of rising from bed during sleep and walking about usually ring during the first third of the major sleep episode.

  B. While sleepwalking, the person has a blank, staring face, is relatively unresponsive to the efforts of others to communicate with him or her, and can be awakened only with great difficulty.

  C. On awakening (either from the sleepwalking episode or the next morning) the person has amnesia for the episode.

D. Within several minutes after awakening from the sleepwalking episode, there is no impairment of mental activity or behavior (although there may initially be a short period of confusion or disorientation).

E. The disturbance is not due to the direct physiological effects of a substance (e.g., a drug of abuse, a medication) or a general medical condition.

(Reprinted, with permission, from *Diagnostic and Statistical Manual of Mental Disorders*, 4th edn., Text Revision. Copyright 2000 Washington, DC: American Psychiatric Association.)

General Considerations

Somnambulism and night terrors are probably of inherited origin. Nightmares are more prevalent in association with anxiety, particularly posttraumatic stress disorder. The etiology of head banging and body rocking is unknown.

Somnambulism and night terrors occur in 2.5–9% of children. Head banging and body rocking occur in 30–40% of children at 9–12 months. Their prevalence drops to about 3% after age 3 years.

Clinical Findings

Nightmares should be distinguished from night terrors. In nightmares the child wakens and recounts a frightening, realistic dream but is consolable. In night terrors the apparently terrified child sits up screaming, sometimes moving about the bedroom, but is not truly awake. When the child is laid down again, he or she returns to sleep. In somnambulism the child walks about the house, unresponsive and blank-faced.

In head banging, the child rhythmically hits his or her head against the crib, sometimes vigorously. In body rocking, the child moves his or her torso rhythmically, sometimes with accompanying vocalizations. These sleep problems affect parents and in extreme cases may so disrupt the parents' sleep that they become exhausted, begin to despair, or are set at odds with one another.

Differential Diagnosis

Somnambulism must be distinguished from nocturnal complex seizures. Complex seizures are usually associated with violent thrashing about and stereotyped movements. Post-traumatic stress disorder should also be considered.

Treatment

A. NIGHTMARES

If nightmares are associated with posttraumatic stress disorder, anxiety disorder, or environmental stress, the cause of the sleep disturbance should be treated or addressed.

B. NIGHT TERRORS & SOMNAMBULISM

The clinician should reassure the parents that the condition is probably a variant of normal development. The child should not be woken but rather should be laid down or led back to bed to sleep. Extraneous sources of stress should be addressed.

C. HEAD BANGING & BODY ROCKING

Isolated case reports have described the use of behavioral techniques (e.g., extinction, reinforcement of nonrocking behavior) to treat these conditions.

Complications/Adverse Outcomes of Treatment

Treatment complications are rare. Most children will improve with time.

Prognosis

Most children who develop a nightmare problem outgrow it. Sleep night terror disorder typically resolves spontaneously in adolescence.

Handford HA, Vgontsas AN: Sleep disturbances and disorders. In: Lewis M (ed). *Child and Adolescent Psychiatry: A Comprehensive Textbook*, 3rd edn. Philadelphia: Lippincott Williams & Wilkins, 2002, pp. 876–888.

Minde K: Sleep disorders in infants and toddlers. *Child Adolesc Psychiatr Clin N Am* 1995;4:589.

Gender Identity Disorder

46

William Bernet, MD

 ESSENTIALS OF DIAGNOSIS

- There are two basic criteria for the diagnosis of gender identity disorder (GID): A strong and persistent cross-gender identification and persistent discomfort about one's assigned sex or a sense of inappropriateness in the gender role of that sex. GID is not simply a child's nonconformity to conventional sex roles but a significant and pervasive disturbance in the child's view of himself or herself. The disturbance is generally severe enough to disrupt both familial and social interactions.

DSM-IV-TR Diagnostic Criteria

Gender Identity Disorder

A. *A strong and persistent cross-gender identification (not merely a desire for any perceived cultural advantages of being the other sex).*

In children, the disturbance is manifested by four (or more) of the following:

1. *repeatedly stated desire to be, or insistence that he or she is, the other sex*
2. *in boys, preference for cross-dressing or simulating female attire; in girls, insistence on wearing only stereotypical masculine clothing*
3. *strong and persistent preferences for cross-sex roles in make-believe play or persistent fantasies of being the other sex*
4. *intense desire to participate in the stereotypical games and pastimes of the other sex*
5. *strong preference for playmates of the other sex*

In adolescents and adults, the disturbance is manifested by symptoms such as a stated desire to be the other sex, frequent passing as the other sex, desire to live or be treated as the other sex, or the conviction that he or she has the typical feelings and reaction of the other sex.

B. *Persistent discomfort with his or her sex or sense of the inappropriateness in the gender role of that sex.*

In children, the disturbance is manifested by any of the following: In boys, assertion that his penis or testes are disgusting or will disappear or assertion that it would be better not have a penis, or aversion toward rough-and-tumble play and rejection of male stereotypical toys, games, and activities; in girls, rejection of urinating in a sitting position, assertion that she has or will grow a penis, or assertion that she does not want to grow breasts or menstruate, or marked aversion toward normative feminine clothing.

In adolescents and adults, the disturbance is manifested by symptoms such as preoccupation with getting rid of primary and secondary sex characteristics (e.g., request for hormones, surgery, or other procedures to physically alter sexual characteristics in such a way as to simulate the other sex) or belief that he or she was born the wrong sex.

C. *The disturbance is not concurrent with a physical intersex condition.*

D. *The disturbance causes clinically significant distress or impairment in social, occupational, or other important areas of functioning.*

302.6   Gender identity disorder in children
302.85   Gender identity disorder in adolescents or adults

(Adapted, with permission, from *Diagnostic and Statistical Manual of Mental Disorders*, 4th edn., Text Revision. Copyright 2000 American Psychiatric Association.)

General Considerations

A. EPIDEMIOLOGY

GID is an infrequent disorder. Boys are referred for evaluation and treatment of GID more often than girls. This may be due, in part, because our society is less tolerant of cross-gender behavior in boys than in girls. In European countries the prevalence of adult GID (which is also called transsexualism) has been estimated as 1 in 30,000 for men and 1 in 100,000 in for women.

B. ETIOLOGY

The etiology of GID is probably multifactorial. Overall, much more attention has been paid to the etiology and treatment of the disorder in boys, most likely owing to the greater social stigma attached to gender-atypical behavior in boys. However, recent studies have examined gender-atypical behaviors in girls as compared with boys. The disorder is located at the extreme of a continuum that begins with mild gender-atypical behavior through gender dysphoria and on to gender identity disturbance.

As with most psychiatric disorders, the etiology is probably best comprehended by a biopsychosocial approach. Research on the biological issues involved in this disorder have not yielded clear conclusions. Animal models suggest that prenatal hormonal influences play a significant role in gender-specific behavior. Although the significance is not clear, it has been found that boys with GID tend to have a higher rate of left-handedness, an excess of brothers to sisters, and a later birth order. It has been proposed that a mother who has multiple sons might produce antibodies to the male fetus resulting in reduced masculinity.

Many psychosocial theories have been proposed. Researchers have suggested a window of psychological vulnerability between age 2 years (when the child establishes gender identity) and age 5 or 6 years (when he or she recognizes that gender assignment is stable over time). Researchers continue to examine the family dynamics for clues concerning the development of this disorder. When young children manifest cross-gender behaviors, most parents are either tolerant toward this behavior or even encouraging it. Some authors suggest that particular children are especially vulnerable to the development of GID in response to trauma. Other children would possibly never exhibit gender-atypical behavior and certainly not GID, regardless of trauma or the family dynamics.

Blanchard R, Zucker KJ, Bradley SJ, Hume CS: Birth order and sibling sex ratio in homosexual male adolescents and probably prehomosexual feminine boys. *Dev Psycho* 1995;31:22–30.

Coates S, Wolfe S: Gender identity disorder in boys: The interface of constitution and early experience. *Psychoanalytic Inquiry* 1995;15:6.

Meyer-Bahlburg HFL: Intersexuality and the diagnosis of gender identity disorder. *Arch Sex Behav* 1994;23:21.

Sandberg DE, et al.: The prevalence of gender-atypical behavior in elementary school children. *J Am Acad Child Adolesc Psychiatry* 1993;32:306.

Zucker KJ: Gender identify development and issues. *Child Adolesc Psychiatric Clin N Am* 2004;13(3):551–568.

Clinical Findings

Boys with GID are markedly preoccupied with activities that are traditionally considered feminine such as dressing in girls' or women's clothes, playing house by role-playing female figures, drawing pictures of beautiful girls, playing with toys such as Barbie dolls, and being interested in female fantasy figures. They avoid competitive sports and display little interest in the cars, trucks, and other activities that are traditionally considered masculine. They may express a wish to be a girl and may pretend to not have a penis.

Girls with GID have a marked preference for masculine appearances and activities. They prefer boys' clothing and short hair and may request to be called by a boy's name. They prefer to play with boys and engage in rough-and-tumble play, contact sports, and traditional boyhood activities. They avoid wearing dresses or other feminine attire. Their role-playing, dreams, and fantasies have masculine themes. A girl with GID may claim that she has a penis or will grow one.

Adults with GID are preoccupied with their desire to live as members of the opposite sex. They adopt the behavior, dress, and mannerisms of the other sex, and may wish to acquire the physical appearance of the other sex through hormonal or surgical treatments. They may spend much time cross-dressed and working on the appearance of being the other sex. Many individuals with this disorder convincingly pass in public as the other sex.

Differential Diagnosis

The differential diagnosis of GID depends on the age of the individual presenting for evaluation. In children, the overriding concern is the significance of the behavior leading to referral and the presence of impairment in social or other important areas of function. Special consideration should be paid to the parents' expectations and concerns. GID represents a profound disturbance in the person's sense of identity, not simply a child's nonconformity to conventional sex-role behavior. During adolescence, the differential diagnosis can be expanded to include a struggle, internally or externally, with homosexual impulses that may or may not be related to gender-atypical behavior.

In contrast to GID, transvestic fetishism occurs in heterosexual men for whom the cross-dressing behavior is for the purpose of sexual excitation. It is important to determine whether an intersex condition exists as this precludes a diagnosis of GID. "Intersex" is a general term that refers to a variety of conditions in which a person is born with mixed or ambiguous sexual anatomy. An intersex condition may be caused by the androgen insensitivity syndrome, congenital adrenal hyperplasia, mixed gonadal dysgenesis, and other disorders.

Regarding comorbidity, there is a predominance of internalizing psychopathology. Children with GID may manifest coexisting separation anxiety disorder, generalized anxiety disorder, and symptoms of depression. Adolescents are at risk for depression and suicidal ideation. Based on Child Behavior Checklist data, it was found that adolescents with GID had more emotional problems than children with GID. The evolution of symptomatology is probably related to the influence of social ostracism and poor peer relationships among teenagers with GID.

Zucker KJ, Bradley SJ: *Gender Identity Disorder and Psychosexual Problems in Children and Adolescents.* New York: Guilford Press, 1995.

Treatment

Treatment of children with GID should address, primarily, problems with social ostracism and conflicts associated with the disorder. Treatment should also be directed at any contributing or comorbid psychopathology. The best results occur when treatment is undertaken early, in a supportive, nonjudgmental but directive frame. Persistent conflicts seem much more likely to occur in children whose primary caregivers either passively or actively encouraged the atypical behaviors. Parents and therapists should be noncritical but clearly supportive of more conventional gender roles.

Most therapists work with the primary short-term goal of reducing gender identity conflict or gender dysphoria. Psychosocial treatments have included individual psychotherapy (to understand and resolve the factors that drive the wish to become the opposite sex) and parent counseling (to help the child feel more comfortable about being his or her biological gender). Parents should set limits on the child's cross-gender behavior and encourage sex-typical activities. Therapist and parents should encourage a same-sex peer group. Treatment has also included behavioral therapy, group therapy, and eclectic combinations of these approaches. There have been no comprehensive studies to show the comparative efficacy of these treatment approaches; however, all may have been beneficial to a degree.

Some therapists have attempted to prevent transsexualism (adult GID) or homosexuality. The development of heterosexual orientation is probably preferred by most of the parents, but there is no strong evidence for the effectiveness of treatment on sexual orientation. When parents request therapy of their child to prevent future homosexuality, the ethical approach is to inform them that it is not known that such treatment is effective. For adolescents and adults, the prevailing opinion is that treatment goals should foster the integration of a homosexual orientation.

Blanchard R, Steiner BW (eds): *Clinical Management of Gender Identity Disorders in Children and Adults.* Washington, DC: American Psychiatric Press, 1990.

Bradley SJ, Zucker KJ: Gender identity disorder: A review of the past 10 years. *J Am Acad Child Adolesc Psychiatry* 1997;36: 872.

Zucker KJ: Gender identity disorder in children and adolescents. In: Gabbard GO (ed). *Treatments of Psychiatric Disorders*, 3rd edn. volume 2, Arlington, VA: American Psychiatric Press, 2001, pp. 2069–2094.

Complications/Adverse Outcomes of Treatment

Treatment may have a bad outcome if therapist, parents, and child do not have approximately the same goals. For example, the parents may be determined that psychotherapy should protect the child or adolescent from becoming homosexual, while the therapist and the child himself may not be addressing that goal at all. It is possible that treatment of a youngster with GID might increase family conflict—as the patient assumes greater autonomy with less compliance to his parents' wishes—rather than reduce family conflict.

An adolescent with GID may use his psychotherapy as a way to insist that he should proceed with contra-sex hormonal treatment in preparation for sex-reassignment surgery. An inexperienced therapist might agree prematurely with that course of action, without fully considering and exploring less intrusive and less permanent options.

Prognosis

When GID is identified in childhood, it frequently remits. Only a very small number of the children referred for GID in childhood will have symptoms that persist as GID of adolescence or adulthood. When GID persists into adolescence and adulthood, it is usually with a homosexual orientation. Even when the GID itself does not persist into adolescence and adulthood, most individuals who previously had childhood GID will have a homosexual orientation as adults. The implication of these data regarding outcome is that early treatment of children with GID may reduce gender dysphoria and future transsexualism, but there is no evidence that early intervention will change homosexual orientation.

When GID is identified in adolescence, it is likely to continue to adulthood. Many adolescents with GID seek sex-reassignment surgery. The implication is that treatment of adolescents with GID is unlikely to change the individual's gender identity or sexual orientation. Treatment during adolescence should probably be geared toward integration and increased self-esteem in gender role and sexual orientation.

Psychological Reactions to Acute & Chronic Systemic Illness in Pediatric Patients

47

Barry Nurcombe, MD

■ PSYCHOLOGICAL REACTIONS TO ACUTE PHYSICAL ILLNESS OR TRAUMA

Regression is a normal reaction to acute physical illness. Physically ill children become more dependent, clinging, and demanding. Younger children may revert to bedwetting and immature speech. Preschool children may interpret the illness as a punishment for something they have done.

Younger children react to hospitalization with protest, if they are separated from, and perceive they have been abandoned by, their parents. Depression and detachment occur subsequently. These serious sequelae can be averted if a parent can stay with the child and help with daily care. Because all modern pediatric hospitals encourage parents to do so, the long-term effects of traumatic separation are seldom seen today.

Adolescents are most affected by acute illness if they see it as shameful, if they are immobilized, or if they have fantastic ideas about the cause or nature of the illness (e.g., that it was caused by masturbation).

Pain complicates adaptation to acute illness. A child's coping can be enhanced if a familiar person is present during a painful procedure; if the procedure is explained ahead of time (e.g., in play); if the medical attendant is truthful, calm, and efficient; and if appropriate reassurance and praise is offered by the physician and the parents after the procedure. If the child does break down emotionally during the procedure, the medical attendant or team must studiously avoid showing irritation or provoking guilt.

Younger children sometimes react to acute burn trauma with dissociation, and delirium may occur as a result of associated fever or tissue breakdown. Badly burned children are subsequently immobilized and exposed to repeated painful procedures (e.g., changes of dressing) and to plastic surgery, which may be required for years. The effect of disfigurement on self-esteem is discussed later in this chapter.

DELIRIUM

 ESSENTIALS OF DIAGNOSIS

DSM-IV-TR Diagnostic Criteria

A. Disturbance of consciousness (i.e., reduced clarity of awareness of the environment) with a reduced ability to focus, sustain, or shift attention.

B. A change in cognition (such as memory deficit, disorientation, language disturbance) or the development of a perceptual disturbance that is not better accounted for by a preexisting, established or evolving dementia.

C. The disturbance develops over a short period of time (usually hours to days) and tends to fluctuate during the course of the day.

D. There is evidence from the history, physical examination, or laboratory findings that the delirium is caused by the direct physiological consequences of (1) a general medical condition; (2) substance intoxication; or (3) substance withdrawal.

(Adapted, with permission, for *Diagnostic and Statistical Manual of Mental Disorders*, 4th edn., Text Revision. Copyright 2000, Washington, DC: American Psychiatric Association.)

General Considerations

Delirium is an acute or subacute, fluctuating, reversible derangement of cerebral metabolism, characterized by (1) impairment of attention, thinking, awareness, orientation, and memory, (2) illusions and hallucinations, and (3) reversal of the sleep–wake cycle. In children, delirium is most often encountered in infectious illness (particularly with fever), trauma (particularly in relation to burns or after cardiotomy), hypoxia, metabolic disturbance (e.g., acidosis, hepatic failure, renal failure), endocrinopathy (e.g., hypoglycemia), or intoxication (e.g., with drugs, pesticides, or heavy metals). In adolescents, withdrawal from illicit drugs or alcohol must be considered.

Clinical Findings

The full diagnostic evaluation of delirium requires physical and neurologic examination; a mental status examination; screening investigations (e.g., blood chemistry, blood count, urinalysis, toxicology screen, blood gases, electrocardiogram, chest X-ray); and discretionary investigations (e.g., electroencephalogram, computed tomography scan, lumbar puncture, specialized blood chemistries) directed by the clinician's diagnostic hypotheses. See Chapter 14 for a more detailed discussion of delirium.

Treatment

The treatment of delirium is directed at the cause. The child psychiatrist is likely to be called on to diagnose it, especially when the cognitive impairment is subtle and delirium has been mistaken for functional psychosis. Agitation can be alleviated with oral or intramuscular haloperidol, with the addition of small doses of lorazepam, if required. Good nursing and the presence of a parent can help to calm the patient.

Complications/Adverse Outcomes of Treatment

Managing disruptive behavior, particularly agitation and combative behavior, is the most challenging aspect of delirium therapy. If this is mismanaged, serious injuries can result.

Prognosis

The prognosis of delirium is dependent on its cause and the ability of the treatment team to prevent future episodes.

■ PSYCHOLOGICAL REACTIONS TO CHRONIC PHYSICAL ILLNESS

 ESSENTIALS OF DIAGNOSIS

DSM-IV-TR Diagnostic Criteria

A. *There is evidence from the history, physical examination, or laboratory findings that the psychiatric disorder is caused by the direct physiological consequences of a general medical condition.*

B. *The disturbance is not better accounted for by another mental disorder*

C. *The disturbance does not occur exclusively during the course of delirium*

(Adapted, with permission, for *Diagnostic and Statistical Manual of Mental Disorders*, 4th edn., Text Revision. Copyright 2000, Washington, DC: American Psychiatric Association.)

General Considerations

The factors that affect a child's response to chronic illness can be classified as follows: (1) factors in the child, (2) factors in the family, (3) factors related to chronic disease in general, and (4) factors related to specific diseases.

A. FACTORS IN THE CHILD

The child's age at the onset of a disease affects his or her psychological reaction. Preschool children are affected by hospitalization if they are separated from their parents. School-aged children are affected by being cut off from their peers and education and by forced immobility. Adolescents are particularly affected if the disease affects their body image or their capacity to relate to peers, especially if heterosexual relationships are interrupted or precluded.

The child's beliefs about the cause, nature, or prognosis of the illness may be inaccurate and interfere with coping. Children with oppositional defiant disorder may transfer their behavior to the medical condition, becoming noncompliant with treatment. This can be a serious problem, for example, in juvenile diabetes, hemophilia, or epilepsy. Other preexisting psychiatric disorders can interfere with coping. Illness can aggravate psychiatric disorders such as anxiety, depression, or disruptive disorders.

B. Factors in the Family

Parents should receive a full explanation of the cause, nature, treatment, and prognosis of the disease. They may have a false, unhelpful sense of responsibility for the illness, particularly if they are carriers of what proves to be a genetic disease. Some parents react initially with denial. Others react by becoming overprotective, by having unrealistic expectations for improvement, by withdrawing, or by rejecting and abandoning the child. Latent tensions between the parents can be aggravated and, at times, separation or divorce precipitated.

Parents with preexisting psychiatric illness, particularly affective disorder, borderline personality disorder, or substance abuse, are likely to have particular difficulty and to need special support. Significant is the quality of the attachment experiences the parents have been able to provide for the child as an infant, before the onset of the disease. If, because of parental inadequacy or extremes of infant temperament or both, the child experienced insecure or disorganized attachment, his or her adaptation to illness may be compromised.

The psychological health of siblings may be overlooked as a result of parental preoccupation with the physically ill child. Siblings may experience deprivation of attention, causing sadness and withdrawal or resentment and acting-out.

C. Factors Related to Chronic Disease in General

Parents find it particularly difficult to cope when the diagnosis is unclear. Similarly, a disease with a hopeless prognosis, such as metastatic osteosarcoma, puts severe stress on the family system. Some chronic diseases (e.g., sickle cell anemia) have intermittent episodes, causing the child and parents to be hypervigilant. Diseases that affect the child's physical appearance or for which the treatment is disfiguring (e.g., the cushingoid appearance caused by corticosteroid treatment) are particularly problematic for adolescents who may become noncompliant with treatment. Diseases that cause severe pain or require invasive treatment (e.g., intravenous chemotherapy for cancer) are also likely to produce adverse psychological reactions. Some treatments can have adverse neurocognitive effects (e.g., cranial irradiation for leukemia).

SPECIFIC DISEASES OR CONDITIONS

ASTHMA

Attacks of asthma can be triggered by a variety of allergic, infectious, physiologic, or psychological factors. Severely asthmatic children are at markedly increased risk of psychological disorder, particularly depression. Affective disorder and family dysfunction increase the risk of a fatal asthmatic attack. The use of corticosteroids and the limitations on activity caused by chronic asthma can impede academic and social functioning.

CYSTIC FIBROSIS

Individuals with cystic fibrosis, a chronic genetic disease, are now surviving into their 30s. Almost all the males are sterile. Pregnancy in women with cystic fibrosis carries a severe risk. One study identified one third of the children with this disease as emotionally disturbed. Eating disorders are more common in adolescents with cystic fibrosis. Family dysfunction and disease severity increase the risk of psychological disorder.

JUVENILE-ONSET DIABETES MELLITUS

Family dysfunction predicts poor diabetic control. About 18% of diabetic adults exhibit emotional disturbance, usually depression or anxiety; and about 50% of severely diabetic adults are so affected. About 36% of children with diabetes are depressed or otherwise disturbed. Fear of hypoglycemia or ketosis, resistance to dietary restrictions, tampering with insulin dosage, and even suicide attempts by insulin overdose have been reported. Poor diabetic control is associated with reading problems and with psychiatric disorder in the child or parent.

LEUKEMIA

Despite improved survival statistics, many children with leukemia exhibit the "Damocles" syndrome, the sense of living on borrowed time, not knowing when a fatal relapse will occur. Bone marrow biopsies, repeated hospitalizations, and chemotherapy can be frightening experiences. Cranial irradiation and intrathecal methotrexate can cause neurocognitive deficits.

HIV ENCEPHALOPATHY

In HIV encephalopathy, the neurologic disease progresses in parallel with the immunodeficiency. The disease follows one of three courses: subacute progressive, plateau type, or static. Subacute encephalopathy is associated with gradual deterioration and loss of function including motor impairment, apathy, loss of facial expression, emotional lability, and loss of concentration. In some patients the disease plateaus for months before the patient finally deteriorates. Other patients exhibit neurocognitive defects that do not progress.

HIV infection acquired from the mother is usually associated with an environment of social deprivation. Parental guilt is a common accompaniment.

Infection caused by contaminated transfusions (e.g., in hemophilia) often provokes parental rage against the source of the contamination. The psychiatrist's task is to keep the child in the mainstream as long as possible, help the family deal with guilt and anger, and prepare the child for the required hospitalization and medical procedures.

SENSORY IMPAIRMENT

When parents are apprised that their child is blind or deaf, they often experience grief. If they become depressed, the child may be affected by relative deprivation of attention. Both blind and deaf children are affected by the difficulty their parents have in establishing joint reference and shared attention (i.e., for parent and child to focus their attention, together, on an object). The prelinguistic games characteristic of normal children and their parents may be replaced by manual gestures.

Hearing adults and children have difficulty making social contact with deaf children. Blind children tend to be even more socially isolated. Although deaf children have been described as egocentric and impulsive, and blind children as introverted and dependent, it is not clear that these generalities are valid.

Blind children exhibit delayed acquisition of classification and conservation skills. Deaf children are slow to conserve; however, many deaf adolescents are capable of formal cognitive operations. Reading and writing are delayed in both groups. There is fierce controversy over whether oral methods or sign language should be used in teaching the deaf, whether oral language should be combined with signing, and whether deaf children should be mainstreamed into schools.

The prevalence of psychiatric disorder among the deaf has been estimated as 2.5–3 times that of those with normal hearing. Increased rates of psychiatric disorder have been found among students who attend residential schools for the deaf. Hearing-impaired children are at risk of physical and sexual abuse. The prevalence of psychiatric disorder among the visually impaired is less certain. One study estimated a prevalence rate of 45% (including 18.6% with mental retardation). There may be an association between retrolental fibroplasia and autism.

CEREBRAL PALSY

Most children with cerebral palsy have three or more disabilities (e.g., cognitive defect, epilepsy, communica-tion disorders, sensory impairment, orthopedic disorders, psychiatric disorder). Between 50% and 75% are mentally retarded. The prevalence of psychiatric disorder is 3–5 times as high as in control groups, but there is no typical psychiatric disorder. Children with organic brain dysfunction are more likely to develop psychiatric disorder. By the age of 4 years, children with cerebral palsy become aware that they are different from their peers, and they become increasingly aware of social rejection and limited prospects. Only 10% marry. By adolescence, their difficulties in forming social relationships and attaining independence are likely to have caused depression, anxiety, lack of confidence, low self-esteem, and in some adolescents, attacks of rage.

EPILEPSY

Epilepsy carries an increased risk of psychiatric disorder (e.g., depression, anxiety, conduct disorder, suicide). The risk is increased if other neurologic abnormalities are present. Epileptic adolescents are particularly affected by the stigma attached to having seizures in public. Phenytoin and phenobarbitone, which are used as anticonvulsants, can dull intellectual performance. There is controversy over the assertion that epilepsy is associated with violent behavior. One study showed that patients with temporal lobe epilepsy had an 85% prevalence of psychiatric disorder, particularly catastrophic rage and hyperkinesis. Another study suggested that the rate of psychiatric disorder in patients with temporal lobe epilepsy is no higher than in patients with other forms of epilepsy. About 10% of children with temporal lobe epilepsy develop a psychotic illness in adolescence or adulthood.

Fritz GK: Common clinical problems in pediatric consultation. In: Fritz GK, et al. (eds). *Child and Adolescent Mental Health Consultation in Hospitals, Schools, and Courts.* Washington, DC: American Psychiatric Press, 1993, pp. 47–66.

Ryan RM, Sundheim STPV, Voeller KKS: Medical diseases. In: Coffey CE, Brumback RA (eds). *Textbook of Pediatric Neuropsychiatry.* Washington, DC: American Psychiatric Press, 1998, pp. 1223–1274.

Williams DT, Pleak RR, Hanesian H: Neurological disorders. In: Lewis M (ed). *Child and Adolescent Psychiatry,* 3rd edn. Philadelphia: Lippincott Williams & Wilkins, 2002, pp. 755–766.

Whitaker AH, Birmaher B, Williams D: Traumatic and infectious brain injury in children. In: Lewis M (ed). *Child and Adolescent Psychiatry,* 3rd edn. Philadelphia: Lippincott Williams & Wilkins, 2002, pp. 431–447.

SECTION IV

Psychiatry in Special Settings

<table>
<tr><td>

Emergency Psychiatry

</td><td>

48

</td></tr>
</table>

Michael J. Sernyak, Jr., MD, & Robert M. Rohrbaugh, MD

Emergency psychiatry encompasses the urgent evaluation and management of patients with active symptoms. The definition of emergency is determined by the ability of the patient or the patient's social environment to tolerate these symptoms. Although these emergency evaluations are most commonly performed in hospital settings, mobile crisis teams permit completion of emergency assessment in community settings.

■ GOALS OF EMERGENCY PSYCHIATRY

The goals of emergency psychiatric care are similar to those of emergency medical–surgical care: (1) triage, (2) expeditious, pertinent assessment, (3) accurate differential diagnosis, (4) management of acute symptoms, and (5) appropriate discharge planning.

Triage

The triage function determines the degree of urgency of the patient's presentation and the initial pathway for evaluation of the patient. The triage clinician must first distinguish between situations that constitute a genuine emergency and those that, although perceived as such by the patient or others, can safely await later assessment.

Next, the triage clinician must correctly identify, among a variety of emergency situations, those that reflect a need for psychiatric evaluation as a first step. This is a critical decision as patients may have both medical and psychiatric complaints or exhibit behaviorial problems that may originate from a medical, neurological or substance induced disorder. A medical evaluation including a brief history of the presenting complaint and physical assessment including vital signs is a critical component of this triage function.

Lastly, the triage clinician must assure the safety of patients until they can be evaluated by a psychiatrist or other mental health professional. In emergency room (ER) settings where patients often present with severe injuries, it is possible to overlook the needs of a well-groomed patient arriving with no obvious disorder. However, this patient may have suicidal or homicidal ideation that can be as life threatening as any other medical emergency and requires immediate attention to ensure the safety of the patient and others.

While initial triage is most commonly undertaken by nursing personnel, the psychiatrist must assume an active role in the training and supervision of those clinicians and in the formulation of standards and clinical criteria applied during the triage "sorting" function. Triage is only as effective as the quality of the standards and the rigor with which they are applied.

Assessment

Assessment of psychiatric patients under emergency circumstances focuses on the need to quickly evaluate the pertinent aspect(s) of the patient's presentation, with special attention to potential life-threatening issues. Although the patient may have had an initial brief medical evaluation and triage to psychiatry, the clinician should continue to be alert to the possibility that the patient has a medical disorder or substance induced disorder underlying their presentation.

The clinician should assemble as much data as possible before addressing the patient directly. For example, if information suggests that the patient may be dangerous to themselves or to others, appropriate security arrangements should be made. For example, the patient may need to have a staff member be assigned to sit with them to assure safety or be searched for potential weapons.

During the initial moments of the direct encounter with the patient, the clinician should form an overall impression of the patient. This impression may include data from sources like the patient's level of consciousness, appearance, willingness to engage with the clinician, apparent mood, psychomotor retardation or agitation and initial conversation. This initial period of direct observation can be helpful in determining whether the patient has been triaged correctly or whether additional medical evaluation or security arrangements are required.

Despite the common pressure to proceed expeditiously, clinicians should attempt to be thorough in both their medical or psychiatric evaluations. Special attention should be focused on recent psychosocial stressors, which may have precipitated the patient's presentation in the ER. These stressors may include disruptions in housing and work or disruptions in important relationships, including romantic relationships, family relationships, and the patient's relationship with their current outpatient clinician. Events like an argument with a family member or friend, or the vacation of an outpatient clinician, can precipitate a patient's presentation for emergency treatment. Clinicians in emergency settings should include information from others in patient's life in their assessment; this collateral information may be quite pertinent to the overall evaluation of the patient.

The emergency assessment must include the presenting history and psychosocial stressors, past and current medical problems, current engagement in medical and psychiatric treatment, current medications and adherence to the medical regimen, history of past and current substance abuse, social history including the patient's living and financial arrangements and current status of significant relationships, physical examination (including neurological screening exam), mental status examination, and screening laboratory workup. This assessment will help determine what other appropriate laboratory, toxicology, or imaging studies should be ordered.

Diagnosis

The pressures of the emergency setting do not allow the detailed diagnostic assessment possible in other settings. However, the clinician should construct a differential

Table 48–1. Differential Evaluation

1 Is the disordered affect, thought, or behavior the product of detectable pathophysiology, especially that associated with a medical problem or substance-induced toxicity?

2 If not, is the disordered affect, thought, or behavior of psychotic quality, especially that associated with schizophrenia or manic states?

3 If not, is the disordered affect, thought, or behavior compatible with some other formal diagnostic entity, especially anxiety states, depression, or personality disorder?

4 If not, is the disordered affect, thought, or behavior contrived to obtain an advantage or to avoid an undesirable consequence (e. g., incarceration)?

diagnosis which can be utilized to guide further emergency evaluation. In constructing this differential diagnosis a high priority must be given to medical, neurological and substance induced etiologies of the presenting complaint. Table 48–1 lists four sequential questions that must be considered in making a differential diagnosis.

Initial Treatment

Treatment interventions, when appropriate as an emergency procedure, will usually follow the diagnostic assessment. However, sometimes the clinician must intervene before gathering all the diagnostic information. This is particularly true when the patient must be kept safe due to concern about being a danger to self or others. In most circumstances, emergency interventions will fall into one or more of four categories: Environmental management, medication, crisis intervention, and education.

A. Environmental Management

As noted above, clinicians must be attentive to providing a safe environment for patients. These interventions often occur before a full evaluation is completed. In addition to ensuring a safe environment, patients may benefit from having diminished stimulation in their environment. Availability of a "quiet room" is often helpful to reducing psychomotor agitation.

At times, modifying the home environment of a patient may avoid a hospitalization. Providing alternative short-term housing during a crisis, respite care for an elderly patient or emergency placement of a child can decrease the patient's symptoms.

B. Medication Interventions

Clinicians in ER settings should be careful about initiating pharmacological interventions for several reasons. First, initial diagnostic impressions may prove inaccurate.

Second, the full laboratory assessment of the patient may not be complete. Third, treatment with medications may produce sedation which can mask other signs of medical illness. Lastly, the clinician in the ER will likely not be treating the patient in follow-up. Therefore, in general, pharmacological interventions should be limited to those needed to help manage the patient in the emergency setting.

Clinicians in the emergency setting utilize medications like benzodiazepines and antipsychotics in order to manage symptoms of psychomotor agitation. The use of benzodiazepines like lorazepam may be appropriate treatment for severe anxiety or for agitation associated with alcohol or sedative withdrawal. Treatment with an antipsychotic like haloperidol is sometimes useful for treating psychomotor agitation in patients with acute psychotic states. When a patient is acutely agitated or threatening these medications can be given intramuscularly to minimize time of onset.

Giving a patient medication to manage symptoms until the patient is seen in outpatient treatment requires careful consideration of several factors including the patient's compliance, issues of safety, and the amount of time before outpatient follow-up care will begin. The possibility that the patient is seeking benzodiazepines or pain medication because of an addiction should be considered before prescription of benzodiazepines or narcotics. In general, patients should not be given more than a few days supply of medication at any one time.

C. CRISIS INTERVENTION

Psychological strategies based on a biopsychosocial understanding of the situation can often de-escalate a crisis. Such techniques include ventilation, identification of alternatives, clarification of interpersonal roles, interpretation of meaning, or simply empathic listening. Meeting with the patient and their family or significant other can help resolve difficulties that may have led to the patient seeking care in an emergency setting.

D. EDUCATION

An important but often overlooked component of treatment in the ER is the opportunity for preventive education. The patient, family members, significant others, and even other caretakers will sometimes benefit greatly from education about the disorder. For example a patient with new onset panic disorder may be able to avoid returning to the ER if sufficiently educated about the nature of their disorder. Clarification of the situation in a way that can avoids unwarranted guilt or confusion will be helpful to all involved. The patient and others important to the patient may avoid a sense of alienation, shame, and hopelessness by better understanding the diagnosed illness, its prevalence, and its prognosis.

Discharge Planning

Discharge planning from a psychiatric emergency depends on the resources that are realistically available. In general, at least four issues must be considered: (1) initial level of care, (2) the patient's willingness to seek treatment, (3) timing of initial follow-up care, (4) interval provisions, and (5) communication with the patient and subsequent caretakers.

A. INITIAL LEVEL OF CARE

As the most restrictive and expensive alternative, 24-hour inpatient care should be utilized only after careful consideration of several factors. Commonly accepted criteria for such care include mental illness associated with imminent danger to self or others, grave impairment of function to a degree that prohibits self-preservation in the most supportive environment available, and diagnostic uncertainty that could result in a lethal outcome.

Less restrictive alternatives include crisis housing with less intensive staff observation, partial or day hospitalization, and intensive or routine outpatient follow-up care. The objective is to provide the least restrictive level of care that meets the patient's clinical needs. The patient's ability to pay for different services is a factor which unfortunately can determine what follow-up care is able to be provided to the patient. In some settings, indigent patients may have access to more services than low-income patients without Title XIX entitlements.

B. THE PATIENT'S WILLINGNESS TO SEEK TREATMENT

A patient presenting for psychiatric treatment may not have been brought to the ER voluntarily. Frequently, the police or the family members bring an individual to the ER for treatment. If a determination is made that the patient requires inpatient level of care, and the patient is unwilling to be admitted, the clinician may need to initiate an involuntary hospitalization process. While the administrative processes vary in each state, licensed physicians are able to involuntarily admit patients who meet standards of suicidality, homocidality, or who are unable to care for themselves due to their mental illness.

In general, patients with psychiatric disorders have the same right to refuse treatment that patients with other medical conditions have. In most instances, if a patient in an ER does not meet legal requirements for involuntary hospitalization and is unwilling to seek outpatient care, the patient's decision must be respected. Patients who report not wanting outpatient treatment should be provided options for accessing care should they change their minds after discharge from the ER.

C. TIMING OF INITIAL FOLLOW-UP CARE

For patients interested in outpatient treatment, the discharge planning should include determination of the clinically permissible time interval before a less restrictive level of care is available. For example, a situation that requires urgent outpatient follow-up care should not be scheduled 2 or 3 weeks later.

D. INTERVAL PROVISIONS

If too much time will elapse before initial follow-up care can be scheduled, the patient and relevant others should be informed of what to do. In most cases, if a scheduled return to the ER is anticipated, the clinician who provided the initial emergency assessment is best prepared to handle return visits.

E. COMMUNICATION WITH THE PATIENT & SUBSEQUENT CARETAKERS

A breakdown in communication with clinicians providing outpatient care often frustrates the patient and can lead to nonadherence with the plan of care developed in the emergency setting. The precise discharge plan should be written out and given to the patient (and, when appropriate, to the family, significant others, and clinicians who will assume the patient's subsequent care). An opportunity to raise questions, seek clarification of details, and better understand the clinical rationale of the discharge plan should be a routine part of this process.

Equally important is, the timely communication with other professional caretakers who are to provide subsequent treatment. This communication should provide enough detail for other clinicians to begin active treatment with the patient. A smooth transition in care gives the patient a reassuring sense of continuity from emergency onset to final initiation of outpatient treatment.

■ SPECIAL CONSIDERATIONS IN EMERGENCY PSYCHIATRY

Four special issues merit special consideration in the setting of emergent psychiatric evaluation: Suicide, homicide and other violence, disaster psychiatry, and the medico–legal aspects of psychiatric evaluation and treatment in the emergency setting.

Suicide

Suicide accounts for about 30,000 deaths each year in the United States. The number of attempted suicides is many times larger. Up to 80% of individuals who commit suicide have seen a physician or other health care personnel within two weeks before their deaths; most often this health care professional was not in the mental health care field. Therefore it is extremely important that all health care professionals be alert to the signals of

Table 48–2. Suicide Risk Factors

Age (especially adolescents and older adults)
Marital status (suicide is more common among single, widowed, or divorced adults)
Sex (females attempt suicide more often than do males, but males succeed more often than do females)
Ethonicity (Caucasians are more likely to commit sucide than Hispanics, African Americans, or Asians)
Economic status (unemployment or economic reverses increase risk)
History of prior attempt
Family history of suicide
Recent separation or loss
Presence of a plan and available means to accomplish it
Lethality of an attempt (more lethal attempts increase risk)
Diagnosis (especially major depression, schizophrenia, alcoholism or other substance dependence, and borderline personality disorder)
Specific symptoms (especially command hallucinations, delusional thinking, and profound depression with hopelessness)
Lack of social support

distress and risk factors for suicide; this is especially true in emergency psychiatry where assessment of patients with suicidal ideation is a common occurrence.

Perhaps the single most important element in the assessment of suicidal risk is constant awareness of the possibility that it exists. The patient may make no direct reference to self-destruction unless asked; this question is of course an essential component of any emergency psychiatric evaluation. Assessment of risk factors known to predispose to suicide is one method to quantify the risk that the patient will attempt suicide (Table 48–2). However, many patients with serious mental illness, especially those with dual diagnosis (mental illness and a substance abuse disorder) will have many of the risk factors known to predispose to suicide. Clinical judgment and the patient's ability to work with the clinician to develop a treatment plan that mitigates certain stresses and risk factors will help determine whether the patient is able to safely leave the emergency evaluation setting or requires inpatient treatment. Clear documentation of the assessment, including risk factor assessment is critical in the evaluations of the suicidal patient.

Homocidal Ideation and Violence

The relationship between violence and mental illness is complex. Although intense media coverage of violence

Table 48–3. Homicide and Other Violence: Clinical and Epidemiologic Factors

Age (violent individuals tend to be young)

Sex (males predominate)

Criminality (some individuals violate social rules without significant psychological impairment)

History (physical or sexual abuse as a child, fire setting, or cruelty to animals)

Proposed victim is a family member or close associate

Environmental influence (violent subcultures beget violence)

Diagnosis (especially manic states, schizophrenia, alcoholism or other substance dependence, conduct disorder, antisocial personality disorder, and intermittent explosive disorder)

Specific symptoms (especially command hallucinations, agitation, and hostile suspiciousness)

perpetrated by patients with mental disorders can lead one to think that this is a common occurrence, it is important to note that more patients with serious mental disorders are more often victims of violence than perpetrators of violence. However, patients with severe mental illness, perhaps especially those with psychotic paranoid component, can act on their delusions that someone is going to hurt them or that they are being told to kill another person. As with the assessment of suicidal ideation, many clinical and epidemiologic factors need to be considered in the assessment of homicidal ideation or violence risk (Table 48–3). The clinician who is called upon to make an emergency assessment must be aware of the legal ramifications (see Chapter 50), he or she is best advised to approach the task with the admonition that justice is served best by thorough, objective, accurate assessment and documentation.

Disaster Psychiatry

In the aftermath of terrorist attacks and natural disasters interest in the psychiatric aspects of response to these events has grown. It is reasonable to expect that in future disasters people, communities, and governments will look to psychiatrists for leadership. While this is a rapidly developing field, some valuable lessons have already been learned. Broadly, successful responses to these situations should be shaped by the type of disaster and the affected populations. These will, of course, vary from situation to situation but an analysis in these terms can help to plan for appropriate initial and enduring responses. Among the different types of disasters are ones without warning (terrorist attacks, earthquakes), ones with some warning,

(hurricanes, floods), and those with potentially longer-term notice (infectious disease outbreaks). The impact of these events can be modified by such variables as intensity and duration of the event, number of people and particular sub-populations affected, degree to which those people are affected, and post-disaster response issues such as ongoing safety and available resources. Following a disaster, initial attention is frequently directed at "new" casualties or the population that is presumed to have suffered psychologically as a result of the disaster. And in fact, survivors of recent disasters have illustrated psychological morbidity associated with these events that have, at times, surprised responders. However, recent experience has also shown the need to address two other critical populations at these times. Responders have observed the pressing, and at times, overwhelming needs of those patients already receiving mental health treatment prior to the disaster. Some groups of patients, such as the severely mentally ill population, are particularly vulnerable to stress and can present in a decompensated state with records that can be inaccessible or destroyed. Lastly, the mental health needs of staff, both mental-health and nonmental-health providers, needs to be carefully monitored as they try to provide services to patients in dire need and under extremely trying circumstances.

Medico–legal Aspects of Psychiatric Care in Emergency Settings

Given the acuity of patient presentations and the frequent risk assessments being completed, attending to the medico–legal aspects of emergency psychiatry is of great importance. Clinicians working in emergency psychiatric settings must have access to legal advice and should have a low threshold to consult with legal counsel. Clear documentation of the patient's history, risk factors, and the clinician's decision-making process (including consultation with other clinicians and with legal counsel), and treatment plan is imperative.

A. INVOLUNTARY PATIENTS

As suggested above, patients may be brought to the ER by the police or by the family because of suicidal ideation, homicidal ideation or due to other aberrant thoughts and behaviors. Once in the emergency setting they may decide they do not want to consent for evaluation or for treatment. In general, if there is suspicion that a patient may be at risk of hurting themselves or others, common law principles would allow holding the patient until a full evaluation can be completed.

As noted above, all states have methods providing for involuntary hospitalization of patients evaluated to be at significant risk of injury to themselves or others. Clinicians working in these settings should be know how to apply these laws and what right of appeal patients may have.

B. CONFIDENTIALITY

Patients have the right to expect clinicians to respect the confidentiality of their communications. There are some circumstances in which common law and case law may support breaching patient confidentiality. One common circumstance involves a patient refusory to allow communication with an outpatient clinician. For example, the clinician may suspect a drug overdose and need to know the medications that the patient was taking. In this clear emergency setting, allowance would generally would be made under common law to proceed with contacting the outpatient clinician. In situations in which there is a less clearly life-threatening situation, the clinician may need to respect the patient's confidentiality and not contact the outpatient clinician.

C. DUTY TO WARN

If a clinician working in an ER believes that a patient poses a significant risk of injury to another person, and the patient leaves the ER before being admitted to the hospital inpatient unit, the ER clinician may be required to warn the individual thought to be at risk. This Duty to Warn stems from California case law, Tarasoff vs. Regents of the University of California (1976). This precedent has not been endorsed in all states.

■ MAJOR CLINICAL SYNDROMES

Patients with a variety of clinical syndromes may present in a health care setting for emergency psychiatric treatment (Table 48–4). The following sections discuss the disorders most commonly requiring emergency treatment.

GERIATRIC CONDITIONS

Assessment

Elderly patients presenting with a psychiatric emergency require careful medical assessment as coexisting medical disorders and medical treatments often precipitate psychiatric presentation. A thorough review of systems, a complete physical examination, and appropriate screening laboratory tests, including a urinalysis, are imperative in this age group. A medically oriented evaluative approach may be more effective than a traditional psychiatric one.

In addition to determining whether the patient may have any sensory deficits, the clinician should speak clearly and slowly to geriatric patients. When a cognitive

disorder is suspected, the clinician should ask short and simple questions in a straightforward manner, should repeat them as necessary and should strongly consider a collateral source to ensure the accuracy of the history.

Common geriatric emergencies include delirium, dementia, depression, and psychosis. Delirium and dementia may coexist with each other and with depression and psychosis (Chapter 14).

Delirium

Because Delirium is characterized by an acute change in mental status, presentation for emergency evaluation is not uncommon. Delirium is characterized by acute changes in concentration, which may be accompanied by other cognitive changes, perceptual changes like hallucinations or delusions and behavior changes like psychomotor retardation or agitation.

Delirium is a medical emergency that has a potentially fatal outcome; the possibility that the patient is delirious should be high on the differential list for all elderly patients presenting in the ER with an acute change in mental status or behavior. As soon as the clinician suspects delirium, a thorough medical evaluation should be initiated to determine the etiology. Urinary tract or other infections, onset or worsening of a medical or neurological condition, and adverse drug interactions, drug side effects (especially anticholinergic side effects) or drug intoxication secondary to an unintentional overdose related to cognitive impairment are all potential causes of delirium.

Dementia

Elderly patients with dementia are often brought to the psychiatric emergency setting with acute psychomotor agitation, including combativeness. If the psychomotor agitation is of new onset, delirium or pain must be suspected and the medical workup initiated. If no medical etiology is found, the possibility that the patient is in pain from constipation, urinary retention, fall or other source should be investigated. If no medical or pain source is identified, the patient may have had onset of a psychotic component to the dementia. If no psychotic component is present, the patient may have been upset by something or someone in the environment and have been unable to express their frustration except through agitation or combativeness. A careful review of the events precipitating the crisis may reveal the environmental issue needing to be changed.

Depression

Depressed elderly patients may minimize mood symptoms but exhibit marked diminishment in interest in activities. Suicidal risk is high in elderly white men

Table 48–4. Clinical Syndromes That May Present as Psychiatric Emergencies

Syndrome	Assessment	Dispositions
Geriatric syndromes	Review of systems Laboratory tests Look for delirium, delirium with dementia, depression, and psychosis	Inpatient care Collaboration with medical team High-potency neuroleptics (e. g., haloperidol, 0.5–1 mg orally or intramuscularly) for agitation
Substance abuse	Look for intoxication or withdrawal	Quiet environment Inpatient care for neuropsychiatric signs Lorazepam (1–2 mg intramuscularly or orally) or haloperidol (5 mg orally or 2 mg intramuscularly) for agitation
Psychosis	New onset versus exacerbation? Rule out substance abuse and medical illness Evaluate for compliance, dangerousness, and ADL	Inpatient care for new-onset psychosis, dangerousness, or severely impaired ADL Collaboration with outpatient team
Depression	Evaluate for suicidal risk, comorbidities, current stressors, and substance abuse	Inpatient care for suicidal risk, agitation, or substance abuse Collaborate with outpatient team
Mania	Evaluate for dangerousness and substance abuse	Inpatient care for psychosis, dangerousness, or substance abuse Lorazepam (1–2 mg intramuscularly) or haloperidol (1–5 mg intramuscularly) for agitation
Catatonia	Two subtypes: withdrawn and excited Look for schizophrenia, mood disorders, and medical disorders (e. g., using amobarbital, 500 mg, 50 mg/min intravenously)	Inpatient care Lorazepam (1–2 mg, intramuscularly or intravenously)
Acute anxiety states	Types include panic disorder, acute stress disorder, posttraumatic stress disorder, conversion states, dissociative states Evaluate for ADL	Inpatient care if ADL markedly impaired Lorazepam (1–2 mg orally or intramuscularly)
Personality disorders	Evaluate for substance abuse, legal history, relationships, "micropsychotic" episodes, mood changes, aggression, and comorbidities	Interdisciplinary treatment Focus on "here and now" issues
Neuroleptic malignant syndrome	Look for sudden onset, autonomic changes, neuromuscular changes, elevated CPK, and leukocytosis	Medical emergency Inpatient care: stop neuroleptic and provide supportive treatment (rehydration, antipyretic) Dantrolene (2–3 mg/kg) or bromocriptine (2.5–10 mg three times daily)

ADL, activities of daily living; CPK, creatine phosphokinase.

living alone and so assessment of risk and construction of a treatment plan must be especially carefully considered for this population.

Psychosis

Presentation with new onset psychosis in the elderly necessitates review for coexisting delirium or dementia. However, recent reports have emphasized that up to 10% of patients with a lifetime history of schizophrenia may have late life onset of illness.

Treatment and Discharge Planning

Because of the high likelihood of a coexisting medical illness, elderly patient presenting in the psychiatry emergency setting are best treated in collaboration with a medical team.

For patients with cognitive disorders, the highly stimulating environment of most ERs are difficult to tolerate. If available, these patients benefit from provision of a quieter, less chaotic environment.

Demented patients who present with psychomotor agitation or combativeness due to a frustration with their environment may be calm upon removal from their environment and transfer to the emergency setting. Clinicians in the ER should work with caregivers to determine what the precipitant might have been and determine how to mitigate that precipitant in the future. When possible, it is preferable for elderly demented patients to be returned to their home environment as admission to hospital itself can predispose the demented patient to worsening of their cognitive status. Knowledge of community resources like respite programs, adult day care, and visiting nurse agencies with psychiatric or dementia care expertise can aid in returning the patient to the community.

If an elderly patient remains agitated and or combative in the emergency setting, clinicians should make efforts to determine whether the individual can be managed with close staff attention, diverting the patient's attention to other topics by talking about family or reading a magazine together. Because of the high incidence of side effects in the elderly, medication management in the emergency setting should be avoided if possible. If medication is necessary to control physical aggression a low dose of an antipsychotic (e.g., haloperidol 1 mg) is usually preferable to benzodiazepines. Low-potency antipsychotics (e.g., thioridazine or chlorpromazine) should be avoided due to anticholinergic side effects, which can worsen or precipitate delirium.

ALCOHOL ABUSE

Assessment

Alcohol-related presentations are among the most common psychiatric emergencies. Presentations to emergency settings are most frequently associated with acute alcohol intoxication and withdrawal, including withdrawal delirium.

The clinical picture of intoxication generally depends on the patient's blood alcohol level (BAL) as determined by a breathalyzer test, but BAL cannot be used exclusively. In most jurisdictions, an individual with a BAL of 0.08–0.1 or greater is considered legally intoxicated. If a patient is intoxicated, the clinician must ascertain whether another chemical in addition to ethanol is related to the clinical presentation. A toxicology screen is essential. An intoxicated state is characterized by a combination of markedly maladaptive behavior or psychological changes and physical changes (e.g., slurred speech, ataxia, nystagmus, stupor, coma) that appear during or after alcohol ingestion.

Alcohol withdrawal delirium typically appears three days after cessation of or reduction in the context of heavy and extended alcohol use. It is characterized by a hyper adrenergic state, agitation, insomnia, gastrointestinal symptoms, hallucinations, hand tremors, and seizures.

Psychotic, mood, and anxiety disorders may be related to alcohol use. A thorough medical evaluation is warranted to exclude physical conditions that resemble intoxication or withdrawal.

Treatment and Discharge Planning

Patients with alcohol abuse often present with denial of their illness and should be interviewed in emergency settings in a manner consistent with the tenets of motivation enhancement. Clinicians should be knowledgeable about the availability of detoxification and treatment facilities in order to provide access to treatment if the patient is motivated. Patients presenting with alcohol abuse should have a physical examination including neurological exam to ensure the patient has not sustained injuries due to a fall or other accident while intoxicated.

A common and complex question is determining when a patient with alcohol intoxication or withdrawal is able to be safely discharged from the ER. After the BAL is below the legal limit for intoxication, the clinician must evaluate whether the patient continues to have significant mental or physical problems related to intoxication. If the patient is no longer acutely intoxicated, screening for other symptoms of psychiatric disorder like depression or psychosis and for the presence of suicidal or homicidal ideation should be completed. As substance abuse raises the risk of suicidal and violent behavior, a patient who exhibits these symptoms need to be evaluated and

Table 48–5. Evidence of Other Drugs of Abuse

Drug	Physical Findings	Psychiatric Findings
Amphetamines	Increased blood pressure, mydriasis	Euphoria, hypervigilance
Cannabis	Tachycardia	Anxiety, social withdrawal
Cocaine	Increased temperature, tachycardia, tremor	Euphoria, hypervigilance
Hallucinogens	Mydriasis, tachycardia, tremor	Anxiety, paranoia
Inhalants	Nystagmus, arrhythmia	Belligerence, apathy
Opioids	Miosis in intoxication, mydtiasis in withdrawal	Agitation, dysphoria
Phencyclidine	Nystagmus, increased blood pressure, arrhythmia	Labile mood, amnesia
Sedative-hypnotics	Decreased respiration, tremor	Aggression, mood lability

managed carefully, including consideration for inpatient treatment.

When possible it is preferable to discharge a patient with alcohol abuse or dependence accompanied by family or friends. Appropriate referral may include an outpatient detoxification or rehabilitation program, partial hospitalization, intensive or routine outpatient treatment, and Alcoholics Anonymous.

■ OTHER DRUGS OF ABUSE

Assessment

Clinical history, specific physical examination findings, and a Toxicology screen may offer evidence of other drugs of abuse (Table 48–5).

Treatment and Discharge Planning

The management of intoxication or withdrawal depends on the specific type of drug (Chapter 15). Associated physical and psychiatric symptoms must be factored into the immediate treatment plan in a manner similar to that described with alcohol abuse.

Chemical restraints (e.g., lorazepam or haloperidol), seclusion, or physical restraints may be needed to manage violent behavior associated with drug intoxication. It is rarely indicated to start opiate detoxification in the ER setting as withdrawl from opiates is not life threatening, and starting these agents may reinforce the idea that the emergency setting can be utilized at times when opiates are not otherwise available. The principles of outpatient referral are the same as for alcohol.

PSYCHOSIS

Assessment

A psychotic state may occur either as a completely new event or as the exacerbation or reactivation of chronic psychotic disorder (see Chapters 16 and 17). The distinction is important because new-onset psychosis frequently warrants hospitalization, whereas the chronic condition often can be managed readily in cooperation with an outpatient team. Because of the high frequency of substance abuse disorders among patients with psychotic disorders, clinicians should strongly suspect substance use as contributing to new onset or exacerbations of psychosis. Assessment should also consider the patient's medical condition; adherence with prior treatment recommendations including psychiatric medications; the severity of impairment in activities of daily living; the patient's dangerousness to self and others; the presence of delusions, command auditory hallucinations, or thought disorder; and impairment of judgment about potentially dangerous situations.

Treatment and Discharge Planning

New onset acute psychotic conditions generally require hospitalization. Command hallucinations with suicidal or homicidal intent or impaired judgment and evidence of dangerous behavior may warrant involuntary hospitalization. Severe psychomotor agitation or threatening behavior may require physical restraint or psychopharmacologic intervention (e.g., haloperidol or lorazepam by mouth or intramuscularly depending on the clinical situation and cooperation of the patient).

Determination of the most appropriate and least restrictive level of care should include consideration of inpatient treatment, partial hospitalization, and outpatient care. When outpatient follow-up care will suffice, attention must be given to appropriate inclusion of the patient's outpatient clinicians, case managers, family members and other caretakers in developing the outpatient care plan. Initiation or adjustment of antipsychotic medication may be indicated after collaboration with the outpatient clinician and necessary laboratory studies are completed.

DEPRESSION

Assessment

A common presentation to the psychiatric ER is a depressed patient with melancholic features and suicidal ideation or behavior (see Chapter 18 and the discussion on suicide earlier in this chapter). In addition to identifying current stressors and probing for a history of depression, the clinician must pay close attention to comorbid conditions such as medical illness, psychosis, substance abuse, anxiety, and personality disorders.

Discharge Planning

As noted previously in this chapter, an inpatient treatment is frequently the most appropriate setting for patients with significant suicidal ideation or attempt. The availability of a vigorous, reliable support system may allow a less restrictive alternative to be considered. Referral for outpatient follow-up care of a depressed patient with suicidal ideation requires forethought about many factors such as safety, availability of supportive monitoring, time interval to next visit, access to help in the event of recurrent emergency, and advisability of medication use. In general, the patient should not be given antidepressant medication in an ER setting as the prescribing clinician will not be able to provide follow-up and there is increasing evidence that some antidepressants may precipitate suicidal ideation, especially in adolescent patients. Small doses of anxiolytics or hypnotics to treat anxiety and insomnia may be utilized to diminish symptoms until the patient is able to connect with outpatient treatment.

MANIA

Assessment

The cardinal features of mania are elevation of mood or irritability and marked increases in goal directed behavior (see Chapter 18). Other frequently associated findings include grandiosity, pressured speech, flight of ideas, insomnia, increased psychomotor activity, social or economic indiscretion, and poor concentration. The manic patient generally does not initiate the search for help, but rather the people around him can no longer tolerate their behavior.

Assessment of the patient with bipolar disorder should include consideration of stimulant ingestion like cocaine, amphetamines, phencyclidine, and other medications like steroids. Cluster B personality disorder may also have mood instability which can be difficult at times to differentiate from bipolar disorder.

Discharge Planning

In the ER, a typical agitated patient with mania warrants immediate intervention. As in the case of acute psychosis, pharmacotherapy (e.g., lorazepam) with or without physical restraint may be required. Valproate or an atypical antipsychotic like olanzepine can be used as an alternative or adjunctively. The primary goal is to contain the patient's agitation as quickly as possible so that the patient may be transferred safely to an inpatient setting.

A clear-cut manic episode, especially if associated with psychotic symptoms, usually warrants inpatient care. A dual-diagnosis program should be considered when mania is associated with chemical abuse or dependence. Proper treatment of such comorbid conditions requires intervention other than the use of mood-stabilizing drugs.

CATATONIA

Assessment

Catatonia is a rarely encountered clinical syndrome characterized by either excitement or withdrawal. The excited type is characterized by extreme purposeless motor activity, the withdrawn type is characterized by negativism, mutism, rigidity, posturing, waxy flexibility, and stupor. Catatonia is an emergency situation that requires immediate assessment to ensure medical problems like encephalitis or other causes of delirium are not present. Neuroleptic malignant syndrome (NMS) (described later in this chapter) merits consideration as a cause of catatonia.

Treatment and Discharge Planning

A thorough medical workup must be pursued in order to ensure significant medical problems are not involved in the presentation. Inpatient care is warranted because dehydration can be a major complication. Lorazepam can bring about quick improvement.

ACUTE ANXIETY STATES

Assessment

Panic attack, acute stress disorder, adjustment disorder, posttraumatic stress disorder, conversion disorder, and dissociative states may lead patients to seek treatment in the ER (see Chapters 19, 20, and 21 for common presenting symptoms for these anxiety disorders).

Clinicians assessing patients presenting with anxiety disorders in emergency settings should be mindful of the events preceding the patient's presentation. For example, a patient with acute anxiety may not reveal to the triage staff that the precipitant for their anxiety was a traumatic event like an assault or a rape. Clinicians in psychiatry emergency settings should be aware of hospital protocols for counseling rape victims and managing evidence collection.

Treatment and Discharge Planning

Many patients with anxiety symptoms respond positively to supportive crisis oriented psychological interventions. Panic and other acute anxiety states respond favorably and quickly to a benzodiazepine such as lorazepam.

Most anxiety disorders can be managed on an outpatient basis with a balanced combination of pharmacotherapy and psychosocial interventions. A marked restriction of activities of daily living or other severe functional impairment may neccesitate inpatient care. Panic disorder patients, in the middle of a panic attack, may have suicidal ideation and have a higher than normal rate of attempting suicide. Reassurance that outpatient treatment can be efficacious and access to a benzodiazepam like lorazepam can usually help avoid inpatient hospitalization for these patients.

PERSONALITY DISORDERS

Assessment

Patients with Cluster B personality disorders frequently present in the ER after committing an impulsive act in the context of an interpersonal difficulty. The assessment of the patient with personality disorder can be made difficult by their mood lability, irritability, and use of defense mechanisms like displacement, projection and splitting.

Treatment and Discharge Planning

Identifying and managing one's own inner reactions to these patients and helping staff maintain therapeutic boundaries are key components to the treatment of patients with Cluster B personality disorders. A "here and now" approach, focused on resolution of the current stressor, is nowhere more important than in this clinical situation. The patient may frustrate clinicians utilizing this approach by refusing to provide permission to contact others important to resolving the presenting complaint. Evaluation of suicidal ideation is difficult in these patients as their mood instability and impulsivity means that a suicide attempt can be precipitated in response to an event that was difficult to predict. Comorbid substance abuse disorders are frequently present and

worsen these patient's impulsivity, making the assessment of suicidality even more difficult.

It is extremely important to be in contact with the patient's treating clinicians and other caregivers in order to enlist them in helping to devise a treatment plan for the patient. Inpatient treatment can be regressive for these patients and so under most circumstances should be avoided. However, at times, inpatient care is unavoidable due to the patient's clinical presentation. Clinicians in emergency settings should have ongoing collaborative relationships with clinical programs like dialectical behavioral treatment programs or case management programs that care for patients with severe personality disorders; these collaborations can minimize the disruptions and staff splitting that can occur when these patients make frequent use of emergency settings.

■ OTHER EMERGENT CONDITIONS

NEUROLEPTIC MALIGNANT SYNDROME

Assesment

NMS is a serious and potentially lethal symptom-complex. In NMS, three sets of symptoms appear very rapidly in response to antipsychotic (neuroleptic) treatment: (1) alteration in level of consciousness, (2) Autonomic symptoms like hyperthermia, tachycardia, labile hypertension, and tachypnea, and (3) neuromuscular symptoms like "lead pipe" muscle rigidity. Elevated creatinine phosphokinase level and leukocytosis are common laboratory findings. While the triad of altered mental status, muscle rigidity, elevated temperature, and hypertension should arouse the clinician's suspicion that NMS is present, the presence of even only one of these elements can be cause for concern. The syndrome can appear at any time, not only shortly after initiation of the antipsychotic.

Clinicians should evaluate the patient for other disorders, especially infections, which might be present.

Treatment

Antipsychotic medication must be stopped at once as NMS is frequently lethal. Supportive treatment like fluids, cooling blankets and medications to maintain blood pressure should be provided in a medical intensive care setting. The prescription of dantrolene or bromocriptine is indicated in situations where the patient is not responding to supportive interventions.

CONCLUSION

As in other fields of medical practice, patients present with urgent psychiatric symptoms that may be life threatening and require emergency evaluation. The first duty of a well-prepared clinician is to recognize which of those situations is more critical than others and then to identify correctly the pertinent problem(s) and to intervene appropriately. Central considerations include whether the patient presents an imminent danger to self or others and whether the patient has grave psychological or behavioral impairment that prevents the patient from living safely in the community.

Common interventions include safety precautions, astute observation, sensitive inquiry, consideration of unsuspected medical conditions, crisis oriented psycho-logical treatment, judicious use of psychopharmacologic agents, and referral to the most appropriate and least restrictive level of follow-up care. Not to be overlooked is the admonition that psychiatric emergency care should always be provided in a respectful manner, no matter how disturbed or disruptive the patient may be.

Allen MH (ed): *Emergency Psychiatry.* Washington, DC: American Psychiatric Press Publishing, Inc., 2002.

Lukens TW, Wolf SJ, Edlow JA, et al.: Clinical policy: Critical issues in the diagnosis and management of the adult psychiatric patient in the emergency room. *Ann Emerg Med* 2006;47(1): 79–99.

Slaby A, Dubin W, Baron D: Other Psychiatric Emergencies. In: Sadock B, Sadock V (eds). *Kaplan and Sadock's Comprehensive Textbook of Psychiatry*, Vol 2. New York: Lippincott Williams and Wilkins, 2005, pp. 2453–2471.

Consultation–Liaison Psychiatry

Catherine Chiles, MD, & Thomas N. Wise, MD

49

INTRODUCTION

Consultation–Liaison Psychiatry is a centuries-old field of medical practice and research that bridges the biological, psychological, and social domains of psychiatric and medical illnesses. Since 2003, it has been recognized by the American Board of Medical Subspecialties as the psychiatric subspecialty *Psychosomatic Medicine*, based upon its historical nomenclature. The practice of *Consultation Psychiatry* usually occurs within general hospital settings. The standard consultation is performed at the request of the primary clinician, and is a neutral collaboration with colleagues and patients in nonpsychiatric settings. Interview techniques in consultations may be open-ended for an individual patient's diagnostic evaluation or structured to screen for psychiatric disorders in a general population. Often a combination of both techniques is utilized. A central role of the consultation psychiatrist is to educate colleagues and patients about the psychiatric presentations or complications of medical illness and about illness behavior. *Liaison Psychiatry* expands the role of the psychiatrist to facilitate comprehensive treatment approaches within a system of care and to enhance communication among disciplines and across divisions in health care systems. The liaison psychiatrist is often a member of a multidisciplinary care team, performing psychiatric screenings, for example in organ transplant surgery or oncology, when the risks of psychiatric comorbidity are expected to be higher.

History of Psychosomatic Medicine and Consultation–Liaison Psychiatry

A. History of Psychosomatic Medicine

In the United States, the historical roots of psychiatry in the general hospital are found in the 1751 charter of the Pennsylvania Hospital, which provided for the care of "persons distempered in mind and deprived of rational faculties." At that time, outpatient psychiatric clinics both in the Philadelphia Hospital and New York's Bellevue Hospital were developed. Reports from these early centers contain themes emphasizing the significant rates of psychiatric disorders in medically ill patients, and the need to integrate services.

In the modern era, the scientific approach to the relationship between psychiatric disorders and medical illness began with early studies in *psychosomatic medicine* which examined the relationship between psychological and medical disorders. Psychosomatic medicine as an area of research began with *psychoanalytic* studies of the mind–body relationship. Beginning in 1900, Sigmund Freud, as a young neurologist, described conversion hysteria as psychological symptoms imbued with deep psychic meaning, which manifested as or *converted* to somatic (physical) illness. In 1910, Sandor Ferenczi related conversion symptoms to the autonomic nervous system. In 1934, Franz Alexander proposed that 'psychosomatic symptoms' were due to prolonged autonomic system arousal linked to repressed psychic conflict. Psychosomatic medicine advanced in the 1940s and 1950s with *psychophysiological* studies such as those by Hans Selye who described the human stress response in relation to adrenocortical hormones. *Sociocultural* researchers Thomas Holmes and Richard Rahe in 1975 linked disease likelihood to the severity and number of stressful life events, and further expanded the psychosomatic medicine framework. Zbigniew Lipowski in 1970 and George Engel in 1977 utilized *systems theory* to examine environmental influences on the mind–body–culture paradigm. All these works have shaped the *biopsychosocial perspective* of psychosomatic medicine extant today.

B. History of Consultation–Liaison Psychiatry

Concurrent with the development of psychosomatic medicine theories, psychiatrists returned to the general hospital they had left during the late 19th century asylum movement. No longer isolated in psychiatric sanatoria or cloistered in consulting rooms, psychiatrists had begun to treat patients in general hospitals. In 1929, George Henry advocated the benefits of general hospital psychiatry that offered consultative services, and was instrumental in the advancement of consultation practices. In addition to the emphasis he placed on the diagnosis and treatment of psychiatric disorders seen in the medically ill, such as delirium, dementia, depression, and anxiety, he recognized that medical students and residents were more likely to utilize psychiatry for patients in medical settings rather than in isolated psychiatric facilities. Psychiatric consultation services developed further with support from the

Rockefeller Foundation and grew with funding from the Psychiatry Education Branch of the National Institutes of Mental Health. By the end of the 20th century, there was a significant cadre of trained consultation–liaison psychiatrists working within hospital settings and medical schools.

C. PSYCHOSOMATIC MEDICINE AS SUBSPECIALTY OF PSYCHIATRY

In May 2003, the American Board of Medical Subspecialties recognized the practice of consultation and liaison psychiatry in the general hospital as a discrete psychiatric subspecialty that requires advanced training and qualification by an examination conducted by the American Board of Psychiatry and Neurology. In recognition of its earliest scientific bases, the subspecialty was named Psychosomatic Medicine by the American Board of Medical Subspecialties to distinguish it from other consult practices in medical subspecialties. In June 2005, the American Board of Psychiatry and Neurology administered the first examination to certify subspecialists in Psychosomatic Medicine. Psychiatric fellowship training programs in *Psychosomatic Medicine* qualify physicians in the *skills and techniques* of consultation–liaison psychiatry within the *domain* of psychosomatic medicine and related research.

Is There a Need for Consultation–Liaison Psychiatry and Psychosomatic Medicine?

A. EVIDENCE FROM NONPSYCHIATRIC SETTINGS

How does the work of a psychiatrist in a nonpsychiatric setting improve patient care? Numerous studies in the past decade have demonstrated that psychiatric consultation contributes to *reduced costs* in health care delivery, and improves *access to mental health care.* Most importantly, psychiatric consultation improves the *detection* of psychiatric illnesses, many of which are life threatening. It is well known that, left undetected and untreated, psychiatric comorbidity increases hospital lengths of stay (and concomitant costs), even when demographics, medical diagnosis, and reasons for admission are taken into account.

Many studies have shown that patient outcome is markedly affected as a consequence of under-recognized or misdiagnosed psychiatric illness in nonpsychiatric settings. In primary care, where most patients with psychiatric illness present, the vast majority of patients do not receive treatment for psychiatric illness. Many factors collude in the limitation of care: Psychiatric symptoms are difficult to distinguish from medical symptoms; patients fear stigma and minimize complaints; time constraints, or inadequate training or the primary physicians' reluctance to stigmatize the patient may impede them from treating psychiatric symptoms.

Studies clearly demonstrate that psychiatric consultation in the hospital lowers morbidity, mortality, length of stay and cost through the earlier recognition and treatment of psychiatric disorders, and has an impact on quality of life measures of self-care. These findings mandate psychiatric education of colleagues, case-finding through psychiatric screening, and expansion of services by the consultation–liaison psychiatrist.

B. EVIDENCE FROM RESEARCH IN PSYCHOSOMATIC MEDICINE

Psychosomatic medicine was first popularized when psychoanalytic theories of mind–body relationships suggested that psychotherapy could modify the course of medical disease. Although speculative, such theories posited that early life experiences (fostering unconscious conflicts) coupled with genetic (biological) vulnerability could cause disease states such as peptic ulcer or asthma. Although many of these ideas were erroneous, there is significant data in both animal and human research to demonstrate an effect of early life experiences on physiology and illness behavior.

Modern psychosomatic research has abandoned much of these early theories, but continues to investigate the role of psychosocial variables in causing or maintaining disease states. It utilizes a variety of empirically based strategies; as an example, structured psychiatric interviews and reliable psychometric inventories are paired with biologic probes and immunologic measures to answer complex questions about the interrelationship between psychosocial and biologic variables.

An example of current research is the study of the biopsychosocial relationship between depression and cardiovascular disease. Landmark research in psychosomatic medicine beginning in the 1980s has revealed that individuals with major depressive disorders have significantly increased mortality risk following uncomplicated myocardial infarction (MI). The depressive episode often predates the acute coronary syndrome and is not a mere "reaction" to the cardiac event. Hostility and anger have been implicated in acute coronary syndromes. Biological factors that play a role in the genesis of coronary artery disease in depressed individuals include reduced heart rate variability, platelet dysfunction, and elevated cytokines. A shared genetic vulnerability for depressive disorders and cardiovascular disease underpins these truly psychosomatic relationships. The advent of sophisticated genetics and molecular biology holds the promise that such relationships will be further elucidated.

Chapter Overview

This chapter will consider the techniques, settings and core concepts of Consultation–Liaison Psychiatry and Psychosomatic Medicine. At present, the general practice of the consultation–liaison psychiatrist includes the recognition and management of the following: (1) the impact of psychiatric disorders on medical illness, (2) comorbid psychiatric and medical disorders, (3) the etiologic role of medical illness in psychiatric disorders, (4) suicidal, homicidal, and violent behavior in medical-surgical settings, (5) legal and ethical principles in the psychiatric care of the medically ill, (6) pharmacological and therapeutic intervention in comorbid illnesses, (7) behavioral responses to medical illness, and (8) the physician–patient relationship.

The chapter will condense Consultation–Liaison Psychiatry and Psychosomatic Medicine into two sections: Clinical Consultations and Core Concepts in Psychosomatic Medicine. The first section on *Clinical Consultations* presents the standard skills and techniques utilized by practitioners in a general hospital, organized as follows: consultation–liaison psychiatry basics; diagnostic evaluation skills; screening techniques to identify psychiatric patients in general populations; consultation treatment; legal issues; emergency assessments; and finally, liaison psychiatry. The second section *on Core Concepts in Psychosomatic Medicine* presents the general conditions that the consultant is likely to encounter. These Core Concepts of diagnosis are based upon the framework proposed by Lipowski in 1967:

1. Psychiatric Disorders Caused by Medical Conditions
2. Psychiatric Disorders Affecting Medical Conditions
3. Psychological Reactions to Medical Illness
4. Somatic Presentations of Psychiatric Disorders

For detailed discussions of specific psychiatric diagnoses and treatments, the reader will be directed to relevant chapters in the book. A concluding section suggests future directions for clinical practice and research in the field of psychosomatic medicine.

■ CLINICAL CONSULTATIONS

Consultation–Liaison Psychiatry Basics

The psychiatric consultant should serve as an ally to patient care provided by the physician (or primary team), the associated health care disciplines, and the system of care. In this alliance, *adaptability* and *diplomacy* enhance the care provided by the psychiatric consultant.

Adaptability is necessitated by the challenge of working in a general hospital. The modern hospital is a busy and crowded environment that usually limits privacy and is often unfamiliar to both patients and mental health professionals. Many hospital floors do not have interview

rooms. Medical treatment rooms are often not conducive to psychiatric interviewing. Evaluations may have to be performed in hospital rooms occupied by other patients. Thus, the consultant must be both practical and flexible. Speaking in a soft voice to allow confidentiality is sometimes the only option. Patients may be critically ill and attached to devices such as intravenous lines, catheters, and respirators. If a patient cannot speak due to a tracheotomy or attachment to a ventilator, a signing board or pad and pen may be necessary. The interview may be interrupted by medical or nursing staff, or by transport personnel for ad hoc procedures. Patients may be obtunded or unable to give a comprehensive history; use of other sources of information is often necessary but raises concern about the right to privacy. Such issues challenge the consultant but also establish the psychiatrist as a physician with unique skills necessary in modern healthcare teams.

Diplomacy in consultation is rarely discussed but inherently useful in practice. It is based upon the following qualities: awareness of the hierarchical and multidisciplinary nature of health care systems; respect for the roles and tasks a provider within a system assumes or is required to perform; regard for the boundaries or limitations of care, whether internal or external to the provider or system, affecting the patient's experience (e.g., economics determining hospital length of stay); and a collaborative or altruistic spirit that bolsters the care by the primary team through education and altered practice patterns. Examples of these qualities are the implementation of psychiatric care for organ transplantation patients and development of psychiatric screening in primary care settings. Consultation psychiatrists are ambassadors for the profession of psychiatry in large health care settings where communication between specialists can be limited.

Diagnostic Evaluation in the General Hospital

Consultations requests may have many origins and serve varied needs for the patient, team and system of care. Requests can be made by the patients, primary providers, multidisciplinary teams, and by the family members. Requests can arise when a physician ponders the clinical status of the patient in regard to mood or affect (e.g., depressed after surgery), cognition (e.g., ability to make medical decisions), or behavior (e.g., agitated or threatening). Requests may seek assistance anywhere along the continuum of diagnosis, evaluation, treatment and management. They may focus on a particular aspect of care, such as suicide risk assessment, or be more general in scope, such as the evaluation of a patient's reaction to medical illness.

Contacting the referring provider is important to understand the broader nature of the consultation request. The personal history of a psychiatric *disorder* may prompt a request for evaluation, although the consultant often is the first psychiatrist to evaluate the patient, even when the patient has a prior history of psychiatric *symptoms*. Some requests are urgent (e.g., "wants to leave against medical advice") in which case contacting the referring clinician can provide important information to expedite the consultation. Often, a simple request such as asking for help in treating depression is really "the tip of the iceberg" heralding broader psychosocial difficulties within the patient and social system. Contacting the referring provider is the best way to elicit the "real story" behind the consultation request.

Collection of behavioral data from primary sources (nurses, medical students) is the next step. Prior to seeing the patient, consultants discuss the patient's status with nursing personnel who know the patient and are able to share observations regarding the patient's clinical status and interaction with family members. Nurses' notes are a trove of information about patient behavior (e.g., "lost returning from the bathroom") that can guide the review. Medical students also can offer keen observations of patient behavior.

Review of medical records can be approached in the manner of detective work. A discerning review of *medical notes* provides clues to the patient's behavior, cognitive status, and physical function. Admission summaries and off-service summaries are concise records from which to obtain a time-line for the hospital course. Pertinent laboratory results and medication records reveal underlying medical conditions or areas that need further investigation. If the consultant is not clear about a medical illness, a review of the condition from available medical texts is done.

The review of medical records should search for *medication that acts on the central nervous system* (CNS), whether intended or as a side effect, and look for possible drug interactions (e.g., through cytochrome isoenzyme substrates and inducers). Substance-induced psychiatric disorders are common, not only for substances of abuse but also for prescribed medications (e.g., steroid-induced psychosis). In addition, a sedating (e.g., benzodiazepine) or activating (e.g., beta-agonist inhaler) medication administered prior to the evaluation can affect the assessment.

Review of pertinent *laboratory investigations* is informative. Metabolic derangements and end-organ disease can affect cognitive status. Awareness of the physiological status can focus the consultation examination and aid in the differential diagnosis. Radiological studies can hone the assessment.

Consent to interview the patient is obtained ideally by the primary team, prior to the consultant's interview,

and this can be verified with the patient. The consultant should obtain permission from the patient to conduct the interview and to communicate findings with the treatment team. The consultant should adopt a neutral stance in order to increase patient participation. This way, the consultant is obtaining consent neither as a member of the medical team nor as a patient advocate. Patients with a prior psychiatric history may anticipate that individual psychiatric treatment is confidential; thus they should be alerted to the consultant's role, particularly the need to confer with the primary team on the patient's behalf.

Diagnostic interviews aim to gather sufficient information to develop an answer to the consultation request. Following the preliminary actions described, the consultant introduces himself or herself as a psychiatric physician. Firstly, ascertain whether the patient has been told that a psychiatric consultation has been requested. If the patient has not been informed, elicit his or her feelings about it and request permission to conduct the interview. Secondly, it is important that the patient be given privacy to speak openly to the psychiatrist. For this reason, it is better if a visitor or family member is excused from the interview. Even when assurances are offered by the patient to allow their involvement, privacy can be presented as a matter of policy for the initial interview. Patients are often in a vulnerable position and unable to ask openly for privacy; the psychiatrist should assume responsibility.

The approach to the interview must be guided by immediate safety concerns in emergent evaluations; this may require restricting the interview to a focus on acute intervention and behavioral management, as is discussed in more detail in II. F. Emergency Consultations (see also Chapter 48). Often, a consultation is requested to assess the patient's level of anxiety or depression. The underlying task may be to assess how the patient is *adjusting to an illness*. A range of inquiries can provide an understanding of the patient's capacity to cope:

When and how was the disease diagnosed?

Were there delays in coming to treatment? Was there patient denial? Were there limitations to access?

How has the patient reacted to the treatment, medical or surgical, and to the primary team?

Have any medications been particularly difficult to take? Have any helped?

What knowledge does the patient have of others with similar disorders?

What has been the psychosocial and financial burden of the disease?

Has the illness forced changes in family roles and responsibilities? Is there a confidante?

Is there a support system? Is there neighborhood/religious/cultural/community support?

Does the patient have an accurate understanding of the prognosis? How does it affect the reaction to the illness?

Are there end-of-life issues that the patient is unable fully to address? Do supports know about the situation?

Some consultations focus on *cognitive capacity* and whether an individual has dementia or delirium. This mandates careful attention to the nursing notes and understanding the effects of the underlying disease process or medication upon the CNS. A careful assessment of mental status is required for all patients, allowing for detection of psychopathological phenomena, affective symptoms, and cognitive integrity. Many patients fluctuate in their ability to attend; serial examinations can provide a more accurate assessment. Some patients are fearful that they will be judged "crazy" if they are experiencing hallucinations (e.g., due to medications such as opioids). Active inquiry about whether the patient has been confused or uncertain about their situation allows them to reveal their cognitive problems. Formal testing for cognitive status via the Folstein Mini-Mental Status Examination (MMSE) provides a baseline cognitive assessment for the initial evaluation; the score is easily recognized by other specialists, and can be followed serially.

General *review of symptoms* from the domains of mood, anxiety, psychosis and substance use should be elicited. Even when they are not the focus of the consultation request, they may inform differential diagnosis and treatment plans. A detailed discussion of the principles of interviewing is discussed elsewhere (see Chapter 4). Frequently, in medically ill patients, symptoms of prior concern to the patient are not reported to the primary team for a variety of reasons, whether omitted by the patient or missed by the team. The psychiatric consultant offers the patient a new opportunity to be heard, and can serve also as a medical translator. If possible, the patient should give verbal consent during the interview to contact other sources of information.

Collateral information is important in situations in which the patient is unable to communicate accurately (e.g., altered consciousness, unreliable historian, cognitive impairments). The sources include spouse, family members, friends, case managers, or outpatient providers. The consultant must protect the patient's privacy; ideally patients can give consent to speak with others, but this is not always possible if the patient is impaired. In emergency situations, collateral information obtained from other sources can be vital, even if the consultant cannot provide information in return. Communication with family members can be essential. Reports from family members may differ from that of the patient

and highlight problems. It is common to see elderly patients who consider that they can return to independent living arrangements while family members report numerous reasons to the contrary. Some patients deny substance abuse while family members contradict them. It is also useful to ascertain the patient's past adherence to treatment.

Consultation reports should summarize the data collected in a clear and legible manner; electronic charting is ideal for cogent communication. If consultations are dictated, put a brief note in the medical record immediately following the consultation with diagnostic or treatment suggestions that can be considered immediately. If time permits, a concise yet thorough summary of findings, expressed in an organized, standard format is indicated (see Fig. 49–1). Differential diagnoses, diagnostic workup, symptomatic treatment and, in most cases, cognitive capacity are documented. When the consultant seeks to narrow the differential diagnosis, it should be communicated to the treatment team that further investigations such as neuroimaging or specialized laboratory investigations are required (see Fig. 49–2).

Recommendations include further testing and medication advice. When psychopharmacologic recommendations are included it is essential to outline side effects that may occur, since the referring provider or treatment team may not be aware of them. The medically ill patient is particularly sensitive to drug side effects, and may tolerate only a reduced dose. Over-sedation may lead to aspiration while eating, and drug–drug interactions can cause toxic side effects. The consultant should warn about possible problems in the consultation report and in person with the consulting provider. Working with nurses and allied health professionals to ascertain the behavioral effects of medications is within the scope of consultation practice. Recommendations to assist with psychiatric disposition and capacity to live independently may rely on collaboration with social work services and liaison with outpatient mental health providers. Recommendations regarding cognitive status may include referral to or liaison with social workers or legal counsel, in accordance with hospital policies and local statutes. Consultation psychiatrists should be informed about the policies and laws that protect patient rights in every setting (see Chapter 50).

Discussions about end-of-life issues commonly arise in the medical setting, often when discussing the patient's coping strategies. Hospitalization itself can evoke fear in a seriously ill patient who is unprepared for death. Others may seek relief from suffering and express a passive wish to die interpreted by staff as suicidality, prompting a psychiatric consultation request. Family histories may reveal an early demise from a condition similar to that of the patient, causing the patient to be concerned about

	Demographic Data
	Reason for Consult
	History of Present Illness
	--- mood/anxiety/psychosis/cognition/substance (review of symptoms)
	--- acute stressors
	--- threats to safety
B	Past Medical History (especially comorbid illnesses)
I	Family History (illnesses that recur in generations)
O	Substance Use History
P	Past Psychiatric History
S	--- challenges to medical adherence
Y	--- prior admissions
C	--- suicidal or violent acts
H	--- psychiatric disorders affecting (or caused) by medical illness
O	--- treatment history
S	Social History
O	--- childhood development, including early losses
C	--- level of education (validity of mental status exam)
I	--- military experience (exposure to trauma)
A	--- marital/family supports (community/religious/cultural)
L	--- socioeconomic stressors (finances/ housing/ access to care)
E	Physical Examination (targeted according to presentation)
X	Vital Signs
A	Laboratory Investigations (see Fig. 49–2)
M	Mental Status Examination
	Impression
	--- differential diagnosis
	--- diagnostic work-up
	--- symptomatic treatment
	--- safety and decision-making capacity assessments
	Recommendations

Figure 49–1. Standard format for consultation note.

the current situation. This psychological connection may not be readily identified by the patient but expressed behaviorally, for example by a refusal of procedures reminiscent of the deceased's medical course. A review of the patient's expectations for the future should be included in the initial diagnostic interview, although rapport should be developed sufficiently for the patient to explore his or her own mortality; premature introduction of a discussion of death may be unnecessarily alarming and better deferred to a follow-up session.

Follow-up of the patient is provided in collaboration with the treatment team, and the frequency of contact determined by the patient's clinical status. For example, a patient experiencing delirium while the team conducts a search for the underlying causes may require daily mental status examinations by the psychiatric consultant to monitor progress. Alternatively, a patient unable to make decisions regarding a procedure may require little or no follow-up once a surrogate decision-maker has been identified. Follow-up after the initial consultation may allow

the consulting psychiatrist to determine whether there should be changes in the initial recommendations. Each contact should be documented.

Screening Techniques to Identify Psychiatric Patients

In comprehensive medical and surgical care, often in outpatient settings, screening for comorbid psychiatric disorders can be time-efficient and cost-effective. Screening tests help nonpsychiatrists to uncover a symptom profile that heralds the need for evaluation by a psychiatrist. Screening tests are not a substitute for a psychiatric interview, but serve as a technique for *early detection.*

Endorsement of psychiatric symptoms may be elicited by self-administered patient questionnaires or by clinician-administered, structured interviews. Although myriad questionnaires are available, the self-administered questionnaire that is well standardized to detect depression, anxiety, and alcohol use in the primary care

CBC/differential
Electrolytes
BUN/creatinine
Glucose
Oxygen saturation
Liver function tests
Electrocardiogram
Chest X-ray
Calcium, Magnesium, Phosphate
Thyroid function tests
Cyanocobalamin/Folate
RPR/VDRL
HIV
Electroencephalogram
Head CT/MRI

Figure 49–2. Common diagnostic laboratories/investigations.

setting is the PRIME-MD Patient Health Questionnaire (PHQ). The PHQ-9 screens for depression and is available through its initial publication. The PHQ-2 is an abbreviated, standardized subset of the PHQ-9 that screens for depression in a general population, with high sensitivity (0.83) and specificity (0.92). The PHQ-2 is often added to a battery of health care questions completed in the outpatient waiting room. The Folstein Mini-mental State Examination (MMSE), a structured, clinician-administered screen for dementia, is available through its initial publication. The MMSE is used in screening for cognitive disorders such as delirium, but is standardized only for dementia. The Mini-Cog is an abbreviated, standardized test that utilizes the 3-object recall item of the MMSE combined with the Clock Drawing Test; it has comparable sensitivity and specificity to the MMSE but taps additional regions in the brain. The CAGE questionnaire, a simple screen for detecting alcohol use is utilized by psychiatric and nonpsychiatric clinicians, and can prompt referral to substance treatment programs (see Chapter 15).

If the patient requires further evaluation after a positive screening questionnaire, referral to the psychiatric consultant is the next step. Patients reluctant to seek care in a psychiatric clinic may agree to evaluation by the consulting psychiatrist who, as a member of the primary care team, avoids the stigma of psychiatric referral. Consultation psychiatrists assist primary physicians who manage general psychiatric disorders directly and reserve referrals to psychiatric care for patients who are acutely ill or require a complicated medication regimen. There are good reasons for these strategies. Even though medical conditions, especially chronic conditions, increase the likelihood of a psychiatric condition, a minority of patients with a psychiatric disorder will be evaluated by mental

health specialists. Moreover, half of all visits to physicians by patients with diagnosable psychiatric disorders occur in primary care clinics, and primary care physicians write most of the prescriptions for antidepressants and anxiolytics.

Psychiatric care provided in the medical setting *in situ* searches for untreated psychiatric patients. Psychiatric care within the setting of primary care closely resembles diagnostic evaluations in the general hospital in that it involves the direct collaboration with the primary provider in the treatment of comorbid medical and psychiatric conditions. However, in response to early detection, whether through screening or by the astute primary provider, psychiatric consultation in primary care settings serves a greater number of psychiatric patients than in general psychiatric settings.

Treatments in Consultation Psychiatry

A. Psychopharmacological Treatments

Special considerations are necessary in the treatment of medically ill patients with psychopharmacologic agents. The pharmacokinetic and pharmacodynamic properties of medications and the underlying clinical status of the patient are germane to the consultant's practice. A search for the cause of psychiatric symptoms is essential, but it also raises concern for the complex variables that affect the medicated, medically ill patient.

Pharmacokinetic changes in *absorption, distribution, metabolism*, and *excretion* often modify choice of agent and dosing regimens. *Absorption* of agents in patients who cannot take oral agents may be possible only via intramuscular, intravenous or rectal routes. Novel routes of administration such as buccal wafer and topical patch offer options for the treatment of patients who cannot swallow. *Distribution* of drugs is altered in patients who are hypovolemic. Antacids, commonly prescribed for hospitalized patients, may slow the distribution and limit the onset of action of oral benzodiazepines. In patients who are chronically ill there is often reduced protein-binding available which can create toxic levels of free agent. *Metabolism* by the liver transforms many psychotropic agents; thus the presence of liver disease mandates reduced dosing. Drug–drug interactions can raise or lower drug level via inhibition or induction of metabolism by cytochrome P450 isoenzymes. Many psychiatric medications have narrow therapeutic indices in which the agent (substrate) has a narrow path for metabolism via a specific isoenzyme; altered function of the isoenzyme, either through its inhibition (immediate) or its induction (delayed) can markedly affect the blood level of the agent. Medical literature and online resources such as micromedex.com can provide this information. *Excretion* via the kidneys is limited in acute and chronic renal failure; patients receiving medication dependent on renal function, such as lithium or bupropion, may require lower dosing. For patients on renal dialysis, lithium must be dosed very carefully. Only a single dose may be required following dialysis since it will not be excreted until the next dialysis.

Pharmacodynamic issues involve the alteration of a drug's intended pharmacologic effect by another drug or mechanism at the site of action. The serotonin syndrome exemplifies this phenomenon. Drugs such as meperidine or dextromethorphan interact with selective serotonin reuptake inhibitors (SSRI) to provoke a potentially fatal syndrome characterized by confusion, ataxia, hyperreflexia, clonus, nausea and hypertension. The putative effects of SSRIs in prolonging bleeding may have clinical consequences. The association of gastrointestinal bleeding in the elderly who are taking serotonin reuptake inhibitors should alert the clinician to minimize such agents in medical settings. Cumulative and excess anticholinergic effects from drugs can cause confusion and decrease bowel and bladder motility in vulnerable patients. Excess sedation in elderly patients can be due to the additive effects of sedatives such as benzodiazepines and hypnotics given together. Independent of sedation, benzodiazepines can increase the risk of falls in the elderly.

The use of medication in the medically ill requires careful attention to all the medications a patient is currently taking, the contribution of underlying medical conditions, possible drug interactions, and possible dosage adjustments. Other variables include *nonadherence* to prescribed medication, and *polypharmacy* in patients treated by several providers. Efforts to simplify medication regimens start with a polite inquiry into the indications for the prescribed agents, especially those suspected of CNS activity. Patients may be overwhelmed by the complexity of pill-taking, which may prompt recommendations that the regimen be streamlined while the patient is hospitalized and thus directly observed. Some hospital units provide "self-medication" programs, allowing the patient to retain some autonomy in self-care. This can serve as an opportunity to further monitor illness behavior.

B. Psychotherapy in the Medically Ill

Psychotherapy for the hospitalized patient is usually brief and supportive. The type of intervention will depend upon the patient's cognitive status, disease state, and treatments. If a patient has had delirium, often there are gaps in memory that can foster fears of embarrassment and distortion of what happened. The psychiatric consultant should inquire about such issues and fill in the periods of time the patient does not recall, replacing misperceptions with accurate information. The patient who has had frightening hallucinations due to opiates or steroids requires reassurance that these were drug effects.

Even when cognitively intact, patients may be depressed and express feelings of helplessness and hopelessness. Patients who have witnessed the unsuccessful resuscitation of a roommate can benefit from gentle inquiry into the emotional sequelae of such an event. *Supportive psychotherapy* includes not only eliciting fears and emotions but also initiating helpful measures. For example, when patients are distressed by the conditions of hospitalization, they may respond to dietary supplementation from home if allowed or from room change when a noisy roommate disturbs sleep. Simple measures like making a wall calendar available or locating eyeglasses can aid adaptation.

Common themes in *brief psychotherapy* are found in the exploration of the patient's ideas about the etiology of the illness, as well as the toll it has taken, and the exposure they have had to others with similar illnesses. Many patients fear discussing these issues with their primary physician. Distortions of causal factors, prognosis and treatment effects should be corrected. This can alleviate anxiety if the patient is overly pessimistic. A contrasting situation occurs when the patient minimizes serious disease or the need for intervention. The diagnosis of denial requires that the patient be told the nature of both disease and treatment. Denial wards off the terror of diagnosis and must be managed slowly and carefully. If denial wards off the implications of disease such that refusal of care is at stake, it is essential to utilize available family supports to understand the factors that promote denial and decide how to intervene.

Long-term psychotherapy is usually conducted in ambulatory or rehabilitation settings. Limited data confirm that this treatment has efficacy for somatic syndromes such as irritable bowel disorder or chronic fatigue syndrome. Cognitive behavioral therapy has been reported as effective for fibromyalgia. Graded exercise can help patients with chronic fatigue syndrome or fibromyalgia, whereas psycho-education is important for patients undergoing treatment for a variety of disorders. Evidence is growing that psychotherapy and psychopharmacological treatment are synergistic in the treatment of depressive disorders, better than either treatment alone. In the context of genetic testing for some diseases such as breast cancer or Huntington disease, the patient needs full knowledge of the risks and benefits of such knowledge. This may generate a role for psychotherapeutic consultation.

C. Electroconvulsive Therapy

Electroconvulsive therapy (ECT) is a first-line treatment in medically ill patients with suicidal depression, psychotic depression, depression during pregnancy, and in medical conditions that cause inanition or risk for cardiovascular collapse. Although generally reserved for refractory disorders and special circumstances, it is the most effective treatment for depressive disorders. The consulting psychiatrist may be in a position to initiate education of patient, family, *and* the patient's provider regarding the indications, potential side effects (retrograde amnesia, elevated blood pressure), and treatment outcomes of ECT. Many patients with a remote history of "shock treatment" require education about recent advances in ECT in order to inform them about the procedure.

Legal Issues in Consultation Psychiatry

The legal issues that arise in consultation psychiatry are most commonly those of confidentiality, competency (decision-making capacity) and whether a patient has a right to die despite attempts to treat. Documentation of the patient's wishes in advance of the need to know often obviates many legal issues. Requests to leave against medical advice are a subset of competency assessments.

Confidentiality is mandated comprehensively by the Health Insurance Portability and Accountability Act. The consultation psychiatrist has a relative exemption from strict confidentiality when sharing information with the health providers who are treating the patient. The consultation note, as well, is exempt from the Health Insurance Portability and Accountability Act confidentiality. When obtaining corollary information from family members, the clinician should attempt to get verbal consent if the patient retains decision-making capacity. In some situations, information the patient divulges should remain confidential. Intimate details of a personal nature with no bearing on the issues that led to the consultation request are confidential and should not be revealed to other medical professionals or in the treatment record. Psychotherapy notes are considered private under the Health Insurance Portability and Accountability Act regulations and separate from the medical record. This does not mean that data from consultation follow up visits that document diagnosis or response to treatment cannot be noted in the progress notes.

Competency is a broad concept that applies to a variety of acts and behavior. It is a legal issue, bestowed at birth. If the patient is impaired, a physician must provide evidence of erosion of competency to the legal system (in probate or "family" courts). Informed consent to a particular procedure or health care intervention, however, focuses upon the individual's ability to make a decision based upon the capacity to understand the information that *must be provided in a clear and understandable manner*; to recognize the options available (including the risks and benefits of each option); to use reason with regard to the information provided by the team; and finally to make a rational decision that is sustained over time. Decisional incapacity, which is determined ultimately by a probate judge or other legal representative, does not automatically indicate incompetence in other activities of living.

Discharges *Against Medical Advice* (AMA) evoke legal fears and risk management concerns. In order to oppose the patient's free will to leave, the consulting psychiatrist must diagnose a condition that impairs judgment, such as delirium, dementia or depression, of such severity that the patient's safety or the safety of others is threatened, either by direct threats to self or others, or by grave disability (unable to obtain food, shelter or clothing). Issues of competency assessment described previously may apply. The challenge is to discriminate *subtly impaired* decisions (due to mental conditions, with or without physical conditions) from *bad* decisions (e.g., marginal capacity to provide for self, homeless, refusing treatment). A rapid assessment of level of risk is required. Often efforts to address the pressing need for discharge reveal the origins of the AMA discharge request. Some patients require social worker assistance with responsibilities such as childcare, housing or work mandates that are valid but impracticable in the face of serious illness. Finally, patients who abuse substances sometimes request abrupt discharge. If no withdrawal state is observed, the consultant can enlist the help of family members to convince the patient to remain in the hospital; however, this is often impossible. In the circumstance where the patient demonstrates capacity to make a decision, albeit inconsistent with what is recommended, the patient retains the right to leave. Clinical status and attempts to contact support systems should be documented.

Right-to-die decisions require that the patient be judged competent and fully understand the nature of the disease state. Impairments in cognition or thought process (e.g., dementia or paranoia) may necessitate transferal of the decision to surrogates. Another complicated issue is of depression that causes a subtle erosion of decisional capacity. The seriously ill patient is often clinically depressed. If depression is aggressively treated, the wish to die may change. Family meetings in concert with the treatment team, and consultation with hospital ethics committees and legal counsel, maximize the opportunity for a fair appraisal of the request to withhold treatment.

Advanced Directives should be reviewed in the patient who has become cognitively compromised. Optimally, a surrogate decision-maker has been identified for a future period of incapacity, and the consulting psychiatrist renders a second opinion to the team declaring that the time has come to utilize or *invoke* it. Advance preparation pays off for these patients as they avoid the legal proceedings of competency. Social workers can assist with documentation of advanced directives; these should be recommended for every patient found to retain the capacity to make such decisions.

Emergency Consultations

A few situations need immediate attention, requiring a rapid assessment of a range of factors, including a scan of the physical situation (e.g., the patient might use medical equipment as a weapon) and the environment (e.g., multiple patient room or intensive care setting). Policies regarding clearing the room of sharp objects and having restraints available on medical and surgical floors, should be in place. However, it may not be routine for staff in the usual medical setting to follow such policies, increasing the need for psychiatric consultant assistance.

Violent patients may be suffering from delirium or substance withdrawal. Such information can be obtained from a review of the medical record, focusing upon the disease status (e.g., presence of a mass lesion in the CNS) or prescribed medication fostering an encephalopathy. In such situations it is imperative that staff and other patients be protected. The concurrent presence of security guards allows safe assessment. The emergency use of psychotropic medication can diffuse these dramatic situations. Involving a family member can be helpful but there may not be sufficient time to allow this.

Suicidal patients become emergencies if there is an attempt at self-harm or if drugs, knives, or weapons are detected that the patient is secretly storing to use for self-harm. Is the behavior a means of attention seeking, is it due to a mood or psychotic disorder, or is it an attempt to assume control when the situation has become so ominous that ending life is preferable to enduring a fantasized medical scenario? Following initial assessment, it is necessary to observe closely the patient who is acutely suicidal but too medically ill to be transferred to a psychiatric unit. Nursing personnel are trained in the monitoring of suicidal patients, but the psychiatric consultant may be sought for management advice. The care of high-risk individuals in such settings is eased by family supports, if available.

Liaison Psychiatry

The liaison psychiatrist is a regular member of a treatment team in transplant programs, cancer centers, or dialysis units. A subspecialized focus of liaison psychiatrists on diseases states (e.g., HIV psychiatry) or medical specialty (e.g., gynecology or pediatrics) has developed in recent years.

Transplantation psychiatry is important due to the psychological stress upon patients and families who undergo life saving procedures or wait on a list for a limited number of available organs. The organ to be transplanted dictates the common psychiatric issues within each procedure. For related-donor kidney transplants, the psychiatric consultant may evaluate both overt and covert family pressures that the putative donor experiences and how the potential recipient feels in response. Treatment adherence is important, especially in patients with diabetes who have not followed diabetic regimens. The essential issue in liver-transplantation recipients who have been substance abusers is their history of abstinence. If potential recipients are still using alcohol or other substances of abuse they need rehabilitation and abstinence before receiving a liver transplant, although candidacy is individualized and may vary according to the scarcity of the organ to be transplanted. Liaison psychiatrists may be called upon to assist with screening to identify latent psychiatric disorders, and to assist with the psychological stressors as discussed. For heart transplantation patients, ongoing support is necessary during the waiting period before an available organ is found. Such patients commonly experience anxiety and depression, and wrestle with mortality.

In *oncology* settings, central issues are depression in the terminally ill, delirious states due to diseases and treatments, and family reactions. In *nephrology* centers, patients who request termination of hemodialysis must be evaluated for delirium and dementia. The treatment of underlying depression may alter the request for cessation of hemodialysis. The role of the psychiatrist in nephrology also focuses upon patients who resist dietary and fluid limitations, often in the context of depression and dementia. The psychiatrist will have many opportunities to teach health professionals to recognize and manage psychiatric disorders in chronic illness and end-of-life care.

■ CORE CONCEPTS IN PSYCHOSOMATIC MEDICINE

Psychiatric Disorders Caused by Medical Conditions

Psychiatric symptoms can occur as a direct consequence of an underlying medical condition. Many examples are catalogued in the *Diagnostic and Statistical Manual of Mental Disorders,* fourth edition, Text Revision. "Mental Disorder Due to a General Medical Condition" is diagnosed when there is evidence that the medical condition caused the psychiatric manifestation of the illness. The categories of psychiatric illness classified in the *Diagnostic and Statistical Manual of Mental Disorders,* fourth edition, Text Revision as caused by or "due to" medical conditions are as follows: Delirium, Dementia, Amnestic Disorder, Catatonia, Personality Change, Psychotic Disorder, Mood Disorder, Anxiety Disorder, Sexual Dysfunction, and Sleep Disorder. Each of these diagnoses is associated with the behavioral phenomena of a *psychiatric disorder*; however, when there is evidence of a causative *medical condition*, the *Diagnostic and Statistical Manual of Mental Disorders*, fourth edition, Text Revision does not regard these "due to" diagnoses as full-fledged *primary* psychiatric disorders. For example, Major Depression should not be diagnosed when there is a known medical etiology, but rather Mood Disorder due to General Medical Condition. Furthermore, the neurovegetative symptoms of Major Depression (see Chapter 18) could also represent a medical symptom (e.g., decreased energy due to depression *or* anemia, *or* both). The confound of medical and psychiatric symptoms identical in their physical expression leaves consultation–liaison psychiatrists in a bit of a quandary.

Most studies have led to the general consensus that all "potentially psychiatric" symptoms of the medical condition should be included in the diagnosis of the psychiatric disorder. In the case of depressive symptoms, for example, this strategy risks the psychiatric diagnosis of patients who do not meet full criteria of Major Depression (false positive), but avoids the failure to diagnose patients who do meet criteria (false negative).

Psychiatric symptoms caused by medical conditions have important implications, not only for diagnosis but also for evaluation, treatment and management of both medical and psychiatric conditions. Detection and diagnosis of the medical cause often relies upon the astuteness of the primary medical clinician; however the patient with psychiatric symptoms might not present to medical care, but rather to a psychiatric setting causing a possible delay in medical diagnosis. The patient with medically-induced psychiatric symptoms who presents to medical settings may be dismissed as not medically ill. Treatment of the presenting psychiatric symptoms, without detection of the underlying medical condition, may actually exacerbate the medical condition. Clinical wisdom suggests that any nonresponder to psychiatric treatment *de facto* merits a review of the medical evaluation obtained at baseline and a repeat or expanded evaluation to search for undetected medical causes. Consultation–liaison psychiatrists identify those patients who elude diagnosis in primary care due to the prominence of the psychiatric presentation. They educate medical and psychiatric colleagues about the medical masquerade, and may be a stalwart force toward completing the medical evaluation of a patient with psychiatric symptoms. The following section will highlight this principle by clinical examples.

A. THE PATIENT WITH CEREBROVASCULAR DISEASE AND DEPRESSION

Stroke, a rapidly occurring disturbance of brain function attributed to vascular disease, is the third leading cause of death in America after heart disease and cancer. The neuropsychiatric complications of stroke include cognitive deficit, and behavioral and emotional dysregulation. Depression following stroke is a frequent and adverse neuropsychiatric sequela of stroke, yet it is undiagnosed by most nonpsychiatric physicians. Depression has a negative impact on the patient's quality of life, not only from a psychosocial standpoint, but also by impeding the recovery of motor function. Depression in the aftermath of stroke (Post-stroke Depression and Post-Stroke Pathological Affect) respond to aggressive treatment but escape detection when interpreted as an "understandable" response to the stroke. Post-stroke Pathological Affect is characterized by emotional dysregulation in which laughter or tears are expressed but are unrelated to mood, and are exacerbated by minor cues. Post-Stroke Pathological Affect can be severely disabling, causing patients to become isolative or agoraphobic. Post-stroke Depression and Post-Stroke Pathological Affect are both responsive to antidepressant treatment (see Chapter 18).

PATIENT VIGNETTE 1

A 59-year-old divorced Caucasian man, right-handed graphic designer, with a history of hypertension, diabetes mellitus and nicotine dependence, was brought to the hospital by his son after the sudden onset of slurred speech and inability to walk. Physical examination revealed aphasia and a dense right-sided paralysis; diagnostic investigations confirmed an ischemic stroke. Mr. S. was stabilized medically for one week and was then referred for physical rehabilitation. Despite aggressive efforts over the ensuing weeks by rehabilitation staff, the patient was increasingly unmotivated for physical therapy, socially isolative, and at times refused to eat. He mentioned in passing to a nursing aide that he would be "better off dead," prompting the team physician to request a psychiatric evaluation. Utilizing a communication board, Mr. S. expressed hopelessness about his career as a graphic designer, and worries about his future financial situation. He also ruminated about past layoffs from work and financially compromising alimony payments. His speech was garbled and a source of immediate frustration. He was unable to write or draw designs with his paretic right hand. After a complete medical workup for additional underlying causes, the patient was started on a low dose of an SSRI. He had an early response to treatment which was followed by improved participation in physical therapy.

PATIENT VIGNETTE 2

An 80-year-old widowed woman, American Indian, tribal elder, and retired casino manager had an extensive history of hypertension, obesity, degenerative joint disease, and chronic obstructive pulmonary disease. Prior to admission, she developed the acute cardiac symptoms of nausea and atypical chest pains. In the emergency room, she had an abnormal electrocardiogram, subsequently undergoing emergency angiography followed by coronary artery bypass graft surgery. Post-operative care was provided in the surgical intensive care unit. Her management was complicated by difficulty in weaning from the respirator, as well as combative behavior despite soft restraints and sedation with parenteral benzodiazepine. Psychiatric consultation was requested to assist with behavior management. Starting with review of the inpatient and outpatient charts that was suggestive of substance abuse, collateral information from family members confirmed that the patient had utilized increasing amounts of long-acting opioid analgesics prescribed by multiple doctors for chronic pain. Of note, a recent episode of pneumonia as a complication of chronic obstructive pulmonary disease had been treated with antibiotics that caused hepatitis and psychiatric side effects. Laboratory investigations revealed metabolic derangements that were in the process of being corrected. Oxygen saturations were low when attempts were made to wean her off the respirator; moreover she had scratched a nurse during one of these episodes. The diagnosis of Delirium due to Multiple Etiologies was made; potential contributors included: (1) hypoxia, (2) opiate withdrawal, (3) psychiatric side effects of medications, (4) drug interaction, and (5) intraoperative cerebral event. A multifaceted approach to her care was recommended: (1) safety assessment (e.g., minimize use of restraints post-sternotomy, implementation of safety monitor), (2) social work consult to document surrogate decision-maker, (3) search for additional reversible etiologies (e.g., vitamin B_{12}, thyroid stimulating hormone, possible head Computerized Tomography if no mental status improvement), (4) minimized use of benzodiazepines for agitation, and (5) possibly morphine to treat pain (degenerative joint disease and surgical wound) and the possible opiate withdrawal.

B. The Patient with Postoperative Delirium

Delirium is an acute cognitive disorder with global impairment in brain function, and fluctuating consciousness and attention. Associated features include hyperactivity, hypoactivity, and reversal of the sleep–wake cycle. Delirium is a common presentation in hospitalized elderly patients, affecting up to 30% of elderly surgical patients. The most common predisposing surgical procedures are emergency hip fracture repair, gastrointestinal surgery, coronary artery bypass grafts, and lung transplants (see Chapter 14).

C. The Patient with Psychosis and Substance Dependence

Psychotic disorders due to medical illness or to substance use can originate from many conditions, such as brain diseases (e.g., seizures, neoplasm, encephalitis, stroke), endocrine disorders (hyper- or hypo-thyroidism, Cushing's syndrome), metabolic disorders (hypoglycemia, hyponatremia, uremia, thiamine deficiency/Korsakoff), and chemicals, including drugs of abuse, medications or toxins. The most common substances that induce psychosis by intoxication are cocaine, amphetamines, and phencyclidine. The most common substances causing psychosis by withdrawal are sedative-hypnotics and alcohol. Psychosis due to general medical conditions or substance-related psychosis can be distinguished from a primary psychotic disorder by fluctuating level of consciousness, focal neurological signs, predominantly visual sensory involvement (e.g., visual hallucinations, illusions), perseverations in thought content, and abnormal vital signs (elevated blood pressure, heart rate) (see Chapter 15).

Psychiatric Disorders Affecting Medical Conditions

Psychiatric disorders may affect compliance with necessary medical treatment or even acceptance of the disease itself. Depression, hopelessness and anhedonia can abet nonadherence to medication, dietary regulation, or ongoing surveillance for the recurrence of disease. Eating disorders are common in diabetic patients and can seriously compromise metabolic regulation. Even defensive mechanisms such as denial, not a psychiatric disorder in itself, can affect a medical condition due to poor compliance. Psychiatric medications with metabolic side effects can induce or interfere with the management of chronic medical conditions, and warrant close monitoring in collaboration with primary providers (see Chapter 18).

PATIENT VIGNETTE 3

A 45-year-old married man, construction worker, with a prior history of gastritis, pancreatitis and anemia, was admitted for lumbar discectomy. Although he denied alcohol consumption during the preoperative visit, by the fourth postoperative day he displayed marked signs of alcohol withdrawal, Delirium Tremens, associated with autonomic instability and frank visual hallucinations. When he began to act in response to the hallucinations by seeking to climb out of bed and talk to an empty chair, psychiatric consultation was requested. Search for reversible causes of the mental status change was completed and did not alter the diagnosis of Delirium Tremens. Treatment with intravenous thiamine, multivitamins, and high doses of an intermediate-acting benzodiazepine led to amelioration of autonomic instability, but the psychotic symptoms persisted until an antipsychotic agent was added. After a protracted hospital course, the patient was referred for substance rehabilitation treatment and outpatient psychiatric care.

PATIENT VIGNETTE 4

A 24-year-old single man was evaluated for noncompliant behavior resulting in recurrent decubitus ulcers. Two years prior to the consultation, he had been involved in a motorcycle accident causing spinal cord injury and paraplegia. Confined to a wheelchair, the patient inconsistently attended rehabilitation. He spent many hours driving around in a van that had been equipped with hand controls. He did not utilize weight shifting or other approaches to minimize decubitus formation and consequently was hospitalized repeatedly. Upon evaluation, the patient was sullen and hostile and initially had nothing to say. Upon further questioning, he was clearly depressed and noted, "Who wouldn't be?" The patient complained that he had recurrent sleep problems. He ruminated about his accident. He began to talk about his loneliness and depression. Background evaluation revealed that the patient had a premorbid personality style involving impulsivity and activity. Social history revealed that he was raised in a single parent family wherein his mother worked many hours to support his older sister and himself. He had dropped out of high school to work. Although his peers often used drugs he did not, but he did enjoy driving recklessly on a motorcycle he had purchased. Following his accident, his friends abandoned him.

After the evaluation, the psychiatric consultant held a few family meetings in which the evidence for depression was clear, as well as additional features of demoralization. The patient felt helpless and hopeless from his accident and saw no way to overcome his injury or life circumstances. Based upon these meetings, the physical therapist introduced him to another patient who had successfully coped with a spinal cord injury. Although the intervention was initially hospital-based, it was many months before he was able to accept his injury better, pursue proper care, and complete his high school education in order to pursue a career in design.

A. NONADHERENCE TO TREATMENT

Nonadherence is particularly common in certain medical illnesses. Psychiatric disorders such as depression or delirium can obstruct proper care. Whether hypertensive medication or more complicated treatments are involved, it is essential to understand the complexity of the regimen and the issues that prevent compliance, financial or psychological. A sense of hopelessness and lack of motivation can be fostered by premorbid characteristics, but also by depressive disorder. Multidisciplinary strategies to encourage compliance include collaboration with case managers, social work service, and primary clinicians who have longstanding relationships with patients. In patients with cognitive deficits, strategies to assist with medication compliance include dose-based pill boxes, simplification of dosing patterns, a switch to long-acting agents or an altered route of administration (e.g., topical patch), and parsimonious prescription patterns that reduce side effects. Written directions at the time of the visit, visiting nurse assistance, case management and the enlisting of family support enhance adherence. Ensuring that underlying psychiatric conditions are adequately treated is important as well; inadequate dosing and inadequate duration are commonly associated with refractory depression in primary care settings, but nonadherence is equally important. In addition, psychotropic agents that interfere with other medications can cause the patient to choose among them.

B. CHRONIC PSYCHIATRIC DISORDER AFFECTING MEDICAL CONDITION

Patients with schizophrenia or bipolar disorder have increased rates of mortality. The shortened lifespan is due to the psychiatric disorder itself, as well as to treatment with medications such as antipsychotic agents, which can induce a metabolic syndrome leading to cardiovascular disease and diabetes. It is essential for the psychiatric

PATIENT VIGNETTE 5

A 52-year-old woman with a 30-year history of schizophrenia and repeated hospital admissions was evaluated in the emergency department for diabetic ketoacidosis. Admission to the hospital for stabilization and diabetes management prompted a psychiatric consultation. She had had a complicated clinical course with multiple hospitalizations and periods of homelessness. At the time of admission, she was living in a group home, maintained on risperidone. On this regimen, she gained 34 pounds and developed Type II diabetes. She was not compliant with a low-carbohydrate diet, and frequently snacked on fast foods. She was episodically not compliant with oral hypoglycemic agents prescribed by her physician. On evaluation, the patient presented as a disheveled, obese woman with hallucinations and delusions who recognized that these phenomena were due to schizophrenia. She was depressed about the impact of the disease upon her life. Treatment involved switching the patient to a medication with less weight gain (such as aripiprazole or ziprasidone) and ongoing checkups by a nurse who visited the group home. Attempts to create an exercise regimen were unsuccessful; nevertheless, the patient continued to take antipsychotic medication and attend a day program.

consultant to work collaboratively with community mental health programs to develop treatment plans that promote health. If antipsychotic agents are utilized, clinicians should monitor the individual's weight and girth on a regular basis to avoid the development of serious metabolic consequences. Psychiatric patients are further at risk for obesity if they are isolated, avoid exercise, and follow sedentary lifestyles. The risks to general health from psychiatric disorders are compounded by the high rates of substance dependence such as cigarette smoking which contributes to cardiovascular disease. Psychiatric consultation can have a role in prevention through education in primary care settings and collaboration with cessation programs.

C. Patient with Depression and Cardiac Disease

Depression is an independent risk factor for ischemic heart disease. It predicts higher morbidity and mortality after uncomplicated MI. For 6 months after the infarction, even up to 5 years, depression has an impact on cardiac mortality, eclipsing standard cardiac variables such as left ventricular ejection fraction. The possible

mechanisms for these phenomena include a three-fold increase in medication nonadherence, shared risk factors (smoking, diabetes, and obesity), lower heart rate variability, chronic inflammation (increased biomarkers such as C-reactive protein), platelet activation, and sympathoadrenal activation due to increased physiological stress. Studies to determine the role of psychiatric treatments aimed at lowering cardiac risk have indicated an improved quality of life, but no clear reversal of increased mortality.

PATIENT VIGNETTE 6

A 49-year-old single man, advertising executive, is admitted to the intensive care unit after the sudden onset of crushing chest pain, with ischemic changes on electrocardiogram. Emergency efforts to treat the patient had no effect on the outcome of a profound MI. He was an active sportsman, community activist and competitor for promotion at the agency where he worked. Within days after his admission to the hospital, he appeared depressed to staff, and had no visitors. Efforts to discuss cardiac rehabilitation were rebuffed as unnecessary by the patient, who stated, "What is the use? The damage is done," causing the medical team to become alarmed. Well-informed about the cardiac mortality risk with comorbid depression, the medical team requested immediate psychiatric consultation. During the interview, the patient expressed depressed mood and a pervasive hopelessness about returning to his productive life. A strong family history of early death due to MI weighed heavily on his mind. Neurovegetative symptoms were prominent, and were predominated by sleep disturbance in which the patient ruminated about the loss of independence. Unable to identify with rehabilitation patients who were older, he eschewed the idea of rehabilitation, or at least his stereotype of it. Search for other reversible etiologies for the depressed mood was negative, and the patient was started on an SSRI antidepressant, to which he responded within days. Social work services mobilized support for the patient, assuring that colleagues from work would be allowed to visit the patient. Outpatient referral to psychiatry was made, to monitor the response to medication, and to encourage compliance with cardiac rehabilitation. As the patient's mood lifted, he began to talk about his social isolation.

Psychological Reactions to Medical Illness

Medical illness creates a crisis. The patient is faced with multiple emotional, physical and financial challenges that can create serious psychological distress. The personal aspects of illness include pain, disability, and loss of function and autonomy due to the disease and or its treatment. Loss of exercise tolerance in congestive heart failure, or pain and dietary limitations in short bowel syndrome, exemplify such challenges. The interpersonal aspects of illness create changes in roles and status such as the ability to be a fully active parent or employee, to be independent and supportive of others. Patients with HIV/AIDS face stigmatization. The patient with terminal cancer may be isolated when supports do not know how to interact with a dying individual. Finally, there is an intrapsychic challenge to disease due to fears of death, disfigurement, and pain. People react differently to the challenges before them in accordance with their coping style, environmental circumstances, and the nature of the disease and its treatment.

Coping with Serious Illness

It is tempting to label a patient's reaction to a life-threatening illness such as cancer as *understandable*. This rarely explains fully the diagnosis of depression; depression due to a medical condition does not always correlate with the level of functional disability or problems in activities of daily living. Although only a minority of patients with cancer develops a formal major depressive disorder, those individuals need effective treatment with both pharmacotherapy and psychosocial support. It is essential to evaluate the level of family support, and the patient's ideas about the disease, knowledge about others with similar health problems, and the availability of community or national support groups.

A. The Hostile Patient

Premorbid personality style often shapes the reaction to a serious illness or hospitalization. The passive patient may tolerate a paternalistic approach, while the patient with obsessional and intellectual defenses will ask questions and seek more information. Patients with hysterical traits may be emotional and require compliments about the courage they display. Patients with borderline traits can split the medical team by idealization and devaluation of its hierarchical members; trainees may be particularly vulnerable to this behavior. Narcissistic patients have the sense that they are particularly important or deserving of preferential treatment. These broad-brushed descriptions are not pathological entities, but they describe coping mechanisms that emerge in stressful situations. Medical illness exaggerates such traits. The physician should

---

PATIENT VIGNETTE 7

A-47-year-old married woman, mother of two adult daughters, found a breast mass during routine self-examination. She quickly sought medical evaluation which revealed she had a breast neoplasm. She was successfully treated with lumpectomy and chemotherapy. Lymph node dissection was negative. Despite these results, she dwelt on the possibility that her neoplasm might return. She experienced frequent crying spells, loss of concentration, sleep difficulties, and fatigue. She had no family history of either mood disorders or breast cancer. Psychiatric evaluation revealed a woman who was sad and cried during the interview. She reported she was having difficulty getting out of bed in the morning and that she could barely manage her work due to problems in concentration. She was not suicidal. She revealed that she believed she developed breast cancer due to promiscuity as a young adult prior to her marriage. In collaboration with her oncologist, the psychiatrist judged that none of her complaints were aspects of her neoplastic disease. The patient was treated with an antidepressant that improved her sleep pattern and fatigue, and psychotherapy that allowed her to ventilate her guilty ruminations about her actions. As the treatment progressed, knowledge about her health dispelled beliefs that these were causal factors. Despite early side effects of nausea, she was encouraged to continue the medication. Over 6 weeks she improved. After 12 weeks, she reported no symptoms of depression. She said she was very lucky to have "caught my cancer so early."

---

not view these behaviors as challenges to professional competence or authority, but as demonstrations of fearfulness and regression during the crisis of illness.

B. The Demoralized Patient

Demoralization does not qualify for a primary psychiatric diagnosis. It is common in medical and surgical settings in the context of a reaction to acute or chronic stress, such as the onset of illness, its treatment (if particularly disabling or disfiguring), or illness that is terminal. The management of demoralization involves promotion of the primary physician's role in soothing the patient's fears about the illness through relevant information about treatment options. Treatment also involves reassurance by the consulting psychiatrist that the patient does not have a psychiatric disorder, but that low mood or

---

PATIENT VIGNETTE 8

A 65-year-old, thrice-married Hispanic man, firearm factory supervisor, with a history of MI at age 58, and emphysema related to nicotine dependence, was admitted to intensive care for cardiac arrhythmia and hematuria. One week prior to admission, he underwent cryo-ablation of a renal carcinoma that had been diagnosed two months prior to admission. During the hospitalization, the insertion of a urinary catheter had been complicated due to an enlarged prostate, and was painful for the patient. Shortly thereafter, the patient began speaking to nurses in a demeaning manner, using expletives and threats to call nursing supervisors. Medical interns, consulting urologists and cardiologists were impugned. Nursing staff avoided him and kept the door of his room closed. He demanded that his needs be prioritized. He was overheard yelling on the telephone, threatening his wife with divorce. Psychiatric consultation was requested. After a chart review and discussion with nursing, the hypothesis was offered that the outward aggression and anger was a mask for fear; his behavior was reframed as a response to medical illness, a life-threatening situation that had placed the patient, who valued being in charge of others at work and in his marriage, in a dependent position. Urological manipulations of his genitalia and use of the bedpan further humiliated him. Initially, at bedside, the psychiatry consultant listened only to his complaints for an extended period. The consultant then encouraged the patient to complain further to the highest authority in hospital administration, regarding his concerns about staff. Although petulant, the patient began to allow a discussion about the threats to his life of the recent diagnosis of cancer, and his cardiac status. (The intensive care setting required to treat the arrhythmia had rekindled worries about his remote cardiac history of MI.) Daily, brief visits by the psychiatry consultant reviewed the stressors in his life, and culminated in the patient's request for an outpatient mental health appointment for marital therapy which was arranged prior to discharge.

PATIENT VIGNETTE 9

A 50-year-old, separated Caucasian man, musician, with no prior history of psychiatric or medical illness, presented to the hospital with generalized fatigue, 35-pound weight loss, and mild depression for the past several months. At the urging of his friends, he agreed to an Emergency Room visit and was surprised by the doctor's plan to admit him. After three days on the general medical unit, a second doctor who had assumed his care after admission informed him that he had pancreatic cancer. The patient reacted calmly and seemed to accept the grim prognosis. Shortly thereafter, he expressed a wish to be discharged against advice, but agreed to a psychiatric consultation for evaluation of his capacity to make that decision. During the psychiatric interview, the patient expressed frustration with the system of care, complaining that the multitude of doctors and nurses, never the same one twice, prevented individualized attention. He was able to repeat the information that the doctor had given him regarding the diagnosis of cancer, but he did not demonstrate an understanding of the recommendations or treatment options. He was appalled at the idea of being a patient as it was not in keeping with his longstanding lifestyle of late nights relishing wine, women, and song. Most shocking to him in this, his only hospital experience, was his first sight in the mirror: a reflection of wasted temporal muscles and hollowed cheeks, in stark contrast to the formerly attractive countenance of which he had been proud. The mirror had been his true love, and now he was betrayed. Acutely demoralized, he held no hope for survival. The psychiatrist requested the primary physician return. He sat down to discuss treatment plans and instilled his hope for future comfort. The patient rescinded the request for discharge, and asked to speak again with the psychiatrist in follow-up.

---

anxiety symptoms are part of a natural response to stress and would be manifested by many patients in similar circumstances.

Somatic Presentations of Psychiatric Disorders

The common presentation of somatic concerns in primary care can be related to psychiatric disorder, most commonly anxiety or depression. Patients with major depression are more likely to present for care in primary care settings, and once there to complain of somatic illness. Chest pain is found in generalized anxiety and panic disorders. Fatigue, headache, and backache are common in major depressive disorders. These psychiatric illnesses are commonly under-recognized in busy outpatient settings. When the psychiatric disorder is identified and effectively treated, the somatic symptoms are alleviated.

Conversely, physical symptoms that are unexplained, not due to other psychiatric disorders such as depression and anxiety, and not intentionally produced, may be due to a somatoform disorder. Somatoform disorders are grouped together because they require the exclusion of medical and substance-induced causes, and are likely to present first to primary care or medical settings. Somatoform disorders include: somatization disorder, conversion disorder, pain disorder, hypochondriasis, and body dysmorphic disorder (see Chapter 22). Psychiatrists consulting to these settings may be asked to assist in the diagnosis and management of these patients who often exasperate caregivers. Strategies include maintaining the patient in primary care settings with one provider, when possible, and encouraging regular appointments that are scheduled at the end of each visit, not on an as-needed basis. In somatization disorder, the consultant may encourage the primary provider to "join in the patient's pessimism" by focusing on symptom management rather than cure.

1. The patient with hypochondriasis

When a patient has persistent fears about symptoms of an illness or beliefs about having an illness, and when no medical illness can be found, "worry" about illness becomes the disease itself: hypochondriasis. In this disorder, worry about illness is not only disabling, it becomes the focus of daily life. The course of illness tends to be chronic, but it has a better prognosis if the onset is acute and brief in duration, with no secondary gain.

■ FUTURE DIRECTIONS

Consultation psychiatry is the bridge between psychiatry and the rest of medicine. As medicine advances, there will be new psychological and emotional challenges for patients requiring the skills and techniques of consultation psychiatrists. Organ transplant technology will evolve into artificial organ transplant; the fear of pandemics such as that generated by SARS will have an emotional toll. These are just two examples that illustrate that there will be an increasing need for psychiatry at the interface with medicine. Consultation psychiatry is already dividing into subspecialized areas to accommodate the expansion of medicine. Consultation–liaison psychiatrists are focusing upon HIV/AIDS, oncology and nephrology as primary interests. Journals and books devoted to these topics complement the general consultation journals. Concurrently, the stresses of hospital life will continue, strained by the forces of economics and health care policies. The shift from hospital-based care to outpatient settings has expanded consultation services into outpatient clinics and specialized care facilities. As new psychiatric treatments emerge, the consult psychiatrist will provide them to patients underserved in nonpsychiatric

---

PATIENT VIGNETTE 10

A 47-year-old married man, practicing attorney, sought emergency evaluation for chest pain. He reported tightness in his chest, which he interpreted as cardiac in origin. After a normal electrocardiogram and laboratory studies, he was reassured. The following day he began to worry that the tests could have been in error, causing increased anxiety. He openly admitted he was a "worrier" but felt that the tightness in his chest was a harbinger of a MI. Repeated medical evaluations found his physical status to be normal. He had no lipid abnormalities, and his blood pressure was normal. He requested that his physician refer him for cardiac catheterization to insure that his coronary arteries were patent. He was referred for a psychiatric evaluation by his internist, after multiple negative medical evaluations for a variety of symptoms that the patient thought indicated cardiac disease. The patient reported that he exercised regularly and kept a careful diet but was preoccupied by the thought he would have a "heart attack." He had no family history of cardiac disease but two of his legal associates had undergone bypass surgery in the previous 3 years. His wife reported that he tended to exaggerate minor viral illnesses or athletic injuries. His developmental history indicated that his mother always worried about his health. She prevented him from participating in normal sports activities when he was in school. Despite this, he became an outstanding tennis player. On full psychiatric evaluation he was anxious and somewhat depressed. He recognized that his fears were not fully realistic but could not get the ideation of cardiac disease out of his head. Treatment involved pharmacological intervention for generalized anxiety with an SSRI, and psychotherapy utilizing cognitive behavioral strategies. Over a period of 6 months he limited calls to his internists to scheduled times and began to feel better. He still worried about cardiac disease when he heard about others with cardiac illness but was able to invoke cognitive strategies that he learned in therapy to reduce his anxiety and prevent maladaptive behavior such as emergency phone calls.

---

settings. Newly recognized as a discrete subspecialty, yet centuries old in practice, psychosomatic medicine has a new role in the ancient art of medicine. Graduate education programs with dedicated fellowship training in psychosomatic medicine will advance the mission to improve patient care. With increasing technologies and advances in biomedical knowledge, this subspecialty will provide the biopsychosocial elements of comprehensive patient care and clinical research to improve clinical outcome and enhance quality of life.

American Psychiatric Association: *Diagnostic and Statistical Manual of Mental Disorders*, 4th edn. Text Revision. Washington, DC: American Psychiatric Publishing, 2000, pp. 13–26.

Borson S, Scanlon J, Brush M, et al.: The Mini-Cog as a screen for dementia: Validation in a population-based sample. *J Am Geriatr Soc* 2003;51:1451–1454.

Chemerinski EC, Robinson RG: The neuropsychiatry of stroke. *Psychosomatics* 2000;41:5–14.

Cozza KL, Scott CA, Jessica RO: *Concise Guide to Drug Interaction Principles for Medical Practice: Cytochrome P450s, UGTs and P-glycoproteins*. Arlington, VA: American Psychiatric Publishing, 2003, pp. 345–369.

Evans D, Charney DS, Lewis L, et al.: Mood disorders in the medically ill: Scientific review and recommendations. *Biol Psych* 2005;58:175–189.

Ewing JA: Detecting alcoholism: The CAGE questionnaire. *JAMA* 1984;252:1905–1907.

Folstein MF, Folstein SE, McHugh R: "Mini-mental state": A practical method for grading the cognitive status of patients for the clinician. *J Psychiatr Res* 1975;12:189–198.

Frasure-Smith N, Lesperance F, Talijic M: Depression following myocardial infarction: Impact on 6 mo survival. *JAMA* 1993;270:1819–1825.

Kroenke K, Spitzer RL, Williams JB: PHQ-15. *Psychsom Med* 2002;64:258–266.

Levenson JL: Introduction. In: Levenson JL (ed). *Textbook of Psychosomatic Medicine*. Arlington, VA: American Psychiatric Publishing, 2005, pp. 19–21.

Lipowski ZJ, Wise TN: History of consultation–liaison psychiatry. In: Wise MG, Rundell JR (eds). *Textbook of Consultation–Liaison Psychiatry: Psychiatry in the Medically Ill*, 2nd edn. Washington: American Psychiatric Publishing, 2002, pp. 3–11.

Lipowski ZJ: Review of consultation–liaison psychiatry and psychosomatic medicine, II: Clinical aspects. *Psychosom Med* 1967;29:201–224.

Masand PS, Christopher EJ, Clary GL, et al.: Mania, catatonia and psychosis. In: Levenson JL (ed). *Textbook of Psychosomatic Medicine*. Arlington: American Psychiatric Publishing, 2005, pp. 242–250.

Powers PS, Santana CA: Surgery. In: Levenson JL (ed). *Textbook of Psychosomatic Medicine*. Arlington, VA: American Psychiatric Publishing, Inc., 2005, pp. 647–656.

Practice Guideline for the Psychiatric Evaluation of Adults, Second Edition, *Am. J. Psychiatry* 163:6(Suppl), 2006, pp. 5–7.

Sadock BJ, Sadock VA: Psychological factors affecting medical condition and psychosomatic medicine. In: Sadock BJ, Sadock VA (eds). *Kaplan and Sadock's Synopsis of Psychiatry*, 9th edn. Philadelphia: Lippincott, Williams and Wilkins, 2003, pp. 824

Slavney PR: Diagnosing demoralization in consultation psychiatry. *Psychosomatics* 1999;40:325–329.

Smith FA, Querques J, Levenson JL, Stern TA: Psychiatric assessment and consultation. In: Levenson JL (ed). *Textbook of Psychosomatic Medicine*. Arlington, VA: American Psychiatric Publishing, 2005, pp. 3–4.

Spitzer RL, Kroenke K, Williams JB: Validation and utility of a self-report version of PRIME-MD: The PHQ primary care study. *JAMA* 1999;282:1737–1744.

Stern TA, Fricchione GL, Cassem NH, Jellinek MS, Rossenbaum JF: *Handbook of General Hospital Psychiatry*, 5th edn. Philadelphia: Mosby Publishing, 2004.

Wise MG, Rundell JR: *Clinical Manual of Psychosomatic Medicine: A Guide to Consultation–liaison Psychiatry*. Arlington: American Psychiatric Publishing, 2005, pp. 1–7, 68–69.

Forensic Psychiatry

William Bernet, MD

■ PSYCHIATRY & THE LAW

Forensic psychiatry is the medical subspecialty, recognized by the American Psychiatric Association since 1991, in which psychiatric expertise is applied to legal issues. The American Board of Psychiatry and Neurology started in 1994 to examine individuals for "added qualifications in forensic psychiatry." There are about 40 1-year fellowship programs in forensic psychiatry accredited by the Accreditation Council for Graduate Medical Education, USA.

There are four divisions of forensic psychiatry. The first pertains to the legal aspects of general psychiatric practice, such as the civil commitment of involuntary patients, the doctrine of informed consent, the requirement to protect third parties from dangerous patients, and matters of privilege and confidentiality.

The second division of forensic psychiatry covers the assessment of mental disability. This includes the evaluation of individuals who have been injured on the job, the assessment of a plaintiff who claims that he or she was injured and is now seeking compensation from a defendant, and the assessment of the competency of individuals to perform specific acts such as making a will.

The most colorful aspect of forensic psychiatry deals with individuals who have been arrested. This division includes the evaluation of competency to stand trial, the evaluation of a person's competency to waive his or her Miranda rights, the assessment of criminal responsibility, evaluations that relate to sentencing, and the treatment of incarcerated individuals.

The fourth division of forensic psychiatry is forensic child psychiatry, which includes child custody evaluations, the evaluation of children who may have been abused, and consultation regarding minors who are involved with juvenile court.

Goldstein AM (ed): *Forensic Psychology.* New York: Wiley, 2003.

Gutheil TG, Appelbaum PS: *Clinical Handbook of Psychiatry and the Law,* 4th edn. Philadelphia: Lippincott Williams & Wilkins, 2006.

Melton GB, Petrila J, Poythress N, Slobogin C: *Psychological Evaluations for the Courts,* 2nd edn. New York: Guilford Press, 1998.

Rosner R (ed): *Principles and Practice of Forensic Psychiatry,* 2nd edn. London: Arnold, 2003.

Simon RI, Gold LH (eds): *Textbook of Forensic Psychiatry.* Washington, DC: American Psychiatric Publishing, 2004.

LEGAL ASPECTS OF PSYCHIATRIC PRACTICE

Professional Liability

Psychiatrists are less likely than other physicians to be sued for professional negligence. However, we live in a litigious society—most psychiatrists will be the subject of at least one professional liability claim during the course of their professional careers.

In a case of professional liability or malpractice, a patient (the plaintiff) sues the psychiatrist (the defendant). In order to prevail legally, the plaintiff must prove each of four elements: (1) The psychiatrist had a duty of care to the patient, (2) there was a breach of the duty to the patient, (3) the patient was injured, and (4) the negligent care was the proximate cause of the patient's injury. That is, if it were not for the negligent act, the injury would not have occurred. At a trial, the plaintiff will attempt to prove each of the four elements by a preponderance of the evidence. Both the plaintiff and the defendant may ask expert witnesses to testify.

Psychiatrists are at risk of being sued in many clinical situations. For example, a psychiatrist may be held responsible when a patient commits suicide if: (1) the suicide was foreseeable, (2) the psychiatrist failed to take a proper history from the patient or other individuals, and/or (3) he or she failed to take appropriate precautions. A psychiatrist may be liable for negligent psychopharmacology if a patient sustains injury as a result of: (1) failure to obtain an adequate history, (2) use of a drug that is not efficacious or not indicated, (3) use of the wrong dosage of medication, or (4) failure to recognize or treat side effects. A particular concern is the occurrence of tardive dyskinesia (a serious side effect caused by certain psychotropic medications), especially if the patient and family members were not warned of the risk and if the psychiatrist did not monitor the patient properly for side effects. A lawsuit may arise out of the use of electroconvulsive therapy if its use was inappropriate or if informed consent was not obtained. A lawsuit may arise out of the use of psychoanalysis if the patient did not give informed consent for this treatment, for example, was not advised of alternative treatments to consider.

Psychiatrists have been sued for engaging in sexual conduct with a patient or with the spouse of a patient. Because it has been clearly stated by professional organizations that sexual activity with patients is a breach of the psychiatric standard of care, the major issue in these cases is to prove that the sexual activity occurred. In some cases patients have made false allegations of sexual conduct against psychiatrists. Even if the sexual activity never occurred, the psychiatrist may have mishandled the case through boundary violations that created the foundation for the false allegations (i.e., through negligent management of the transference).

Informed Consent

Informed consent refers to the continuing process through which a patient understands and agrees to the evaluation and treatment proposed by the physician or other mental health professional. Although informed consent is a concept that all psychiatrists claim to endorse, many practitioners do not understand what the concept means or give only lip service to its implementation.

There are three components to informed consent: mental competency, adequate information, and voluntariness. The assessment of competency is discussed later in this chapter.

Regarding the disclosure of adequate information, this generally means the patient should know the nature and purpose of the proposed treatment, the potential benefits and risks, and the alternative treatments that may be considered. The states have set different criteria for the amount of information that a physician should disclose. Some states have adopted the rule that a physician should disclose the amount of information that a **reasonable physician** would disclose in a similar situation. Most states have adopted a more progressive rule, that a physician should disclose the information that a **reasonable patient** would want to know about the proposed treatment. Regarding the requirement for giving consent voluntarily, this means the patient should not be coerced or offered inducements by the physician, other members of the treatment team, or family members.

Informed consent is more than just a signature on a form. As treatment progresses there should be a continuing dialogue regarding the nature of the treatment and its possible side effects. In some circumstances, such as starting a psychotic patient on neuroleptic medication, the patient will be able to discuss these topics coherently only after treatment has begun. In some cases informed consent should involve a discussion with close family members as well as the patient. When a chronically suicidal patient is being discharged from the hospital, for instance, it is useful for the immediate family to understand both the pros and cons of the discharge and for all parties (i.e., patient, family, and psychiatrist) to share and accept the inherent risks.

Civil Commitment

In some circumstances, psychiatric patients are hospitalized involuntarily. The legal bases for involuntary or civil commitment are the principle of *parens patriae* (i.e., the government may act as "father of the country" to protect individuals who are unable to take care of themselves) and the police power of the state (i.e., the government has the authority to protect society from dangerous individuals). Psychiatrists participate in this process by evaluating patients as to whether they meet criteria for civil commitment. Although the specific procedures vary from state to state, the criteria for involuntary commitment generally include all of the following: (1) The patient has a serious psychiatric disorder, such as a psychosis or bipolar disorder, (2) there is significant risk that the patient will harm himself or others, and (3) hospitalization is the least restrictive alternative. In some jurisdictions, civil commitment is hard to justify (requiring an overt act rather than mere risk of danger) or less difficult to justify (allowing civil commitment if the patient is not likely to take care of basic personal needs).

The Rights of Patients

On many occasions, hospitalized psychiatric patients and institutionalized mentally retarded persons have been railroaded, warehoused, and abused. As a result, state and federal courts and legislators have declared that patients have specific rights. For example, the right to treatment means that civilly committed mental patients have a right to individualized treatment. Likewise, patients also have the right to refuse treatment. That is, a patient who is civilly committed may still be competent to decide whether to agree to use psychotropic medication. If the psychiatrist proposes to use medication even though the patient refuses, he or she should follow the appropriate local procedures. Such procedures may include referring the question to a treatment review committee or asking the court to appoint a guardian for the patient.

In some jurisdictions, psychiatric patients have the following rights: to receive visitors; to send uncensored mail; to receive uncensored mail from attorneys and physicians, although other mail may be examined before being delivered; to confidentiality; to have medical records available to authorized individuals; and to a written statement outlining these rights. An important patient right is that seclusion and mechanical restraint will not be used unless required for the patient's medical or treatment needs. Seclusion and restraint may not be used for punishment or for the convenience of staff.

Confidentiality

Psychiatric patients have a right to be assured that information they have related in therapy will not be revealed to other individuals. The American Medical Association has promulgated ethical principles for many years, and these principles include the importance of confidentiality. The American Psychiatric Association has published both general principles and detailed guidelines regarding patient confidentiality. In some states, the medical licensing act or a separate statute defines the physician's obligation to maintain patient confidentiality.

In 1996, the United States Congress passed the Health Insurance Portability and Accountability Act and in 2001, the U.S. Department of Health and Human Services implemented "Standards for Privacy of Individually Identifiable Health Information" (the "Privacy Rule"), which created national standards to protect individuals' medical records and other personal health information. The federal government took an important medical principle (Hippocrates said, "Whatsoever things I see or hear concerning the life of men, which ought not to be noised abroad, I will keep silence thereon, counting such things to be sacred secrets.") and created a very detailed set of rules. Many providers responded by becoming unnecessarily legalistic and restrictive in the way they handle protected healthcare information.

The issue of confidentiality in clinical practice is complex. In some situations, confidentiality should be given great importance; but in other situations, it is therapeutically important to share information with other clinicians or people involved in the patient's daily life. For example, the treatment of chronically ill patients may require continuing collaboration with the individual's family members and close friends. The sharing of clinical information is almost always done with the patient's knowledge and consent. In treating a minor, the importance of confidentiality will depend on the patient's age and developmental level, his or her psychopathology, his or her relationship with the parents, and the specific topic in question. For example, most therapists would maintain confidentiality regarding an adolescent's sexual activities and occasional drug usage that might be considered part of youthful experimentation. However, therapists would want parents to become aware of a teenager's sexual promiscuity, pregnancy, serious delinquent behavior, and serious substance abuse. The expectation of confidentiality is not absolute.

Table 50–1. Exceptions to Confidentiality

The patient himself or herself.
Emergency circumstances to prevent a serious and imminent threat to the health or safety of a person or the public.
After a general consent is given, an individual's treatment providers can exchange health information for the purpose of carrying out treatment or health care operations.
Family members and close personal friends to the extent the information is directly relevant to that person's involvement with the individual's care.
Trainees can discuss their patients' psychotherapy with supervisors.
Information from an individual's psychotherapy can be disclosed to defend oneself in a legal action brought by the individual.
Reporting disease and injury to authorized public health authority.
Reporting victims of abuse, neglect, or domestic violence as required by law.
Reporting adverse events to the Food and Drug Administration.

Table 50–1 lists some of the many exceptions to confidentiality in clinical and forensic practice, which are mentioned in the Privacy Rule that followed from the Health Insurance Portability and Accountability Act. Clinicians have a strong impulse to discuss case material with colleagues, and these conversations sometimes occur in elevators, cafeterias, and other public places where they can be overheard by strangers. The urge to discuss cases occurs because clinical material is both extremely interesting (so the therapist wants to tell about it in order to show off in some way) and extremely anxiety provoking (so the therapist wants to find reassurance by sharing the case with a colleague). If a psychiatrist is concerned or puzzled about a clinical issue, he or she should confer in a formal setting with a consultant or a supervisor.

The clinician should be aware that any written record may later be read by the patient or by many other people. The wise psychiatrist will protect himself or herself from future chagrin by always keeping this in mind when he or she dictates an evaluation or writes a progress note. Prospective patients should know the limits of confidentiality. One way that therapists can ensure patient understanding of such limits is to provide them with an office brochure that explains that the therapist values confidentiality very highly but that particular exceptions to confidentiality exist.

The right to confidentiality continues after a patient's death, but it must be balanced against the family's right to certain information. After a patient's suicide, for instance, it may be appropriate for the patient's therapist to meet with family members and close friends and for all of them (i.e., including the therapist) to try to make sense of what happened. That meeting might involve the therapist's sharing certain kinds of information with the family (e.g., the diagnosis of bipolar disorder, the affection the deceased expressed toward a spouse), but it need not involve extensive or detailed revelations.

Privilege

Confidentiality and privilege are related concepts because they both assert the privacy of information that one person has shared with another. "Confidentiality" is a broad concept that prohibits professionals from revealing information about a client to anyone. "Privilege"—a narrower concept—describes specific types of information that may not be disclosed in a legal setting. Privileged information is almost always confidential; not all the confidential information is privileged.

A person has the right of testimonial privilege when he or she has the right to refuse to testify or to prevent another person from testifying about specific information. For instance, a woman may claim privilege and refuse to testify about conversations she had with her attorney because such discussions are considered private under the concept of attorney-client privilege. Likewise, a man may claim that his therapy is covered by physician-patient privilege and prevent the psychiatrist from testifying about him. On the other hand, the man may waive the right to physician-patient privilege and allow his psychiatrist to testify. It is up to the patient, not the psychiatrist, to make that decision. The psychiatrist should ordinarily go ahead and testify if the patient has waived his right to privilege.

Protection of Third Parties

Occasionally, a patient may reveal that he or she has murderous feelings toward a particular other person. The psychiatrist should assess, of course, the cause and the seriousness of these feelings. In addition, the psychiatrist should devise a treatment plan to protect the other person (i.e., the third party). Ideally, the psychiatrist and patient should cooperate in devising a safety plan. For example, a psychiatrist was treating a patient who had chronic schizophrenia and who expressed thoughts of hurting his parents. The psychiatrist and the patient agreed to a joint telephone call to the parents to inform them of the danger, the patient's medication was adjusted, and the patient signed a written statement that

he would not visit the parents until the crisis had been resolved.

If the psychiatrist and patient cannot agree on a safety plan or if it is clinically inappropriate to attempt such an agreement, the psychiatrist must take steps unilaterally to protect the third party. For example, an acutely paranoid man has told his psychiatrist that he intends to take revenge against his former boss. The psychiatrist protects both the patient and the boss by arranging for the patient's involuntary commitment to an inpatient facility.

Warning a potential victim is usually done with the patient's knowledge, if not with his or her permission. But this is not always possible. For example, an extremely angry and jealous man, who has been threatening his wife, has eloped from a supposedly secure inpatient program. It is no longer possible to discuss the issue therapeutically. The psychiatrist immediately notifies the wife and also the police.

State legislatures have adopted a variety of laws and local courts have held a variety of opinions, so psychiatrists should become familiar with the local standards. There could be contradictory practices as a professional moves from one state to another. Some states have laws that protect mental health professionals from liability if they disclose in good faith confidential information to the patient's intended victim.

American Psychiatric Association: *Opinions of the Ethics Committee on the Principles of Medical Ethics with Annotations Especially Applicable to Psychiatry.* Washington, DC: American Psychiatric Association, 2001.

American Psychiatric Association: *The Principles of Medical Ethics with Annotations Especially Applicable to Psychiatry.* Washington, DC: American Psychiatric Association, 2001.

Department of Health and Human Services: Standards for Privacy of Individually Identifiable Health Information, at www.hhs.gov/ocr/hipaa/finalreg.html

Grisso T, Appelbaum PS: *Assessing Competence to Consent to Treatment: A Guide for Physicians and Other Health Professionals.* New York: Oxford University Press, 1998.

Simon RI, Sadoff RL: *Psychiatric Malpractice: Cases and Comments for Clinicians.* Washington, DC: American Psychiatric Press, 1992.

ASSESSMENT OF MENTAL DISABILITY

There are several circumstances in which psychiatrists evaluate individuals to determine degree of disability, if any. These circumstances include claims under workers' compensation programs; personal injury lawsuits; and evaluations to determine mental competence to perform specific acts.

Disability & Workers' Compensation

The Social Security Administration provides financial benefits for individuals who are not able to work at any occupation for at least 12 months because of a serious physical condition or psychiatric illness. Through the Department of Veterans Affairs, the federal government provides benefits to veterans who are partially or fully disabled because of a service-related condition. Individual states administer workers' compensation programs that provide defined and limited compensation to individuals who were injured during the course of their employment. Finally, some people have individual or group disability insurance policies and apply for benefits from an insurance company.

Individuals who are seeking disability benefits or workers' compensation should be evaluated in a thorough and systematic manner. The clinician should carefully read the referral information because the agency or company may be asking the evaluator to address very specific questions. In some cases the cause or the date of onset of the illness may be very important. In other cases the issue may be whether the person can currently engage in a particular occupation.

In addition to a thorough interview and mental status examination, a psychiatric disability evaluation may include the following: psychological testing, neuropsychological assessment, review of medical and psychiatric records, review of military and employment records, and interviews of family members and other informants. The evaluator should actively consider the possibility of malingering or of the exaggeration of either psychological (e.g., depression, anxiety, fearfulness) or cognitive (e.g., problems with memory and concentration) symptoms. The American Medical Association has published guidelines for the assessment of physical and mental disability.

Personal Injury

Personal injury litigation is part of a large domain called tort law, the law of civil wrongs. A person who injures another can be arrested and tried (under criminal law) or sued (under tort law). A successful tort action requires proof of the four elements mentioned previously: (1) a duty was owed to the plaintiff by the defendant, (2) the duty was breached, (3) an injury occurred, and (4) the breach of duty directly caused the injury.

Courts allow plaintiffs to be compensated for both physical and psychological injuries. If a person was severely injured physically, it is easy to see how he or she may have sustained psychological damage as well. In some circumstances courts will allow compensation for psychological injury even when no physical injury occurred at all. This may happen when the plaintiff was so close to the incident (within the "zone of danger") that he or she could have been physically injured or when the plaintiff was not in the zone of danger but observed a close relative being injured.

Psychiatrists become involved in these cases by evaluating whether a plaintiff has been psychologically injured and whether the injury was the direct result of the negligent act by the defendant. The evaluator should interview the plaintiff carefully and ask the referring attorney to collect information from other sources (e.g., school records in children, military records in adults) in order to compare the person's psychological and social functioning before and after the alleged trauma. Several psychiatric conditions may follow a serious trauma: posttraumatic stress disorder, generalized anxiety disorder, phobias, panic disorder, adjustment disorder, dysthymia, and major depression. The evaluator should clarify whether the condition antedated the alleged trauma, whether other psychological stressors could have caused the symptoms, and whether there was a direct relationship between the alleged injury and the psychiatric disorder.

It is common for a psychiatrist to be asked to take on multiples roles with the same patient—for example, treating an individual and also describe the person's mental condition for some legal or administrative purpose. This is the problem of dual agency (Strasburger 1997). For example, a psychiatrist may already have a treatment relationship with an individual who is injured on the job and subsequently requires an evaluation to support his claim for workers' compensation benefits. It is usually preferable for the psychiatrist to avoid taking on both roles, but recommend that the patient have a separate, independent medical evaluation for purposes of the claim for benefits. An independent medical evaluation is an examination by a physician who evaluates, but does not provide care for, the individual. Although the problem of dual agency is an important issue for psychiatrists and psychologists, it is not so much an issue for other medical specialists. For example, orthopedic surgeons and neurologists may be ideally suited to provide both treatment and forensic evaluation for the same individual.

Competence

In psychiatry, competence refers to a person's mental ability to perform or accomplish a particular task. Some writers make a distinction: "mental capacity" is assessed by a physician or a mental health professional, while "mental competency" is a legal finding determined by a court. Although the details of the competency evaluation will depend on the circumstances (Table 50–2) of the case, the general principles are the same. There are four functional abilities to consider in assessing competence (Grisso and Appelbaum 1998):

Table 50–2. Circumstances in which Competency is an Issue

In criminal law
to waive Miranda rights
to stand trial
to testify
to be executed
In civil law
to write a will
to make a contract
to vote or hold office
to mange one's own funds
to care for a child
In medical practice
to consent to surgery or electroconvulsive therapy
to refuse surgery or electroconvulsive therapy

A. THE ABILITY TO EXPRESS A CHOICE

For example, an elderly woman who is making a will must be able to communicate her intentions either verbally, in writing, or in some other manner. It may be important to interview the person on two or three occasions to make sure her choice remains consistent.

B. THE ABILITY TO UNDERSTAND RELEVANT INFORMATION

For example, the elderly woman must understand that she is meeting with her attorney and they are preparing a legal document. She must know the extent of her property and who the potential heirs are.

C. THE ABILITY TO APPRECIATE THE SIGNIFICANCE OF THAT INFORMATION FOR ONE'S OWN SITUATION

For example, the woman who is drafting her will must realize that her children will not receive anything if she puts her entire estate in a trust fund for her cats.

D. THE ABILITY TO REASON WITH REGARD TO THAT INFORMATION ENGAGING IN A LOGICAL WEIGHING OF OPTIONS

If the woman decides to leave her estate to her children—and not to the trust fund for her cats—the evaluator should assess whether her decision was made in a rational manner. A person who makes the "right decision" for the wrong reason, such as a delusion, would not be competent.

American Medical Association: *Guides to the Evaluation of Permanent Impairment,* 6th edn. Chicago: AMA Press, 2008.

Grisso T, Appelbaum PS: *Assessing Competence to Consent to Treatment: A Guide for Physicians and Other Health Professionals.* New York: Oxford University Press, 1998.

Rogers R (ed): *Clinical Assessment of Malingering and Deception,* 2nd edn. New York: Guilford Press, 1997.

Strasburger LH, Gutheil TG, Brodsky A: On wearing two hats: Role conflict in serving as both psychotherapist and expert witness. *Am J Psychiatry* 1997;154:448–456.

INDIVIDUALS WHO HAVE BEEN ARRESTED

Forensic psychiatrists sometimes evaluate individuals who have been arrested and are awaiting trial. Usually, it is the defense attorney who is concerned about the defendant's mental competency to go to trial and his or her state of mind at the time of the alleged offense.

Competency to Stand Trial

In order to be competent to stand trial, the defendant must understand the charges that have been brought against him or her and the nature of the legal proceedings. For example, the defendant needs to understand the roles of the defense attorney, prosecuting attorney, judge, and jury. The defendant must be aware of the possible outcome of the legal proceedings (e.g., release to the community, imprisonment, capital punishment). Finally, the defendant must be able to cooperate with his or her attorney, disclose to the attorney the facts regarding the case, and testify relevantly.

If the defendant is found not competent to stand trial, the court will arrange for psychiatric treatment in the jail or at a state psychiatric facility. In some cases a defendant becomes competent following psychotropic medication or psycho-educational intervention. A person, who is permanently incompetent, such as a severely retarded individual, may never go to trial. He or she may simply be released or, if dangerous to self or others, civilly committed.

Competency to Waive Miranda Rights

Almost every U.S. citizen has heard the admonition: "You have the right to remain silent. Anything you say can and will be used against you in a court of law. You have the right to be speak to an attorney, and to have an attorney present during any questioning. If you cannot afford a lawyer, one will be provided for you at government expense." If the police have taken a person into custody, they must advise the person of his or her Miranda rights prior to interrogation. They must not continue to question a person who has asserted her right to remain silent or has requested an attorney. A person who has not been taken into custody may be questioned by police without any Miranda warning.

Forensic psychiatrists sometimes evaluate whether a criminal defendant was mentally competent to waive his Miranda rights after being arrested and prior to questioning by police. That is, whether the individual waived his Miranda rights in a knowing, intelligent, and voluntary manner. In general, "knowing" means the person is aware of what is happening and the possible consequences of making a statement to police; "intelligent" means the person has weighed the pros and cons in a logical manner; and "voluntary" means the lack of coercion. These criteria are comparable to the components of informed consent, in that "knowing" for the Miranda waiver is equivalent to "disclosure of adequate information" of informed consent, and "intelligent" for the Miranda waiver approximates the ability to reason in a logical manner that is required for informed consent.

Some people are particularly vulnerable in the sense that they are overly willing to waive their Miranda rights. For example, individuals with mental retardation may not understand the gravity of the situation and may be overly compliant in following the request of the police officer to answer questions. People with serious psychiatric disorders may be so mentally disorganized they are incapable of exercising good judgment when they are arrested. Children and adolescents who have been arrested may simply assume that they should be obedient and do what the police officer wants them to do.

Criminal Responsibility

A person who has committed a crime is not held responsible for his or her behavior if he or she was legally insane at the time the crime was committed. In this sense, "insanity" is a legal term that implies a severe mental disorder or a significant degree of mental retardation. The courts have applied several standards to define criminal insanity. The most common are the M'Naghten rule and the American Law Institute test.

The **M'Naghten rule** provides for only a *cognitive test* for the insanity defense. That is, the person is held not responsible for a crime if "the party accused was labouring under such a defect of reason, from disease of the mind, as not to know the nature and quality of the act he was doing; or, if he did know it, that he did not know he was doing what was wrong."

The **American Law Institute test** provides for both a *cognitive* and a *volitional test.* That is, a defendant would not be responsible for criminal conduct "if at the time of such conduct as a result of mental disease or defect he lacks substantial capacity to appreciate the criminality of his conduct or to conform his conduct to the requirements of the law."

Insanity is determined by a person's mental functioning, not by a specific diagnosis. To be considered insane, however, the defendant must have a serious psychiatric condition such as bipolar disorder, paranoid schizophrenia, or another severe mental disorder. Some jurisdictions explicitly state in their insanity statute that "mental disease or defect" does not include any disorder that is manifested simply by antisocial conduct.

If a judge or jury finds a defendant not guilty by reason of insanity, the person does not go to prison. Nor does he or she go home. Usually the disposition is to a secure inpatient facility to determine if the person can be civilly committed to either hospital or outpatient treatment. Some states provide an alternative outcome, in that the defendant can be found guilty but mentally ill. That is, the defendant had a mental illness at the time of the alleged offense, but it was not severe enough to acquit him or her. The defendant found guilty but mentally ill goes to prison, where treatment is presumably available.

Diminished Capacity

Like insanity, the concept of diminished capacity also refers to the defendant's mental condition at the time of the alleged offense. In order to convict a defendant, the prosecution must prove that a criminal act occurred (referred to as the "actus reus") and that the perpetrator of the act had a particular mental state (referred to as the "mens rea"). For some crimes, it is simply required that the actor has the mental state of "knowing" what he or she is doing. For some crimes, it is required that the actor have the mental state of "intending" what he or she is doing, a higher level of mental activity than simply knowing. For some forms of first-degree murder, it is required that the actor has the mental state of "premeditation," a higher level of mental activity than either intending or knowing. States have various definitions for these terms.

Some states allow mental health professionals to testify regarding a person's capacity to form a particular mental state at the time of the alleged offense. For example, a forensic psychiatrist might be asked to evaluate whether a man who was very intoxicated by both alcohol and cocaine was mentally capable of premeditating a crime when he violently killed another person in a bar fight. If a judge or jury finds the defendant was not capable of premeditation and therefore did not commit first-degree murder, the person is not usually acquitted and sent home. Usually, the person is found guilty of a lesser-included offense such as second-degree murder or voluntary manslaughter. A successful insanity defense is exculpatory and the person is found not guilty of any crime. A successful diminished capacity defense usually means the person is found guilty of a crime with a shorter sentence.

Prison Psychiatry

American jails and prisons have much higher proportions of mentally ill and mentally retarded individuals than are found in the general population. Forensic psychiatrists provide treatment to these individuals, who may have serious conditions manifested by chronic depression, violent and aggressive behavior, and overt psychosis.

Perlin ML: *The Jurisprudence of the Insanity Defense*. Durham, NC: Carolina Academic, 1998.

Rogers R: *Conducting Insanity Evaluations*, 2nd edn. New York: Guilford, 2000.

Scott CL, Gerbasi JB (eds): *Handbook of Correctional Mental Health*. Washington, DC: American Psychiatric Publishing, 2005.

FORENSIC CHILD PSYCHIATRY

The interface between child psychiatry and the law is a very young discipline. The forensic child psychiatrist is likely to be consulted regarding child custody disputes, child maltreatment (such as physical, sexual, and psychological abuse), minors involved in the juvenile justice system, and personal injury (see page 715).

Child Custody Evaluation

When parents divorce and disagree regarding the custody of the child, mental health professionals sometimes evaluate the family and make recommendations to the court. Since the 1920s, lawmakers and courts have emphasized "the best interests of the child," which implies that the needs of the child override the rights of either parent. The American Academy of Child and Adolescent Psychiatry (1997) developed practice parameters for child custody evaluations.

In conducting these evaluations, it is best to have access to all members of the family, including both parents. In some circumstances the psychiatrist may conduct a one-sided evaluation by interviewing only one parent and the child. In such a case the psychiatrist may make only limited observations and recommendations, such as commenting on the psychiatric condition of one parent and his or her relationship with the child. Usually the psychiatrist would not be able to make any recommendations regarding custody because he or she had no way of evaluating the relative merits of the mother and father.

Typically, the psychiatrist has an initial conference with both parents together (if this is not too disruptive); meets with each parent individually in order to complete a psychiatric evaluation and to assess each person's parenting attitudes and skills; and meets twice with the child, so that each parent can bring the child for an appointment at least once. The psychiatrist may find it helpful to collect information from outside sources such as grandparents, babysitters, the pediatrician, and teachers. It is important to speak to previous and current psychotherapists of the child and of the parents.

Decisions regarding custody are guided by the best interests of the child, but there are no standard guidelines for the specific factors that should be taken into consideration and what weight should be given to each factor. The following factors are generally considered important: parental attitudes and parenting skills; which parent has been more involved with day-to-day child rearing; continuity of placement (it is usually presumed preferable to maintain the status quo unless there is good reason to change it) the physical health of the parents the mental health of the parents (psychiatric diagnosis is less important than the person's parenting skills in the present and the future) substance abuse by the parents the relative merits of the two households (e.g., whether the parent has remarried) allegations of physical or sexual abuse the child's attachment to the parents and the child's preference, if he or she articulates a definite preference for reasons that seem valid.

Child Maltreatment

Psychiatrists in private practice, as well as those employed by courts or other agencies, see children who are alleged to have been psychologically, physically, or sexually abused. The purpose of the evaluation may be to assist the court in determining what happened to the child, to make recommendations regarding placement or treatment, or to offer an opinion on the termination of parental rights. The evaluation of a child, who is alleged to have been maltreated, is described in Chapter 42.

Juvenile Justice

Forensic child psychiatrists may consult with the juvenile justice system to evaluate a juvenile's competency to go to trial and his or her state at the time of the alleged offense, if an insanity defense is being considered. Psychiatrists can also assist the court in determining if a juvenile, who has been accused of committing an unusually serious offense, should be tried as an adult ("waiver to adult court"), the risk the child presents of violent or sexual offending, the reasons for the child's behavior, and the best disposition.

American Academy of Child and Adolescent Psychiatry: Practice parameters for psychiatric custody evaluations. *J Am Acad Child Adolesc Psychiatr* 1997;36(Suppl 10):57S.

Bernet W: Child custody evaluations. Child and Adolescent Psychiatric Clinics of North America 2002;11:781–804.

Grisso T: *Forensic Evaluation of Juveniles*. Sarasota, FL: Professional Resource Exchange, 1998.

Grisso T, Vincent G, Seagrave D (eds): *Mental Health Screening and Assessment in Juvenile Justice*. New York: Guilford Press, 2005.

Table 50–3. Outline for Typical Forensic Report

Identifying information: for example, names and birth dates.

Background information: a brief chronology of the situation and a statement about the circumstances of the referral and the specific purpose of the evaluation.

Procedure for this evaluation: an explanation of the various meetings which were held, the psychological testing utilized, and the outside information that was collected. It may be appropriate to state specifically that the evaluee gave informed consent for the evaluation.

Observations: a systematic presentation of the data that was collected during the evaluation.

Conclusions: a list of specific statements that the psychiatrist believes are supported by his or her data.

Recommendations: these follow logically from the conclusions.

Appendixes: associated information, such as psychological testing.

Qualifications of the evaluator: may be a curriculum vitae.

Nurcombe B, Partlett DJ: *Child Mental Health and the Law.* New York: Free Press, 1994.

Schetky DH, Benedek EP (eds): *Principles and Practice of Child and Adolescent Forensic Psychiatry.* Washington, DC: American Psychiatric Publishing, 2002.

THE PSYCHIATRIST IN COURT

The Written Report

The report should be carefully written. It will be read by several people and the reader will tend to attach great significance to particular sentences or phrases. Probably the best approach is to make the report detailed enough for the reader to understand fully the procedure that was followed and the basis for the conclusions and recommendations but not to include every scintilla of data. Table 50–3 offers an outline of a typical forensic report.

Role Definition

There are many times when the psychiatrist must keep straight in his or her own mind, and for others, both who is the client and what precisely is the psychiatrist's role in the current situation. The client may be the person the psychiatrist is examining or it may be somebody else. The psychiatrist may have the role of therapist or simply that of an evaluator. In forensic work, any confusion regarding the psychiatrist's role will be magnified and highlighted by the legal process and will compromise his or her work, whether the psychiatrist is intending to be a therapist, an evaluator, a consultant, or an administrator.

The Problem of Bias

Psychiatrists and other mental health professionals may not realize how easily and how often they become biased in their work with patients and families. Despite all that is known about unconscious processes (such as countertransference) and conscious motivations (such as greed and the desire for popularity or fame), it is common for therapists to base their conclusions on preconception rather than on the data that have been presented. Bias is more prevalent in forensic cases because the evaluator may be exposed to anger, threat, deceit, tragedy, innuendo, hypocrisy, flattery, or inducement. It is extremely important for the psychiatrist to be aware of his or her own motivations, as well as the agenda of the other professionals involved in the case.

Bias is a distorting glass through which the evaluator views the situation. For example, an evaluator who is a very strong believer in law and order may always interpret the facts to support criminal responsibility rather than a finding of not guilty by reason of insanity. The psychiatrist who enters a case with a particular bias is likely to change a situation despite a belief that he or she is studying it objectively. For example, an evaluator predisposed to find child abuse may interview children in such a suggestive manner that the children allege abusive acts that did not occur.

Several safeguards against bias are available. The psychiatrist should try to be aware of his or her own conscious and unconscious motivations. It may be helpful if the psychiatrist says something like this to himself or herself: "My job is not to win this case. My task is to help the court by collecting accurate and pertinent data and organizing it in a way that is scientifically and medically valid." Another safeguard against bias is for the psychiatrist to carefully indicate in the written report the reasons for his or her conclusions, so that the court will truly understand the basis for the opinion.

Some forensic psychiatrists misuse their expertise by manipulating the court into believing something that may not be true. Sometimes, unscrupulous psychiatrists use obfuscating jargon in order to cloak shaky reasoning with a false air of certainty.

Degrees of Certainty

An important aspect of legal decisions is the standard of proof or the level of certainty that must be established in order for a particular decision or verdict to be reached. There are several levels of certainty.

The least exacting level of certainty to achieve is **probable cause.** In criminal law, probable cause is the set of circumstances sufficient to lead a reasonable man to suspect the person arrested had committed a crime. In psychiatric practice, that may be a sufficient level of certainty to report a suspected instance of child abuse.

In civil cases the side that prevails is the one that establishes a **fair preponderance of the evidence.** This can be expressed roughly as being 51% certain.

In some cases that involve psychiatric evidence, the level of certainty is **clear and convincing proof,** which is proof necessary to persuade by a substantial margin, and more than a bare preponderance. In most states civil commitment, paternity suits, and legal insanity must be proven to a degree that is clear and convincing. In most circumstances, the proof that child abuse has occurred or that parental rights should be severed must be clear and convincing.

Criminal cases require proof that is **beyond a reasonable doubt,** which means that the jury is satisfied to a moral certainty that every element of a crime has been proven. The term means that no reasonable alternative could explain the evidence. To convict a specific person

---

Table 50–4. Important Cases in Forensic Psychiatry

Addington v. Texas, 441 U.S. 418 (1979). The U.S. Supreme Court found that the standard of proof for civil commitment is at least "clear and convincing evidence."

Ake v. Oklahoma, 470 U.S. 68 (1985). The U.S. Supreme Court said that an indigent defendant who raised the question of insanity has the right to a court-appointed psychiatrist to perform an evaluation and assist the defense in preparation of an insanity defense.

Canterbury v. Spence, 464 F.2d 772 (1972). The U.S. Court of Appeals for the District of Columbia stated that the proper criterion for informed consent is that the physician should warn the patient of all potential risks that a reasonable patient would want to know.

Daubert v. Merrell Dow, 61 U.S.L.S. 4805, 113 S.Ct. 2786 (1993). The U.S. Supreme Court held that judges in federal courts should consider factors such as the following when determining whether scientific evidence is relevant and reliable: whether the theory or technique can be and has been tested; whether it has been subjected to peer review and published; its error rate; and whether it has been generally accepted within the relevant scientific community.

Dillon v. Legg, 441 P.2d 912 (1968). The Supreme Court of California found that a person could be awarded damages for psychological injury that was caused by witnessing the physical injury of a close relative.

Dusky v. United States, 362 U.S. 402 (1960). The Supreme Court defined the test for competency to stand trial: whether the defendant "has sufficient present ability to consult with his lawyer with a reasonable degree of rational understanding – and whether he has a rational as well as a factual understanding of the proceedings against him."

In re Gault, 387 U.S.1 (1967). The U.S. Supreme Court defined the due process rights of a juvenile who has been arrested: written and timely notice of the charges; protection against self-incrimination; defense counsel; and right to cross-examination.

Landeros v. Flood, 551 P.2d 389 (1976). The Supreme Court of California established the standard of care for diagnosing the battered child syndrome, which was "whether a reasonably prudent physician examining this plaintiff . . . would have been led to suspect she was a victim of the battered child syndrome . . . and would have promptly reported his findings to appropriate authorities . . . ."

Miranda v. Arizona, 384 U.S. 436 (1966). The U.S. Supreme Court stated that the admissibility in evidence of any statement given during custodial interrogation of a suspect would depend on whether the police provided the suspect with four warnings: that a suspect "has the right to remain silent, that anything he says can be used against him in a court of law, that he has the right to the presence of an attorney, and that if he cannot afford an attorney one will be appointed for him prior to any questioning if he so desires."

Rennie v. Klein, 720 F.2d 266 (1983). The Third Circuit Court of Appeals found that civilly committed patients have a constitutional right to refuse treatment.

Tarasoff v. Regents of the University of California, 551 P.2d 334 (1976). The California Supreme Court found that the therapist of a dangerous patient "bears a duty to exercise reasonable care to protect the foreseeable victim of that danger."

Wyatt v. Aderholt, 503 F.2d 1305 (1974). The Fifth Circuit Court of Appeals said that civilly committed patients "unquestionably have a constitutional right to receive such individual treatment as will give each of them a realistic opportunity to be cured or to improve his or her mental condition."

of child abuse would require proof beyond a reasonable doubt.

One of the most puzzling terms in forensic psychiatry is **reasonable degree of medical certainty.** When a physician testifies in court, he or she is frequently asked if his or her opinions are given with a reasonable degree of medical certainty. Unfortunately, there is no specific meaning for that term. At one time or another, physicians have taken it to mean about the same as "beyond a reasonable doubt," the same as "clear and convincing," and even the same degree of certainty as "preponderance of the evidence." It has been proposed that reasonable medical certainty is a level of certainty equivalent to that which a physician uses when making a diagnosis and starting treatment. The implication is that the degree of certainty depends on the clinical situation. For example, the diagnosis of syphilis is accomplished with almost 100% certainty because there is a reliable laboratory test for that purpose. The determination that a patient has posttraumatic stress disorder as a result of a specific event can be made with considerably less certainty.

Brodsky SL: *The Expert Witness: More Maxims and Guidelines for Testifying in Court.* Washington, DC: American Psychological Association, 1999.

Gutheil TG: *The Psychiatrist in Court: A Survival Guide.* Washington, DC: American Psychiatric Press, 1998.

Rappeport J: Reasonable medical certainty. Bull Am Acad Psychiatry Law 1985;13:5.

Ziskin J, Faust D: *Coping with Psychiatric and Psychological Testimony.* Los Angeles: Law and Psychology Press, 1995.

CONCLUSION

Forensic psychiatry is an unusual medical specialty because of the diverse clinical situations and the broad scope of practice that it encompasses. For instance, a forensic evaluation might involve a very young child (regarding child maltreatment), a very old person (regarding competency to make a will), or anybody in between. The forensic practitioner must be familiar not only with the clinical literature but also with the applicable law and important legal precedents. Several important legal cases have influenced both the practice of law and the practice of psychiatry (Table 50–4).

In addition, it is challenging to apply psychiatric expertise to legal situations—both through written reports and oral testimony—in a manner that is evenhanded and unbiased. Finally, forensic psychiatrists experience a wealth of human relationships and a variety of roles. They may consult with clients and evaluees in the office, in the hospital, in jail, on death row, and in the corporate boardroom. After conducting an evaluation, they frequently take on the role of teacher or lecturer, as they explain their findings to family members, attorneys, and perhaps a judge and jury. The diversity of forensic psychiatry gives this medical specialty its own blend of suspense, accomplishment, and satisfaction.

Index